Compliments of

Bio-Research

Laboratories Ltd.

Arthur!
Not for every day use -
unless Rover is into
field trials in the tropics

George J Losos

George Losos

10th Dec 1986

INFECTIOUS TROPICAL DISEASES OF DOMESTIC ANIMALS

George J. Losos

INFECTIOUS TROPICAL DISEASES OF DOMESTIC ANIMALS

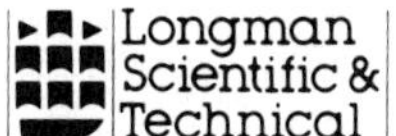

PUBLISHED IN ASSOCIATION WITH THE INTERNATIONAL DEVELOPMENT RESEARCH CENTRE
CANADA

Longman Scientific & Technical,
Longman Group UK Limited
Longman House, Burnt Mill, Harlow
Essex CM20 2JE, England
Associated companies throughout the world

Published in the United States of America by Churchill Livingstone Inc., New York

First Published 1986

British Library Cataloguing in Publication Data

Losos, George J.
Infectious tropical diseases of domestic animals.
1. Communicable diseases in animals
2. Veterinary tropical medicine
I. Title
636.089'69'00913 SF781

ISBN 0-582-40408-8

Library of Congress Cataloging-in-Publication Data

Losos, George.
Infectious tropical diseases of domestic animals.
"Published in association with the International Development Research Centre, Canada."
Bibliography: p.
1. Communicable diseases in animals – Tropics.
2. Domestic animals – Diseases – Tropics. 3. Veterinary tropical medicine. I. Title.
SF781.L63 1986 636.089'69'0913 85–13372
ISBN 0–582–40408–8

Printed and Bound in Great Britain at
The Bath Press, Avon

This book is dedicated to my family, Gudrun, Yvonne and Jan for their enthusiasm and support.

Foreword

I have taken one basic scientific theme in my approach to the pathogenesis of tropical diseases. This in turn affects all other consideration on the disease such as control and economic significance. The theme is as follows:

'Most human beings, indeed probably all living things, carry throughout life, a variety of microbial agents potentially pathogenic for them. Under most conditions, these pathogenes do not manifest their presence by either symptoms or lesions; only when something happens which upsets the equilibrium between host and parasite does infection evolve into disease. In other words, infection in many cases is the normal state; it is only disease which is abnormal.' (René J. Dubos, *Biochemical Determinants of Microbial Diseases*, Harvard University Press, Cambridge, Massachusetts, 1954)

In the tropics, possibly more than anywhere else, understanding of indigenous diseases is dependent on making a clear distinction between mere infections and infections causing diseases.

I wrote the text to provide an introductory single source of the information available, and a reasonably comprehensive bibliography on twenty-five diseases of domestic animals which are of major importance in tropical and sub-tropical climates. The need for a single monograph is obvious to anyone who has experience with these diseases, particularly to those who work in the developing countries.

Each chapter has been reviewed by a scientist who has an in-depth knowledge of the subject. The comments and suggestions have, for the most part, been incorporated. Unfortunately, the subject has been reviewed only up to 1982–83; the next three years were required to finish writing the manuscript and for its publication.

I hope that this monograph will be useful to those interested in tropical diseases of domestic animals.

GEORGE J. LOSOS, D.V.M., M.V.Sc., Ph.D.

Past Associations:

UNIVERSITY OF IBADAN, IBADAN

EAST AFRICAN TRYPANOSOMIASIS
RESEARCH ORGANIZATION, TORORO, UGANDA

VETERINARY RESEARCH DEPARTMENT
KENYA AGRICULTURAL RESEARCH INSTITUTE
FORMERLY: EAST AFRICAN VETERINARY RESEARCH
ORGANIZATION, MAGUGA, KENYA

Present Association:

BIO-RESEARCH LABORATORIES INC.
87 SENNEVILLE ROAD
SENNEVILLE, QUEBEC
CANADA
H9X 3R3

Contents

Acknowledgments

I thank the many African colleagues for the opportunity to work in their countries, for their valuable assistance in enabling me to gain experience and obtain information necessary to write this book.

I am most grateful to Dr Walter Masiga, the former Director of the Veterinary Research Department of the Kenya Agricultural Research Institute for initiating the financial support through the joint Kenya-IDRC project on Trypanosomiasis.

Additional support was provided by the International Development Research Center to complete the book. I am most grateful to Mrs Marilyn Campbell at IDRC who had the patience and faith throughout the protracted period required to finish the text. I received enthusiastic support from the library staff at the Ontario Veterinary College who greatly helped in gathering of the information.

I wish to thank Mrs Jean Henderson for her dedication in typing and checking of the manuscript.

I would like to acknowledge the assistance of the following reviewers who provided most valuable suggestions and corrections.

Dr D. F. Mahoney	– Babesiosis
Dr T. Dolan	– Theileriosis
Dr L. Goodwin	– Trypanosomiasis
Not reviewed	– Leishmaniasis
Dr H. Mirchamsy	– African Horse Sickness
Dr W. R. Hess	– African Swine Fever
Dr T. E. Walton	– Bluetongue
Dr. T. D. St. George	– Ephemeral Fever
Dr T. E. Walton	– Equine Arboviral Encephalitides
Dr F. G. Davies	– Lumpyskin Disease
Dr D. F. Mahoney	– Nairobi Sheep Disease
Dr R. C. Rowland	– Peste des Petits Ruminants
Dr F. G. Davies	– Pox Diseases
Dr R. F. Sellers	– Rift Valley Fever
Dr G. Scott	– Rinderpest
Dr R. N. Gourlay	– Contagious Bovine and Carpine Pleuropneumonia

Dr D. H. Lloyd – Dermatophilosis
Dr G. R. Carter – Hemorrhagic Septicemia
Dr G. G. Wagner – Anaplasmosis
Dr R. D. Smith – Ehrlichiosis
Dr J. L. Du Plessis – Heartwater
Dr D. Behymer – Q Fever
Dr G. S. Nelson – Filariasis
Dr T. W. Schillhorn von Veen – Fascioliasis
Dr J. M. Preston – Schistosomiasis

Dr. D Behymer
School of Veterinary Medicine
Dept. of Epidemiology and
Preventive Medicine
University of California, Davis
Davis, CA 95616
USA

Dr G. R. Carter
Division of Pathobiology and
Public Practice
Virginia-Maryland Regional
College of Veterinary Medicine
Virginia Tech
Blacksburg, VA 24061
USA

Dr F. G. Davies
Senior Veterinary Research
Officer
Dept. of Veterinary Services
Veterinary Research Laboratory
P.O. Kabete
Kenya, Africa

Dr T. Dolan
British Technical Co-operation
Projects
Overseas Development
Administration
Veterinary Research Department
Kenya Agricultural Research
Institute
Maguga
P.O. Box 32
Kikuyu, Kenya

Dr J. L. Du Plessis
Veterinary Research Institute
P.O. Onderstepoort 0110
South Africa

Dr Len Goodwin
Shepperlands Farm
Park Lane
Finchampstead, Berks RG11 4QF
England

Dr R. N. Gourlay
Agricultural Research Council
Institute for Research on Animal
Diseases
Comptom, Nr Newbury,
Berkshire RG16 ONN
England

Dr William R. Hess
Research Microbiologist
US Department of Agriculture
Science and Education
Administration Agricultural
Research
Northeastern Region
Plum Island Animal Disease
Center
Post Office Box 848
Greenport, NY 11944
USA

Dr D. H. Lloyd
Dept. of Microbiology and
Parasitology
The Royal Veterinary College
University of London
Royal College Street
London, NW1 OTU
England

Dr D. F. Mahoney
Chief of Division
CSIRO
Division of Tropical Animal
Science

Private Bag No. 3
P.O. Indooroopilly, Queensland 4068
Australia

Dr H. Mirchamsy
Associate Director
Institut d'Etat des Sérums et Vaccins Razi
B.P. 656
Teheran, Iran

Professor G. S. Nelson
Head, Dept. of Parasitology
Liverpool School of Tropical Medicine
Pembroke Place
Liverpool L3 5QA
England

Dr J. M. Preston
Merck Sharp & Dohme Ltd
Hertford Road
Hoddesdon, Herts EN11 9BU
England

Dr Alan C. Rowland
Department of Veterinary Pathology
Royal (Dick) School of Veterinary Studies
Veterinary Field Station
Easter Bush,
Roslin,
Midlothian,
Scotland

Dr T. W. Schillhorn Von Veen
Veterinary Clinical Center
College of Veterinary Medicine
Michigan State University
East Lansing, MI 48824
USA

Dr Gordon R. Scott
University of Edinburgh
Royal (Dick) School of Veterinary Studies
Centre for Tropical Veterinary Medicine
Easterbush, Roslin,
Midlothian EH25 9RG
Scotland

Dr R. F. Sellers
Director
The Animal Virus Research Institute
Pirbright, Woking
Surrey GU24 0NF
England

Dr Ronald D. Smith
Associate Professor
College of Veterinary Medicine
University of Illinois
Urbana, IL 61801
USA

Dr T. D. St. George
CSIRO
Division of Tropical Animal Science
Private Bag No. 3,
P.O. Indooroopilly, Queensland 4068
Australia

Dr G. G. Wagner
Center for Tropical Animal Health
College of Veterinary Medicine
Texas A&M University
College Station, TX 77843
USA

Dr Thomas E. Walton
Arthropod-borne Animal Diseases Research
US Department of Agriculture
P.O. Box 25327
Denver Federal Center
Denver, CO 80225
USA

PART

I

PROTOZOAL DISEASES

Chapter

1

Babesiosis

CONTENTS

INTRODUCTION

Babesioses are a group of tick-borne diseases caused by several species of protozoa in the genus *Babesia*. These organisms are capable of infecting all species of domestic animals, and are also found in some game animals which serve as reservoirs of infection. The term 'babesiosis' is used to designate an infection in which a period of rapid growth and multiplication results in clinical disease, while 'babesiasis' refers to a subclinical infection that recurs in animals which have recovered from acute disease and exist in the carrier state. In nature, acute, chronic, or inapparent type of disease syndrome are found, depending on the particular species. The acute syndrome is characterized by fever, anemia, hemoglobinuria, jaundice, and variable mortality. The chronic syndromes are poorly defined clinically and are associated with anemia and variable weight loss, while the carrier state is asymptomatic. The major economic impact of the disease is felt in relation to the morbidity and mortality among domestic ruminants; the greatest losses occur when fully susceptible animals are introduced into enzootic areas. Indigenous animals in enzootic areas are normally protected by natural infections early in life, and the degree of protection depends on the level of early infection.

Literature

The most comprehensive reviews to date on the economic importance, range of host susceptibilities, life cycles in the vector and mammalian hosts, *in vitro* culture methods, transmission, pathogenesis, chemotherapy, immunology, and vaccination have been published in a monograph edited by Ristic and Kreier (1981). The literature also contains reviews on babesiosis in domestic animals (Mahoney 1979); on nonspecific resistance, immunity, immunology, and pathogenesis (Zwart and Brocklesby 1979); and on infections in man, wild and laboratory animals (Ristic and Lewis 1979).

ETIOLOGY

The speciation of *Babesia* is difficult because of the incomplete knowledge of many of the isolates, particularly those infecting wild animals. The domestic animals and the *Babesia* species they are most commonly infected with are listed as follows:

Cow: *B. bigemina, B. bovis, B. divergens, B. major.*
Horse: *B. caballi, B. equi.*
Sheep: *B. foliata, B. motasi, B. ovis.*
Goat: *B. motasi, B. ovis, B. taylori.*
Pig: *B. perroncitoi, B. trautmanni.*
Dog: *B. canis, B. gibsoni.*
Cat: *B. felis.*

Literature

Levine *et al.* (1980) listed 71 species in the genus *Babesia* of which only 18 were found in domestic animals. The babesiosis in various species of animals was reviewed by Purnell (1981), who summarized the most pertinent aspects of the epizootiology, morphology, life cycle, and clinical syndromes. Purnell also described the species found in the camel, water buffalo, and reindeer. Ristic and Lewis (1979) discussed the babesioses in man and wild and laboratory animals and presented a comprehensive list of the species of *Babesia* isolated from wild and domestic mammals. A symposium on human babesiosis was held in 1980 in which reports on various aspects of human babesiosis (Hoare 1980) and on the occurrence of the disease in North America (Ruebush 1980) and in Europe (Garnham 1980) were presented.

Life cycle in the vector

The life cycle of *Babesia* in the tick is more complicated than that which occurs in the vertebrate host since it involves the intracellular development of various parasitic stages. After the female tick is engorged with infected blood, a sexual part of the life cycle (although as yet not described) probably starts in the gut lumen prior to the penetration of the ookinetes into the epithelial cells of the gut. Asexual stages have been clearly demonstrated. Two or three cycles of primary schizogony produce large populations of vermicules which through the hemolymph invade various tissues and organs, including the oocytes in the ovary and the alveolar tissue of the salivary gland. In the latter tissue the organisms undergo secondary schizogony and produce infective particles (sporozoites). This multiplication of the organism within the ticks encompasses the full developmental cycle between the initial infection in the tick and the subsequent induction of infection in the next vertebrate host. Some *Babesia* species are adapted to transstadial transmission through larvae to nymphs and from nymphs to adults in the two- and three-host ticks, whereas others invade the ovaries for the transovarial transmission to ensure their propagation by succeeding generations of ticks.

Literature

The life cycle in the tick has been reviewed by Ristic *et al.* (1981) and Friedhoff (1981). *Babesia* do not arbitrarily infect any tick stage or tick tissue, but have a specific life cycle in various tick stages depending on the species of *Babesia* and tick involved. The *B. bovis* and *B. bigemina* infections in *Boophilus microplus* have been the best studied and are typical of the life cycle of *Babesia* in the vector. The morphology of other *Babesia* species observed in the tick vectors is similar to that of *B. bovis* and *B. bigemina* in *B. microplus*, but there are some significant differences. There is confusion regarding the terms 'trophozoite' and 'merozoite', which have been applied to both the blood and tick stages of *Babesia* despite considerable morphological differences apparent in these stages. The rapid digestion of blood in the gut of the tick causes the release of the intraerythrocytic piroplasms. There is evidence that sexual stages also occur in the midgut of *B. microplus*. Only a small proportion of the blood forms survive digestion and continue the tick cycle. Schizonts, also called 'fission bodies', proceed to develop in the cells of the gut wall. These cells eventually rupture and release the vermicules into the midgut. The vermicules then penetrate the epithelium, invade the hemolymph, and migrate to the ovary where they penetrate the immature ova. These vermicules also localize in the salivary glands. A second cycle has been described in which vermicules invade the cells of the Malpighian tubules and infect the hemolymph to repeat the intestinal schizogonous cycle. This results in the release of a secondary population of vermicules which then infects the ova.

The life cycle of *B. bigemina* in *B. microplus* was investigated during the first 24 hours after infection. Most of the forms observed in the bovine erythrocytes were destroyed during digestion and only certain oval or spherical bodies survived and developed. Invasion of the epithelial cells of the intestine transpired at about 24 hours, and reproduction occurred by multiple fission. Mature vermicules were released into the hemolymph approximately 72 hours after infection, and by day 4 some of these vermicules invaded the cells of the Malpighian tubules and of the hemolymph. Other vermicules invaded the ova of the tick and underwent a similar life cycle in the cells of the gut walls of the developing larvae. The final cycle took place in the salivary glands of the nymph; forms infective for the vertebrate host appeared 8 to 10 days after larval attachment (Riek 1964).

In *B. decoloratus* infected by transovarian passage with *B. bigemina*, primary schizogony occurred as a continuous repetitive process in all three stages of the tick's life cycle. The primary schizonts and the vermicules produced by them were observed in the gut epithelium, hemocytes, muscle, and peritracheal cells. Secondary schizogony, which led to the formation of infective forms, occurred mainly in the salivary glands but was also observed in the cortex of the synganglion. Mature infective forms were observed only in the nymphal and adult ticks (Potgieter and Els 1977a, b).

The structure of *B. bovis* in the gut epithelium of *B. microplus* was investigated by Potgieter *et al.* (1976). Friedhoff and Buscher (1976) proposed that sexual reproduction in *B. bigemina* was possible. The differentiation of *B. major* and *B. bigemina* by examination of the vermicules in the tick hemolymph was attempted, and it was shown that the vermicules of *B. major* were significantly larger than those of *B. bigemina* (Morzaria and Brocklesby 1977; Morzaria *et al.* 1978). The fine structure of *B. bigemina* in the ovaries of *B. microplus* and *B. decoloratus* was studied (Friedhoff and Scholtyseck 1969). The development of small pyriform infective particles of *B. bovis* in the granule-secreting cells of the salivary glands of *B. microplus* took place through a process of schizogony and resulted in the formation of many particles (Potgieter and Els 1976; Weber and Friedhoff 1979). The electron-microscopic study of the development of *B. bovis* in the salivary glands of *Rhipicephalus bursa* was undertaken (Moltmann *et al.* 1982). The developmental forms of an avirulent vaccine strain and an unmodified virulent strain of *B. bovis* in the tick *B. microplus* differed with respect to the structure and the number of parasites detectable at each phase of the life cycle (Stewart 1978). The tick-infective strain was seen in the hemolymph and ova of ticks and in the larval progeny. It appeared that continuous blood passaging resulted in the selection of parasites incapable of penetrating the gut epithelial cells of the tick. Wright *et al.* (1983) have recently demonstrated that avirulent *Babesia bovis* lacks a protease enzyme and is incapable of being transmitted by ticks.

Only limited additional information is available on the life cycle of *Babesia* which infect other species of domestic animals such as sheep, horses, and dogs. Merozoites and fission bodies were detected in the gut, hemolymph, epidermis, muscles, Malpighian tubules, ovaries, and eggs of *R. bursa* transovarially infected with *B. ovis* (Friedhoff 1969). The development of *B. ovis* infective particles from large schizonts in the salivary glands of *R. bursa* was studied (Friedhoff *et al.* 1972). The salivary glands of *R. bursa* ticks infected with *B. ovis* were examined for DNA, RNA, proteins, lipids, and polysaccharides of merozoite origin (Weber and Friedhoff 1971). The development of *B. caballi* was studied in the cells of the Malpighian tubules, hemolymph and ovaries of *Dermacentor nitens*; the ovarian cells contained parasites multiplying by fission (Holbrook *et al.* 1968a). Light and/or electron microscopy was used to observe the development of *B. canis* sporozoites in the salivary glands (Schein *et al.* 1979) and in the gut (Mehlhorn *et al.* 1980) of *D. reticulatus*.

Life cycle in the vertebrate host

Babesial organisms enter the bloodstream of the mammalian host after inoculation by infected ticks and multiply in the erythrocytes. *Babesia* are pleomorphic and may assume round, oval, elongate, amoeboid, or bizarre shapes. They also appear as pyriform bodies arranged in pairs or in multiples of two. Two groups of *Babesia* are distinguished according to the size of the intraerythrocytic forms. The 'small' species are characterized by pyriform bodies between 1.0 and 2.5 μm long and include *B. bovis* (synonyms: *B. argentina* and *B. berbera*), *B. divergens, B. equi, B. ovis, B. perroncitoi, B. gibsoni,* and *B. felis*. The 'large' species are differentiated by pyriform bodies between 2.5 and 5.0 μm long and include *B. bigemina, B. major, B. caballi, B. motasi, B. trautmanni* and *B. canis*. The asexual life cycle in the vertebrate is a form of schizogony, with the merozoites occurring as pyriform bodies and the trophozoites appearing as single forms. The process of entering the erythrocyte is rapid and commences with the indentation of the red blood cell membrane by the blunt end of the merozoite. The parasite then rapidly penetrates the cell and the cell membrane closes behind it. There is no evidence for host cell membrane around the newly entered parasite. Multiplication is by binary fission and one cycle of division in the cell requires approximately 8 hours.

Literature

The invasion of erythrocytes by merozoites and their behavior inside the cells was reviewed (Rudzinska 1981). Merozoites and trophozoites are the two developmental forms of *Babesia* which occur in the erythrocyte. The ultrastructure of merozoites, the process of transformation to trophozoites, and the method of multiplication of *B. bigemina* were studied. After penetration of an erythrocyte, merozoites developed into trophozoites through a schizogonous transformation process (Potgieter and Els 1977a, b). Further ultrastructural studies of the erythrocytic forms of *B. bigemina, B. divergens,* and *B. ovis* revealed that there are species-specific differences with respect to the intracellular location of the parasite and the shape of the merozoites, the number, shape, and size of the rhoptries and the localization of food vacuoles, the shape, size, and structure of the spheroid bodies, and the presence of Maurer's clefts (Friedhoff and Scholtyseck 1977). *Babesia* species seem to feed by means of a special organelle which is composed of tightly coiled double membranes located partly inside and partly outside the parasite (Rudzinska 1976). The feeding mechanism in the extracellular *B. microti* was investigated and it was suggested that hemoglobin is pinocytosed (Langreth 1976), but unlike malaria *Babesia* does not have hemoglobin feeding vacuoles of hemozoin. The intraerythrocytic development of *B. caballi* and *B. equi* involved the transformation of an anaplasmoid, or round, body to a ring-like form which became amoeboid.

The cellular division of these species began with a process resembling budding; ultimately, each *B. caballi* organism gave rise to two pyriform parasites, while *B. equi* formed four pyriform bodies (Holbrook *et al.* 1968b). *Babesia caballi* and *B. equi* are dissimilar with respect to the length of the incubation period and the degree of parasitemia observed; these disparities might be related to certain differences in the ultrastructures of the two organisms (Simpson *et al.* 1967). The mature forms of *B. equi* in *Rhipicephalus evertsi* collected from zebras were substantially smaller than those of other *Babesia* species (Young and Purnell 1973). The ultrastructural differences between the intraerythrocytic stages of *B. gibsoni* and *B. canis* are not qualitative but quantitative; i.e. some organelles, especially the endoplasmic reticulum, are better developed in *B. canis* (Buttner 1968). However, the intraerythrocytic forms of *B. canis* and *B. caballi* were found to have similar ultrastructures (Simpson *et al.* 1963). The intraerythrocytic forms of *B. gibsoni* were investigated (Ray and Idnani 1947).

Biochemistry

Because optimal *in vitro* methods of growing *Babesia* have not been established, there is very little information available on the metabolism and biochemistry of these organisms.

Literature

Wright (1981) reviewed the biochemical characteristics of *Babesia* and the physiochemical reactions in the host. He concluded that very little is known about the biochemistry of these parasites and summarized the available information on babesial protein and carbohydrate metabolism. Weber (1980) studied the structure and cytochemistry of *B. bigemina* and *B. bovis* found in the hemolymph of the ticks *B. microplus* and *R. bursa*.

Tissue culture

The cultivation of *Babesia* in erythrocytes and the *in vitro* development of the parasites in the organs and tissues of ticks are systems which have only recently been developed and are not yet optimal for research or practical applications.

Literature

The absence of a method for *in vitro* propagation of *Babesia* has long complicated efforts to study these organisms. *Babesia bovis* was cultured in suspensions of bovine erythrocytes incubated at 37 °C in Medium 199 with 50% bovine serum. The medium was stirred and replaced every 24 hours and subcultured (Erp *et al.* 1978). The results of attempts to optimize suspension culture methods for the *in vitro* cultivation of *B. bovis* indicated that the pH markedly influenced the growth rate and that growth improved with increasing complexity of the medium (Erp *et al.* 1980b).

The persistent multiplication of the parasite in short series of subcultures suggested that a method of continuous culture was feasible (Erp *et al.* 1978). Using a culture method based on the candle jar technique, *B. bovis, B. bigemina,* and *B. rodhaini* were found to multiply within host red blood cells and were maintained for up to 96 hours. Regular changes of medium and subculture at 24-hour intervals were essential for optimal parasite survival (Timms 1980). The infectivity of *B. bovis* obtained from continuous *in vitro* cultures was comparable to that of infected bovine blood, and there was no alteration in the morphology of *Babesia* maintained *in vitro* for extended periods of time (Erp *et al.* 1980a). Merozoites deprived of carbon dioxide accumulated in the medium rather than in new erythrocytes and retained their infectivity (Levy and Ristic 1980). *Babesia bovis* was passaged between continuous *in vitro* cultures and splenectomized calves. The cultured *Babesia* organisms were identical morphologically to erythrocytic forms and showed no loss of infectivity or virulence (Erp *et al.* 1980a, b). Short-term *in vitro* multiplication of *B. bovis* was achieved with the development of suspension cultures. The use of spinner flask cultures permitted the continuous growth of the organisms *in vitro,* but the large volumes and extensive manipulation required by these cultures, coupled with the organisms' relatively slow growth under these conditions, limited the utility of this method. These shortcomings were eliminated by the development of the micro-aerophilous stationary phase culture system. This system was considered optimal because a high yield of organisms with good growth characteristics was produced using micro-titer culture plates. The suspension cultures of *B. bovis* and *B. canis,* and the stationary cultures of *B. bovis* were reviewed (Levy *et al.* 1981). Bovine erythrocytes parasitized with *B. major* were fused with human HeLa cells by means of Sendai virus. *Babesia major* parasites entered the HeLa cell cytoplasm and, in some cases, underwent multiplication over a period of 3 days (Irvin and Young 1979a). The replacement of Hanks' balanced salt solution by sorbitol in saline increased the survival of *B. microti* during cryopreservation (Gray and Phillips 1981). An *in vitro* technique for measuring the uptake of [^{3}H]-hypoxanthine by erythrocytic forms could be of practical value in assessing the infectivity of stored blood and of cultures of *Babesia* species infective for cattle and mice (Irvin and Young 1979b).

The *in vitro* development of *Babesia* in the tick organ and tissue preparations was described. The developmental stages of *B. bigemina* were observed to survive for long periods of time in an infected *Boophilus annulatus* organ maintained in culture; the sequential isolation of various developmental phenomena is not possible in this kind of system because of the parasites' continuous type of life cycle

(Hadani 1981). Undifferentiated embryonic cells derived from *B. bovis*-infected *B. microplus* tick eggs which had been incubated for 8 to 10 days at 26 °C and for 80 hours at 37 °C caused clinical disease in calves (Ronald and Cruz 1981). The ultraerythrocytic forms of *B. bovis* which were inoculated into cultures of *B. microplus* embryonic cells invaded the tick cells and multiplied for up to 48 hours (Bhat *et al.* 1979).

Laboratory animals and man

The limitations of existing culture techniques have stimulated the search for methods by which babesial species pathogenic for domestic animals could be adapted to laboratory rodents. Although rodents are susceptible to infection with specific babesial species, laboratory rodents are in general resistant to persistent infection with species natural to other hosts. Humans and monkeys under certain conditions, e.g. in postsplenectomy hosts, are susceptible to infection with *Babesia* organisms, particularly *B. microti*, the natural parasite of rodents, which may cause severe clinical syndromes and death.

Literature

Intraperitoneally injected *B. bovis*, *B. bigemina*, *B. equi*, and *B. caballi* (but not *B. trautmanni*) were able to establish infections in suckling mice. The piroplasms were observed for 2 to 4 days but did not invade the murine erythrocytes (Dennig 1962). Mice congenitally deficient in T-lymphocytes did not remain infected with *B. divergens* or *B. major* for long periods of time, although the former organism persisted for 10 days and the latter for 1 day (Irvin *et al.* 1978a). Mongolian gerbils could be infected with *B. divergens* by the intraperitoneal inoculation of infected bovine blood. The parasite retained its infectivity for splenectomized calves after two gerbil passages (Lewis 1979; Lewis and Williams 1979).

Cases of human babesiosis and babesiasis were reported in the USA (Ristic *et al.* 1971) and in England (Coombs 1977) respectively. The old and modern literature on the occurrence of human babesiosis in the USA, Yugoslavia, Ireland, Mexico, France, Russia, and Scotland was reviewed (Brocklesby 1979). Teutsch *et al.* (1980) described the disease induced by *B. microti* in splenectomized human patients. The infections caused by *B. microti* in a variety of species of splenectomized nonhuman primates were investigated (Moore and Kuntz 1981). The experimental infection of nonsplenectomized rhesus monkeys (*Macaca mulatta*) with *B. microti* was characterized by a prepatent period of 15 to 46 days and parasitemia which persisted for at least 90 days and, in one case, as long as 559 days after inoculation (Ruebush *et al.* 1979). *Babesia microti* could also be transmitted to rhesus monkeys via the tick *Ixodes dammini*; the parasitemia persisted for 15 to 17 months (Ruebush *et al.* 1981).

EPIZOOTIOLOGY

Incidence

The arthropod vectors of *Babesia* are all hard ticks of the family Ixodidae. In general, each species of *Babesia* is associated with a single vector species; e.g. in Europe *B. bovis* infects cattle through *Rhipicephalus bursa*, but *B. divergens* is transmitted by *Ixodes ricinus*. The vector associated with any given parasite may differ from region to region. For example, in Australia and South America the vector of *B. bovis* is *B. microplus*, whereas in Europe it is *R. bursa*. In horses the vector of *B. equi* in Central America is *Dermacentor nitens*, whereas in Europe the vector is *D. marginatus*.

The epizootiological investigation of babesiosis involves the determination of disease distribution and frequency among individually managed animals (e.g. dogs) and animal groups (e.g. herds of ruminants). The control of disease in individual animals is relatively simple and depends on the identification of the organism and effective drug treatment. The evaluation of the epizootiology of babesiosis in a herd is more complex, requiring consideration of the host, the *Babesia* species, and the vector. These three parameters must be known before effective long-term control measures can be instituted. Accurate figures showing the extent of the economic losses due to babesiosis are not available in many countries.

Literature

Most of the literature available on the incidence of babesiosis is concerned with species which infect cattle, and the majority of the reports from tropical climates were from Australia. A few brief reviews on tick-borne diseases of domestic animals in Australia (Anon. 1970) and on protozoan diseases transmitted by the cattle tick *B. microplus* (Pierce 1956) have been published. Barnett (1974a, b) reviewed the economic aspects of tick-borne disease control in the UK and of protozoal tick-borne diseases of livestock in the rest of the world. In the latter review, Barnett defined the epizootiological factors which have to be considered when planning control measures against protozoal tick-borne diseases as follows: (1) the presence of ticks and diseases which cause damage and loss; (2) the presence of ticks in an area where the disease is enzootic and controlled; and (3) the absence of both ticks and diseases in a region where they could become established. Joyner and Donnelly (1979) discussed the epizootiology of babesiosis in Australia and the UK and presented a general descriptive mathematical model.

In New South Wales, Australia, is a quarantine area with very little tick fever while in Queensland, where ticks are relatively uncontrolled, the incidence of tick fever is endemic in most properties within the tick zone. The incidence of clinical and subclinical infections in New South Wales between 1964 and 1970 was ascertained by means of serological studies, examination of blood films and transmission tests. Of the 544 herds tested, 55 were found to contain subclinical infection with *B. bovis*, 25 with *B. bigemina*, and 6 with mixed infections; in any one herd the highest number of *B. bovis* and *B. bigemina* infections detected was four and two, respectively. The incidence of subclinically infected herds ranged from 3.8 to 19.1% (Curnow 1973b). In a short review of the epizootiology of *B. bovis* and *B. bigemina* in Australia, Callow (1979) described the difference between the species with respect to the transmission, incidence, and severity of the infections and discussed disease control through vaccination. Positive complement fixation (CF) reactions indicated that the incidence of *B. bovis* and *B. bigemina* was from 0.5 to 1% in New South Wales and 77 to 81% in Queensland (Australia) (Curnow 1973c). Ninety-two percent of all the outbreaks of babesiosis in Queensland from 1966 to 1976 were caused by *B. bovis*, and 70% of the outbreaks occurred in the *B. microplus* enzootic zone (Copeman *et al.* 1978). The incidence of clinical babesiosis in cattle in Queensland between 1947 and 1963 was examined; 90% of the cases were found to be due to *B. bovis* (Johnston 1968). A subclinical infection rate from 3.8 to 19.1% was detected in New South Wales using the CF test, thick blood smear techniques, and transmission tests (Curnow 1973b). The incidence of *Babesia* infection in Droughtmaster and Hereford herds of calves in Queensland was investigated (Johnston 1967). It was found that the rate of infection with *B. bovis* was significantly lower in the Droughtmaster herd than in the Herefords, but the incidence of *B. bigemina* infections was similar in both herds.

The occurrence of *B. bovis* in cattle in Sri Lanka was reported (Bandaranayake 1961). In Colombia, morphologic and immunologic methods were used to identify the existing *Babesia* species. Sensitive and practical serological tests for the diagnosis of latent *Babesia* infections were investigated and a system of chemoprophylaxis was evaluated (Todorovic 1976a). Serological surveys were conducted to determine the incidence of *B. bigemina* (92 to 93%) and *B. bovis* (12 to 44%) and subtropical infections in the tropical regions of Colombia (Corrier *et al.* 1978). The indirect fluorescent antibody (IFA) and CF tests were used to ascertain the relative incidence of *B. bigemina* and *B. bovis* in Guyana. Using the IFA test, it was determined that 80 and 61% of the sera examined were positive for *B. bigemina* and *B. bovis* respectively, while the corresponding incidence data obtained with the CF test were 40 and 60% (Applewhaite *et al.* 1981). Information regarding cases of babesiosis among domestic animals and humans, serological methods of diagnosis, and various vaccination procedures was published in a report on the research programs under way at the Mexican National Institute of Animal Research (Osorno 1978). The occurrence of babesiosis and *B. microplus* infestation in northern Mexico was reported (Thompson *et al.* 1980).

The occurrence of tick-borne diseases of domestic animals in northern Nigeria between 1923 and 1966 was discussed. It was noted that *B. bigemina* infections occurred in cattle undergoing rinderpest immunization and in animals suffering from trypanosomiasis. Babesiosis was considered to be one of the most significant diseases in imported breeds of cattle and in those maintained under intensive systems of management (Leeflang 1977). The results of the research conducted on tick-borne diseases in northern Nigeria between 1966 and 1976 were summarized; it was concluded that most of the tick-borne organisms caused inapparent infections, but could induce clinical diseases when conditions were adverse to the host (Leeflang and Ilemobade 1977). Brain smears made from 313 cattle slaughtered in northern Nigeria indicated that approximately 10 and 0.7% of the animals were infected with *B. bovis* and *B. bigemina* respectively (Folkers *et al.* 1967). In another Nigerian study, *B. bovis* was observed in 7.2% of 694 animals examined for cerebral babesiosis (Ajayi 1978). On the basis of serological tests, the incidence of *B. bigemina* in Botswana was found to be 78% (Mehlitz and Ehret 1974).

Purnell (1977a) described the incidence of bovine babesiosis in the European Community and discussed the need for routine serological screening of cattle being moved within the region. *Babesia divergens*, *B. bovis*, and *B. major* occur within the European Community, but *B. divergens* is the principal cause of babesiosis. The control of blood protozoa in Iran was reviewed (Hooshmand-Rad 1974), and the epizootiology of *B. bovis* in Indonesia was investigated (Holz 1960).

Roberts *et al.* (1962) quoted Henning (1956) on the distribution of equine babesiosis in Africa; the prevalence of the disease in southern and eastern Europe, the USSR, India, the Philippines, Asia, Central America and northern parts of South America was also investigated. Donnelly *et al.* (1980a) researched the incidence of antibodies to *B. equi* and *B. caballi* in horses reared in Oman. It was discovered through use of the IFA test that approximately 90% and 40 to 60% of the animals tested were infected with *B. equi* and *B. caballi* respectively; the corresponding incidence rates obtained with the CF test were 70% and 30 to 40%. The discrepancies between the two tests were probably due to the greater sensitivity of the IFA test and the faster decay of the antibodies detected by the CF test. Using these serological techniques, it was also determined that 77.1 and 11.4% of the racehorses imported into Kuwait developed serum antibodies to *B. equi* and *B. caballi* respectively. The antibody titers detected with the IFA test persisted for longer periods of time than those obtained with the CF test (Donnelly *et al.* 1980b). A total of 115 cases of equine babesiosis from a population of approximately 6000 in South Africa and Zimbabwe were investigated to establish whether such factors as season, sex, coat color, and age influenced the incidence of the disease. It was found that the distribution of the cases was significantly related to these factors (Littlejohn and Walker 1979). The introduction of equine babesiosis to the USA and the epizootiology of the disease were described by Sippel *et al.* (1962). Taylor *et al.* (1969) listed the incidence of *B. caballi* in the various states between 1962 and 1969. Some clinical signs were of assistance in differentiating the diseases produced by

B. equi and *B. caballi*. *Babesia equi* caused intermittent fever, whereas the fever induced by *B. caballi* was persistent. Similarly, hemoglobinuria was common in horses with *B. equi* but rare with *B. caballi* infections. In the USA, equine babesiosis was an epizootic disease caused solely by *B. caballi*, while in South Africa the disease was enzootic and was caused by either *B. caballi* or *B. equi* (Retief 1964). A tentative diagnosis of *B. equi* was made in the USA in 1965 (Knowles *et al.* 1966).

Babesia gibsoni was reported to be very widespread in India and in southeast Asia, extending from India, Sri Lanka, Malaysia, China to Japan (Seneviratna 1965a, b). *Babesia canis* infections have been observed in Africa, Asia, Brazil, Europe, Puerto Rico, the Panama Canal Zone, and the USA (Rokey and Russell 1961). *Babesia canis* is also present in Australia. The overall incidence of babesiosis in dogs in Uganda was about 1.9% (Bwangamoi and Isyagi 1973). *Babesia canis* was transmitted from the domestic dog to the wild dog (*Lycaon pictus*) and black-backed jackal (*Canis mesomelas*) and was also successfully retransmitted from the wild carnivores to the domestic dog (van Heerden 1980). A case of *B. trautmanni* infection occurred in the Central African Republic (Itard 1964).

Transmission

The arthropod vectors of *Babesia* are hard ticks of the family Ixodidae. Each species of *Babesia* is transmitted by a single tick species which varies from one region to another, thereby causing differences in the epizootiology of babesial diseases. Transmission occurs when an infected tick feeds on a susceptible host. There are four stages in the life cycle of the vector. Adult ticks feed and mate on the host. The engorged female then lays between 1000 and 5000 eggs that hatch into larvae which actively seek a new host. The larvae of three-host ticks feed on a new host until they become engorged and drop to the ground to molt into nymphs. These nymphs repeat the cycle with another new host and ultimately molt into either male or female adults. In the case of two-host tick species of the genus *Hyalomma*, the engorged larvae stay on the host and molt into nymphs which then feed and drop engorged to the ground. One-host ticks such as *Boophilus* species undergo both their larval and nymphal molts on the same host. The infectivity of the larvae, nymphs, and adults varies depending upon whether the tick is a one-, two-, or three-host species.

Babesia parasites are generally transmitted transovarially; i.e. the organisms invade the eggs and thus infect the new generation of larvae. This transovarial, or vertical, transmission enables infections to be disseminated to a large number of the progeny. Transovarial transmission occurs in one-, two-, and three-host ticks, but horizontal, or transstadial, transmission may also take place. Generally, the infection in ticks does not survive for more than one generation; however, it has been shown that certain babesial species may survive through a number of generations of ticks, indicating that tick populations may remain carriers for extended periods of time when susceptible mammalian hosts are not available.

The number of ticks in the environment is an important factor which affects the epizootiology of babesiosis. In areas where tick populations are large, the incidence is stable; the organism persists in the environment and rarely causes clinical cases. In areas adjacent to these enzootic zones, tick reproduction may be suppressed by unfavorable climatic conditions, and the resultant fluctuations in the tick population engender outbreaks of babesiosis. The incidence of babesiosis stabilizes in an enzootic area when the inoculation rate is sufficient to infect all calves before their resistance disappears between 6 and 9 months of age. The rate of transmission of *B. bovis* by *B. microplus* is different in European and Zebu x European cattle subjected to various levels of tick challenge. When tick-control methods are sparingly used, a minimal inoculation rate is required to produce stability in the European cattle grazing on pastures favorable to tick reproduction. Instability occurs in those herds of European cattle after the tick population has been reduced in pastures by dipping and after the infection rate in ticks has been decreased by unfavorable environmental conditions. The Zebu x European cattle do not generate inoculation rates in the tick population above the minimum required for stability, even when tick-control measures are not initiated because of the low rates of infection in ticks and the high resistance of Zebu crosses to ticks.

Literature

Friedhoff and Smith (1981) discussed in detail the transmission of *Babesia* by ticks and the complexity of the transmissions which were dependent on the host, babesial, and tick species involved. In a review of the literature pertaining to the pathogenesis of babesiosis and to the factors involved in nonspecific resistance and immunity to the disease, Zwart and Brocklesby (1979) presented a table in which the methods of transmitting *Babesia* species between domestic and wild mammals were summarized. The epizootiological features of *B. bovis* transmission were discussed by Mahoney *et al.* (1981a).

There has been a great deal of information available on the transmission of *B. bovis* and *B. bigemina*, the two species which infect cattle, but relatively little is known about the other babesial species. The susceptibility of *B. microplus* females to infection with *B. bigemina* and *B. bovis* was restricted to the last 24 hours of the normal 21-day period the ticks spend on the host. If the parasitemia was not high just prior to detachment, the ticks may not become infected. The transmission of *Babesia* by the one-, two-, and three-host ticks was described by Friedhoff and Smith (1981). The nymphs and adults of *B. microplus*, a one-host tick, transmitted *B. bigemina*. The occurrence of continuous transstadial and transovarial infections throughout an entire generation has not been shown. The progeny of infected adults were not infective, when the ticks were fed either on a nonbovine host or on a host treated with chemotherapeutic agents. Infected *B. microplus* larvae were not infective, while infected nymphs and adults were capable of transmitting the disease. The males of *B. microplus* could transmit *B. bigemina*, but it has not been proved conclusively that the female ticks transmitted the infection. The extent to which nymphs and females of *B. microplus* transmitted *Babesia* to other hosts by attaching or reattaching has not been established. There was no evidence which indicated that larvae or nymphs could acquire the infection by ingesting infected blood. The transmission of *B. bovis* by *B. microplus* differed from that of *B. bigemina* since the parasite was transmitted exclusively by the larval stage of the tick. The larvae lost the infection after transmission; hence the nymphs and adults that developed from these larvae were not infective.

The most important vector of *Babesia* among the two-host ticks is *R. bursa*. It was shown that various *Babesia* species (e.g. *B. ovis*) could be maintained through many generations of ticks. The engorged females were infective a few hours prior to detachment. After the female was infected, the eggs, larvae, nymphs, and adults acquired the parasite both transovarially and transstadially. The infected larvae and nymphs did not transmit the infection but the adults were able to do so. Although other babesial strains were transmitted by the nymphs, it appeared that the adults of *R. bursa* were the most important agents in the transmission of the disease. The infection persisted throughout the life of the female tick. Among the three-host ticks, e.g. *I. ricinus*, *Haemaphysalis punctata*, and *R. sanguineous*, only the engorged female acquired the organism, but all of the stages were infective.

The efficiency of transmission of *Babesia* was influenced by the environmental temperature and the age and strain of the tick. The quantitative aspects of the transmission of *Babesia* have not been extensively studied. The morphological changes of *B. bigemina* and *B. bovis* in the gut of the engorged female ticks were investigated. The ingested erythrocytic forms developed into rayed forms, the *Strahlenkorper*. The latter were transformed in the epithelial cells of the gut to fission bodies which finally released the club-shaped bodies known as vermicules or kinetes.

A number of investigations have further defined the various aspects of transmission of *B. bigemina* and *B. bovis* by *B. microplus*. After transovarian transmission, the infectivity of *B. bovis* terminated at the end of the larval stage, but *B. bigemina* did not become infective until midway through the nymphal stage of the tick. Thereafter, *B. bigemina* was continuously transmitted by the nymphal and adult stages; replete females and males were infective for up to 35 days (Callow and Hoyte 1961a; Callow 1968a, 1979). *Babesia bigemina* and *B. bovis* were capable of uninterrupted development in the organs of ticks, and both transstadial and transovarial transmissions occurred. Hadani (1981) observed that there were concurrent babesial life cycles within a given stage of the tick's life cycle, so that vermicules, schizonts, and infective particles were simultaneously present in the tissues. The maintenance of a colony of *B. microplus* infected with *B. bigemina* was described (Thompson 1976).

The stimulus of feeding was required for *Babesia* to become infective for cattle. Infective *B. bovis* parasites were shown to develop in unfed larval ticks. In addition, it was found that *B. bovis* and *B. bigemina* could develop in incubated tick eggs, and infective *B. bigemina* matured in unfed larval ticks maintained at 37 °C (Dalgliesh and Stewart 1978). Different methods were used to determine the infection rates in tick populations exposed to these species of *Babesia*. The infection rates were ascertained by direct microscopic examination of the various stages and then compared with the infectivity of the ticks for cattle, which was determined by feeding small groups of larvae on susceptible calves. A close correlation was found between larval infectivity and the *Babesia* infection rate, measured by the examination of smears of tick larvae made about 24 to 48 hours after attachment to the host (Mahoney and Mirre 1971).

The concept that babesial organisms persist in tick populations without undergoing part of the life cycle in the vertebrate host was investigated. The results of experiments involving the transmission of *B. bovis* by *B. microplus* indicated that the larvae of the next generation of ticks did not become infected unless the protozoan went through its life cycle in the vertebrate host. Only the larvae which originated from infected eggs were infective for cattle (Mahoney and Mirre 1979). *Babesia bigemina* infection in *B. microplus* was not eliminated when the ticks were fed on ovine, caprine, and equine hosts, even though these nonbovine hosts were shown to carry the organism in their blood while the ticks fed (Callow 1965).

The interactions among *B. bovis*, *B. microplus*, and the vertebrate host have been extensively investigated, but there have been relatively few published studies on the transmission of other babesial species to various domestic animals by other tick species. In Kenya, *B. bigemina* was shown to be transmitted by *B. decoloratus* (Morzaria *et al.* 1977). The larvae of infected adult *B. decoloratus* transmitted *B. bigemina* to cattle and played a role in the epizootiology of babesiosis in Nigeria (Akinboade *et al.* 1981). A successful method for the rearing of *I. ricinus* was described by Donnelly and Peirce (1975), who applied the procedure in a study of the transmission of *B. divergens*. These researchers demonstrated that both parasitemic and carrier hosts were infective only to the adult stages of the tick. It was found that *B. major* was transovarially transmitted to *Haemaphysalis punctata* ticks; splenectomized calves which acquired the protozoan from these ticks developed a mild disease (Brocklesby and Sellwood 1973). The hereditary transmission of *B. caballi* in *D. nitens* was investigated (Roby *et al.* 1964). The reliability of tick transmission of equine babesiosis was examined by subjecting the unfed larvae and nymphs of *Hyalomma*, *Rhipicephalus*, and *Dermacentor* species to low temperature and humidity. *Hyalomma* species were xerothermic, while *Dermacentor* species were hydrophilic and psychrophilic. Because both *B. caballi* and *B. equi* resist wide thermal deviations in the vector ticks, transmission can occur in both temperate and tropical regions (Enigk 1950).

There have been a number of reports on the intrauterine transmission of *Babesia*. Klinger and Ben-Yossef (1972) described a case of *B. bovis* infection in a bovine fetus. Intrauterine transmission of *B. bovis* was also observed in a calf which was born normally but showed intravascular hemolysis and nervous involvement 24 hours after birth (De Vos *et al.* 1976).

INFECTION

In much of the research on babesial infections, a common method of inducing the disease involves passaging infected blood; the vector cycle of the parasite is used infrequently. However, transmission by serial passaging of infected blood changes the infectivity for ticks, pathogenicity, virulence, immunogenicity, drug resistance, and, to some degree, the morphology of the organisms.

Babesial infections start with the invasion of the erythrocyte by the organism. The merozoites penetrate the red blood cells by a process which can be divided into the following steps: (1) contact between the protozoan and the red blood cells; (2) orientation of the protozoan so that the organelles (rhoptries and granules) are in apposition with the cell membrane; (3) membrane fusion; (4) rhoptry release; (5) invagination of the red cell membrane; and (6) entry.

The number of organisms injected affects the time of onset of parasitemia and the nature of the clinical signs. Generally, a large number of piroplasms are observed in cases with severe clinical syndromes. The level and duration of parasitemia depends on the species of *Babesia* and on the susceptibility of the host. For example, the parasitemia levels caused by *B. bovis* in acute fatal, severe nonfatal, and mild cases range from 0.01 to 0.2%, while the acute syndromes caused by *B. bigemina* are associated with levels exceeding 10%. The parasitemia levels measured in dogs with fatal or nonfatal *B. gibsoni* infections may be as high as 45 and 14% respectively, whereas the parasitemia fluctuates considerably in subacute, chronic cases. Parasitemia is lowest in the carrier state. Following recovery from patent disease, subclinical infections may last for several years. Relapses are associated with the resurgence of the parasitemia which may occur every 3 to 8 weeks in single infections. In a field situation where there is repeated exposure to challenge, the incidence of detectable parasitemia is higher than that found in single infections, fluctuates widely, and gradually decreases over a period of years. In enzootic areas, the incidence and level of patent parasitemia decline as an animal ages since it is constantly exposed to reinfection by all of the antigenic types found in a particular habitat. Under these natural field conditions, babesiosis may occur as a single infection or as a multiple infection involving more than one *Babesia* species. The manifestation of the clinical signs of babesiosis may be complicated by the presence of symptoms induced by concurrent infections with other blood parasites; e.g. *Trypanosoma, Anaplasma,* and *Ehrlichia*.

It is necessary to enumerate the babesial organisms in order to determine the level and fluctuation of the parasitemia and thereby define the various host–parasite relationships. The accuracy of these estimates depends on the distribution of organisms in the circulating blood. There are some species (e.g. *B. bovis*) which localize in the blood vessels of the brain; hence, the parasitemia observed in the peripheral circulation may not reflect the actual level of infection.

The virulence of the organism can be changed by either mechanical passaging of infected blood through splenectomized calves or irradiation. Rapid passages of blood have resulted in the development of avirulent strains which can be used in immunization procedures. The investigation of the various behavioral properties of the organisms depends on the use of cryopreservation, which ensures the stability of the specimens during prolonged laboratory manipulations.

Literature

Boophilus microplus injects *B. bigemina* into the bovine 8 to 9 days after the larvae attach to the host. Since piroplasms were already present in the erythrocytes 9 to 13 days after infection, pre-erythrocytic schizogony probably did not occur (Hoyte 1961, 1965). The mechanisms involved in the penetration of the erythrocytes by *Babesia* have been investigated in laboratory rodents. The results of several experiments indicated that complement-induced modifications of either the rat erythrocyte or the *B. rodhaini* cell membrane facilitated the penetration process. The C3b receptor, which is present on both red blood cells and *B. rodhaini*, appears to be involved in this process (Ward and Jack 1981). Further investigations showed that the ability of *B. rodhaini* to penetrate human red cells depends on factors of the alternative complement pathway, ionic magnesium, and the third and fifth components of complement. The requirement of complement for the invasion of erythrocytes suggests that the babesial parasites have developed a novel mechanism for exploiting the host's immune system (Chapman and Ward 1977).

The *Babesia* multiply by binary fission, and it was found that the multiplication rates of *B. bovis* and *B. bigemina* in cattle were similar (Wright and Goodger 1977). The doubling time of both species was about 8 hours (Mahoney and Goodger 1972; Mahoney *et al.* 1973a; Wright and Kerr 1975). Thus the parasite doubling time for *B. bigemina* was in accord with that observed for *B. bovis* and with the estimate of Hoyte (1961) that *B. bigemina* multiplied tenfold in 24 hours. *Babesia bovis* multiplied approximately twentyfold every 24 hours for the first 6 days of infection (Wright and Goodger 1977). In *B. canis* infections, the initial transient parasitemia which developed lasted for 3 to 4 days and was followed by a second peak of parasitemia 2 weeks after infection; subsequent relapses occurred at irregular and unpredictable intervals (Ewing 1965b).

Some species of *Babesia* may differ with respect to their patterns of distribution in the circulating blood. *Babesia bovis* could be readily demonstrated in bovine brain smears, while *B. bigemina* was rarely observed in brain capillaries. An examination of cattle from enzootic areas revealed that 299 out of 458 brains were positive for *B. bovis*. The organisms in the brain capillaries do not stain as clearly; hence, it was difficult to differentiate morphologically between *B. bovis* and *B. bigemina* (Callow and Johnston 1963). Also *B. bovis* in capillaries is as large as *B. bigemina* which is the real problem in differential diagnosis.

The age of the host influences its susceptibility to infection and therefore affects the incidence of disease in a population of animals. Infections by *B. bovis* increased with age from about 6 months; in 6-, 12-, and 18-month-old calves, the rates were 49.2, 56.9, and 69.1% respectively (Callow *et al.* 1976a). This was confirmed by Mahoney (1979), who found that the incidence of *B. bovis* in infected environments rose from zero at birth to a maximum at 1 to 2 years of age and then declined, while in *B. bigemina* infections the incidence was maximal among calves 6 to 12 months of age. Among native calves living in an enzootic area of Colombia, the mean age of first infection with *Anaplasma* and *Babesia* was 11 weeks. There was an initial significant decrease in the packed cell volume (PCV) which returned to preinfection levels within 4 weeks (Corrier and Guzman 1977).

A computer model used to simulate the occurrence of detectable parasitemia with *B. bovis* in *Bos taurus* cattle was based on an immunological mechanism proposed to account for the fluctuations in the levels of detectable parasitemia in chronically infected animals. The epizootiological model developed as a possible explanation for the pattern of age-associated prevalence of parasitemia in enzootic herds, can be summarized as follows. Since a population of *B. bovis* has the genetic potential to produce a finite number of different antigens on the surface of a parasitized erythrocyte, a random sample of this antigenic pool will be expressed each time an animal becomes infected. The likelihood of detectable parasitemia in a young animal rises in proportion to the number of superinfections contracted because, given a large pool, the probability that any antigen will be repeated during the early infections acquired by a calf is low. However, as the animal is progressively exposed to the entire antigenic pool, an increasing number of parasite antigens are recognized and destroyed by the immunological defenses of the host. Thus, the frequency of detectable parasitemia declines in parallel with the exhaustion of the new antigenic types (Ross and Mahoney 1974).

The duration of an infection varies with the species of *Babesia* and the susceptibility of the host. After a single infection with either *B. bigemina* or *B. bovis*, recurrences of parasitemia were observed for 1.5 to 2 years. Following infection with *B. bovis* or *B. bigemina*, cattle were infective to ticks for up to a year and for only 4 to 7 weeks respectively. Cattle were shown to be parasitized by *B. bovis* 13 months after infection irrespective of whether they had been subsequently tick-free or tick-infested (Johnston and Tammemagi 1969). The duration of latent infection and immunity was investigated in Droughtmaster and Hereford cattle following natural infection with *B. bovis* and *B. bigemina*. The Droughtmaster cattle were 3/8 to 5/8 Brahman × British beef bred. The animals underwent a natural challenge for 3 years and were monitored for 3 additional years. *Babesia bovis* infections in Herefords were more persistent than those in the Droughtmasters. Both the Hereford and Droughtmaster cattle showed a marked degree of resistance to infection with a heterologous strain of *B. bovis* (Johnston *et al.* 1978). In *Bos taurus* calves which acquired infection with *B. bovis* and *B. bigemina* before 5 to 7 months of age, relapsing parasitemia with *B. bovis* was observed more frequently than that with *B. bigemina* over a period of 2 years (Mahoney *et al.* 1973b). In splenectomized calves with chronic *B. divergens* infections, the relapsing parasitemia occurred on average every 14.7 days (Trees 1978).

The accurate and precise enumeration of *Babesia* is essential for the determination of fluctuations in the parasitemia levels, which in turn are related to various aspects of host–parasite interactions. The accurate counting of piroplasms is particularly important in research and vaccination procedures. In the direct enumeration techniques, parasites were counted either in thick smear preparations of measured quantities of blood or in wet preparations of diluted blood in a counting chamber. A direct technique in which erythrocytes were fixed in gluteraldehyde and diluted to 1/1000 in water combined the accuracy of the thick film technique with the convenience of using diluted blood to reduce the number of parasites in heavily infected samples. In a commonly used indirect method, the number of piroplasms was computed from the total number of erythrocytes and the percentage of infected erythrocytes counted on a stained slide. There were errors in the estimates of the parasitemia levels because the distribution of erythrocytes and organisms in thin blood smears prepared from heavily infected bovine blood was not random (Parker 1973). A newer method involved labeling the deoxyribonucleic acid (DNA) intraerythrocytic *Babesia* with fluorescent bisbenzimidazole dye (33258 Hoechst). The labeled cells were sorted on a fluorescence-activated cell sorter on the basis of cell fluorescence. This method could be used for the separation of infected and uninfected red blood cells for biochemical and immunochemical studies (Howard and Rodwell 1979). Gluteraldehyde-fixed blood stained with 33258 Hoechst and dispensed as 1 mm^3 droplets onto microscope slides provided accurate estimates of parasitemia when a direct counting method was used (Rodwell and Howard 1981).

The storage of infective materials, e.g. blood and tick tissues, in a stable state (referred to as stabilates) is central to much of the standardization of research on vaccination methods. Some of the labile behavioral properties of the organism can be affected by laboratory manipulation. For example, differences in the infectivity of *B. bovis* were detected after the organisms were incubated for 24 hours in plasma and serum. The *Babesia* were less viable following incubation in serum than in plasma, and the differences in viability were related to the presence of glucose in plasma and its absence in the serum when these diluents were conventionally prepared (Farlow 1976). There were no changes observed in the virulence and behavior of *Babesia* contained in bovine and porcine blood which has been stored at −79 °C and supplemented with 7% (v/v) glycerol (Barnett 1964). Stabilates were prepared from nymphs of *B. decoloratus* ticks infected with *B. bigemina* (Morzaria *et al.* 1977). Subcutaneous and intravenous inoculates of homogenates of whole *B. microplus* larvae infected with *B. bovis* were also found to be infective for cattle (Mahoney and Mirre 1974).

There is a relatively good correlation between the size of the inoculating dose of organisms and the levels of parasitemia, the time of onset, and the severity of the clinical syndromes, which may range from acute disease of a few days' duration to carrier states lasting several years. The titration (using doses of 2.94×10^{10}, 2.94×10^{7} and 2.94×10^{4} of parasitized erythrocytes) of *B. major* piroplasms in intact calves resulted in a linear increase in the length of the prepatent period to the onset of the disease (Purnell *et al.* 1979c). When *B. divergens* was titrated in splenectomized calves, a linear relationship was observed between the infective doses (10^5 to 10^9 organisms) and the onset of disease. The minimum dose required to produce patent disease or resistance to homologous challenge in the inoculated animals was 10^3 parasites (Purnell *et al.* 1977a). Kemron *et al.* (1964) also found a direct relationship between the number of piroplasms in the inoculum and the course of the reaction in vaccinated intact cattle, but in splenectomized cattle a severe reaction with high mortality was observed irrespective of the dose used. The blood obtained from 'latent' chronic carriers failed to infect consistently, but when it did produce an infection the incubation period was protracted and the reaction was usually mild.

In cattle infected with *B. bovis*, fever, anemia, and the level of parasitemia were correlated and could be used to measure the intensity of the host–parasite interaction (Callow and Pepper 1974). A positive correlation was also established between the level of parasitemia caused by *B. bigemina* and a rise in body temperature; fever peaked when the parasitemia was 22% (Pandey and Mishra 1978a). The reaction of calves to five isolates of *B. divergens* was also compared on the basis of parasitemia, fever, and hematological parameters. The principal component analysis of these data indicated that the responses could be characterized in two dimensions which were used to determine the relative pathogenicity of each isolate (Purnell *et al.* 1976).

The virulence of *Babesia* organisms depends on the species and the strain and can be changed by laboratory procedures involving serial transmission through infected blood or ticks. The virulence of *B. divergens* isolated from infected animals during the reaction and carrier phases was investigated in splenectomized calves. Parasitological, hematological, and clinical parameters were used to evaluate the response in hosts which were infected with high and low doses of parasites collected 10 to 196 days after infection. The only significant differences between the groups were those related to the parasite dose; e.g. the prepatent periods to detectable parasites in the blood smears and to a febrile response. The parasites harvested from the donor animal 196 days after inoculation apparently lost their virulence (Purnell *et al.* 1978b). A marked loss of virulence of *B. bovis* in intact cattle resulted after 11 blood passages through splenectomized calves, although the latter were severely affected. This method has enabled the preparation of a safe living vaccine for the control of babesiosis. The attenuation was reversed by passaging through intact cattle; the parasite became virulent again at passage 5. The selection for particularly immunogenic antigens, against an immunosuppressive effect, for a lower multiplication rate, or for a combination of these features could decrease the virulence (Callow *et al.* 1979b). Serial passage of two strains of *B. bovis* through splenectomized calves also reduced the organisms' pathogenicity for replete female *B. microplus*. The attenuated strains infected a higher proportion of ticks and produced comparable numbers of morphologically similar parasites in the hemolymph, but killed fewer ticks. It was suggested that the attenuated strains lost the factor which caused pathological effects on the gut cells of infected ticks (Dalgliesh *et al.* 1981b).

Another method used for reducing the lower virulence of *Babesia* involved irradiation. After *B. bovis* was attenuated by 35 krad of gamma irradiation, the organisms caused only mild effects in susceptible animals. The multiplication rates and the maximum parasitemias were similar for the irradiated and nonirradiated parasites. It was concluded that irradiation had selected an avirulent parasite population (Wright *et al.* 1980a). It was determined that *B. major* and *B. divergens* were susceptible to the effects of irradiation at doses of 40 krad and above by cultivating the organisms *in vitro* in the presence of [^{3}H]-hyoxanthine for 24 hours after they had been exposed to a ^{60}C source and then measuring their incorporation of the tritiated purine (Irvin and Young 1979b).

Further investigations of the properties of virulent and avirulent strains were undertaken. Two virulent strains of *B. bovis* were rendered avirulent as follows: one was exposed to 35 krad of gamma irradiation and the other was passaged through splenectomized calves. The parent strains caused a fatal disease in splenectomized calves and intact cattle, while a nonfatal disease was observed in intact cattle which received the avirulent parasites. Preparations of disrupted parasites were obtained from the four parasite populations. It was found that the virulent strains contained high levels of protease, whereas the avirulent strains contained insignificant amounts. The doubling times and the maximum parasitemias were the same for the four parasite populations (Wright *et al.* 1981a).

Mixed infections with two or three *Babesia* species and with other hemoparasites have been observed. The three species, *B. bigemina, B. bovis,* and *B. major* may appear together as a mixed infection and their incidence seems to be related to the size and the activity of the tick population at various altitudes. *Babesia bigemina* could be separated from other blood parasites by rapid passages through splenectomized calves because of its ability to multiply rapidly. *Babesia bigemina* was found in thin smears 24 to 57 hours after calves were inoculated with relatively small numbers of parasites (Bishop *et al.* 1973). Dual infection of *B. canis* and *Ehrlichia* species (e.g. *E. canis*) caused severe anemia of the normocytic-cormochromic type, suggesting destruction of red blood cells and impairment of erythropoiesis. Infection by either of the two pathogens alone resulted in lowered mortality (Ewing and Buckner 1965). Splenectomized calves with a dual infection of *B. divergens* and *E. phagocytophila* had less marked hematological changes than those inoculated with either organism separately. The *Babesia* infection appeared to be suppressed by the *Ehrlichia* pathogens (Purnell *et al.* 1977b). A mixed infection of *B. caballi* and *B. equi* was indicated by the size, mode of multiplication, and number of parasites in the infected erythrocytes of an equine blood sample (Ristic *et al.* 1964).

CLINICAL SIGNS

There is wide variation in the clinical signs of babesiosis because some species are not pathogenic and, within any one species, there are strain differences with respect to virulence. In addition, the age, breed, and level of environmental stress affect the susceptibility of a particular host. In general, the organisms are first observed in the blood 8 to 16 days after vector-transmitted infection and the increase in parasitemia is accompanied by fever of 41 to 45.5 °C. The animals become listless, anorectic, dehydrated, and weak, and their coats roughen. Muscle trembling and grinding of teeth occur. Hemoglobinemia, hemoglobinuria, and jaundice subsequently develop. The feces may be dry yellow and at times bloodstained. In diseases caused by *B. bovis* and *B. canis,* signs of terminal central nervous system involvement are paddling of limbs, ataxia, mania, and coma. The clinical signs displayed by horses infected with *B. caballi* include pyrexia, sluggishness, depression, thirst, lacrimation, anorexia, nasal discharge, and swelling of the eyelids. Icterus and hemorrhages are observed in the mucous membranes. Hemoglobinuria is evident and the animals may be constipated or diarrheic. As the disease progresses, the animals become weaker and more emaciated, stagger, and develop cutaneous edema of the lower abdomen, thorax and groin. Recovery from the acute phase is characterized by the clearance of the parasite from the peripheral blood and the rapid return of appetite and normal temperature. The animals either remain asymptomatic or develop a milder, more chronic syndrome. In the latter case, an increase in the levels of parasitemia occurs several times over a period of 1 to 3 weeks, with the recurrence of clinical signs characterizing the acute phase. The carrier state is often asymptomatic.

Literature

The severity of the responses was measured in Holstein × Friesian calves infected either by the injection of infected blood or by the application of infected *B. microplus* larvae. Tick-induced infections produced severe responses even when relatively small numbers of infected ticks were applied, while infected blood caused only parasitemia and mild subclinical reactions. The severity of tick-induced reactions was due to the large number of infective particles injected rather than to the greater virulence of tick-derived organisms (Smith *et al.* 1978). The converse was also thought to be true. It did not appear to matter what dose was injected the course of infection was the same and at lower doses the prepatent period was longer (Wright *et al.* 1980a). The severity of the response was related to the age of the animals, with higher fever and more morbidity and mortality occurring among the older calves. No relationship was observed between the parasitemia, the decrease in the PCV, and mortality in tick-induced infections (Smith *et al.* 1978). Aged cows, 2-year-old steers, yearlings, and 5- to 6-month-old calves were used to determine whether resistance to infection with *B. bovis* is age-related. It was found that the aged cows were highly susceptible, whereas the steers and yearlings experienced milder reactions and the calves had innate resistance. The animals in the age groups showing reduced susceptibility were found to develop peak parasitemia, temperature, and anemia before the more susceptible age groups (Trueman and Blight 1978). Acute babesiosis was caused by *B. bigemina* in exotic and crossbred cattle (Dwivedi *et al.* 1976) and by *B. bovis* in very young exotic calves (Roychoudhury *et al.* 1976).

The symptoms of the disease caused by *B. canis* and *B. gibsoni* in dogs, direct and serological diagnostic techniques, therapy, and prophylaxis were discussed (Dennig *et al.* 1980). The incubation period of experimental *B. gibsoni* infections varied with the mode of infection. Anemia was the only consistent sign; it increased steadily over a 2- to 4-week period, after which the animal either died or recovered. The fever was variable and did not correlate with parasitemia. The anemia was macrocytic and there was an obvious hematopoietic response. Splenomegaly, hepatomegaly, listlessness, and anorexia were frequently observed. In contrast to the acute disease caused by *B. canis*, icterus and hemoglobinuria were extremely rare, even in severe syndromes. There was no evidence indicating that *B. gibsoni* tended to localize in the brain: the pathogenesis of the disease was more related to the progressive anemia. Resistance followed infection and latent parasitemia was observed for approximately 3 years. Parasitemia could recur in recovered animals, but the number of infected erythrocytes seldom exceeded 1% (Groves 1968; Groves and Dennis 1972). The occurrence of *B. canis*-induced cerebral babesiosis in dogs in Kenya was reported (Piercy 1947; Purchase 1947). The clinical syndromes and pathology caused by *B. gibsoni* and *B. canis* infections in 100 dogs were studied. In the 21 dogs examined at postmortem, there was central nervous system involvement characterized by proliferation of glial cells, perivascular infiltrates, and hemorrhage. These changes occurred during the final stages of the infection (Reube 1954).

A historical review of feline babesiosis was presented (Futter and Belonje 1980a). The clinical symptoms of experimental and natural feline babesiosis included lethargy, anorexia, and anemia with occasional icterus, while fever was not a feature of the disease (Futter and Belonje 1980b).

PATHOGENESIS

There are two principal mechanisms by which babesial organisms cause cellular and tissue injury. The primary mechanism involves the development of intravascular hemolysis, which is directly proportional to the parasitemia. The hemolysis causes anoxia and secondary inflammatory lesions in various organs, especially the kidneys and liver. These effects are variable depending on the babesial species, the virulence of the strain, and the breed and age of the host. The circulating blood and the vascular system are initially affected, while other solid organs and tissues develop lesions later in the disease. The secondary mechanism causes electrolytic changes, complement activation, coagulation disorders, and the release of pharmacologically active compounds which results in vascular malfunctions and hypotensive shock.

Lesions

At postmortem examination, the animals which had succumbed to the acute syndrome show congestion of various organs and tissues, particularly the spleen, brain, lungs, and skeletal muscle. Jaundice, dark red urine, thick granular bile, and subepicardial and subendocardial hemorrhages are also present. In the milder syndrome, the carcass is pale and slightly icteric, and the organs show varying degrees of congestion.

Central nervous system lesions are characteristic of *B. bovis* and *B. canis* infections. The parasitized red blood cells concentrate in the brain capillaries where they adhere to each other and to the endothelium by means of deformations of, and strand-like processes on, their membranes. The 'stickiness' of the parasitized erythrocytes has been attributed to membrane changes induced by parasite-derived enzymes and/or the secretion of antigens.

The destruction of erythrocytes occurs in parallel with parasite multiplication and often exceeds that which may be attributed to the maturing organisms. The PCVs, red blood cell counts, and hemoglobin values decrease by more than 50% of preinfection levels. The osmotic fragility of both infected and noninfected red blood cells is either increased or decreased depending on the babesial species involved. During the acute hemolytic phase, the anemia is normocytic and then becomes macrocytic with the appearance of reticulocytes and a rise in the mean corpuscular volume. Leukocyte counts fall slightly at first, but in the postacute phase there is a two- to threefold increase over normal values due to the lymphocytosis. The hematological changes which accompany the anemia include increased levels of serum glutamic oxalacetic transaminase (SGOT) and serum glutamic pyruvic transaminase (SGPT), alkaline phosphatase, unconjugated bilirubin, blood urea nitrogen (BUN), and, in the late stages of infection, a decrease of calcium. The rise in BUN precedes the increases in SGOT and in bilirubin and the onset of hemolysis by 1 to 2 days. The whole blood-clotting time, partial thromboplastin time, and prothrombin time are prolonged, and the numbers of platelets are reduced. The plasma fibrinogen is modified and becomes associated with fibrin monomer in the formation of a cold precipitable complex, cryofibrin. The serum kinin-forming enzyme, kallikrein, is activated several days before the parasites reach detectable levels in the peripheral blood. This results in shock and a fall in the PCV before the effects of erythrocyte destruction by parasites are evident.

The role of circulating antigens in the production of anemia has not been completely determined. The predominant pathogenic effect of these antigens probably arises as a result of the formation of complexes with circulating antibody and complement which localize in the kidneys and cause glomerulonephritis. This reaction depletes complement levels, releases anaphlatoxin, and contributes to the shock. The autoimmune sensitization of erythrocytes does not appear to be responsible for the erythrophagocytosis observed in domestic animals. The red blood cell destruction usually parallels increasing parasitemia, so that the phagocytosis of noninfected erythrocytes is probably related to alterations in the shape of the erythrocytes, osmotic fragility, and increased reticuloendothelial activity.

Literature

The pathogenesis of bovine babesiosis was reviewed by Mahoney (1979), Wright (1981), and Zwart and Brocklesby (1979). The pathogenesis of canine syndromes was also extensively studied, and many significant findings resulted from investigations on the rodent forms of babesiosis.

Babesia invade red cells by a process which might involve complement-induced modification of erythrocyte and/or parasite membranes. The experimental evidence indicated that a complement-induced alteration of the erythrocyte was the most probable mechanism, but other red cell membrane determinants could also be essential factors in the penetration process (Jack and Ward 1981). On the basis of the mean corpuscular diameter of both infected and noninfected red blood cells in *B. bigemina*-infected splenectomized calves, new erythrocytes were preferentially parasitized (Wright and Kerr 1974). However, in *B. hylomysci* infections in mice, the older, mature erythrocytes were preferentially parasitized (Hussein 1976). *Babesia bigemina* and *B. bovis* caused cytoplasmic stippling, intensification of the cell margin, and alteration of the color of parasitized erythrocytes (Saal 1964). Erythrocytes infected with *B. bovis* were more resistant to lysis than normal cells from either infected or noninfected animals. Unparasitized erythrocytes were markedly fragile on the last day of infection, and spherocytosis was observed in all of the infected red cells. In contrast, *B. bigemina*-infected erythrocytes were larger and more fragile than uninfected erythrocytes from parasitized animals and from control animals (Wright 1973d). Two proteolytic enzymes released into the circulation by *B. bigemina* and *B. bovis* were thought to contribute to the fragility of the red blood cells (Wright and Goodger 1973).

Babesia bovis and *B. bigemina* caused a macrocytic, hypochromic, hemolytic anemia, but up to and during the acute hemolytic process, there was normocytic, normochromic anemia. After the acute hemolytic phase ended, the macrocytosis occurred and corresponded to the appearance of reticulocytes. A terminal leukocytosis was also observed once the acute hemolytic phase had passed (Wright 1973c).

The hematological reactions of splenectomized calves infected with irradiated and nonirradiated *B. bovis* and nonirradiated *B. bigemina* were similar with respect to the decreases in PCV and mean corpuscular hemoglobin concentration (MCHC), and the increases in mean corpuscular volume (MCV), reticulocytes, nucleated red cells, and macrocytes. Osmotic fragility increased in both *B. bovis* and *B. bigemina* infections. The initial reduction in leukocyte levels was followed by leukocytosis during which the lymphocyte numbers increased and the neutrophil population decreased (Wright 1973c). The hematological responses to *B. bigemina* infection were studied in splenectomized purebred Sahiwal cattle or Channel Island × Zebu crosses and nonsplenectomized purebred Ayrshire cattle. The changes observed in the hematological parameters were comparable to those reported by other workers (Lohr *et al.* 1977). In calves infected with *B. bigemina* there were significant decreases in the hemoglobin, PCV, and total erythrocyte in addition to a gradual fall in the blood glucose level. A leukocytosis characterized by neutrophilia and lymphopenia was also reported (Pandey and Mishra 1977b). It was suggested that the decrease in erythrocytic sodium and the increase in potassium observed during the course of *B. bigemina* infection in cattle resulted from the anemia rather than the presence of the parasites. However, these changes can be ascribed to erythropoiesis; young erythrocytes had levels of sodium reduced and potassium elevated (Timms and Murphy 1980).

On postmortem examination lesions were less obvious in animals with *B. bigemina* than in those with *B. bovis* infections. There was paleness of the subcutaneous tissue and mucous membranes, enlargement of the liver, distention of the gall bladder, and urinary bladder, congestion of the kidneys and edema of the lungs. Histologically, there was diffuse coagulative necrosis in the liver, epithelial degeneration of the renal tubules, and edema of the lungs, brain, and heart (Pandey and Mishra 1977a).

In those syndromes characterized by muscle wasting, weakness, and recumbency, degeneration of skeletal and cardiac muscles was observed. The levels of plasma creatine kinase, lactate dehydrogenase, and creatinine also rose and showed highly significant increases terminally. These changes developed as a result of anoxia (Wright *et al.* 1981b). Hydropic and vesicular degeneration of liver cells was observed in cases of bovine babesiosis (Merino *et al.* 1976).

The pathological changes in the liver and kidney were further examined in splenectomized calves with *B. bovis* and *B. bigemina* infections. Renal lesions preceded hepatic damage by 1 to 2 days. The concentrations of BUN increased two to four times, SGOT increased four times and unconjugated bilirubin increased eight to ten times, while conjugated bilirubin levels fell terminally. Bromosulfalein fractional clearance levels fell in severe *B. bovis* infections, but were unaltered in syndromes caused by *B. bigemina*. The concentration of potassium fell in the serum and rose in the urine. In all severe cases, hepatic centrilobular and midzonal degeneration and necrosis were observed. Vascular stasis was observed only in *B. bovis* infections. Degeneration was also found in the convoluted and collecting tubules, with glomerular shrinkage occurring in moderate and severe cases (Wright 1972b). The renal malfunctions which developed in splenectomized calves with a hypotensive syndrome caused by *B. bovis* were characterized by reductions in urinary volume, urinary kinin, kallikrein, and electrolytes. Proteinuria consisting of hemoglobin (15 to 20%) and albumin (70 to 75%) was also observed. Fibrin degradation products, fibrinogen-like products, and haptoglobin were not detected in the urine (Wright and Goodger 1979).

Extensive blood stasis occurred only in severe syndromes caused by *B. bovis*. The packing of parasitized erythrocytes was most marked in the capillaries of the gray matter of the brain and in the kidneys. This was accompanied by variable degrees of centrilobular necrosis of the liver and biliary retention. Renal degeneration with cast formation was also observed. Hemosiderin deposits and erythrophagocytosis were present in macrophages of the liver, lymph nodes, lungs, and, to a lesser extent, in the spleen and kidneys. Mobilization of lymphocytes and hyperplasia of the reticuloendothelial system were noted. Plasma cells accumulated in the spleen, liver, and kidneys (Rogers 1971b).

Babesia bovis has been found to be the primary cause of various forms of bovine cerebral babesiosis; central nervous system involvement in *B. bigemina* infections is rarely seen (Tchernomoretz 1943; Zlotnik 1953). Atypical cases of cerebral babesiosis were associated with intercurrent viral and rickettsial infections (Uilenberg 1965). The examination of a relatively high number of capillaries in brain smears was an accurate diagnostic procedure for detecting *B. bovis* infections (Leeflang 1972).

The lesions in the brain and kidneys in terminal cases of *B. bovis* infection were associated with a parasitemia above 90%. Although the numbers of parasitized erythrocytes in the venous blood seldom exceeded 1 to 2% in acute cases, parasitemia in the brain capillaries varied from 5% in mild cases to 96% in acute terminal cases. In these cerebral forms of babesiosis, the gray and white matter of the brain was congested, with the tissue having a uniformly pinkish color. There was also histological evidence of perivascular, perineuronal, and interstitial edema. The prognosis should be guarded once acute nervous signs have begun or should a drop in temperature occur unaccompanied by a drop in parasitemia (Callow and McGavin 1963). The erythrocytes isolated from the cerebral cortex of *B. bovis*-infected calves were stellate in appearance and connected by fine strands to each other and to the capillary endothelium, which showed degeneration and necrosis once intravascular agglutination occurred (Potgieter and Els 1979; Wright 1972a). The fibrin-like reactions observed histochemically were the result of sludged erythrocytes packed together and did not stick to each other or to the capillary endothelium as they did in the brain, although their margins were distorted and twisted into bizarre shapes (Wright 1973b).

The lesions in canine babesiosis are representative of those caused by *Babesia* in other animals (Malherbe 1956). *Babesia canis* infections in splenectomized and intact dogs caused pathological changes characteristic of hemolytic disease (Dorner 1969). The anemia in acute babesiosis was in part mediated by beta-globulin-associated antigen which became bound to erythrocytes. The majority of these red blood cells were removed rapidly from the peripheral circulation. The antisera to this antigen selectively agglutinated and eventually disintegrated erythrocytes containing mature parasites. The activity of the antibodies against the infective erythrocytes indicated that the antigens were elaborated primarily by infected erythrocytes and that the antibody activity was directed at the erythrocytes rather than at the parasites (Sibinovic *et al.* 1969a). Erythrocytes parasitized by *B. canis* were phagocytosed by neutrophils (Simpson 1974). The increases observed in the serum levels of total lactate dehydrogenase (LDH), malate dehydrogenase (MDH), and isoenzyme fractions of LDH (LDH_1 and LDH_2) in *B. gibsoni* infections were correlated to the lysis of red blood cells, and increased concentration of LDH_3 were associated with damage to the spleen (Ruff *et al.* 1971). Dogs infected with *B. canis* developed accumulations of parasitized red blood cells in the brain, eyes, and periorbital tissues as well as in the spleen, kidneys, skeletal muscles, intestine, and lymph nodes. Degenerative, hemorrhagic, and necrotic lesions were found in the brain, skeletal muscles, and lymphoid tissues (Basson and Pienaar 1965). In dogs, *B. gibsoni* caused a hemolytic macrocytic anemia associated with enlargement of the spleen and liver and fluctuating fever. Hemoglobinuria was not observed, but histologically the disease was characterized by hemosiderin deposits in the liver, spleen, bone marrow, and other reticuloendothelial cells (Seneviratna 1965b). In severe cases there is both hepatic and renal malfunction with necrotic and degenerative lesions (Seneviratna 1965a).

In acute *B. canis* infections, bilirubinemia, bilirubinuria, and urobilinuria occurred. The centrilobular areas of the liver were affected; the changes ranged from congested to patent necrosis (Gilles *et al.* 1953). Serum glutamic pyruvic transaminase activity (Malherbe 1956) and serum alkaline phosphatase activity (Malherbe 1965c) indicated that liver damage developed in early cases manifesting only moderate anemia. The appearance of unconjugated bilirubin in the plasma of early acute cases signified that extensive hemolysis had occurred (Malherbe 1965d). There was also a progressive malfunction of the kidneys (Malherbe 1966). Dogs infected with *B. gibsoni* had increased levels of BUN, bilirubin, alkaline phosphatase, and SGOT prior to death (Fowler *et al.* 1972). Metabolic acidosis developed in dogs with fatal as well as nonfatal *B. canis* infection. In the fatal infections, the acidosis was uncompensated and was considered a result of the anemic shock (Button 1979).

In experimental and natural cases of feline babesiosis, there was a rapid drop in the hematocrit, hemoglobin, and erythrocyte count. The total serum proteins remained unchanged, but there was a definite increase in gamma globulin and a decrease in alpha and beta globulins. In most cases liver function was essentially normal, although function tests occasionally indicated hepatic dysfunction. Renal function was unaffected. Bile stasis and hepatic necrosis were observed on postmortem examination (Futter *et al.* 1980c and 1981).

There are relatively few reports on the pathology of equine babesiosis. In a report on an outbreak of *B. equi* in imported mares, clinical disease was characterized by high fever, petechial hemorrhages, anemia, and icterus. Postmortem examination revealed hepatomegaly, and hemorrhages with generalized icterus (Gautam and Dwivedi 1976). In *B. equi* infections there was generally a wide variation in the leukograms, with monocytosis and eosinopenia constituting the most common alterations. Plasma fibrinogen increased early in the infection and was sustained throughout the clinical disease (Rudolph *et al.* 1975). *Babesia caballi* caused decreases in the red blood cell count, hemoglobin concentration, and hematocrit within 1 to 4 days after infection, and free bilirubin increased immediately after inoculation. In the animals that died, active erythrophagocytosis was present in the lymph nodes, spleen, liver, and lungs (Allen *et al.* 1975a). The phagocytosis of erythrocytes infected with *B. equi* occurred in the Kupffer's cells of the hepatic sinusoids, and degenerate parasites were present in phagocytic vacuoles (Simpson 1970).

A number of significant contributions to the understanding of the pathogenesis of babesiosis have been made using rodent infections. The syndromes observed in rodent models have many features in common with those seen in domestic animals. *Babesia hylomysci* infection in mice was characterized by fever, anorexia, anemia, hemoglobinuria, and icterus; atypical signs of respiratory, circulatory, digestive, and nervous tissue malfunction were also evident. The main histological lesions were degenerative and necrotic changes in the liver (Hussein 1977a). Hemoglobinuria was associated with hemosiderin deposits in the tubular epithelium of the kidney. In addition, tubular necrosis and infarction were observed (Hussein 1977b). In the early stages of *B. microti* and *B. hylomysci* infections, the spleen controlled the excessive multiplication of the organisms. Erythrophagocytosis of infected and uninfected red blood cells was detected in the spleen and bone marrow and rarely in blood smears (Hussein 1979). *Babesia rodhaini* caused hemolytic anemia, reticuloendothelial hyperplasia, and focal, and sometimes midzonal, necrosis of the liver in mice (Paget *et al.* 1962). In rats infected with *B. rodhaini*, the anemia was not proportional to the degree of parasitemia and was macrocytic in character, and spherocytosis developed as the infection progressed. Hemagglutinins were present in the sera and were associated with the onset of erythrophagocytosis in the spleen. It was concluded that the anemia was related to splenomegaly, erythrophagocytosis, and serum autohemagglutinins and not directly to parasitemia (Schroeder *et al.* 1966). Todorovic *et al.* (1967) also found that the spleen was the site of intense erythrophagocytic activity. In addition, *B. rodhaini*-infected rats developed kidney lesions characterized by acute proliferative glomerulitis. The presence of glomerular deposits of IgG and the third component of complement indicated immune complex-induced nephritis (Annable and Ward 1974; Chapman and Ward 1976a).

Coagulation disturbances

Coagulation disturbances play a significant role in the pathogenesis of some forms of babesiosis caused by *B. bovis*. These disorders are characterized by the development of disseminated intravascular coagulation and the presence of fibrinogen-like proteins. The coagulation process is probably started by thrombin activation due to the release of thromboplastin-like substances from lysed erythrocytes and to the activation of kallikrein.

Literature

The disseminated intravascular coagulation which was observed in splenectomized calves with acute *B. bovis* infections occurred with massive pulmonary edema and widespread fibrin thrombi in the capillaries and large vessels of the lung, in the capillaries of the renal glomeruli, and in the hepatic sinusoids. The prolongation of the prothrombin time and the pathological levels of the fibrinogen degradation products were related to these histological changes (Dalgliesh *et al.* 1976). A positive protamine sulfate test proved a reliable method for the detection of intravascular coagulation based upon findings in animals which had histopathological changes indicative of disseminated intravascular coagulation (Dalgliesh *et al.* 1977). Classical disseminated intravascular coagulation was not demonstrated in *B. bigemina* infection of cattle; fibrinogen degradation products were not constantly detected in the plasma and there was no evidence of fibrinolysis or fibrin deposition (Goodger and Wright 1977a). However, disturbances in the coagulation system were detected by assaying the plasma of splenectomized calves infected with *B. bigemina*. There were changes in the thrombin time, reptilase-R time, whole blood clotting time, one-stage prothrombin time determination, partial thromboplastin time, and fibrinogen, calcium, and thrombocyte levels. These changes were most marked during days 6 to 7 when the parasitemia was highest and were associated with massive intravascular hemolysis. The plasma kallikrein levels fell and the level of activated kallikrein rose slightly. A progressive fall in plasma fibrinogen levels and the appearance of a soluble fibrin were also observed (Wright and Goodger 1977).

Two substances were isolated from the sera of *B. bovis*-infected calves; one was immunologically identical with bovine fibrinogen, and the other was a pigmented macromolecular complex containing a number of proteins found in normal tissues (Mahoney and Goodger 1969).

Plasma obtained from cattle dying from infection with *B. bovis* formed a cold precipitable gel when stored at 4 °C. This gel was comprised of fibrinogen-like proteins with a wide molecular weight spectrum (Goodger 1975). The cryofibrinogen complex formed in the plasma primarily consisted of fibrinogen and soluble fibrin and contained proteins from both the erythrocytes and the piroplasms (Goodger 1977; Goodger *et al.* 1978; Goodger and Wright 1977a, b). The size and chain structure of fibrinogen and the fibrinogen-like proteins were consistent with the assumption that fibrin cross-linking and subsequent fibrinolysis were not important in the pathogenesis of the infection. The structures of these proteins indicated that the blood was in a hypercoagulable state due mainly to the enhanced production of hydrogen-bonded fibrin and offset partly by slight inhibition of chain cross-linking (Goodger and Wright 1979). The plasma and serum of *B. bovis*-infected cattle contained proteins which reacted with protamine sulfate and ethanol to form gels. The sizes and chain structures of these proteins indicated that they were intermediates in the conversion of fibrinogen into cross-linked fibrin. It was suggested that the proteins resulted from thrombin activation and not fibrinolysis (Goodger *et al.* 1980a). Wright *et al.* (1979) demonstrated that the fibrin stains were not specific and that fibrin deposits did not occur in *B. bovis* infections. The thrombi observed were sequestered cells and not cross-linked fibrin deposits. It was also suggested that babesial enzyme–fibrinogen complexes contributed to the pathogenesis of the disease by causing sludging and adhesion of the erythrocytes to blood vessel walls (Goodger *et al.* 1980b). Saline eluates from erythrocytes of cattle infected with *B. bovis* contained fibrinogen, plasminogen, and IgG_2. These proteins could be associated with the removal of erythrocytes from the circulation and contributed to the processes of coagulation and fibrinolysis during infection (Goodger 1978).

Coagulation disturbances have also been observed in babesiosis in other species. In horses acutely infected with *B. caballi*, there were rapid decreases in platelet numbers and an elevation of fibrinogen levels in the plasma. The clot retraction *in vitro* was impaired, indicating that *B. caballi* infection causes alterations in the clotting factor levels (Allen *et al.* 1975b). Disseminated intravascular coagulation was observed in dogs with severe *B. canis* infections. Thrombocytopenia occurred in both the mild and severe syndromes. Fibrin microthrombi associated with edema and hemorrhage were detected primarily in the brain, kidneys, and heart (Moore and Williams 1979). The experimental infection of rats with *Plasmodium chabaudi*, *B. rodhaini*, and *Trypanosoma lewisi* resulted in the stimulation of elevated levels of antibody to fibrinogen/fibrin-related products (Thoongsuwan *et al.* 1979).

Pharmacologically active substances

The kallikrein and kinin systems are involved in the pathogenesis of the intravascular changes which result in blood vessel dilatation and permeability, vascular stasis, and circulatory failure. The release of proteolytic enzymes from the organisms is associated with the activation of plasma prekallikrein. This, in turn, probably causes the release of other active substances which contribute to the malfunctions observed in the circulating blood and the vasculature.

Literature

Plasma kinin and its precursor enzyme, kallikrein, were the inflammatory agents involved in the intravascular disturbances which characterize babesiosis (Wright and Kerr 1977; Wright and Mahoney 1974). In acute *B. bovis* infection, only kinin was initially released. This then triggered a sequence of events including the release of other pharmacologically active agents which acted both independently and synergistically in the production of vasodilatation, capillary permeability, edema, vascular stasis, and tissue anoxia. These effects resulted in profound hypotension and vascular collapse (Wright, 1973a, 1977, 1978). The purification of an esterase from *B. bovis* resulted in two fractions which differed in their ability to activate bovine plasma prekallikrein. The active fraction was associated with a fibrinogen-like substance and caused fibrin formation *in vitro*. The activation of bovine plasma prekallikrein *in vitro* by purified fractions of *B. bovis* with high esterase activity suggested that the *in vivo* activation of bovine plasma prekallikrein was probably due to the activity of proteolytic enzymes released from the parasites (Wright 1975). Serum carboxypeptidase B (SCPB) levels were determined in splenectomized and nonsplenectomized cattle infected with virulent and avirulent strains of *B. bovis*, and in splenectomized cattle infected with a virulent form of *B. bigemina*. Since SCPB inactivates anaphylatoxins and kinins, the enzyme's activity was considered an indication of the concentrations of these vasodilatory substances in the circulation. The SCPB levels fell in the hosts of the virulent *B. bovis* strains and were unaltered in the animals with the avirulent *B. bovis* and *B. bigemina* infections. The relatively small variation in the SCPB levels observed in *B. bigemina* and avirulent *B. bovis* infections indicated that the vasodilatory substances were not produced in consistently large amounts. This finding supported earlier observations that these infections did not normally involve extensive activation of the kallikrein and coagulation systems (Wright *et al.* 1980b). Three groups of splenectomized calves were infected with *B. bovis*. Trasylol (Bayer Pharmaceuticals), a proteinase inhibitor, was administered intravenously to early and late treatment groups, starting 3 and 8 days postinfection respectively. It was found that the levels of activated kallikrein in the plasma were significantly lower in the early treatment group, which also showed significantly higher levels of plasma kallikrein inhibitor. No significant differences in the total plasma kallikrein levels were seen among the three groups. The PCVs in the two treated groups remained significantly higher than those in the control animals (Wright and Kerr 1975).

IMMUNOLOGY

Antigens

An important characteristic of *Babesia* infections is the long duration, which indicates that the organisms can survive in the host in spite of the immunological responses. This ability is partly due to the antigenic variation which occurs with each succeeding parasitemia during chronic phases of infection. The variant populations revert to one antigenic type after infecting the tick, but this basic strain antigen is also variable. Antigenic variation can be predicted using a mathematical model to simulate parasitemia patterns; organisms infecting herds have the potential to produce apparently 100 different antigenic types. Neither tests for cross-immunity nor serological methods can define whether common protective antigens are shared between different species of *Babesia*. These tests cannot determine whether cross-immunity between two species capable of infecting the same host species depends on the presence of soluble antigen or live organisms. Evidence of cross-immunity has been accumulated from field observations: animals that recover from infection with one strain are more resistant to homologous challenge than to heterologous challenge. The investigation of *Babesia* antigens is complicated by the lack of optimal systems of culturing the parasites. At present, cultivation requires the harvesting of organisms from infected blood, which results in the contamination of antigens with host protein in spite of the various methods used to purify the material. The recent advances in the *in vitro* cultivation of the organism in tick tissues and in blood may enable the obtainment of purified antigens.

Literature

Mahoney and Goodger (1981) reviewed the method used in the isolation of the organisms and their products from the erythrocytes and the plasma. The separation is difficult because of the parasites association with the host-cell cytoplasm. A significant advance in the preparation of antigen for serological testing was made by using the French pressure cell method to rupture infected erythrocytes (Amerault *et al.* 1978). Soluble antigens were found in the serum of cattle heavily infected with *B. bovis* or *B. bigemina* (Mahoney 1966), and their possible biological significance was reviewed (Ferris *et al.* 1968). Ristic *et al.* (1981) reviewed the more recent work on the characterization of *Babesia* antigens which have been obtained from erythrocyte and tick tissue cultures. The authors also discussed the biological significance of the different babesial forms found in each tick stage.

Outbreaks of babesiosis in previously immune cattle following their transfer from one locality to another indicated the existence of different strains of *Babesia*. Serological tests showed that there were antigenic differences among four stabilates of *B. bigemina* derived from a single purified isolate and propagated as acute and chronic, blood-borne and tick-borne infections (Thompson *et al.* 1977, 1978a). The slide agglutination test was used to demonstrate antigenic differences between isolates of *B. bigemina* (Curnow 1973d). Using this test, it was demonstrated that the *B. bovis* organisms obtained at relapses in one animal were antigenically different from one another; however, when these parasites were transmitted through the tick *B. microplus* they reverted to a common antigenic type. Serologically distinct strains were also demonstrated in the field, indicating that a multiplicity of strain-specific antigens exist (Curnow 1973a).

Antigenic cross-reactions were shown between *B. bovis* and two human malarial parasites (Ludford *et al.* 1972). Strain-specific antigens were also demonstrated in laboratory rodents with *B. rodhaini* infections (Thoongsuwan and Cox 1973). Three types of antigen were detected in the plasma of calves infected with *B. bovis*. The first was an autoantigen which was associated with polymeric haptoglobin complexes. It stimulated the formation of precipitating antibodies which were not specific for babesial infection and it was not associated with the development of acquired immunity. The second category was comprised of cattle blood-group antigens which caused the production of lysins for homologous but not autologous erythrocytes. It was unlikely that these antigens influenced the development of acquired immunity. The third group probably originated in the organisms and induced partial protection against different strains of *B. bovis*. This effect was indicated by a delay in the time required for the parasitemia to reach detectable levels (Mahoney and Goodger 1972).

Several radiolabeling probes were used in studies on the composition of erythrocyte membranes. These methods revealed that the surface glycoproteins of *B. bovis*-infected cells were very similar to those of the uninfected red cells. One observation of practical importance was that quantitative and qualitative differences existed between uninfected animals in the major surface proteins identified by these techniques (Howard *et al.* 1980). The soluble component obtained from *B. bovis*-infected erythrocytes contained at least two distinct antigens which were species-specific. One was found on the internal rim of the erythrocytic membrane, and the other was located in the internal stromata of the infected erythrocytes (Goodger 1973a). A crude soluble hemagglutination antigen derived from a mixture of *B. bovis* organisms and infected erythrocyte stromata contained fibrinogen. Since all of the antigenic activity was associated with the fibrinogen component, it was suggested that the antigen was either a babesial moiety complexed with fibrinogen or an altered fibrinogen molecule (Goodger 1971, 1976). Soluble antigen was extracted from *B. bovis*-infected erythrocytes by sonic disintegration. After fractionation of the soluble material by the precipitation of fibrinogen-like proteins, the precipitate was found to contain babesial antigens that were located on the stroma of infected cells. The other fraction was not heavily contaminated with antigenic material from erythrocytes (Mahoney *et al.* 1981b).

A crude suspension of *B. bovis* and *B. bigemina* parasites was prepared by distilled water lysis of infected erythrocytes for use in a routine CF test. Cross-absorption tests indicated that *B. bovis* and *B. bigemina* CF reactions each consisted of a major species-specific component (Mahoney 1967a). A soluble precipitating antigen which was extracted from plasma and hemolysate could be used for diagnostic tests in *B. bigemina* infections (Goldman and Bukovsky 1975). Immunochemical analyses of soluble antigens derived from *B. bovis* which had been cultured using the improved microaerophilous stationary system demonstrated that at least three antigens were released into the medium (James *et al.* 1981b). Antigens were observed in the sera of horses, dogs, and rats with *Babesia* infections. The results obtained from sucrose density gradient centrifugation, paper electrophoresis, and analytical ultracentrifugation indicated that each antigen was composed of two fractions with complex structures (Sibinovic *et al.* 1965, 1967a). The presence of these soluble antigens in the sera of animals with acute babesiosis was correlated with the emergence and duration of parasitemia. These serum antigens were significant immunizing substances and were not species-specific in their serological or immunological properties (Sibinovic *et al.* 1967b).

Serology

A number of serological tests using antigens prepared from the parasitized erythrocytes, plasma, serum, and tissues of animals afflicted with acute babesiosis have been studied. The most commonly used techniques are the fluorescent antibody (FA), agglutination, precipitation, and CF tests. These serological methods must be applied with a full appreciation of their purposes and limitations. Relatively simple and standardized techniques are necessary for practical purposes. The majority of serological tests are not suitable for the detection of early stages of infection with the parasitemia appearing before antibodies become detectable. Antibodies can be detected before the peak of parasitemia in a primary response using the radioimmunoassay (D. F. Mahoney personal communication). Also, none of the serological tests will be negative within a relatively short time after infection has terminated by autosterilization or chemotherapy. Although cross-reactions occur among various species of *Babesia*, there are significant differences in titers between homologous and heterologous sera, but not if the species are closely similar. The presence of the cross-reaction does not affect the value of the technique when it is carefully conducted using antigen isolated from heavily parasitized blood, and with a proper control system, minimal erros in accuracy and specificity occur. For example, except for the first few weeks of a primary *B. bigemina* infection no cross-reactivity occurs between it and *B. bovis*. The immunofluorescent technique uses intraerythrocytic parasites as antigen rather than extracts and has been reported to be more sensitive than the CF test. The limitations of the IFA test result from the subjective nature of the interpretation and the lack of specificity due to reaction to extraneous antigen when a whole parasite is used. Gel precipitation appears to be a useful technique for the characterization of babesial antigens, but its practical application has not been demonstrated. The agglutination reactions such as the hemagglutination, capillary, slide, and card techniques provide sensitive methods of detecting antibodies. The results obtained from the CF test vary to a certain degree with the antigens used. The antigenic components of erythrocytes can lead to errors.

Literature

Carson and Phillips (1981) discussed the immunological responses of the mammalian hosts to *Babesia*. The authors reviewed the use of various serological tests for the diagnosis of *Babesia* in different species of animals (Zwart and Brocklesby 1979). A comprehensive review of the serological tests included a table in which the babesial species, sources of antibody and antigen, and references for each technique were listed (Todorovic 1975a). The author described the application of the more commonly used serological methods; e.g. the CF, gel precipitation, agglutination, and FA tests, and the conditions under which they were used.

The IFA test is widely used and has been shown to be highly specific and accurate but not very sensitive. In *B. bigemina* infection, a correlation was established between protective antibodies and those detected by immunofluorescence. Sera analyzed by the IFA test were positive very soon after the prepatent period; the responses peaked at 21 days after infection and gradually decreased thereafter. However, a minimum positive response could still be detected 18 to 24 months after a single experimental infection (Ross and Lohr 1968). The blood dried on filter paper was compared with sera as sources of antibody to *B. bigemina* for use in the IFA test. Good correlation was found between the antibody titers of sera and dried blood samples (Burridge *et al.* 1973). Using the IFA test, significant differences were observed between the *B. bigemina* antibody titers of the dams and calves; the titers of the latter were higher. These results indicated that part of the natural resistance of calves in the field might be due to passive immunization which occurred at a young age (Ross and Lohr 1970). This test was also useful in assessing the efficacy of vaccination (Goldman and Pipano 1974). The IFA test was an accurate measure of the infection rates in a herd of cattle after a natural outbreak of *B. divergens* infection (Donnelly *et al.* 1972). In splenectomized calves and intact adult cattle infected with *B. divergens*, the IFA titers appeared after peak parasitemia and maximum titers were observed 35 days after infection. It was concluded that the absence of a spleen did not inhibit the IFA response (Trees 1978). The direct FA test was also a reliable indicator of current infection with *B. bovis* but did not differentiate between various strains (Johnston *et al.* 1973).

An *in vitro* agglutination test of erythrocytes infected with *B. bovis* was highly specific for each isolate and enabled the investigation of antigenic variation in *B. bovis* infections (Curnow 1968). The capillary-tube agglutination test was shown to be a sensitive method of detecting positive sera. Cross-reactions could not be demonstrated when the test was conducted using specific antisera from animals recently recovered from *B. divergens* infection (Lohr and Ross 1969).

Complement-fixing antibodies were detectable in the sera of *B. bovis*- or *B. bigemina*-infected animals for 7 and 4 months respectively. Thereafter the positive sera declined, and it was shown in proven carriers of both infections that the complement-fixing antibody tended to fall below the diagnostic levels before the infection was eliminated. Calves born in enzootic areas were likely to have a weak CF antibody response to primary infection after receiving colostrum from their mothers. However, following the relatively short period in which the passively acquired antibody would be lost, these calves should have the ability to produce CF antibody titers sufficient for diagnostic purposes if reinfection occurred (Mahoney 1964). However, more recently antibodies have been detected in uninfected calves for up to 6 months using the radioimmunoassay (D. F. Mahoney personal communication). Use of the CF test allowed earlier detection of antibodies to *B. divergens* and *B. major* in the sera of experimentally infected cattle than either the enzyme-linked immunosorbent assay (ELISA) or the IFA test, but the titers obtained by the CF test were consistently lower than those detected with the other two tests. The ELISA was preferable to the IFA test since it was less subject to operator error and more adaptable for field use (Bidwell *et al.* 1978). Through use of the indirect immunofluorescence and the indirect hemagglutinaction tests, antibody formation to *B. divergens* was observed a few days earlier than with the ELISA (Weiland *et al.* 1980).

An intradermal skin test was used to demonstrate a delayed cutaneous hypersensitivity reaction in *B. equi* infection in donkeys. A skin response was elicited in vaccinated, infected and carrier intact, and splenectomized animals. The results of a leukocyte migration inhibition test indicated that cell-mediated immunity was correlated with protection (Banerjee *et al.* 1977).

In laboratory animals, the IFA technique, using specific anti-mouse Ig, IgM, and IgG, showed that antibody levels were correlated with the parasitemia until the crisis, and then continued to rise more slowly until the parasite disappeared. Eventually, an elevated plateau was achieved. The IgM levels increased until the crisis, and then rose when the parasites disappeared from the blood (Cox and Turner 1970). *Babesia microti* infections in mice caused a depression of the IgM and IgG responses, although cell-mediated immunity was not affected (Purvis 1977). The classical complement pathway was activated during the course of *B. rodhaini* infection in rats. Depletion of the whole hemolytic complement and various complement components occurred. The complement levels varied inversely with the developing parasitemia (Chapman and Ward 1976b).

Immunity

The resistance to infection is dependent upon the following mechanisms: (1) innate immunity, in which physiological factors render the host unsuitable for the multiplication of the organisms; (2) natural immunity, in which basic host defense processes assist in the removal of invading organisms; and (3) acquired immunity, in which protection is completely reliant on specific immunologic responses. The natural and acquired immunity function together to establish a level of resistance to *Babesia* infection.

Babesial organisms are generally host-specific, but cross-infections can occur under certain circumstances in which the resistance of the host is altered; e.g. splenectomy. These natural nonspecific protective factors reflect the relatively narrow host specificity ascribed to each *Babesia* species and include age and genetic factors which affect the resistance of a particular breed within a species. Concurrent infections with other organisms also influence the susceptibility to *Babesia* infections and affect the severity of the resultant clinical syndromes. For example, *Bos indicus* cattle and recurrence of high parasitemia is less frequent in the chronic phase of infection. Although pups are highly susceptible to *B. canis* infection, it is generally true that the young of other domestic animals, particularly ruminants, are relatively resistant. Passive protection from the infected cow to the calf reinforces this natural immunity which is most effective between 4 and 7 months of age.

In acquired immunity, the reaction to intracellular pathogenic organisms depends on the interaction between the parasite and the host and is related to the host species, the physiological state of the host, and the species and strain of the parasite. The immune response is related to the development of protection as well as to the pathogenesis of the disease. Babesial organisms are found only in mammalian erythrocytes, a microenvironment which protects them from some of the host's defense mechanisms. The immune system controls the parasitemia by destroying the parasites and suppressing the multiplication of the organisms. The circulating antibodies prevent penetration of extracellular *Babesia* forms, and the cytophilic antibodies, or opsonins, enhance the uptake of the parasites and the parasitized cells by the phagocytes. Phagocytosis and cell-mediated immunity may play a role in host resistance to *Babesia*. The spleen has an important function in the development of acquired immunity and, to a varying degree, in the suppression of infection in chronically infected, partially protected animals. Splenectomy not only increases the susceptibility to babesiosis but enables cross-species infection as well. The functions of the spleen include the following: (1) removal of the parasites from the infected cells by a process of 'pitting'; (2) phagocytosis; and (3) antibody production. The spleen is essential for the host's survival, particularly in the initial infection when phagocytosis and early production of antibody are necessary to counter parasite proliferation. Splenectomy removes the individual variation between animals with respect to susceptibility to babesiosis and amplifies the differences in acquired immunity on subsequent challenge.

Although the mechanisms that eliminate *Babesia* from the blood are not totally known, antibodies have an important role. Specific agglutinogens on the surface of the infected erythrocytes are probably the primary targets for the antibody action. The immunological reaction on the cell surface promotes phagocytosis of infected cells and alters the membrane permeability resulting in a change of internal environment or possibly the entry of parasiticidal antibodies. The latter effects are not certain because the reaction of antibodies with infected erythrocytes during the period when organisms were being removed from the blood did not reduce the parasites' viability on subinoculation, thus indicating that they were not irreversibly damaged.

Species-specific antibodies occur against most *Babesia* species, but a direct correlation between these detectable antibodies and protection has not been established. However, passive protection can be induced by the transfer of antibodies to offspring, presumably via colostrum from the mother, and to splenectomized calves providing that (1) the donors of the antiserum were hyperimmunized by multiple infections; and (2) the infection was from the same parasite strain as that used to stimulate antibody production. The antibodies rise to an early peak and thereafter decline. The length of the period during which these antibodies are detectable depends on the serological test used. Different classes of immunoglobulins, both IgG and IgM, have the antibabesial antibodies to some species of *Babesia*. This protection is strain-specific, and despite the fact that variations in protective antigens occur between strains, there is little effect on the protective efficiency of the host immune response. These interstrain differences in antibody specificity are observed in cases of cross-immunity when different strains infect animals. It appears that the mechanism of cross-immunity depended more on the priming of the hosts immune system by the protective antigen, which promotes a rapid secondary response against heterologous strains. Thus, the antibody to the variant antigen may be only part of the protection; a more important component would be the rapid antibody response to each new antigenic variant caused by the effect on the immune system of the antigen–antibody complexes formed at the time the preceding variant strain was eliminated.

Recovery from the acute phase of infection results in immune responses which prevent the occurrence of disease on subsequent challenge with the same species. This resistance does not prevent the entry and restricted multiplication of the parasites on subsequent challenge, particularly if an infection involves different strains of the organisms. Under natural conditions, infections become superimposed on one another without causing clinical disease to develop in the host. Clinical responses sometimes occur after reinfection with a different strain, and the host has a slight fever and low parasitemia. Stress may also precipitate the breakdown of immunity, resulting in weak immunological responses which cannot prevent the extensive multiplication of the organisms. The acquired immunity to *B. bigemina* is investigated by challenging splenectomized and intact cattle, either with the original infecting (homologous) strain or with one which they have never previously encountered (heterologous). The result of the challenge depends on which strain is used and whether the challenged animal is a carrier. The following range of responses are observed: complete sterile immunity in homologously challenged, self-cured animals, partial susceptibility and asymptomatic parasitemia in heterologously challenged carrier animals, and full susceptibility in heterologously challenged, self-cured animals.

Literature

Bos indicus cattle and their crosses are resistant to a number of diseases, including babesiosis, and adverse environmental conditions relative to breeds imported from Europe. For example, Droughtmaster cattle carry ten times fewer ticks than cattle of the British breeds, and Zebu-type cattle are also very resistant to babesiosis. These features are important with respect to the development of cattle industries in the tropics (Francis 1966). Sahiwal cattle possessed higher innate resistance to *B. bigemina* than Charolais cattle. Splenectomized Sahiwal cattle were highly susceptible to infection, irrespective of the age of the animal or the interval between splenectomy and challenge (Lohr 1973). Following *B. bigemina* infections, the average maximum parasitemias and decreases in PCV in Boran cattle were 0.35 and 19.0% respectively; corresponding changes in Ayrshire cattle were 2.3 and 42% (Lohr *et al.* 1975). No significant correlation was established between the susceptibility of Zebu-type and Hereford cattle to *B. bovis* and the erythrocyte adenosine triphosphate levels (Bachmann *et al.* 1976). No definite relationship could be demonstrated between the frequencies of various hemoglobin types and the severity of the parasitemia in Zebu-type cattle (Bachmann *et al.* 1977). The Murrah buffalo (*Bubalus bubalis*) was shown to be refractory to infection by *B. bigemina;* asymptomatic infection was established only in splenectomized calves (Roychoudhury and Gautam 1979).

Hereford cattle of various ages were experimentally infected with *B. bovis* to demonstrate the age-related differences in innate resistance. The reactions of 18-month and 2-year-old steers was significantly greater than those of 2- to 6-month-old calves, but less than those of aged cows which were highly susceptible. The age groups showing reduced susceptibility reached peak parasitemia, temperature, and anemia before the less resistant cattle (Trueman and Blight 1978). Six-month-old Holstein Friesian calves infected with *B. bigemina* did not develop clinical signs and had a relatively low (0.6%) parasitemia, while 1-year-old calves had typical clinical signs and a parasitemia of 6.6%. The infection persisted for 22 months in both groups (Latif *et al.* 1979). The 3- to 6-week-old progeny of cows immunized against *B. bovis* did not develop clinical signs after challenge by infected ticks, although they became infected (Hall 1960, 1963). However, cows and calves were found to be equally susceptible to infection with *B. divergens* (Brocklesby *et al.* 1971a).

The acquired immunity, whether passive or active, depended on the relationship between the immunizing and challenging organisms (Callow 1967). The existence of premunition and the occurrence of different strains of *B. bigemina* were discussed (Uilenberg 1970). Cows which were immunized against *B. bigemina* during mid-pregnancy and again in late pregnancy transmitted the resultant antibodies to their calves through the colostrum. The passive acquired immunity protected the calves against challenge with the homologous strain, while challenge with the heterologous strain caused a high-level infection; the reactions were of comparable severity to those experienced by calves from unimmunized cows (Hall *et al.* 1968). Using the indirect immunofluorescence technique, it was found that the colostrum of cows infected with *B. bigemina* or *B. bovis* contained higher titers of antibodies than the serum, but after 1 to 3 days, the titers in the colostrum were lower than those in the serum. The antibodies in calves persisted from 7 to 148 days (Weisman *et al.* 1974). Antibabesial antibodies were passively transferred by serum from carriers of *B. bovis* and protected highly susceptible calves. Donors which had experienced four or more superinfections produced higher serum antibody levels than those which had had a single infection (Mahoney 1967b).

The degree of immunity to *B. bigemina* following drug cure, self-cure, or persistence of infection differed. A high level of immunity occurred in self-cured animals, and an appreciable degree of immunity to challenge was observed in drug-cured animals 28 weeks after infection (Callow *et al.* 1974a; Callow 1968b). Sterile immunity to homologous strain challenge was demonstrated in animals with *B. bigemina* infection (Callow 1964), and was also thought to play a part in the resistance of cattle to reinfection with *B. divergens* (Joyner and Davies 1967). British-breed cattle infected with *B. bovis* for 13 months and challenged with the homologous strain were resistant to infection, while those challenged with the heterologous strain became infected (Johnston and Tammemagi 1969). It was observed that prior infection with *B. bigemina* or *B. bovis* did not significantly reduce the susceptibility or the severity of responses of cattle to tick-borne infection with the heterologous species. The carrier infections were not activated during the heterologous species challenge, nor was the severity of the challenge-induced disease aggravated (Smith *et al.* 1980). Primary infection with *B. bovis* altered the level of resistance of the host to the tick *B. microplus*, with more ticks maturing on infected than on uninfected cattle. Therefore, cattle infected with *Babesia* either naturally or by vaccination might subsequently suffer more tick worry than those not infected (Callow and Stewart 1978).

The innate and acquired forms of resistance have been investigated in laboratory rodents. Rats that recovered from a variety of anemia-inducing infections, e.g. trypanosomiasis, babesiosis, and malaria, acquired nonspecific cross-resistance which was manifested as a reduction in the parasitemia associated with enhanced survival following heterologous challenge (Thoongsuwan *et al.* 1978). Spleen function in controlling *B. rodhaini* infections of mice was studied by the intravenous injection of large doses of parasites sufficient to give immediate parasitemias. Normal, actively immune, or passively immunized hosts were challenged with homologous and heterologous strains. It was found that (1) the spleen did not affect the multiplication of organisms in normal hosts; (2) passively immunized hosts controlled the multiplication of homologous strains as effectively as actively immunized hosts; and (3) the spleen did not have a significant role in controlling parasite multiplication during the early stages of infection. However, the subsequent response of the host to infection is largely dependent on the spleen which is primed to respond to antigenic variants of the parasite by forming antibodies that restrict multiplication (Roberts *et al.* 1972). The transfer of T-lymphocytes from the lymph nodes and spleens of mice infected with *B. microti* produced immunity which was characterized by lower parasitemia in the recipient mice (Ruebush and Hanson 1980a). The resistance to and recovery from primary *B. microti* infection in mice was modulated by T lymphocytes, and suppressed B cell function and normal T cell function were correlates of the infection (Ruebush and Hanson 1980b). Babesiosis in man has also been associated with the removal of the spleen (Teutsch *et al.* 1980).

VACCINATION

Infected blood

The immunization of cattle against babesiosis involves transmitting the organisms by the inoculation of infected blood, and when necessary, subsequent treatment with a babesiacidal drug to prevent severe illness or death. The critical requirement of immunization is the standardization of virulence of the organisms in the infected blood used as vaccine. Attenuation of babesial virulence is achieved by continuous passage through splenectomized calves. This is only practised up to about 23 passages; after that immunogenicity falls. The vaccine is viable when maintained at 4 °C for a few days, and cryopreservation is used for storage and transport. The prevention of severe reactions to vaccines that contain *Babesia* species which are not readily attenuated is accomplished by the administration of depot-forming babesiacidal drugs.

Literature

Purnell (1979) reviewed the current blood vaccines using infection and chemotherapy against organisms in the families Babesiidae and Theileriidae. The development of alternative vaccines involving the use of irradiated parasites, nonspecific immunization, passage through an unusual host, and dead antigen was discussed. Methods of vaccination against bovine babesiosis, particularly those used against *B. bovis* in Australia, were described by Callow (1977). The *Babesia* strains used in the successful Australian vaccination procedures were immunogenic over a wide geographical area. After laboratory manipulation, these vaccine strains were of reduced virulence and were incapable of being spread by ticks (Callow 1976). However, strains must be tick transmissible to retain sufficient immunogenicity. A vaccine against *B. bovis* was prepared by the serial passage of infected blood through splenectomized calves (Callow and Mellors 1966). The virulence of *B. bigemina* could also be reduced by seven syringe passages through splenectomized calves, and the resultant vaccine caused a mild infection in the recipient animals (Dalgliesh *et al.* 1981a). The collection and sterilization of large volumes of bovine serum for use as a diluent in the preparation of the vaccines against babesiosis were described (Rodwell *et al.* 1980).

The blood obtained from cattle latently infected with *B. bovis* was compared to that drawn from animals undergoing a primary clinical reaction to the organism, and differences with respect to infectivity and virulence were found. The carrier blood caused mild or inapparent reactions, while blood from the reacting donors was highly infective and caused severe responses (Callow and Tammemagi 1967). However, Wright *et al.* (1982) showed that virulent organisms after 1 year in chronically infected cattle are still as virulent as at time of infection 12 months previously. After repeated blood passage in cattle, *B. bovis* vaccine strains lost their infectivity for *B. microplus* ticks. The vector proved incapable of transmitting a primary infection which had been established from a chronic infection of 11 months' duration. The loss of infectivity for ticks was attributed to qualitative rather than to quantitative changes in the organisms (Dalgliesh and Stewart 1977b). A subcutaneous dose consisting of 1×10^6 parasitized erythrocytes was necessary to insure infection after vaccination with *B. bovis*, but when an intravenous route was used, less than ten organisms were necessary to infect the animals. A *B. bovis* strain, which was maintained by needle passage and used routinely to produce vaccine, was safe due to its low virulence, but it induced poor protection to challenge with field isolates. Animals infected with this attenuated strain and subsequently challenged with a heterologous field strain were solidly immune when challenged with yet other field strains. The field strains, although more virulent, conferred a high degree of immunity to heterologous challenge (De Vos 1978). The infected blood used for vaccines maintained optimum infectivity for a relatively short time when stored at 4 °C, and for optimal preservation vaccines had to be stored in a frozen state (Pipano 1978).

The efficacy of various blood vaccination procedures was investigated under different field and laboratory challenges. In a large experiment, 60 calves, 3 to 6 months of age, were vaccinated against *B. bovis* by a variety of methods which included tick infestation, inoculation of virulent organisms obtained from early infection, inoculation of organisms attenuated by passage through splenectomized calves, and injection of commercially available, live, attenuated vaccine. All vaccinated animals were strongly immune to challenge with a heterologous strain of *B. bovis* 4 years after vaccination, and there were no differences in the immunogenicity of the *B. bovis* populations used to induce immunity (Mahoney *et al.* 1979a). Cattle which were repeatedly vaccinated with *B. bovis* and kept at a low level of infestation with *B. microplus* were shown to be resistant to heterologous challenge (Rogers 1971a). Following vaccination with *B. bovis*, the incidence of clinical babesiosis in about 1000 breeding cattle under natural challenge was about 1% in vaccinated animals and 18% in unvaccinated groups. Increasing the number of vaccinations did not increase protection (Emmerson *et al.* 1976). Over 90% of the cattle not previously exposed to ticks and more than 30% of the cattle previously exposed developed fever when inoculated with a vaccine containing 10^7 to 10^8 *B. bovis* per dose (Dalgliesh 1968). Splenectomized calves infected with *B. major* were not resistant to challenge with *B. divergens;* however, *B. divergens* conferred good protection against subsequent challenge with *B. major* (Brocklesby *et al.* 1976). It was proposed that the concentrations of fibrinogen, kininogen, and bradykinin, and the production of soluble fibrin, cryofibrinogen, and high molecular weight fibrinogen complexes reflected the severity of the infection and could be used to assess the efficacy of immunization techniques (Goodger *et al.* 1981). Vaccination of cattle with *B. bovis* using a whole blood vaccine caused the development of blood group antibodies. These antibodies are important because they induce hemolytic disease in newborn calves which absorb incompatible blood group antibodies from colostrum. The level of antibody was dependent on the time elapsed since vaccination, the number and frequency of the vaccinations, and the intrinsic capacity of the animal to develop these antibodies (Dimmock 1973).

Dead antigen

A number of different vaccination procedures have been devised which utilize either killed organisms or various antigenic components derived from parasitized erythrocytes, plasma, serum, and infected tissues. Although the experimental findings have been varied, there is good evidence to suggest that dead material can be used to induce protection against heterologous *Babesia* challenge. It is concluded that these killed antigen vaccines may induce sufficient protection in animals newly exposed to natural challenge in enzootic areas to enable them to survive the initial infection and develop solid acquired immunity to the disease.

Literature

Cattle inoculated subcutaneously with killed antigen which had been prepared by mixing disrupted *B. bovis*-infected erythrocytes with Freund's complete adjuvant were immunized against heterologous strain challenge. The protection was comparable to that induced by subclinical infection. In contrast, antigen prepared from the plasma of infected cattle was weakly immunogenic (Mahoney and Wright 1976). Animals which were injected with freeze-dried suspensions of *B. bovis,* either subcutaneously in Freund's complete adjuvant or intravenously in distilled water, also developed a degree of immunity to challenge with homologous strain (Mahoney 1967c). Further work showed that calves which were injected intramuscularly with antigens from the erythrocytes and plasma of cattle infected with *B. bigemina* and *B. bovis* acquired a high degree of sterile immunity to experimental and field challenges, irrespective of whether or not the vaccine had been admixed with Freund's complete adjuvant. Antigens obtained from the sera provided more protection than those from the erythrocytes (Todorovic *et al.* 1973a). Splenectomized calves inoculated with a vaccine which contained antigen derived from *B. bigemina* organisms and erythrocytic stroma and Freund's complete adjuvant were also protected against the development of severe clinical signs following challenge (Kuttler and Johnson 1980). Clinical observations and serological testing established that immunity occurred in cattle which had been inoculated twice with a vaccine containing dead antigen from *B. bigemina*-infected erythrocytes and Freund's complete adjuvant (Lohr 1978). Splenectomized calves which were injected on several occasions with lyophilized plasma from an animal infected with *B. divergens* showed limited protection to isologous and homologous challenges (Purnell and Brocklesby 1977). Approximately 3 weeks after challenge, a stong anamnestic response was observed in cattle which had been vaccinated with culture-derived soluble *B. bovis* antigens. Serum IgG and IgM levels increased after vaccination and challenge (James *et al.* 1981a). Mice injected with BCG developed nonspecific immunity to rodent forms of babesiosis, but this vaccine failed to protect calves against infection with *B. divergens* (Brocklesby and Purnell 1977).

With the recent advances in *in vitro* techniques for the cultivation of *Babesia*, there are good possibilities of developing a more standardized vaccine utilizing soluble and insoluble components. Both corpuscular and soluble fractions of *B. bovis* from supernatant fluids obtained during routine medium exchange of blood cultures produced specific antibabesial antibodies in calves. The corpuscular antigens contained intra- and extraerythrocytic merozoites, and the surface coat adhered loosely to the plasma membranes of the parasites (Gravely *et al.* 1979). The calves which were vaccinated with Freund's incomplete adjuvant and the soluble antigen obtained from the supernatants of erythrocyte cultures developed some resistance to challenge. These animals had reduced fever, less severe PCV reduction, and lower mortality and were able rapidly to eliminate parasites from the circulation (Smith *et al.* 1979). Filtered, freeze-dried soluble antigens prepared from supernatant fluids from cultures of *B. bovis* and reconstituted with saponin adjuvant protected challenged cattle against severe clinical response and death. Serum from vaccinated cattle caused thickening of the merozoite surface coat, aggregation and lysis of merozoites *in vitro*. These effects were similar to those caused by serum from immune carrier animals, suggesting that the protective antigen present in the culture supernates was merozoite surface coat antigen (Kuttler *et al.* 1982; Smith *et al.* 1981).

Vaccination has not been extensively used in species of animals other than cattle. Killed antigens prepared from the *B. equi*-infected erythrocytes and plasma of a splenectomized donkey protected against homologous challenge. Although a mild parasitemia developed, there were no changes in the hematological parameters and fever did not develop (Singh *et al.* 1981). Dogs acquired immunity to *B. canis* only after infection with live parasites and not with killed antigens. This protection was evident even when CF tests were negative and parasites could not be demonstrated by passage (Schindler *et al.* 1966).

Babesia rodhaini and the less virulent *B. microti* infections in rodents are useful models with which to study the immune response to babesiosis. It was found that nonspecific immunity could be induced in mice by injecting intraerythrocytic protozoa, *Mycobacterium bovis* (bacillus-Calmette-Guérin, BCG), *Corynebacterium parvum*, and muramyl dipeptide, a microbial extract which was the smallest unit capable of replacing mycobacterial cell wall as adjuvant. These micro-organisms and synthetic substances stimulate very effective and long-lasting nonspecific immunity to rodent babesiosis, causing the death of the intracellular parasites at the height of the first parasitemia. The parasites which were not killed continued to persist at low levels of parasitemia. These methods of vaccination could prove applicable to domestic animals (Cox 1980). It was postulated that BCG confers protection against *B. microti* and *B. rodhaini* infections by increasing the release of non-antibody soluble mediators which cause the death of the organisms inside the erythrocytes. This effect occurred before a specific antibody response was evoked. Since nonspecific and specific mechanisms are involved in providing protection against babesiosis, an effective vaccine could combine an adjuvant with an attenuated organism to induce both types of immunity (Clark *et al.* 1976, 1977a, b).

Irradiated organisms

The irradiation of organisms in either the tick or mammalian host causes a reduction in their infectivity and virulence. When susceptible animals are inoculated with these organisms, the ensuing infection may be mild or asymptomatic and induce varying degrees of immunity to homologous and heterologous challenges. Experimental vaccines produced by exposing infected blood to ionizing radiation contain organisms which multiply at the same rate (8-hour) as the virulent parent strain and are avirulent. Further research is necessary to define the usefulness of this approach under field conditions.

Literature

The radiation and isotopic techniques utilized in the production of vaccines against *Babesia* and *Theileria* were reviewed, and it was concluded that some success has been achieved by employing radiation to modify tick or mammalian stages of the parasite for use as potential vaccines (Irvin *et al.* 1979a). After exposure to between 20 and 50 krad, *B. bovis* had reduced rates of multiplication in the host and caused mild infections that left strong immunity to reinfection. Parasites whose multiplication was completely inhibited by radiation did not protect splenectomized calves against challenge infection; the inoculant behaved immunologically as antigen from killed organisms (Mahoney *et al.* 1973a). *Babesia bovis* irradiated at 35 krad showed reduced pathogenicity. The parasite multiplication rates and maximum parasitemias were similar in groups of cattle which had received either irradiated or nonirradiated blood; however, the latter induced changes in the coagulation and kinin systems (Wright *et al.* 1980a). In a further group of experiments it was shown that cattle vaccinated with a single dose of irradiated *B. bovis* were immune to virulent heterologous challenge 12 months later. Moreover, these organisms reisolated after 12 months in carrier animals had not reverted to a virulent or tick-transmissible state after that period (Wright *et al.* 1982, 1983). Calves inoculated with *B. bigemina* irradiated at 48 and 60 krad acquired resistance which was sufficient to suppress parasite multiplication and to prevent the development of otherwise severe clinical infections due to challenge with nonirradiated organisms (Bishop and Adams 1974).

In a further effort to develop an irradiated vaccine against *B. divergens* and *B. major*, a number of experiments were undertaken to study the effect of radiation on the infectivity of the piroplasms. Infected blood was harvested from a donor calf when the parasitemia reached levels of 5 to 10%. The infected blood was then irradiated at doses of 24 to 40 krad. When this material was injected into splenectomized and intact calves, it was apparent that a reduction in the pathogenicity of the organisms had occurred. The prepatent period was prolonged, and only a mild reaction was observed. The animals which were inoculated with piroplasms irradiated at 36 and 40 krad had no overt reactions. On challenge, the animals which had mild reactions were solidly immune, and those with no reactions had limited protection. Although the results of these laboratory experiments are encouraging, it has to be shown whether cattle inoculated with irradiated vaccines can withstand unlimited challenge with infected ticks in the field (Purnell *et al.* 1980a). A series of experiments leading towards the field trial of an irradiated blood-derived vaccine against *B. divergens* was undertaken. Calves inoculated intravenously with infected blood irradiated at 24 to 32 krad mounted the required immune response without developing clinical disease. In a field trial the vaccinated calves were protected against field challenge (Purnell *et al.* 1979b). Animals receiving *B. divergens* irradiated at 24, 28, and 32 krad had a mild reaction and were immune to heterologous and homologous challenges (Lewis *et al.* 1979, 1980a). Higher doses of radiation reduced the ability of the parasites to induce resistance to challenge (Purnell *et al.* 1978a). Cattle immunized against *B. divergens* which had been irradiated at 30 krad were also resistant to developing clinical disease upon challenge with a heterologous strain in the field (Taylor *et al.* 1980).

It was concluded that the protective effect of an irradiated *B. divergens* vaccine was due to the combined inoculation of large numbers of dead parasites killed by irradiation and a small number of the remaining live organisms (Purnell and Lewis 1981). Calves inoculated with *B. major*-infected blood irradiated at 23 to 35 krad developed minimal reactions, and upon challenge with homologous parasites all animals were immune. The reactions in immunized animals were minimal; parasitemia became briefly patent, fever was absent, and there was no apparent effect on the hematological parameters (Purnell *et al.* 1979a).

Infection and treatment method

Babesiacidal compounds are used either to control the development of severe clinical signs without complete elimination of the organisms or to induce sterilization, and in both cases result in an immune state. These babesiacidal agents must be used cautiously in vaccination procedures because the elimination of the organism in the early stages of infection would impair the subsequent development of immunity.

Literature

Aliu (1980) described the chemoimmunization of ruminants against *Babesia, Anaplasma, Theileria* and *Cowdria* species and suggested that these methods could be used widely, particularly when susceptible animals were introduced into enzootic areas. The vaccine used in cattle in South Africa contained both *B. bovis* and *B. bigemina*, and it was shown that chemotherapy with imidocarb could control reactions (Taylor and McHardy 1979). The degree of immunity developed by cattle infected with *B. bovis* and then sterilized with imidocarb was dependent on the duration of prior infection. Partial immunity occurred in cattle sterilized during the primary infection, and a high level of immunity was observed in animals that, before sterilization, had been carriers following two infections with different strains (Callow *et al.* 1974b). Immunity to *B. bigemina* infection also depends on the clinical reaction phase. The total clearance of parasites by chemotherapy in the early stages of the reaction prevented the establishment of immunity and animals were susceptible to reinfection (Pipano *et al.* 1972). A single dose of 0.5 to 1 mg/kg of pentamidine caused recovery of splenectomized calves infected with *B. bigemina*. Since the dose required to cause sterilization was at least five times as great as the therapeutic dose, the drug could be used for chemoimmunization (Pipano *et al.* 1979). The development of sterile immunity following treatment with Berenil at a dose of 6 mg/kg required contact of sufficient duration between *B. bigemina* and the host. This was demonstrated by the fact that carrier animals treated with 10 mg/kg of Berenil survived challenge (Dwivedi and Gautam 1976). The control of anaplasmosis and babesiosis by the immunization of cattle with fully virulent *Anaplasma marginale, B. bovis*, and *B. bigemina* is possible when the postinfection reactions are controlled by chemotherapy. Chemoprophylaxis was found to be a less effective method of controlling these diseases. Animals treated during the acute stage of the infection showed weight gains not significantly different from those of immunized cattle. Both methods were found to be advantageous for cattle raised in areas where anaplasmosis and babesiosis are endemic (Thompson *et al.* 1978b).

DIAGNOSIS

Parasitological methods

The diagnosis of babesiosis can be accomplished by the direct method of identifying the presence of organisms in the blood and by the indirect method of detecting antibodies via serological tests. The definitive diagnosis of babesiosis is made by demonstrating the organisms. Blood obtained at postmortem from the peripheral circulation, kidney, heart, spleen, or liver is examined on smears stained with Giemsa. Thick smears from the peripheral blood are used to detect low concentrations of organisms. In blood smears the species are differentiated on the basis of their morphology. Microscopic examination of blood may not be an efficient technique in the early and chronic stages of the disease when the parasitemia is low or absent, and necessitating the inspection of a number of samples taken over a period of time. In *B. bovis* and *B. canis* infections, brain smears are particularly important. In cattle, *B. bovis* and *B. bigemina* are detected in kidney smears for up to 8 hours, and in brain smears for up to 24 hours after death. However, when an examination is conducted more than 1 hour after the death of the animal, identification of the particular species is difficult because the organisms undergo morphological changes.

Literature

The procedures used for the diagnosis of babesiosis were reviewed by Todorovic and Carson (1981). Due to the low levels of parasitemia which are caused by different species of *Babesia,* diagnosis by the examination of thin blood films is difficult. The examination of thick blood films is a more reliable and practical method for detecting babesial organisms. In this technique, the lysis of the erythrocytes and the staining of the piroplasms enable the inspection of larger volumes of blood (Mahoney and Saal 1961). A method was described for preparing a combination of thin and thick blood films on the same slide (Bishop and Adams 1973). Differential diagnosis of *B. bovis* and *B. bigemina* was made using blood and brain smears. *Babesia bigemina* was larger than *B. bovis,* and the latter was concentrated in the capillaries up to ten times more than in the peripheral blood. This difference between capillary and peripheral blood was a distinctive characteristic of the species. It was noted that *B. bovis* was larger in the capillaries than in the peripheral blood and therefore seems to be comparable in size to *B. bigemina* (Hoyte 1971).

The accuracy of the direct fluorescent antibody and Giemsa staining techniques in the postmortem diagnosis of babesiosis was compared. Using Giemsa stain, *B. bovis* was detected in smears of heart, lung, and kidney immediately and up to 8 hours after death, while the organisms were demonstrated in the brain even after 28 hours. The direct FA technique detected *B. bovis* in heart and lung smears up to 12 hours, in the kidney up to 16 hours, and in the brain up to 28 hours after death. *Babesia bigemina* was detected in Giemsa-stained smears of the heart, lung, and kidney immediately after death, but by 1 hour postmortem, its morphology resembled that of *B. bovis*. A few erythrocytes inside and outside the brain capillaries were parasitized with organisms resembling *B. bovis* up to 16 hours after death. The direct FA test was capable of detecting *B. bigemina* in heart and lung smears for 12 hours, and in kidney films for 16 hours after death. A few infected red blood cells inside and outside capillaries were also seen in brain smears 16 hours after death. Organ smears could be stored for 5 days at 22 °C. Both babesial species were still detectable by the Giemsa and direct antibody staining techniques after organ smears were stored at 22 °C for 5 days (Johnston *et al.* 1977).

Babesia bigemina and *B. bovis* could also be stained in fixed smears with acridine orange and demonstrated by fluorescence microscopy. This method was more sensitive; the organisms were identified in 64 times higher dilutions than with Giemsa-stained thin smears and in 16 times higher dilutions than with Giemsa-stained thick films (Winter 1967). In *B. caballi* infection in horses, the red blood cells containing parasites were found in the region just below the buffy coat when the blood was centrifuged. This procedure increased the numbers of organisms and made their direction easier (Watkins 1962). It was shown that venous blood was more suitable than capillary blood for making diagnosis of *B. canis* infections (Ewing 1965a).

Serological methods

Serological tests were developed for the diagnosis of babesiosis because examination of smears was not optimal for the detection of subclinical infections. These tests are capable of identifying current infections as well as antibodies to *Babesia* species and to substances antigenically related to *Babesia* species. The serological tests which are available include CF, IFA, labeled anti-complement FA, indirect hemagglutination, latex particle agglutination, and agglutination of parasites. Not all of these tests are useful diagnostic methods, and some are used only in specialized areas of research. The techniques most commonly used are the CF, FA, hemagglutination, and agglutination tests. These serological methods are potentially useful in epizootiological surveys and for the evaluation of the enzootic status of herds. The CF test is used in the diagnosis of *B. bigemina*, *B. bovis*,

B. caballi, *B. equi*, *B. canis*, and *B. ovis* infections. In cattle, it is highly specific, showing no more than 2% false positive reactions. Weak cross-reactions occur between different *Babesia* species and are detectable only during a brief period immediately following recovery from the acute phase. Antibodies can be detected for only a few months in spite of the persistence of subclinical infections; therefore, it is not an efficient diagnostic method in enzootic areas. This test can detect equine antibodies to *B. caballi* throughout the period of infection. The IFA test is used to detect infections in cattle, horses, and dogs. In cattle, it is highly sensitive, giving a detection rate of 97 to 98% in subclinically infected animals and a false positive rate of 3 to 4%. The cross-reactions between the different species of *Babesia* are weak. The IFA test is one of the preferred diagnostic methods, but requires stringent standardization to ensure accuracy. Indirect hemagglutination has been used in the diagnosis of *B. bovis* and *B. bigemina*. In the case of *B. bovis*, the procedure gives a low false positive rate of 0.5% and a high sensitivity of 97.5% in experimental animals, whereas with *B. bigemina*, the detection decreased to about 80% under field conditions. The indirect hemagglutination test is technically more difficult to perform than other procedures and requires further adaptation for use in other species. Agglutination tests have been developed for the field diagnosis of both *B. bovis* and *B. bigemina*. Although there are some differences in its sensitivity to the two types of infections, the test is very useful under field conditions because of its rapidity and simplicity.

Literature

Various serological tests have been used in surveys to determine the incidence of antibodies in populations of animals and for the differentiation of various species of *Babesia*. Todorovic and Carson (1981) described the various serological tests used to monitor the immunological responses to *Babesia* and presented tables in which the serodiagnostic tests for bovine as well as for other types of babesiosis were listed. Mahoney (1979) evaluated the more commonly used diagnostic serological tests. The development of practical tests required relatively simple techniques, objective interpretation, low cost, sensitivity, a high level of specificity, and reproducibility under field conditions (Todorovic 1975a).

Fluorescein-conjugated globulins were prepared from the sera of animals recovered from acute infections with *B. bovis*, *B. bigemina*, *B. canis* and *B. rodhaini*. This technique revealed features of the parasitized erythrocyte that were not observed in Giemsa-stained blood smears; namely, the periphery of erythrocytes infected with *B. bovis* and *B. canis* and the granules in the erythrocytes parasitized by *B. bigemina* showed specific fluorescence. The granules were stained to a lesser extent in *B. bovis* and *B. canis* infections (Ludford 1969). A comparison between the use of dried blood on filter paper and serum for antibody titers was conducted using the indirect fluorescent antibody test. Good correlation was demonstrated under experimental and field conditions; there were no differences in the sensitivity or specificity of these methods. The filter paper technique had practical advantages for field use because it was more easily handled and could be stored at different temperatures (Todorovic and Garcia 1978).

Based on the result of immunofluorescent tests conducted with bovine antisera, Australia, South Africa, the UK, Federal Republic of Germany, and Holland were identified as belonging to the following four species: *B. bovis, B. bigemina, B. divergens*, and *B. major* (Goldman and Rosenberg 1974). Considerable cross-reactivity among *Babesia* species occurred, but species could be differentiated by the higher titers in homologous tests than in heterologous tests (Anderson *et al.* 1980). The IFA technique was used to determine the antigenic differentiate relationships among *B. bigemina, B. bovis, B. major*, and *B. divergens*; titers against the heterologous antigens were consistently lower than those obtained with homologous antigens. This finding indicated that species-specific common antigens existed (Leeflang and Perié 1972). High titers and specificity were maintained after *B. major*- or *B. divergens*-infected calves recovered (Joyner *et al.* 1972). The test showed that strains of *B. bovis* from South America, Mozambique, and Australia were serologically similar. This similarity of strains from widely separated geographical areas was considered evidence of the homogeneity of this organism throughout the world. The practical implication of these findings is that cattle could be immunized with a single vaccine before being shipped to various enzootic areas (Callow 1976, Callow *et al.* 1981). Immunofluorescent methods indicated that the *Babesia* species in Japan was serologically different from *B. major, B. bigemina*, and *B. bovis* (Fujinaga *et al.* 1980), while the IFA test was used to identify *B. major* in the UK (Brocklesby *et al.* 1971b).

Under field conditions in Colombia, the IFA test detected *B. bovis* antibodies an average of 4 weeks earlier than the CF test. Both serological tests were capable of differentiating *B. bovis* from *B. bigemina* infections, but in some cases cross-reactions were observed. The IFA test had advantages over the CF test in its simplicity, economy, and rapidity (Todorovic and Long 1976). It was found that the CF and IFA tests were both effective in detecting specific antibodies against *B. bigemina* during the first 84 days of infection. Thereafter, the CF antibody titers dropped below reliable levels, whereas the IFA titers could still be detected at significant levels even though they had also decreased (Kuttler *et al.* 1977). In *B. bigemina* and *B. bovis* infections, the CF test detected homologous antibodies within 7 to 21 days. These antibodies were detectable from the time parasitemia was observed in thick smears to the time when parasites could not be detected by the direct method. The antigen appeared to possess species specificity and showed only a limited reaction with heterologous antibodies (Mahoney 1962).

The card agglutination test detected antibodies simultaneously with the onset of the first *B. bigemina* parasitemia. The reaction persisted for up to 3 months, or long after the disappearance of the organisms. There was an excellent correlation between the results of the card agglutination test and those of the CF test. Because of its simplicity and specificity, the card agglutination test may be useful under field conditions (Todorovic and Kuttler 1974). The CF and capillary-tube agglutination tests were used to differentiate *B. bigemina* from a large *Babesia* species frequently infecting cattle in Japan (Minami *et al.* 1979).

A rapid slide agglutination test detected antibody in conjunction with the first appearance of *B. bovis* parasites in thin blood smears. Positive reactions in plasma from animals with natural infections were confirmed by blood smears and the IFA and CF tests. The test was used to diagnose *B. bovis* infection in animals under 2 years of age and detected 80 to 90% of the infections among older animals. The false-positive rate was 3.0% (Goodger and Mahoney 1974b; Lopez and Todorovic 1978).

An indirect hemagglutination test was developed for the diagnosis of *B. bovis* and was found to be of equal sensitivity to the CF test. The indirect hemagglutination test was observed to have fewer false-positive reactions (Curnow and Curnow 1967). The sensitivity of the hemagglutination test for differentiating *B. bigemina* from *B. bovis* was improved by using antigen derived from the lysate of infected erythrocytes. The lysate contained species-specific antigens. By comparing the cross-reactions of antigens from both species, it was possible to differentiate between the two species without using the inhibition techniques which would be needed to distinguish between *B. bovis* infection and mixed infection (Goodger 1973b). The passive hemagglutination test eliminated most nonspecific reactions and was highly specific and sensitive (Goodger and Mahoney 1974a). The bentonite agglutination and passive hemagglutination tests required less antigen than the gel precipitation test and were more rapid (Sibinovic *et al.* 1969a).

The IFA test was found to be both sensitive and specific for the diagnosis of *B. equi* infections in horses (Callow *et al.* 1979a). The IFA test was also specific for the detection of antibody in carrier horses experimentally infected with *B. caballi*. There was no cross-reaction with *B. equi*, and although strong positive reactions were easily detectable, considerable experience was required to differentiate weak positive reactions from negative ones (Madden and Holbrook 1968). The precipitation test detected comparable responses in horses during the acute and subclinical phases of *B. caballi* infection. Although a one-step fluorescein labeled antibody-inhibition test was useful in the detection of the carrier state, it appeared to be more suitable for research purposes rather than for routine diagnosis (Ristic and Sibinovic 1964). The serological responses of *B. caballi*-infected horses were evaluated by CF testing. It was discovered that CF antibody titers persisted longer than did the animals' ability to transmit the infection. The latter was determined by subinoculating erythrocytes into susceptible animals. The CF test was highly specific for differentiating *B. caballi* infections from *B. equi* (Frerichs *et al.* 1969a). The correlation between the CF test and the card agglutination test indicated that the latter required further standardization in order to be used in serological surveys of babesiosis in horses (Amerault *et al.* 1978). A capillary-tube agglutination test for detecting *B. equi* and *B. caballi* infections was developed and recommended for field diagnosis because of its simplicity, specificity, and economy (Anon. 1963; Singh *et al.* 1978).

The IFA test was both sensitive and reproducible in the diagnosis of *B. gibsoni* infections in dogs (Anderson *et al.* 1980). Using antigens from *B. rodhaini*, antibodies to *B. canis* and *B. gibsoni* could be detected by means of the IFA test and the ELISA (Weiland and Kratzer 1979). The CF test was also of value in identifying *B. canis* infection (Schindler and Dennig 1962).

CHEMOTHERAPY

The large species of *Babesia* are more sensitive to chemotherapy than the small ones, but no treatment can be relied upon to provide a complete cure. The successful treatment of babesiosis is dependent on the drug's toxicity for the host and efficacy against a particular species of *Babesia*. Babesiacides are effective in bringing about clinical remission of the disease, but the prognosis is poor for animals treated *in extremis* or for those cases showing central nervous system involvement. The aim of the treatment is to promote clinical recovery from acute infection and to allow some organisms to persist; asymptomatic infection results in the susbsequent development of resistance. The chemotherapy of babesiosis is largely dependent upon the use of the following drugs: quinuronium (5,5′-methylene bis-salicylate), amicarbilide (3,3′-diamidinocarbanilide diisethionate), diminazene (4,4′-diamidinodiazoaminobenzene diaceturate), phenamidine and imidocarb [3,3′-bis (2-imidazolin-2-yl) carbanilide].

Diminazene is used to treat babesiosis in all species of animals and is one of the two drugs known to have an effect on *B. gibsoni*. Phenamidine is active against *B. gibsoni* but is not widely used in other species. Amicarbilide is clinically effective against babesial species which parasitize cattle and horses. Clinical signs of toxicity were observed in calves only at doses four to six times higher than those used for treatment. Imidocarb is a prophylactic drug that renders the progeny of infected ticks which have fed on treated animals incapable of transmitting *B. bovis* and probably also *B. bigemina*. Although recent restrictions have been placed on the marketing of imidocarb because of toxic residues in animals, it is an efficient drug in horses and cattle. It is most effective against *B. caballi* and less active in *B. equi* and *B. bovis* infections. The compound can eliminate carrier *B. bovis* infections but not carrier *B. equi* infections. The dipropionate derivative of the drug is less toxic than the dihydrochloride salt. Drug resistance is relatively easily induced with all of the commonly used compounds. Advances in the understanding of the pathogenesis of babesiosis indicate that supportive therapy which could alleviate the shock and the coagulation dysfunctions would be beneficial.

Literature

The chemotherapy of babesiosis, theileriosis, and anaplasmosis was reviewed, and the therapeutic effects of three babesiacidal compounds (amicarbalide, diminazene, and imidocarb) in various species of domestic animals were discussed in detail (Joyner 1981; Joyner and Brocklesby 1973). Dennig (1974) described the chemotherapeutics of babesiosis and theileriosis in cattle. In an article on the chemotherapy of the major tropical parasitic diseases of man, Van den Bossche (1978) briefly discussed antimalarial, antitrypanosomal, antileishmanial, antischistosomal, antinematodal, and anticestodal drugs. He concluded that good drugs are now available for some of the serious parasitic organisms that infect people living in tropical and subtropical regions. It will be necessary to conduct large-scale clinical trials with most of the drugs or with combinations of drugs in order to determine the most effective treatment regimens. Conditions in the tropics should be improved with respect to the utilization of pharmaceutical products so that the potential of new compounds and existing efficacious drugs can be maximally exploited. These conclusions also apply to the situation on many of the tropical diseases of domestic animals, particularly babesiosis and trypanosomiasis.

Imidocarb is the drug of choice in the prophylaxis of bovine babesiosis. Calves which were given an intramuscular dose of 2 mg/kg of imidocarb dihydrochloride 46 days before receiving a lethal dose of *Babesia*-infected blood did not develop acute disease. An intravenous injection of the same dose 20 days prior to challenge also conferred protection. Calves treated intravenously with 3 mg/kg of imidocarb 21 days prior to exposure resisted tick-borne challenge, and the resistance was evident for 15 weeks of field exposure (Todorovic *et al.* 1973b). The prophylactic effect was observed when the compound was administered subcutaneously at a dose of 2 mg/kg 33 days before exposure to *B. bovis* and was more pronounced when the animals were treated 24, 23, and 13 days before exposure. Prophylaxis did not interfere with the normal development of acquired immunity to *B. bovis*. Animals which received this dose were also strongly resistant to infection with *B. bigemina* 12 weeks after treatment (Callow and McGregor 1970). A subcutaneous dose of 2 mg/kg given at the time of field exposure to *B. bovis* and *B. bigemina* prevented the development of clinical signs but allowed the production of antibodies. Treatment at 36 days before exposure was less effective (Roy-Smith 1971). The prophylactic use of imidocarb dihydrochloride resulted in a 2.5% failure of protection in cattle challenged with *B. divergens* under field conditions (Haigh and Hagan 1974).

Imidocarb dihydrochloride was also found to have therapeutic activity. *Babesia bigemina*-infected calves were sterilized with a subcutaneous dose of 1 mg/kg (Hashemi-Fesharki 1975). Concurrent carrier infections of *B. bigemina* and *B. bovis* were eliminated by 5 or 10 intramuscular injections of 2.5 mg/kg given at 48-hour intervals (Adams and Todorovic 1974b). Single intramuscular injections of 1.0, 2.0, and 2.5 mg/kg of imidocarb were effective against *B. bigemina* and concurrent infections of *B. bigemina* and *B. bovis,* but these doses inhibited the development of immunity (Adams and Todorovic 1974a). Splenectomized calves with acute *B. bigemina* infections were also sterilized with subcutaneous doses of 0.4 to 0.6 mg/kg. Severe infections due to *B. bovis* were readily controlled with imidocarb at doses of 1 to 20 mg/kg, while *B. bigemina* infections were successfully treated with doses of 0.4 to 20 mg/kg. The compound was active when given both subcutaneously and intravenously (Callow and McGregor 1970). Imidocarb dihydrochloride administered subcutaneously or intramuscularly at dose levels down to 1 mg/kg and intravenously at dose levels as low as 0.125 mg/kg suppressed both the multiplication of the parasites and the development of anemia in acute infections caused by *B. bigemina* (Brown and Berger 1970). A subcutaneous or intramuscular dose of 1 mg/kg of imidocarb dihydrochloride controlled very severe acute disease caused by *B. bigemina* and *B. bovis* (Todorovic *et al.* 1973b). Tolerance to imidocarb was induced in *B. bovis* by transmitting the parasite from infected ticks in a series of non-splenectomized calves which had been treated prophylactically at 2 mg/kg. As the number of exposures to imidocarb increased, the animals became more readily infected. Subsequently, a 3 mg/kg dose did not eliminate subclinical infections with exposed parasites, while a dose of 1 mg/kg controlled acute infections with either tolerant or intolerant organisms (Dalgliesh and Stewart 1977a). At doses of less than 6 mg/kg, imidocarb dihydrochloride did not eliminate *B. ovis* infections in splenectomized lambs. However, the subcutaneous administration of 2 mg/kg for 3 days caused sterilization. Toxicity was observed after a single injection of 10 mg/kg (Hashemi-Fesharki 1977).

Imidocarb dipropionate at 5 mg/kg was prophylactic against *B. bigemina* infections for 30 days after treatment. Calves challenged 65 days after treatment developed a mild parasitemia (Dwivedi *et al.* 1977). It was suggested that imidocarb dipropionate could be used prophylactically at doses of 3.6 mg/kg within 14 days of challenge with *B. divergens,* and a repeat dose of the drug was not recommended because it prevented the establishment of the parasite and thus the development of immunity (Purnell *et al.* 1980b). A dose of 2.4 mg/kg was also prophylactic when given up to 26 days before infection with *B. bigemina* (Purnell *et al.* 1981b). When a dose of 5 mg/kg was administered 14 or 28 days before exposure to ticks, it prevented the development of clinical babesiosis due to *B. bovis* or *B. bigemina*. The larval progeny of ticks reared on calves receiving this treatment were infected. Treatment at 42 days before exposure was less effective. The administration of the drug 14 days before and 14 days after exposure rendered the next generation of larvae incapable of transmitting *Babesia* infection. Subcutaneous doses of imidocarb dipropionate at 2 mg/kg eliminated *B. bigemina* infection (Dwivedi *et al.* 1977).

Toxicity with very low mortality was observed at doses of 10 mg/kg of imidocarb hydrochloride, but animals which received total subcutaneous or intramuscular doses of 25 to 35 mg as repeated daily doses of 5 to 10 mg/kg died of accumulated toxicity 8 to 14 days later (Brown and Berger 1970). Mortality occurred in calves that were treated with 10 intramuscular injections of the compound at 2.5 mg/kg (Adams and Todorovic 1974b). Intravenous injections of 3 mg/kg caused acute toxicity in calves which showed clinical signs of respiratory problems, excessive salivation, muscular tremors, incoordination, urination, defecation, and prostration. The signs were milder when injections were subcutaneous or intramuscular (Todorovic *et al.* 1973b). No toxic effects were observed with imidocarb dihydrochloride at the subcutaneous dose of 1 mg/kg, and only mild transient side effects were observed at 5 and at 10 mg/kg (Hashemi-Fesharki 1975). Signs of toxicity were observed after intravenous injections of 10 and 20 mg/kg, but there was no mortality. The clinical signs of toxicosis were mild or absent with subcutaneous doses of 2 and 10 mg/kg, but not at 1 mg/kg (Callow and McGregor 1970). In dogs, imidocarb dipropionate administered intravenously at doses of 1 to 6 mg/kg produced hypotension which was prevented by atropine at 3 mg/kg (Rao *et al.* 1980).

A subcutaneous 1 g dose of a 20% suspension of the quinuronium compound, 5,5′-methylene bis salicylate in arachis oil had a prophylactic effect when administered to calves 7 to 30 days prior to challenge with *B. bovis*. Acute toxic effects were induced at doses of 2 g per animal, and fatal nephritis subsequently developed (Newton and O'Sullivan 1969). Quinuronium sulfate at a dose of 1 mg/kg arrested the development of *B. divergens* infection when the drug was administered at the time of onset of fever or hemoglobinuria, and treated animals remained carriers (Purnell *et al.* 1981a). The intravenous injection of 1 mg/kg of quinuronium methylsulfate caused a fall in blood pressure in sheep, while larger doses caused more marked hypotension and inhibition of respiratory movement. The drug also induced hypersecretion of gastric acid in the rat and of saliva in sheep. Amicarbalide isethionate, by comparison, was weakly active. It was concluded that the toxic effects produced by therapeutic doses of quinuronium might be attributed to cholinesterase inhibition, the symptoms of which were largely prevented by atropine. Severe intoxication with quinuronium produces irreversible cardiovascular and respiratory depression (Eyre 1967). Quinuronium was shown to be a potent inhibitor of circulating cholinesterases in the horse, sheep, cow, rabbit, pig, rat, guinea pig, chicken, and dog, while amicarbalide was less active (Eyre 1966).

There is less information available on the use of amicarbalide in cattle. Amicarbalide at a dose of 5 mg/kg was active against

B. divergens and was well tolerated at 40 mg/kg (Lucas 1960). In a series of chemotherapeutical trials involving splenectomized cattle infected with *B. bigemina*, amicarbalide at 10 mg/kg was effective but immunity did not develop, whereas at 7.5 mg/kg premunity developed and some fatal relapses occurred (Barnett 1965).

Diminazene diaceturate administered intramuscularly at a dose of 8 mg/kg, and acriflavin (5% solution) given intravenously at a dose of 15 ml per animal were effective against *B. bigemina* infections in calves; diminazene caused sterilization of blood, while acriflavin caused remission of clinical signs but did not eliminate the parasites (Pandey and Mishra 1978b). At a dose of 3.5 mg/kg, the drug eliminated *B. bigemina* organisms, and at 5 mg/kg, a sterile cure was achieved (Barnett 1965).

A number of other drugs have been tested in bovine babesiosis with varying degrees of success. Pentamidine at a dose of 0.5 to 1 mg/kg resulted in clinical recovery of splenectomized calves with acute infections of *B. bigemina*, but a dose of 5 mg/kg did not sterilize intact carriers (Pipano *et al.* 1979). Phenamidine isethionate (8 to 13.5 mg/kg) and quinuronium sulfate (1 mg/kg) both effectively controlled *B. bigemina* infections and allowed premunity to develop (Barnett 1965). Primaquine phosphate at a dose of 0.5 mg/kg could be used prophylactically against *B. bigemina* (Purnell *et al.* 1981b). An *in vitro* test for screening drugs for activity against *Babesia* involved monitoring the uptake of [^{3}H]-hypoxanthine; compounds which reduced the uptake by about 75% were considered to be active (Irvin and Young 1977, 1978).

Amicarbalide is the drug of choice in the treatment of equine babesiosis. Four doses of 8.8 mg/kg of amicarbalide administered at 24-hour intervals were effective in eliminating *B. caballi* but not *B. equi*, whereas four doses of 10 mg/kg given at 72-hour intervals were effective against *B. equi* in about 50% of the cases (Carbrey *et al.* 1971). When the drug was administered at a dose of 8.8 mg/kg for 2 consecutive days, it was effective against *B. caballi* but not *B. equi*. A delayed anaphylactic-type reaction with respiratory and digestive disturbances was observed after treatment (Kirkham 1969).

Imidocarb dipropionate administered at a dose of 5 mg/kg and repeated after 72 hours caused degeneration of *B. equi* parasites in the erythrocytes of horses. Sequential degenerative changes in the parasites included dilatation of the nuclear cisterns and clumping of chromatin, dissolution of the nuclear envelope and passage of nuclear material into the cytoplasm, and vacuolation of cytoplasm and compression of the chromatin to the periphery of the cell (Simpson and Neal 1980). After treatment, crystalline inclusions were observed in erythrocytes parasitized with *B. equi* (Simpson *et al.* 1980). Imidocarb dipropionate administered intramuscularly at 5 mg/kg and repeated after 48 hours was effective in donkeys. However, a single intramuscular dose of 5 or 2 mg/kg was only partially effective against *B. equi* (Singh *et al.* 1980). When *B. caballi*-infected horses were treated with imidocarb dipropionate at doses of 0.5 to 8.0 mg/kg injected intramuscularly twice at intervals, the parasites were eliminated (Frerichs and Holbrook 1974). There have been reports of local and systemic toxicity in horses treated with imidocarb. Two doses of 15.99± 1.49 mg/kg separated by 24 hours constituted the LD50 of imidocarb; mortalities occurred within 6 days of the first injection. The mortalities were attributed to acute renal cortical tubular necrosis and acute periportal hepatic necrosis (Adams 1981). The systemic toxic reactions observed in horses given 8 mg/kg consisted of moderate dyspnea, severe colic, and excessive gut motility. The toxic signs were minimal at doses up to 2 mg/kg (Frerichs and Holbrook 1974). At the site of injection of 16 or 32 mg/kg, there was hemorrhagic necrosis of the skeletal muscle surrounded by extensive edema. Coagulative necrosis and mineralization of the skeletal muscle, which was encapsulated by fibrous tissue, were evident in animals treated with smaller doses. The size of the lesion corresponded with the dosage (Adams 1981).

Groups of horses were successfully treated by the intramuscular administration of diminazene diaceturate at a dose of 5 mg/kg, phenamidine isethionate (40% solution) at 1 ml/45 kg, or amicarbalide isethionate at 180 mg/100 kg for 2 consecutive days (Bryant *et al.* 1969). An intramuscular dose of 12 mg/kg of diminazene diaceturate which was repeated after 24 hours controlled the rising parasitemia of *B. equi* infection in splenectomized donkeys. The drug was more effective in the early stages of the disease and had a prophylactic effect for 30 to 35 days (Singh *et al.* 1980). A dose of 8.8 mg/kg of phenamidine isethionate injected intramuscularly into multiple sites (no more than 2 ml per site) cleared *B. caballi* and *B. equi* infections. Diminazene given at 11 mg/kg for 2 consecutive days was also effective against *B. caballi* and *B. equi* (Kirkham 1969).

Babesia canis infection in the dog may be manifested as a mild syndrome or as an acute, rapidly fatal disease characterized by disseminated intravascular coagulation. These forms of the disease were treated differently; severe infections required supportive therapy which included intravenous fluids, heparin, and blood transfusions (Moore and Williams 1979). Imidocarb at a dose of 3 mg/kg sterilized *B. canis* infections and was prophylactic for at least 6 weeks, while a dose of 1 mg/kg protected dogs for 30 days against clinical disease but allowed infections to occur (Euzéby *et al.* 1980a, b, 1981). Diminazene diaceturate at 50 mg/kg exerted a prophylactic effect against *B. canis* for about 40 days. Animals which were treated with subcurative doses usually became premune and ultimately developed immunity (Bauer 1966). Diminazene aceturate given at 11 mg/kg in two doses 5 days apart was found to be effective against *B. gibsoni* infections (Fowler *et al.* 1972). Treatment with 5 to 7 mg/kg of diminazene diaceturate given subcutaneously or intramuscularly resulted in clinical cure and a stable long-lasting premunity. However, four doses of 10 mg/kg did not eradicate *B. gibsoni* parasites (Bauer 1967). Phenamidine isethionate administered at doses of 16.5 mg/kg for 2 consecutive days effectively controlled the clinical disease induced by *B. gibsoni* but did not eliminate the parasitemia (Groves and Vanniasingham 1970).

The semi-synthetic antibiotic ceporin 7-(2-thienyl acetamido)-3-(1-pyridylmethyl)-3-cephem-4-carboxylic acid betaine, given at a dose of 40 mg/kg had a rapid curative effect in *B. felis*-infected cats (Dorrington and du Buy 1966).

The toxicity of the diamidines in dogs and cattle has been established. Multiple doses of diminazene aceturate (3.5 or 10.5 mg/kg) or phenamidine (15 or 20 mg/kg) were used to induce diamidine poisoning in dogs. Dogs which received these treatments showed nervous symptoms including imbalance, rolling movements, extensor rigor, opisthotonus, nystagmus, and terminal paralysis. Death resulted from the hemorrhagic and malacic lesions in the cerebellum, midbrain, and thalamus. Comparable lesions were not observed in the brains of cattle. Degenerative lesions, mainly of a fatty nature, occurred in the liver, kidneys, myocardium, and skeletal muscles of some dogs (Naudé *et al.* 1970).

The chemotherapy of rodent forms of babesiosis has been investigated. Imidocarb dihydrochloride had greater babesiacidal effect in *B. rodhaini* infections in mice and rats than amicarbalide, diminazene diaceturate, and quinuronium sulfate. Imidocarb and amicarbalide had comparable prophylactic effects in mice (Beveridge 1969). The prolonged administration of an interferon inducer delayed death due to experimental *B. rodhaini* infection by a day (Brocklesby and Harradine 1973). Several members of a series of 1-(chlorophenoxyalkaloxy)-4,6-diamino-1,2-dihydro-2,2-dimethyl-1,3,5-triazine hydrobromides (I) have shown marked suppressive activity against *B. rodhaini* infections in mice (Knight 1981).

CONTROL

The methods which are undertaken to control babesiosis include treatment, vaccination, and tick eradication. These methods should be adopted for particular epizootiological situations, e.g. infected ticks are introduced into *Babesia*-free areas; susceptible animals are introduced into *Babesia*-infested areas; and tick infestation is temporarily reduced in an infected area by either natural or artificial means. The general principles of epizootiology which must be applied in order to control the disease efficiently are as follows: (1) the use of quantitative methods to evaluate a situation; (2) the determination of the probability of host infection; and (3) the measurement of all the parameters involved in the maintenance of an organism in the environment. The determination of the severity of the challenge and the recognition of factors which govern the enzootic stability in the absence of disease outbreaks are also important in the control of babesiosis. The prevention of disease in developing unstable enzootic situations entails identifying the animals at immediate risk, establishing the duration of protection required, and delineating the zones of maximal and minimal risk.

Literature

The application of qualitative and particularly quantitative epizootiological principles to the control of bovine babesiosis in cattle was reviewed (Mahoney 1974; Mahoney and Ross 1972). Purnell (1979) briefly discussed the use of vaccination in the control of tick-borne diseases like babesiosis, theileriosis, and heartwater. He concluded that, with careful application and monitoring, these relatively unsophisticated methods could be effective against all the major tick-borne diseases of cattle. Todorovic (1974) investigated several methods for diagnosing and controlling babesiosis in Colombia, South America. Serological tests were used to determine (1) whether sterile immunity was attained after calves were vaccinated with killed babesial organisms; (2) whether a state of premunition existed after calves were exposed to virulent *Babesia* species and a chemotherapeutic agent; and (3) whether chemoprophylaxis by use of a babesiacide having long residual activity was possible. The epizootiological conditions in enzootic areas will dictate the method of choice. In areas heavily populated with *B. microplus* the combination of premunition and therapy should be used; in areas where the tick population is controlled, or in areas where cattle are at constant risk of tick exposure, vaccination with dead antigen or chemoprophylaxis is indicated. Hourrigan (1976) described the control and eradication of bovine babesiosis in the USA and included a discussion of the control measures undertaken in the quarantined areas of Texas.

BIBLIOGRAPHY

Adams, L. G., 1981. Clinicopathological aspects of imidocarb dipropionate toxicity in horses, *Res. vet. Sci.*, **31**: 54–61.

Adams, L. G. and Todorovic, R. A., 1974a. The chemotherapeutic efficacy of imidocarb dihydrochloride on concurrent bovine anaplasmosis and babesiosis. I. The effects of a single treatment, *Trop. Anim. Hlth Prod.*, **6**: 71–8.

Adams, L. G. and Todorovic, R. A., 1974b. The chemotherapeutic efficacy of imidocarb dihydrochloride on concurrent bovine anaplasmosis and babesiosis. II. The effects of multiple treatments, *Trop. Anim. Hlth Prod.*, **6**: 79–84.

Ajayi, S. A., 1978. A survey of cerebral babesiosis in Nigerian local cattle, *Vet. Rec.*, **103**: 564.

Akinboade, O. A., Dipeolu, O. O. and Adetunji, A., 1981. Experimental transmission of *Babesia bigemina* and *Anaplasma marginale* to calves with the larvae of *Boophilus decoloratus, Zbl. Vet. Med.*, **B28**: 329–32.

Aliu, Y. O., 1980. Chemo-immunization of ruminants against *Babesia, Anaplasma, Theileria,* and *Cowdria* species, *Vet. Res. Communications*, **4**: 99–106.

Allen, P. C., Frerichs, W. M. and Holbrook, A. A., 1975a. Experimental acute *Babesia caballi* infections. I. Red blood cell dynamics, *Exp. Parasitol.*, **37**: 67–77.

Allen, P. C., Frerichs, W. M. and Holbrook, A. A., 1975b. Experimental acute *Babesia caballi* infections. II. Response of platelets and fibrinogen, *Exp. Parasitol.*, **37**: 373–9.

Amerault, T. E., Roby, T. O., Rose, J. E. and Frerichs, W. M., 1978. Recent advances in serologic diagnosis of anaplasmosis and babesiosis. In *Tick-borne Diseases and their vectors*, ed. J. K. H. Wilde. Lewis Reprints (Tonbridge), pp. 121–9.

Anderson, J. F., Magnarelli, L. A. and Sulzer, A. J., 1980. Canine babesiosis: indirect fluorescent antibody test for a North American isolate of *Babesia gibsoni, Am. J. vet. Res.*, **41**(12): 2102–5.

Annable, C. R. and Ward, P. A., 1974. Immunopathology of the renal complications of babesiosis, *J. Immunol.*, **112**(1): 1–8.

Anon., 1963. New test for diagnosis of equine piroplasmosis, *J. Am. vet. med. Ass.*, **142**: 679.

Anon., 1970. Tick-borne diseases of domestic animals in Australia. I. Tick toxaemias, *Bull. Off. int. Epiz.*, **73**(1–2): 121–9.

Applewhaite, L. M., Craig, T. M. and Wagner, G. G., 1981. Serological prevalence of bovine babesiosis in Guyana. *Trop. Anim. Hlth Prod.*, **13**: 13–18.

Bachmann, A. W., Campbell, R. S. F., Johnston, L. A. Y. and Yellowlees, D., 1977. Bovine haemoglobin types and their possible relationship to resistance to babesiosis: an experimental study, *Z. Tropenmed. Parasitol.*, **28**: 361–6.

Bachmann, A. W., Johnston, L. A. Y., Jones, P. N. and Campbell, R. S. F., 1976. Erythrocyte adenosine triphospate levels in cattle infected with *Babesia argentina, Z. Tropenmed. Parasitol.*, **27**: 372–6.

Bandaranayake, A., 1961. A note on the occurrence of *Babesia argentina* in cattle in Ceylon, *Ceylon vet. J.*, **9**: 51–4.

Banerjee, D. P., Singh, B., Gautam, O. P. and Sarup, S., 1977. Cell-mediated immune response in equine babesiosis, *Trop. Anim. Hlth Prod.*, **9**: 153–8.

Barnett, S. F., 1964. The preservation of *Babesia bigemina, Anaplasma centrale* and *Anaplasma marginale* by deep freezing, *Vet. Rec.*, **76** (1): 4–8.

Barnett, S. F., 1965. The chemotherapy of *Babesia bigemina* infection in cattle, *Res. vet. Sci.*, **6**: 397–415.

Barnett, S. F., 1974a. Economical aspects of tick-borne diseases control in Britain, *Bull. Off. int. Epiz.*, **81**(1–2): 167–82.

Barnett, S. F., 1974b. Economical aspects of protozoal tick-borne diseases of livestock in parts of the world other then Britain, *Bull. Off. int. Epiz.*, **81**(1–2): 183–96.
Basson, P. A. and Pienaar, J. G., 1965. Canine babesiosis: a report on the pathology of three cases with special reference to the 'cerebral' form, *J. S. Afr. vet. med. Ass.*, **36**(3): 333–41.
Bauer, F., 1966. Treatment of *Babesia canis* infection with Berenil, *Z. Tropenmed. Parasitol.*, **17**: 390–6.
Bauer, F., 1967. Chemotherapy of *Babesia gibsoni* infection in the dog, *Zbl. Vet. Med.*, **B14**: 170–8.
Beveridge, E., 1969. Babesicidal effect of basically substituted carbanilides. II. Imidocarb in rats and mice: toxicity and activity against *Babesia rodhaini, Res. vet. Sci.*, **10**: 534–9.
Bhat, U. K. M., Mahoney, D. F. and Wright, I. G., 1979. The invasion and growth of *Babesia bovis* in tick tissue culture, *Experienta*, **35**(6): 752–3.
Bidwell, D. E., Turp, P., Joyner, L. P., Payne, R. C. and Purnell, R. E., 1978. Comparisons of serological tests for *Babesia* in British cattle, *Vet. Rec.*, **103**: 446–9.
Bishop, J. P. and Adams, L. G., 1973. Combination thin and thick blood films for the detection of *Babesia* parasitemia. *Am. J. vet. Res.*, **34**(9): 1213–14.
Bishop, J. P. and Adams, L. G., 1974. *Babesia bigemina*: immune response of cattle inoculated with irradiated parasites, *Exp. Parasitol.*, **35**: 35–43.
Bishop, J. P., Adams, L. G., Thompson, K. C. and Corrier, D. E., 1973. The isolation, separation, and preservation of *Babesia bigemina, Trop. Anim. Hlth Prod.*, **5**: 141–5.
Brocklesby, D. W., 1979. Human babesiosis, *J. S. Afr. vet. med. Ass.*, **50**(4): 302–7.
Brocklesby, D. W., Harness, E. and Sellwood, S. A., 1971a. The effect of age on the natural immunity of cattle to *Babesia divergens, Res. vet. Sci.*, **12**: 15–17.
Brocklesby, D. W. and Harradine, D. L., 1973. The effect of an interferon inducer on experimental mouse piroplasmosis (*Babesia rodhaini* infection), *Res. vet. Sci.*, **14**: 397–8.
Brocklesby, D. W., Harradine, D. L. and Young, E. R., 1976. *Babesia major* in Britain: cross-immunity trials with *Babesia divergens* in splenectomized calves, *Res. vet. Sci.*, **21**: 300–2.
Brocklesby, D. W. and Purnell, R. E., 1977. Failure of BCG to protect calves against *Babesia divergens* infection, *Nature*, **265**: 343.
Brocklesby, D. W. and Sellwood, S. A., 1973. *Babesia major* in Britain: tick transmitted infections in splenectomised calves, *Res. vet. Sci.*, **14**: 47–52.
Brocklesby, D. W., Zwart, D. and Perié, N. M., 1971b. Serological evidence for the identification of *Babesia major* in Britain, *Res. vet. Sci.*, **12**: 285–7.
Brown, C. G. D. and Berger, J., 1970. Chemotherapy of experimental *Babesia bigemina* infections with imidocarb

dihydrochloride, *Trop. Anim. Hlth Prod.*, **2**: 196–203.

Bryant, J. E., Anderson, J. B. and Willers, K. H., 1969. Control of equine piroplasmosis in Florida. *J. Am. vet. med. Ass.*, **154**(9): 1034–6.

Burridge, M. J., Kimber, C. D. and McHardy, N., 1973. Detection of antibodies to *Babesia bigemina* in dried blood samples using the indirect fluorescent antibody test, *Ann. trop. Med. Parasitol.*, **67**(2): 191–5.

Buttner, D. W., 1968. Vergleichende untersuchung der feinstruktur von *Babesia gibsoni* und *Babesia canis*, *Z. Tropenmed. Parasitol.*, **19**: 330–42.

Button, C., 1979. Metabolic and electrolyte disturbances in acute canine babesiosis, *J. Am. vet. med. Ass.*, **175**(5): 475–9.

Bwangamoi, O. and Isyagi, A. O., 1973. The incidence of filariasis and babesiosis in dogs in Uganda, *Bull. epiz. Dis. Afr.*, **21**: 33–7.

Callow, L. L., 1964. Strain immunity in babesiosis, *Nature*, **204**: 1213–14.

Callow, L. L., 1965. *Babesia bigemina* in ticks grown on non-bovine hosts and its transmission to these hosts, *Parasitology*, **55**: 375–81.

Callow, L. L., 1967. Sterile immunity, coinfectious immunity and strain differences in *Babesia bigemina* infections, *Parasitology*, **57**: 455–65.

Callow, L. L., 1968a. The infection of *Boophilus microplus* with *Babesia bigemina*, *Parasitology*, **58**: 663–70.

Callow, L. L., 1968b. A note on homologous strain immunity in *Babesia argentina* infections, *Aust. vet. J.*, **44**: 268–9.

Callow, L. L., 1976. Tick-borne livestock diseases and their vectors. 3. Australian methods of vaccination against anaplasmosis and babesiosis, *World Anim. Rev.*, **18**: 9–15.

Callow, L. L., 1977. Vaccination against bovine babesiosis. In *Immunity to Blood Parasites of Animals and Man*, eds L. H. Miller, J. A. Pino, J. J. McKelvey Jr. Plenum Press (New York), pp. 121–49.

Callow, L. L., 1979. Some aspects of the epidemiology and control of bovine babesiosis in Australia, *J. S. Afr. vet. med. Ass.*, **50**(4): 353–6.

Callow, L. L., Emmerson, F. R., Parker, R. J. and Knott, S. G., 1976a. Infection rates and outbreaks of disease due to *Babesia argentina* in unvaccinated cattle on 5 beef properties in south-eastern Queensland, *Aust. vet. J.*, **52**: 446–50.

Callow, L. L. and Hoyte, H. M. D., 1961a. Transmission experiments using *Babesia bigemina*, *Theileria mutans*, *Borrelia* sp. and the cattle tick, *Boophilus microplus*, *Aust. vet. J.*, **37**: 381–90.

Callow, L. L. and Hoyte, H. M. D., 1961b. The separation of *Babesia bigemina* from *Babesia argentina* and *Theileria mutans*, *Aust. vet. J.*, **37**: 66–70.

Callow, L. L. and Johnston, L. A. Y., 1963. *Babesia* spp. in the brains of clinically normal cattle and their detection by a brain smear technique. *Aust. vet. J.*, **39**: 25–31.

Callow, L. L., Kanhai, G. K. and Vandenberghe, A., 1981. Serological comparison of strains of *Babesia bovis* occurring in Australia and Mozambique, *Trop. Anim. Hlth Prod.*, **13**: 79–82.

Callow, L. L. and McGavin, M. D., 1963. Cerebral babesiosis due to *Babesia argentina, Aust. vet. J.*, **39**: 15–21.

Callow, L. L. and McGregor, W., 1969. Vaccination against *Babesia argentina* infection in cattle during chemoprophylaxis with a quinuronium compound, *Aust. vet. J.*, **45**: 408–10.

Callow, L. L. and McGregor, W., 1970. The effect of imidocarb against *Babesia argentina* and *Babesia bigemina* infections of cattle, *Aust. vet. J.*, **46**: 195–200.

Callow, L. L., McGregor, W., Parker, R. J. and Dalgliesh, R. J., 1974a. Immunity of cattle to *Babesia bigemina* following its elimination from the host, with observations on antibody levels detected by the indirect fluorescent antibody test, *Aust. vet. J.*, **50**: 12–15.

Callow, L. L., McGregor, W., Parker, R. J. and Dalgliesh, R. J., 1974b. The immunity of cattle to *Babesia argentina* after drug sterilisation of infections of varying duration, *Aust. vet. J.*, **50**: 6–11.

Callow, L. L., McGregor, W., Rodwell, B. J., Rogers, R. J., Fraser, G. C., Mahoney, D. F. and Robertson, G. M., 1979a. Evaluation of an indirect fluorescent antibody test to diagnose *Babesia equi* infection in horses, *Aust. vet. J.*, **55**: 555–9.

Callow, L. L. and Mellors, L. T., 1966. A new vaccine for *Babesia argentina* infection prepared in splenectomised calves, *Aust. vet. J.*, **42**: 464–5.

Callow, L. L., Mellors, L. T. and McGregor, W., 1979b. Reduction in virulence of *Babesia bovis* due to rapid passage in splenectomised cattle, *Int. J. Parasitol.*, **9**: 333–8.

Callow, L. L. and Pepper, P. M., 1974. Measurement of and correlations between fever, changes in the packed cell volume and parasitaemia in the evaluation of the susceptibility of cattle to infection with *Babesia argentina, Aust. vet. J.*, **50**: 1–5.

Callow, L. L., Quiroga, Q. C. and McCosker, P. J., 1976b. Serological comparison of Australian and South American strains of *Babesia argentina* and *Anaplasma marginale, Int. J. Parasitol.*, **6**: 307–10.

Callow, L. L. and Stewart, N. P., 1978. Immunosuppression by *Babesia bovis* against its tick vector, *Boophilus microplus, Nature*, **272**: 818–19.

Callow, L. L. and Tammemagi, L., 1967. Vaccination against bovine babesiosis. Infectivity and virulence of blood from animals either recovered from or reacting to *Babesia argentina, Aust. vet. J.*, **43**: 249–56.

Carbrey, E. A., Avery, R. J., Knowles, R. C. and Sash, S. C., 1971.

Drug therapy of equine babesiasis, *J. Am. vet. med. Ass.*, **158**: 1889.

Carmichael, J., 1956. Treatment and control of babesiosis, *Ann. N.Y. Acad. Sci.*, **46**: 147–51.

Carson, C. A. and Phillips, R. S., 1981. Immunologic response of the vertebrate host to *Babesia*. In *Babesiosis*, eds M. Ristic, J. P. Kreier. Academic Press (New York), pp. 411–43.

Chapman, W. E. and Ward, P. A., 1976a. Changes in C3 metabolism during protozoan infection (*Babesia rodhaini*) in rats, *J.Immunol.*, **116**(5): 1284–8.

Chapman, W. E. and Ward, P. A., 1976b. The complement profile in babesiosis, *J. Immunol.*, **117**(3): 935–8.

Chapman, W. E. and Ward, P. A., 1977. *Babesia rodhaini*: requirement of complement for penetration of human erythrocytes, *Science*, **196**: 67.

Claessens, J. and Spruyt, J., 1959. Un cas de nuttalliose dans la province de Kiva, *Bull. Agric. Congo Belge*, **50**: 1075–82.

Clark, I. A., Cox, F. E., and Allison G. A. C., 1976. Protection of mice against *Babesia* and *Plasmodium* with BCG, *Nature*, **259**: 309–11.

Clark, I. A., Cox, F. E. G. and Allison, A. C., 1977a. Protection of mice against *Babesia* spp. with killed *Corynebacterium parvum*, *Parasitology*, **74**: 9–18.

Clark, I. A., Richmond, J. E., Wills, E. J. and Allison, A. C., 1977b. Intra-erythrocytic death of the parasite in mice recovering from infection with *Babesia microti*, *Parasitology*, **75**: 189–96.

Coombs, W. G., 1977. Bovine babesiasis: a case reported in Devon, England, *Can. vet. J.*, **18**: 193–5.

Copeman, D. B., Tuemaun, F. and Hall, W. T. K., 1978. The prevalence of babesiosis and anaplasmosis in Queensland from 1966 to 1976. In *Tick-borne Diseases and their Vectors*, ed. J. K. H. Wilde. Lewis Reprints (Tonbridge), pp. 133–6.

Corrier, D. E., Gonzalez, E. F. and Betancourt, A., 1978. Current information on the epidemiology of bovine anaplasmosis and babesiosis in Colombia. In *Tick-borne Diseases and their Vectors*, ed. J. K. H. Wilde. Lewis Reprints (Tonbridge), pp. 114–20.

Corrier, D. E. and Guzman, S., 1977. The effect of natural exposure to *Anaplasma* and *Babesia* infections on native calves in an endemic area of Colombia, *Trop. Anim. Hlth Prod.*, **9**: 47–51.

Cox, F. E. G., 1980. Non-specific immunization against babesiosis. *Isotope and Radiation Research on Animal Diseases and Their Vectors*, proceedings of a symposium, Vienna, 7–11 May 1979, jointly organized by the IAEA and FAO. International Atomic Energy Agency (Vienna, Austria), IAEA-SM-240/14, pp. 95–104.

Cox, F. E. G. and Turner, S. A., 1970. Antibody levels in mice infected with *Babesia microti*, *Ann. trop. Med. Parasitol.*, **64**(2): 167–73.

Cox, F. E. G. and Wedderburn, N., 1972. Enhancement and prolongation of *Babesia microti* infections in mice infected with oncogenic viruses, *J. gen. Microbiol.*,**72**: 79–85.

Curnow, J. A., 1968. *In vitro* agglutination of bovine erythrocytes infected with *Babesia argentina, Nature,* **217**: 267–8.
Curnow, J. A., 1973a. Studies on antigenic changes and strain differences in *Babesia argentina* infections, *Aust. vet. J.,* **49**: 279–83.
Curnow, J. A., 1973b. Studies on the epizootiology of bovine babesiosis in north-eastern New South Wales. *Aust. vet. J.,* **49**: 284–9.
Curnow, J. A., 1973c. Studies on the epizootiology of bovine babesiosis in common border areas of New South Wales and Queensland, *Aust. vet. J.,* **49**: 294–7.
Curnow, J. A., 1973d. The use of a slide agglutination test to demonstrate antigenic differences between *Babesia bigemina* parasites, *Aust. vet. J.,* **49**: 290–3.
Curnow, J. A. and Curnow, B. A., 1967. An indirect haemagglutination test for the diagnosis of *Babesia argentina* infection in cattle, *Aust. vet. J.,* **43**: 286–90.

Dalgliesh, R. J., 1968. Field observations on *Babesia argentina* vaccination in Queensland, *Aust. vet. J.,* **44**: 103–4.
Dalgliesh, R. J., Callow, L. L., Mellors, L. T. and McGregor, W., 1981a. Development of a highly infective *Babesia bigemina* vaccine of reduced virulence, *Aust. vet. J.,* **57**: 8–11.
Dalgliesh, R. J., Dimmock, C. K., Hill, M. W. M. and Mellors, L. T., 1976. *Babesia argentina*: disseminated intravascular coagulation in acute infections in splenectomized calves, *Exp. Parasitol.,* **40**: 124–31.
Dalgliesh, R. J., Dimmock, C. K., Hill, M. W. M. and Mellors, L. T., 1977. The protamine sulphate test as a screening test for intravascular coagulation in experimental *Babesia bovis* infections, *Res. vet. Sci.,* **23**: 105–8.
Dalgliesh, R. J. and Stewart, N. P., 1977a. Tolerance to imidocarb induced experimentally in tick-transmitted *Babesia argentina, Aust. vet. J.,* **53**: 176–80.
Dalgliesh, R. J. and Stewart, N. P., 1977b. Failure of vaccine strains of *Babesia bovis* to regain infectivity for ticks during long-standing infections in cattle, *Aust. vet. J.,* **53**: 429–31.
Dalgliesh, R. J. and Stewart, N. P., 1978. The extraction of infective *Babesia bovis* and *Babesia bigemina* from tick eggs and *B. bigemina* from unfed larval ticks, *Aust. vet. J.,* **54**: 453–4.
Dalgliesh, R. J. and Stewart, N. P., 1979. Observations on the morphology and infectivity for cattle of *Babesia bovis* parasites in unfed *Boophilus microplus* larvae after incubation at various temperatures, *Int. J. Parasitol.,* **9**: 115–20.
Dalgliesh, R. J., Stewart, N. P. and Duncalfe, F., 1981b. Reduction in pathogenicity of *Babesia bovis* for its tick vector, *Boophilus microplus,* after rapid blood passage in splenectomized calves, *Z. Parasitenkd.,* **64**: 347–51.

Dennig, H. K., 1962. Experimental transmission of *Babesia bovis, B. bigemina, B. equi, B. caballi* and *B. trautmanni* to unweaned mice, *Z. Tropenmed. Parasitol.*, **13**: 472.

Dennig, H. K., 1974. Chemotherapy of protozoal tick-borne diseases, *Bull. Off. int. Epiz.*, **81**(1–2): 103–21.

Dennig, H. K., Centurier, C., Gobel, E. and Weiland, G., 1980. Canine babesiosis and its importance in the Federal Republic of Germany and West Berlin, *Berl. Münch. Tierarztl. Wschr.*, **93**: 373–9.

De Vos, A. J., 1978. Immunogenicity and pathogenicity of three South African strains of *Babesia bovis* in *Bos indicus* cattle, *Onderstepoort J. vet. Res.*, **45**(2): 119–24.

De Vos, A. J., Imes, G. D. and Cullen, J. S. C., 1976. Cerebral babesiosis in a new-borne calf, *Onderstepoort J. vet. Res.*, **43**(2): 75–8.

Dimmock, C. K., 1973. Blood group antibody production in cattle by a vaccine against *Babesia argentina, Res. vet. Sci.*, **15**: 305–9.

Donnelly, J., Joyner, L. P. and Crossman, P. J., 1972. The incidence of *Babesia divergens* infection in a herd of cattle as measured by the indirect immunofluorescent antibody test, *Res. vet. Sci.*, **13**(6): 511–14.

Donnelly, J., Joyner, L. P., Graham-Jones, O. and Ellis, C. P., 1980a. A comparison of the complement fixation and immunofluorescent antibody tests in a survey of the prevalence of *Babesia equi* and *Babesia caballi* in horses in the Sultanate of Oman, *Trop. Anim. Hlth Prod.*, **12**: 50–60.

Donnelly, J., Joyner, L. P. and Frank, C., 1980b. Quantitative epidemiological studies on the prevalence of babesiosis in horses in Kuwait, *Trop. Anim. Hlth Prod.*, **12**: 253–8.

Donnelly, J. and Peirce, M. A., 1975. Experiments on the transmission of *Babesia divergens* to cattle by the tick *Ixodes ricinus, Int. J. Parasitol.*, **5**: 363–7.

Dorner, J. L., 1969. Clinical and pathological features of canine babesiosis. *J. Am. vet. med. Ass.*, **154**(6): 648–52.

Dorrington, J. E. and du Buy, W. J. C., 1966. Ceporan: efficacy against *Babesia felis, J. S. Afr. vet. med. Ass.*, **37**(1): 93.

Dwivedi, S. K. and Gautam, O. P., 1976. Immunity to *Babesia bigemina* in calves after babesicidal treatment during acute and carrier stages, *Indian J. Anim. Sci.*, **46**(12): 627–9.

Dwivedi, S. K. and Gautam, O. P., 1978. A note on indirect haemagglutination test for evaluating experimental babesiosis, *Indian J. Anim. Sci.*, **48**: 148–9.

Dwivedi, S. K. and Gautam, O. P., 1979. A note on capillary-tube-agglutination test for the diagnosis of experimental babesiosis in calves, *Indian J. Anim. Sci.*, **49**: 395–6.

Dwivedi, S. K. and Gautam, O. P., 1980. Experimental studies on passive immunization against *Babesia bigemina* infection in calves, *Indian J. Anim. Sci.*, **50**: 169–72.

Dwivedi, S. K. and Gautam, O. P., 1980. Changes in serum–protein patterns in experimental babesiosis in calves, *Indian J. Anim. Sci.*, **50**: 241–6.

Dwivedi, S. K., Gautam, O. P. and Banerjee, D. P., 1977. Therapeutic and prophylactic activity of imidocarb dipropionate against *Babesia bigemina* infection in splenectomized bovine calves, *Indian vet. J.*, **54**: 697–702.

Dwivedi, S. K., Sharma, S. P. and Gautam, O. P., 1976. Babesiosis: clinical cases in exotic and cross-bred cattle, *Indian vet. J.*, **53**: 469–72.

Emmerson, F. R., Knott, S. G. and Callow, L. L., 1976. Vaccination with *Babesia argentina* in 5 beef herds in south-eastern Queensland, *Aust. vet. J.*, **52**: 451–4.

Enigk, K., 1950. The influence of climate on the incidence of piroplasmosis in horses, *Z. Tropenmed. Parasit.*, **2**: 401–10.

Enigk, K., Friedhoff, K. and Wirahadiredja, S., 1964. I. Susceptibility of domestic and wild ruminant to *Theileria ovis*. II. Host specificity of *Babesia motasi* and *Babesia ovis*, *Z. parasitenkd.*, **24**: 276–87, 309–18.

Erp, E. E., Gravely, S. M., Smith, R. D., Ristic, M., Osorno, B. M. and Carson, C. A., 1978. Growth of *Babesia bovis* in bovine erythrocyte cultures, *Am. J. Trop. Med. Hyg.*, **27**(5): 1061–64.

Erp, E. E., Smith, R. D., Ristic, M. and Osorno, B. M., 1980a. Continuous *in vitro* cultivation of *Babesia bovis*, *Am. J. vet. Res.*, **41**(7): 1141–2.

Erp, E. E., Smith, R. D., Ristic, M. and Osorno, B. M., 1980b. Optimization of the suspension culture method for *in vitro* cultivation of *Babesia bovis*, *Am. J. vet. Res.*, **41**(12): 2059–62.

Euzéby, J., Dubor, M., Gauthey, M. and Moreau, Y., 1980a. Immunology of *Babesia* infections. Trial (in dogs and cattle) of chemo-immunization (with imido-carb), *Bull. soc. Sci. Vét. Méd. Comp. de Lyon*, **82**: 137–42.

Euzéby, J., Moreau, Y., Chauve, C., Gevrey, J. and Gauthey, M., 1980b. Effect of imidocarb on *Babesia canis*, the causal agent of canine piroplasmosis in Europe, *Bull. acad. vét. de France*, **53**: 475–80.

Euzéby, J., Moreau, Y., Gauthey, M. and Dubor, M., 1981. Experiments on the antipiroplasmic properties of imidocarb on *Babesia divergens* and *Babesia canis*, agents of bovine and canine piroplasmosis in Europe, *Bull. soc. sci. vét. et Comparée*, **83**(3): 129–34.

Ewing, S. A., 1965a. Evaluation of methods used to detect *Babesia canis* infections in dogs, *Cornell Vet.*, **56**: 211–20.

Ewing, S. A., 1965b. Method of reproduction of *Babesia canis* in erythrocytes, *Am. J. vet. Res.*, **26**: 727–33.

Ewing, S. A. and Buckner, R. G., 1965. Manifestations of babesiosis, ehrlichiosis, and combined infections in the dog, *Am. J. vet. Res.*, **26**: 815–28.

Eyre, P., 1966. The anticholinesterase activity of the babesicidal agents quinuronium and amicarbalide and the influence of pyridine 2-aldoxime methiodide, *Res. vet. Sci.*, **7**: 161–7.

Eyre, P., 1967. Some pharmacodynamic effects of the babesicidal agents quinuronium and amicarbalide, *J. Pharm. Pharmac.*, **19**: 509–19.

Farlow, G. E., 1976. Differences in the infectivity of *Babesia* incubated in plasma and serum and the role of glucose in prolonging viability, *Int. J. Parasitol.*, **6**: 513–16.

Ferris, D. H., Todorovic, R. and Ristic, M., 1968. Significance and application of babesial and plasmodial ectoantigens to comparative medicine, *J. Am. vet. med. Ass.*, **153**(12): 1888–96.

Folkers, C., Kuil, H. and Perié, N. M., 1967. The prevalence of *Babesia bovis* (*Babesia argentina*) in the brains of slaughter cattle in northern Nigeria, *Bull. epiz. Dis. Afr.*, **15**: 359–61.

Fowler, J. L., Ruff, M. D., Fernau, R. C. and Ferguson, D. E., 1972. Biochemical parameters of dogs infected with *Babesia gibsoni, Cornell Vet.*, **62**: 412–25.

Francis, J., 1966. Resistance of zebu and other cattle to tick infestation and babesiosis with special reference to Australia: an historical review, *Br. vet. J.*, **122**: 301–7.

Frerichs, W. M. and Holbrook, A. A., 1974. Treatment of equine piroplasmosis (*B. caballi*) with imidocarb dipropionate. *Vet. Rec.*, **95**: 188–9.

Frerichs, W. M., Holbrook, A. A. and Johnson, A. J., 1969a. Equine piroplasmosis: complement-fixation titers of horses infected with *Babesia caballi, Am. J. vet. Res.*, **30**(5): 697–702.

Frerichs, W. M., Holbrook, A. A. and Johnson, A. J., 1969b. Equine piroplasmosis: production of antigens for the complement fixation test, *Am. J. vet. Res.*, **3**: 1337–41.

Friedhoff, K. T., 1969. Lichtmikroskopische Untersuchungen uber die Entwicklung von *Babesia ovis* (Piroplasmidea) in *Rhipicephalus bursa* (Ixodoidea) 1). Die Entwicklung in weiblichen Zecken nach der Repletion, *Z. Parasitenkd.*, **32**: 191–219.

Friedhoff, K. T., 1981. Morphologic aspects of *Babesia* in the tick (*Boophilus*). In *Babesiosis*, eds M. Ristic, J. P. Kreier. Academic Press (New York), pp. 143–69.

Friedhoff, K. T. and Buscher, G., 1976. Rediscovery of Koch's 'Strahlenkorper' of *Babesia bigemina, Z. Parasitenkd.*, **50**: 345–47.

Friedhoff, K. T. and Scholtyseck, E., 1969. Feinstrukturen der Merozoiten von *Babesia bigemina* im Ovar von *Boophilus microplus* und *Boophilus decoloratus, Z. Parasitenkd.*, **32**: 266–83.

Friedhoff, K. T. and Scholtyseck, E., 1970. Feinstrukturen und Entwicklung erythrocytarer studien von *Babesia bigemina, B. divergens*, und *B. ovis, Z. Parasitenkd.*, **37**: 7.

Friedhoff, K. T. and Scholtyseck, E., 1977. Fine structural identification of erythrocytic stages of *Babesia bigemina*,

B. divergens, and *B. ovis*, *Protislogica*, XIII(2): 195–204.

Friedhoff, K. T., Scholtyseck, E. and Weber, G., 1972. Die feinstruktur der differenzierten merozoiten von *Babesia ovis* in den speicheldrusen weiblicher zecken, *Z. Parasitenkd.*, **38**: 132–40.

Friedhoff, K. T. and Smith, R. D., 1981. Transmission of *Babesia* by ticks. In *Babesiosis*, eds M. Ristic, J. P. Kreier. Academic Press (New York), pp. 267–321.

Fujinaga, T., Minami, T. and Ishihara, T., 1980. Serological relationship between a large *Babesia* found in Japanese cattle and *Babesia major*, *B. bigemina* and *B. bovis*, *Res. vet. Sci.*, **29**: 230–4.

Futter, G. J. and Belonje, P. C., 1980a. Studies on feline babesiosis. 1. Historical review (*Babesia felis*), *J. S. Afr. vet. med. Ass.*, **51**: 105–6.

Futter, G. J. and Belonje, P. C., 1980b. Studies on feline babesiosis. 2. Clinical observations, *J. S. Afr. vet. med. Ass.*, **51**: 143–6.

Futter, G. J., Belonje, P. C. and Van den Berg, A., 1980c. Studies of feline babesiosis. 3. Haematological findings, *J. S. Afr. vet. med. Ass.*, **51**: 271–80.

Futter, G. J., Belonje, P. C., Van den Berg, A. and Van Rijswijk, A. W., 1981. Studies on feline babesiosis. 4. Chemical pathology; macroscopic and microscopic post mortem findings, *J. S. Afr. vet med. Ass.*, **52**: (1): 5–14.

Garnham, P. C. C., 1980. Human babesiosis: European aspects, *Trans. R. Soc. Trop. Med. Hyg.*, **74**(2): 153–5.

Gautam, O. P. and Dwivedi, S. K., 1976. Equine babesiosis: a severe outbreak in a stud farm at Hissar, *Indian vet. J.*, **53**: 546–5.

Gilles, H. M., Maegraith, B. G. and Horner Andrews, W. H., 1953. The liver in *Babesia canis* infection, *Ann. trop. Med. Parasit.*, **47**: 426–30.

Goldman, M. and Bukovsky, E., 1975. Extraction and preliminary use for diagnosis of soluble precipitating antigen from *Babesia bigemina*, *J. Protozool.*, **23**(2): 262–4.

Goldman, M. and Pipano, E., 1974. Serological response in field cattle immunised against *Babesia berbera*, *Trop. Anim. Hlth Prod.*, **6**: 123–7.

Goldman, M. and Rosenberg, A. S., 1974. Immunofluorescence studies of the small *Babesia* species of cattle from different geographical areas, *Res. vet. Sci.*, **16**: 351–4.

Gonzalez, E. F., Todorovic, R. A. and Thompson, K. C., 1976. Immunization against anaplasmosis and babesiosis. Part I. Evaluation of immunization using minimum infective doses under laboratory conditions. *Z. Tropenmed. Parasitol.*, **27**: 427–37.

Goodger, B. V., 1971. Preparation and preliminary assessment of purified antigens in the passive haemagglutination test for

bovine babesiosis, *Aust. vet. J.*, **47**: 251–6.
Goodger, B. V., 1973a. *Babesia argentina*: intraerythrocytic location of babesial antigen extracted from parasite suspensions, *Int. J. Parasitol.*, **3**: 387–91.
Goodger, B. V., 1973b. Further studies of haemagglutinating antigens of *Babesia bigemina*, *Aust. vet. J.*, **49**: 81–4.
Goodger, B. V., 1975. A cold precipitable fibrinogen complex in the plasma of cattle dying from infection with *Babesia argentina*, *Z. Parasitenkd.*, **48**: 1–7.
Goodger, B. V., 1976. *Babesia argentina*: studies on the nature of an antigen associated with infection, *Int. J. Parasitol.*, **6**: 213–16.
Goodger, B. V., 1977. *Babesia argentina*: observations on the immunogenicity of the cryofibrinogen complex, *Z. Parasitenkd.*, **53**: 47–52.
Goodger, B. V., 1978. *Babesia bovis* (=*argentina*): changes in erythrophylic and associated proteins during acute infection of splenectomized and intact calves, *Z. Parasitenkd.*, **55**: 1–8.
Goodger, B. V. and Mahoney, D. F., 1974a. Evaluation of the passive haemagglutination test for the diagnosis of *Babesia argentina* infection in cattle, *Aust. vet. J.*, **50**(6): 246–9.
Goodger, B. V. and Mahoney, D. F., 1974b. A rapid slide agglutination test for the herd diagnosis of *Babesia argentina* infection, *Aust. vet. J.*, **50**(6): 250–4.
Goodger, B. V. and Wright, I. G., 1977a. Acute *Babesia bigemina* infection: changes in fibrinogen catabolism, *Z. Parasitenkd.*, **53**: 53–61.
Goodger, B. V. and Wright, I. G., 1977b. *Babesia bovis* (*argentina*): observations of coagulation parameters, fibrinogen catabolism and fibrinolysis in intact and splenectomized cattle, *Z. Parasitenkd.*, **54**: 9–27.
Goodger, B. V. and Wright, I. G., 1979. *Babesia bovis* (*argentina*): analysis of fibrinogen-like proteins during infection, *Z. Parasitenkd.*, **60**: 211–20.
Goodger, B. V., Wright, I. G., Mahoney, D. F. and McKenna, R. V., 1978. *Babesia bovis* (*argentina*): components of the cryofibrinogen complex and their contribution to pathophysiology of infection in splenectomized calves, *Z. Parasitenkd.*, **58**: 3–13.
Goodger, B. V., Wright, I. G., Mahoney, D. F. and McKenna, R. V., 1980a. *Babesia bovis* (*argentina*): studies on the composition and the location of antigen associated with infected erythrocytes, *Int. J. Parasitol.*, **10**: 33–6.
Goodger, B. V., Wright, I. G. and Mahoney, D. F., 1980b. *Babesia bovis* (*argentina*): analysis of paracoagulation proteins in acutely infected cattle, *AJEBAK*, **58** (Pt 2): 179–88.
Goodger, B. V., Wright, I. G. and Mahoney, D. F., 1981. The use of pathophysiological reactions to assess the efficacy of the immune response to *Babesia bovis* in cattle, *Z. Parasitenkd.*, **66**: 41–8.

Gravely, S. M., Smith, R. D., Erp, E. E., Canto, G. J., Aikawa, M., Osorno, B. M. and Ristic, M., 1979. Bovine babesiosis: partial purification and characterization of blood culture-derived *Babesia bovis*, *Int. J. Parasitol.*, **9**: 591–8.

Gray, G. D. and Phillips, R. S., 1981. Use of sorbitol in the cryopreservation of *Babesia*, *Res. vet. Sci.*, **30**: 388–9.

Groves, M. G., 1968. *Babesia gibsoni* in a dog, *J. Am. vet. Med. Assn.*, **153**: 689–94.

Groves, M. G. and Dennis, G. L., 1972. *Babesia gibsoni*: field and laboratory studies of canine infections, *Exp. Parasitol.*, **31**: 153–9.

Groves, M. G. and Vanniasingham, J. A., 1970. Treatment of *Babesia gibsoni* infections with phenamidine isethionate, *Vet. Rec.*, **86**: 8–10.

Hadani, A., 1981. *In vitro* development of *Babesia* and *Theileria* parasites in organs and tissues of ticks. In *Babesiosis*, eds M. Ristic, J. P. Kreier. Academic Press (New York), pp. 225–66.

Haigh, A. J. B. and Hagan, D. H., 1974. Evaluation of imidocarb dihydrochloride against redwater disease in cattle in Eire, *Vet. Rec.*, **94**: 56–9.

Hall, W. T. K., 1960. The immunity of calves to *Babesia argentina* infection, *Aust. vet. J.*, **36**: 361–6.

Hall, W. T. K., 1963. The immunity of calves to tick-transmitted *Babesia argentina* infection, *Aust. vet. J.*, **39**: 386–9.

Hall, W. T. K., Tammemagi, L. and Johnston, L. A. Y., 1968. Bovine babesiosis: the immunity of calves to *Babesia bigemina* infection, *Aust. vet. J.*, **44**: 259–64.

Hashemi-Fesharki, R., 1975. Studies on imidocarb dihydrochloride in experimental *Babesia bigemina* infection in calves, *Br. vet. J.*, **131**: 666–72.

Hashemi-Fesharki, R., 1977. Studies on imidocarb dihydrochloride in experimental *Babesia ovis* infection in splenectomized lambs, *Br. vet. J.*, **133**: 609–14.

Hashemi-Fesharki, R. and Uilenberg, G., 1981. *Babesia crassa* n.sp. (Sporozoa, Babesiidae) of domestic sheep in Iran, *Vet. Quarterly*, **3**(1): 1–8.

Henning, 1956. Redwater, Texas fever, rooi-water. In *Animal Diseases in South Africa, Being an Account of the Infectious Diseases of Domestic Animals*. Central News Agency (South Africa), pp. 537–61.

Hildebrandt, P. K., 1981. The organ and vascular pathology of babesiosis. In *Babesiosis*, eds M. Ristic, J. P. Kreier. Academic Press (New York), pp. 439–73.

Hill, M. W. M. and Bolton, B. L., 1966. Canine *Babesia* in Queensland, *Aust. vet. J.*, **42**: 84–6.

Hoare, C. A., 1980. Comparative aspects of human babesiosis, *Trans. R. Soc. Trop. Med. Hyg.*, **74**(2): 143–8.

Holbrook, A. A., Anthony, D. W. and Johnson, A. J., 1968a.

Observations on the development of *Babesia caballi* (Nuttall) in the tropical horse tick *Dermacentor nitens* Neumann, *J. Protozool.*, **15**(2): 391–6.

Holbrook, A. A., Johnson, A. J. and Madden, P. A., 1968b. Equine piroplasmosis: intraerythrocytic development of *Babesia caballi* (Nuttall) and *Babesia equi* (Laveran), *Am. J. vet. Res.*, **29**(2): 297–303.

Holz, J., 1960. *Babesia berbera* infection in cattle in Indonesia, *Berl. Münch. Tierarztl. Wschr.*, **73**: 448–51.

Hooshmand-Rad, P., 1974. Blood protozoan diseases of ruminants, *Bull. Off. int. Epiz.*, **81**(9–10): 779–92.

Hourrigan, J. L., 1976. Bovine piroplasmosis – cattle fever. Tick control and eradication, *Bull. Off. int. Epiz.*, **85**(5–6): 685–94.

Howard, R. J. and Rodwell, B. J., 1979. *Babesia rodhaini, Babesia bovis,* and *Babesia bigemina*: analysis and sorting of red cells from infected mouse or calf blood by flow fluorimetry using 33258 Hoechst, *Exp. Parasitol.*, **48**: 421–31.

Howard, R. J., Rodwell, B. J., Smith, P. M., Callow, L. L. and Mitchell, G. F., 1980. Comparison of the surface proteins and glycoproteins on erythrocytes of calves before and during infection with *Babesia bovis. J. Protozool.*, **27**(2): 241–7.

Hoyte, H. M. D., 1961. Initial development of infections with *Babesia bigemina, J. Protozool.*, **8**: 462–6.

Hoyte, H. M. D., 1965. Further observations on the initial development of infections with *Babesia bigemina, J. Protozool.*, **12**: 83–5.

Hoyte, H. M. D., 1971. Differential diagnosis of *Babesia argentina* and *Babesia bigemina* infections in cattle using thin blood smears and brain smears, *Aust. vet. J.*, **47**: 248–50.

Hussein, H. S., 1976. *Babesia hylomysci* in mice: preference for erythrocytes of a particular age-group and pathogenesis of the anaemia, *Z. Parasitenkd.*, **50**: 103–8.

Hussein, H. S., 1977a. The pathology of *Babesia hylomysci* infection in mice. I. Clinical signs and liver lesion, *J. Comp. Pathol.*, **87**: 161–7.

Hussein, H. S., 1977b. The pathology of *Babesia hylomysci* infection in mice. II. Kidney lesion, *J. Comp. Pathol.*, **87**: 169–75.

Hussein, H. S., 1979. *Babesia microti* and *Babesia hylomysci*: spleen and phagocytosis in infected mice, *Exp. Parasitol.*, **47**: 1–12.

Irvin, A. D., 1973. *Babesia thomasi* from rock hyraces in Kenya, *J. Parasitol.*, **59**(1): 203–4.

Irvin, A. D., Brocklesby, D. W. and Purnell, R. E., 1979a. Radiation and isotopic techniques in the study and control of piroplasms of cattle: a review, *Vet. Parasitol.*, **5**: 17–28.

Irvin, A. D. and Young, E. R., 1977. Possible *in vitro* test for screening drugs for activity against *Babesia* and other blood protozoa, *Nature*, **269**: 407–9.

Irvin, A. D. and Young, E. R., 1978. Comparison of the effect of drugs on *Babesia in vitro* and *in vivo, Res. vet. Sci.*, **27**: 211–14.

Irvin, A. D. and Young, E. R., 1979a. Introduction and multiplication of bovine *Babesia* in human cells, *Res. vet. Sci.*, **27**: 241–3.

Irvin, A. D. and Young, E. R., 1979b. Further studies on the uptake of titrated nuclei acid precursors by *Babesia* spp. of cattle and mice, *Int. J. Parasitol.*, **9**: 109–14.

Irvin, A. D., Young, E. R. and Adams, P. J. V., 1979b. The effects of irradiation on *Babesia* maintained *in vitro, Res. vet. Sci.*, **27**: 200–4.

Irvin, A. D., Young, E. R. and Osborn, G. D., 1978a. Attempts to infect T-lymphocyte-deficient mice with *Babesia* species of cattle, *Res. vet. Sci.*, **25**: 245–6.

Irvin, A. D., Young, E. R. and Purnell, R. E., 1978b. The *in vitro* uptake of tritiated nucleic acid precursors by *Babesia* spp. of cattle and mice, *Int. J. Parasitol.*, **8**: 19–24.

Itard, J., 1964. Porcine piroplasmosis: natural *Piroplasma trautmanni* Knut and du Toit, 1921, infection (Central African Republic), *Red. Elev. Med. vét. Pays trop.*, **17**(2): 221–31.

Jack, R. M. and Ward., P. A., 1981. Mechanisms of entry of *Plasmodia* and *Babesia* into red cells. In *Babesiosis*, eds M. Ristic, J. P. Kreier. Academic Press (New York), pp. 445–57.

James, M. A., Kuttler, K. L., Levy, M. G. and Ristic, M., 1981a. Antibody kinetics in response to vaccination against *Babesia bovis, Am. J. vet. Res.*, **42**(11): 1999–2001.

James, M. A., Levy, M. G. and Ristic, M., 1981b. Isolation and partial characterization of culture-derived soluble *Babesia bovis* antigens, *Infect. Immun.*, **31**(1): 358–61.

Johnston, L. A. Y., 1967. Epidemiology of bovine babesiosis in northern Queensland, *Aust. vet. J.*, **43**: 427–31.

Johnston, L. A. Y., 1968. The incidence of clinical babesiosis in cattle in Queensland, *Aust. vet. J.*, **44**: 265–7.

Johnston, L. A. Y., Leatch, G. and Jones, P. N., 1978. The duration of latent infection and functional immunity in Droughtmaster and Hereford cattle following natural infection with *Babesia argentina* and *Babesia bigemina, Aust. vet. J.*, **54**: 14–18.

Johnston, L. A. Y., Pearson, R. D. and Leatch, G., 1973. Evaluation of an indirect fluorescent antibody test for detecting *Babesia argentina* infection in cattle, *Aust. vet. J.*, **49**: 373–7.

Johnston, L. A. Y. and Tammemagi, L., 1969. Bovine babesiosis: duration of latent infection and immunity to *Babesia argentina, Aust. vet. J.*, **45**: 445–9.

Johnston, L. A. Y., Trueman, K. F. and Pearson, R. D., 1977. Bovine babesiosis: comparison of fluorescent antibody and Giemsa staining in post-mortem diagnosis of infection, *Aust. vet. J.*, **53**: 222–6.

Joyner, L. P., 1981. The chemotherapy of protozoal infections of veterinary importance. *J. Protozool.*, **28**(1): 17–19.

Joyner, L. P. and Brocklesby, D. W., 1973. Chemotherapy of anaplasmosis, babesiasis, and theileriasis, *Adv. Pharmacol. Chemo.*, **11**: 321–55.

Joyner, L. P. and Davies, S. F. M., 1967. Acquired resistance to *Babesia divergens* in experimental calves, *J. Protozool.*, **14**(2): 260–2.

Joyner, L. P. and Donnelly, J., 1979. The epidemiology of babesial infections. In *Advances in Parasitology*, eds W. H. R. Lumsden, R. Muller, J. R. Baker. Academic Press (London), vol. 17, pp. 115–40.

Joyner, L. P., Donnelly, J., Payne, R. and Brocklesby, D. W., 1972. The indirect fluorescent antibody test for the differentiation of infections with *Babesia divergens* or *Babesia major*, *Res. vet. Sci.*, **13**(6): 515–18.

Kemron, A., Hadani, A., Egyed, M., Pipano, E. and Neuman, M., 1964. Studies on bovine piroplasmosis caused by *Babesia bigemina*. III. The relationship between the number of parasites in the inoculum and the severity of the response, *Refuah Vet.*, **21**: 112–16.

Kirkham, W. W., 1969. The treatment of equine babesiosis, *J. Am. vet. med. Ass.*, **155**(55): 457–60.

Klinger, Y. and Ben-Yossef, H., 1972. A case of intra-uterine infection with *Babesiella berbera*, *Refuah Vet.*, **29**(2): 73–4.

Knight, D. J., 1981. *Babesia rodhaini* and *Plasmodium berghei*. A highly active series of chlorophenoxyalkoxy-substituted diamino-dihydrotriazines against experimental infections in mice, *Ann. trop. Med. Parasitol.*, **75**(1): 1–6.

Knowles, R. C., Mathis, R. M., Bryant, J. E. and Willers, K. H., 1966. Equine piroplasmosis, *J. Am. vet. med. Ass.*, **148**(4): 407–10.

Kuttler, K. L., Adams, L. G. and Todorovic, R. A., 1977. Comparisons of the complement-fixation and indirect fluorescent antibody reactions in the detection of bovine babesiasis, *Am. J. vet. Res.*, **38**(2): 153–6.

Kuttler, K. L., Graham, O. H. and Trevino, J. L., 1975. The effect of imidocarb treatment on *Babesia* in the bovine and the tick *Boophilus microplus*, *Res. vet. Sci.*, **18**: 198–200.

Kuttler, K. L. and Johnson, L. M., 1980. Immunization of cattle with a *Babesia bigemina* antigen in Freund's complete adjuvant, *Am. J. vet. Res.*, **41**(4): 536–8.

Kuttler, K. L., Levy, M. G., James, M. A. and Ristic, M., 1982. Efficacy of a nonviable culture-derived *Babesia bovis* vaccine, *Am. J. vet. Res.*, **43**(2): 281–4.

Langreth, S. G., 1976. Feeding mechanisms in extracellular *Babesia microti* and *Plasmodium lophurae*, *J. Protozool.*, **23**(2): 215–23.

Latif, B. M. A., Said, M. S. and Ali, S. R., 1979. Effect of age on the immune response of cattle experimentally infected with *Babesia bigemina*, *Vet. Parasitol.*, **5**: 307–14.

Leeflang, P., 1972. Diagnosis of *Babesia argentina* infections in cattle using brain smears, *Aust. vet. J.*, **48**(2): 72.

Leeflang, P., 1977. Tick-borne diseases of domestic animals in northern Nigeria. I. Historical review, 1923–1966, *Trop. Anim. Hlth Prod.*, **9**: 147–52.

Leeflang, P. and Ilemobade, A. A., 1977. Tick-borne diseases of domestic animals in northern Nigeria. II. Research summary, 1966 to 1976, *Trop. Anim. Hlth Prod.*, **9**: 211–18.

Leeflang, P. and Perié, N. M., 1972. Comparative immunofluorescent studies on 4 *Babesia* species of cattle, *Res. vet. Sci.*, **13**: 342–6.

Levine, N. D., Corliss, J. O., Cox, F. E. G., Deroux, G., Grain, J., Honigberg, B. M., Leedale, G. F., Loeblich, A. R. III, Lom, J., Lynn, D., Merinfield, E. G., Page, F. C., Poijansky, G., Sprague, V., Vavra, J. and Wallace, F. G., 1980. A newly revised classification of protozoa. *J. Protozool.*, **27**(1): 37–58.

Levy, M. G., Erp, E. and Ristic, M., 1981. Cultivation of *Babesia*. In *Babesiosis*, eds M. Ristic, J. P. Kreier. Academic Press (New York), pp. 207–23.

Levy, M. G. and Ristic, M., 1980. *Babesia bovis*: continuous cultivation in a microaerophilous stationary phase culture, *Science*, **207**: 1218–20.

Lewis, D., 1979. Infection of the Mongolian gerbil with the cattle piroplasm *Babesia divergens*, *Nature*, **278**: 170–1.

Lewis, D., Francis, L. M. A., Purnell, R. E. and Young, E. R., 1981. The effect of treatment with imidocarb dipropionate on the course of *Babesia divergens* infections in splenectomized calves, and on their subsequent immunity to homologous challenge, *J. Comp. Path.*, **91**: 285–92.

Lewis, D., Purnell, R. E. and Brocklesby, D. W., 1978. Immunization of cattle against *Babesia* species using irradiated piroplasms, *Parasitology*, **77**: xliv.

Lewis, D., Purnell, R. E. and Brocklesby, D. W., 1979. *Babesia divergens*: immunisation of splenectomised calves using irradiated piroplasms, *Res. vet. Sci.*, **26**: 220–2.

Lewis, D., Purnell, R. E. and Brocklesby, D. W., 1980a. *Babesia divergens*: protection of intact calves against heterologous challenge by the injection of irradiated piroplasms, *Vet. Parasitol.*, **6**: 297–303.

Lewis, D., Purnell, R. E. and Young, E. R., 1980b. The effects of Imizol on *Babesia divergens* infections in splenectomized calves, *Parasitology*, **81**: vi–vii.

Lewis, D. and Williams, H., 1979. Infection of the Mongolian gerbil with the cattle piroplasm *Babesia divergens*, *Nature* **278** (5700): 170–1.

Littlejohn, A. and Walker, E. M., 1979. Some aspects of the

epidemiology of equine babesiosis, *J. S. Afr. vet. med. Ass.*, **50**: 308–10.

Lohr, K. F., 1973. Susceptibility of non-splenectomized and splenectomized Sahiwal cattle to experimental *Babesia bigemina* infection; *Zbl. Vet. Med.*, **B20**: 52–6.

Lohr, K. F., 1978. Immunization of splenectomized calves against *Babesia bigemina* infection by use of a dead vaccine – a preliminary report. In *Tick-borne Diseases and Their Vectors*, ed. J. K. H. Wilde. Lewis Reprints (Tonbridge), pp. 398–404.

Lohr, K. F., Ashford, W. A., Higgs, J., Meyer, H. and Otieno, P. S., 1977. Haematological reactions to experimental *Babesia bigemina* infection in splenectomised and non-splenectomised cattle, *Zbl. Vet. Med.*, **B24**: 508–16.

Lohr, K. F., Otieno, P. S. and Gacanga, W., 1975. Susceptibility of Boran cattle to experimental infections with *Anaplasma marginale* and *Babesia bigemina*, *Zbl. Vet. Med.*, **B22**: 842–9.

Lohr, K. F. and Ross, J. P. J., 1969. A capillary tube-agglutination test for the detection of *Babesia bigemina* antibodies, *Z. Tropenmed. Parasit.*, **20**: 287–92.

Lopez, V. G. and Todorovic, R. A., 1978. Rapid latex agglutination (RLA) test for the diagnosis of *Babesia argentina*, *Vet. Parasitol.*, **4**: 1–9.

Lucas, J. M. S., 1960. The chemotherapy of experimental babesiasis in mice and splenectomized calves, *Res. vet. Sci.*, **1**: 218–25.

Ludford, C. G., 1969. Fluorescent antibody staining of four *Babesia* species, *Exp. Parasitol.*, **24**: 327–35.

Ludford, C. G., Hall, W. T. K., Sulzer, A. J. and Wilson, M., 1972. *Babesia argentina*, *Plasmodium vivax* and *P. falciparum*: antigenic cross-reactions, *Exp. Parasitol.*, **32**: 317–26.

Madden, P. A. and Holbrook, A. A., 1968. Equine piroplasmosis: indirect fluorescent antibody test for *Babesia caballi*, *Am. J. vet. Res.*, **29**: 117–23.

Mahoney, D. F., 1962. Bovine babesiosis: diagnosis of infection by a complement fixation test. *Aust. vet. J.*, **38**: 48–52.

Mahoney, D. F., 1964. Bovine babesiosis: an assessment of the significance of complement fixing antibody based upon experimental infection, *Aust. vet. J.*, **40**: 369–75.

Mahoney, D. F., 1966. Circulating antigens in cattle infected with *Babesia bigemina* or *B. argentina*, *Nature*, **211**: 422.

Mahoney, D. F., 1967a. Bovine babesiosis: preparation and assessment of complement fixing antigens, *Exp. Parasitol.*, **20**: 232–41.

Mahoney, D. F., 1967b. Bovine babesiosis: the passive immunization of calves against *Babesia argentina* with special reference to the role of complement fixing antibodies, *Exp. Parasitol.*, **20**: 119–24.

Mahoney, D. F., 1967c. Bovine babesiosis: the immunization of cattle with killed *Babesia argentina*, *Exp. Parasitol.*, **20**: 125–9.

Mahoney, D. F., 1969. Bovine babesiasis: a study of factors concerned in transmission, *Ann. trop. Med. Parasitol.*, **63**(1): 1–14.
Mahoney, D. F., 1972. Immunity response to hemoprotozoa. II. *Babesia* spp. In *Immunity to Animal Parasites*, ed. E. J. L. Soulsby. Academic Press (New York), pp. 301–41.
Mahoney, D. F., 1974. The application of epizootiological principles in the control of babesiosis in cattle. *Bull. Off. int. Epiz.*, **81**(1–2) 123–38.
Mahoney, D. F., 1979. *Babesia* of domestic animals. In *Parasitic Protozoa*, ed. J. P. Kreier. Academic Press (New York), vol. IV, pp. 1–52.
Mahoney, D. F., 1981. Immunization against blood-derived antigens of *Babesia*. In *Babesiosis*, eds M. Ristic, J. P. Kreier. Academic Press (New York), pp. 475–83.
Mahoney, D. F. and Goodger, B. V., 1969. *Babesia argentina*: serum changes in infected calves, *Exp. Parasitol.*, **24**: 375–82.
Mahoney, D. F. and Goodger, B. V., 1972. *Babesia argentina*: immunogenicity of plasma from infected animals, *Exp. Parasitol.*, **32**: 71–85.
Mahoney, D. F. and Goodger B. V., 1981. The isolation of *Babesia* parasites and their products from blood. In *Babesiosis*, eds M. Ristic, J. P. Kreier. Academic Press (New York), pp. 323–35.
Mahoney, D. F., Goodger, B. V., Kerr, J. D. and Wright, I. G., 1979b. The immune response of cattle to *Babesia bovis* (syn. *B. argentina*). Studies on the nature and specificity of protection, *Int. J. Parasitol.*, **9**: 297–306.
Mahoney, D. F., Goodger, B. V. and Wright, I. G., 1980. Changes in the haemolytic activity of serum complement during acute *Babesia bovis* infection in cattle, *Z. Parasitenkd.*, **62**: 39–45.
Mahoney, D. F. and Mirre, G. B., 1971. Bovine babesiasis: estimation of infection rates in the tick vector *Boophilus microplus* (Canestrini), *Ann. trop. Med. Parasitol.*, **65**: 309–17.
Mahoney, D. F. and Mirre, G. B., 1974. *Babesia argentina*: the infection of splenectomized calves with extracts of larval ticks (*Boophilus microplus*), *Res. vet. Sci.*, **16**: 112–14.
Mahoney, D. F. and Mirre, G. B., 1979. Note on the transmission of *Babesia bovis* (syn. *B. argentina*) by the one-host tick *Boophilus microplus*, *Res. vet. Sci.*, **26**: 253–4.
Mahoney, D. F. and Ross, D. R., 1972. Epizootiological factors in the control of bovine babesiosis, *Aust. vet. J.*, **48**: 292–8.
Mahoney, D. F. and Saal, J. R., 1961. Bovine babesiosis: thick blood films for the detection of parasitemia, *Aust. vet. J.*, **37**: 44–7.
Mahoney, D. F. and Wright, I. G., 1976. *Babesia argentina*: immunization of cattle with a killed antigen against infection with a heterologous strain, *Vet. Parasitol.*, **2**: 273–82.
Mahoney, D. F., Wright, I. G. and Goodger, B. V., 1979a. Immunity in cattle to *Babesia bovis* after single infections with parasites of various origin. *Aust. vet. J.*, **55**: 10–12.
Mahoney, D. F., Wright, I. G. and Goodger, B. V., 1981b. Bovine

babesiosis: the immunization of cattle with fractions of erythrocytes infected with *Babesia bovis* (syn. *B. argentina*), *Vet. Immunol. Immunopathol.*, **2**: 145–56.

Mahoney, D. F., Wright, I. G., Goodger, B. V., Mirre, G. B., Sutherst, R. W. and Utech, K. B. W., 1981a. The transmission of *Babesia bovis* in herds of European and Zebu × European cattle infested with the tick, *Boophilus microplus*, *Aust. vet. J.*, **57**: 461–9.

Mahoney, D. F., Wright, I. G. and Ketterer, P. J., 1973a. *Babesia argentina*: the infectivity and immunogenicity of irradiated blood parasites for splenectomized calves, *Int. J. Parasitol.*, **3**: 209–17.

Mahoney, D. F., Wright, I. G. and Mirre, G. B., 1973b. Bovine babesiosis: the persistence of immunity to *Babesia argentina* and *B. bigemina* in calves (*Bos taurus*) after naturally acquired infection, *Ann. trop. Med. Parasit.*, **67**(2): 197–203.

Malherbe, W. D., 1956. The manifestations and diagnosis of *Babesia* infections. *Ann. N.Y. Acad. Sci.*, **64**: 128–46.

Malherbe, W. D., 1965a. Clinico-pathological studies of *Babesia canis* infection in dogs. I. The influence of the infection in bromosulphalein retention in the blood, *J. S. Afr. vet med. Ass.*, **36**(1): 25–30.

Malherbe, W. D., 1965b. Clinico-pathological studies of *Babesia canis* infection in dogs. II. The influence of the infection on plasma transaminase activity, *J. S. Afr. vet. med. Ass.*, **36**(2): 173–6.

Malherbe, W. D., 1965c. Clinico-pathological studies of *Babesia canis* infection in dogs. III. The influence of the infection on plasma alkaline phosphatase activity, *J. S. Afr. vet. med. Ass.*, **36**(2): 179–82.

Malherbe, W. D., 1965d. Clinico-pathological studies of *Babesia canis* infection in dogs. IV. The effect on bilirubin metabolism. *J. S. Afr. vet. met. Ass.*, **36**(4): 569–73.

Malherbe, W. D., 1966. Clinico-pathological studies of *Babesia canis* infection in dogs. V. The influence of the infection on kidney function, *J. S. Afr. vet. med. Ass.*, **37**(3): 261–4.

Malhotra, D. V., Gautam, O. P. and Banerjee, D. P., 1979. Note on chemotherapeutic trials against *Babesia-equi* infection in donkeys, *Indian J. Anim. Sci*, **49**(1): 75–7.

McCosker, P. J., 1981. The global importance of babesiosis (*Babesia bovis, Babesia bigemina, Boophilus* ticks). In *Babesiosis*, eds M. Ristic, J. P. Kreier. Academic Press (New York), pp. 1–24.

Mehlhorn, H., Schein, E. and Voigt, W. P., 1980. Light and electron microscopic study on developmental stages of *Babesia canis* within the gut of the tick *Dermacentor reticulatus*, *J. Parasitol.*, **66**: 220–8.

Mehlitz, D. and Ehret, R., 1974. Serological investigations on the prevalence of anaplasmosis and piroplasmosis in cattle in Botswana, *Z. Tropenmed. Parasit.*, **25**: 3–10.

Merino, N., Garcia, G. and Villanueva, J., 1980. Post mortem detection of healthy cattle carrying *Babesia argentina* by histological examination of brain impression smears, *Revista de Salud Animal*, **2**: 79–89.

Merino, N., Rodriguez, O. N., Torroella, E. and Renaud, J., 1976. Histopatologica comparada del higado en la Anaplasmosis y la Babesiosis Bovina, *Rvta. Cub. Cienc. Vet.*, **7**: 9–14.

Minami, T., Yamabe, K., Hayashi, S. and Ishihara, T., 1979. Serological relationship of a Japanese *Babesia* species and *Babesia bigemina* by the complement fixation and capillary-tube agglutination tests, *Vet. Parasitol.*, **5**: 29–38.

Moltmann, U. G., Mehlhorn, H. and Friedhoff, K. T., 1982. Electron microscopic study on the development of *Babesia ovis* (Piroplasmia) in the salivary glands of the vector tick *Rhipicephalus bursa*, *Acta trop.*, **39**: 29–40.

Moore, D. J., 1979. Therapeutic implications of *Babesia canis* infection in dogs, *J. S. Afr. vet med. Ass.*, **50**(4): 346–352.

Moore, D. J., and Williams, M. C., 1979. Disseminated intravascular coagulation: a complication of *Babesia canis* infection in the dog, *J. S. Afr. vet. med. Ass.*, **50**(4): 265–75.

Moore, J. A. and Kuntz, R. E., 1981. *Babesia microti* infections in nonhuman primates, *J. Parasitol.*, **67**(3): 454–56.

Morzaria, S. P., Bland, P. and Brocklesby, D. W., 1978. Ultrastructure of *Babesia major* vermicules from the tick *Haemaphysalis punctata* as demonstrated by negative staining, *Z. Parasitenkd.*, **55**: 119–26.

Morzaria, S. P. and Brocklesby, D. W., 1977. A differential diagnostic criterion for *Babesia major* and *Babesia bigemina* vermicules from tick haemolymph, *Z. Parasitenkd.*, **52**: 241–43.

Morzaria, S. P., Young, A. S. and Hudson, E. B., 1977. *Babesia bigemina* in Kenya: experimental transmission by *Boophilus decoloratus* and the production of tick-derived stabilates, *Parasitology*, **74**: 291–8.

Naudé, T. W., Basson, P. A. and Pienaar, J. G., 1970. Experimental diamidine poisoning due to commonly used babecides, *Onderstepoort J. vet. Res.*, **37**(3): 173–84.

Neitz, W. O., 1956. Classification, transmission, and biology, of piroplasms of domestic animals, *Ann. N.Y. Acad. Sci.*, **64**: 56–111.

Newton, L. G. and O'Sullivan, P. J., 1969. Chemoprophylaxis in *Babesia argentina* infection in cattle, *Aust. vet. J.*, **45**: 404–7.

Osorno, E. M., 1978. *Babesia* infections in Mexico (horse, cattle, sheep, dog, man). *Veterinaria (Mexico)*, **9**: 203–18.

Paget, G. E., Alcock, S. J. and Ryley, J. F., 1962. The pathology of *Babesia rodhaini* infections in mice, *J. Pathol. Bacteriol.*, **84**: 218–20.

Pandey, N. N. and Mishra, S. S., 1977a. Studies on the pathological changes in *Babesia bigemina* infection in indigenous cow calves, *Zbl. Vet. Med.* **B24**: 522–8.

Pandey, N. N. and Mishra, S. S., 1977b. Studies on the haematological

changes and blood glucose level in *Babesia bigemina* infection in indigenous cow calves, *Indian vet. J.*, **54**: 880–3.
Pandey, N. N. and Mishra, S. S., 1978a. Studies on the clinical symptoms and percentage of parasitaemia in experimental *Babesia bigemina* infection in cow calves, *Indian vet. J.*, **55**: 139–43.
Pandey, N. N. and Mishra, S. S., 1978b. Comparative efficacy of Berenil, Acriflavin and Sulfadimethoxine in *Babesia bigemina* infection in indigenous cow calves, *Indian vet. J.*, **55**: 144–8.
Parker, R., 1973. A direct counting technique for estimating high parasitaemias in infections of *Babesia argentina, Babesia bigemina* and *Plasmodium berghei, Ann. trop. Med. Parasitol.*, **67**(4): 387–90.
Pierce, A. E., 1956. Protozoan diseases transmitted by the cattle tick, *Aust. vet. J.*, **32**: 210–15.
Piercy, S. E., 1947. Hyper-acute canine *Babesia* (tick fever), *Vet. Rec.*, **59**(44): 612–13.
Pipano, E., 1978. Immunization of cattle with *Babesia bigemina* vaccine stored in the frozen state. In *Tick-borne Diseases and their Vectors*, Proc. Int. Conf., Edinburgh 1976, ed. J. K. H. Wilde. Centre for Tropical Veterinary Medicine (Edinburgh, UK), pp. 389–90.
Pipano, E., Jeruham, I. and Frank, M., 1979. Pentamidine in chemoimmunisation of cattle against *Babesia bigemina* infection, *Trop. Anim. Hlth Prod.*, **11**: 13–16.
Pipano, E., Weisman, Y., Raz, A. and Klinger, I., 1972. Immunity to *Babesia bigemina* in calves after successful babesicidal treatment of a previous infection. *Refuah Vet.*, **29**(1): 1–8.
Potgieter, F. T. and Els, H. J., 1976. Light and electron microscopic observations on the development of small merozoites of *Babesia bovis* in *Boophilus microplus* larvae, *Onderstepoort J. vet. Res.*, **43**(3): 123–8.
Potgieter, F. T. and Els, H. J., 1977a. The fine structure of intraerythrocytic stages of *Babesia bigemina, Onderstepoort J. vet. Res.*, **44**(3): 157–67.
Potgieter, F. T. and Els, H. J., 1977b. Light and electron microscopic observations on the development of *Babesia bigemina* in larvae, nymphae, and non-replete females of *Boophilus decoloratus, Onderstepoort J. vet. Res.*, **44**(4): 213–31.
Potgieter, F. T. and Els, H. J., 1979. An electron microscopic study of intra-erythrocytic stages of *Babesia bovis* in the brain capillaries of infected splenectomized calves, *Onderstepoort J. vet. Res.* **46**: 41–9.
Potgieter, F. T., Els, H. J. and van Vuuren, A. S., 1976. The fine structure of merozoites of *Babesia bovis* in the gut epithelium of *Boophilus microplus, Onderstepoort J. vet. Res.*, **43**(1): 1–10.
Purchase, H. S., 1947. Cerebral babesiosis in dogs, *Vet. Rec.*, **59**: 269–70.
Purnell, R. E., 1977a. Bovine babesiosis in the European community, *Vet. Sci. Comm.*, **1**: 289–96.
Purnell, R. E., 1977b. *Babesia divergens* in splenectomized calves – titration of infective dose, *Res. vet. Sci.*, **23**: 124.
Purnell, R. E., 1977c. *Babesia divergens* in splenectomized calves –

immunogenicity of lyophilised plasma from an infected animal, *Res. vet. Sci.*, **23**: 255.

Purnell, R. E., 1979. Tick-borne diseases of cattle – a case for pragmatism? *Vet. Rev.*, **25**: 56–62.

Purnell, R. E., 1981. Babesiosis in various hosts. In *Babesiosis*, eds M. Ristic, J. P. Kreier. Academic Press (New York), pp. 25–63.

Purnell, R. E. and Brocklesby, D. W., 1977. *Babesia divergens* in splenectomised calves: immunogenicity of lyophilised plasma from an infected animal, *Res. vet. Sci.*, **23**: 255–6.

Purnell, R. E., Brocklesby, D. W., Hendry, D. J., Stark, A. J. and Young, E. R., 1977a. *Babesia divergens* in splenectomised calves: titration of the infective dose, *Res. vet. Sci.*, **23**: 124–5.

Purnell, R. E., Brocklesby, D. W., Kitchenham, B. A. and Young, E. R., 1976. A statistical comparison of the behaviour of five British isolates of *Babesia divergens* in splenectomized calves, *J. Comp. Path.*, **86**: 609–14.

Purnell, R. E., Brocklesby, D. W. and Stark, A. J., 1978a. Protection of cattle against *Babesia major* by the inoculation of irradiated piroplasms, *Res. vet. Sci.*, **3**: 388–90.

Purnell, R. E., Brocklesby, D. W., Stark, A. J. and Young, E. R., 1978b. Reactions of splenectomized calves to the inoculation of blood containing *Babesia divergens* from an infected animal during its reaction and carrier phases, *J. Comp. Path.*, **88**: 419–23.

Purnell, R. E. and Lewis, D., 1981. *Babesia divergens*: combination of dead and live parasites in an irradiated vaccine, *Res. vet. Sci.*, **30**: 18–21.

Purnell, R. E., Lewis, D. and Brocklesby, D. W., 1979a. *Babesia major*: protection of intact calves against homologous challenge by the injection of irradiated piroplasms, *Int. J. Parasitol.*, **9**: 69–71.

Purnell, R. E., Lewis, D. and Brocklesby, D. W., 1980a. Bovine babesiosis. Protection of cattle by the inoculation of irradiated piroplasms, *Isotope and Radiation Research on Animal Diseases and Their Vectors*, proceedings of a symposium, Vienna, 7–11 May 1979, jointly organized by the IAEA and FAO. International Atomic Energy Agency (Vienna, Austria), IAEA-SM-240/14, pp. 77–94.

Purnell, R. E., Lewis, D., Brocklesby, D. W. and Taylor, S. M., 1979b. Bovine babesiosis: steps towards an irradiated vaccine. *J. S. Afr. vet. med. Ass.*, **50**(4): 339–44.

Purnell, R. E., Lewis, D. and Young, E. R., 1980b. Investigations on the prophylactic effect of treatment with imidocarb dipropionate on *Babesia divergens* infections of splenectomised calves, *Br. vet. J.*, **136**: 452–6.

Purnell, R. E., Lewis, D. and Young, E. R., 1981a. Quinuronium sulphate for the treatment of *Babesia divergens* infections of splenectomised calves, *Vet. Rec.*, **108**: 538–9.

Purnell, R. E., Rae, M. C. and Deuk, S. M., 1981b. Efficacy of imidocarb dipropionate and primaquine phosphate in the prevention of tick-borne disease in imported Hereford heifers in

South Korea, *Trop. Anim. Hlth Prod.*, **13**: 123–7.

Purnell, R. E., Stark, A. J., Lewis, D. and Brocklesby, D. W., 1979c. Titration of *Babesia major* piroplasms in intact calves, *Br. vet. J.*, **135**: 44–9.

Purnell, R. E., Young, E. R., Brocklesby, D. W. and Hendry, D. J., 1977b. The haematology of experimentally-induced *B. divergens* and *E. phagocytophilia* infection in splenectomised calves, *Vet. Rec.*, **100**: 4–6.

Purvis, A. C., 1977. Immunodepression in *Babesia microti* infections, *Parasitology*, **75**: 197–205.

Rao, K. S., Sharma, L. D., Sabir, M. and Bhattacharyya, N. K., 1980. Studies on some pharmacological actions of imidocarb dipropionate, *Indian vet. J.*, **57**: 283–7.

Ray, H. N. and Idnani, J. A., 1947. Observations on the forms of *Babesia gibsoni* (Patton) in the dog; with a note on the systematic position of the parasite, *Indian J. vet. Sci.*, **13**: 267–73.

Retief, G. P., 1964. A comparison of equine piroplasmosis in South Africa and the United States, *J. Am. vet. med. Ass.*, **145**: 912–16.

Reube, U., 1954. Symptoms and pathology of *Babesia* infection in dogs, *Z. Tropenmed. Parasit.*, **5**: 451–69.

Riek, R. F., 1964. The life cycle of *Babesia bigemina* (Smith and Colborne, 1893) in the tick vector *Boophilus microplus* (Canestrini), *Aust. J. Agric. Res.*, **15**: 802–21.

Riek, R. F., 1966. The life cycle of *Babesia argentina* (Lignieres, 1903) (Sporozoa: Piroplasmidea) in the tick vector *Boophilus microplus* (Canestrini), *Aust. J. Agric. Res.*, **17**: 247–54.

Ristic, M., 1976. Immunologic systems and protection in infections caused by intracellular blood protista, *Vet. Parasitol.*, **2**: 31–47.

Ristic, M., Conroy, J. D., Siwe, S., Healy, G. R., Smith, A. R. and Huxsoll, D. L., 1971. *Babesia* species isolated from a woman with clinical babesiosis, *Am. J. trop. Med. Hyg.*, **20**(1): 14–22.

Ristic, M., Kakoma, I. and Smith, R. D., 1981. Characterization of *Babesia* antigens derived from cell cultures and ticks. In *Babesiosis*, eds M. Ristic, J. P. Kreier. Academic Press (New York), pp. 337–80.

Ristic, M. and Kreier, J. P. (eds), 1981. *Babesiosis*. Int. Conf. on Malaria and Babesiosis (1979, Mexico City, Mex.). Academic Press (New York), vol. XV, 589 pp.

Ristic, M. and Lewis, G. E. Jr, 1979. *Babesia* in man and wild and laboratory-adapted mammals. In *Parasitic Protozoa*, ed. J. P. Kreier. Academic Press, (New York), vol. IV, pp. 53–76.

Ristic, M., Oppermann, J., Sibinovic, S. and Phillips, T. N., 1964. Equine piroplasmosis – a mixed strain of *Piroplasma caballi* and *Piroplasma equi* isolated in Florida and studied by the fluorescent antibody technique, *Amer. J. vet. Res.*, **25**(104): 15–23.

Ristic, M. and Sibinovic, S., 1964. Equine babesiosis: diagnosis by a precipitation in gel and by a one-step fluorescent antibody-inhibition test, *Am. J. vet. Res.*, **25**: 1519–26.

Roberts, E. D., Morehouse, L. G., Gainer, J. H. and McDaniel, H. A., 1962. Equine piroplasmosis, *J. Am. vet. med. Ass.*, **141**(11): 1323–9.

Roberts, J. A., Kerr, J. D. and Tracey-Patte, P., 1972. Function of the spleen in controlling infections of *Babesia rodhaini* in mice, *Int. J. Parasitol.*, **2**: 217–26.

Roby, T. O., Anthony, D. W., Holbrook, A. A. and Thornton, C. W. Jr, 1964. The hereditary transmission of *Babesia caballi* in the tropical horse tick, *Dermacentor nitens* Neumann, *Am. J. vet. Res.*, **25**: 494–9.

Rodwell, B. J. and Howard, R. J., 1981. A fluorescent method for counting *Babesia*, *Anaplasma*, *Plasmodium*, and *Trypanosoma* following DNA staining with 33258 Hoechst (Bisbenzimide), *Ann. trop. Med. Parasit.*, **75**(2): 123–9.

Rodwell, B. J., Timms, P. and Parker, R. J., 1980. Collection and sterilization of large volumes of bovine serum and its use in vaccines against bovine babesiosis and anaplasmosis, *AJEBAK*, **58** (Pt 2): 143–7.

Rogers, R. J., 1971a. The acquired resistance to *Babesia argentina* of cattle exposed to light infestation with cattle tick (*Boophilus microplus*), *Aust. vet. J.*, **47**: 237–41.

Rogers, R. J., 1971b. Observations on the pathology of *Babesia argentina* infections in cattle, *Aust. vet. J.*, 242–7.

Rokey, N. W. and Russell, R., 1961. Canine babesiasis (piroplasmosis) – a case report, *J. Am. vet. med. Ass.*, **138**(12): 635–8.

Ronald, N. C. and Cruz, D., 1981. Transmission of *Babesia bovis*, using undifferentiated embryonic cells from *Boophilus microplus* tick eggs, *Am. J. vet. Res.*, **42**(3): 544–5.

Ross, J. P. J. and Lohr, K. F., 1968. Serological diagnosis of *Babesia bigemina* infection in cattle by the indirect fluorescent antibody test, *Res. vet. Sci.*, **9**: 557–62.

Ross, J. P. J. and Lohr, K. F., 1970. Transfer and persistence of antibodies to *Babesia bigemina* and *Anaplasma marginale* acquired via the colostrum, *Z. Tropenmed. Parasit.*, **21**: 401–11.

Ross, D. R. and Mahoney, D. F., 1974. Bovine babesiasis: computer simulation of *Babesia argentina* parasite rates in *Bos taurus* cattle, *Ann. trop. Med. Parasit.*, **68**: 385–92.

Roychoudhury, G. K. and Gautam, O. P., 1979. Experimental studies on the pathogenicity of *Babesia bigemina* in buffalo calves, *Trop. Anim. Hlth Prod.*, **11**: 91–3.

Roychoudhury, G. K., Kalita, C. C. and Roychoudhury, R. K., 1976. Babesiosis in exotic calves, *Indian vet. J.*, **53**: 364–7.

Roy-Smith, F., 1971. The prophylactic effects of imidocarb against *Babesia argentina* and *Babesia bigemina* infections of cattle, *Aust. vet. J.*, **47**: 418–20.

Rudolph, W., Correa, J., Zurita, L. and Manley, W., 1975. Equine piroplasmosis: leukocytic response to *Babesia equi* (Laveran, 1901) infection in Chile, *Br. vet. J.*, **131**: 601–9.

Rudzinska, M. A., 1976. Ultrastructure of intra-erythrocytic *Babesia microti* with emphasis on the feeding mechanism, *J. Protozool.*, **23**(2): 224–33.

Rudzinska, M. A., 1981. Morphologic aspects of host–cell parasite relationships in babesiosis. In *Babesiosis*, eds M. Ristic, J. P. Kreier. Academic Press (New York), pp. 87–141.

Ruebush, M. J. and Hanson, W. L., 1980a. Transfer of immunity to *Babesia microti* of human origin using T lymphocytes in mice, *Cell. Immunol.*, **52**: 255–65.

Ruebush, M. J. and Hanson, W. L., 1980b. Thymus dependence of resistance to infection with *Babesia microti* of human origin in mice, *Am. J. Trop. Med. Hyg.*, **29**(4): 507–15.

Ruebush, T. K. II, 1980. Human babesiosis in North America, *Trans. R. Soc. Trop. Med. Hyg.*, **74**(2): 149–52.

Ruebush, T. K. II, Collins, W. E., Healy, G. R. and Warren, M., 1979. Experimental *Babesia microti* infections in non-splenectomized *Macaca mulatta*, *J. Parasitol.*, **65**(1): 144–6.

Ruebush, T. K. II, Piesman, J., Collins, W. E., Spielman, A. and Warren, M., 1981. Tick transmission of *Babesia microti* to rhesus monkeys (*Macaca mulatta*), *Am. J. Trop. Med. Hyg.*, **30**(3): 555–9.

Ruff, M. D., Fowler, J. L., Matsuda, K. and Fernau, R. C., 1971. *Babesia gibsoni*: influence of infection on serum enzymes of dogs, *Southeast Asian J. trop. Med. Public Hlth.*, **2**(3): 297–307.

Saal, J. R., 1964. Giemsa stain for the diagnosis of bovine babesiosis. II. Changes in erythrocytes infected with *Babesia bigemina* and *B. argentina*, *J. Protozool.*, **11**: 582–5.

Schein, E., Mehlhorn, H. and Voigt, W. P., 1979. Electron microscopical studies on the development of *Babesia canis* (Sporozoa) in the salivary glands of the vector tick *Dermacentor reticulatus*, *Acta trop.*, **36**: 229–41.

Schindler, R. and Dennig, H. K., 1962. Demonstration of *Babesia* antibodies by the complement fixation reaction, *Z. Tropenmed. Parasit.*, **13**: 480–8.

Schindler, R., Wokatsch, R. and Schroder, G., 1966. Immunity and serologic reaction against *Babesia canis* in dogs after immunization with a soluble antigen, *Z. Tropenmed. Parasit.*, **17**: 226–40.

Schroeder, W. F., Cox, H. W. and Ristic, M., 1966. Anaemia, parasitaemia, erythrophagocytosis, and haemagglutinins in *Babesia rodhaini* infection, *Ann. trop. Med. Parasit.*, **60**: 31–8.

Seneviratna, P., 1965a. Studies of *Babesia gibsoni* infections of dogs in Ceylon, *Ceylon vet. J.*, **13**(1): 1–6.

Seneviratna, P., 1965b. The pathology of *Babesia gibsoni* (Patton, 1910) infection in the dog, *Ceylon vet. J.*, **13**(4): 107–10.

Sibinovic, K. H., MacLeod, R., Ristic, M., Sibinovic, S. and Cox, H. W., 1967a. A study of some of the physical, chemical and serologic properties of antigens from sera of horses, dogs, and rats with acute babesiosis, *J. Parasitol.*, **53**(5): 919–23.

Sibinovic, K. H., Milar, R., Ristic, M. and Cox, H. W., 1969a. *In vivo* and *in vitro* effects of serum antigens of babesial infection and their antibodies on parasitized and normal erythrocytes, *Ann. trop. Med. Parasit.*, **63**(3): 327–36.

Sibinovic, K. H., Ristic, M., Sibinovic, S. and Phillips, T. N., 1965. Equine babesiosis: isolation and serologic characterization of a blood serum antigen from acutely infected horses, *Am. J. vet. Res.*, **26**: 147–53.

Sibinovic, K. H., Sibinovic, S., Ristic, M. and Cox, H. W., 1967b. Immunogenic properties of babesial serum antigens, *J. Parasitol.*, **53**(6): 1121–9.

Sibinovic, S., Sibinovic, K. H. and Ristic, M., 1969b. Equine babesiosis: diagnosis by bentonite agglutination and passive hemagglutination tests, *Am. J. vet. Res.*, **30**(5): 691–5.

Simpson, C. F., 1970. Electron microscopic comparison of *Babesia* spp. and hepatic changes in ponies and mice, *Am. J. vet. Res.*, **31**: 1763–8.

Simpson, C. F., 1974. Phagocytosis of *Babesia canis* by neutrophils in the peripheral circulation, *Am. J. vet. Res.*, **35**(5): 701–4.

Simpson, C. F., Bild, C. E. and Stoliker, H. E., 1963. Electron microscopy of canine and equine *Babesia*, *Am. J. vet. Res.*, **24**: 408–14.

Simpson, C. F., Kirkham, W. W. and Kling, J. M., 1967. Comparative morphologic features of *Babesia caballi* and *Babesia equi*, *Am. J. vet. Res.*, **28**: 1693–7.

Simpson, C. F. and Neal, F. C., 1980. Ultrastructure of *Babesia equi* in ponies treated with imidocarb, *Am. J. vet. Res.*, **41**(2): 267–71.

Simpson, C. F., Taylor, W. J. and Kitchen, H., 1980. Crystalline inclusions in erythrocytes parasitized with *Babesia equi* following treatment of ponies with imidocarb, *Am. J. vet. Res.*, **41**(8): 1336–40.

Singh, B., Banerjee, D. P. and Gautam, O. P., 1980. Comparative efficacy of diminazene diaceturate and imidocarb dipropionate against *Babesia equi* infection in donkeys, *Vet. Parasitol.*, **7**: 173–9.

Singh, B., Banerjee, D. P., Gautam, O. P. and Malhotra, D. V., 1978. A capillary tube agglutination test for equine babesiosis, *Indian vet. J.*, **55**: 677–9.

Singh, B., Gautam, O. P. and Banerjee, D. P., 1981. Immunization of donkeys against *Babesia equi* infection usine killed vaccine, *Vet. Parasitol.*, **8**: 133–6.

Sippel, W. S., Cooperrider, D. E., Gainer, J. H., Allen, R. W., Mouw, J. E. B. and Teigland, M. B., 1962. Equine piroplasmosis in the United States, *J. Am. vet. med. Ass.*, **141**(6): 694–8.

Smith, R. D., Carpenter, J., Cabrera, A., Gravely, S. M., Erp, E. E., Osorno, M. and Ristic, M., 1979. Bovine babesiosis: vaccination against tick-borne challenge exposure with culture-derived *Babesia bovis* immunogens, *Am. J. vet. Res.*, **40**(12): 1678–82.

Smith, R. D., James, M. A., Ristic, M., Aikawa, M. and Vega y Murguia, C. A., 1981. Bovine babesiosis: protection of cattle with culture-derived soluble *Babesia bovis* antigen, *Science*, **212**: 335–8.

Smith, R. D., Molinar, E., Larios, F., Monroy, J., Trigo, F. and Ristic, M., 1980. Bovine babesiosis: pathogenicity and heterologous species immunity of tick-borne *Babesia bovis* and *B. bigemina* infections, *Am. J. vet. Res.*, **41**: 1957–65.

Smith, R. D., Osorno, B. M., Brener, J., Rosa, R. De La and Ristic, M., 1978. Bovine babesiosis: severity and reproducibility of *Babesia bovis* infections induced by *Boophilus microplus* under laboratory conditions, *Res. vet. Sci.*, **24**: 287–92.

Smith, R. D. and Ristic, M., 1981. Immunization against bovine babesiosis with culture-derived antigens. In *Babesiosis*, eds M. Ristic, J. P. Kreier. Academic Press (New York), pp. 485–507.

Stewart, N. P., 1978. Differences in the life cycles between a vaccine strain and an unmodified strain of *Babesia bovis* (Babes, 1889) in the tick *Boophilus microplus* (Canestrini), *J. Protozool.*, **25**(4): 497–501.

Taylor, R. J. and McHardy, N., 1979. Preliminary observations on the combined use of imidocarb and *Babesia* blood vaccine in cattle, *J. S. Afr. vet. med. Ass.*, **50**: 326–9.

Taylor, S. M., Kenny, J., Purnell, R. E. and Lewis, D., 1980. Exposure of cattle immunised against redwater to tick-induced challenged in the field: challenge by a heterologous strain of *Babesia divergens*, *Vet. Rec.*, **106**: 385–7.

Taylor, W. M., Bryant, J. E., Anderson, J. B. and Willers, K. H., 1969. Equine piroplasmosis in the United States – a review, *J. Am. vet. med. Ass.*, **155**(6): 915–19.

Tchernomoretz, I., 1943. Blocking of the brain capillaries by parasitized red blood cells in *Babesiella berbera* infections in cattle, *Ann. trop. Med. Parasit.*, **37**: 77–9.

Tella, A. and Maegraith, B. G., 1965. Physiopathological changes in primary acute blood-transmitted *Malaria* and *Babesia* infections. I. Observations on parasites and blood-cells in rhesus monkeys, mice, rats, and puppies, *Ann. trop. Med. Parasit.*, **59**: 135–46.

Teutsch, S. M., Etkind, P., Burwell, E. L., Sato, K., Dana, M. M., Fleishman, P. R. and Juranek, D. D., 1980. Babesiosis in post-splenectomy hosts, *Am. J. Trop. Med. Hyg.*, **29**(5): 738–41.

Thompson, G. D., Medellin, J. A., Trevino, G. S. and Wagner, G. G., 1980. Bovine babesiosis in northern Mexico, *Trop. Anim. Hlth Prod.*, **12**: 132–6.

Thompson, K. C., 1976. A technique to establish a laboratory colony of *Boophilus microplus* infected with *Babesia bigemina*, *Vet. Parasitol.*, **2**: 223–9.

Thompson, K. C., Todorovic, R. A. and Hidalgo, R. J., 1977. Antigenic variation of *Babesia bigemina*, *Res. vet. Sci.*, **23**: 51–4.

Thompson, K. C., Todorovic, R. A. and Hidalgo, R. J., 1978a. The immune responses to antigenic variants of *Babesia bigemina* in the bovine, *Res. vet. Sci.*, **24**: 234–7.

Thompson, K. C., Todorovic, R. A., Mateus, G. and Adams, L. G., 1978b. Methods to improve the health of cattle in the tropics: immunisation and chemoprophylaxis against haemoparasitic infections, *Trop. Anim. Hlth Prod.*, **10**: 75–81.

Thoongsuwan, S. and Cox, H. W., 1973. Antigenic variants of the haemosporidian parasite, *Babesia rodhaini*, selected by *in vitro* treatment with immune globulin, *Ann. trop. Med. Parasit.*, **67**: 373–85.

Thoongsuwan, S., Cox, H. W. and Patrick, R. A., 1978. Immunoconglutinin associated with nonspecific acquired resistance in malaria, babesiosis, and other anemia-inducing infections, *J. Parasitol.*, **64**(6): 1050–6.

Thoongsuwan, S., Cox, H. W. and Rickman, W. J., 1979. Antibody to fibrinogen/fibrin products (Anti-F) in malaria, babesiosis, and trypanosomiasis of rodents, *J. Parasitol.*, **65**(3): 426–9.

Timms, P., 1980. Short term cultivation of *Babesia* species, *Res. vet. Sci.*, **29**: 102–4.

Timms, P. and Murphy, G. M., 1980. Erythrocytic Na^+ and K^+ changes during *Babesia bigemina* infection in cattle, *Res. vet. Sci.*, **29**: 367–9.

Todorovic, R. A., 1973. Bovine babesiosis: its diagnosis and control, *Proc. VII Panamerican Congress Vet. Med. Zootechnics, Bogota, Colombia*, pp. 23–8, 38–9.

Todorovic, R. A., 1974. Bovine babesiasis: its diagnosis and control, *Am. J. vet. Res.*, **35**(8): 1045–52.

Todorovic, R. A., 1975a. Serologic diagnosis of babesiosis: a review, *Trop. Anim. Hlth Prod.*, **7**: 1–14.

Todorovic, R. A., 1975b. The premunition of adult cattle against babesiosis and anaplasmosis in Colombia, South America, *Trop. Anim. Hlth Prod.*, **7**(3): 125.

Todorovic, R. A., 1976a. Comparison of indirect fluorescent antibody (IFA) with complement fixation (CF) tests for diagnosis of *Babesia* spp infections in Colombian cattle, *Z. Tropenmed. Parasit.*, **27**(2): 169–81.

Todorovic, R., 1976b. Bovine babesiosis in Colombia, *Vet. Parasitol.*, **2**: 97–109.

Todorovic, R. A. and Carson, C. A., 1981. Methods for measuring the immunological response to *Babesia*. In *Babesiosis*, eds M. Ristic, J. P. Kreier. Academic Press (New York), pp. 381–410.

Todorovic, R., Ferris, D. and Ristic, M., 1967. Roles of the spleen in acute plasmodial and babesial infections in rats, *Exp. Parasitol.*, **21**: 354–72.

Todorovic, R. and Garcia, R., 1978. Comparison of dried blood on filter paper and serum techniques for the diagnosis of bovine babesiosis utilizing the indirect fluorescent antibody (IFA) test, *Z. Tropenmed. Parasit.*, **29**: 88–94.

Todorovic, R. A., Gonzalez, E. F. and Adams, L. G., 1973a. Bovine babesiosis: sterile immunity to *Babesia bigemina* and *Babesia argentina* infections, *Trop. Anim. Hlth Prod.*, **5**: 234–45.

Todorovic, R. A., Gonzalez, E. F. and Adams, L. G., 1974a. Bovine babesiosis: co-infectious immunity to *Babesia bigemina* and *Babesia argentina* infections, *Exp. Parasitol.*, **35**: 351–8.

Todorovic, R. A., Gonzalez, E. F. and Adams, L. G., 1975a. *Babesia bigemina, Babesia argentina*, and *Anaplasma marginale*: co-infectious immunity in bovines, *Exp. Parasitol.*, **37**: 179–92.

Todorovic, R. A. and Kuttler, K. L., 1974. A babesiosis card agglutination test, *Am. J. vet. Res.*, **35**(10): 1347–50.

Todorovic, R. A. and Long, R. F., 1976. Comparison of indirect fluorescent antibody (IFA) with complement fixation (CF) tests for diagnosis of *Babesia* spp. infections in Colombian cattle, *Z. Tropenmed. Parasit.*, **27**(2): 169–82.

Todorovic, R. A., Lopez, L. A., Lopez, A. G. and Gonzalez, E. F., 1974b. Bovine babesiosis and anaplasmosis: control by premunition and chemoprophylaxis, *Exp. Parasitol.*, **35**: 675–8.

Todorovic, R. A., Lopez, L. A., Lopez, A. G. and Gonzalez, E. F., 1975b. Bovine babesiosis and anaplasmosis: control by premunition and chemoprophylaxis, *Exp. Parasitol.*, **37**: 92–104.

Todorovic, R. A. and Tellez, E. H., 1974. The premunition of adult cattle against babesiosis and anaplasmosis in Colombia, South America, *Trop. Anim. Hlth Prod.*, **7**: 125–31.

Todorovic, R. A., Vizcaino, O. G., Gonzalez, E. F. and Adams, L. G., 1973b. Chemoprophylaxis (Imidocarb) against *Babesia bigemina* and *Babesia argentina* infections, *Am. J. vet. Res.*, **34**(9): 1153–61.

Trees, A. J., 1978. Indirect fluorescent antibody levels in experimental *Babesia divergens* infections of cattle, *Res. vet. Sci.*, **24**: 126–8.

Trueman, K. F. and Blight, G. W., 1978. The effect of age on resistance of cattle to *Babesia bovis*, *Aust. vet. J.*, **54**: 301–5.

Uilenberg, G., 1965. Pathogenesis of cerebral forms of *Babesia* infections in cattle in Madagascar, *Rev. Elev. Méd. vét. Pays trop.*, **18**(1): 83–8.

Uilenberg, G., 1970. Notes on babesiosis and anaplasmosis of cattle in Madagascar. V. A. Immunity and premunition. B. Epidemiology, *Rev. Elev. Méd. vét. Pays trop.*, **23**(4): 439–54.

Van den Bossche, H., 1978. Chemotherapy of parasitic infections, *Nature*. **273**: 626–30.

van Heerden, J., 1980. The transmission of *Babesia canis* to the wild dog *Lycaon pictus* (Temminck) and black-backed jackal *Canis mesomelas* (Schreber), *J. S. Afr. vet. med. Ass.*, **51**: 119–20.

Ward, P. A. and Jack, R. M., 1981. The entry process of *Babesia* merozoites into red cells, *Am. J. Pathol.*, **102**(1): 109–13.

Watkins, R. G., 1962. A concentration and staining technique for diagnosing equine piroplasmosis, *J. Am. vet. med. Ass.*, **141**(11): 1330–2.

Weber, G., 1980. Ultrastructures and cytochemistry pellicle and apical complexes of kinetes of *Babesia bigemina* and *Babesia ovis* in hemolymph and ovary of ticks, *J. Protozool.*, **27**(1): 59–71.

Weber, G. and Friedhoff, K., 1971. Lichtmikroskopische Untersuchungen uber die Entwicklung von *Babesia ovis* (Piroplasmidea) in *Rhipicephalus bursa* (Ixodoidea). II. Cytochemische Untersuchungen an differenzierten Merozoiten in den Speicheldrusen weiblicher Zecken, *Z. Parasitenkd.*, **35**: 218–33.

Weber, G. and Friedhoff, K., 1979. Electron microscopic detection of initial and some subsequent developmental stages of *Babesia bigemina* in salivary glands of ticks, *Z. Parasitenkd.*, **58**: 191–4.

Weiland, G. and Kratzer, I., 1979. Serologic investigation into canine piroplasmosis by means of indirect fluorescent antibody test and enzyme-linked immunosorbent assay, *Berl. Münch. Tierarztl. Wschr.*, **92**: 398–400.

Weiland, G., Reif, L., Schmidt, M. and Boch, J., 1980. Serodiagnostic investigations on *Babesia divergens* infections in cattle, *Berl. Münch. Tierarztl. Wschr.*, **93**: 261–4.

Weisman, J., Goldman, M. and Pipano, E., 1974. Passive transfer of maternal antibodies against *Babesia* to newborn calves, *J. Protozool.*, **21**(3): 466.

Winter, H., 1967. Diagnosis of babesiasis by fluorescence microscopy, *Res. vet. Sci.*, **8**: 170–4.

Wright, I. G., 1972a. An electron microscopic study of intravascular agglutination in the cerebral cortex due to *Babesia argentina* infection, *Int. J. Parasitol.*, **2**: 209–15.

Wright, I. G., 1972b. Studies on the pathogenesis of *Babesia argentina* and *Babesia bigemina* infections in splenectomised calves, *Z. Parasitenkd.*, **39**: 85 102.

Wright, I. G., 1973a. Plasma kallikrein levels in acute *Babesia argentina* infections in splenectomised and intact calves, *Z. Parasitenkd.*, **41**: 269–80.

Wright, I. G., 1973b. Ultrastructural changes in *Babesia argentina*-infected erythrocytes in kidney capillaries, *J. Parasitol.*, **59**(4): 735–6.

Wright, I. G., 1973c. Observation on the haematology of experimentally induced *Babesia argentina* and *B. bigemina* infections in splenectomised calves, *Res. vet. Sci.*, **14**: 29–34.

Wright, I. G., 1973d. Osmotic fragility of erythrocytes in acute *Babesia argentina* and *Babesia bigemina* infections in splenectomised *Bos taurus* calves, *Res. vet. Sci.*, **15**: 299–305.

Wright, I. G., 1974. The activation of kallikrein in acute *Babesia argentina* infections of splenectomised calves, *Z. Parasitenkd.*, **43**: 271–8.

Wright, I. G., 1975. The probable role of *Babesia argentina* esterase in the *in vitro* activation of plasma prekallikrein, *Vet. Parasitol.*, **1**: 91–6.

Wright, I. G., 1977. Kinin, kininogen, and kininase levels during acute *Babesia bovis* (= *B. argentina*) infection of cattle, *Br. J. Pharmac.*, **61**: 567–72.

Wright, I. G., 1978. Biogenic amine levels in acute *Babesia bovis* infected cattle, *Vet. Parasitol.*, **4**: 393–8.

Wright, I. G., 1981. Biochemical characteristics of *Babesia* and physiochemical reactions in the host. In *Babesiosis*, eds M. Ristic, J. P. Kreier. Academic Press (New York), pp. 171–205.

Wright, I. G. and Goodger, B. V., 1973. Proteolytic enzyme activity in the intra-erythrocytic parasites *Babesia argentina* and *Babesia bigemina*, *Z. Parasitenkd.*, **42**: 213–20.

Wright, I. G. and Goodger, B. V., 1977. Acute *Babesia bigemina* infection: changes in coagulation and kallikrein parameters, *Z. Parasitenkd.*, **53**: 63–73.

Wright, I. G. and Goodger, B. V., 1979. Acute *Babesia bovis* infections: renal involvement in the hypotensive syndrome, *Z.Parasitenkd.*, **59**: 115–19.

Wright, I. G., Goodger, B. V. and Mahoney, D. F., 1980a. The irradiation of *Babesia bovis*. 1. The difference in pathogenicity between irradiated and non-irradiated populations, *Z. Parasitenkd.*, **63**: 47–57.

Wright, I. G., Goodger, B. V. and Mahoney, D. F., 1981a. Virulent and avirulent strains of *Babesia bovis*: the relationship between parasite protease content and pathophysiological effect of the strain, *J. Protozool.*, **28**(1): 118–20.

Wright, I. G., Goodger, B. V., McKenna, R. V. and Mahoney, D. F., 1979. Acute *Babesia bovis* infection: a study of the vascular lesions in kidney and lung, *Z. Parasitenkd.*, **60**: 19–27.

Wright, I. G. and Kerr, J. D., 1974. The preferential invasion of young erythrocytes in acute *Babesia bigemina* infections of splenectomised calves, *Z. Parasitenkd.*, **43**: 63–9.

Wright, I. G. and Kerr, J. D., 1975. Effect of Trasylol on packed cell volume and plasma kallikrein activation in acute *Babesia argentina* infection of splenectomised calves, *Z. Parasitenkd.*, **46**: 189–94.

Wright, I. G. and Kerr, J. D., 1977. Hypotension in acute *Babesia bovis* (= *B. argentina*) infections of splenectomized calves, *J. Comp. Path.*, **87**: 531–7.

Wright, I. G. and Mahoney, D. F., 1974. The activation of kallikrein in acute *Babesia argentina* infections of splenectomised calves, *Z. Parasitenkd.*, **43**: 271–8.

Wright, I. G., Mahoney, D. F. and Goodger, B. V., 1980b. Serum carboxypeptidase B levels during acute and mild *Babesia bovis* and acute *Babesia bigemina* infections of cattle, *Z. Parasitenkd.*, **63**: 191–4.

Wright, I. G., Mahoney, D. F., Mirre, G. B., Goodger, B. V., and

Kerr, J. D., 1982. The irradiation of *Babesia bovis*. II. The immunogenicity of irradiated blood parasites for intact cattle and splenectomised calves, *Vet. Immunol. Immunopath.*, **3**: 591–601.

Wright, I. G., McKenna, R. V. and Goodger, B. V., 1981b. Acute *Babesia bovis* infections: plasma creatine kinase, lactate dehydrogenase and creatinine levels and associated muscle damage, *Z. Parasitenkd.*, **64**: 297–302.

Wright, I. G., Mirre, G. B., Mahoney, D. F. and Goodger, B. V., 1983. Failure of *Boophilus microplus* to transmit irradiated *Babesia bovis*, *Res. vet. Sci.*, **34**: 124–5.

Young, A. S. and Purnell, R. E., 1973. Observations on *Babesia equi* in the salivary glands of *Rhipicephalus evertsi*, *Bull. epiz. Dis. Afr.*, **21**: 377–83.

Zlotnik, I., 1953. Cerebral piroplasmosis in cattle, *Vet. Rec.*, **65**(40): 642–3.

Zwart, D. and Brocklesby, D. W., 1979. Babesiosis: non-specific resistance, immunological factors and pathogenesis. In *Advances in Parasitology*, eds W. H. R. Lumsden, R. Muller, J. R. Baker. Academic Press (London), vol. 17, pp. 49–113.

Chapter

2

Theileriosis

CONTENTS

INTRODUCTION

Theilerioses are a group of tick-borne diseases of cattle, water buffalo, sheep, goats, and occasionally, of wild ruminants caused by species of protozoa in the genus *Theileria*. In the various species of hosts the *Theileria* can cause either asymptomatic infection or disease syndromes which may be acute, chronic, or mild. The theilerioses of greatest importance in veterinary medicine are the diseases caused in cattle by *Theileria parva, T. lawrencei, T. annulata,* and *T. mutans*. In sheep and goats the infections are caused by *T. hirci* and *T. ovis*, while a variety of *Theileria* and *Theileria*-like organisms cause infections in several African members of the family Bovidae, particularly the buffalo (*Syncerus caffer*) and eland (*Taurotragus oryx*); these wild species may play a role in the epizootiology of the disease in cattle.

In Africa the most important form of theileriosis is caused by *Theileria parva* and is commonly referred to as East Coast fever (ECF). It is now known that ECF is not a single disease entity with a uniform etiological agent but a complex of syndromes caused by antigenically similar organisms; in the host, some of these organisms display behavior characteristic of *T. lawrencei*, while others resemble *T. parva*, or are of an intermediate type. Some strains of *T. lawrencei* can be transformed by tick passage through cattle into organisms which behave like typical *T. parva*. However, for epidemiological reasons it is still convenient to retain *T. lawrencei* as a separate species indicating its buffalo origin.

East Coast fever is a usually fatal disease of cattle caused by *T. parva* or *T. lawrencei*, and characterized by pyrexia, malaise, anorexia, lacrimation, digestive disturbances, emaciation, dyspnea, swelling of the superficial and internal lymph nodes, enlargement of the spleen and liver, lymphoid infiltration of the kidneys, and ulceration of the abomasum; recovered animals have solid and sterile immunity. *Theileria annulata* infection results in peracute, acute, subacute, or chronic disease of cattle characterized by clinical signs and lesions comparable to those observed in *T. parva* infections with additional occurrence of anemia, icterus, and hemoglobinuria. Theileriosis caused by *T. mutans* is a mild form of disease characterized by pyrexia, anorexia, and varying degrees of anemia.

Ovine and caprine theilerioses caused by *T. hirci* are either acute, subacute, or chronic diseases characterized by dominant clinical signs and lesions comparable to those observed in *T. parva* infections of cattle with the additional occurrence of icterus and transitory hemoglobinuria. *Theileria ovis* causes a mild disease in sheep and goats which is rarely characterized by pyrexia, swelling of superficial lymph nodes, and mild anemia.

Literature

Our knowledge of the theilerioses has been summarized in a number of good reviews and symposia. Neitz (1957) presented an exhaustive review of the literature pertaining to various forms of theileriosis including historical accounts of laboratory research and fieldwork, classification, speciation, geographic distribution, comparison of clinical signs, pathology and chemotherapy. It forms the most comprehensive body of information available on the topic. The author emphasized the differences among the various types of theilerioses and presented theilerioses as a complex of diseases with the diverse syndromes having many similarities but also important distinctions. Wilde reviewed studies which were undertaken subsequent to the work summarized by Neitz (1957) and particularly referred to the work which was undertaken in two research laboratories in Kenya (Wilde *et al.* 1966; Wilde 1967). In a 1977 article, Purnell provided a detailed description of the individual experiments conducted in the Kenyan investigations, and focused on the development of technology, tick transmission, level of infection in ticks, tick infectivity, parasite development in the vertebrate host, vaccination procedures, and serological diagnosis. The techniques that were developed were critical to the study of the complex life cycle of *Theileria* and demonstrated the effects of various factors on the tick-organism relationship with respect to infectivity and virulence. The review was based largely on the work carried out by the UNDP–FAO Immunological Research on Tick-borne Diseases and Tick Control Project which became operational at the laboratories of the East African Veterinary Research Organization (Kenya) in 1967. This work was assessed by Brocklesby (1978) and included the following major areas of research: collection of parasites from ticks, preservation of triturated tick supernates, chemoprophylaxis, tissue culture, serology, establishment of *T. parva* in laboratory animals, cell fusion, and chemotherapy. The more recent review by Barnett (1978) was intended to augment and update the previously published major review articles, and emphasized the classification of various *Theileria* = isolates and the host-parasite interaction in disease. Theileriosis in cattle caused by *T. mutans* was reviewed by Saidu (1982).

ETIOLOGY

Classification

Theileria organisms have the following classification:

Phylum/Apicomplexa
Class/Sporozoa
Subclass/Piroplasma
Order/Piroplasmida
Family/Theileriidae
Genus/*Theileria*

There are two other genera, *Haematoxenus* and *Cytauxzoon,* which have been recognized, although not universally accepted, in infections involving *Theileria*-like organisms, particularly in wild game in Africa.

Literature

The question of speciation of various isolates of *Theileria* is as yet unresolved. Classification of an organism as a specific species depends on epizootiological, pathogenetic, behavioral, morphological, immunological, and biochemical properties. As more information becomes available, and as new techniques are used in the identification of *Theileria,* so the methods used in differentiation of species change, resulting in a continued reevaluation of species classification (Neitz and Jansen 1956). Of particular promise has been the recent definition of isoenzyme patterns in various isolates.

The most recent classification of *Theileria* was presented by Levine *et al.* (1980). These authors recognize two genera, *Theileria* and *Haematoxenus,* and synonymized the third genus *Cytauxzoon* with *Theileria*. The genus *Cytauxzoon* has not been found in domestic animals but commonly occurs in wild ungulates in Africa; while the piroplasms are indistinguishable from those of *Theileria* in cattle, the site and development of schizonts are different. Although available knowledge of the life cycle and host specificity has indicated that *Cytauxzoon* is a separate entity, its classification has not yet been clearly established and debate continues over the issue of whether it should be included in the genus *Theileria* (Brocklesby 1978).

The genus *Haematoxenus* was created to include intraerythrocytic organisms in cattle in Madagascar. These entities, given the name *Haematoxenus veliferus,* can be differentiated from those of *Theileria* species by the presence of a delicate rectangular veil on the side of the Giemsa-stained erythrocytic piroplasms. Also, antigens prepared from the piroplasms of *H. veliferus* did not cross-react serologically either with antisera from *T. parva* or *T. mutans* infected animals. The species *H. separatus* was described in sheep (Uilenberg and

Schreuder 1976b). Two splenectomized sheep in Kenya were found to be infected with piroplasms identical to *T. ovis* and *H. separatus* (Young and Mchinja 1977). Further examination of piroplasms of *H. veliferus* revealed that the veil had a crystal-like structure and stained with benzidine like hemoglobin. Since comparable veil-like structures have been observed in other *Theileria* species, it was proposed that the genus *Haematoxenus* was synonymous with the genus *Theileria* (Vorstenbosch *et al.* 1978). Differentiation of species within a genera is more of an art than a science and is based on a number of biological properties such as pathogenicity, pathogenesis, species of vector, and to some extent antigenic similarities. The morphological similarity among the members of the genera *Theileria* makes their differentiation difficult. Morphological characteristics may be helpful in certain stages of life-cycle infection, but are not acceptable as a definition of speciation. The current terminology used is related to three biological races of bovine *Theileria*: *T. parva, T. annulata,* and *T. mutans*. Within the groups there are biological and immunological differences which have led researchers to grant some members of the group species status. However, on an immunological basis alone it is difficult to know where racial or strain differences stop and species differences begin; hence, the question of antigenic structure in systematic classification is problematic (Barnett 1978).

Brocklesby (1978) was of the opinion that there are four species of *Theileria* which include *T. parva, T. annulata, T. mutans,* and *T. sergenti.* He reviewed the classification of other species of *Theileria* and pointed out that there were observable differences between *T. sergenti* and *T. annulata* on the basis of serology and xenodiagnosis. The author concluded that transmission of the different species of *Theileria* was related to passage through different species of ticks, i.e. *Rhipicephalus* species transmitted *T. parva, Haemaphysalis* species transmitted *T. sergenti, Hyalomma* species transmitted *T. annulata,* and *Amblyomma* species transmitted *T. mutans.* In South Africa theileriosis was attributed to four species or subspecies of *Theileria* on the basis of serological tests and epidemiology (Lawrence 1979).

In Africa the importance of *T. lawrencei* in the etiology of theileriosis has been reemphasized in the more recent research. It was considered a separate species on the basis of cross-immunity studies, although the validity of this method of speciation was not generally recognized. The development of the parasite in the salivary glands of ticks is similar to that of *T. parva* but the infection rate is lower. The level of parasitosis in the lymphoid system of the mammalian host is also lower than that found in *T. parva* infections, with the microschizonts and piroplasms being absent or scanty (Purnell 1977). Passage of *T. lawrencei* through cattle demonstrated the lability of the bovine *Theileria* species in Africa: increase in the piroplasm, microschizont, and macroschizont populations, and an increase in the average size of macroschizonts resulted in a parasitosis indistinguishable from that caused by *T. parva* (Barnett and Brocklesby 1966a). Similar observations were made after an organism which was believed to be

T. mutans was passed through *R. appendiculatus*; the resultant changes rendered the organism indistinguishable from *T. parva*. In order to overcome some difficulties in taxonomy it was proposed that there may be several strains of a single species which exhibit different biological host–parasite interactions (Brocklesby 1969).

The diversity of the *Theileria* species causing infections and diseases in Africa was further exemplified by the isolation of atypical organisms from cattle and game animals. An isolate from cattle (designated as *T. githunguri*) was characterized by the production of low numbers of macroschizonts and an absence of microschizonts and piroplasms. In addition, the animals experienced only a mild clinical reaction to infection. This atypical strain was antigenically distinct from *T. parva*, *T. lawrencei*, and *T. mutans*, but shared some antigens with *T. parva* and *T. lawrencei* (Burridge *et al.* 1974a). Farmers and veterinarians have implicated the eland in the epizootiology of cattle theilerioses in East and Central Africa. It was shown that the eland harbours *Theileria* species infective for cattle (Grootenhuis *et al.* 1977). A *Theileria* species isolated from eland, designated as *T. taurotragi*, had low pathogenicity for eland and cattle, although mortality in the eland has been associated with infection. Cattle recovered from this organism were fully susceptible to *T. parva* challenge (Grootenhuis *et al.* 1979). Further comparisons of *T. taurotragi* and one isolate of *T. parva* of low pathogenicity from Tanzania showed that the two organisms had many characteristics in common including immunological and infectivity properties, which indicated that they may be two strains of the same species adapted to different hosts (Grootenhuis *et al.* 1981).

Because taxonomic and immunological differences are insufficient to identify species, additional criteria such as enzyme complements in protozoa can be used to distinguish species and strains. Isoelectric focusing of blood containing piroplasms of *T. parva* showed bands of glucose phosphate isomerase activity (Meer *et al.* 1981). Isoenzyme variation in the piroplasms was detected in the respective patterns of glucose phosphate isomerase of *T. parva* and *T. annulata*. The differences between these two species were confirmed using antigens from bovine lymphoblastoid cell lines; strains of *T. annulata* from different geographical areas had major differences in their isoenzyme patterns, whereas no differences were observed between strains from the same geographical area (Melrose *et al.* 1980). Glucose phosphate isomerase provided a means of identifying species of parasites in ticks and showed the differences between vector cell activity and the organism's activity in the salivary glands of *H. anatolicum anatolicum* and *R. appendiculatus*; differences were detected between *T. parva* and *T. annulata* as well as between two strains of *T. annulata* (Melrose *et al.* 1981). *Theileria parva* and *T. lawrencei* could be clearly differentiated from *T. annulata* on the basis of three enzymes: glucose phosphate isomerase, glyceraldehyde phosphate dehydrogenase, and aldolase. The *T. parva* and *T. lawrencei* patterns were alike except for those of glucose phosphate isomerase (Musisi *et al.* 1981a, b).

The classification of *T. mutans* from different geographical regions has not yet been fully established. There are geographical differences in the species of ticks transmitting the *T. mutans*-like organisms. The South African and East African isolates were serologically identical; however, serological and morphological comparisons of organisms from Australia and Britain with those of Africa showed that the Australian and European organisms were not *T. mutans*. The Australian and European isolates were related serologically and morphologically (Uilenberg *et al.* 1976a; Uilenberg 1977). Two other strains of nonpathogenic *Theileria* isolated in Tanzania produced low numbers of macroschizonts and were serologically unrelated to *T. mutans*. Sera from infected animals had low titers to *T. parva* schizont antigens in the indirect fluorescent antibody (IFA) test, but the animals were still fully susceptible to *T. parva* challenge (Uilenberg *et al.* 1977b). *Theileria mutans* from Britain and *T. sergenti* from Japan were serologically indistinguishable using the IFA test (Joyner *et al.* 1979). The main difference between the two parasites appears to be in their pathogenicity, i.e. the Japanese organisms can cause clinical anemia and occasionally death, while the British isolates do not cause clinical disease.

Life cycle in the vector

The life cycles of various *Theileria* species in the tick are probably similar. For example, *R. appendiculatus* larvae and nymphs ingest the piroplasms of *T. parva* from infected cattle; after engorgement, they detach from the host animal and molt to the next instar. During this time the organisms undergo stages of development in the intestine and hemolymph with final localization in the salivary glands. When the tick attaches itself to a new host and begins feeding, the parasites mature into infective particles which are then inoculated into new hosts. Light and electron microscopy has shown that the different species of *Theileria* start gamogony in the gut of the vector soon after its detachment from the vertebrate host. This induces kinete formation, which may begin either before or after the molt of the tick nymphs depending on the species of *Theileria* involved. These forms leave the intestinal cells, invade the hemolymph, and finally penetrate the salivary glands where sporozoite formation takes place.

Literature

The complete life cycle of *T. parva* in *R. appendiculatus* is not known. A small proportion (not more than 0.0001%) of the ingested piroplasms develops into the young, intermediate, and mature forms found in the salivary glands of the adult tick (Purnell 1977). The development of *T. parva* in the salivary glands was studied with the electron microscope (Mugera and Munyua 1973).

Schein (1975) described the life cycle of *T. annulata* in the midgut and hemolymph of *H. anatolicum excavatum*. Bhattacharyulu *et al.*

(1975a) detailed the development of *T. annulata* in the gut and salivary glands of *H. anatolicum anatolicum*. Gamogony of *T. annulata* occurs within the intestine of *H. anatolicum excavatum* nymphs with the formation of microgamonts and macrogamonts and stages indicative of gametic fusion. The resulting zygotes in the intestinal cells undergo differentiation to kinetes, a motile stage, while leave the intestinal cells and finally localize in the salivary glands where sporozoites (infective particles) are produced (Mehlhorn and Schein 1976a, b, 1977; Mehlhorn *et al.* 1979). Fully differentiated kinetes of *T. annulata* were observed in the hemolymph and salivary glands of engorged *H. anatolicum excavatum* nymphs 17 to 20 days after the vectors fed; in the salivary glands, the kinetes were transformed into fission bodies that grew and divided, resulting in the development of sporozoites (Schein and Friedhoff 1978).

Early work had shown that the development of *T. mutans* in the gut and hemolymph of *A. variegatum* occurred as follows: the sexual stage appears between days 5 to 7 and zygotes and kinetes are observed in the gut from days 29 and 30 respectively. These developmental stages were similar to those of *T. annulata* and *T. parva*, but there were marked differences in their relative sizes and times of development. The infective particles of *T. mutans* in *A. variegatum* were found to be considerably larger than those of *T. parva* in *R. appendiculatus* (Purnell *et al.* 1975a, b).

The sexual cycle of *T. taurotragi* was identified in the intestinal lumen of *R. appendiculatus* (Young *et al.* 1980), and gamogony of *T. ovis* was observed in the gut of *R. evertsi evertsi* nymphs (Mehlhorn *et al.* 1979). *Theileria velifera* was shown to have stages in the gut and hemolymph of *A. variegatum* characteristic of the genus *Theileria* (Warnecke *et al.* 1979). The sexual cycle of *Theileria* in ticks increases the incidence of the emergence of new antigenic variants in the parasite population. It may thus be possible to manipulate the sexual cycle by genetic recombination techniques in order to produce new clones which are devoid of virulence factors but retain traits required for the development of an effective vaccine (Irvin and Boarer 1980).

Life cycle in the mammalian host

The life cycle of *Theileria* in the mammalian host has been investigated in detail primarily in infections caused by *T. parva*; however, many of the features are probably common to other forms of theileriosis. The mammalian host contracts the infection when the feeding tick injects infective particles contained in its saliva. These infective particles are nucleated sporozoites about 1.5 μm in diameter. Four days after the injection of infective particles, macroschizonts develop in the lymphoblastoid cells (large lymphocytes and lymphoblasts) in the local drainage lymph nodes and then disseminate throughout the lymphoid system. The first visible stages of schizonts are found 5 to 8 days after injection and appear as small round bodies 2 μm in diameter with a round nucleus and a pale-staining area of the cytoplasm. The early infection is associated with the proliferation of lymphoblastoid cells which often do not appear to contain the organisms. The macroschizonts are 2 to 16 μm in diameter and contain on the average eight irregularly shaped nuclei, each about 1 μm in size. The surrounding cytoplasm is paler than that of the host lymphoblastoid cells, which have reddish-purple nuclei with Giemsa stain. In smears made of infected tissues, there are large numbers of free macroschizonts which probably result from the rupture of parasitized cells. The macroschizont population increases progressively and the infection rate in lymphoblastoid cells varies greatly from animal to animal and from strain to strain. The release of merozoites from intracellular macroschizonts has not been observed, although it has been established that the macroschizont divides into two approximately equal masses during the mitosis of the host cell. Approximately 14 days after tick attachment, the macroschizonts give rise to microschizonts which have 50 to 120 small dense round nuclei; these micromerozoites are then released and invade the erythrocytes to form piroplasms. The degree of parasitemia is generally proportional to the host survival time. The piroplasms in red blood cells are rod-shaped, round, oval, or anaplasma-like with the cytoplasm staining light blue and the nucleus staining reddish purple with Giemsa stain. *Theileria parva* and *T. lawrencei* piroplasms are morphologically indistinguishable from those of *T. mutans*. The piroplasms of *T. annulata* are comparable to those of the other three species except that multiplication occurs within the erythrocytes. The morphology of *T. ovis* is indistinguishable from that of *T. hirci* and comparable to that of *Theileria* observed in cattle; division is intraerythrocytic. *Theileria* piroplasms have a diversity of shape which generally would distinguish them from *Babesia* organisms, but individual piroplasms of the two genera cannot be differentiated.

Literature

It was concluded from a number of experiments designed to investigate the initial stages of the life cycle in the host that *T. parva* infective particles from the tick or macroschizonts came into contact with bovine leukocytes and became closely associated with these cells either at the site of injection by the tick or in the local drainage lymph nodes (Brown *et al.* 1969). Initial electron-microscopic studies of *T. parva*-infected cells in lymph nodes did not reveal the presence of infective particles in association with all cells undergoing hyperplasia (Jarrett and Brocklesby 1966). More recently, however, it was shown that sporozoites of *T. parva* incubated with leukocytes attached rapidly to the cells; penetration resulted in changes in cellular morphology marked by increasing amounts of cytoplasm and enlargement of the Golgi apparatus. Macroschizonts were observed by the third day, and multiple infections were frequent and up to eight schizonts were found per cell (Stagg *et al.* 1981). It has been suggested that the transformed cells were T-lymphocytes (Roelants *et al.* 1977), and more specifically, that a discrete subpopulation of T-lymphocytes which had a receptor for the *T. parva* infective particles was susceptible to this transformation (Pinder *et al.* 1981). These transformed lymphocytes became parasitized lymphoblastoid cells which proliferate. *Theileria* infection of lymphoblastoid cells *in vitro* is eradicated by treatment with a naphthoquinone derivative, but the fact that the cellular proliferation is not inhibited until several days after the parasite has been eliminated indicates that the once-infected cells did not revert to small lymphocytes (Pinder *et al.* 1981).

Because the break-up of the macroschizonts into uninuclear components has not been observed, it has been suggested that the multiplication of the macroschizonts occurs in association with the mitosis of the infected cell (Brocklesby 1970). Additional experimental work in cell culture verified this hypothesis. Lymphocyte cultures infected with sporozoites of *T. parva* developed small mononuclear trophozoites after 2 days which then differentiated into typical macroschizonts. After further passage, the schizonts resembled those seen in lymphoblastoid cell lines persistently infected with macroschizonts (Kurtti *et al.* 1981). *In vitro* the nuclear particles of *T. parva* divided at the same rate as the host cell, but the mean number of parasite particles and the percentage of infected cells remain constant. During division of the host cell, the schizonts were closely associated with the mitotic apparatus and were pulled apart and distributed to both daughter cells (Hulliger *et al.* 1966). The division of macroschizonts was synchronized: the association of the parasites with the microtubules of the centriole during interphase and their subsequent orientation with the mitotic spindle formed by the microtubules resulted in a passive but often uneven division of the macroschizonts into the two infected daughter cells (Stagg *et al.* 1980). It was shown that lymphoblastoid cells infected with either *T. parva, T. lawrencei,* or *T. annulata* had cytoplasmic tubules which joined the parasites to the host cell centriole during cellular mitosis, and there was no evidence that the host cell developed any reaction to the parasite (Musisi *et al.* 1981a, b). The microschizonts were produced in cultures of macroschizonts incubated at 40 °C. The high temperature appeared to slow or impede cellular mitosis, while the *Theileria* particles continued multiplying by binary fission (Hulliger *et al.* 1966).

Macroschizont-infected cells were detected simultaneously in the spleen and prescapular lymph nodes following inoculation of a *T. parva* stabilate in front of the ear, thus indicating wide dissemination of the organisms throughout the body (Shatry *et al.* 1981). A large variation in the degree of parasitosis was observed among the different tissues and the numbers of macroschizonts could vary with strains from different regions (Barnett *et al.* 1961). The microstructure of the multiplying nuclei in the schizonts was described and it was concluded that the course of schizogony in *Theileria* was similar to that in other plasmodia (Büttner 1967a). *Theileria mutans* macroschizonts were detected in the local drainage lymph nodes from the eighth day of infection and were distinguishable from those of *T. parva* and *T. lawrencei* by their larger size, more irregular shape, and greater number of nuclei; they were also detectable in circulating mononuclear cells. The macroschizont phase lasted 6 days, and microschizont production was detected from day 12 onward with piroplasms dividing in the blood by binary or quarternary fission (Young *et al.* 1978a). The morphology of the macroschizonts and merozoites of *T. parva, T. lawrencei, T. annulata,* and *T. mutans* was studied with light and electron microscopy. It was concluded that the terms 'macroschizont' and 'microschizont', based on light microscopy studies alone and indicating that two different types of schizont occurred, were inaccurate because each schizont developed through both of these morphological forms; during the phase of nuclear division it appeared as a macroschizont and later during formation of merozoites as a microschizont (Schein *et al.* 1978). Electron microscopy revealed that erythrocytic *T. annulata* piroplasms existed in two different forms, i.e. slender, comma-shaped stages, and spherical stages (Schein *et al.* 1977a, b). A single unit membrane of the *T. parva* piroplasm was found to separate the organism from the surrounding cytoplasm of the host cell, and nutrients were absorbed by pinocytosis (Büttner 1966).

Tissue culture

The *in vitro* growth of the various species of *Theileria* pathogenic for cattle has been of primary importance to the advancement of theileriosis research. The principles of establishing and maintaining *Theileria*-infected culture systems are basically the same for *T. parva* and *T. annulata,* but the former is more difficult to establish. Infected lymphoblastoid cell lines can be established either by harvesting parasitized cells from cattle or by inoculating infected particles obtained from ticks into lymphocyte cultures. These cell lines can be maintained via techniques comparable to those used in the culture of neoplastic cell lines.

Literature

Brown (1979) presented a comprehensive review of the propagation of *Theileria* and included the history of the development of the *in vitro* culture method. The author provided a detailed description of the technical procedures involved in the selection of infected ticks, collection of isolates from the field, establishment and infection of the cultures, preparation of ground-up tick supernatant, chromosome preparations, and cryopreservation of the cultures. A summary of the recent advances in *in vitro* techniques of *Theileria* propagation was presented by Cox (1976).

In initial attempts to grow *T. parva,* the culture was maintained for

14 days (Brocklesby and Hawking 1958). The first continuous cultures of *T. annulata* and *T. parva* macroschizonts were successfully grown using infected tissues and normal spleen implants (Tsur 1953; Tsur *et al.* 1966). *Theileria annulata*-infected lymphoid cells were cultivated by obtaining lymph node fluid and pulp by biopsy at the time there was fever (Hooshmand-Rad and Hashemi-Fesharki, 1968, Hooshmand-Rad, 1975). Lymphoblastoid cell lines infected with *T. parva* were also established from lymph nodes biopsied from cattle, and a feeder layer of bovine embryonic spleen cells was used (Malmquist and Brown 1974).

Using these systems, *T. parva, T. lawrencei,* and *T. annulata* were then cultivated in bovine lymphocytes associated with baby hamster kidney cells (Hulliger *et al.* 1964; Hulliger 1965). Cultivation *in vitro* of bovine spleen cell lines infected with *T. parva* enabled the establishment of culture systems which could be subcultured without any need of feeder layers (Malmquist *et al.* 1970). After the disappearance of the original parasitized spleen cells, the lymphoblastoid cells continued to grow in the suspension culture. Initially the cells needed monolayers of feeder cells, but they later underwent continuous multiplication cycles without feeder layers and could be maintained for a long period of time (Moulton *et al.* 1971). Cultures of lymphoblastoid cells isolated from cattle infected with *T. parva* were comparable to those obtained by infecting normal lymphocytes with sporozoites *in vitro* (Kurtti *et al.* 1981). Irradiation of *T. parva*-infected lymphoblastoid cells in culture inhibited cell division but not the parasite division resulting in an increase of schizont nuclear particles to several hundred (Irvin *et al.* 1975a). Other species of *Theileria* have also been grown in tissues derived from sheep and game animals; *T. hirci* in ovine lymphoid cells independent of fibroblasts Hooshmand-Rad and Hawa 1975); *T. lawrencei* in lymphoblastoid cells derived from buffalo (*Syncerus caffer*) and grown on a feeder layer of bovine embryo spleen cells (Stagg *et al.* 1974); and *C. taurotragi* in cells from eland (*T. oryx*) (Stagg *et al.* 1976).

Other culture systems have also been used in attempts to establish *in vitro* the different phases of the life cycle observed in the mammalian host and vector. The intraerythrocytic stage of *T. parva* was established *in vitro* with the appearance of microschizonts, micromerozoites, and piroplasms in short-term cultures (Danskin and Wilde 1976a, b). Merozoites of *T. parva* and *T. lawrencei* were propagated *in vitro* in enriched media, and limited multiplication was thought to have taken place with the development of piroplasms in red blood cells introduced into the media (Nyindo *et al.* 1978). Organ cultures from *R. appendiculatus* supported the development *in vitro* of salivary stages of *T. parva;* the backless tick explant technique was simpler and gave better results than excised salivary glands (Bell 1980).

In an effort to produce parasitized mouse cell lines, *T. parva* was integrated into the cytoplasm of the heterokaryons induced by Sendai virus and derived from *T. parva*-infected lymphoblastoid cells and

Ehrlich ascites tumor cells (Smith *et al.* 1976). A variety of techniques was employed in an attempt to increase the fusion percentage and harvest of heterokaryons (Irvin *et al.* 1976). Live bovine virus was used to join bovine and lymphoid cells infected with *T. parva* to mouse heart and baby hamster kidney cells. The heterokaryons contained macroschizonts which were also observed in the cells of nonbovine origin. The schizonts underwent varying degrees of development with some evidence of microschizont formation and massive atypical parasite aggregations (Irvin *et al.* 1975b). Irvin *et al.* (1976) reviewed the application of cell fusion techniques in the study of *Theileria* and concluded that the organisms were readily transferred to different species using the fusion technique. It was concluded that the invasion of cells was dependent on the cell surface and that the internal cell environment of different species was compatible with the survival of the organisms.

Laboratory animals

The adaptation of *T. parva* to laboratory animals was proposed as another possible method of achieving attenuation of the organism and to facilitate much of the basic research required. A variety of laboratory animals has been used in trying to establish infection, and with the exception of irradiated and athymic mice, all of the species tested were unsuitable.

The lack of success in infecting mice, chick embryos, rabbits, and guinea pigs, and the use of cortisone, ethyl stearate, and splenectomy was reported (Guilbride 1963). Bovine lymphoid cells infected with *T. parva* also did not grow in newborn and normal mice on subcutaneous injection, in hamster cheek pouches, or in the anterior chamber of rabbits' eyes (Irvin *et al.* 1972a).

The successful propagation of *T. parva* was achieved in irradiated mice. Mice receiving whole-body irradiation developed tumor-like masses of *T. parva*-infected lymphoid cells at the site of subcutaneous inoculation which persisted for 17 days and then were gradually rejected (Irvin *et al.* 1972b, 1974). These parasitized lymphoblastoid cells of bovine origin in murine tumors were transferable to other irradiated mice and could be reestablished in tissue culture (Irvin *et al.* 1973a). Parasitized cells isolated from cattle with *T. parva* infections readily caused tumor-like masses in irradiated athymic mice. The lesions developed 8 to 9 days after inoculation and continued to grow until the animal died. Although the infected bovine lymphoid cells were disseminated throughout the body, they were confined to the blood vessels and did not cause metastatic masses (Irvin *et al.* 1975c, d). Piroplasms of *T. parva* were observed in erythrocytes of tumor-bearing mice (Irvin *et al.* 1975d) and were detected in erythrocytes after the intraperitoneal inoculation of mice with irradiated bovine lymphoid cells (Irvin *et al.* 1977a). Further investigation in this laboratory model established that *T. parva*-infected bovine lymphoblastoid cells grew tumor-like masses at the site of subcutaneous inoculation in neonatal and adult mice immunosuppressed by irradiation, thymectomy, or injection of antilymphocyte serum. The establishment of the lesion was dependent on the degree of immunosuppression which was most marked in the irradiated thymectomized neonatal mice. Following passage between animals there was no evidence of adaptation to growth in mice, although in some systems an indefinite passage could be achieved (Irvin *et al.* 1977b).

Biochemistry

There is very little known about the metabolic processes of Theileriidae.

Literature

Biochemical activity related to the respiratory enzymes was investigated in the sporozoites in tick salivary glands (Weber 1980). Histochemical changes that occurred in the cells of the salivary glands infected with *T. parva* indicated that phosphate and folate enzymes were utilized in the synthesis of nuclei acids (Martins 1978). The defect in purine metabolism observed in *T. parva*-infected cells indicated that folate antagonists may have a therapeutic application (Irvin and Stagg 1977).

EPIZOOTIOLOGY

Domestic animals

On the basis of the quantitative relationship between the tick infestation rate and the incidence of disease, regions are designated as either recently or permanently enzootic, epizootic, or disease free. The incidence of infection, the severity of the disease syndromes, and the economic importance of theileriosis in cattle, sheep, and goats vary considerably from one geographical region to another. Accurate estimates of costs of either the preventative and control measures or losses from disease outbreaks are not available from any region. The most dramatic effect of theilerial infections is observed when exotic cattle are introduced into an enzootic area. In enzootic areas in Africa it is possible to keep Zebu stock, but the mortality may be very high in exotic animals and in Zebu cattle imported from tick-free areas.

Literature

The economic importance of theileriosis in cattle was reviewed by Barnett (1974). The occurrence of *T. parva* is largely restricted to those regions which are suitable for the survival of *R. appendiculatus*. In these regions the infections in indigenous cattle populations are seen in calves; the adults which survive are immune (Yeoman 1966a, b). Neitz (1957) listed theileriosis in Africa in areas associated with infestation by *R. appendiculatus* and included Zaïre, Zambia, Kenya, Zimbabwe, Malawi, Angola, Lesotho, Tanzania, Uganda, the Union of South Africa and Zanzibar. Since then other countries in eastern and southern Africa have been included.

Theileria annulata is distributed throughout North Africa, parts of Europe, the Middle and Far East, and the USSR and is transmitted by the tick of the genus *Hyalomma* (Barnett 1974).

Theileria mutans occurs in Africa, North and South America, Asia, Australia, and Europe, and the countries in which it has been reported up to 1957 were listed by Neitz (1957). Because *T. mutans* is endemic and so ubiquitous, it complicates the investigation of other theilerial species. It is morphologically indistinguishable from other *Theileria* and readily transmitted by blood and tissues.

Theileria hirci is reported in Asia, Africa, and Europe, where in enzootic areas the young lambs and kids contract a relatively mild form of the disease which renders mature animals immune. The mortality rate in sheep is relatively low at 16% in infected cases. The distribution of *T. ovis* is comparable to that of *T. hirci*.

The epizootiology, economic importance, and major research programs into control were presented in a monograph by Henson and Campbell (1977) which included national reports from Kenya, Uganda, Tanzania, Zanzibar, Pemba, Rwanda, Burundi, Mozambique, Somalia, Zambia, India, Iran, Turkey, Egypt, and Pakistan. However, only some of these reports provided any information (and this was often very general) on the losses from, and economic importance of, various forms of theileriosis. The number of ECF cases in Kenya was estimated to be 50 000 to 70 000 out of a cattle population of 9.7 million (Duffus 1977). In Malawi, an estimated 165 000 of 250 000 calves died of ECF in 1976 (Moodie 1977). Oteng (1970) and Taylor (1954) reported on the epizootiology of theileriosis in Uganda up to 1970, and the losses in exotic cattle were appraised by Okao and Oteng (1973). The main economic losses in Uganda occurred as a result of the 50% mortality rate in calves, unthriftiness in 5 to 10% of the calves recovered from clinical infections, mortality in adults which ranged as high as 90%, and unthriftiness of adults recovered from infection. The occurrence of additional clinical sequelae not commonly observed was noted and included turning sickness, unthriftiness in recovered cattle, and skin conditions (Oteng 1976). The distribution of *R. appendiculatus* and theileriosis in Tanzania was reviewed (Robson *et al*. 1961). The epizootiology of theileriosis in Tanzania was reported in 1968 by McCulloch (1968) and McCulloch *et al*. (1968). McCulloch (1964) reported on the outbreak of theileriosis in Tanzania and pointed out the difficulty of identifying species from parasitological and pathological examination. Out of a population of 13 000 calves born in Zanzibar and Pemba, 4000 calves were lost (Hofstedt 1977), while in Burundi the estimated death rate from theileriosis is between 10 and 30% in cattle up to 4 years of age (Bonaventure 1977).

There is even less accurate information on the losses caused by *T. annulata*. A report from India contained morbidity and mortality data for the estimated 179 million head of cattle in 1972, as well as information on the past and present research programs. It was pointed out that vaccination against rinderpest using goat-adapted virus resulted in a flare-up of latent protozoal and rickettsial infections (Gill *et al.* 1976a, b, 1977). In the Sudan it was reported that the mortality rates from *T. annulata* were 20 to 25% in adult cattle and 15% in calves in an overall population of 22 million head (Shommein 1977). Purnell (1978) reviewed the hazards to cattle in countries of the northern Mediterranean littoral. The distribution of *T. annulata* extends in a wide belt of tropical and subtropical zones from Portugal, Spain, and Morocco in the west to China in the east. Infection spread to the countries in the northern Mediterranean littoral from the west through Morocco and from the east through the Middle East. The incidence of *Hyalomma* species of ticks was determined in Turkey, Greece, Albania, Yugoslavia, Italy, France, and Spain.

There is little information available in the literature on the other forms of the theileriosis. The occurrence of *Theileria* in goats was reported in Sierra Leone for the first time in 1974. Reliable evidence obtained from serological tests indicated that *T. mutans* and *T. velifera* were present in Nigeria. But it was emphasized that the identification of *T. annulata* based solely on the morphology of the piroplasms as reported by a group of workers from Ibadan was unreliable and cast doubt on the claim that this species occurred in West Africa (Perié *et al.* 1979). Leeflang, summarizing the findings of work conducted in Nigeria, confirmed that *T. mutans* was present (Leefland and Ilemobade 1977). Tayama (1975) and Kitaoka (1970) provided brief reviews of the *Theileria* that occur in Japan.

Game animals

Various wild members of the family Bovidae which have a habitat in rhipicephaloid tick-infested zones are known commonly to harbor intraerythrocytic theilerial and *Theileria*-like piroplasms in the genera *Cytauxzoon* and *Haematoxenus*. The African buffalo (*S. caffer*) has been definitely implicated in the epizootiology of theileriosis syndrome in East Africa. The eland (*Taurotragus* or *Pattersonianus*) has some significance in the transmission of the disease while the wildebeest (*Connochaetes taurinus*) has been suspected but not implicated.

Literature

The confused taxonomy of the group of protozoa which causes the development of piroplasms in wild animals was discussed and it was pointed that the organisms are extremely common and that the taxonomy continues to evolve. The *Theileria*-like organisms in the African antelopes probably belong the genus *Cytauxzoon* (Barnett and Brocklesby 1968). The hemaprotozoa in the wild members of the order Artiodactyla were surveyed in East Africa and it was found that 65% of these animals were infected with intraerythrocytic piroplasms of Theileriidae, with schizonts being found in the reticulated giraffe and Coke's hartebeest (Brocklesby and Vidler 1965, 1966). Investigations using *T. parva* and *T. mutans* antigens revealed that the sera of game animals reacted only with *T. parva* antigens. The *Theileria* organisms found in the erythrocytes of these animals could not be transmitted to splenectomized calves by the inoculation of blood (Löhr and Meyer 1974).

The African buffalo was conclusively implicated in the epizootiology of theileriosis in Kenya (Barnett and Brocklesby 1959). The literature on the buffalo acting as a reservoir of classical ECF and *T. lawrencei* infection was surveyed (Brocklesby and Barnett 1966a). The literature on theileriosis of the African buffalo and the cytauxzoonoses in wild animals was also reviewed (Burridge 1975). During the early stages of work on theileriosis in buffalo, the organism was named *T. barnetti*, but the designation has not been subsequently used (Brocklesby 1965a). *Haematoxenus* and *Theileria* were commonly found in African buffalo in Uganda (Young *et al.* 1973). In 13 areas of East Africa the incidence of theilerial piroplasms and antibodies in 245 buffalo as detected by the indirect fluorescent antibody test was 50 and 97.1% respectively. *Haematoxenus* species was detected in the blood of 56 of these buffalo (Young *et al.* 1978b). African buffalo remained infective carriers of *T. lawrencei* for 5 years and could also be infected with *H. veliferus* and *T. mutans* from cattle (Schreuder *et al.* 1977).

Theileria lawrencei sporozoites underwent the complete life cycle in the buffalo with final piroplasms appearing which were infective for ticks; the development of schizonts but not piroplasms in cattle led to the proposal that cattle could not serve as reservoirs for the infection to the vectors (Neitz 1958). However, in more recent studies, *R. appendiculatus* transmitted *T. lawrencei* from buffalo to cattle and between cattle. The buffalo was shown to be a carrier for 26 months and the efficiency of transmission by ticks to cattle was higher than that between cattle. The infection rate in the salivary glands was much lower than that of *T. parva* and was probably related to the small number of *T. lawrencei* piroplasms observed in both buffalo and cattle (Young and Purnell 1973). When engorged nymphs of *R. appendiculatus* were collected from wild African buffalo and transmitted serially through four buffalo calves, one calf died and the others reacted clinically (Brocklesby and Barnett 1966b). Of six African buffalo exposed to *T. parva*, some animals became infected and a proportion of these developed a clinical response (Barnett and Brocklesby 1966b), whereas *Theileria* infections from buffalo were readily transmitted through the *R. appendiculatus* ticks to cattle and caused fatal infections (Burridge 1975). Nymphal *R. appendiculatus* ticks fed on buffalo transmitted a lethal infection to cattle which had relatively few lymphocytes parasitized with macroschizonts when neither microschizonts nor piroplasms were detectable (Young *et al.* 1973).

The characteristics of the infection caused by new *Theileria* species isolated from eland and designated *T. taurotragi* were examined in both eland and cattle (Grootenhuis *et al.* 1979). Earlier work did not indicate that the eland was significant in the transmission of disease to cattle, although it was proposed that it could play an important role in the transmission of *Theileria* in wild animals (Brocklesby 1965a, b). An organism classified as *C. taurotragi* was reported to cause a fatal infection in young eland; schizonts were present in liver, lung, and lymph nodes, and infections were also found in *R. appendiculatus* and *R. pulchellus* ticks removed from a dead eland in a natural field case (Brocklesby 1962a). Studies of the structure of the intraerythrocytic forms of the *Theileria* in eland confirmed the presence of the bar and veil (Young *et al.* 1978a). The *Theileria* species from naturally infected eland was transmitted transstadially by *R. appendiculatus* to susceptible eland (Grootenhuis *et al.* 1977). In more recent studies of transmission to cattle, *R. appendiculatus* ticks from a number of eland were applied to cattle and induced mild infections which resulted in low numbers of schizonts and piroplasms. These infections stimulated the production of antibodies which reacted with schizont antigens of a *Theileria* species isolated from eland and designated *Githunguri*, but not with other theilerial antigens (Young *et al.* 1977a). However, in earlier experiments *R. appendiculatus* and *R. simus* nymphs fed on seven parasitemic eland developed salivary gland infection but did not transmit the organism to cattle (Irvin *et al.* 1972c).

There is less information available on theilerial infections in other game species. The blue wildebeest (*Connochaetes taurinus*) was found to harbour *T. gorgonis* infection (Brocklesby and Vidler 1961), and the ultrastructure of *T. gorgonis* was investigated (Smith *et al.* 1974). Splenectomy caused an exacerbation of the parasitemia which resulted in death in some wildebeest. Transmission by blood passage and by tick to cattle failed (Purnell *et al.* 1973a). Theilerial piroplasms and *Haematoxenus* organisms were detected in 44.7 and 2.3% of impala (*Aepyceros melampus*) respectively (Irvin *et al.* 1973b). Theilerial parasites isolated from naturally infected impala could be passaged to a *Theileria*-free impala but not to splenectomized steer (Grootenhuis *et al.* 1979).

Cytauxzoon species have been identified in African ungulates and constitute one of the genera of protozoa listed in the family Theileriidae. The genus *Cytauxzoon* is distinguished from other Theileria by the occurrence of schizogony in histiocytes rather than lymphocytes. Recently a *Cytauxzoon*-like agent, *C. felis*, has been observed to cause fatal disease in cats in southwestern Missouri in the USA (Wagner 1976). Four cases were reported with clinical signs of fever, dehydration, and pale and icteric mucous membranes. In addition to the mucous membrane changes observed clinically at post mortem, there was petechial and ecchymotic hemorrhage in the serosal membranes of thoracic and abdominal organs, orange-brown liver, enlargement of lymph nodes which were either congested or hemorrhagic and edematous, and enlargement of the spleen. Histiological analysis revealed a marked accumulation of parasitized reticuloendothelial cells containing cytoplasmic schizonts with large numbers of merozoites in varying stages of replication in the spleen, lungs, liver, and kidneys. The disease could be experimentally passaged through cats by the administration of fresh or frozen blood or infected tissues. The induced illness was consistently fatal within 20 days. *Cytauxzoon felis* infection was also successfully transmitted to the Florida bobcat (*Lynx rufus floridanus*) and passaged back to domestic cats (Kier *et al.* 1982a). However, in these experiments domestic cats did not develop clinical signs, although parasitemia was evidenced. Subsequent challenge with *Cytauxzoon* inoculum of domestic cat origin caused fatal disease in all experimental animals. Thirty-two domestic and wild species had been used in the study of *Cytauxzoon* transmission and only the bobcat was found susceptible to infection (Kier *et al.* 1982b).

Transmission

At least seven species of *Rhipicephalus* and *Hyalomma* have been shown to transmit *T. parva* under experimental conditions. *Rhipicephalus appendiculatus* is widely distributed in enzootic regions of central, eastern, and southern Africa, and is considered to be the chief vector. The other species of *Rhipicephalus*, although much less important, probably play a significant role in maintaining the infection in nature, but there is no evidence that *Hyalomma* species transmit the infection under natural conditions. Stage-to-stage transmission within the same generation is observed in all vectors, but transovarian transmission does not take place. The infection is not always sustained throughout the entire life span of the tick with temperature affecting the infectivity. Artificial transmission can be achieved with infected tissues from ECF-infected cattle by intravenous injection of spleen and lymph gland material; there are reports that intradermal and subcutaneous methods may also be used.

At least six *Hyalomma* species are capable of transmitting *T. annulata*. Infections are easily transmissible to cattle via blood and organ suspensions injected by any route. The cosmopolitan nature of *T. mutans* suggests that several genera and species are involved in its transmission, with *Haemaphysalis* and *Amblyomma* species possibly being most prevalent. Infections are readily transmitted mechanically by piroplasms.

Literature

In epizootic regions of ECF severe losses occurred when the average vector infestation may be as low as one to four adult ticks per animal, and sporadic outbreaks could occur when the rate was less than one tick per animal, thus indicating that a quantitative relationship existed between the average rate of infestation and the epizootiological situation in different zones (Yeoman 1966a). It was found that sheep were good hosts of *R. appendiculatus* in heavily infested areas, but at low density of infestation they carried fewer ticks than did calves. Goats were poor hosts of the adult ticks and good hosts of the nymphs; there was no evidence that other domestic animals were important hosts (Yeoman 1966b). The large spotted genet (*Genetta tigrina*) was capable of carrying and feeding *R. appendiculatus* ticks which were subsequently infective for cattle (Purnell *et al.* 1970a).

The distribution of tick vectors of theileriosis in eastern and Central Africa was briefly reviewed (Wilson 1953). *Rhipicephalus carnivoralis* was shown to be capable of transmitting *T. parva* under experimental conditions, and the organisms were demonstrated in the salivary glands (Brocklesby *et al.* 1966). *Rhipicephalus evertsi* successfully transmitted experimental *T. parva* (Uilenberg and Schreuder 1977) and two additional species, *R. pulchellus* and *R. carnivoralis,* were also shown to transmit the organism under experimental conditions. Because the distribution of *A. variegatum* often coincides with the occurrence of *R. appendiculatus* the former organism has been considered on epizootiological grounds to be a possible vector of *Theileria* (Yeoman 1968).

An important contribution to the work on transmission of *T. parva* and *T. lawrencei* to cattle was made in Kenya by the establishment of a 2 ha experimental paddock containing a monitored population of *R. appendiculatus* ticks infected with *T. parva* (Purnell *et al.* 1975b). A similar paddock infested with *T. lawrencei*-infected *R. appendiculatus* ticks was also established by maintaining two parasitized buffalo on the premises. The transmission of *T. lawrencei* from buffalo to cattle was first noted 7 to 8 months after introduction of the buffalo. This delay was accounted for by the slow buildup of the tick population and the lower rates of infection in the ticks. After exposure, the mortality of cattle became progressively more rapid as the tick population increased (Young *et al.* 1977b).

The correlation between the distribution of the genus *Hyalomma* and the occurrence of *T. annulata* infections in the countries of the northern Mediterranean littoral was discussed (Purnell 1978). The transmission of *T. annulata* by *H. excavatum* in Egypt was recorded (Daubney and Sami Said 1950). The transstadial transmission of *T. annulata* through common ixodid ticks infecting Indian cattle was determined, and variable efficiency of transmission was shown to occur with *H. anatolicum anatolicum, H. dromedarii,* and *H. marginatum isaaci* (Bhattacharyulu *et al.* 1975a, b). *Hyalomma anatolicum anatolicum* was also shown to infect cattle and buffalo (Gautam 1976). The distribution of *H. asiaticum asiaticum,* a three-host tick and a vector of *T. annulata,* was described in Iran (Mazlum 1968). The transmission of *T. annulata* experimentally by the three-host tick *H. excavatum* and the two-host tick *H. detritum* was reported in Israel (Samish and Pipano 1978).

Theileria mutans was successfully transmitted by *A. variegatum* but not by *R. appendiculatus,* a species which has been shown to transmit the southern African type of *T. mutans*. These findings suggested that the *Theileria* from southern and eastern Africa are different species (Uilenberg *et al.* 1974, 1976a, b). Earlier experimental and field observation of *T. mutans* transmitted by *R. appendiculatus* and *R. evertsi* indicated that these tick species were not important vectors (Purnell *et al.* 1970b). Macroschizonts morphologically characteristic of *T. mutans*, originally isolated from buffalo, were observed after the experimental transmission of *T. mutans* in cattle by *A. gemma* (Paling *et al.* 1981). *Theileria mutans* was also experimentally transmitted by *H. punctata* (Brocklesby *et al.* 1975).

Theileria hirci was transmitted by *H. anatolicum anatolicum* (Hooshmand-Rad and Hawa 1973a). *Theileria ovis* was successfully transmitted by *R. evertsi mimeticus* and *R. bursa* and several other species of ticks have been incriminated as vectors (Jansen and Neitz 1956; Neitz 1972).

Theileria annulata could be readily transmitted via blood and tissues from clinical cases, while *T. parva* was difficult to transmit in this way (Barnett 1974). The infections were similar irrespective of whether they were established via intravenous, subcutaneous, or intraperitoneal routes (Neitz 1956). The piroplasm stage of *T. ovis* was shown to be infective for a number of species of deer which had been splenectomized (Enigk *et al.* 1964).

INFECTION

Artificial infection of ticks

Methods for infecting ticks with *Theileria*, mostly *T. parva*, were developed in laboratories for use in experimental systems involving induction of infection and storage of the organisms. The reduction of the number of infective forms in the inoculant by dilution decreases the incidence of fatal infection. A threshold of infection can thus be established on the basis of the number of infective particles in the inoculant. Cryopreservation at −70 °C is used for maintaining infective tick tissues, mammalian tissues, and cell cultures. These preserved materials are known as stabilates and can be maintained unchanged for several years.

Theileria parva undergoes a maturation cycle in the tick salivary glands which is induced by feeding ticks on mammalian hosts for several days. Immature ticks fed on parasitemic cattle produced infective stages in their next instar resulting in adults becoming infective; this cycle is responsible for maintenance of the disease in the field. Infection rates of *T. parva* in adult *R. appendiculatus* ticks were higher than in the nymphs; the adults had approximately three times as many infected acini. Considerable variability in infection rates of tick batches fed as nymphs were detected when they were fed on cattle with comparable parasitemias. Adult ticks which had fed as nymphs on animals which had a rising or peak parasitemia were more heavily infected than those whose juvenile forms were fed when the parasitemia was decreasing. The age of the molted tick and prolonged starvation at room temperature are known to affect the infectivity of ticks. The fact that the organism disappears if infected ticks are fed on immune cattle or animals not susceptible to theileriosis indicates that infections can be eliminated. The organisms in nymphal and adult stages of the tick disappear when a meal is not obtained for about a year or when the vectors are exposed to continuous high temperature during the period of molting.

Literature

The rearing of *R. appendiculatus* under experimental conditions for the transmission of *T. parva* has been described (Bailey 1960). One of the first attempts at artificial induction was made by using capillary tubes containing blood infected with *T. parva* to feed nymphal *R. appendiculatus* ticks. The nymphs which were initially partially fed on rabbits and subsequently engorged by the capillary tube method then became infected (Purnell 1970). A capillary tube feeding technique was also used for the collection of infective particles from ticks (Purnell and Joyner 1967). Another method of infecting ticks involved the injection of blood infected with *T. parva* into nymphs of *R. appendiculatus* (Jongejan *et al.* 1980). Engorged *A. variegatum* nymphs which had fed on rabbits when they were percutaneously injected also transmitted *T. mutans* after molting; *R. appendiculatus* transmitted *T. parva* under the same experimental conditions (Schreuder and Uilenberg 1976). A comparison between the various artificial feeding methods and the injection of ticks showed that the latter technique was simpler and as efficient as the former (Walker *et al.* 1979a).

The salivary gland stimulants, pilocarpine nitrate and arecoline hydrobromide, were the most effective parasympathomimetic drugs when injected per anus into female *R. appendiculatus* ticks and caused salivation which enabled the collection of infective particles (Purnell *et al.* 1969). The effect of salivary stimulants was also investigated on isolated preparations of *T. parva*-infected normal parasite-free salivary glands from *R. appendiculatus* (McCall 1978). A somewhat unusual method involved feeding nymphal *R. appendiculatus* ticks on splenectomized rabbits which had received 20 ml of infected bovine blood; this procedure resulted in a high infection rate in the tick salivary glands (Purnell *et al.* 1974). A bizarre method involving an isolated rabbit head perfused with *T. parva*-infected bovine blood was also reported to infect ticks (Irvin *et al.* 1970).

The maintenance of *T. parva* infection by passaging the organism through cattle via *R. appendiculatus* under laboratory conditions was effective provided that the level of parasitemia which developed at the beginning of the disease was sufficiently high to enable nymphs to acquire a high degree of infectivity. Acute syndromes were not effective because of the short period of patent disease, while mild reactions were often associated with low levels of parasitemia (Branagan 1969). Nymphal ticks developed high rates of infection when they were applied to cattle with a maximal parasitemia (Purnell 1977). However, it has been shown that when nymphal ticks were fed on cattle, the subsequent infection rates in adults had no correlation with the parasitemia of the cattle at the time of nymphal engorgement (Irvin *et al.* 1981), but there was approximately three times as many infected acini in adult ticks as in nymphs (Purnell *et al.* 1971). In terms of the percentage of ticks infected and the numbers of acini involved, female ticks consistently demonstrated higher rates of infection than the male ticks infected and the numbers of acini involved (Irvin *et al.* 1981). The development of *T. parva* in the salivary glands of *R. appendiculatus* was related to the feeding process of the ticks. Maximum numbers of organisms were present at 3 to 5 days after attachment with 30.5 to 42% of the ticks being infested (Purnell and Joyner 1968; Joyner and Purnell 1968).

Experiments were undertaken to determine the most suitable day on which infected ticks could be harvested for the collection of sporozoites. Adult *R. appendiculatus* ticks infected as nymphs by feeding on African buffalo were then fed on rabbits and subsequently ground up. The most infective supernatant fluid was produced from ticks fed for 5 to 6 days and it was found that the presence of mature ticks coincided with infectivity (Young *et al.* 1975). Also, adult ticks fed as nymphs on *T. parva*-infected cattle and then on rabbits had a maximal number of parasites 4 to 5 days after attachment (Purnell *et al.* 1970c). Adult female *R. appendiculatus* ticks infected with *T. parva* and pre-fed on rabbits for 4 days were observed to release parasites for at least 6 hours by a subsequent *in vitro* feeding method (Joyner *et al.* 1972). Maximum infectivity was observed in *A. variegatum* nymphs infected with *T. mutans* after feeding on rabbits for 3 to 7 days (Young 1977).

Lewis (1950) described how temperature, starvation of the tick, and duration of infection in the vector affected the infectivity and virulence of the parasite. The literature on the cyclic development and longevity of *T. parva* in *R. appendiculatus* was reviewed, and it was observed that the ticks became noninfective between 34 and 40 weeks after molting and that they transmitted the parasite within 24 hours after being placed on the host (Martin *et al.* 1964). The molting behavior of nymphal *R. appendiculatus* was greatly influenced by temperatures between 18 and 37 °C; some temperatures were detrimental to infectivity since they influenced the rate of development and the numbers of the early stages of *T. parva* in the ticks (Young and Leitch 1981). Infective forms were induced by exposing ticks to 37 °C, but the production of sporozoites was not as efficient as that obtained by feeding ticks on rabbits. However, the induction of infective stages by higher temperature could be of importance under field conditions (Young *et al.* 1979). There was no difference in the infection rate in adults when parasite maturation was stimulated either by incubation at 37 °C or by feeding on rabbits (Irvin *et al.* 1981).

The infection rate in *T. mutans* in ticks is consistently lower than that of *T. parva*, but the developmental stages cannot be differentiated from those of *T. parva.* Salivary gland stages of *T. lawrencei* could not be morphologically differentiated from those of *T. parva* and were detected after the ticks had fed for 4 to 5 days. The number of ticks showing parasites from buffalo and cattle was 5.9 and 2.1% respectively. After continued passage through cattle, the infectivity of all *Theileria* for ticks increases considerably.

Enumeration of infected acini has been undertaken in both smears and sections of salivary glands. The presence of mature parasites in the salivary glands of *R. appendiculatus* ticks infected with *T. parva* could be correlated with infectivity for cattle; the highest infectivity was prepared from ticks fed for about 5 days on rabbits (Purnell *et al.* 1973b). The simple technique of cutting thin sections on a cryostat and staining with Giemsa stain was as efficient in demonstrating theilerial parasites as the standard histological procedure which entails imbedding in paraffin wax (Kimber and Purnell 1972). Rapid, simple methods using methyl green pyronin stain enabled quantitative assessment of both *T. parva* and *T. annulata* in *R. appendiculatus* and *H. anatolicum* respectively. Considerable variation in the incidence and intensity of infections in infected ticks required large samples to be examined to define accurately the infectivity in a given population of ticks (Walker *et al.* 1979b; Irvin *et al.* 1981). Developing stages of *T. parva* in nymphal *R. appendiculatus* ticks were more efficiently examined by the indirect rather than the direct fluorescent antibody (FA) technique (Kimber *et al.* 1973).

The most critical step in the research on infectivity and virulence of *Theileria* was the cryopreservation of infective organisms harvested from ticks. The use of these stabilates enabled the standardization of the challenge techniques (Purnell 1977). The standardization was required because the quantity of infected material obtained from individual ticks or batches of ticks varied considerably (Cunningham *et al.* 1973a). Both rabbits and cattle were used in a basic standardized method developed to provide feeding adequate for the induction of optimal numbers of infective particles from ticks (Bailey 1960). The harvesting of infective particles by *in vitro* feeding techniques or by grinding ticks in a suitable medium was the first stage in obtaining infective material which could be standardized. Various substrates were investigated for diluting and maintaining *T. parva* infective particles obtained from *R. appendiculatus* by the capillary tube feeding method. This infected material could then be maintained at –80 °C or –196 °C over prolonged periods of time without loss of viability (Cunningham *et al.* 1973b).

Similar methods of stabilate preparation have also been used to preserve *T. annulata* organisms. Unfed nymphs, adults, and ground-up tissue suspensions of *H. anatolicum* induced clinical theileriosis in calves, and there was a direct correlation between the infectivity of ticks and the volume of *T. annulata*-infected blood which was engorged (Srivastava and Sharma 1978). Adult *H. excavatum* ticks became infective after minimal feeding of 2 days either on cattle or rabbits. In the absence of blood meals, an environmental temperature of 37 °C and a high relative humidity of 95% were sufficient biological stimuli for the development of infective stages (Samish 1977a, b). Ground-up tick supernate prepared from unfed adult ticks was not infective; the highest infectivity was observed from the 3-day pre-fed ticks (Singh *et al.* 1979a). Nymphs of *H. anatolicum* infected with *T. annulata* were obtained by interrupted feeding of larvae on rabbits which then feed well on cattle (Hosie and Walker 1979).

Radiation was used in addition to dilution methods in attempts to decrease the virulence of infective particles. Increasing doses of radiation resulted in decreases in the infection rate of ticks and in the number of parasite masses observed in infected ticks. No normal parasites were observed at doses higher than 4 krad (Purnell *et al.* 1972a, b). Molting nymphs and adults were able to survive irradiation better than unfed and engorged nymphs (Purnell *et al.* 1973c). Higher doses of radiation increased the number of parasites which were destroyed in suspensions of *T. parva* (Cunningham *et al.* 1973c).

Infectivity and virulence

The range of mammalian hosts for *Theileria* is significant in the epizootiology of these diseases because of the possible existence of carriers in game animals. A number of species are probably susceptible to *T. parva* and *T. mutans* infections, while *T. annulata* appears to be limited to cattle and water buffalo.

The interaction between the mammalian host and the theilerial organism depends on the susceptibility of the host, the virulence of the strain of *Theileria*, and the intensity of the challenge dose. There is no evidence that *Bos taurus* is inherently more susceptible to theilerial infections than *B. indicus*. When either species is reared for generations in an enzootic situation there is a reduction in the susceptibility, as shown by the reduced severity of disease. Therefore, the wide variation in the degree of innate resistance displayed among the races of cattle in enzootic areas is dependent on the development of resistance by local selection of individuals rather than on any specific genetic factor. Thus Zebu (*B. indicus*) cattle exhibit a high natural resistance to *T. parva* in enzootic regions where the infection occurs in calfhood. Zebu calves contract theilerial infections and develop a premune state which is reflected in a relatively low incidence of mortality and a comparatively mild clinical syndrome in adult cattle. However, severe losses occur in calves and mature animals of all breeds which are introduced into enzootic areas. There is a wide variation in the virulence of *T. annulata* strains which has been observed between different countries as well as within any one enzootic region. A similar situation also appears to exist with *T. parva* and *T. mutans* infections, although the evidence is not as well documented. There is little known about the variation and virulence of *T. hirci* and *T. ovis* species.

Literature

The infectivity and virulence of various species of *Theileria* in domestic ruminants has been discussed by Barnett (1978). *Theileria parva* and *T. lawrencei* both infect the African buffalo (*S. caffer*) and the Asian water buffalo (*Bubalus bubalis*). *Theileria annulata* has not been shown to parasitize the African buffalo although it can infect the Asian water buffalo and the American bison (*Bison bison*). The severity of the clinical signs varies with the host and theilerial species involved. Titration experiments have demonstrated that the quantum of infective material determines whether the infection becomes established and what course the disease will take (Wilde 1966a, 1967).

In clinical syndromes the multiplication of the organisms after the infection was exponential with high temperature. The prepatent period was dependent on the dose of infective particles introduced. After the initial stage of active multiplication in nonfatal cases the organism persisted in small numbers in various tissues for a long period of time, resulting in premunition which could last throughout the entire life of the host; alternatively, the organism could die out following a variable length of infection. Occasionally the host–parasite interaction resulted in premunition which was unbalanced; recrudescence of parasite multiplication then caused clinical signs and mortality (Barnett 1978).

With the exception of the host–parasite interaction which takes place at the site of the tick bite, successive stages of the life cycle have been studied (Purnell 1977). In an *in vitro* experiment, infective particles became associated with white blood cells and the infectivity of this parasitized infected blood depended on the acceptance of the white blood cells by the new host (Brown *et al.* 1969). Five to fifteen days after the infective ticks were applied to the ears, macroschizonts of *T. parva* were found in the parotid lymphatic glands; a rise in temperature soon followed. The rapid appearance of the organisms in lymphoid organs suggested that their dissemination was hematogenous (Shatry *et al.* 1981).

The quantitative aspect of progression of infections was first thoroughly studied by Jarrett *et al.* (1969). *Theileria parva* grew exponentially from day 11 to 21, but probably also from the start of the growth phase, with a tenfold increase in macroschizonts occurring every 3 days. This exponential phase of replication was by small macroschizonts with one to six nuclei; larger schizonts developed later and were followed subsequently by the appearance of microschizonts and piroplasms which was time- but not dose-dependent. The growth rate of the organisms was independent of the size of the dose. There appeared to be a fixed number of cell divisions during the exponential phase of multiplication, and when the number of schizonts produced reached a certain level (7×10^9), they were detectable in the prescapular lymph nodes at a ratio of parasitized to nonparasitized lymphoblastoid cells of 1 per 100. Subsequently the infection rate in cells increases, giving rise to widespread dissemination of infection. The mean time of the tenfold cycle reflected the virulent properties of the organisms and the severity of the syndrome produced. The mean nuclear schizont number at any given time depended on the infecting dose and the inherent prolificacy of a particular strain. Partially immune hosts were able to withstand the primary infection because parasite replication was suppressed and the macroschizonts never became sufficiently numerous to cause either severe or fatal disease. Further quantitative studies of *T. parva* in cattle supported observations that the prepatent period, time to onset of febrile response, and time to death of the animal was dose-related, but contradicted other observations by showing that time of development of piroplasms was not time-dependent. Also, contrary to previous observations, it was proposed that the multiplication rate of macroschizonts was dose-dependent (Radley *et al.* 1974).

Neitz (1957) summarized the available information on the quantitative aspects of infection with other species of *Theileria*. Schizonts of *T. annulata* can be observed in various tissues and organs, and in fairly large numbers in the peripheral blood when the clinical signs are evident. In *T. hirci* macroschizonts have also been observed in very large numbers in different tissues. Cattle recovered from infection with *T. annulata* suffered a relapse within 3 weeks of splenectomy. Relapses have also been reported to occur either idiopathically or as a result of concurrent infection with other agents, e.g., *Babesia*, *Anaplasma*, and foot-and-mouth virus. It is difficult to demonstrate the presence of *T. mutans* but a splenectomy in pre-immune animals causes a relapse in 3 weeks; 50% of the red blood contained organisms, while only small numbers of schizonts were detectable in the spleen and lymph nodes. However, in severe cases larger numbers of schizonts could be found. The recrudescence of virulence of a nonvirulent strain of *T. annulata* was accomplished by passaging the organisms through cattle by ticks. Reduction of the virulence was brought about by serial blood passages through cattle (Sharma 1976).

The differences in susceptibility and resistance of various breeds of cattle to any of the theilerial infections has not been clearly demonstrated. The definition of resistance to *T. parva* infection is difficult because a large number of animals with appropriate controls was required (Guilbride and Opwata 1963). A similar situation exists with other species of *Theileria*. It was proposed that the difference in the resistance to *T. parva* demonstrated by the *Bos indicus* and *B. taurus* types could be related to the possession of an HbC hemoglobin type with lower levels of glucose-6-phosphate dehydrogenase being associated with resistance (Burdin and Boarer 1972).

In performing research on *Theileria* infection in cattle, it is often necessary to eliminate other organisms that are present in the blood of animals which are asymptomatic carriers. *Theileria mutans* was separated from *Babesia* species by the rapid subpassage of infected blood through cattle (Callow and Hayte 1961). In a mixed infection of *A. marginale* and *T. mutans*, the former could be eliminated by imidocarb treatment (Kuttler and Craig 1975).

CLINICAL SIGNS

East Coast fever is an often fatal tick-borne disease clinically characterized by pyrexia, malaise, anorexia, lachrymation, digestive disturbances, emaciation, dyspnea, and swelling of superficial and internal lymph nodes. The severity of the clinical response to *T. parva* infection depends on the intensity and duration of the challenge. The incubation period varies from 8 to 25 days (mean incubation time 13 days) depending on the degree of virulence of the particular strain involved and the resistance of the host. Attenuation of *T. parva* infection has been associated with prolonged starvation of tick nymphae and adults and with the exposure of engorged larvae and nymphae to continuous high temperatures (31 to 38 °C) for the full period of molting. *Bos taurus* and *B. indicus* cattle reared in zones free of *T. parva* are highly susceptible to infection. Calves and immature cattle possess a greater degree of resistance than mature animals. Although the calf mortality rate varies between 5 and 50%, up to 75% of infected calves may mature. The low mortality in calves may be observed both at low and high tick infestations. The Asian water buffalo and the African buffalo are susceptible to natural *T. parva* infection; the African species is highly resistant to the development of any clinical signs, while the Asian buffalo presents symptoms that are similar to those observed in cattle.

Theileria parva causes acute, subacute, mild, and inapparent syndromes. In the acute form fever ranges from 40 to 41.6 °C and may be continuous or interrupted. Clinical symptoms usually appear a few days after the initial rise in temperature and include inappetence, cessation of rumination, ocular and nasal discharge, swelling of eyelids, ears, cervical regions, enlargement of superficial lymph nodes, increased pulse rate, general weakness, and icterus. Diarrhea may occur about a week after the initial rise in temperature and may contain blood and mucus. The animals rapidly become emaciated and recumbent, and the respiration is accelerated with dyspnea and cough. In the terminal stage a frothy discharge often exudes from the nostrils. In the subacute form, which is encountered most often in calves and in partially immune animals, the symptoms are comparable to, but less severe than, those in the acute form; although recovery usually occurs, it may take several weeks for the effects of the infection to disappear totally. The mild form is characterized by listlessness and swelling of the superficial lymph nodes; these symptoms are not as marked as those in the more serious forms of the disease and persist for 3 to 7 days. Inapparent infections are symptomless and difficult to detect.

There is evidence that strains may differ in their interaction with the host. The properties of a given strain may result in syndromes which have uncommon symptoms such as jaundice, skin lesions, and signs of central nervous system involvement. 'Turning sickness', a syndrome which occurs in *T. parva* and possibly *T. mutans* infections and characterized by signs of central nervous system involvement, results from the localization of the organisms in the central nervous system. The organisms are not totally limited to the brain; macroschizonts are present in other tissues and appear transiently in the blood as these animals are infective to ticks. In enzootic areas this syndrome is observed in animals that appear to have partial immunity which prevents the development of an overt systemic infection. It is observed in cattle which had been moved within enzootic areas and are challenged by different strains.

There is little known about the disease caused by *Theileria* in various game animals. Occasionally, mortality is associated with the presence of large numbers of theilerial organisms in the tissues.

The syndromes caused by *T. lawrencei* are classified as peracute, acute, subacute, and mild. The peracute form is occasionally found, and the clinical signs observed are similar to those generally seen in *T. parva* infections with the additional occurrence of keratitis and muscle tremors in *T. lawrencei* infections. Death occurs within 3 to 4 days of the initial rise in temperature. The acute syndrome is the predominant form encountered; most clinical signs are comparable to those seen in *T. parva* infections, with the additional development of keratitis and photophobia. Corneal opacity is often observed in the latter stages of *T. lawrencei* infection and in some cases of *T. parva* infection. Paresis of the hindquarters occasionally develops. The subacute form is encountered in about 10% of affected animals; the signs are less obvious than in the more acute forms and the animals usually recover. The major clinical signs of the mild form of the disease are low fever, listlessness, and moderate swelling of lymph nodes. These symptoms may persist for 3 to 5 days, after which the animal makes a full recovery.

Diseases caused by *T. annulata* are peracute, acute, subacute, and chronic. The peracute form is characterized by symptoms comparable to those observed in *T. parva* infections with the additional observation of rare central nervous system symptoms. Anemia is commonly associated with hemaglobinuria, bilirubinemia and bilirubinuria. Compared to the acute form, the symptoms of the subacute and chronic diseases are less severe and occur over a longer period of time. Occasionally, the animals may develop symptoms that are either chronic or mild, but then the acute form evolves and death ensues.

Theileria mutans infections are usually symptomless or mild; however, acute forms of the disease occur on massive exposure to ticks in an enzootic region. The rare severe cases are characterized by intermittent fever, listlessness, and swelling of superficial lymph nodes. Heavy tick infestation may result in extensive inflammation and necrosis of the ears. The animals may also show anorexia, drooling, lachrymation, ophthalmia, marked loss of condition, diarrhea, anemia, and icterus. In the mild form slight anemia develops and there is rapid recovery.

Theileria hirci causes malignant theileriosis in sheep and goats which may be acute, subacute, or chronic. In the acute form there is fever with death following rapidly. The animals develop listlessness, malaise, nasal discharge, hyperemia of the conjunctiva, pallor of visible mucous membranes, icterus in advanced cases, tachycardia, dyspnea, and edema of the throat. The superficial lymph nodes are swollen and hemaglobinuria is frequently observed. In subacute and chronic cases the course of the disease is protracted and the symptoms which occur are comparable to those found in the acute form except that they are less marked. In the chronic form which may follow the acute syndrome, there may be pronounced anemia, listlessness, emaciation, and weakness.

Benign ovine and caprine theilerioses caused by *T. ovis* has been observed only in splenectomized animals. These cases exhibit fever, moderate swelling of the lymph nodes, and mild anemia, and then rapidly recover.

Literature

Although ECF has often been referred to in the literature as a fatal disease suggesting that death is the invariable outcome, there has been ample evidence that less severe syndromes are common. Despite the fact that in some regions of Africa 95% of all cattle infected with *T. parva* die, it has been documented that in some areas up to 25% of infected animals may recover (Shannon 1973). On the other hand, syndromes have been observed to be so severe that typical lesions did not develop (Aruo 1977). An examination of the medical records of animals naturally infected with *T. parva* revealed that there were no clinical signs which could be used in prognosis since symptoms ranged from mild to severe among 20 recovered cases (Shannon 1977). Under experimental conditions in drug trials, the morbidity and mortality rates of high-grade cattle exposed to *T. parva* were 87.6 and 95% respectively (Brocklesby *et al.* 1961). Experimental infection of similar cattle with *T. parva* showed that the incubation period averaged 14 days and the reaction period averaged 12 days with a remission of fever occurring in 12% of the cases. A strain of *T. parva* was isolated which caused a mortality rate of only 23%; the mortality rate was related to the number of ticks used in inducing the infection (Barnett and Brocklesby 1961). The virulence was increased by passage of the organism through cattle under experimental conditions (Brocklesby and Bailey 1968). Another strain of *T. parva* which was isolated from a wild tick population and passaged through cattle via *R. appendiculatus* and *R. kochi* caused mortality in only 25% of infected cattle; the death rate was proportional to the number of ticks used to induce infection. Since a number of animals became carriers after recovery, it has been suggested that survivors constitute a potential source of *T. parva* infection (Barnett and Brocklesby 1966c).

Experimentally induced *T. parva* and *T. lawrencei* infections were compared in cases where the syndromes were similar and the respective time courses of the diseases and mortality rates were the same. The characteristics which differentiated *T. lawrencei* infection from that of *T. parva* were signs of central nervous system involvement and complete anorexia in the latter. The enlargement of the peripheral lymph nodes in *T. lawrencei* infection persisted until the time of death, while in *T. parva* infection the initial enlargement was followed by a decrease in the size. A hundredfold increase of the dose used to induce *T. parva* infections reduced the time of onset for the majority of clinical signs and the duration of syndromes which terminated in death (Jura and Losos 1980).

Theileria annulata infection in indigenous calves was characterized by temperature elevation, enlargement of lymph nodes, and anemia; hemaglobinuria and severe jaundice were occasionally observed (Sharma and Gautam 1971). In exotic breeds the disease was characterized by fever, swelling of superficial lymph nodes, and marked anemia accompanied by hemaglobinuria (Gautam *et al.* 1970). *Theileria annulata* infection of Friesian cattle imported to Iraq from Europe caused a mortality rate of 29%, but the mortality in crossbred adults was only 0.3% (Yousif 1969). In Syria *T. annulata* infection in imported European cattle caused high mortality, but all locally bred cattle recovered (Giesecke and Weisenhütter 1965). An outbreak of *T. annulata* infection in Afghanistan was reported to have had an 80% incidence in 1- to 3-month-old calves with mortality at 50% (Bulman *et al.* 1979). The characteristics of the syndromes caused by a tick-transmitted virulent strain of *T. annulata* were also studied in crossbred calves (Srivastava and Sharma 1976a).

Three cases of acute fatal *T. mutans* infections were described in southeast Queensland, Australia. The characteristic signs were fever, anorexia, increased respiratory rate, pale and icteric mucous membranes, brown or red urine, anemia, and icterus (Rogers and Callow 1966). A pathogenic strain of *T. mutans* isolated in East Africa also caused a hemolytic syndrome marked by anemia and jaundice. Macroschizonts and microschizonts were observed in only 1 of 18 animals, but piroplasms were present in large numbers (Irvin *et al.* 1972c).

There has been increasing evidence that, under certain field conditions, *T. parva, T. lawrencei, T. annulata*, and *T. mutans* could result in syndromes which are characterized by signs of central nervous system involvement. In the old literature bovine cerebral theileriosis ('turning sickness') was defined as a fatal nervous condition which was characterized by circling or turning movements and an afebrile course (Schulz and Schutte 1957). According to reports, turning sickness usually occurred sporadically, but sometimes became epizootic and was responsible for significant economic losses. On certain farms, the syndrome was enzootic: it was found in calves 2 to 6 months of age more commonly than in adult animals and was associated with heavy tick infestation. A detailed description of the clinical signs of turning sickness was presented by Mettam and Carmichael (1936). In acute cases of turning sickness the onset was reported to be sudden – apparently healthy animals developed violent nervous symptoms such as spinning and turning in one direction until they became dizzy and then collapsed. The recumbent animal was comatose, showed very profuse salivation, twitching, trembling of muscles, and hyperesthesia. The duration of these violent clinical signs lasted up to 3 minutes. The eyelids were wide open with congestion of conjunctiva and pupillary dilatation. Between these fits the animals were observed to be depressed but the temperatures were normal. In the less acute syndromes the symptoms were milder and included the animals pushing their heads against solid objects. In both the acute and milder forms, the animals could be temporarily or permanently blind. In the chronic cases the animals were unthrifty, in poor condition, and blind as a result of corneal opacities. Recovery was not observed in those cases with typical clinical signs.

Cerebral theileriosis has been reported to occur in various regions of Africa. In a report of two cases from South Africa, macroschizonts were occasionally found in the peripheral blood, the superficial lymph nodes, and the spleen, but piroplasms were uncommon (Flanagan and Le Roux 1957). *Theileria mutans* was the suspect causative agent in another case from this region; theilerial schizonts were found in the blood vessels of the central nervous system, particularly those in the spinal cord (Tustin and Heerden 1979). Five more cases of bovine cerebral theileriosis in South Africa were described; in these animals thrombosis of the splenic blood vessels was associated with the presence of schizonts (Rensburg 1976). In a more recent report, an outbreak of disease in Masai cattle in Kenya was characterized by nervous signs and by the absence of piroplasms from the blood; schizonts were either absent or extremely rare in lymph nodes, spleen, liver, and lungs, but were present in the brain in very large numbers. Serological evidence supported the opinion that the etiologic agent was probably *T. parva* and not *T. mutans* (Giles *et al.* 1978).

Cerebral theileriosis caused by *T. annulata* was reported to occur infrequently, but schizonts have been observed in impression smears of the brain (Srivastava and Sharma 1976b). Nervous symptoms were observed during terminal stages of a disease caused by *T. annulata*, and schizonts were demonstrated in impression smears of the brain and tissues (Sharma and Gautam 1973).

Another relatively unusual clinical manifestation of theileriosis is the development of skin lesions. The occurrence of cutaneous lesions was associated with *Theileria* infestation for some time (Grimpret 1953). More recently, it was shown in experimental *T. parva* infections that three of five calves developed skin eruptions due to intradermal nodules containing numerous schizonts, and demodectic mites were also observed in the nodules of some of the cases (Uilenberg and Zwart 1979). In *T. annulata* infection in calves, numerous subcutaneous and intramuscular nodules were found scattered throughout the body, and bilateral exophthalmia also occurred (Baharsefat *et al.* 1977).

Sheep and goats were reported to be asymptomatic in *T. ovis*-induced theileriosis, while *T. hirci* infections caused severe illness (Raghvachari and Reddy 1956). Natural infection of sheep with *T. hirci* in enzootic areas resulted in a morbidity rate of 100% and a mortality of approximately 90%. This high morbidity and mortality in animals probably already exposed to *T. hirci* suggested the existence of antigenically different strains in different localities. The animal husbandry practices in countries such as Iraq involve the movement of sheep from one area to another in search of pasture during different seasons. Thus, newborn lambs might contract *T. hirci* infection due to strains that differed from those which challenged their dams (Hooshmand-Rad and Hawa 1973b; Hooshmand-Rad 1976).

PATHOLOGY

The pathogenesis of various forms of theileriosis is dependent either on the macroschizonts or on microschizont and piroplasm, or on the piroplasm alone. These injurious stages of the parasite vary with the theilerial species, e.g. macroschizonts appear to be the most pathogenic form of *T. parva*, *T. annulata* macroschizonts and piroplasms are associated with injurious mechanisms, and in *T. mutans* infections only the piroplasms cause tissue injury. In *T. parva* infections, pathogenesis is dependent either directly or indirectly on the effects of the schizont on the lymphoblastoid cells. The pathogenesis of *T. lawrencei* may differ from that of *T. parva* because the severity of the disease is not directly related to the number of schizonts which are observed. In *T. annulata* infection, there is destruction of the red blood cells by piroplasms in addition to the effects of the macroschizonts which result in bilirubinemia and bilirubinuria. In contrast, the mechanisms of injury in *T. mutans* and *T. sergenti* infections appear to be entirely associated with the proliferation of the piroplasms which cause anemia and sometimes jaundice in the very severe cases.

The development of lesions in the fatal cases of *T. parva* is dependent on the duration of the disease and on the strain. For example, in addition to causing extensive lymphoid organ hyperplasia, certain strains in South Africa have been reported to induce the development of pseudo-infarcts in the kidneys, which is consistently observed in eastern Africa. The macroscopic lesions in acute and subacute syndromes are similar in the diseases caused by *T. parva*, *T. lawrencei*, and *T. annulata*. The pathological picture is dominated by the changes which occur in the three components of the lymphoid system: the major lymphoid organs, the peripheral lymphoid tissues in various other organs and tissues, and the lymphocytes in the circulation.

On external observation, the carcass is usually emaciated with a variable amount of froth escaping from the nostrils. Enlargement of the peripheral lymph nodes varies in degree, and there may be evidence of diarrhea containing blood and mucus.

In the thoracic cavity there is hydrothorax and hydropericardium, and the lungs are distended, discolored, solid in texture, and filled with a large quantity of fluid which exudes from the bronchi and parenchyma. Stable froth is present in the bronchi and trachea. The visceral and parietal pleurae may have petechiae or ecchymotic hemorrhages. Similar hemorrhages may be present in the visceral and parietal peritonea.

In the abdominal cavity the liver is increased in size, friable, and often brownish-yellow in color with the gall bladder being markedly distended. The spleen is usually enlarged and soft with prominent Malpighian corpuscles. The internal lymph nodes are swollen and often show varying degrees of hemorrhage and necrosis. The kidneys may be pale, congested, or brown in color, and frequently have either small hemorrhagic or larger greyish-white nodules. The abomasum usually has multiple ulcers which on occasion are also found throughout the entire length of the small intestine in the enlarged Peyer's patches.

Microscopically, the lesions in the major lymphoid organs comprise proliferating lymphoblastoid cells and varying amounts of necrosis. Infected cells disseminate in the lung with resultant interstasial pneumonia and effusion of fluids into the alveolar tissue. In the peripheral lymphoid system, the different tissues and organs exhibit varying degrees of lymphoblastoid cell infiltration, which occurs with and without necrosis and is observed most often in the liver, kidneys, and the gastrointestinal tract and rarely in the heart, skeletal muscle, and nervous tissue.

In acute and chronic cases of *T. hirci* infection, the lesions are basically the same as those observed in bovine theileriosis. There is emaciation, marked anemia, and a variable degree of icterus. The liver may be increased in size, soft, friable, and yellowish-brown in color. The spleen may be enlarged and the lymph nodes may be enlarged and hemorrhagic.

Literature

The first lesion develops at the site of inoculation of the parasite. The infective stages of *T. parva* were observed to be associated with both granulocytes and lymphoid cells at the site of inoculation (Kimeto 1978). The changes in the lymph nodes draining the site of infection became apparent in 3 to 4 days (before the onset of pyrexia), with an increase in mitosis and the appearance of lymphoblastoid cells. Cell destruction occurred with the continued proliferation of schizonts and the infiltration of neutrophils and macrophages (Wilde 1963). The sequential changes in the local lymph nodes consisted of an initial multiplication of lymphocytes and reticular cells which was soon complicated by the degeneration and necrosis of these lymphocytes. This process resulted in the development of large areas of necrosis. In those animals which survived a few days longer, there was some evidence of regenerative lymphocytic proliferation. Comparable changes were observed in other lymph nodes (Barnett 1960). There was some variation in the frequency, size, and distribution of the changes observed in the lymph nodes in various parts of the body. In the early phase of infection, lymphocytic cells were depleted due to the loss of small immature lymphocytes; large- and medium-sized lymphoid cells increased in number and became clusters of necrotic lymphoid cells which coalesced to form large areas of necrosis. Fluid exudate and fibrin accumulation in varying amounts were associated with the lymphocytic necrosis.

Variations in the condition of the spleen were comparable to those observed in the lymph nodes (de Kock 1957). In cattle dying of *T. parva* infection, the spleens were small, which indicated that they were depleted of lymphocytes. A depletion of lymphocytes occurred from the nodules, and there was disruption and destruction of lymphocytopoietic centres (Barnett 1960). The spleen was enlarged in 21 of the 54 naturally infected animals, shrunken in 5, and normal in 28 (Bwangamoi *et al.* 1971).

In the myeloid tissue the development of granulocytic series was arrested, bone marrow cells were destroyed, and the percentage of lymphocytes was increased (Wilde 1966b). The severe panleukopenia could not be correlated with the level of parasitemia. The injection of *Hyalomma pertussis* bacteria was known to cause a marked increase in the number of lymphocytes and neutrophils in circulating blood. However, it did not prevent the development of leukopenia when it was administered before infection, during the incubation period, or during patent disease (Wilde 1963). It was concluded that the myeloid tissue changes occurred in three phases: a transient stage of stimulation, a prolonged destruction, and an increase in the immature cells of all series. It was suggested that these changes were the result of a diffusible toxin liberated by the parasite (Barnett 1960). Large numbers of parasitized lymphoblasts were present in the paracortical zone, sinuses, and medullary cords; in *T. parva* infections nonspecific changes have been reported to occur in the lymph nodes. These changes were characterized by germinal center development and regression, paracortical hyperplasia, and plasmacytosis. Free schizonts were numerous during the latter phases of the disease, and terminal necrosis was common (DeMartini and Moulton 1973a). Lymph from tracheal and thoracic ducts contained increased numbers of large lymphocytes as the result of the presence of antigenically stimulated lymphoblasts and variable numbers of parasitized lymphoblasts from the central lymph (DeMartini and Moulton 1973b). There were significant differences in the hematological changes observed in *T. parva* and *T. lawrencei* infections, e.g. a high terminal peripheral blood lymphocytosis and a depression of bone marrow erythropoiesis occurred in the latter disease (Hill and Matson 1970; Maxie *et al.* 1982). *Theileria lawrencei* and *T. parva* caused panleukopenia and hypoproteinemia; in addition, the latter infection was associated with mild normocytic, normochronic, nonresponsive anemia. Disseminated intravascular coagulation was observed in both types of infections and was regarded as an important intermediate development causing death (Maxie *et al.* 1982).

Lesions in various organ and tissue systems were often associated with the peripheral component of the lymphoid system which consisted of lymphoid infiltration and nodules in the connective tissue stroma. In addition to other macroscopic lesions commonly observed in ECF, macroscopic lymphoid aggregates (the so-called pseudo-infarcts) were observed in the gall bladder, heart, and small intestine of naturally infected cattle in Kenya (Bwangamoi *et al.* 1971). The erosion and ulcers in the mucous membranes of the gastrointestinal tract resulted from localized superficial necrosis associated with extensive proliferation of lymphoblastoid cells in the propria. Lymphoblastoid cell infiltration varied in severity in the kidney and resulted in nodular or diffuse accumulations; the infiltrations in the liver were mainly periportal. In the lungs lymphoblastoid cells aggregated around the bronchi and related blood vessels and were diffusely disseminated throughout the parenchyma (de Kock 1957). In addition to the other changes often observed in *T. parva* infections, 6 out of 27 afflicted cattle demonstrated lymphocytic infiltration of the blood vessels of the brain (Munyua *et al.* 1973). Perivascular lymphoblastoid cell infiltrations were more commonly observed in *T. lawrencei* infection than in *T. parva* and were associated with clinical signs of central nervous system malfunction (Losos and Jura in preparation). The occasionally observed skin eruptions were due to intradermal nodules which contained numerous theilerial schizonts and macroscopic infiltrations of lymphoblastoid cells. These eruptions have to be differentiated from the lesions caused by demodectic mites (Uilenberg and Zwart 1979).

In acute cases of turning sickness the lesions were hemorrhagic, while in chronic syndromes there was necrosis, atrophy, fibrosis, and cavity formation, with the lesions being most prominent in the white matter of one or both of the cerebral hemispheres. The occurrence of other gross and histological lesions characteristic of theileriosis was usually rare. The predominant microscopic lesion in the brain and pia mater consisted of a partial or complete blockage of the smaller arteries and arterioles by dense masses of lymphoblastoid cells infected with schizonts. In chronic cases the schizonts were less common and sometimes difficult to find. It was noticed that schizonts quickly disappeared from tissues which were undergoing decomposition. These emboli were responsible for extensive blocking of the blood vessels over large areas of the brain and gave rise to vascular thrombosis. This was accompanied by increased numbers of cells in the adventitial tissue which caused perivascular cuffing. Increases in globulin and total protein were observed in cerebrospinal fluid (Carmichael and Jones 1939). It was concluded that cerebral forms of theileriosis were due to either thrombosis of blood vessels in the brain by parasitized lymphocytes, or to perivascular infiltrations of these cells. The latter lesions are more commonly observed, particularly in those infections caused by *T. lawrencei* and some strains of *T. parva* (Losos and Jura in preparation).

The macroscopic and microscopic lesions caused by *T. annulata* were comparable to those produced by *T. parva* and *T. lawrencei* with the additional finding of anemia accompanied by icterus in acute cases (Neitz 1957). The intracellular development of *Theileria* was recorded in a variety of cells (Vulchovski and Pavlov 1970). However, this does not conform with the generally accepted belief that theilerial infections are limited to lymphocytes. *Theileria annulata* schizonts were present in the lymphoblastoid cells of an unusual ocular lesion in cattle which was characterized by swelling of the eyelids and ulceration of the conjunctiva (Khalid and Jawad 1967). Anemia, thrombocytopenia, and leukopenia developed without regenerative changes in the bone marrow and were observed before the appearance of piroplasms (Laiblin 1978). In the acute phase of both acute and chronic *T. annulata* infections, hypoproteinemia was accompanied by increases in the alpha and beta globulin fractions; in the chronic phase these fractions became almost normal but the gamma globulin component increased significantly (Dhar and Gautam 1979). In both chronic and acute *T. annulata* infection, the serum concentration of bilirubin was increased while that of calcium was decreased; no changes occurred in the serum sodium and potassium levels (Dhar and Gautam 1977a). The variable degree of icterus was associated with the liver being enlarged, discolored yellow, and friable. There was accompanying anemia with an erythrocytic infection rate of 15%, and schizonts were observed in the smears from the liver (Hooshmand-Rad and Hawa 1973b). The hepatic damage was indicated by changes in the activity of the enzymes glutamic oxalactic transaminase, sorbitol dehydrogenase, and aldolase and an increase in bilirubin levels during the latter stage of the disease. There was no apparent involvement of the kidney (Laiblin *et al.* 1978).

In acute cases of *T. mutans* infection, anemia and jaundice were observed (Irvin *et al.* 1972c), and changes in the blood consisted of poikilocytosis, anisocytosis, polychromocia, metachromucia, vasophilic granulation, and macrocytosis (Saidu 1981). The macroscopic and microscopic lesions observed were described by Saidu (1982) and differed from those recorded in *T. parva* and *T. lawrencei* infections. The lesions were found in the lymph nodes, liver, spleen, and kidneys. Although lymphoid cell hyperplasia occurred in the infiltrations, the lesions were not severe and there was no necrosis, thus suggesting that the pathogenesis of *T. mutans* infection is primarily associated with parasitism of the red blood cells.

IMMUNOLOGY

Antigens

Piroplasm and schizont antigens have been used in the investigation of theilerial infections. Antigenically different strains are recognized in *T. parva* and *T. annulata* and consist of antigenic components common to all strains and other components which are strain-specific. Antigenic diversity probably occurs in all forms of theileriosis.

Literature

The study of theilerial antigens is dependent on the methods used in the preparation of the antigens and on the standardization of these techniques. A number of methods have been used to isolate and identify both piroplasm and macroschizont antigens. The piroplasm antigen of *T. parva* was isolated by sonication or by French pressure cell disruption and was partially separated from the erythrocyte antigen by differential ammonium sulphate precipitation. It had a wide molecular weight range of 4 to 20 million and a sedimentation coefficient of 7 to 15*S* (Wagner *et al*. 1974b). A three-stage method used to separate macroschizonts from intact host cells resulted in a collection of relatively pure macroschizonts (Nyormoi *et al*. 1981). A bovine lymphoid cell culture infected with *T. parva* had no specific parasite antigen on the surface detectable by either the FA technique or by antibody-dependent cell-mediated cytotoxicity. The infected cells had a common antigen with normal thymic lymphocytes and possessed a transplantation antigen (Duffus *et al*. 1978). Serologically specific antigens of *T. parva* were extracted from schizonts and shown to have a molecular weight in the region of 200 000 to 400 000 and a sedimentation coefficient of approximately 7*S* (Wagner *et al*. 1974a). The agar-gel precipitation test showed that a number of antigens were common to the blood and lymph nodes of *T. parva*-infected animals (Gourlay and Brocklesby 1967). Further investigation of each type of antigen revealed that the precipitating antigens of *T. parva* schizonts and piroplasms shared the same specificity and had considerable molecular heterogeneity which was considered a result of the preparative methods. The fact that these antigens contained large amounts of deoxyribonucleic acid indicated that both were of nuclear origin. The antigens were weakly antigenic and their reactivity with humoral antibodies from recovered animals was low (Allsopp *et al*. 1977).

Serology

Of major importance to the work on theileriosis is the availability of reliable serological tests. Several different tests have been developed in order to diagnose infection, define species and strains, monitor serological responses, and assess immunity. Complement fixation (CF), indirect immunofluorescence, capillary agglutination and indirect hemagglutination are some of the methods commonly employed. The IFA technique is the most useful. The efficient serological diagnostic test depends on the availability of suitable antigens and the reproducibility of the technique. For example, schizont antigens derived from tissue cultures are preferred to piroplasm antigens because their greater specificity and reliability enable greater standardization of tests.

Literature

Using the single radial immunodiffusion test, it was shown that cattle dying of *T. parva* infection had a marked reduction in the concentrations of IgM and protein designated as *7S* alpha$_1$ with an accompanying decrease in the levels of IgG$_1$ but not of IgG$_2$. In cattle recovered from severe infection, the drop in the titers of the three immunoglobulins and the protein occurred during the peak of clinical reaction, and the immunoglobulin levels returned to preinfection levels within 5 days. The Ig$_1$ and IgM titers continued to rise after recovery and peaked by day 28; thereafter, they fell slowly to preinfection levels. Cattle recovered from mild infections had negligible changes in their Ig$_1$ and Ig$_2$ titers but did have a rise in IgM and a slight fall in *7S* alpha$_1$ (Spooner *et al.* 1973). In severe cases of *T. parva*-induced infection there was sequential production of IgM and *7S* Ig antibody (Wagner *et al.* 1975). Specific classes of IgM and IgG of antibodies appeared 18 to 36 days after infection of cattle with *T. annulata* and persisted up to 120 days (Goldman and Pipano 1978). The IgM and IgG antibodies were detected in calves with *T. sergenti* infection by means of the IFA test (Takahashi *et al.* 1976).

The IFA test was regarded as a more reliable method of predicting immunity in cattle infected with *T. parva* and was a more efficient tool for diagnosing infection than the method involving the demonstration of schizonts in Giemsa-stained lymph node biopsy smears (Burridge 1971). The collection of blood on filter paper was found to be as efficacious as the use of serum in the routine serological screening of cattle by means of the IFA test (Burridge and Kimber 1972a, b; Kimber and Burridge 1972). Differences in the sensitivity of the test were observed with respect to schizont and piroplasm antigens; antibody titers demonstrable for a longer period of time when schizont antigens were used (Burridge and Kimber 1972b). Significant antibody titers to *T. parva* cell culture schizont antigen were demonstrated 12 to 73 weeks after infection with a mean of 29.7 weeks while titers to the piroplasm antigen were detected 7 to 25 weeks after infection with a mean of 13.5 weeks (Burridge and Kimber 1973a). The colostrum of cows immune to *T. parva* contained a higher concentration of antibodies to schizont and piroplasm antigens than that observed in the sera of these animals (Burridge and Kimber 1973b). The IFA technique showed that cattle with mechanically or cyclically induced *T. mutans* infection had antibody titers against piroplasm antigen which persisted for periods of over 1 year. However, an antibody response to schizont antigens was elicited only in animals with tick-induced infections obtained from lymph node biopsy material (Kimber and Young 1977). Antibodies against *T. sergenti* were detected by the IFA and CF tests; the former was shown to be more sensitive in surveys of infected cattle (Fujinaga and Minami 1981). Peak antibody titers were detected 24 days after *T. hirci* infection using schizont antigens from cultures of lymphoblastoid cells (Hawa *et al.* 1976). The detection of serum antibodies to intraerythrocytic parasites by means of immunofluorescence was often made difficult by the presence of extensive background fluorescence. Because the animal which donated the antigen had hemolytic anemia, antigens were released into the plasma; hence, the FA stained other intracellular components as well as the parasites (Löhr and Ross 1968).

Other serological tests have also been found to be useful. Hemagglutination inhibition, indirect hemagglutination, agar-gel precipitation, capillary tube agglutination, CF and conglutinating complement absorption proved to be more reliable methods of examining latent *T. annulata* infections than the examination of blood smears (Dhar and Gautam 1977b, c, d). Complement-fixing antibodies to tissue culture schizonts were detected in the sera of *T. annulata*-infected or vaccinated animals for up to 100 days (Hooshmand-Rad and Hashemi-Fesharki 1971). Using *T. parva* piroplasm antigens, an indirect hemagglutination test was developed to detect antibodies in *T. parva* infections (Duffus and Wagner 1974b). Conglutination and conglutinating complement-absorption tests were also used to detect *T. parva* infections in cattle, but these techniques were difficult to standardize and of questionable utility (Cawdery *et al.* 1968). The piroplasm antigen was used in the enzyme-linked immunosorbent assay to detect antibodies to *T. parva* and *T. annulata,* and the patterns of antibody production were comparable to those detected by the IFA test (Gray *et al.* 1980).

Antibody response to *Theileria* parasites can be measured by titration against various known theilerial antigens including those of *T. annulata, T. parva, T. lawrencei,* and *T. mutans.* The antigens of cell culture schizonts give greater specificity than piroplasm antigens in the indirect fluorescent antibody test (Burridge *et al.* 1974b). When tested by indirect immunofluorescence, the antigens of *T. lawrencei* and *T. parva* mutually cross-react with the sera of cattle recovering from these two infections, thus indicating a close antigenic relationship (Burridge *et al.* 1973; Lawrence 1977; Schindler *et al.* 1969a). *Theileria parva, T. annulata,* and *T. mutans* could be differentiated serologically when homologous antigens were used in the CF and IFA tests (Schindler and Wokatsch 1965). Schizont antigen prepared from cultured lymphoid cells infected with *T. parva* was effective and no serological cross-reaction was detected with sera from cattle infected with *T. mutans* piroplasms (Burridge and Kimber 1972b). The IFA antibody test could detect some cross-reactions between *T. parva* and *T. mutans* antigens at lower titers in infected cattle, while the CF test was more efficient in differentiating single mixed infections (Schindler and Mehlitz 1969).

The capillary tube agglutination test could also be used to distinguish the piroplasm antigens of *T. parva* and *T. mutans,* and cross-reactivity was noted only with undiluted sera. The simplicity of this test makes it useful for laboratory and field application (Ross and Löhr 1972). *Theileria mutans* was serologically distinguishable from other East African species of *Theileria* by indirect immunofluorescence (Kimber and Young 1977). Using the IFA test, *T. gorgonis* was found to be antigenically distinct from *T. parva, T. lawrencei* and *T. mutans* (Burridge and Kimber 1973c). There was no cross-reaction between *H. veliferus* and either *T. parva* or *T. mutans* in the IFA test. A theilerial species in Britain was distinguishable from *T. mutans* isolated from eastern and southern Africa on the basis of antibody specificity in the IFA test (Morzaria *et al.* 1977). The British *T. mutans* was indistinguishable from the Japanese *T. sergenti* (Joyner *et al.* 1979). Complement fixation was used to differentiate *T. parva* and *T. annulata. Theileria annulata* antigens did not cross-react with those of *T. parva* or *T. mutans* (Dhar and Gautam 1977f). The enzyme-linked immunosorbent assay also indicated a closer antigenic similarity between *T. parva* and *T. annulata* than between either one of these species and *T. mutans, T. sergenti,* and *T. velifera* (Gray *et al.* 1980).

Immunity

Cattle and buffalo are the only mammals that do not have a strong innate resistance to *T. parva*. Young cattle are more resistant to theileriosis in areas where the disease is enzootic. The immunity is relatively stable, wanes slowly with age, and is not influenced by the virulence of *T. parva* challenge. In calves from immune dams, decreasing natural resistance to disease with age is not correlated with the waning passive immunity derived from colostrum since calves from susceptible dams are more resistant at 1 month of age than at 4 months of age. It is proposed that cattle living for generations in enzootic areas have undergone a process of selection; the resultant population possesses greater resistance which is most highly developed in calves. Persistence of immunity in enzootic areas is dependent on constant reinfection with the various strains in the enzootic area. The immunity to *T. parva* is almost certainly stimulated by the microschizont rather than the piroplasm. Premunition is usually established in the animals that recover from theilerial infection. Small numbers of piroplasms persist in these animals, which therefore become a source of infection for ticks for years and possibly for life. The resistance to challenge with homologous strains of *Theileria* is almost total, but this wanes slowly over a period of years with the animals surviving reexposure to comparable antigenic strains. However, challenge with heterologous strains usually results in diseases of varying clinical severity and incidence of mortality.

Immunization processes with live organisms which generate resistance for prolonged periods of time always present the possibility of creating a carrier state which may be infective for ticks. This situation varies with different species of *Theileria* and changes with the adaptation of a species to a host. The cross-immunity between *T. parva* and *T. lawrencei* is partially effective; *T. lawrencei* induces a greater protection against *T. parva* than vice versa. Cattle which recover from

T. mutans infection and sheep and goats which survive *T. ovis* infection develop durable premunition with piroplasms persisting throughout life. Young calves 6 to 7 months of age are resistant to *T. annulata* infection, while animals that recover from natural infections of *T. annulata* have durable immunity which decreases after 3 years. Reinfection of immune and partially immune cattle results in nonfatal disease which varies in severity depending upon the strain and the extent of challenge. Antigenically different strains occur in enzootic areas and have some antigenic components in common and others which are strain-specific.

There are other factors which influence the effectiveness of the acquired immunity. In the older literature it was reported that the breakdown of premunition with *T. annulata* occurred following immunization against rinderpest, and a relatively severe systemic reaction to the vaccine subsequently developed. Other severe stresses or heavy reinfestations by *Theileria* can also result in the breakdown of the resistance, thus causing clinical disease and the occasional death.

There is ample evidence that humoral immunologic responses are not directly associated with acquired immunity. Although some workers have reported the therapeutic effect of administering whole blood from recovered animals in cases of *T. annulata* infection, the immune factor is probably cellular and acts against either the parasitized host cell or the intracellular parasite. Some investigators have also suggested that the immune factor is not only cellular but is also produced within the parasitized cell.

Literature

The importance of humoral and cellular immunologic responses in producing resistance were summarized by Allison and Eugui (1980). Although antibodies to various parasite antigens could be detected by a number of serological methods, there was no evidence regarding their significance in the development of immunity. The cellular reactions which occurred in some forms of theileriosis, e.g. the dissemination of infected lymphoid cells throughout the body and the proliferation of clones of specific cytotoxic cells able to lyse xenogeneic and allogeneic infected cells, would appear to have a more direct role in the development of resistance.

The administration of immune serum or concentrated globulins did not affect either the establishment of infection or, in cattle infected with a *T. parva* stabilate, the clinical hematological changes or the mortality rate (Muhammed *et al.* 1975). Also, hyperimmune serum had no therapeutic value with respect to the course of disease caused by *T. annulata* (Dhar and Gautam 1978), although in the older literature there were statements regarding the beneficial effect of whole blood. Bovine antisera against the transplantation antigens could initiate the destruction of the cultured cells by normal bovine mononuclear cells in antibody-dependent cell-mediated cytotoxicity. It was considered that an anamnestic response against these transplantation antigens was responsible for the defective immunity that exists in cattle recovering from *T. parva* infections (Duffus *et al.* 1978).

Because immunity could not be directly related to the action of antibodies and could not be transferred between twins through the thoracic duct leukocytes, it was suggested that resistance might be associated with cell-mediated mechanisms. In *T. parva* infections cytotoxicity was mediated by the lysis of allogeneic parasitized cells and xenogeneic uninfected cells (Eugui and Emery 1981). The autologous mixed leukocyte reaction indicated that the cell-mediated immunity occurred at the later stages of infection and was associated with the continued multiplication of infected lymphoblasts (Emery and Morrison 1980). Using sensitized peripheral leukocytes, migration inhibition of cultured bovine lymphoblastoid cells was found to persist for 8 months after *T. parva* infection (Muhammed *et al.* 1975). The Rosette test was used to investigate cellular immunological responses (Duffus and Wagner 1974a).

The resistance to lethal challenge with *T. parva* was established by transferring 5 to 9 × 10^{10} syngeneic thoracic duct leukocytes from one chimeric bovine twin to another, thus indicating that the circulating lymphocytes conferred resistance (Emery 1981). Lymphoblastoid cells infected with *T. parva* express antigens recognized by effector cells which are involved in the cell-mediated cytotoxicity functions. These cytotoxic cells kill *Theileria*-transformed cells and the effector cells may be used to measure the immunity mechanism (Pearson *et al.* 1979). The effector cells which caused the cytotoxicity against parasitized autologous lymphocytes were T-lymphocytes rather than either antibody-dependent cellular toxicity or macrophages (Emery *et al.* 1981b). The migration of cultured bovine lymphoblastoid cells was inhibited *in vitro* by the peripheral leukocytes obtained from cattle vaccinated against *T. parva,* and this phenomenon could be associated with limiting the dissemination of infected lymphocytes throughout the body in immune cattle (Muhammed 1975). The study of autologous mixed lymphocyte reactions and the examination of specific and nonspecific cytotoxicity against cultured leukocytes obtained from lethal and nonlethal infections have led to the conclusion that the control of infection is associated with specific cell-mediated responses mounted against parasite-induced antigens in combination with polymorphic host antigens on the leukocyte membrane (Emery *et al.* 1981a).

The immunity of *T. annulata* was comparable to that acquired against *T. parva,* with resistance developing in the animals which recovered from infections involving homologous but not heterologous strains; the administration of gamma globulin obtained from field cases did not affect the course of the disease (Hooshmand-Rad 1976). Peripheral lymphocytes from *T. annulata*-infected cattle inhibited the migration of macrophages, thus indicating that sensitized lymphocytes are the effector cells of cell-mediated immunity. Using different Rosette techniques, it was shown that both T and B-lymphocytes were stimulated during *T. annulata* infections (Rehbein *et al.* 1981). The migration of peripheral leukocytes collected from cattle carrying *T. annulata* was inhibited by the presence of piroplasm antigen, and the fact that these animals were sensitized to this antigen indicated that sensitized leukocytes persisted in recovered animals (Singh *et al.* 1977). It was concluded that lymphoid cells containing *Theileria* schizonts undergo antigenic changes and are destroyed by immune lymphoid cells (Hooshmand-Rad 1976).

VACCINATION

A number of methods have been used to immunize cattle against the various forms of theilerioses. The intravenous administration of suspension of spleen and lymph nodes from infected animals causes 25% mortality but the survivors are immune. The difficulty of this method, which was the first to be tried, instigated the development of simpler methods of harvesting and preserving infective particles from ticks and macroschizonts from tissue cultures. Using these techniques, considerable effort is being made to immunize cattle against the different theilerioses. The development of a vaccine is based on the principle that immunogenesis is caused by infections in which the organism becomes established without causing pronounced clinical signs; dead organisms are not effective in generating immunity.

Vaccination with titrated doses of infective particles produces unacceptable variation in the immune response. This may be due in part to an inadequate dispersion of the infective particles during the dilution of the suspension. Irradiation modifies the course of infection by sublethally damaging the organisms, thus decreasing their virulence. They are capable of establishing an infection but cannot multiply sufficiently to cause clinical disease. Increasing doses of radiation slowed the development of the parasite in the ticks. This technique is not satisfactory because of the narrow safety margins between sublethal and lethal infections.

Cattle can be immunized by a method based on suppressing the parasite virulence chemoprophylactically; four daily treatments of oxytetracycline are effective against a variety of stabilated *T. parva* strains. Protection was conferred against challenge by homologous and by other strains, but not all strains of *T. parva*. A single laboratory strain of *T. parva* is not suitable for the development of a monovalent chemoprophylactic vaccine; other strains have to be incorporated and a 'cocktail' of different strains is used. Animals immunized with the 'cocktail' have a mild or inapparent reaction to heterologous challenge. This method appears to be an effective form of vaccination against a variety of heterologous East African strains of *Theileria*. However, under experimental conditions, the vaccinated animals are often challenged by a single, normally lethal dose of tick-derived infected stabilate, whereas in the field the continuous challenge could influence the efficacy of this type of vaccination. Further investigations of the effects of continuous challenge on vaccinated cattle in experimentally infected paddocks show that the cattle are protected against very severe homologous challenge. The successful application of this vaccination technique in the field depends on the selection of appropriate strains of *Theileria* in a particular enzootic area. Although there are definite indications that the method engenders resistance to challenge under certain circumstances in the field, it is not consistently successful. The utilization of local strains provides the safest vaccines because it enhances the probability of selecting the appropriate strains of *Theileria* and prevents the introduction of theilerial strains which have been isolated from other areas. The application of a universal vaccine, i.e. one that is composed of the strains found throughout various enzootic areas, will depend on further investigations of its efficacy under field challenge, preferably in the absence of carrier states which further complicate the epizootiology of theileriosis.

Tissue culture methods for vaccinating against *T. parva* and *T. annulata* have been developed. Cattle inoculated with a minimum dose of 10^7 tissue culture lymphoblasts parasitized with *T. parva* macroschizonts become infected. The organism completes its bovine life cycle with the development of macroschizonts, microschizonts, and intraerythrocytic piroplasms. The responses to this form of vaccination with *T. parva* are variable and include animals which do not react, those which react severely and recover, and a few which die. The inoculation of *T. annulata*-infected tissue culture lymphoblasts induces infections which are limited to the development of macroschizonts.

The tissue culture method is effective and widely used with *T. annulata* infections. Partial or complete attenuation of virulence of *T. annulata* schizonts is achieved by cultivation. Low passages of cultured cells cause clinical theileriosis; schizonts appear in the lymph nodes and liver and piroplasms develop later in the peripheral blood. Further passages reduce the virulence and cause complete attenuation without clinical signs, and schizonts and piroplasms are usually absent. However, some strains continue to produce schizonts but not piroplasms even after 300 or more passages. Stress may induce clinical theileriosis in the animals infected with these strains. The attenuated schizonts appear to have the same immunological properties as the virulent schizonts. There is no cross-immunity to infections engendered by schizonts and piroplasms. Immunization with living macroschizonts protects against tick-derived infection, but the resistance is never absolute and infected immunized animals show some parasites and fever. Vaccines can be maintained and stored in a frozen state for long periods of time; the shelf life at 4 °C is 3 to 4 days. The tissue culture method is safe in all breeds of cattle, including pregnant cows, and protection varies with the age and breed. Adult cattle of most breeds are protected by vaccination with the exception of adult Friesian dairy cows which develop clinical signs. The reinfection of immunized cattle enhances their resistance to any subsequent severe challenge.

Literature

Neitz (1964) reviewed the immunization procedures using *T. parva* and concluded that sterile immunity did not exist and piroplasms were always present although often in extremely low numbers. This latent form of infection was responsible for the recrudescence of diseases on farms where several years had elapsed between outbreaks. Based on field observation in enzootic areas, animals exposed to *T. parva* and *T. mutans* appeared to acquire solid immunity to local theilerial strains despite evidence of the existence of immunologically different strains (Robson *et al.* 1981). Cattle experimentally vaccinated with *T. parva* by a variety of methods and challenged subsequently at various periods of time (up to 43 months) had a gradual increase in the mild febrile reaction which was related to the time after vaccination and indicated a progressive loss of resistance. The extent of the immunity was not related to the severity of the initial reaction. It was concluded that, on an antigenic basis, only one species of *Theileria* is essentially involved in the epizootiology of the disease referred to as ECF. The species has two strains, the phylogenetically older *T. lawrencei*, and its variant *T. parva*, which had adapted to cattle. Therefore, vaccines for use in all parts of East Africa must include as many antigenic variants of *T. lawrencei* as possible (Löhr 1978).

Some of the attempts at vaccination using infected tissues and irradiation were partially successful. Cattle vaccinated intravenously with macroschizonts obtained from lymph nodes of *T. parva*-infected animals developed partial protection against tick-derived challenge with homologous strains (Pirie *et al.* 1970). Vaccination with splenic material from animals infected with *T. parva* also produced significant amounts of immunity (Brocklesby *et al.* 1965). Radiation at doses of 20 and 30 krad reduced the virulence of *T. parva* in infested *R. appendiculatus* ticks, thus subclinical infection was produced (Munyua *et al.* 1973). Since there was no conclusive evidence that infective particles which survived irradiation were attenuated, this method was not useful in the development of a vaccination procedure (Cunningham *et al.* 1973d). Immunization of cattle with bacillus-Calmette-Guérin, a *Mycobacterium bovis* vaccine, was ineffective in providing nonspecific resistance to *T. parva* infection (Dolan *et al.* 1980a).

The immunization of cattle against theileriosis via lymphoblastoid cell lines transformed by *T. parva* required a definite quantity of cells and passage of a specific *T. parva*-infected cell line to induce effective immunity to tick-derived homologous challenges (Brown *et al.* 1978). The effectiveness of tissue culture appeared to be dependent on the lymphocyte antigens. Normal lymphocyte antigen was compared to the antigens from lymphoblastoid cell lines infected with *T. parva* and *T. annulata*. The phenotypes of the lymphoblastoid cell lines were identical to the antigens observed in the animal that donated cells which originated the cell line. Histocompatibility differences were more relevant to *T. parva*-infected cell lines than in those parasitized by *T. annulata*. Approximately one-tenth as many *T. annulata*-infected cells as *T. parva*-infected cells are required to initiate effective immunity. It was suggested that the lymphocyte antigens also played a role in the acceptability of the *T. parva*-infected cell lines by vaccinated cattle (Spooner and Brown 1980).

The most successful vaccinations against *T. parva* have involved infection and treatment methods. The early work on the use of tetracyclines was reviewed by Brocklesby and Bailey (1965). It was subsequently shown that immunization by chemoprophylaxis was possible against a variety of *T. parva* strains. Solid immunity developed against homologous challenges, but incomplete immunity arose against heterologous laboratory challenges, resulting in the occurrence of mild to severe clinical reactions (Radley *et al.* 1975a, c). The method involved the simultaneous injection of infective particles of *T. parva* derived from *R. appendiculatus* ticks and oxytetracycline. Injection of N-pyrrolidinomethyl tetracycline at doses of 5 mg/kg q.i.d. starting on the day of infection minimized the clinical reaction observed with other tetracyclines and resulted in 100% immunity to homologous challenge (Brown *et al.* 1977a).

The combination of three strains in a 'cocktail' and treatment was partially successful in engendering an immunity which withstood some heterologous challenges in the field but none with *T. lawrencei* (Radley 1978). Further cross-immunity trials using *T. parva* and *T. lawrencei* strains showed that partial protection was only obtained against heterologous laboratory challenges, particularly against *T. lawrencei*, which would have to be included in a multiple-strain vaccine to be applicable in the field (Radley *et al.* 1975b).

The chemoprophylactic method of immunization was improved by the application of long-acting tetracycline in a single injection. It was shown that cattle immunized with a 'cocktail' consisting of two *T. parva* strains and one *T. lawrencei* variant withstood experimental challenge against field isolates of *T. parva*. The immunized cattle had either mild or inapparent reactions (Dolan *et al.* 1980b). It was also proposed that immunization by similar methods could prevent the development of the high parasitemia caused by natural tick-borne infections of pathogenic *T. mutans* (Uilenberg *et al.* 1976b, 1977a). It was concluded that cattle immunized against *T. parva* were not protected against challenge with *T. lawrencei* (Cunningham *et al.* 1974). However, even with this liability, it was considered that the infection and treatment method of bovine vaccination would prove to be of great value in controlling ECF (Cunningham 1978).

Additional research was undertaken using two experimental paddocks infested with *R. appendiculatus* ticks which carried either *T. parva* or *T. lawrencei*. Cattle that had been immunized by chemoprophylaxis and exposed to *T. parva*-infected ticks in an experimental paddock for 60 days survived the challenge (Radley *et al.* 1975d). The results of sequentially exposing vaccinated and control cattle to these experimentally infected paddocks led to the conclusion that the feeding of parasitized ticks on immune cattle over a period of time caused the loss of infection in the tick population (Radley *et al.* 1978).

Because of the incomplete cross-immunity between *T. parva* and *T. lawrencei* and the difficulty of immunizing against *T. lawrencei* itself, an immunization method was developed in which a combination of three theilerial strains, including a *T. lawrencei* variant, was administered in a so-called 'cocktail'. This technique provided incomplete protection against tick-borne *T. lawrencei* challenge in an experimental paddock infected by *T. lawrencei*, resulting in severe clinical reactions and 55% fatality in the vaccinated cattle. It was concluded that field immunization of cattle against *T. lawrencei* would be difficult due to the apparent number of antigenic variants of the parasite emanating from the buffalo population (Radley *et al.* 1979). Cattle immunized against *T. lawrencei* isolated from an experimental paddock were subsequently exposed to challenge in the same experimental paddock and survived without showing clinical signs. However, on one occasion a particular isolate from the paddock failed to protect fully against subsequent challenge and half of the animals died. This finding indicated that different immunogenic types of *T. lawrencei* occur in the buffalo, and the development of an effective vaccine for *T. lawrencei* may be hindered as a result (Young *et al.* 1977b). Further investigations involving the infection and chemoprophylaxis technique demonstrated that more than one antigenic type of *T. lawrencei* existed in the paddock. These antigenic types continued to mutate over a period of years. Therefore, in an epizootiological situation where *T. lawrencei* played a role, the antigenic types involved would have to be identified before successful vaccinations could be developed (Young *et al.* 1978c).

The next step in the development of a successful vaccine entailed exposing cattle which had been immunized against a strain of *T. parva* to field challenge. Although all vaccinated and control animals died in the first attempt, some protective effects of the immunization were evident. The deaths were attributed to a strain of *T. parva* which differed immunologically from the vaccination strain; moreover, the animals were coinfected with a pathogenic variant of *T. mutans* (Snodgrass *et al.* 1972). However, cattle vaccinated against three strains of *T. parva* and exposed to a massive and continued challenge of *T. parva* and *T. mutans* in an enzootic field condition were partially protected; deaths occurred approximately 70 days after exposure, while control cattle died after a period of 25 days (Robson *et al.* 1977). Another group of cattle immunized against strains of *T. parva* by the infection and treatment method was exposed to a site in Tanzania where there was a continuous influx of infected ticks from different regions of the country as a result of the importation of tick-infested cattle. In this situation, the infection and treatment method of immunization was found to be effective in preventing mortality (Uilenberg *et al.* 1977a). Uilenberg reviewed the results of these field trials and concluded that the infection and treatment method conferred a high degree (90 to 100%) of protection against moderate natural challenge with *Theileria* under field conditions, which ensured exposure to a wide variety of strains from different enzootic areas (Uilenberg *et al.* 1976b).

Vaccination against *T. annulata* had been initially attempted by the transfer of infected blood after serial passage through cattle. Strains which produced mild reactions were not as immunogenic as virulent strains and were less efficacious in protecting against field challenge; however, the latter caused unacceptable levels of morbidity and mortality. There has been little evidence that immunized animals could withstand tick-transmitted infections of varying intensities. More recently, it has been observed that cattle immunized with even moderately virulent strains and subsequently challenged with homologous or heterologous strains suffered severe reactions and died (Barnett 1978). In *T. annulata*-infected cattle, there was a correlation between the quantum of infection and the ensuing reaction, i.e. mild reactions were caused by one or two tick dose levels and severe responses were produced by a minimum of ten tick dose levels (Gill *et al.* 1977). Using three different strains of *T. annulata*, it was shown that increasing the quanta of infection did not reduce the incubation or prepatent periods. Although a minimum number of quanta was necessary for the establishment of infection and for the development of resistance, increasing the dose levels beyond this required minimum did not raise the level of protection (Hashemi-Fesharki 1978).

The virulence and immunogenicity of cultured *T. annulata* schizonts were described by Pipano (1979). Vaccines composed of *T. annulata*-infected tissue culture cells did not induce clinical signs or the appearance of piroplasms, and the animal's immune response could be measured by the FA test (Pipano and Cahana 1968; Pipano *et al.* 1969). *Theileria annulata* from the 80th to 200th passages through bovine lymphoid cells caused no clinical signs of theileriosis when injected into cattle (Pipano *et al.* 1973). Organisms grown in tissue culture lost the capacity to induce erythrocytic forms in cattle in parallel with the loss of virulence (Pipano and Israel 1971). In autologous systems, consisting of reinoculation of schizont-infected lymphocytes back into the original donor of the cells, macroschizonts were transferred to cells of the recipient host (Hooshmand-Rad 1976). A vaccine prepared from bovine lymphocytes infected with completely avirulent macroschizonts was cryopreserved and administered at doses of 2×10^6 macroschizonts. This vaccine induced an immune response which withstood challenge by *Theileria*-infected *H. detritum*, although transient fever and the rare schizont were detected in the liver. Under field conditions this vaccine provided sufficient protection to imported European breeds of cattle to ensure their survival in enzootic areas (Pipano 1975), and protected against severe tick challenge (Gill *et al.*

1976a). In enzootic areas, vaccination with attenuated cultured schizonts was successful and resulted in a high degree of protection against tick-transmitted challenge of most breeds of cattle. The one exception was adult Friesian cattle which, unlike other breeds, could succumb to field infection after vaccination (Pipano *et al.* 1981).

The infection and treatment methods used to combat *T. parva* infections were also found to be effective against *T. annulata*. Tick-induced theilerial infection and treatment with chlortetracycline at a dose of 16 mg/kg for 8 days prevented the development of severe clinical signs and induced solid resistance of severe homologous challenge (Gill *et al.* 1976a). A successful vaccination was prepared using one tick stabilate and simultaneous treatment with chlortetracycline administered orally at a dose of 16 mg/kg for 8 days (Gill *et al.* 1977). Another method involved vaccination with two or five tick-derived stabilates of *T. annulata* and simultaneous treatment either with one or two subcutaneous injections of long-acting oxytetracycline at 20 mg/kg or with chlortetracycline given orally at 16 mg/kg for 8 days; complete or partial suppression of clinical signs resulted. The effect of one dose of long-acting oxytetracycline was comparable in efficacy to eight treatments with chlortetracycline, while two doses of oxytetracycline almost completely suppressed the development of clinical responses (Gill *et al.* 1978). The intramuscular administration of rolitetracycline at 5 mg/kg on days 0 to 3 postinfection also resulted in the production of a relatively mild clinical reaction and the development of durable immunity to severe homologous challenge (Jagdish *et al.* 1979). It was also shown that treatment with 10 to 20 mg/kg of oxytetracycline for 2 to 12 days after infection engendered solid resistance to homologous stabilate challenge (Pipano *et al.* 1981). The immunological relationships among five strains of *T. annulata* were investigated in cross-immunity trials. It was found that using infection and treatment method protection was conferred against severe homologous challenge, and varying degrees of protection were produced against heterologous challenge (Gill *et al.* 1980).

Other methods of vaccination against *T. annulata* have proved less successful. Killed schizonts with Freund's adjuvant protected against blood challenge but not against the infective particles from ticks. Although serum antibodies could be demonstrated by the immunofluorescent test, there was no correlation between antibody titers and extent of protection (Pipano *et al.* 1977). Washed infected bovine erythrocytes injected intravenously were not infective or immunogenic (Srivastava and Sharma 1976c). Tissue cultures of bovine lymphocytes irradiated at 5 and 10 kR caused a relatively mild disease with low parasitemia, mortality, and morbidity, and induced resistance to tick-derived homologous challenge (Srivastava and Sharma 1977a). Stabilates prepared from the supernate material of infective ground-up ticks and irradiated at 6 or 10 krad caused a minimal clinical reaction, no mortality, and resistance to subsequent tick-derived homologous challenge (Singh *et al.* 1979b). Although these techniques result in less severe diseases with longer incubation periods, the reproducibility of these methods of immunoprophylaxis have not been established (Srivastava and Sharma 1977b).

CHEMOTHERAPY

There are a few drugs and administration regimes which have been proposed as effective treatments, but their efficacy has not been substantiated. Considerable effort has been made in the search for antitheilerial drugs. It is only recently that a few compounds have been shown to be effective against *T. parva in vitro* and *in vivo*. Tetracyclines are effective only when administered at the time of infection and thereafter for a variable period of time, depending on the formulation of the compound. Menoctone and hydroxynaphthoquinone have antischizont activity in addition to their antimalarial and anticoccidial effects. Methotrexate (amethopterin), a folate antagonist with wide application in cancer therapy, suppresses schizont development *in vitro*, but is only marginally effective *in vivo*. In cattle menoctone is very effective against experimentally induced *T. parva* infection, but when it is used prophylactically, schizont development is markedly suppressed leaving the cattle fully susceptible to subsequent challenge. In its therapeutic application, the drug rapidly arrests the development of schizonts, causing subsequent stages of the life cycle to occur only in low numbers.

Literature

Neitz (1957) surveyed the results of treatments with compounds in use at that time. Although considerable numbers of drugs were administered during the course of a theilerial infection, none proved effective. The one exception was Aureomycin: a dose of 100 mg/kg administered repeatedly during the incubation period of *T. parva* infection proved to be a schizonticide capable of suppressing nuclear division but was ineffective against the piroplasms. Thus, clinical disease failed to develop but solid immunity was produced. Tetracycline possessed the same prophylactic properties and Aureomycin. When administered together during the clinical course, Aureomycin and Tetramycin at doses of 10 mg/kg and pamaquin at 1 mg/kg exerted some effect, although fairly severe symptoms still developed. The daily administration of single antibiotics for 10 to 17 days had no effect. In a short review of the testing of 170 chemotherapeutic agents in East Africa, the therapeutic effects of tetracycline administered during the incubation period were confirmed, and results were tabulated (Wilde *et al.* 1966). The chemotherapy of piroplasmosis and theileriosis in farm animals in the USSR was reviewed by Mack (1957), who concluded that as yet there were no drugs which consistently influenced recovery from *T. annulata* infection, although the combination of some drugs appeared to give better results than single drugs. The efficacy of these drugs could not be adequately assessed because the conditions under which they were administered varied considerably, and insufficient numbers of cattle were used.

Tissue cultures of *T. annulata* have been used in the screening of compounds for their chemotherapeutic activity. Forty compounds, including antimalarials, trypanocides, and antibiotics, were tested and found to be inactive (Hawking 1958). A large number of compounds, including antimalarials, anticoccidials, antibabesials, and menoctone, were tested *in vitro* for their actions against *T. parva* and *T. annulata*. Only menoctone and methotrexate showed significant activities (McHardy 1978a; McHardy *et al.* 1976). In an *in vitro* study of the effect of naphthoquinones on *T. parva* infection, it was observed that the antischizont activity was associated with a 2-hydroxyl moiety (Boehm *et al.* 1981).

Further research was undertaken to determine the mode of action of the tetracyclines and to establish regimens. Daily treatment with 15 mg/kg of oxytetracycline hydrochloride (Terramycin) suppressed the development of fever in *T. parva* starting with the day that infected ticks were placed on cattle and continuing for a period of 28 days. The chemotherapy failed to cure established cases when treatment was commenced on the first day of fever (Brocklesby and Bailey 1962). Oxytetracycline at a dose of 15 mg/kg daily for 5 days was effective when administered either on the day when parasites were first detected or when there was an onset of fever (Brown *et al.* 1977b). Terramycin therapy in *T. annulata* infection had no therapeutic value when it was administered at 12 mg/kg for several days during the incubation period, at the beginning of the clinical syndrome, and at the height of parasitemia and fever (Hashemi-Fesharki and Shad-Del 1974). However, clinical cases of *T. annulata* treated with 10 to 15 mg/kg of oxytetracycline daily for 4 to 6 days were cured, and supportive treatment also proved beneficial (Singh *et al.* 1980). The injection of 5 mg/kg of menoctone on the first day of fever or at the time when macroschizonts were first detected, followed by five daily doses of 1 mg/kg arrested the development of the disease and returned temperature to normal; schizonts began degenerating within 48 hours of the first injection (McHardy *et al.* 1976). Menoctone administered intravenously at doses of 2.5 mg/kg and 5 mg/kg on day 0 of infection and then daily for 9 days at 0.5 mg/kg and 0.1 mg/kg was found to be effective (Dolan and McHardy 1978).

Other compounds have been tried more recently, primarily in *T. annulata* infections. The subcutaneous administration of imidocarb dihydrochloride at a dose of 1.2 mg/kg to Friesian cattle with subacute *T. annulata* infections resulted in clinical improvement within 1 month of treatment and a subsequent disappearance of the parasites from peripheral blood (El-Abdin *et al.* 1976). Two separate treatments, which involved the administration of multiple doses of amodiaquinine hydrochloride at 10 mg/kg orally and imidocarb diproprionate at

3 mg/kg subcutaneously during clinical disease, retarded mortality and reduced parasitemia, pyrexia, dyspnea, and tachycardia (Sharma *et al.* 1977). Imidocarb diproprionate administered at a single prophylactic dose of 2.4 mg/kg 15 days prior to vaccination prevented the development of theileriosis (El-Refaii and Michael 1976). Imidocarb diproprionate at a dose of 1.2 mg/kg was also effective in reducing the parasitemia in *T. sergenti* infections by about 80% (Purnell and Rae 1981), but amicarbalide isethionate (3;3′diamidinocarbanalide diisethionate) was not an effective treatment of the disease caused by *T. parva* (Brocklesby 1961). Oxytetracycline and chloroquine have been used in clinical cases of theileriosis, but the efficacy of these treatments remains to be determined. Resochin diphosphate had no therapeutic or prophylactic value in the treatment of *T. annulata* infection (Laiblin and Müller 1977). The administration of chloroquine phosphate in doses of 1200 to 2800 mg intramuscularly, together with intravenous or intramuscular doses of 3 g of quinine dihydrochloride once a day for 4 days provided some beneficial effect in the treatment of *T. annulata* infections in exotic and crossbred cattle (Anjaria *et al.* 1976). The administration of halofuginone at a single dose of 1.2 to 2 mg/kg was effective against experimentally induced *T. parva* and *T. annulata* infections, resulting in a decrease of fever and an absence of schizonts within 3 to 4 days of treatment (Voigt and Heydorn 1981). *Theileria annulata*-infected cattle and buffalo were cured of disease by berenil at doses of 7 to 10 mg/kg and 10 to 12 mg/kg respectively (Mahmoud *et al.* 1956).

DIAGNOSIS

Diagnosis of theilerial infections is made either by identification of the organisms or by detection of the antibodies. There are no pathognomonic clinical signs by which theilerial infections can be readily identified, particularly in subacute, chronic, and asymptomatic syndromes. The diagnosis of theileriosis can be confirmed only by the demonstration of piroplasms and schizonts in blood and lymph node smears, but there is no means of distinguishing the various theilerial species by their morphology. In making a differential diagnosis of the various forms of theilerioses, the epizootiology, symptomatology, pathology, and incidence of piroplasms and macroschizonts are taken into account. The presence of erythrocytic piroplasms may be difficult to interpret: a few piroplasms of *T. mutans* and *T. ovis* are often present in normal animals, while piroplasms are rare in all stages of *T. lawrencei* infection and may be absent or rare in acute fatal cases of *T. parva* and *T. annulata*. If death occurs about the time of microschizont formation, piroplasms would appear in the blood. There are no certain morphological criteria by which piroplasms of different species can be identified. The piroplasms of *Theileria* species are also difficult to differentiate from those observed in certain species of *Babesia*.

Serum antibodies appear as early as 5 days after infection, and their detection varies with the serological test used. Serological tests can be used to identity theilerial species, to screen animals for their susceptibility, and to survey the extent of exposure to infection in an enzootic situation. The IFA test is the serological method of choice.

Literature

The differentiation of the erythrocytic form of *Babesia* and *Theileria* in stained blood smears may be a problem in making a field diagnosis, but the presence of bacillary-, rod-, or bayonet-shaped parasites is strongly suggestive of *Theileria* (Barnett 1957). *Theileria lawrencei* in cattle was differentiable from *T. parva* because the microschizonts were smaller (5 μm vs. 8 μm), and intraerythrocytic piroplasms were absent (Brocklesby 1966). The IFA test has been used most extensively in the work on *T. parva* and other African species. This test was also more reliable for detecting latent *T. annulata* infection in cattle than the examination of blood smears (Dhar and Gautam 1977e). The presence of antibodies indicated prior exposure to theilerial antigens, which could persist for considerable periods of time and could not be directly related to a patent infection.

CONTROL

The control of theileriosis involves the control of the tick vector, chemotherapy, isolation of the wild animal host, and vaccination. Prophylactic measures include the elimination of ticks, quarantine measures, and the immunization of cattle. The elimination of ticks is accomplished only by regular sytematic dipping or spraying and may require additional careful hand-dressing because, in heavily infested regions, dipping alone may not keep the animals entirely tick-free. Quarantine measures have to be employed since recovered domestic and game animals may serve as reservoirs.

Literature

Wilde (1978) reviewed the methods used in the control of theileriosis in Africa. During the first period (up to the middle of 1950), prophylactic measures centered on the elimination of the vector. This was an effective approach, but it had to be supplemented by strict quarantine measures. Heroic methods of immunization, primarily by the use of material from infected animals, were also undertaken during this period, but had only limited success since the effects of the methods were unpredictable and mortality rates were high. During the next period, an extensive search for useful chemotherapeutic agents was undertaken, and the efficacy of the tetracyclics was determined. Immunization techniques and chemotherapeutic agents were investigated during the third period. An artificial immunization method was developed using the principle of infection and treatment; long-acting tetracycline destroyed the parasite in the early stages of its life cycle in the host. This method is not an optimal field vaccine for the following reasons. The vaccination procedures are cumbersome and could present logistical difficulties under wide-scale field applications. The lack of standardization of these procedures could also be a serious disadvantage under field conditions. The occurrence of antigenic variants among the *Theileria* requires a mixture of different strains in the vaccine. Wilde concluded that the infection and treatment method of vaccination has to be refined and used with discretion. Another method of immunization involved the injection of cultures of lymphoblasts transformed by macroschizonts. This method would have to be further refined, standardized, and tested to determine its efficacy under field conditions. The latest developments in chemotherapy show great promise.

Cunningham (1978) reviewed the work which was undertaken to develop methods of immunization against theileriosis in East Africa. He concluded that if the antigenic types of *T. parva* are limited in number and can be isolated and identified, chemoprophylactic vaccination can be used effectively to control the disease.

Pipano (1976) reviewed the basic principles of control of *T. annulata*. Epizootiological studies have not been carried out over large areas during the last two to three decades. Wild animals did not play any role in the epizootiology, and cattle and possibly water buffalo were the main reservoirs of infection. Various degrees of innate resistance have been reported for different breeds. Each developmental stage of *T. annulata* elicited a homologous immune response that may provide little or no protection against infection with other stages. Antigenic variation and wide differences in virulence have been observed in isolates from the field. The variability of virulence was related to the rate of replication rather than to the antigenic structure. In summary, Pipano believed that tissue culture vaccines provide significant protection against *T. annulata* infections.

BIBLIOGRAPHY

Allison, A. C. and Eugui, E. M., 1980. Theileriosis. Cell-mediated and humoral immunity, *Am. J. Pathol.*, **101**: 114–20.

Allsop, B. A., Kariavu, C. G., Matthews, K. P. and Wagner G. G., 1977. Purification and characterization of precipitating antigens from *Theileria parva*, *J. gen. Microbiol.*, **100**: 319–28.

Anjaria, J. V., Jhala, V. M. and Shersingh, 1976. Chloroquine phosphate in treatment of theileriosis in exotic and crossbred cattle: a clinico-pharmacological approach, *Gujarat Agric. Univ. Res. J.*, **1**: 119–24.

Aruo, S. K., 1977. The clinical and pathological picture of East Coast fever in European breeds of cattle in Uganda, *Bull. Hlth Prod. Afr.*, **25**: 223–7.

Baharsefat, M., Ahourai, P., Amjadi, A. R., Arhabi, I. and Hashemi-Fesharki, R., 1977. Unusual cases of *Theileria annulata* infection in calves, *Arch. Inst. Razi*, **29**: 47–58.

Bailey, K. P., 1960. Notes on the rearing of *Rhipicephalus appendiculatus* and their infection with *Theileria parva* for experimental transmission, *Bull. epiz. Dis. Afr.*, **8**: 33–43.

Barnett, S. F., 1957. Theileriasis control, *Bull. epiz. Dis. Afr.*, **5**: 343–57.

Barnett, S. F., 1960. Connective tissue reactions in acute fatal East Coast fever (*Theileria parva*) of cattle, *J. Infect. Dis.*, **107**: 253–82.

Barnett, S. F., 1974. Economical aspects of protozoal tick-borne diseases of livestock in parts of the world other than Britain, *Bull. Off. int. Epiz.*, **81**: 183–96.

Barnett, S. F., 1978. *Theileria*. In *Parasitic Protozoa*, ed. J. P. Kreier. Academic Press (New York), vol. IV, pp. 77–113.

Barnett, S. F. and Brocklesby, D. W., 1959. *Theileria lawrencei* in Kenya, *Bull. epiz. Dis. Afr.*, **7**: 345–7.

Barnett, S. F. and Brocklesby, D W., 1961. A mild form of East Coast fever, *Vet. Rec.*, **73**: 43–4.

Barnett, S. F. and Brocklesby, D. W., 1966a. The passage of *Theileria lawrencei* (Kenya) through cattle, *Br. vet. J.*, **122**: 396–401.

Barnett, S. F. and Brocklesby, D. W., 1966b. The susceptibility of the African buffalo (*Syncerus caffer*) to infection with *Theileria parva* (Theiler, 1904), *Br. vet. J.*, **122**: 379–86.

Barnett, S. F. and Bocklesby, D. W., 1966c. Recent investigation into Theileriidae of cattle and buffalo in Africa: a mild form of East Coast fever (*Theileria parva*) with persistence of infection, *Br. vet. J.*, **122**: 361–70.

Barnett, S. F. and Brocklesby, D. W., 1968. Some piroplasms of wild mammals, *Symp. zool. Soc. Lond.*, **24**: 159–76.

Barnett, S. F., Brocklesby, D. W. and Vidler, B. O., 1961. Studies on macroschizonts of *Theileria parva*, *Res. vet. Sci.*, **2**: 11–18.

Bell, L. J., 1980. Organ culture of *Rhipicephalus appendiculatus* with maturation of *Theileria parva* in tick salivary glands *in vitro*, *Acta trop.*, **37**: 319–25.

Bhattacharyulu, Y., Chaudri, R. P. and Gill, B. S., 1975a. Studies on the development of *Theileria annulata* (Dschunkowsky and Luhs, 1904) in the tick – *Hyalomma anatolicum anatolicum* (Koch, 1844), *Ann. Parasit.*, **50**: 397–408.

Bhattacharyulu, Y., Chaudri, R. P. and Gill, B. S., 1975b. Transstadial transmission of *Theileria annulata* through common ixodid ticks infesting Indian cattle, *Parasitology*, **71**: 1–7.

Boehm, P., Cooper, K., Elphick, J. P., Hudson, A. T. and McHardy, N., 1981. *In vitro* activity of 2-alkyl-3-hydroxy-1, 4-naphthaquinones against *Theileria parva, J. Med. Chem.*, **24**: 295–9.

Bonaventure, M., 1977. Country reports: Burundi. In *Theileriosis*, eds J. B. Henson, M. Campbell. IDRC (Ottawa), **086e**, pp. 37–8.

Branagan, D., 1969. The maintenance of *Theileria parva* infections by means of the ixodid tick, *Rhipicephalus appendiculatus, Trop. Anim. Hlth Prod.*, **1**: 119–30.

Brocklesby, D. W., 1961. Amicarbalide in East Coast fever, *Vet. Rec.*, **73**: 1454.

Brocklesby, D. W., 1962a. *Cytauxzoon taurotragi* Martin and Brocklesby, 1960, a piroplasm of the eland (*Taurotragus oryx pattersonianus* Lydekker, 1906), *Res. vet. Sci.*, **3**: 334–44.

Brocklesby, D. W., 1962b. The febrile reaction in fatal East Coast fever – a review of 150 cases, *Bull. epiz. Dis. Afr.*, **10**: 49–54.

Brocklesby, D. W., 1965a. A new theilerial parasite of the African buffalo (*Syncerus caffer*), *Bull. epiz. Dis. Afr.*, **13**: 325–30.

Brocklesby, D. W., 1965b. Evidence that *Rhipicephalus pulchellus* (Gerstacker, 1873) may be a vector of some piroplasms, *Bull. epiz. Dis. Afr.*, **13**: 37–44.

Brocklesby, D. W., 1966. Theileriidae of the buffalo in East Africa, *Proc. 1st Int. Congr. Parasitol.*, **1**: 274–6.

Brocklesby, D. W., 1969. The lability of a bovine *Theileria* species, *Exp. Parasitol.*, **25**: 258–64.

Brocklesby, D. W., 1970. The development of *Theileria parva* in bovine tissues, *Proc. 2nd Int. Congr. Parasitol.*, Washington, pp. 35–6.

Brocklesby, D. W., 1978. Recent observations on tick-borne protozoa. In *Tick-borne Diseases and their Vectors*, ed. J. K. H. Wilde. Lewis Reprints (Tonbridge) pp. 263–86.

Brocklesby, D. W. and Bailey, K. P., 1962. Oxytetracycline hydrochloride in East Coast fever (*Theileria parva* infection), *Br. vet. J.*, **118**: 81–5.

Brocklesby, D. W. and Bailey, K. P., 1965. The immunization of cattle against East Coast fever (*Theileria parva* infection) using tetracyclines: a review of the literature and reappraisal of the method. *Bull. epiz. Dis. Afr.*, **13**: 161–8.

Brocklesby, D. W. and Bailey, K. P., 1968. A mild form of East Coast fever (*Theileria parva* infection) becoming virulent on passage through cattle, *Br. vet. J.*, **124**: 236–8.

Brocklesby, D. W., Bailey, K. P., Jarrett, W. F. H., Martin, W. B., Miller, H. R. P., Nderito, P. and Urquhart, G. M., 1965. Experiments in immunity to East Coast fever, *Vet. Rec.*, **77**: 512.

Brocklesby, D. W., Bailey, K. P. and Vidler, O. B., 1966. The transmission of *Theileria parva* (Theiler, 1904) by *Rhipicephalus carnivoralis* Walker, 1965, *Parasitology*, **56**: 13–14.

Brocklesby, D. W. and Barnett, S. F., 1966a. The literature concerning Theileriidae of the African buffalo (*Syncerus caffer*), *Br. vet. J.*, **122**: 371–8.

Brocklesby, D. W. and Barnett, S. F., 1966b. The isolation of *Theileria lawrencei* (Kenya) from a wild buffalo (*Syncerus caffer*) and its serial passage through captive buffaloes, *Br. vet. J.*, **122**: 387–95.

Brocklesby, D. W., Barnett, S. F. and Scott, G. R., 1961. Morbidity and mortality rates in East Coast fever (*Theileria parva* infection) and their application to drug screening procedures, *Br. vet. J.*, **117**: 529–31.

Brocklesby, D. W., Harradine, D. L. and Morzaria, S. P., 1975. *Theileria mutans*: experimental transmission by *Haemaphysalis punctata*, *Z. Tropenmed. Parasit.*, **26**: 295–302.

Brocklesby, D. W. and Hawking, F., 1958. Growth of *Theileria annulata* and *T. parva* in tissue culture, *Trans. Roy. Soc. trop. Med. Hyg.*, **52**: 414–20.

Brocklesby, D. W. and Vidler, O. B., 1961. Haematozoa of the blue wildebeest, *Bull. epiz. Dis. Afr.*, **9**: 245–9.

Brocklesby, D. W. and Vidler, O. B., 1965. Some parasites of East African wild animals, *E. Afr. Wildl. J.*, **3**: 120–2.

Brocklesby, D. W. and Vidler, O. B., 1966. Haematozoa found in wild members of the order *Artiodactyla* in East Africa, *Bull. epiz. Dis. Afr.*, **14**: 285–99.

Brown, C. G. D., 1979. Propagation of *Theileria*. In *Practical Tissue Culture Applications*, eds K. Maramorosch and H. Hirumi. Academic Press (London), pp. 223–54.

Brown, C. G. D., Bailey, K. P., Branagan, D., Corry, G., Cunningham, M. P., Joyner, L. P. and Purnell, R. E., 1969. *Theileria parva*: the importance of leukocytes in the establishment of the parasite in cattle. In *Progress in Protozoology, Proc. 3rd Int. Congr. Protozool.*, Leningrad, p. 26.

Brown, C. G. D., Bailey, K. P., Branagan, D., Corry, G. L., Cunningham, M. P., Joyner, L. P. and Purnell, R. E., 1978. *Theileria parva*: significance of leukocytes for infecting cattle, *Exp. Parasitol.*, **45**: 55.

Brown, C. G. D., Burridge, M. O., Cunningham, M. P. and Radley, D. E., 1977b. The use of tetracyclines in the chemotherapy of experimental East Coast fever (*Theileria parva* infection of cattle), *Z. Tropenmed. Parasit.*, **28**: 513–20.

Brown. C. G. D., Cunningham, M. P., Dirimi, I. M., Morzaria, S. P., Musoke, A. J. and Radley, D. E., 1977a. Immunization against East Coast fever (*Theileria parva* infection of cattle) by infection and treatment: chemoprophylaxis with n-pyrrolidinomethyl tetracycline, *Z. Tropenmed. Parasit.*, **28**: 342–8.

Bulman, G. M., Arzo, G. M. and Nassimi, M. N., 1979. An outbreak of tropical theileriosis in cattle in Afghanistan, *Trop. Anim. Hlth Prod.*, **11**: 17–20.

Burdin, M. L. and Boarer, C. D. H., 1972. Glucose 6-phosphate dehydrogenase levels and haemoglobin types of cattle in East Africa in relation to resistance to East Coast fever, *Vet. Rec.*, **90**: 299–302.

Burridge, M. J., 1971. Application of the indirect fluorescent antibody test in experimental East Coast fever (*Theileria parva* infection of cattle), *Res. vet. Sci.*, **12**: 338–41.

Burridge, M. J., 1975. The role of wild mammals in the epidemiology of bovine theilerioses in East Africa, *J. Wildl. Dis.*, **11**: 68–75.

Burridge, M. J., Brown, C. G. D., Crawford, J. G., Kirimi, I. M., Morzaria, S. P. and Payne, R. C., 1974a. Preliminary studies on an atypical strain of bovine *Theileria* isolated in Kenya, *Res. vet. Sci.*, **17**: 139–44.

Burridge, M. J., Brown, C. G. D., Cunningham, M. P. and Morzaria, S. P., 1972. Duration of immunity to East Coast fever (*Theileria parva* infection of cattle), *Parasitology*, **63**: 511–15.

Burridge, M. J., Brown, C. G. D. and Kimber, C. D., 1974b. *Theileria annulata*: cross-reactions between a cell culture schizont antigen and antigens of East African species in the indirect fluorescent antibody test, *Exp. Parasitol.*, **35**: 374–80.

Burridge, M. J. and Kimber, C D., 1972a. The indirect fluorescent antibody test for experimental East Coast fever (*Theileria parva* infection of cattle). Detection of antibodies to schizonts in dried blood samples, *Z. Tropenmed. Parasit.*, **23**: 327–31.

Burridge, M. J. and Kimber, C. D., 1972b. The indirect fluorescent antibody test for experimental East Coast fever (*Theileria parva* infection of cattle). Evaluation of a cell culture schizont antigen, *Res. vet. Sci.*, **13**: 451–5.

Burridge, M. J. and Kimber, C. D., 1972c. A pathogenic theilerial syndrome of cattle in the Narok district of Kenya. II. Serological studies, *Trop. Anim. Hlth Prod.*, **4**: 230–6.

Burridge, M. J. and Kimber, C. D., 1973a. Duration of serological response to the indirect fluorescent antibody test of cattle recovered from *Theileria parva* infection, *Res. vet. Sci.*, **14**: 270–1.

Burridge, M. J. and Kimber, C. D., 1973b. Studies on colostral antibodies to *Theileria parva* using the indirect fluorescent antibody test, *Z. Tropenmed. Parasit.*, **24**: 305–8.

Burridge, M. J. and Kimber, C. D., 1973c. Serological studies on *Theileria gorgonis* using the indirect fluorescent antibody test, *Z. Tropenmed. Parasit.*, **24**: 186–91.

Burridge, M. J., Kimber, C. D. and Young, A. S., 1973. Use of the indirect fluorescent antibody technique in serologic studies of *Theileria lawrencei* infections in cattle. *Am. J. vet. Res.*, **34**: 897–900.

Burridge, M. J. and Odeke, G. M., 1973. *Theileria lawrencei*: infection in the Indian water buffalo, *Bubalus bubalis*, *Exp. Parasitol.*, **34**: 257–61.

Büttner, D. W., 1966. Uber die feinstrukture der erythrozytaren formen von *Theileria mutans*, *Z. Tropenmed. Parasit.*, **17**: 397–406.

Büttner, D. W., 1967a. Electron microscopic studies of the multiplication of *Theileria parva* in cattle, *Z. Tropenmed. Parasit.*, **18**: 245–68.

Büttner, D. W., 1967b. Die feinstruktur der merozoiten von *Theileria parva*, *Z. Tropenmedizin*, **18**: 224–44.

Bwangamoi, O., Frank, H., Munyua, W. K. and Wandera, J. G., 1971.

Gross lesions in natural bovine East Coast fever at Kabate, *Bull. epiz. Dis. Afr.*, **19**: 271–7.

Callow, L. L. and Hayte, H. M. D., 1961. The separation of *Babesia bigemina* from *Babesia argentina* and *Theileria mutans*, *Aust. vet. J.*, **37**: 66–70.

Carmichael, J. and Jones, E. R., 1939. The cerebrospinal fluid in the bovine: its composition and properties in health and disease, with special reference to 'turning sickness', *J. Comp. Path.*, **52**: 222–8.

Cawdery, M. J. H., McAnulty, E. G., Ross, H. M. and Simmons, D. J. C., 1968. *Theileria parva*: possible serological test for East Coast fever, *Exp. Parasitol.*, **23**: 234–7.

Cox, F. E. G., 1976. *Theileria* in the laboratory, *Nature*, **26**: 276.

Cunningham, M. P., 1978. Vaccination of cattle against East Coast fever: an appraisal of nine years' work at EAURO. In *Tick-borne Diseases and their Vectors*, ed. J. K. H. Wilde. Lewis Reprints (Tonbridge), pp. 330.

Cunningham, M. P., Bailey, K. P., Brown, C. G. D., Joyner, L. P. and Purnell, R. E., 1973a. Infection of cattle with East Coast fever by inoculation of the infective stage of *Theileria parva* harvested from the tick vector *Rhipicephalus appendiculatus*, *Bull. epiz. Dis. Afr.*, **21**: 235–8.

Cunningham, M. P., Brown, C. G. D., Burridge, M. J., Dargie, J. D., Musoke, A. J. and Purnell, R. E., 1973d. East Coast fever of cattle: ^{60}Co irradiation of infective particles of *Theileria parva*, *J. Protozool.*, **20**: 298–300.

Cunningham, M. P., Brown, C. G. D., Burridge, M. J., Irvin, A. D., Kirimi, I. M., Purnell, R. E., Radley, D. E. and Wagner, C. G., 1974. Theileriosis: the exposure of immunized cattle in a *Theileria lawrencei* enzootic area, *Trop. Anim. Hlth Prod.*, **6**: 39–43.

Cunningham, M. P., Brown, C. G. D., Burridge M. J., Musoke, A. J. and Purnell, R. E., 1973c. Some effects of irradiation on the infective stage of *Theileria parva* harvested from infected ticks. In *Isotopes and Radiation in Parasitology*. IAEA (Vienna), vol. III, pp. 145–53.

Cunningham, M. P., Brown, C. G. D., Burridge M. J. and Purnell, R. E., 1973b. Cryopreservation of infective particles of *Theileria parva*, *J. Protozool.*, **20**: 298–300.

Danskin, D. and Wilde, J. K. H., 1976a. The effect of calf lymph and bovine red blood cells on *in vitro* cultivation of *Theileria parva*-infected lymphoid cells, *Trop. Anim. Hlth Prod.*, **8**: 175–85.

Danskin, D. and Wilde, J. K. H., 1976b. Simulation *in vitro* of bovine host cycle of *Theileria parva*, *Nature*, **261**: 311–12.

Daubney, R. and Sami Said, M., 1950. Egyptian fever in cattle: the transmission of *Theileria annulata* (Dschunkowsky and Luhs 1904) by *Hyalomma excavatum*, (Koch, 1844), *Parasitology*, **40**: 249–60.

de Kock, G., 1957. Studies on the lesions and pathogenesis of East Coast fever (*Theileria parva* infection) in cattle with special reference to the lymphoid tissue, *Onderstepoort J. vet. Res.*, **27**: 431–53.

DeMartini, J. C. and Moulton, J. E., 1973a. Responses of the bovine lymphatic system to infection by *Theileria parva*. I. Histology and ultrastructure of lymph nodes in experimentally infected calves, *J. Comp. Path.*, **83**: 281–98.

DeMartini, J. C. and Moulton, J. E., 1973b. Responses of the bovine lymphatic system to infection by *Theileria parva*. II. Changes in the central lymph in experimentally infected calves, *J. Comp. Path.*, **83**: 299–306.

Dhar, S. and Gautam, O. P., 1977a. Some biochemical aspects of *T. annulata* infection in cattle, *Indian J. Anim. Sci.*, **47**: 169–72.

Dhar, S. and Gautam, O. P., 1977b. *Theileria annulata* infection of cattle. I. Complement-fixation and conglutinating-complement-absorption tests for serodiagnosis, *Indian J. Anim. Sci.*, **47**: 389–94.

Dhar, S. and Gautam, O. P., 1977c. *Theileria annulata* infection in cattle. II. Capillary-tube-agglutination test for serodiagnosis, *Indian J. Anim. Sci.*, **47**: 458–62.

Dhar, S. and Gautam, O. P., 1977d. *Theileria annulata* infection in cattle. III. Haemagglutination-inhibition, indirect haemagglutination and agar-gel-precipitation tests for serodiagnosis, *Indian J. Anim. Sci.*, **47**: 566–70.

Dhar, S. and Gautam, O. P., 1977e. Indirect fluorescent-antibody test for diagnosis in cattle infected with *T. annulata*, *Indian J. Anim. Sci.*, **47**: 720–3.

Dhar, S. and Gautam, O. P., 1977f. Species differentiation of *Theileria* of cattle by means of complement fixation test, *Indian vet. J.*, **54**: 21–4.

Dhar, S. and Gautam, O. P., 1978. A note on the use of hyperimmune serum in bovine tropical theileriasis, *Indian vet. J.*, **55**: 738–40.

Dhar, S. and Gautam, O. P., 1979. Serum proteins in experimental *Theileria annulata* infection in cattle, *Indian J. Anim. Sci.*, **49**: 511–16.

Dolan, T. T., Brown, C. G. D. and Cunningham, M. P., 1980a. The effect of immunization with BCG on *Theileria parva* infection in cattle, *Res. vet. Sci.*, **28**: 132–3.

Dolan, T. T., Brown, C. G. D., Cunningham, M. P., Morzaria, S. P., Radley, D. E. and Young, A. S., 1980b. East Coast fever. 4. Further studies on the protection of cattle immunized with a combination of theilerial strains, *Vet. Parasitol.*, **6**: 325–32.

Dolan, T. T. and McHardy, N., 1978. The chemotherapy of experimental *Theileria parva* infection. In *Tick-borne Diseases and their Vectors*, ed. J. K. H. Wilde. Lewis Reprints (Tonbridge), pp. 318–23.

Duffus, W. P. H., 1977. Country reports: Kenya. In *Theileriosis*, eds.

J. B. Henson, M. Campbell. IDRC (Ottawa), **086e**, pp. 28–30.

Duffus, W. P. H., Preston, J. M. and Wagner, G. R., 1978. Initial studies on the properties of a bovine lymphoid cell culture line infected with *Theileria parva, Clin. exp. Immunol.*, **34**: 347–53.

Duffus, W. P. H. and Wagner, G. R., 1974a. The specific immune response in the lymph nodes of cattle undergoing *Theileria parva* infection, as determined by the Rosette test, *Parasitic Zoonoses Clin. Exp. Studies*, pp. 85–95.

Duffus, W. P. H. and Wagner, G. R., 1974b. Immunochemical studies on East Coast fever: III. Development of an indirect haemagglutination assay using *Theileria parva* piroplasm and antigen, *J. Parasitol.*, **60**: 860–5.

Duffus, W. P. H. and Wagner, G. R., 1980. Comparison between certain serological tests for diagnosis of East Coast fever, *Vet. Parasitol.*, **6**: 313–24.

El-Abdin, Y. Z., Hamza, S. M. and El-Refaii, A. H., 1976. Some biochemical studies on 'Imidocarb' in Friesian cattle infected with *Theileria annulata, Egypt. J. Vet.*, **13**: 77–84.

El-Refaii, A. H. and Michael, S. A. 1976. The application of imidocarb diproprionate for the control of *Theileria annulata* infection in Egyptian cattle used for testing rinderpest vaccine, *Br. vet. J.*, **132**: 363–8.

Emery, D. L., 1981. Adoptive transfer of immunity to infection with *Theileria parva* (East Coast fever) between cattle twins, *Res. vet. Sci.*, **30**: 364–7.

Emery, D. L., Eugui, E. M., Nelson, R. T. and Tenywa, T., 1981a. Cell-mediated immune responses to *Theileria parva* (East Coast fever) during immunization and lethal infections in cattle, *Immunology*, **43**: 323–36.

Emery, D. L., Jack, R. M. and Tenywa, T., 1981b. Characterization of the effector cell that mediates cytotoxicity against *Theileria parva* (East Coast fever) in immune cattle, *Infect. Immun.*, **32**: 1301–4.

Emery, D. L. and Morrison, W. I., 1980. Generation of autologous mixed leukocyte reactions during the course of infection with *Theileria parva* (East Coast fever) in cattle, *Immunology*, **40**: 229–37.

Enigk, K., Friedhoff, K. and Wirahadiredja, S., 1964. *Theileria ovis*. II. Host specificity of *Babesia motasi* and *Babesia ovis, Z. Parasitenkd.*, **24**: 309–18.

Eugui, E. M. and Emery, D. L., 1981. Genetically restricted cell-mediated cytotoxicity in cattle immune to *Theileria parva, Nature*, **290**: 251–4.

Flanagan, H. O. and Le Roux, J. M. W., 1957. Bovine cerebral theileriosis – a report on two cases occurring in the Union, *Onderstepoort J. vet. Res.*, **27**: 453–61.

Fujinaga, T. and Minami, T., 1981. Indirect fluorescent antibody and complement fixation tests in the diagnosis of bovine theileriosis and babesiosis in Japan, *Vet. Parasitol.*, **8**: 115–26.

Gautam, O. P., 1976. Bovine theileriosis in India, *Haryana Vet.*, **15**: 77–87.

Gautam, O. P., 1978. *Theileria annulata* infection in India. In *Tick-borne Diseases and their Vectors*, ed. J. K. H. Wilde. Lewis Reprints (Tonbridge), pp. 374–6.

Gautam, O. P., Kalra, D. S. and Sharma, R. D., 1970. Theileriosis in exotic breeds and a Sahival calf, *Indian vet. J.*, **47**: 78–83.

Giesecke, W. and Wiesenhütter, E., 1965. Treatment of *Theileria annulata* infections of cattle in Syria, *Berl. Münich. Tierartzl. Wschr.*, **78**: 123–5.

Giles, N., Davis, F. G., Duffus, W. P. and Heinonen, R., 1978. Bovine cerebral theileriosis, *Vet. Rec.*, **102**: 313.

Gill, B. S., 1978. Chemoprophylaxis with tetracycline drugs in the immunization of cattle against *Theileria annulata* infection, *Int. J. Parasitol.*, **8**: 467.

Gill, B. S., Bansal, G. C., Bhattacharyulu, Y., Kaur, D., and Singh, A., 1980. Immunological relationship between strains of *Theileria annulata* (Dschunkowsky and Luhs, 1904), *Res. vet. Sci.*, **29**: 93–7.

Gill, B. S. and Bhattacharyulu, Y., 1977. Country reports: Bovine theileriosis in India. In *Theileriosis*, eds J. B. Henson, M. Campbell. IDRC (Ottawa), **086e**, pp. 8–11.

Gill, B. S., Bhattacharyulu, Y. and Kaur, D., 1976a. Immunization against bovine tropical theileriosis (*Theileria annulata* infection), *Res. vet. Sci.*, **21**: 146–9.

Gill, B. S., Bhattacharyulu, Y., Kaur, D. and Singh, A., 1976b. Vaccination against bovine tropical theileriosis (*Theileria annulata*), *Nature*, **264**: 355–6.

Gill, B. S., Bhattacharyulu, Y., Kaur, D. and Singh, A., 1977. Immunization of cattle against tropical theileriosis (*Theileria annulata* infection) by 'infection-treatment' method, *Ann. Rech. Vet.*, **8**: 285–92.

Gill, B. S., Bhattacharyulu, Y., Kaur, D. and Singh, A., 1978. Chemoprophylaxis with tetracycline drugs in the immunization of cattle against *Theileria annulata* infection, *Int. J. Parasitol.*, **8**: 467–9.

Gill, H. S., Bhattacharyulu, Y. and Gill, B. S., 1980. Attempts to transmit *Theileria ovis* through the ticks *Haemaphysalis bispinosa* and *Rhipicephalus haemaphysaloides*, *Trop. Anim. Hlth Prod.*, **12**: 61.

Goldman, M. and Pipano, E., 1978. Specific IgM and IgG antibodies in cattle immunized or infected with *Theileria annulata*, *Z. Tropenmed. Parasit.*, **29**: 85–7.

Gourlay, R. N. and Brocklesby, D. W., 1967. Preliminary experiments with antigens of *Theileria parva* (Theiler, 1904), *Brit. vet. J.*, **123**: 533–40.

Gray, M. A., Brown C. G. D., Luckins A. G. and Rae, P. F., 1980.

Evaluation of an enzyme immunoassay for serodiagnosis of infections with *Theileria parva* and *T. annulata*, *Res. vet. Sci.*, **29**: 360–6.

Grimpret, J. M., 1953. Symptomes cutanes de la theileriose bovine, *Bull. Acad. vet. Fr.*, **26**: 535–7.

Grootenhuis, J. G., Dolan, T. T., Stagg, D. A. and Young, A. S., 1979. Characteristics of *Theileria* species (eland) infections in eland and cattle, *Res. vet. Sci.*, **27**: 59–68.

Grootenhuis, J. G., Haller, R. D., Kerstad, L., Morrison, W. I., Murray, M., Sayer, P. D. and Young, A. S., 1980. Fatal theileriosis in eland (*Taurotragus oryx*) – pathology of natural and experimental cases, *Res. vet. Sci.*, **29**: 219–29.

Grootenhuis, J. G., Kanhai, G. K., Paling, R. W. and Young, A. S., 1977. Experimental tick transmission of *Theileria* species between eland, *J. Parasitol.*, **63**: 1127–9.

Grootenhuis, J. G., Uilenberg, G. and Young, A. S., 1981. The relationship between *Theileria taurotragi* from eland and *Theileria* sp. (Idobogo) from cattle, *Vet. Parasitol.*, **8**: 39–47.

Guilbride, P. D. L., 1963. Attempts to adapt *Theileria parva* to laboratory animals, *Bull. epiz. Dis. Afr.*, **11**: 283–7.

Guilbride, P. D. L. and Opwata, B., 1963. Observations on the resistance of Jersey/Nganda calves to East Coast fever (*Theileria parva*), *Bull. epiz. Dis. Afr.*, **11**: 289–98.

Hashemi-Fesharki, R., 1978. Quantitative studies of three different strains of *Theileria annulata* in experimental calves. In *Tick-borne Diseases and their Vectors*, ed. J. K. H. Wilde. Lewis Reprints (Tonbridge), pp. 357–64.

Hashemi-Fesharki, R. and Shad-Del, F., 1974. The therapeutic value of oxytetracycline hydrochloride (Terramycin) in cattle infected experimentally with *Theileria annulata*, *Trop. Anim. Hlth Prod.*, **6**: 119–21.

Hawa, N., Bakir, F. A. and Latif, B. M. A., 1976. Application of the indirect fluorescent antibody test for diagnosis of *Theileria hirci* infection of sheep: using cell culture schizont antigen, *Trop. Anim. Hlth Prod.*, **8**: 97–101.

Hawking, F., 1958. Chemotherapeutic screening of compounds against *Theileria annulata* in tissue culture, *Br. J. Pharmacol.*, **13**: 458–60.

Hawking, F., 1963. Chemotherapy of theileriosis. In *Experimental Chemotherapy*, eds R. J. Schnitzer, F. Hawking. Academic Press (New York and London), vol. 1, pp. 625–32.

Henson, J. B. and Campbell, M., (eds), 1976. Theileriosis. IDRC (Ottawa), **086e**.

Hill, R. R. H. and Matson, B. A., 1970. The haematology of experimental *Theileria lawrencei* infection, *J. S. Afr. vet. med. Ass.*, **41**: 275–84.

Hofstedt, L. 1977. Country reports: Zanzibar and Pemba. In

Theileriosis, eds J. B. Henson, M. Campbell. IDRC (Ottawa), **086e**, pp. 31–2.

Hooshmand-Rad, P., 1975. The growth of *Theileria annulata* infected cells in suspension culture, *Trop. Anim. Hlth Prod.*, **7**: 23–8.

Hooshmand-Rad, P., 1976. The pathogenesis of anaemia in *Theileria annulata* infection, *Res. vet. Sci.*, **20**: 324–9.

Hooshmand-Rad, P., 1978. A study on the mechanism of immunity in theileriosis due to *Theileria annulata*. In *Tick-borne Diseases and their Vectors*, ed., J. K. H. Wilde. Lewis Reprints (Tonbridge), pp. 365–70.

Hooshmand-Rad, P. and Hashemi-Fesharki, R., 1968. The effect of virulence on cultivation of *Theileria annulata* strains in lymphoid cells which have been cultured in suspension, *Arch. Inst. Razi*, **20**: 85–9.

Hooshmand-Rad, P. and Hashemi-Fesharki, R., 1971. Complement-fixing antibodies in cattle experimentally uninfected with *Theileria annulata* or vaccinated with tissue cultures, *Br. vet. J.*, **127**: 244–50.

Hooshmand-Rad, P. and Hawa, N. J., 1973a. Transmission of *Theileria hirci* in sheep by *Hyalomma anatolicum anatolicum*, *Trop. Anim. Hlth Prod.*, **5**: 103–9.

Hooshmand-Rad, P. and Hawa, N. J., 1973b. Malignant theileriosis of sheep, *Trop. Anim. Hlth Prod*, **5**: 97–102.

Hooshmand-Rad, P. and Hawa, N. J., 1975. Cultivation of *Theileria hirci* in sheep lymphoid cells, *Trop. Anim. Hlth Prod.*, **7**: 121–2.

Hosie, B. D. and Walker, A. R., 1979. The production of nymphs of *Hyalomma anatolicum anatolicum* for experimental infection with *Theileria annulata*, *Trop. Anim. Hlth Prod.*, **11**: 181–5.

Hulliger, L., 1965. Cultivation of three species of *Theileria* in lymphoid cells *in vitro*, *J. Protozool.*, **12**: 649–55.

Hulliger, L., Brown, C. G. D., Turner, L. and Wilde, J. K. H., 1964. Mode of multiplication of *Theileria* in cultures of bovine lymphocytic cells, *Nature*, **203**: 728–30.

Hulliger, L., Brown, C. G. D. and Wilde, J. K. H., 1966. Transition of developmental stages of *Theileria parva in vitro* at high temperature, *Nature*, **211**: 328–9.

Irvin, A. D. and Boarer, C. D. H., 1980. Some implications of a sexual cycle in *Theileria*, *Parasitology*, **80**: 571–9.

Irvin, A. D., Boarer, C. D. H., Dobbelaere, D. A. E., Mahan, S. M., Masake, R. and Ocama, J. G. R., 1981. Monitoring *Theileria parva* infection in adult *Rhipicephalus appendiculatus* ticks, *Parasitology*, **82**: 137–47.

Irvin, A. D., Brown, C. G. D., Burridge, M. J., Cunningham, M. P., Musosi, A. J., Pierce, M. A., Purnell, R. E. and Radley, D. E., 1972d. A pathogenic theilerial syndrome of cattle in the Narok District of Kenya. 1. Transmission studies, *Trop. Anim. Hlth Prod.*, **4**: 220–9.

Irvin, A. D., Brown, C. G. D. and Crawford, J. G., 1972a. Attempts to grow culture cells, infected with *Theileria parva*, in laboratory animals, *Res. vet. Sci.*, **13**: 589–90.

Irvin, A. D., Brown, C. G. D., Crawford, J. G., Kanhai, G. K. and Kimber, C. D., 1974. Response of whole-body irradiated mice to inoculation of *Theileria parva*-infected bovine lymphoid cells, *J. Comp. Path.*, **84**: 291–300.

Irvin, A. D., Brown, C. G. D. and Cunningham, M. P., 1972b. Growth of *Theileria parva*-infected bovine lymphoid cells in irradiated mice, *Nat. phys. Sci.*, **230**: 106–7.

Irvin, A. D., Brown, C. G. D. and Cunningham, M. P., 1973a. Studies on *Theileria parva* in whole-body irradiated mice. In *Isotopes and Radiation in Parasitology*. IAEA (Vienna), vol. III, pp. 155–9.

Irvin, A. D., Brown, C. G. D., Kanhai, G. K., Rowe, L. W., Stagg, D. A., 1975b. Hybrid cells, infected with *Theileria parva*, formed by fusion of hamster and mouse cells with parasitized bovine lymphoid cells. *Res. vet. Sci.*, **19**: 142–51.

Irvin, A. D., Brown, C. G. D., Kanhai, G. K. and Stagg, D. A., 1977b. Establishment of *Theileria parva*-infected bovine tissue culture in Swiss and athymic (nude) mice, *Vet. Parasitol.*, **3**: 141–60.

Irvin, A. D., Brown, C. G. D., Stagg, D. A., 1975a. *Theileria parva*: effects of irradiation on a culture of parasitized bovine lymphoid cells, *Exp. Parasitol.*, **38**: 64–74.

Irvin, A. D. *et al.* 1975c. Comparative growth of bovine lymphsarcoma cells and lymphoid cells infected with *Theileria parva* in athymic (nude) mice, *Nature*, **255**: 713.

Irvin, A. D., Kanhai, G. K., Omwoyo, P. L. and Payne, R. C., 1977a. *Theileria parva* piroplasmosis in mice, and its attempted transmission with *Rhipicephalus appendiculatus* ticks, *Z. Tropenmed. Parasit.*, **28**: 507–12.

Irvin, A. D., Kanhai, G. K. and Stagg, D. A., 1975d. Heterotransplantation of *Theileria parva*-infected cells to athymic mice, *Nature*, **253**: 549–50.

Irvin, A. D., Kanhai, G. K. and Stagg, D. A., 1976. Attempts to produce *Theileria parva*-infected mouse cells using cell fusion techniques, *Res. vet. Sci.*, **21**: 197–204.

Irvin, A. D., King, J. M., Peirce, M. A. and Purnell, R. E., 1972c. The possible role of the eland (*Taurotragus oryx*) in the epidemiology of East Coast fever and other bovine theilerioses, *Vet. Rec.*, **91**: 513–17.

Irvin, A. D., Omwoyo, P., Peirce, M. A. and Purnell, R. E., 1973b. Blood parasites of the impala (*Aepyceros melampus*) in the Serengeti National Park, *Vet. Rec.*, **93**: 200–3.

Irvin, A. D., Peirce, M. A. and Purnell, R. E., 1970. Infection of *Rhipicephalus appendiculatus* ticks with *Theileria parva*, using a rabbit's head perfusion technique, *Res. vet. Sci.*, **11**: 493–5.

Irvin, A. D. and Stagg, D. A., 1977. *Theileria parva*: purine and pyrimidine metabolism and the action of folate antagonists in parasitized bovine lymphoid cells, *Exp. Parasitol.*, **41**: 172–85.

Jagdish, S., Dhar, S., Gautam, O. P. and Singh, D. K., 1979. Chemoprophylactic immunization against bovine tropical theileriosis, *Vet. Rec.*, **104**: 140–2.

Jansen, B. C. and Neitz, W. O., 1956. The experimental transmission of *Theileria ovis* by *Rhipicephalus evertsi, Onderstepoort J. vet. Res.*, **27**: 3–6.

Jarrett, W. F. H. and Brocklesby, D. W., 1966. A preliminary electron microscopic study of East Coast fever (*Theileria parva* infection), *J. Protozool.*, **13**: 301–10.

Jarrett, W. F. H., Crighton, G. W. and Pirie, H. M., 1969. *Theileria parva*: kinetics of replication, *Exp. Parasitol.*, **24**: 9–25.

Jongejan, F., Franssen, F. F., Perié, N. M. and Uilenberg, G., 1980. Artificial infection of *Rhipicephalus appendiculatus* with *Theileria parva* by percutaneous injection, *Res. vet. Sci.*, **29**: 320–4.

Joyner, L. P., Brocklesby, D. W., Irvin, A. D., Payne, R. C., and Takahashi, K., 1979. Serological comparison of British *Theileria mutans* and Japanese *T. sergenti, Res. vet. Sci.*, **26**: 387–8.

Joyner, L. P., Brown, C. G. D., Cunningham, M. P. and Purnell, R. E., 1972. The duration of emission of infective particles of *Theileria parva* by infected ticks fed artificially, *Res. vet. Sci.*, **13**: 402–3.

Joyner, L. P. and Purnell, R. E., 1968. The feeding behaviour on rabbits and *in vitro* of the ixodid tick *Rhipicephalus appendiculatus* Neumann, 1901, *Parasitology*, **58**: 715–23.

Jura, W. G. Z. and Losos, G. J., 1980. A comparative study of the disease in cattle caused by *Theileria lawrencei* and *Theileria parva*. I. Clinical signs and parasitological observations, *Vet. Parasitol.*, **7**: 275–86.

Khalid, K. and Jawad, K. K., 1967. Unusual lesions in *Theileria annulata* infection in a calf, *Vet. Rec.*, **81**: 76–8.

Kier, A. B., Morehouse, L. G. and Wagner, J. E., 1982b. Experimental transmission of *Cytauxzoon felis* from bobcats (*Lynx rufus*) to domestic cats (*Felis domesticus*), *Am. J. vet. Res.*, **43**: 97–101.

Kier, A. B., Wagner, J. E. and Wightman, S. R., 1982a. Interspecies transmission of *Cytauxzoon felis, Am. J. vet. Res.*, **43**: 102–5.

Kimber, C. D. and Burridge, M. J., 1972. The indirect fluorescent antibody test for experimental East Coast fever (*Theileria parva* infection of cattle). Evaluation of dried blood samples as a source of antibody, *Res. vet. Sci.*, **13**: 133–5.

Kimber, C. D. and Purnell, R. E., 1972. A rapid technique for the detection of theilerial parasites in the salivary glands of the tick *Rhipicephalus appendiculatus, Res. vet. Sci.*, **13**: 393–5.

Kimber, C. D., Purnell, R. E. and Sellwood, S. A., 1973. The use of fluorescent antibody techniques to detect *Theileria parva* in the salivary glands of the tick *Rhipicephalus appendiculatus, Res. vet. Sci.*, **14**: 126–7.

Kimber, C. D. and Young, A. S., 1977. Serological studies on strains of *Theileria mutans* isolated from cattle in East Africa using the indirect fluorescent antibody technique, *Ann. trop. Med. Parasit.*, **71**: 1–10.

Kimeto, B. A., 1976. Ultrastructure of blood platelets in cattle with East Coast fever, *Am. J. vet. Res.*, **37**: 443–7.

Kimeto, B. A., 1978. Histopathologic and electron microscopic studies of cutaneous lesions in calves with experimentally induced East Coast fever (Theileriosis), *Am. J. vet. Res.*, **39**: 1117–22.

Kimeto, B. A., 1980. Fine structure of *Theileria parva* in the bovine skin, *Vet. Parasitol.*, **7**: 25–32.

Kitaoka, S., 1970. Ticks and tick-borne diseases in Japan, *Bull. Off. int. Epiz.*, **73**: 115–19.

Kurtti, T. J., Buscher, G., Irvin, A. D. and Munderloh, U. G., 1981. *Theileria parva*: early events in the development of bovine lymphoblastoid cell lines persistently infected with macroschizonts, *J. Parasitol.*, **52**: 280–91.

Kuttler, K. L. and Craig, T. M., 1975. Isolation of a bovine *Theileria*, *Am. J. vet. Res.*, **36**: 323–5.

Laiblin, C., 1978. Clinical investigations in cattle experimentally infected with *Theileria annulata*. II. Haematological investigations, *Berl. Münch. Tierzartl. Wschr.*, **91**: 48–50.

Laiblin, C., Baysu, N. and Muller, M., 1978. Clinical investigations in cattle experimentally infected with *Theileria annulata*. I. Clinico-chemical investigations enzyme and bilirubin activity in blood, *Berl. Münch. Tierarztl. Wschr.*, **91**: 25–7.

Laiblin, C. and Müller, M., 1977. (Therapy and prophylaxis of *Theileria annulata* in steers with Resochin). Untersuchungen zur therapie und prophylaxe der *Theileria annulata* erkrankung des rindes mit Resochin 'Bayer', *Berl. Münch. Tierarztl. Wschr.*, **90**: 234–7.

Lawrence, J. A., 1977. The serological relationship between *Theileria parva* (Muguga) and *Theileria lawrencei* from Rhodesia cattle, *Vet. Rec.*, **100**: 470–1.

Lawrence, J. A., 1979. The differential diagnosis of the bovine theilerias of Southern Africa, *J. S. Afr. vet. med. Ass.*, **50**: 311–33.

Leeflang, P. and Ilemobade, A. A., 1977. Tick-borne diseases of domestic animals in Northern Nigeria. II. Research summary, 1966–1978, *Trop. Anim. Hlth Prod.*, **9**: 211–18.

Levine, D., Corliss, J. O., Cox, F. E. G., Deroux, G., Grain, J., Honigberg, B. M., Leedale, G. F., Loeblich, A. R. III., Lom, J., Lynn, D., Merinfields, E. G., Page, F. C., Paljansky, G., Sprague, V., Vaura, J. and Wallace, F. G., 1980. A newly revised classification of protozoa, *J. Protozool.*, **27**: 37–58.

Lewis, E. A., 1950. Conditions affecting the East Coast fever parasite in ticks and cattle, *East Afr. Agric. J.*, **16**: 65–77.

Löhr, K. F., 1978. A hypothesis on the role of *Theileria lawrencei* in the epizootiology of East Coast fever and its importance in attempting vaccination. In *Tick-borne Diseases and their Vectors*, ed. J. K. H.

Wilde. Lewis Reprints (Tonbridge), pp. 315–17.
Löhr, K. F. and Meyer, H., 1974. Game theilerioses – a serological investigation, *Z. Tropenmed. Parasit.*, **25**: 288–92.
Löhr, K. F., Meyer, H. and Ross, J. P. J., 1974. Detection in game of fluorescent and agglutination antibodies to intraerythrocytic organisms, *Z. Tropenmed. Parasit.*, **25**: 217–26.
Löhr, K. F. and Ross, J. P. J., 1968. Improvement of the indirect fluorescent antibody test for the diagnosis of diseases caused by intraerythrocytic parasites, *Tropenmed. Parasit.*, **19**: 427–30.
Losos, G. J. and Jura, W. G. Z., in preparation.

Mack, R., 1957. Chemotherapy of piroplasmosis and theileriosis of farm animals in the USSR, *Vet. Rev. Annot.*, **3**: 57–68.
Mahmoud, A. H., Awad, F. I., Haiba, M. H. and Zafer, S. A. W., 1956. Die wirksamkeit von Berenil bei subklinischen fallen von theileriose bei rindern und buffeln, *Z. Tropenmed. Parasit.*, **7**: 282–5.
Malmquist, W. A. and Brown, C. G. D., 1974. Establishment of *Theileria parva*-infected lymphoblastoid cell lines using homologous feeder layers, *Res. vet. Sci.*, **16**: 134–5.
Malmquist, W. A., Nyindo, M. B. A. and Brown, C. G. D., 1970. East Coast fever: cultivation *in vitro* of bovine spleen cell lines infected and transformed by *Theileria parva*, *Trop. Anim. Hlth Prod.*, **2**: 139–45.
Martin, H. M., Barnett, S. F. and Vidler, O. B., 1964. Cyclic development and longevity of *Theileria parva* in the tick *Rhipicephalus appendiculatus*, *Exp. Parasitol.*, **15**: 527–55.
Martins, M. I., 1978. Histochemical studies on salivary glands of unfed and feeding *Rhipicephalus appendiculatus* during the development of *Theileria parva*. In *Tick-borne Diseases and their Vectors*, ed. J. K. H. Wilde. Lewis Reprints (Tonbridge), pp. 336–42
Maxie, M. G., Dolan, T. T., Flowers, M. J., Jura, W. G. Z. and Tabel, H., 1982. A comparative study of the diseases in cattle caused by *Theileria parva* or *T. lawrencei*: II. Haematology, clinical chemistry, coagulation studies and complement, *Vet. Parasitol.*, **10**: 1–19.
Mazlum, Z., 1968. *Hyalomma asiaticum asiaticum* Schulse and Schlottke, 1929. Its distribution, host's seasonal activity, life cycle, and role in transmission of bovine theileriosis in Iran, *Acarologia*, **10**: 437–42.
McCall, H., 1978. Effect of salivary stimulants on isolated preparations of *Theileria parva*-infected and non-infected salivary glands of *R. appendiculatus*. In *Tick-borne Diseases and their Vectors*, ed. J. K. H. Wilde. Lewis Reprints (Tonbridge), pp. 343–50.
McCulloch, B., 1964. An outbreak of theileriosis in Tanganyika, *Bull. epiz. Dis. Afr.*, **12**: 63–6.
McCulloch, B., 1968. A study of East Coast fever, drought and social obligations, in relation to the need for economic development of the livestock industry in Sukumaland, Tanzania, *Bull. epiz. Dis. Afr.*, **16**: 303–26.

McCulloch, B., Kalaye, W. J., Mbasha, E. M. S., Suda, B. Q. J. and Tungaraza, R., 1968. A study of the life history of the tick *Rhipicephalus appendiculatus* – the main vector of East Coast fever – with reference to its behaviour under field conditions and with regard to its control in Sukumaland, Tanzania, *Bull. epiz. Dis. Afr.*, **16**: 477–500.

McHardy, N., 1978a. *In vitro* studies on the action of Menoctone and other compounds on *Theileria parva* and *Theileria annulata* (in cattle), *Ann. trop. Med. Parasit.*, **72**: 501–11.

McHardy, N., 1978b. An *in vitro* screen for compounds active against *Theileria* spp. In *Tick-borne Diseases and their Vectors*, ed. J. K. H. Wilde. Lewis Reprints (Tonbridge), pp. 334–5.

McHardy, N., Haigh, A. J. B. and Dolan, T. T., 1976. Chemotherapy of *Theileria parva* infection, *Nature*, **261**: 698–9.

Mchinja, S. J., Omwoyo, P. and Young, A. S., 1977. Effects of oxytetracycline on *Theileria parva*: inoculation of rabbits on which infected *Rhipicephalus* are feeding, *Bull. Anim. Hlth Prod. Afr.*, **25**: 158–61.

Meer, P. van der, Bergh, S. G. van den, Perié, N. M., Spanjer, A. A. M. and Uilenberg, G., 1981. Isoenzyme studies on *Theileria* (protozoa, sporozoa). Enzyme activity associated with erythrocytic stage, *Vet. Quarterly*, **3**: 61–5.

Mehlhorn, H., 1975. Electron microscope studies on developmental stages of *Theileria annulata* (Dschunkowsky and Luhs, 1904) in the intestine and haemolymph of *Hyalomma anatolicum excavatum* (Koch, 1844), *Z. Parasitenkd.*, **48**: 137–50.

Mehlhorn, H. and Schein, E., 1976a. Elektonennukroskopische untersuchungen an Entwicklungsstadien von *Theileria parva* (Theiler, 1904) in Dam der ubertrogerzecke *Hyalomma anatolicum excavatum* (Koch, 1844), *Z. Tropenmed. Parasit.*, **27**: 180–92.

Mehlhorn, H. and Schein, E., 1976b. Fine structure of *Theileria*, *Z. Parasitenkd.*, **50**: 203.

Mehlhorn, H. and Schein, E., 1977. Electron microscopic studies of the development of kinetes in *Theileria annulata* (Dschunkowsky and Luhs, 1904) (sporozoa, piroplasmea), *J. Protozool.*, **24**: 249–57.

Mehlhorn, H., Schein, E. and Warnecke, M., 1978. Electron microscopic studies on the development of kinetes of *Theileria parva* (Theiler, 1904) in the gut of the vector tick *Rhipicephalus appendiculatus* Neumann, 1901, *Acta trop.*, **35**: 123–36.

Mehlhorn, H., Schein, E. and Warnecke, M., 1979. Electron-microscopic studies on *Theileria ovis* Ridhain 1916: development of kinetes in the gut of the vector tick, *Rhipicephalus evertsi evertsi* (Neumann, 1897), and their transformation within cells of the salivary glands, *J. Protozool.*, **26**: 377–85.

Melrose, T. R. and Brown, C. G. D., 1979. Isoenzyme variation in piroplasms isolated from bovine blood infected with *Theileria annulata* and *T. parva*, *Res. vet. Sci.*, **27**: 379–81.

Melrose, T. R., Brown, C. G. D. and Sharma, R. D., 1980. Glucose phosphate isomerase isoenzyme patterns in bovine lymphoblastoid cell lines infected with *Theileria annulata* and *T. parva*, with an improved enzyme visualisation method using meldola blue, *Res. vet. Sci.*, **29**: 298–304.

Melrose, T. R., Brown, C. G. D. and Walker, A. R., 1981. Identification of *Theileria* infections in the salivary glands of *Hyalomma anatolicum anatolicum* and *Rhipicephalus appendiculatus* using isoenzyme electrophoresis, *Trop. Anim. Hlth Prod.*, **13**: 70–8.

Mettam, R. W. M. and Carmichael, J., 1936. Turning sickness, a protozoan encephalitis of cattle in Uganda. Its relationship with East Coast fever, *Parasitology*, **28**: 254–83.

Mohammed, A. N., 1978. Prevalence and experimental transmission of bovine piroplasms in northern Nigeria. In *Tick-borne Diseases and their Vectors*, ed. J. K. H. Wilde. Lewis Reprints (Tonbridge), p. 149.

Moodie, P. A., 1977. Country reports: Malawi. In *Theileriosis*, eds J. B. Henson, M. Campbell. IDRC (Ottawa), **086e**, pp. 25–7.

Morrison, W. I., Buscher, G., Cook, R. H., Emery, D. L., Masake, R. A., Murray, M. and Wells, P. W., 1981. *Theileria parva*: kinetics of infection in the lymphoid system of cattle, *Exp. Parasitol.*, **52**: 248–60.

Morzaria, S. P., Brocklesby, D. W., Kimberley, C. D. and Young, A. S., 1977. The serological relationship of a British *Theileria* with other *Theileria* species using the indirect fluorescent antibody, *Res. vet. Sci.*, **22**: 330–3.

Moulton, J. E., Krauss, H. H. and Malmquist, W. A., 1971. Growth characteristics of *Theileria parva* infected bovine lymphoblast cultures, *Am. J. vet. Res.*, **32**: 1365–70.

Mugera, G. M. and Munyua, W. K., 1973. A study of developmental stages of *Theileria parva* by electron microscopy, *Bull. epiz. Dis. Afr.*, **21**: 51–66.

Muhammed, S. I., 1975. The effect of leukocytes from cattle immunized against East Coast fever on the migration of bovine lymphoblasts infected with *Theileria parva*, *Zbl. Vet. Med.*, **22**: 455–60.

Muhammed, S. I., Johnson, L. W. and Lauerman, L. H., 1975. Effect of humoral antibodies on the course of *Theileria parva* infection (East Coast fever) of cattle, *Am. J. Vet. Res.*, **36**: 399–402.

Muhammed, S. I., Lauerman, L. H. and Wagner, G. G., 1974. Leukocyte migration inhibition as a model for the demonstration of sensitized cells in East Coast fever, *Immunology*, **27**: 1033–7.

Munyua, W. K., Bitakarmire, P. K. and Mugera, G. M. 1973. Pathogenesis and pathology of East Coast fever induced by irradiated ticks, *Bull. epiz. Dis. Afr.*, **21**: 75–85.

Munyua, W. K. and Wamakima, D. N., 1979. Serum transaminase activities in the bovine experimentally infected with East Coast fever (*Theileria parva* infection), *Bull. Anim. Hlth Prod. Afr.*, **27**: 253–6.

Musisi, E. L., Bird, R. G., Brown, C. G. D. and Smith, M., 1981a. The fine structural relationship between *Theileria* schizonts and

infected bovine lymphoblasts from cultures, *Z. Parasitenkd.*, **65**: 31–42.
Musisi, F. L., Brown. C. G. D., Kilgour, V. and Morzaria, S. P., 1981b. Preliminary investigations on isoenzyme variants of lymphoblastoid cell lines infected with *Theileria* species, *Res. vet. Sci.*, **30**: 38–43.

Neitz, W. O., 1956. Review of the theilerioses, *Bull. epiz. Dis. Afr.*, **4**: 215–17.
Neitz, W. O., 1957. Theilerioses, gonderioses and cytauxzoonoses. A review, *Onderstepoort J. vet. Res.*, **27**: 275–461.
Neitz, W. O., 1958. Can Corridor-disease recovered cattle serve as reservoirs of *Gonderia lawrencei*?, *Bull. epiz. Dis. Afr.*, **6**: 151–4.
Neitz, W. O., 1964. The immunity in East Coast fever, *J. S. Afr. vet. med. Ass.*, **35**: 5–6.
Neitz, W. O., 1972. The experimental transmission of *Theileria ovis* by *Rhipicephalus evertsi mimeticus* and *R. bursa*, *Onderstepoort J. vet. Res.*, **39**: 83–5.
Neitz, W. O. and Jansen, B. C., 1956. A discussion on the classification of the Theileriidae, *J. vet. Res.*, **27**: 7–18.
Nyindo., M. B. A., Kaminjolo, J. S., Lule, M. and Wagner, G. G., 1978. East Coast fever: cultivation *in vitro* of cell-free schizonts and merozoites of *Theileria parva* and their immunogenicity to cattle, *Vet. Res.*, **39**: 37.
Nyormoi, O., Bwayo, J. J. and Hirumi, H., 1981. *Theileria parva*: isolation of macroschizonts from *in vitro* propagated lymphoblastoid cells in cattle, *Exp. Parasitol.*, **52**: 303–12.

Okao, E. T. and Oteng, A. K., 1973. An appraisal of the factors causing losses to newly introduced exotic cattle (*Bos taurus*) into Uganda, *Bull. epiz. Dis. Afr.*, **21**: 193–205.
Oteng, A. K., 1970. Epidemiology of East Coast fever in Uganda: a review, *Proc. 2nd Int. Congr. Parasitol.*, Washington, **2**: 456–7.
Oteng, A. K., 1971. Growth and multiplication of the piroplasms of the Australian *Theileria mutans* in bovine erythrocytes, *Bull. epiz. Dis. Afr.*, **19**: 223–42.
Oteng, A. K., 1976. Fever: a critical factor in the pathogenesis of East Coast fever (*Theileria parva* infection) in cattle. In *Pathophysiology of Parasitic Infection*, ed. E. J. L. Soulsby. Academic Press (New York and London), pp. 211–19.

Paling, R. W., Grootenhuis, J. G. and Young, A. S., 1981. Isolation of *Theileria mutans* from Kenyan buffalo and transmission by *Amblyomma gemma*, *Vet. Parasitol.*, **8**: 31–7.
Pearson, T. W., Lundin, L. B., Dolan, T. T. and Stagg, D. A., 1979.

Cell-mediated immunity to *Theileria*-transformed cell lines, *Nature*, **28**: 678–80.
Perié, N. M., Schreuder, B. E. C. and Uilenberg, G., 1979. *Theileria mutans* in Nigeria, *Res. vet. Sci.*, **26**: 359–62.
Pinder, M., Kar, S., Lundin, L. B., Roelants, G. E. and Withey, K. S., 1981. Proliferation and lymphocyte stimulatory capacity of *Theileria*-infected lymphoblastoid cells before and after elimination of intracellular parasites, *Immunology*, **44**: 51–60.
Pinder, M., Roelants, G. E. and Withey, K. S., 1981. *Theileria parva* parasites transform a subpopulation of T lymphocytes, *J. Immunol.*, **127**: 389–90.
Pipano, E., 1970. Immune response in calves to varying numbers of attenuated schizonts of *Theileria annulata*, *J. Protozool.*, **17**: 31.
Pipano, E., 1974. Immunological aspects of *Theileria annulata* infection, *Bull. Off. int. Epiz.*, **81**: 139–59.
Pipano, E., 1975. Immunization against *Theileria annulata* infection. In *20th World Veterinary Congress* (summaries). Thessalonika (Greece), vol. 1, pp. 188–9.
Pipano, E., 1976. Control of bovine theileriosis and anaplasmosis in Israel, *Bull. Off. int. Epiz.*, **86**: 55–9.
Pipano, E., 1979. Virulence and immunogenicity of cultured *Theileria annulata* schizonts, *J. S. Afr. vet. med. Ass.*, **50**: 332–3.
Pipano, E., 1980. Immunization against intracellular blood protozoans of cattle, *Prog. Clin. Biol. Res.*, **47**: 301–14.
Pipano, E. and Cahana, M., 1968. Measurement of the immune response to vaccine from tissue cultures of *Theileria annulata* by the fluorescent antibody test, *J. Protozool.*, **15**: 45.
Pipano, E. and Cahana, M., 1969. Fluorescent antibody test for the serodiagnosis of *Theileria annulata*, *J. Parasitol.*, **55**: 765.
Pipano, E., Cahana, M., David, E., Feller, B. and Shabat, Y., 1969. A serological method for assessing the response to *Theileria annulata* immunization, *Refuah Vet.*, **26**: 145–8.
Pipano, E., Cohen, R. and Klopper, U., 1973. Inoculation of cattle with bovine lymphoid cell lines, *Res. vet. Sci.*, **20**, 388–9.
Pipano, E., Friedhoff, K. T., Goldman, M. and Samish, M., 1977. Immunization of cattle against *Theileria annulata* using killed schizont vaccine, *Vet. Parasitol.*, **3**: 11–22.
Pipano, E. and Israel, V., 1971. Absence of erythrocyte forms of *Theileria annulata* in calves inoculated with schizonts from a virulent field strain grown in tissue culture, *J. Protozool.*, **18**: 37.
Pipano, E., Kriegel, Y., Samish, M. and Yeruham, I., 1981. Immunization of Friesian cattle against *Theileria annulata* by the infection-treatment method, *Br. vet. J.*, **137**: 416–20.
Pipano, E. and Shkap, V., 1979. Attenuation of two Turkish strains of *Theileria annulata*, *J. Protozool.*, **26**: 80A.
Pirie, H. M., Crighton, G. W. and Harrett, W. F. H., 1970. Studies on vaccination against East Coast fever using macroschizonts, *Exp. Parasitol.*, **27**: 343–9.
Purnell, R. E., 1970. Infection of the tick *Rhipicephalus appendiculatus*

with *Theileria parva* using an artificial feeding technique, *Res. vet. Sci.*, **11**: 403–5.

Purnell, R. E., 1977. East Coast fever of cattle: some recent research in East Africa *Theileria*, *Adv. Parasitol.*, **15**: 83–132.

Purnell, R. E., 1978. *Theileria annulata* as a hazard to cattle in countries on the northern Mediterranean littoral, *Vet. Sci. Commun.*, **2**: 3–10.

Purnell, R. E., Bailey, K. P., Branagan, D., Joyner, L. P. and Radley, D. E., 1970c. Technique for harvesting the infective particles in saliva of the tick *Rhipicephalus appendiculatus*. In *Isotopes and Radiation in Parasitology*. IAEA (Vienna), vol. II, pp. 99–103.

Purnell, R. E., Boarer, C. D. H. and Peirce, M. A., 1971. *Theileria parva*: comparative infection rates of adult and nymphal *Rhipicephalus appendiculatus*, *Parasitology*, **62**: 349–53.

Purnell, R. E., Branagan, D. and Brown, C. G. D., 1970b. Attempted transmissions of some piroplasms by *Rhipicephalid* ticks, *Trop. Anim. Hlth Prod.*, **2**: 146–50.

Purnell, R. E., Branagan, D. and Radley, D. E., 1969. The use of parasymphathomimetic drugs to stimulate salivation in the tick *Rhipicephalus appendiculatus*, and the transmission of *Theileria parva* using saliva obtained by this method from infected ticks, *Parasitology*: **59**: 709–918.

Purnell, R. E., Brown, C. G. D., Burridge, M. J., Cunningham, M. P., Kirimi, I. M. and Ledger, M. A., 1973b. East Coast fever: correlation between the morphology and infectivity of *Theileria parva* developing in its tick vector, *Parasitology*, **66**: 539–44.

Purnell, R. E., Brown, C. G. D., Irvin, A. D., Ledger, M. A., Payne, R. C., Radley, D. E., Schiemann, B. and Young, A. S., 1973a. Attempted transmission of *Theileria gorgonis*, Brocklesby and Vidler, 1961, from blue wildebeest (*Connochaetes taurinus*) to cattle, *Z. Tropenmed. Parasit.*, **24**: 181–5.

Purnell, R. E., Cunningham, M. P., Musisi, F. L. and Payne, R. C., 1975b. The establishment of an experimental field population of *Theileria parva*-infected ticks, *Trop. Anim. Hlth Prod.*, **7**: 133–7.

Purnell, R. E., Dargie, J. D., Gilliver, B., Irvin, A. D. and Ledger, M. A., 1972a. Some effects of irradiation on the tick *Rhipicephalus appendiculatus*, *Parasitology*, **64**: 429–40.

Purnell, R. E., Dargie, J. D., Irvin, A. D. and Ledger, M. A., 1973c. Co-irradiation of the tick *Rhipicephalus appendiculatus*, In *Isotopes and Radiation in Parasitology*, IAEA (Vienna), vol. III, pp. 139–44.

Purnell, R. E., Irvin, A. D., Kimber, C. D., Omwoyo, P. L. and Payne, R. C., 1974. East Coast fever: further laboratory investigations on the use of rabbits as vehicles for infecting ticks with theilerial piroplasms, *Trop. Anim. Hlth Prod.*, **6**: 145–51.

Purnell, R. E. and Joyner, L. P., 1967. Artificial feeding technique for *Rhipicephalus appendiculatus* and the transmission of *Theileria parva* from the salivary secretion, *Nature*, **216**; 484–5.

Purnell, R. E. and Joyner, L. P., 1968. The development of *Theileria parva* in the salivary glands of the tick *Rhipicephalus appendiculatus*, *Parasitology*, **58**: 725–32.

Purnell, R. E., Ledger, M. A. and Obatre, J. B., 1972b. Some effects of irradiation on *Theileria parva* in the salivary glands of the tick *Rhipicephalus appendiculatus*, *Parasitology*, **65**: 23–6.

Purnell, R. E., Musoke, A. and Peirce, M. A., 1970a. Carnivores as vehicles for ticks carrying disease agents: a possible role of the large-spotted genet, *Genetta tigrina* in the epizootiology of East Coast fever, *Trop. Anim. Hlth Prod.*, **2**: 87–9.

Purnell, R. E. and Rae, M. C., 1981. The use of imidocarb diproprionate for the treatment of *Theileria sergenti* infection of cattle, *Austr. vet. J.*, **57**: 224–6.

Purnell, R. E., Young, A. S., Mwangi, J. M. and Payne, R. C., 1975a. Development of *Theileria mutans* (Aitong) in the tick *Amblyomma variegatum* compared to that of *T. parva* (Muguga) in *Rhipicephalus appendiculatus*, *J. Parasitol.*, **61**: 725–9.

Radley, D. E., 1978. Chemoprophylactic immunization against East Coast fever. In *Tick-borne Diseases and their Vectors*, ed. J. K. H. Wilde. Lewis Reprints (Tonbridge), pp. 324–9.

Radley, D. E., Brown, C. G. D., Burridge, M. J., Cunningham, M. P., Kirimi, I. M., Purnell, R. E. and Young, A. S., 1975a. East Coast fever: 1. Chemoprophylactic immunization of cattle against *Theileria parva* (Muguga) and five theilerial strains, *Vet. Parasitol.*, **1**: 35–41.

Radley, D. E., Brown, C. G. D., Burridge, M. J., Cunningham, M. P., Musisi, F. L., Purnell, R. E. and Young, A. S., 1975b. East Coast fever: 2. Cross-immunity trials with a Kenya strain of *Theileria lawrencei*, *Vet. Parasitol.*, **1**: 43–50.

Radley, D. E., Brown, C. G. D., Burridge, M. J., Cunningham, M. P., Peirce, M. A. and Purnell, R. E., 1974. East Coast fever: quantitative studies of *Theileria parva* in cattle, *Exp. Parasitol.*, **36**: 278–87.

Radley, D. E., Brown, C. G. D., Cunningham, M. P., Kimber, C. D., Musisi, F. L., Payne, R. C., Purnell, R. E., Stagg, S. M. and Young, A. S., 1975c. East Coast fever: 3. Chemoprophylactic immunization of cattle using oxytetracycline and a combination of theilerial strains, *Vet. Parasitol.*, **1**: 51–60.

Radley, D. E., Brown, C. G. D., Cunningham, M. P., Kimber, C. D., Musisi, F. L., Purnell, R. E. and Stagg, S. M., 1975d. East Coast fever: challenge of immunized cattle by prolonged exposure to infected ticks, *Vet. Rec.*, **96**: 525–7.

Radley, D. E., Cunningham, M. P., Dolan, T. T., Grootenhuis, J. G., Morzaria, S. P. and Young, A. S., 1979. Further studies on the immunization of cattle against *Theileria lawrencei* by infection and chemoprophylaxis, *Vet. Parasitol.*, **5**: 117–28.

Radley, D. E., Newson, R. M., Cunningham, M. P. and Punyua, D. K., 1978. Effects of prolonged exposure of *T. parva* immunized cattle in experimentally infected paddock. In *Tick–borne Diseases and their Vectors*, ed. J. K. H. Wilde. Lewis Reprints (Tonbridge), pp. 297–301.

Raghvachari, K. and Reddy, A. M., 1956. Acute theileriasis in sheep, *Indian vet. Sci.*, **26**: 123–4.

Rehbein, G., Ahmed, J. S., Horchner, F., Schein, E. and Zweygarth, E., 1981. Immunological aspects of *Theileria annulata* infection in calves. I. E, EA, and EAC rosettes forming cells in calves infected with *T. annulata*, *Z. Tropenmed. Parasit.*, **32**: 101–4.

Rensburg, I. B. J. van, 1976. Bovine cerebral theileriosis: a report on five cases with splenic infarction, *J. S. Afr. vet. med. Ass.*, **47**: 137–41.

Ristic, M., 1967. The vertebrate development cycle of *Babesia* and *Theileria*. In *Biology of Parasites*, ed. E. J. L. Soulsby. Academic Press (New York), pp. 128–41.

Robson, J., Brown, C. G. D., Kamya, E. P., Odeke, G. M. and Pedersen, V., 1977. East Coast fever immunization trials in Uganda: field exposure of Zebu cattle immunized with three isolates of *Theileria parva*, *Trop. Anim. Hlth Prod.*, **9**: 219–31.

Robson, J., Odeke, G. M., Pedersen, V. and Uilenberg, G., 1981. Theileriosis in Uganda. Parasitological and serological responses in cattle continually exposed to natural infection, *Trop. Anim. Hlth Prod.*, **13**: 1–11.

Robson, J., Ross, J. L. P. J. and Yeoman, G. H., 1961. *Rhipicephalus appendiculatus* and East Coast fever in Tanganyika, *E. Afr. med. J.*, **38**: 206–14.

Roelants, G. E., Buscher, G., London, J., Mayor-Withey, K. S., Rovis, L. and Williams, R. O., 1977. On the transformation of lymphocytes by *Theileria*, an intracellular parasite. In *Protides of Biological Fluids*, ed. H. Peters. Pergamon (London), pp. 743–5.

Rogers, R. J. and Callow, L. L., 1966. Three fatal cases of *Theileria mutans* infection, *Aust. vet. J.*, **42**: 42–6.

Ross, J. P. and Löhr, K. F., 1972. A capillary tube agglutination test for detection and titration of *Theileria parva* and *Theileria mutans* antibodies in bovine serum, *Res. vet. Sci.*, **13**: 405–10.

Saidu, S. N. A., 1981. Bovine theileriosis in Nigeria. M.Sc. thesis, Ahmadu Bello Univ. (Zaria, Nigeria), pp. 48–114.

Saidu, S. N. A., 1982. Bovine theileriosis due to *Theileria mutans*: a review, *Vet. Bull.*, **52**: 451–9.

Samantaray, S. N., Bhattacharyulu, Y. and Gill, B. S., 1980. Immunization of calves against bovine tropical theileriosis (*Theileria annulata*) with graded doses of sporozoites and irradiated sporozoites, *Int. J. Parasitol.*, **10**: 355–8.

Samish, M., 1977a. Infective *Theileria annulata* in the tick without a blood meal stimulus, *Nature*, **270**: 51–2.

Samish, M., 1977b. Transmission of *Theileria annulata* by *Hyalomma excavatum* under various environmental conditions, *J. Protozool.*, **24**: 67A–68A.

Samish, M., 1978. Development of infectivity in *Hyalomma detritum* (Schulze, 1919) ticks infected with *Theileria annulata* (Dschunkowsky and Luhs, 1904), *Parasitology*, **77**: 375.

Samish, M. and Pipano, E., 1978. Transmission of *Theileria annulata* by two and three host ticks of genus *Hyalomma* (Ixodidae). In *Tick-borne Diseases and their Vectors*, ed. J. K. H. Wilde. Lewis Reprints (Tonbridge), pp. 371–2.

Schein, E., 1975. On the life cycle of *Theileria annulata* (Dschunkowsky and Luhs, 1904) in the midgut and haemolymph of *Hyalomma anatolicum excavatum* (Koch, 1844), *Z. Parasitenkd.*, **47**: 165–7.

Schein, E., 1976. Developmental stages of *Theileria annulata* in *Hyalomma anatolicum excavatum*, *Z. Parasitenkd.*, **50**: 205–6.

Schein, E. and Friedhoff, K. T., 1978. Light microscopic studies on the development of *Theileria annulata* (Dschunkowsky and Luhs, 1904) in *Hyalomma anatolicum excavatum* (Koch, 1844). II. The development in haemolymph and salivary glands, *Z. Parasitenkd.*, **56**: 287–303.

Schein, E., Kirmse, P. and Warnecke, M., 1977a. Development of *Theileria parva* (Theiler, 1904) in the gut of *Rhipicephalus appendiculatus* (Neumann, 1901), *Parasitogy*, **75**: 309–16.

Schein, E., Mehlhorn, H. and Warnecke, M., 1977b. Fine structural study on the erythrocytic stages of *Theileria annulata* (Dschunkowsky, Luhs, 1904), *Z. Tropenmed. Parasit.*, **28**: 349–60.

Schein, E., Mehlhorn, H. and Warnecke, M., 1978. Electron microscopic studies on the schizogony of four *Theileria* species of cattle (*T. parva*, *T. lawrencei*, *T. annulata* and *T. mutans*), *Protistologica*, **14**: 337–48.

Schein, E. and Voigt, W. P., 1979. Chemotherapy of bovine theileriosis with halofuginone, *Acta trop.*, **36**: 391–4.

Schein, E. and Warnecke, M., 1976. Developmental stages of *Theileria parva* in the intestine of ticks, *Z. Parasitenkd.*, **50**: 211.

Schindler, R., Matson, B. and Mehlitz, D., 1969a. Serological and immunological studies on *Theileria lawrencei* infection in cattle, *Z. Tropenmed. Parasit.*, **20**: 162–83.

Schindler, R. and Mehlitz, D., 1968. Serologische untersuchungen bei der *Theileria parva* infektion des rindes, *Z. Tropenmed. Parasit.*, **19**: 316–29.

Schindler, R. and Mehlitz, D., 1969. Serologische untersuchungen bei der *Theileria mutans* infektion des rindes, *Z. Parasitenkd.*, **20**: 459–73.

Schindler, R., Mehlitz, D. and Wissenhutter, E., 1969b. The use of serological methods in the epidemiological study of East Coast fever in Tanzania, *Berl. Münch. Tierarztl. Wschr.*, **62**: 6–10.

Schindler, R. and Wokatsch, R., 1965. Attempts at differentiation of *Theileria* species from cattle by serological tests, *Z. Tropenmed, Parasit.*, **16**: 17–23.

Schreuder, B. E. C., Silayo, R. S. and Uilenberg, G., 1976. Studies on Theileriidae (sporozoa) in Tanzania. VI. Second field trial on immunization against cattle theileriosis, *Z. Tropenmed. Parasit.*, **27**: 26–34.

Schreuder, B. E. C., Tondeur, W. and Uilenberg, G., 1977. Studies on Theileriidae (sporozoa) in Tanzania. VIII. Experiments with African buffalo (*Syncerus caffer*), *Z. Tropenmed. Parasit.*, **28**: 367–71.

Schreuder, B. E. C. and Uilenberg, G., 1976. Studies on Theileriidae (sporozoa) in Tanzania. V. Preliminary experiments on a new method for infecting ticks with *Theileria parva* and *Theileria mutans*. *Z. Tropenmed. Parasit.*, **27**: 422–6.

Schulz, K. C. A. and Schutte, J. R., 1957. 'Turning sickness.' Bovine theileriosis in the Rustenberg district. *J. S. Afr. vet. med. Ass.*, **28**: 279–89.

Shannon, D., 1973. The mortality rate in East Coast fever, *Vet. Rec.*, **92**: 213.

Shannon, D., 1977. Field cases of East Coast fever in grade cattle in Uganda, *Trop. Anim. Hlth Prod.*, **9**: 29–35.

Sharma, L. D., Bhattacharya, N. K., Sabir, M. and Sharma, N. N., 1977. Effect of amodiaquine hydrochloride and imidocarb diproprionate in experimental theileriosis in bull-calves, *Indian vet. J.*, **54**: 979–83.

Sharma, L. D., Bhattacharya, N. K. and Sabir, M., 1980a. Effect of diethylcarbamazine citrate on clinical haematological and biochemical aspects in experimental theileriasis in bull-calves, *Vet. res. J.*, **3**: 91–5.

Sharma, L. D., Bhattacharya, N. K. and Sabir, M., 1980b. Effect of amodiaquine hydrochloride and imidocarb diproprionate on certain haematological and biochemical parameters in *Theileria annulata* infected crossbred calves, *Vet. res. J.*, **3**: 117–19.

Sharma, N. N., 1976. Recrudescence of virulence in an 'avirulent strain' of *Theileria annulata*, *Parasitologica*, **38**: 253–7.

Sharma, N. N., 1979. Haematological observations in bovine theileriosis, anaplasmosis and in mixed infections, *Indian J. Parasitol.*, **3**: 153–5.

Sharma, N. N., Kaushik, K. C., Raisinghani, P. M. and Yadav, S. S., 1979. Studies on incidence and control of theileriosis in Jersey cattle, *Indian vet. Med. J.*, **3**: 187–91.

Sharma, R. D. and Gautam, O. P., 1971. Theileriasis. II. Clinical cases in indigenous calves, *Indian vet. J.*, **48**: 83–91.

Sharma, R. D. and Gautam, O. P., 1973. Cerebral theileriosis in a Hariani calf, *Indian vet. J.*, **50**: 823–39.

Shatry, A. M., Wilson, A. J., Varma, S. and Dolan, T. T., 1981. Sequential study of lymph nodes and splenic aspirates during *Theileria parva* infection in calves, *Res. vet. Sci.*, **30**: 181–4.

Shommein, A. M., 1977. Country reports: Theileriosis in the Sudan. In *Theileriosis*, eds J. B. Henson, M. Campbell. IDRC (Ottawa), **086e**, pp. 46–8.

Singh, B., Anantwar, L. G., Bhonsle, V. G. and Samad, A., 1980. Chemotherapeutic activity of oxytetracycline against clinical cases of *Theileria annulata* infection in exotic and cross-bred cattle, *Indian vet. J.*, **57**: 849–52.

Singh, D. K., Dhar, S., Gautam, O. P. and Jagdish, S., 1979a. Infectivity of ground-up tick supernates prepared from *Theileria annulata* infected by *Hyalomma anatolicum anatolicum*, *Trop. Anim. Hlth Prod.*, **11**: 87–90.

Singh, D. K., Gautam, O. P. and Jagdish, S., 1977. Cell-mediated immunity in tropical theileriosis (*Theileria annulata* infection), *Res. vet. Sci.*, **23**: 391–2.

Singh, D. K., Gautam, O. P. and Jagdish, S., 1979b. Immunization against bovine tropical theileriosis using ^{60}Co-irradiated infective particles of *Theileria annulata* (Dschunkowsky and Luhs, 1904) derived from ticks, *Am. J. vet. Res.*, **40**: 767–9.

Smith, K., 1976. An ultrastructural study of heterokaryons derived from *Theileria parva* infected bovine lymphoblasts and Ehrlich ascites tumour cells, *Res. vet. Sci.*, **21**: 205–14.

Smith, K., Bland, P., Brocklesby, D. W., Brown, C. G. D., Payne, R. C. and Purnell, R. E., 1974. The fine structure of intra-erythrocytic stages of *Theileria gorgonis* and a strain of *Anaplasma marginale* isolated froom wildebeest (*Connochaetes taurinus*), *Z. Tropenmed. Parasit.*, **25**: 293–300.

Smith, K., Irvin, A. D. and Stagg, D. A., 1976. An ultrastructural study of heterokaryons derived from *Theileria parva*-infected bovine lymphoblasts and Ehrlich ascites tumour cells, *Res. vet. Sci.*, **21**: 205–14.

Snodgrass, D. R., Bergman, J. R., Bowyer, W. A., Daft, J., Trees, A. J. and Wall, A. E., 1972. East Coast fever: field challenge of cattle immunized against *Theileria parva* (Muguga), *Trop. Anim. Hlth Prod.*, **4**: 142–51.

Splitter, J. E., 1950. *Theileria mutans* associated with bovine anaplasmosis in the United States, *J. Am. vet. Med. Ass.*, **117**: 134–5.

Spooner, R. L. and Brown, C. D. G., 1980. Bovine lymphocyte antigens (BoLA) of bovine lymphocytes and derived lymphoblastoid lines transformed by *Theileria parva* and *Theileria annulata*, *Parasit. Immunol.*, **2**: 163–74.

Spooner, R. L., Brown, C. G. D., Burridge, M. J. and Penhale, W. J., 1973. Some serum globulin changes in East Coast fever, *Res. vet. Sci.*, **13**: 368–74.

Srivastava, P. S. and Sharma, N. N., 1976a. Characteristics of a tick-transmitted virulent strain of *Theileria annulata* (Dschunkowsky and Luhs, 1904) in crossbred calves, *Pantnagar J. Res.*, **1**: 83–8.

Srivastava, P. S. and Sharma, N. N., 1976b. Note on bovine cerebral theileriosis in crossbred calves *Theileria annulata*, *Pantnagar J. Res.*, **1**: 147–50.

Srivastava, P. S. and Sharma, N. N., 1976c. Infectivity and immunogenicity of washed bovine erythrocytes in crossbred calves infected with *Theileria annulata* (Dschunkowsky and Luhs, 1904), *Pantnagar J. Res.*, **1**: 70–2.

Srivastava, P. S. and Sharma, N. N., 1977a. Studies on the potential immunoprophylaxis using *Theileria annulata* attenuated by cobalt-60 irradiation in bovine lymphocytes, *Vet. Parasitol.*, **3**: 23–31.

Srivastava, P. S. and Sharma, N. N., 1977b. Potential of immunoprophylaxis using cobalt-60 irradiated *Theileria annulata* in salivary gland suspensions of the tick *Hyalomma anatolicum, Vet. Parasitol.*, **3**: 183–8.

Srivastava, P. S. and Sharma, N. N., 1978. Studies on the infectivity of *Theileria annulata* infected nymphs, adults and ground tissues of the tick *Hyalomma anatolicum, Vet. Parasitol.*, **4**: 83–9.

Stagg, D. A., Brown, C. G. D., Crawford, J. G., Kanhai, G. K. and Young, A. S., 1974. *In vitro* cultivation of *Theileria lawrencei*-infected lymphoblastoid cell lines derived from a buffalo (*Syncerus caffer*), *Res. vet. Sci.*, **16**: 125–7.

Stagg, D. A., Brown, C. G. D., Kanhai, G. K. and Young, A. S., 1976. The establishment of *Theileria*-infected cell lines from an eland (*Taurotragus oryx*, Lydekker 1906), *Res. vet. Sci.*, **20**: 122–6.

Stagg, D. A., Chasey, D., Dolan, T. T., Morzaria, S. P. and Young, A. S., 1980. Synchronization of the division of *Theileria* macroschizonts and their mammalian host cells, *Ann. trop. Med. Parasit.*, **74**: 263–5.

Stagg, D. A., Dolan, T. T., Leitch, B. L. and Young, A. S., 1981. The initial stages of infection of cattle cells with *Theileria parva* sporozoites *in vitro, Parasitology*, **83**: 191–7.

Takahashi, K., Isayama, Y., Shimizu, Y. and Yamashita, S., 1976. Serological response to the indirect fluorescent antibody test of cattle infected with *Theileria sergenti, Br. vet. J.*, **132**: 112–17.

Tayama, H., 1975. Studies on the life of bovine *Theileria* species of Japan – with special reference to growth and multiplication of parasite inhabiting the blood in the body of cattle, *Kitasato Arch. Exp. Med.*, **48**: 107–20.

Taylor, J. I., 1954. East Coast fever in Uganda. *Bull. epiz. Dis. Afr.*, **2**: 391–2.

Tsur, I., 1953. *Theileria annulata* et *Leishmania* en cultur de tissu, *Proc. XVth Int. Congr., Stockholm*, pp. 26–36, 162–3.

Tsur, I. and Adler, S., 1963. Growth of *Theileria annulata* schizonts in monolayer tissue cultures, *J. Protozool.*, **10**: 36.

Tsur, I. and Adler, S., 1965. The cultivation of lymphoid cells and *Theileria annulata* schizonts from infected bovine blood, *Refuah Vet.*, **22**: 62.

Tsur, I., Adler, S., Pipano, E. and Senft, Z., 1966. Continuous growth of *Theileria annulata* schizonts in monolayer tissue cultures, *Proc. 1st. Congr. Parasitol.*, **1**: 266–7.

Tustin, R. C. and Heerden, J. van, 1979. Bovine cerebral theileriosis (Turning sickness) with spinal cord involvement, *J. S. Afr. vet. med. Ass.*, **50**: 49–51.

Uilenberg, G., 1977. Biological differences between African *Theileria mutans* (Theiler, 1906) and two benign species of *Theileria* of cattle in Australia and Britain, *Aust. vet. J.*, **53**: 271–3.

Uilenberg, G., Franssen, F. F., Jongejan, F. and Perié, N. M., 1980. Chemotherapy of cattle theileriosis with halofuginone and anticocoidian, *Rev. Elev. Med. vet. Pays trop.*, **33**: 33–43.

Uilenberg, G., Mpangala, C., Sanga, H. J. N., Silayo, R. S., Tatchell, R. J. and Tondeur, W., 1977a. Studies on Theileriidae (sporozoa) in Tanzania. X. A large scale field trial on immunization against cattle theileriosis, *Z. Tropenmed. Parasit.*, **28**: 499–506.

Uilenberg, G., Mpangala, C. and Schreuder, B. E. C. 1976a. Studies on Theileriidae (sporozoa) in Tanzania. III. Experiments on the transmission of *Theileria mutans* by *Rhipicephalus appendiculatus* and *Amblyomma variegatum* (Acarina, Ixododae), *Z. Tropenmed. Parasit.*, **27**: 323–8.

Uilenberg, G., Mpangala, C., Schreuder, B. E. C. and Tondeur, W., 1977b. Studies on Theileriidae (sporozoa) in Tanzania. IX. Unidentified bovine theileriae, *Z. Tropenmed. Parasit.*, **28**: 494–8.

Uilenberg, G., Pedersen, V. and Robson, J., 1974. Some experiments on the transmission of *Theileria mutans* (Theiler, 1906) and *Theileria parva* (Theiler, 1904) by the ticks *Amblyomma variegatum* (Fabricius, 1794) and *Rhipicephalus appendiculatus* (Neumann, 1901) in Uganda, *Z. Tropenmed. Parasit.*, **25**: 207–15.

Uilenberg, G. and Schreuder, B. E. C., 1976a. Studies on Theileriidae (sporozoa) in Tanzania. I. Tick transmission of *Haematoxenus veliferus*, *Z. Tropenmed. Parasit.*, **27**: 106–11.

Uilenberg, G. and Schreuder, B. E. C., 1976b. Further studies on *Haematoxenus separatus* (sporozoa, theileriidae) of sheep in Tanzania, *Rev. Elev. Med. vet. Pays trop.*, **29**: 119–26.

Uilenberg, G. and Schreuder, B. E., 1977. Studies on theileriidae (sporozoa) in Tanzania. VII. Additional note on the transmission of *Theileria parva*, *Z. Tropenmed. Parasit.*, **28**: 181–4.

Uilenberg, G., Schreuder, B. E. C. and Silayo, R. S., 1976b. Studies on Theileriidae (sporozoa) in Tanzania. IV. A field trial on immunization against East Coast fever (*Theileria parva* infection of cattle), *Z. Tropenmed. Parasit.*, **27**: 329–36.

Uilenberg, G. and Zwart, D., 1979. Skin nodules in East Coast fever, *Res. vet. Sci.*, **26**: 243–5.

Voigt, W. P. and Heydorn, A. O., 1981. Chemotherapy of sarcosporidiosis and theileriosis in domestic animals, *Zbl. Bakt. Hyg.*, **250**: 256–9.

Vorstenbosch, C. J. A. H. van, Dijk, J. E. van and Uilenberg, G., 1978. Erythrocytic forms of *Theileria velifera*, *Res. vet. Sci.*, **24**: 214–21.

Vulchovski, Y. A. and Pavlov, N., 1970. Pathology of *Theileria annulata* infection, *Vet. Sci.*, **7**: 55–69.

Wagner, G. R., Akwabi, C., Burridge, M. J., Duffus, W. P. H. and Lule, M., 1975. The specific immunoglobulin response in cattle to *Theileria parva* (Muguga) infection, *Parasitology*, **70**: 95–102.

Wagner, G. R., Brown, C. G. D., Crawford, J. G., Duffus, W. P. H., Kimber, C. D. and Lule, M., 1974a. Immunochemical studies on East Coast fever: I. Partial segregation and characterization of the *Theileria parva* schizont antigen, *J. Parasitol.*, **60**: 848–53.

Wagner, G. R., Duffus, W. P. H., Kimber, C. D. and Lule, M., 1974b. Immunochemical studies on East Coast fever: II. Partial segregation and characterization of the *Theileria parva* piroplasm antigen, *J. Parasitol.*, **60**: 854–9.

Wagner, J. E., 1976. A fatal cytauxzoonosis-like disease in cats, *J. Am. vet. med. Ass.*, **168**: 585–8.

Wagner, J. E., Ferris, D. H., Hansen, R. D., Kier, A. B., Maring, E., Morehouse, L. G. and Wightman, S. R., 1980. Experimentally induced cytauxzoonosis-like disease in domestic cats, *Vet. Parasitol.*, **6**: 305–11.

Walker, A. R., Bell, L. J., Brown, C. G. D. and McKeller, S. B., 1979a. Artificial infection of the tick *Rhipicephalus appendiculatus* with *Theileria parva*, *Res. vet. Sci.*, **26**: 264–5.

Walker, A. R., Bell, L. J., Brown, C. G. D. and McKellar, S. B., 1979b. Rapid quantitative assessment of *Theileria* infection in ticks, *Trop. Anim. Hlth Prod.*, **11**: 21–6.

Walker, A. R., Leitch, B. L. and Young, A. S., 1981. Assessment of *Theileria* infections in *Rhipicephalus appendiculatus* ticks collected from the field, *Z. Parasitenkd.*, **65**: 63–9.

Warnecke, M., Schein, E., Uilenberg, G. and Voigt, W. P., 1979. On the life cycle of *Theileria velifera* (Uilenberg, 1964) in the gut and haemolymph of the tick vector *Amblyomma variegatum* (Fabricius, 1794), *Z. Tropenmed. Parasit.*, **30**: 318–22.

Warnecke, M., Schein, E., Uilenberg, G., Voigt, W. P. and Young, A. S., 1980. Development of *Theileria mutans* (Theiler, 1906) in the gut and the haemolymph of the tick *Amblyomma variegatum* (Fabricius, 1794), *Z. Parasitenkd.*, **62**: 119–25.

Weber, G., 1980. Ultrastructural demonstration of succinic dehydrogenase and cytochrome oxidase activity in sporozoites of *Babesia ovis* and *Theileria annulata* (Apicomplexa: Piroplasmea) in salivary glands of tick vectors (*Rhipicephalus bursa, Hyalomma anatolicum excavatum*, *J. Parasitol.*, **66**: 904–13.

Wilde, J. K. H., 1963. Attempts to induce leukocytosis in normal cattle and in cattle with East Coast fever, *Bull. epiz. Dis. Afr.*, **11**: 415–26.

Wilde, J. K. H., 1966a. Observations on the bone marrow of cattle treated with some therapeutic substances, *Res. vet. Sci.*, **7**: 225–9.

Wilde, J. K. H., 1966b. Changes in bovine bone marrow during the course of East Coast fever, *Res. vet. Sci.*, **7**: 213–24.

Wilde, J. K. H., 1967. East Coast fever, *Adv. vet. Sci.*, **11**: 207–59.

Wilde, J. K. H., 1978. Tick-borne protozoa. In *Tick-borne Diseases and their Vectors*, ed. J. K. H. Wilde. Lewis Reprints (Tonbridge), pp. 287–92.

Wilde, J. K. H., Brown, C. G. D., Gall, D., Hulliger, L. and MacLeod, W. G., 1968. East Coast fever: experiments with the tissues of infected ticks, *Br. vet. J.*, **124**: 196–208.

Wilde, J. K. H., Brown, C. G. D. and Hulliger, L., 1966. Some recent East Coast fever research, *Bull, epiz. Dis. Afr.*, **14**: 29–35.

Wilson, S. G., 1950a. An experimental study of East Coast fever in Uganda. I. A study of the type of EAC reaction produced when the number of infected ticks is controlled, *Parasitology*, **40**: 195–214.

Wilson, S. G., 1950b. An experimental study of East Coast fever in Uganda. III. A study of the East Coast fever reactions produced when infected ticks 31 days old are fed on susceptible calves in limited numbers over a period of three weeks, *Parasitology*, **40**: 23–35.

Wilson, S. G., 1953. A survey of the distribution of tick vectors of East Coast fever in East and Central Africa, *Proc. XVth Int. Vet. Congr., Stockholm*, **1**: 287–90.

Yeoman, G. H., 1966a. Field vector studies of epizootic East Coast fever. I. A quantitative relationship between *R. appendiculatus* and the epizooticity of East Coast fever, *Bull. epiz. Dis. Afr.*, **14**: 5–27.

Yeoman, G. H., 1966b. Field vector studies of epizootic East Coast fever. II. Seasonal studies of *R. appendiculatus* on bovine and non-bovine hosts in East Coast fever enzootic and epizootic free areas, *Bull. epiz. Dis. Afr.*, **14**: 113–40.

Yeoman, G. H., 1968. Field vector studies of epizootic East Coast fever. VI. The occurrence of *Amblyomma variegatum* and *A. lepidum* in the East Coast fever zones, *Bull. epiz. Dis. Afr.*, **16**: 183–203.

Young, A. S., 1977. *Theileria mutans* – infectivity for cattle of parasites derived from pre-fed *Amblyomma variegatum* nymphs, *Z. Tropenmed. Parasit.*, **28**: 521.

Young, A. S., Branagan, D., Brown, C. G. D., Burridge, M. J., Cunningham, M. P. and Purnell, R. E., 1973. Preliminary observations on a theilerial species pathogenic to cattle isolated from buffalo (*Syncerus caffer*) in Tanzania, *Br. vet. J.*, **129**: 382–9.

Young, A. S., Brocklesby, D. W., Dolan, T. T., Flowers, M. J., Grootenhuis, J. G., Smith, K., 1978a. Structures associated with *Theileria* parasites in eland erythrocytes, *Ann. trop. Med. Parasitol.*, **72**: 443–54.

Young, A. S., Brown, C. G. D., Burridge, M. P., Cunningham, M. P., Payne, R. C. and Purnell, R. E., 1977b. Establishment of an experimental field population of *Theileria lawrencei*-infected ticks maintained by African buffalo (*Syncerus caffer*), *J. Parasitol.*, **63**: 903–7.

Young, A. S., Brown, C. G. D., Burridge, M. J., Grootenhuis, J. G., Kanhai, G. K., Purnell, R. E. and Stagg, D. A., 1978b. Incidence of theilerial parasites in East Africa buffalo (*Syncerus caffer*), *Z. Tropenmed. Parasit.*, **29**: 281–8.

Young, A. S., Burridge, M. J. and Payne, R. C., 1977c. Transmission of a *Theileria* species to cattle by the Ixodid tick, *Amblyomma Cohaerens*, Donitz 1909, *Trop. Anim. Hlth Prod.*, **9**: 37–45.

Young, A. S., Brown, C. G. D., Cunningham, M. P. and Radley, D. E., 1978c. Evaluation of methods of immunizing cattle against *Theileria lawrencei*. In *Tick-borne Diseases and their Vectors*, ed. J. K. H. Wilde. Lewis Reprints (Tonbridge), pp. 293–366.

Young, A. S., Grootenhuis, J. G., Kanhai, G. K., Kimber, C. D. and Stagg, D. A., 1977a. Isolation of a *Theileria* species from eland (*Taurotragus oryx*) infective for cattle, *Z. Tropenmed. Parasit.*, **27**: 185–94.

Young, A. S., Grootenhuis, J. G., Leitch, B. L. and Schein, E., 1980. The development of *Theileria – Cytauxzoon taurotragi* (Martin and Brocklesby, 1960) from eland in its tick vector *Rhipicephalus appendiculatus*, *Parasitology*, **81**: 129–44.

Young, A. S., Irvin, A. D. and Woodford, M. J., 1973. *Haematoxenus* species from Ugandan buffalo (*Syncerus caffer*), *J. Wildl. Dis.*, **9**: 94–8.

Young, A. S., Kimber, C. D., Payne, R. C. and Purnell, R. E., 1975. Correlation between the morphology and infectivity of *Theileria lawrencei* developing in the tick *Rhipicephalus appendiculatus*, *Parasitology*, **71**: 27–34.

Young, A. S. and Leitch, B. L., 1981. Epidemiology of East Coast fever: some effects of temperature on the development of *Theileria parva* in the tick vector, *Rhipicephalus appendiculatus*, *Parasitology*, **83**: 199–211.

Young, A. S., Leitch, B. L. and Omwoyo, P. L., 1979. Induction of infective stages of *Theileria parva* by exposure of host ticks to high temperatures, *Vet. Rec.*, **105**: 531–3.

Young, A. S. and Mchinja, S. J., 1977. Observations on *Heamatoxenus separatus* (Uilenberg and Andreasen, 1974) in the erythrocytes of Kenyan sheep, *Res. vet. Sci.*, 387–8.

Young, A. S. and Purnell, R. E., 1973. Transmission of *Theileria lawrencei* (Serengeti) by the Ixodid tick, *Rhipicephalus appendiculatus*, *Trop. Anim. Hlth Prod.*, **5**: 146–52.

Yousif, B. N., 1969. *Theileria annulata* infection in Friesian cattle imported to Iraq from Europe, *Vet. Rec.*, **84**: 360–3.

Chapter

3

Trypanosomiases

CONTENTS

INTRODUCTION

Trypanosomiases are a group of diseases in man and animals caused by five well-differentiated subgenera which include ten less well-defined species in the genus *Trypanosoma*. Either one, two, or more species invading the host simultaneously or sequentially produce infections. The resulting diseases are made up of syndromes ranging from mild, virtually asymptomatic forms lasting for years, to fulminating diseases of a few days' duration. Although similarities exist between the diseases caused by different species in some of the clinical and pathological manifestations, many of the underlying host–parasite interactions are significantly different. These similarities and differences in the pathogenesis are of practical importance not only in the diagnosis and control, but also in research. Therefore, the descriptions of the trypanosomiases which follow are divided according to the subgenera, and where necessary, subdivided further according to either the species of trypanosomes or host, to emphasize the differences. For the purpose of discussion, the diseases are grouped into: the African tsetse-transmitted trypanosomiases, the more cosmopolitan disease commonly known as surra caused by *Trypanosoma evansi, T. equiperdum* limited to dourine of horses and donkeys, and *T. cruzi* which is primarily a zoonosis in South America causing Chagas' disease in man.

Literature

A great deal of literature has been published on trypanosomal parasitisms of reptiles, birds, and mammals. The pathogenic species of veterinary and medical importance make up a relatively small group within the numerous species of trypanosomes which infect but do not cause overt injury to the mammalian hosts which are usually wild animals. This nonpathogenic designation is a relative one; under certain, although rare, circumstances the host may be injured (D'Alesandro 1979). From a practical standpoint, nonpathogenic species have to be differentiated from the pathogenic, for example *Trypanosoma rangeli* in Chagas' endemic areas may require serologic, morphologic, and behavioral examinations before it can be differentiated from *Trypanosoma cruzi* (D'Alesandro 1976). A broader knowledge of the host–parasite interactions including nonpathogenic infections is useful in understanding the pathogenic mechanisms of trypanosomiases. One of the most authoritative reference books on pathogenic and nonpathogenic trypanosomes was published by Wenyon in 1926. Since then, a number of excellent monographs have been published of various aspects of trypanosomal infections of man and animals. These include texts on trypanosomes of mammals by Hoare (1972), the African tsetse-transmitted trypanosomiases of veterinary and medical importance edited by Mulligan (1970), the ecology and epidemiology of African trypanosomiasis by Ford (1971), and more recently the biology of Kinetiplastidae edited by Lumsden and Evans (1976), and Lumsden *et al.* (1979). In addition, symposia were published on trypanosomiasis and leishmaniasis with special reference to Chagas' disease (Ciba Foundation 1970), new approaches to research on Chagas' disease (Pan American Health Organization 1976), and pathogenicity of trypanosomes (Losos and Chouinard 1979). The more recently published reviews were on African animal trypanosomiases (Leach 1973), the problems of tsetse-fly infestation in relation to rural economy were discussed (MacLennan 1980), and the recent research on *T. evansi* dealing with cultivation, morphology, pathogenesis, diagnosis, and chemotherapy by Mahmoud and Gray (1980), and Losos (1980). A short but very comprehensive summary covering morphology, taxonomy, biochemistry, cultivation, host–parasite interactions, diagnosis, and control of *T. cruzi* was published by Fife (1978).

ETIOLOGY

Classification

Pathogenic trypanosomes in the genus *Trypanosoma* are divided into two sections, Salivaria and Stercoraria, according to their development in the vector and transmission by either the saliva or by fecal contamination of the wound caused by bite of the vector. Each section is subdivided into subgenera and species, and a practical classification of trypanosomes of veterinary and medical importance is as follows:

Salivaria
Subgenus *Duttonella*
Species *Trypanosoma vivax*
Subgenus *Nannomonas*
Species *Trypanosoma congolense, T. simiae*

Subgenus *Trypanozoon*
Species *Trypanosoma brucei, T. rhodesiense, T. gambiense, T. evansi,* and *T. equiperdum*
Subgenus *Pycnomonas*
Species *Trypanosoma suis*

Stercoraria
Subgenus *Schizotrypanum*
Species *Trypanosoma cruzi*

Literature

The above classification is an abbreviated form of that presented by Hoare (1972) and serves as a practical breakdown of pathogenic trypanosomes of veterinary and medical importance. Because trypanosomes do not appear to have a sexual cycle, differentiation of species depends on their structural and behavioral characteristics. Speciation is difficult because there is no uniformity in the choice of criteria for attributing an organism to a particular species; the decision is left to the judgement of the worker (Hoare 1972). Minor morphological differences between subpopulations in a species could be regarded as indicating subspecies, while differences in some characteristic as showing either biologically or physiologically distinct strains or races. Therefore, a species may be regarded as containing a number of subpopulations which differ within the relatively narrow bounds of the biological criteria which define the species, and are responsible for some of the diversity in the host–parasite interactions. As Hoare (1972) pointed out, his classification, which was even more complicated than the one given above, is already a compromise between a purely academic approach to taxonomy and the demands for a practical breakdown for veterinary and medical workers. An extensive review by Gibson *et al.* (1980) discussed the application of the numerical analysis of enzyme polymorphism, a most valuable new technique in the studies of the epidemiology and taxonomy of trypanosomes in the subgenus *Trypanozoon*. This technique of digestion of the deoxyribonucleic acid (DNA) with selected restriction endonucleases followed by the electrophoretic analysis of the fragment yielded characterisitic patterns that could be used for the intrinsic characterization of isolates (Morel and Simpson 1980). Using restricted enzyme analysis of kinetoplast DNA (kDNA) *T. brucei* could not be differentiated from *T. rhodesiense* but quantitative differences were observed between different stocks of these trypanosomes (Borst *et al.* 1981). The isoenzyme marker, a slow alanine aminotransferase pattern, identified *T. gambiense* in pigs and dogs in Liberia, but there was a lack of correspondence between the characteristic *T. gambiense* isoenzyme pattern and resistance to human sera (Gibson *et al.* 1978). The electrophoretic mobilities and activities on the 11 enzymes of bloodstream and culture forms of *T. brucei* were compared (Kilgour 1980a). Biochemical characterization of *T. cruzi* and *T. rangeli* using isoenzyme separation by cellulose acetate electrophoresis revealed a high level of intraspecific polymorphism (Kreutzer and Sousa 1981).

Morphology and motility

In Giemsa-stained blood smears, the subgenera are distinguished by their size, shape, location and size of kinetoplast, position of nucleus, and the attachment and length of flagellum. In wet mounts, the type of motility and locomotion are also useful in differentiating subgenera. *Trypanosoma vivax* has a fluttering movement resulting in a rapid darting linear locomotion. *Trypanosoma congolense* is stationary and has a slow intermittent twisting movement, while *T. brucei* and other species in the subgenus *Trypanozoon* have a rapid twisting motion with a relatively slow forward locomotion.

Literature

In the past, much attention has been given to morphology of trypanosomes in the vertebrate and invertebrate hosts to identify species and subgenera, demonstrate stages of life cycles, and relate structure to function. Although morphology readily identified subgenera, attempts to relate minor structural differences with biological behavior, such as host-specificity, severity of disease, and differences due to geographic distribution have been generally inconclusive and are currently not used. This also applied to speciation within a subgenus as with attempts to separate *T. uniforme* from *T. vivax* (Hoare 1972) and divide *T. congolense* into the short *congolense* and the long *dimorphon* types associated with mild and severe syndromes respectively (Godfrey 1960, 1961). Morphological identification of species in the subgenus *Trypanozoon* have also been unsuccessful. These methods, using routine Giemsa-stained preparations, having inherent inconsistencies in the morphology of trypanosomes brought about by the variability of techniques used, making differentiation based on minor morphological differences difficult.

On the basis of morphology, the life cycles of various species have been described in the invertebrate host. In the vertebrate host the course of development, or the life cycle, has not been determined for *T. congolense* and *T. vivax*, but with *T. brucei* and the related species affecting man considerable work has been undertaken and has been reviewed by Ormerod (1979). These *brucei*-like species have been described as having stumpy, intermediate, and long slender forms in the circulating blood representing functionally different variants as demonstrated by their infectivity for tsetse flies and animals (Ashcroft 1957; Balber 1972; Wijers 1959; Wijers and Willett 1960; Ellis *et al.* 1980). Another feature of pleomorphism studied was cytoplasmic liquid containing granules (Ormerod 1958; Ormerod and Page 1967). The morphology of *T. brucei* isolated from lymph nodes at different stages of infection was monomorphic and resembled the slender forms of the bloodstream and did not consist of pleomorphic populations found in the bloodstream (Tanner *et al.* 1980). The absence of a kinetoplast in *T. evansi* had also been thought – but no longer – as differentiating it from *T. brucei* (Hoare 1949) and has been studied in relation to chemotherapy (Killick-Kendrick 1964). Recent studies have shown that during a *T. congolense* parasitemia there is considerable variation of morphological types, including the two forms reported by Godfrey (1960) (Nantulya *et al.* 1978).

Further studies have been undertaken on the ultrastructural morphology of blood, vector, and cultural forms of *T. brucei* (Brown *et al.* 1973; Steiger 1973; Vickerman 1962, 1970; Nyindo *et al.* 1980; Ito *et al.* 1981), as well as quantitative morphometric studies (Hecker *et al.* 1972, 1973). Fewer investigations are available on the other Salivarian species, *T. equiperdum* (Anderson *et al.* 1956), *T. congolense* (Vickerman 1969), and *T. vivax* (Muhlpfordt 1975). The ultrastructure of *T. cruzi* organelles and their relation to function, and the association of pleomorphism of blood trypomastigotes with strain, infectivity, and course of infection has been reviewed by Brener (1973).

Biochemistry

Studies of biochemistry of pathogenic trypanosomes determine the cellular composition, metabolism, and function. Improvement of existing methods through either chemotherapy or immunization depends on determining biochemical differences between the host cells and trypanosomes which could be exploited to develop new drugs and immunization procedures. These studies also provide information as to how trypanosomes injure the host, as for example with the detection and analysis of the toxic factor in trypanosomes. However, the role of this factor in development of lesions has so far not been determined. Many of the metabolic pathways in trypanosomes have been defined and are used to direct the development of new chemotherapeutic agents. The biochemical composition of the cell wall of trypanosomes has also been studied extensively to determine the antigens which enable the trypanosomes to escape the host's immunologic defense mechanisms.

Literature

The relevance of information on the biochemistry of trypanosomes to practical control has been considered by Newton and Burnett (1972) and Williamson (1976), who state that although much information is available on the basic structure, chemical composition, and metabolism, this knowledge has not been fully utilized in the improvement of control through either chemotherapy or vaccination. Various aspects of trypanosomal biochemistry and metabolism have been published as chapters of textbooks. Comprehensive reviews are available on peculiarities of trypanosomatid flagellates (Newton 1968), the comparative studies of DNA of Kinetoplastidae (Newton and Burnett 1972), the oxidative metabolism of trypanosomes (Bowman and Flynn 1976), and on the metabolism of *T. cruzi* (von Brand 1967, 1973).

A more recent brief review of the current work in the biochemistry of *T. brucei* and *T. cruzi* concluded that there is an outstanding need for more refined microtechnique in biochemical investigations to fill the enormous gaps which exist in our knowledge of the biochemistry (Kilgour 1980a, b). Trypanosomes have a number of intriguing attributes of scientific interest; mitochondrial DNA is the most bizarre in nature consisting of large networks of cantenated circles, glycolysis is unique in that it is organized in separate organelles (the glycosomes), trypanosomes suppress mitochondrial biogenesis, trypanosomes share some typical aspects of eukaryotic genone organization, and antigenic variation (Borst *et al.* 1981). In studies identifying trypanosomes the digestion of the kDNA fraction with selected restriction endonucleases followed by electrophoretic analysis of the fragments yielded patterns that could be used to characterize various populations of trypanosomes such as stocks, strains, and clones (Morel and Simpson 1980). The kinetoplast DNA of normal and mutant *T. brucei* has been investigated (Stuart and Gelvin 1980), and *T. gambiense* was compared to that of the kDNA of *T. equiperdum* (Riou and Barrois 1981). The kDNA and ribonucleic acid (RNA) of bloodstream and procyclic culture forms of *T. brucei* (Simpson and Simpson 1980), and the effects on the growth, structure, and metabolism of the inhibition of the replicative DNA synthesis by hydroxurea were undertaken (Brun 1980). Restriction cleavage maps of kDNA minicircles from *T. equiperdum* (Riou and Barrois 1979; Barrois *et al.* 1981) and a comparative study characterizing the molecular components in the kinetoplast–mitochondrial DNA of dyskinetoplastic and natural isolates of *T. equiperdum* (Riou and Saucier 1979) were studied.

The glycolysis of trypanosomes has been investigated and included the following: the glycolysis of *T. brucei* (Visser and Opperdoes 1980) and *in vitro* metabolite studies in simple medium (Brohn and Clarkson 1980); the isolation of intact glycosomes from *T. brucei* by gradient centrifugation (Opperdoes 1981); the inhibition of glycolysis in bloodstream forms of *T. brucei* in the development of chemotherapy (Clarkson *et al.* 1981); the inhibition of anaerobic metabolism of glucose in *T. brucei* by glycerol (Hammond and Bowman 1980a); purification and characterization of pyruvate kinase in *T. brucei* and its role in regulation of glycolysis and its role in the adenosine triphosphate synthesis in *T. brucei* investigated in the anaerobic glucose metabolism (Hammond and Bowman 1980b; Flynn and Bowman 1980); the hexokinase and phosphofructokinase activity in regulation and of glycolysis in *T. brucei* (Nwagwu and Opperdoes 1982); the determination of the electron transport chain in respiration of *T. brucei* (Njogu *et al.* 1980); the oxygen uptake of *T. brucei* and *T. vivax* (Isoun and Isoun 1981); the preparation and properties of a multi-enzyme complex catalyzing part of the glycolytic pathway (Oduro *et al.* 1980a, b); the effect of oligomycin on glucose utilization and calcium transport in *T. brucei* and *T. evansi* in both normal and dyskinetoplastic strains (Miller and Klein 1980).

The more recent research into the biochemistry of trypanosomes included the following studies: the characterization by enzymatic markers of subcellular fraction from bloodstream forms of *T. brucei* (Rovis and Baekkeskov 1980); review and discussion of polyamines and their biosynthesis as a possible target in chemotherapy (Bacchi *et al.* 1979; Bacchi 1981); examination by electrophoresis of the peptidase of *T. brucei* (Letch and Gibson 1981); the activation of adenylate cyclase in *T. brucei* by calcium ions (Voorheis and Martin 1980, 1981); the malate dehydrogenase in *T. brucei* (Falk *et al.* 1980); characterization and assay of the hydrolases in *T. brucei* (Steiger *et al.* 1980); isolation and partial characterization of calcium-dependent andoribonuclease of *T. brucei* (Gbenle and Akinrimisi 1981); the uptake of purine bases and nucleosides (James and Born 1980); uptake of fatty acids by bloodstream forms of *T. brucei* (Voorheis 1980), comparison of pyrazolopyrimidine metabolism in *T. brucei* with that of *T. cruzi* and *Leishmania* (Berens *et al.* 1980).

The biochemical aspects of *T. cruzi* were reviewed by Gutteridge and Rogerson (1979) and Gutteridge (1981) and it was concluded that although there were no marked morphological differences between intracellular amastigotes, trypomastigotes, and epimastigotes, there were no significant qualitative biochemical differences associated with these changes. The following biochemical research has also been undertaken recently: on acid hydrolases (Avila *et al.* 1979), common proteinase in epimastigote, trypomastigote, and amastigote of different strains (Rangel *et al.* 1981), and the respiratory terminals of *T. cruzi* epimastigotes (Carneiro and Caldas 1982).

Culture techniques

Basic studies of structure, function, metabolism, and nutrition of trypanosomes require techniques for growing the organisms in large numbers *in vitro* culture systems. In order to study the various stages observed in the vector and mammalian host, a number of cultures are used ranging from simple media to invertebrate and vertebrate organ cultures. Species of pathogenic and nonpathogenic trypanosomes vary in their ability to grow in artificial media. The Salivarian pathogens are relatively more diffficult to cultivate than the Stercorarian trypanosomes, and growth is usually limited to the one stage, the noninfective invertebrate form of the vector life cycle. The practical application in the field of culture techniques is limited to *T. cruzi*, and is used as one of a number of diagnostic techniques.

Literature

In research, several culture techniques are used to grow various forms of pathogenic trypanosomes. These vary in complexity and include relatively simple culture fluids, i.e. defined media with known chemical composition, more complex semi-defined media containing blood or tissue extracts, and cell and organ cultures of invertebrate and vertebrate tissues. Pathogenic trypanosomes do not grow well, as compared to nonpathogens, in defined media. In order for culture forms to express required biological functions such as infectivity which is vital to many forms of research, cell and organ cultures from tsetse flies and mammals are used. The use of the relatively simple media for Salivarian and Stercorarian trypanosomes has been reviewed (Taylor and Baker 1968; Tobie 1964; Trager and Krassner 1967). The majority of studies on these using cultural techniques in Salivarian trypanosomes have been on *T. brucei* with a few on *T. congolense* and have been summarized by Baker (1970). Because these methods are not suitable for some biochemical studies, a new simplified semi-defined medium was developed (Cross and Manning 1973). A continuous dialysis technique capable of maintaining concentrated suspensions of bloodstream *T. brucei* for 2 hours without loss of viability was developed to study metabolism (Fairlamb and Bowman 1980b). The short-term *in vitro* metabolic study in a simple medium at high cell densities of trypanosomes has been used (Brohn and Clarkson 1980). Morphological transformation in a semi-defined medium permits biochemical and physiological study of transformation of the bloodstream to procyclic trypomastigotes and mitochondrial biogenesis (Bienen *et al.* 1981). The transformation of *T. brucei* bloodstream forms to procyclic culture forms in the semi-defined medium involved stumpy and intramediate forms changing to procyclic forms, whereas the slender forms died (Ghiotto *et al.* 1979). Citrate and *cis*-aconitate stimulate transformation of *T. brucei* in cultures from blood forms to procyclic forms (Brun and Schonenberger 1981).

The morphological transformation of bloodstream trypomastigotes to procyclic trypomastigotes of *T. brucei* occurred on a different time scale than biochemical transformation (Bienen *et al.* 1980). A correlation between the morphological types, intramediate and short stumpy forms, and the level of cyclic 3′,5′-adenosine monophosphate were studied (Mancini and Patton 1981). In all of these methods the biological behavior of the trypanosomes is limited, and the important feature of infectivity is quickly lost after a short time of *in vitro* growth.

Better growth (Cunningham 1973, 1977; Steiger *et al.* 1977) and improved infectivity of *T. brucei* were obtained in tsetse-fly tissue and organ cultures, and the infectivity was related to the invasion of cultured salivary glands (Cunningham and Honigberg 1977). Infective *T. brucei* developed in culture of tsetse-fly head–salivary gland explants inoculated with bloodstream trypanosomes and were morphologically similar to metacyclic stages found in tsetse flies with the characteristic surface coat (Gardiner *et al.* 1980a). Noninfective procyclic forms of *T. brucei* cultivated in head–salivary glands, alimentary tract, and abdominal body wall explant of tsetse flies transformed into infective metacyclic stages (Cunningham *et al.* 1981; Cunningham and Taylor 1979). Culture procyclic forms of *T. rhodesiense* and

T. congolense fed artificially to tsetse flies established infections which developed to mature metacyclic trypanosomes capable of infecting small mammalian hosts (Evans 1979). Metacyclic trypanosomes of different stocks grown in tsetse head–salivary gland explant cultures produced antibodies in rabbits which were used to identify serotypes from various geographical areas (Jones *et al.* 1981). Culture-derived trypanosomes were used in serological studies of *T. brucei* and *T. gambiense* infection in rabbits (Jones *et al.* 1981; Jenni and Brun 1981). The culture of *T. congolense* in a tsetse-fly culture system was achieved by Steiger *et al.* (1977). Infective *T. brucei* metatrypomastigotes have also been reported in culture of tsetse-fly salivary gland with bovine embryonic spleen feeder layer (Nyindo *et al.* 1978). Schneider (1979) reviewed the cultivation of the invertebrate stages of Salivarian trypanosomes in tsetse-fly tissues and presented the various systems in a table. The author described the initiation, evaluation, and characteristics of these tsetse-fly cell lines and presented a detailed description of the equipment and materials required, and a detailed outline of the protocols required for initiating primary cultures and for maintaining and subculturing, including the use of antibiotic and antifungal agents, sterilizing solution, and balanced salt solutions, for different types of culture media.

A more recent important development has been the growth of large numbers of infective blood trypomastigote forms of *T. brucei* in bovine fibroblast cells (Hirumi *et al.* 1977), and *T. rhodesiense* in Chinese hamster lung cells (Hill *et al.* 1978). The dyskinetoplast *T. brucei* was cultured in fetal tissue cultures (Stuart 1980; Stuart and Gelvin 1980). *Trypanosoma brucei, T. rhodesiense,* and *T. gambiense* have been grown on yet another tissue culture system consisting of a feeder layer of fibroblast-like cells from rabbits or voles. Metacyclic forms from tsetse flies and bloodstream forms were used to initiate the cultures. The bloodstream forms so maintained were infective for mice and could be transmitted through tsetse flies. *In vitro* cloning with single bloodstream forms and metacyclic forms could also be achieved with high efficiency (Brun *et al.* 1981).

Another approach has been taken with *T. congolense* by putting infected dermal explants from the site of tsetse-fly bite into a medium, which resulted in multiplication of infective blood forms for periods of up to 21 days, but these could not be subpassaged into cultures of fibroblast-like cells (Gray *et al.* 1979, 1981). Successful cultivation of infective forms of *T. congolense* was established by incorporating infected tsetse proboscis together with bovine dermal collagen explant. Primary and subpassaged cultures showed a variety of morphologically different developmental forms of *T. congolense* closely resembling those described in tsetse flies (Gray *et al.* 1981). Successful *in vitro* maintenance and culture of *T. vivax* has seldom been reported. In semi-defined media, multiplication up to 96 hours occurred (Isoun and Isoun 1974a, b) and the development of an infective polymorphic population, including a metacyclic form, in tsetse fly organ culture was observed (Trager 1959, 1975).

A comprehensive review by Hirumi (1979) emphasized the technical details for the *in vitro* cultivation of animal-infective forms of salivarian trypanosomes and their application. In monophasic and diphasic media, bloodstream forms rapidly transformed into forms similar to those observed in the vector, and these multiplying trypanosomes were not infective for mammals. Cocultivation with vector organs, tissues, and cells has been achieved in primary cultures of *T. vivax, T. brucei,* and *T. congolense*. These host cell-free and the tsetse-fly tissue systems did not support the growth of the blood-form trypomastigotes. This was achieved by Hirumi *et al.* (1977) using bovine fibroblast-like feeder cells to grow typical bloodstream forms of *T. brucei* which were highly infective for mammals. This culture system was applied in the research on the cyclic development of the trypanosomes, *in vitro* cloning and antigenic variation (Hirumi 1979), and possible *in vitro* attenuation of animal-infective forms.

Trypanosoma cruzi, although less exacting in its *in vitro* growth requirements, has also not been grown successfully in totally defined medium. Recently a new chemically defined medium, but with fetal calf serum has been proposed (O'Daly 1975). Many different semi-defined media have been used and these have been reviewed by Brener (1973). The infectivity of cultures, which depends on the presence of metacyclic forms, can be maintained for very long periods of time. The complex tissue culture of variety of human and animal cell lines are readily susceptible to infection by metacyclic forms.

The culture systems now available for pathogenic trypanosomes, particularly the cell cultures of infective *T. brucei* blood forms, appear not to be adaptable to the two most important trypanosomes transmitted by the tsetse fly, *T. vivax* and *T. congolense*. The successful development of *T. brucei* culture systems depended on taking into consideration the preferential tissue microenvironment of this species, the connective tissues, and the use of fibroblasts in the culture. A similar approach to culturing other species could prove rewarding, e.g. the use of endothelial cells and capillary cultures with *T. congolense*. This field of research is rapidly developing and further advances with other species of trypanosomes should occur.

EPIZOOTIOLOGY

Transmission

Transmission of trypanosomes depends on their subgenera and species, and includes cyclic and mechanical transmission by insect vectors, ingestion, transplacental infection, and contact with infected mammalian host. Most species are spread by more than one method, but when insect vectors are involved they usually play the most important role.

Salivarian trypanosomes, except for *T. evansi* and *T. equiperdum*, are disseminated by at least 34 species, subspecies, or races of tsetse flies belonging to the genus *Glossina*, which are divided on the basis of their evolution, geographic distribution, and habitat into three groups: *fusca*, *palpalis*, and *morsitans*. About half of these species are of veterinary and medical importance. Trypanosomes ingested by the tsetse fly from a parasitemic host undergo a life cycle of up to 20 days, during which they undergo morphological changes, multiplication, tissue migration, and final localization in the mouth parts. The four subgenera have different distribution in the tsetse fly. *Duttonella* is confined to the proboscis, *Nannomonas* is found in the proboscis and midgut, while *Trypanozoon* and *Pyenomonas* are present in the midgut and salivary glands. These localizations are used to identify the types of infections. The incidence of infection in a population of tsetse flies depends on a number of factors including environmental temperature, availability of preferential food host, species of flies, and the age of the tsetse-fly population. Young flies feeding for the first time on infected blood are more apt to become infected than if infected blood is taken in subsequent to a noninfective first blood meal, although flies may remain infective throughout life and each bite does not necessarily cause infection in the host. The efficiency of transmission to livestock by flies depends on climate, and feeding habits of the tsetse-fly species in a particular area. In addition, the strain of trypanosomes carried by the tsetse flies may vary in its infectivity for a mammalian host species. Therefore, an accurate measure of challenge in an enzootic area is difficult, requiring taking into consideration climate and the peculiarities, both qualitative and quantitative, of the populations of hosts, tsetse flies, and trypanosomes. For this reason, in practice the severity of challenge is usually ascertained by the frequency with which treatment with the trypanocide, Berenil, is required to eliminate injections. A measure of challenge is necessary because it affects the regime of prophylactic trypanocidal drugs which have to be used.

Trypanosoma cruzi is the other species transmitted cyclically, and there are around ten important species of triatomine bugs in the epidemiology of Chagas' disease in man. Many more of more than 50 species of triatomine bugs known to be infected are probably involved in the transmissions of *T. cruzi* and *cruzi*-like organisms between wild animals. In enzootic areas of chronic disease in man, which is comparable to the chronic carrier state in dogs and cats, 20% of bugs may be infected, while from an acute disease produced in laboratory animals 100% become infected. The life cycle in the bugs is from 5 to 16 days and involves morphological transformation and multiplication in the gut, with final localization of the infective metacyclics in the rectum where they remain for the life of the vector.

Mechanical transmission on the mouthparts of flies in the genera *Stomoxys* and *Tabanus* is the second most important mode of transmission. In the Salivarian group transmitted by tsetse flies, only *T. vivax* is considered to be spread beyond the confines of the tsetse belts by this method. In South America, however, biting flies have spread this infection throughout the continent. *Trypanosoma evansi* is transmitted primarily by these biting flies. Transfer from one mammalian host to another is dependent on the time between feeding on an infected host and subsequently biting a susceptible host, and infectivity is highest minutes after feeding, decreases rapidly, and is lost within 8 hours. The severity of the challenge is governed by the density of these fly populations and the incidence of infection in animals.

Transfer of infection caused by some species of trypanosomes can also occur through contact between infected and susceptible animals. *Trypanosoma equiperdum* is transmitted venereally between horses. *Trypanosoma evansi* is transferred by the saliva from infected vampire bats during feeding on cattle and horses. Bats are more effectual than biting flies because the trypanosomes multiply in their tissues and infections are maintained for long periods of time. Another form of contact transmission occurs through ingestion of meat from animals infected with *T. evansi* and *T. brucei.* It is probably of considerable importance in some natural situations involving wild carnivore in Africa. *Trypanosoma evansi* has also caused outbreaks of trypanosomiasis in carnivore in zoological gardens. Ingestion of milk from an infected dam is yet another possible mode of transmission. Finally, transplacental infections do occur with *T. brucei, T. vivax*, and *T. cruzi*, but the importance of this mode of transmission in trypanosomiasis of livestock has not been determined.

Literature

Comprehensive general reviews are available for the tsetse-transmitted varieties (Ford 1971) and for *T. cruzi* (Hoare 1972). The efficacy of transmission of pathogenic trypanosomes by tsetse flies in a particular enzootic area is dependent on a number of variable qualitative and quantitative factors relating to the species of tsetse flies and of hosts, and the species and strains of trypanosomes. A complex situation also occurs with *T. cruzi* and *cruzi*-like organisms involving many species of mammalian hosts and triatomine bugs, and different infectivity of the various strains. The mechanical transmission of *T. vivax* in Africa has been thought to be responsible for its spread from the tsetse-fly belts. Wells (1972) reviewed the evidence for this in the literature and concluded that proof of mechanical transfer playing a major role is inconclusive. Leeflang (1975) proposed that on the periphery of tsetse-fly belts low densities of tsetse flies still transmit *T. vivax*.

With the other salivarian species, *T. brucei* has been transmitted experimentally by flies in the genera *Tabanus* and *Stomoxys* (Dixon *et al.* 1971). Chaudhuri *et al.* (1965) and Yutuc (1949) showed that some species of these flies were more efficient than others in the transfer of *T. evansi*, and summarized the older literature on the subject. The classification of the oriental horsefly vectors of *T. evansi* has been revised (Burger and Thompson 1981). The role of the vampire bat in transmission of this species in South America has been reviewed by Hoare (1965). Following ingestion of infected blood a generalized infection occurs, and is followed by a carrier state with trypanosomes being present in the saliva. The ability of certain of the Salivarian trypanosomes to penetrate the mucous membrane and cause systemic infection is best shown by *T. equiperdum*, but *T. evansi* and *T. brucei* are also infective through ingestion of infected meat which, depending on temperature, may be infective for periods of up to 66 hours (de Jesus 1951, 1962; Moloo *et al.* 1973; Soltys *et al.* 1973). Congenital infections have been demonstrated in infected man with the Salivarian species (Buyst 1976). There are only single references to transplacental infections with *T. vivax* and *T. evansi* (Ikede and Losos 1972d; Abdel-Latif 1963c) in domestic animals. In man, 2 to 4% of infected mothers transmit *T. cruzi* infections to children (Bittencourt 1976). The literature on transplacental transmission of trypanosomes in natural and experimental infections has been reviewed in various species of animals, including man, infected with different species of trypanosomes (Ogwu and Nuru 1981).

Incidence

Worldwide, regional, and local distributions vary with the different types of trypanosomiases and are related in most cases to the presence of the insect vectors: tsetse flies, other biting flies, and reduviid bugs. The one exception is *T. equiperdum* which is transmitted venereally. The regional and local incidence of infections and diseases and their economical impact on livestock production are governed in turn by many other factors such as prevalence of carriers in domestic and wild animals, density of vector populations, and local husbandry practices such as annual migration of livestock. The variability of these factors determines the local epizootiological situation and governs the methods used for the implementation of efficient control measures. The key to the effective control of trypanosomiases is thorough knowledge of the local enzootic situation. Unfortunately, up-to-date and accurate information of practical use is often not available. Therefore, improvement of existing, and implementation of new, control programs must often begin by obtaining more information on regional distribution, local incidence prevalence of vectors, and by relating the problem of trypanosomiasis to the economics of the local livestock industry which has to support the control measures.

In Africa the most important forms of trypanosomiases, in their impact on livestock production, are caused by the Salivarian species transmitted by tsetse flies, which infest vast regions totalling about 10 million km^2 where tsetse flies greatly limit livestock production. The remarkably efficient transmission, with trypanosomes multiplying in the tsetse-fly tissues and large numbers of highly infective forms awaiting transmission through the bite, becomes devastating when infected flies swarm around livestock. All forms of domestic animals are susceptible, with the exception of poultry, to infections by one or more of the species. The most important type of trypanosomiases are caused by *T. congolense* and *T. vivax* in cattle. The incidence of these species in other animals varies and depends on the local prevalence of the other species of livestock in tsetse-fly-infested areas. The incidence of *T. congolense* and *T. vivax* infections is different between East and West Africa. Although both species are found, *T. vivax* is more important in the West and *T. congolense* in the East. However, the less prevalent species may occasionally cause a high incidence of severe disease with high mortality. One of the most important features of the tsetse-fly-transmitted trypanosomiases of cattle is frequently multiple infection, occurring simultaneously or sequentially, of *T. congolense, T. vivax,* and *T. brucei*. This adds to the complexity of the problem, affecting the methods which have to be used in diagnosis and chemotherapy. Although *T. brucei* is prevalent in cattle and small ruminants, it is usually regarded as causing low morbidity. However, because it is difficult to detect in the blood and is masked by higher parasitemias of concomitant infections with the other two species, its importance may be underestimated, especially as a reservior of *T. rhodesiense* infections for man.

Trypanosoma evansi and *T. equiperdum* are closely related to *T. brucei* in many biological features. *Trypanosoma evansi* infects all those domestic species susceptible to tsetse-transmitted varieties as well as water buffalo. On the basis of morphology, geographic distribution, and type of disease it causes, *T. evansi* probably originated from *T. brucei* in the most northern boundaries of tsetse-fly-infested zones of Africa. It has been proposed that camels became infected and spread the organisms to Asia by caravans and military campaigns. Further spread during the early part of this century throughout Asia, and more recently to South America, occurred from India by exported livestock. The epizootiology is characterized by an initial high incidence of morbidity and mortality followed by reduction in the incidence of infection and severity of disease. The same pattern is observed locally, either when a new focus of infection occurs or when susceptible animals are introduced into an enzootic area where the disease smolders along at a low rate in the indigenous livestock. Another Salivarian species, *T. vivax,* has also shown ability to break out of Africa, and has spread to South America with the importation of infected cattle. Its epizootiology appears to be comparable to that of *T. evansi,* in that the initial high morbidity and mortality has now been replaced in the enzootic regions by a lower incidence of milder syndromes. The remaining species in the Salivarian group, *T. equiperdum,* is on the worldwide basis a parasite of the past, its importance linked to the horse-drawn era. It is mechanically transmitted by coitus, and spread by movement of infected, but asymptomatic, horses. This relatively simple epizootiology, combined with an efficient diagnostic method, enabled its early eradication from most parts of the world. It now persists in regions where horses are numerous and veterinary services inadequate. Unfortunately there are few reports of its prevalence, but it is known to occur in North and South Africa and parts of Asia and South America.

An integral part of the epizootiology of all forms of trypanosomiasis is the carrier state, which is an infection of domestic and wild animals characterized by either mild or asymptomatic response. The carrier animals are the most effective means by which enzootic conditions are maintained. In comparison, the infections in the acute syndromes terminating in death are self-limiting and play a short-term role in the spread of the disease in epizootics. The most effective carriers of Salivarian trypanosomes are the wild animals. Domestic species are also important reservoirs with those trypanosomiases of livestock characterized by either chronic disease or an asymptomatic infection, e.g. caused by *T. evansi* and *T. brucei* in cattle. With the tsetse-transmitted species, the rich African wild game fauna provides a vast reservoir of infection. The role each species of wild animal plays depends on its susceptibility to infection by various species of trypanosomes and on the food-host preferences of different species of flies. The other Salivarian trypanosome, *T. evansi*, is also carried by various wild animals but they probably play a minor role in comparison to the importance of the reservoirs of the chronic syndromes caused in domestic animals. *Trypanosoma cruzi* causes infections in 100 to 150 species of wild animals in South America, and these species are carriers while the diseases occur in man, dog, and cat. These infections are of limited importance in veterinary medicine. The prevalence of disease of dogs and cats is low although the incidence of infections may be high. Natural disease and death have rarely been reported in dogs, and they have occurred outside the recognized Chagasaic endemic areas. The role played by other domestic species is not clear. Indications are that they may be infected experimentally but the incidence in nature is rare.

Literature

The amount of information available on the geographic distribution, regional and local incidence, and economic importance varies greatly with different types of animal trypanosomiases. Most has been published on the tsetse-transmitted varieties, with very little up-to-date information on *T. evansi* and *T. equiperdum*. The *FAO Year Book* lists annually and on a country basis the prevalence of the different forms of trypanosomiasis. Based on this information available for 1974, Finelle (1974) published a brief summary on the world distributions of various forms of trypanosomiases. Often the best sources of information on the local and regional situation are the reports of the veterinary services.

The most complete account of the epizootiology and ecology of tsetse-fly-transmitted trypanosomiasis of man and animals in various regions of Africa was the monograph by Ford (1971). The epizootiology of livestock trypanosomiasis was also presented by Willett

(1970) for Central and East Africa and by MacLennan (1970) for West Africa, who underlined the regional differences which exist, the prevalence of the different species of trypanosomes, the role of wild animals and different species of tsetse, husbandry practices, and the importance of trypano-tolerant breeds. From West Africa there were additional reports on the Nigerian situation which were representative of the whole region. The characteristic cattle production practices consist of raising of animals in the Sahel zones in the North and their movement south to markets in the tsetse-infested zones. Infection rates of up to 70% were found in cattle trekked for 1 or 2 months (Killick-Kendrick and Godfrey 1963; Godfrey *et al.* 1965; Yesufu and Mshelbwala 1973). Along these cattle routes high infection rates, up to 90%, have been recorded in tsetse flies (Jordan 1965; Riordan 1977). In recent years, a lower incidence in cattle has resulted from the increased use of lorry transport (Kilgour and Godfrey 1978). In Liberia, a serological survey of N'Dama cattle, pigs, dogs, sheep, and goats indigenous to tsetse-fly-infested rain forest showed that the infection rate with pathogenic trypanosomes were 80.4% in N'Dama cattle, 76.0% in pigs, 48.5% in dogs, 35.1% in goats, and 28.1% in sheep (Mehlitz 1979). The incidence of infection in the Zebu breed was compared with trypano-tolerant Baoulè and shown to be 12.3% versus 2.5% and the parasitemias were higher in the former (Haase *et al.* 1980). An authoritative review of the impact of trypanosomiasis on livestock practices in West Africa was published by Wilson *et al.* (1963).

In East Africa, numerous surveys have been undertaken on the incidence of infection in livestock, tsetse flies, and particularly in wild animals because of their prevalence and importance as reservoirs. The surveys in wild animals from 1900 onwards have been summarized (Ashcroft *et al.* 1959; Lumsden 1962). A complete checklist of the wild species known to be infected with Salivarian trypanosomes has been compiled by Hoare (1972). Surveys using parasitological and serological tests have been reported from Botswana (Dräger and Mehlitz 1978), Uganda (Reid *et al.* 1970a, b; Burridge *et al.* 1970) and Tanzania (Geigy *et al.* 1971). These formed part of the investigations which included determining rates in cattle and tsetse flies (Moloo *et al.* 1971; Moloo and Kutuza 1974; Mwambu and Mayende 1971; Wain *et al.* 1970). A high infection rate in tsetse flies was reported from Zambia (Okiwelu 1977). Only two reports, one from Kenya and the other from Nigeria, are available on the incidence, up to 80%, of infections in sheep and goats indigenous to enzootic areas (Griffin and Allonby 1979a; Kramer 1966). The importance of trypanosomiasis in these species has been virtually neglected in many control programs, and yet the financial loss from reduced weight gain and death amounted to 36.2 and 62.9 Kenya shillings per head for goats and sheep due to natural trypanosomiasis under a low tsetse-fly challenge. Seasonal incidence of trypanosomiasis and the trypano-tolerance of indigenous breeds were important factors to be considered when initiating small stock improvement programs in trypanosomiasis-endemic areas (Griffin and Allonby 1979b).

Surveys of trypanosome infections in animals and vectors are a part of the evaluation of the economic importance of trypanosomiasis in livestock production, which includes losses due to reduced production and the expenditures required for control. There were two FAO reports, one summarized in general terms economic problems of animal trypanosomiasis (Finelle 1974), and the other presented information compiled by a panel on costings of various control measures, and the impact of trypanosomiasis on the livestock industry of Botswana, Ivory Coast, Nigeria, Upper Volta, Benin, Chad, Ethiopia, Mali, Somalia, and Zambia (FAO/UNDP 1977). The economic and ecological effects of trypanosomiasis in southern Nigeria and southern Cameroon have been assessed on the basis of the prevalence of different species of *Glossina* (Jordan 1961). Also in Nigeria, the role of migrating pasturalists in the spread of human and animal trypanosomiasis, and the relation of this form of husbandry to animal production has been considered (Aliu 1975; Adekolu-John 1978; Esuoroso 1974). In a recent study, human trypanosomiasis caused by *T. gambiense* in the Ivory Coast occurred most frequently among men in the age group 10 to 30 years (Stanghellini and Duvallet 1981). A great deal of international interest has been focused on alleviating the problem of livestock trypanosomiasis in Africa. Whether control is undertaken on regional or local levels, its success depends on taking into consideration the variable social, economic, and ecological features in different parts of Africa.

Preventative control measures have involved the eradication of tsetse flies. Over the years various methods have been tried, often at great expense. The history of tsetse-fly eradication from Africa is full of failures of programs undertaken in isolation, with no regard for the social changes which must accompany these schemes. In recent seminars this problem has been discussed in the light of the availability of new methods, relevance of laboratory research, and the scope of the current campaigns in Africa (Jordan 1976; Langley 1977; Hadaway 1977). The theme of these discussions has been that integrated rural development must go hand in hand with tsetse-fly eradication, which is possible only in limited areas and must be related to cost (Jordan 1978). Newly reclaimed land must be settled and developed quickly to prevent the tsetse-flies from coming back. The difficulties of controlling and eradicating tsetse flies by any one method has drawn attention to the need for an integration of known methods, such as bush clearing and insecticide application, with new methods e.g. biological control, which are as yet to be developed (Laird 1977). It would appear from the current opinions that tsetse-fly control will be possible only if new methods are developed to supplement the old, and if eradication programs are fully supported by immediate rural development of reclaimed land – a difficult solution, even if all the resources of technology is available, in the many countries of Africa which are undergoing political and economic changes.

Among the furor to free Africa from trypanosomiasis, Ormerod

(1976) dissented and claimed droughts as a possible result of vastly increased livestock populations, because of widespread use of efficient control methods. This provocative article was important only in that it drew attention to environmental damage caused by overgrazing in poorly managed livestock production. To propose, however, to control the numbers of cattle in Africa by losses through morbidity and mortality from trypanosomiasis is totally unacceptable.

From the confines of tsetse-fly belts of Africa, *T. vivax* moved during the last century to Mauritius, the West Indies, and South America. Two factors were responsible: the exportation of cattle from Africa to increase tropical animal production in these regions, and the ease of mechanical transmission of *T. vivax*. Already on the African continent, *T. vivax* has been incriminated on extensive circumstantial evidence that it was spread mechanically by other biting flies. The subject was evaluated by Wells (1972) who concluded that there was insufficient evidence that transmission other than by tsetse flies occurred in regions bordering tsetse-fly-infested areas. Outside the African continent, *T. vivax* was transmitted by biting flies and became widely disseminated, with initial infections resulting in a high incidence of morbidity and mortality in cattle. The literature on the epizootiology in South America and the Caribbean Islands was summarized by Shaw and Lainson (1972). More recent serological surveys have shown an incidence from 10 to 54% of positive reactors in cattle in El Salvador, Costa Rica, Colombia, Ecuador, Peru, Brazil, and Paraguay (Wells *et al.* 1970, 1977), and Venezuela (Clarkson *et al.* 1971b). In spite of this widespread incidence, there has been very little literature on the severity of the diseases these infections cause, and on their economic importance (Clarkson 1976a).

The most cosmopolitan parasite in the Salivarian group, *T. evansi*, has a wide distribution throughout the Old and New Worlds and was thought to have originated in Africa (Hoare 1957). With its original introduction, the disease has high morbidity and mortality which subsequently – because of chemotherapy or continued exposure of livestock to the organism – became less frequent and less severe. Very few surveys have been undertaken on the incidence and virtually no information is available on the economic importance. In enzootic areas where camels are indigenous, they have the highest infection rates and have been recorded as 41% in Egypt (Abdel-Latif 1958), 36% in Ethiopia (Pegram and Scott 1976), 30% in Chad (Gruvel and Balis 1965), 27% in northern Nigeria (Godfrey and Killick-Kendrick 1962), and 12% in Iraq (Awkati and Al-Khatib 1972). Less information is available on the incidence in other species. In Iraq, infections were not detected in cattle, buffaloes, horses, donkeys, sheep, goats, and dogs, although 12% of camels were infected (Awkati and Al-Khatib 1972). In India in an outbreak of the disease, 29% of cattle and 37% of water buffalo were infected (Mandal *et al.* 1977). As with the tsetse-transmitted varieties, the wild animal reservoirs play an important role and have been listed by Hoare (1972). In South America, the capybara (*Hyderochoerus hyderochaeris*) has been singled out as particularly important with an infection rate of 27% (Morales *et al.* 1976). Cattle, a species which often does not develop clinical signs, was considered as a source of infection for other species (Boehringer 1977). On the last Salivarian species, *T. equiperdum*, very little up-to-date information is available. Maps summarizing the world distributions were published by Finelle (1976) and distribution in southern Africa from 1955 to 1975 by Barrowman and van Vuuren (1976). The situation in South America was evaluated by Clarkson (1976a). Caporale *et al.* (1980) described an outbreak of dourine in 1975 in Italy and stated that in 1975 dourine was known to occur in Syria, Morocco, Algeria, Libya, USSR, Ethiopia, Senegal, Botswana, Lesotho, South Africa, Saudi Arabia, Nepal, Laos, and Iran. In Italy the survey undertaken in the Abruzzi region showed an average prevalence rate in the horses and donkeys of 7.4% in a population of about 5000 animals.

The literature available on the epizootiology of *T. cruzi* and *cruzi*-like trypanosomes is based on the investigations on the epidemiology of Chagas' disease in men. The subject is extremely complex involving a region extending from the USA to Argentina, up to 150 species of wild and domestic animals, and about 80 species of triatomine bugs. The more recent reviews were by Hoare (1972), Zeledòn (1974), a symposium (Pan American Health Organization 1976), and Miles (1979). The identification of *cruzi*-like trypanosomes as *T. cruzi*, i.e. infective for man, in the vector and reservoir animals in an endemic area is circumstantial, depending on the contact between man, vector, and reservoir host. Brener (1976), in the summary of the Pan American Health Organization symposium, noted that *T. cruzi* is 'actually a biologic complex of parasitic populations that circulate in nature among humans, domestic animals, wild reservoirs, and sylvatic and domiciliary vectors'. The heterogeneity of *T. cruzi* in the view of understanding its epidemiology and zoonosis has been discussed by Miles (1979). The differences between various isolates of *T. cruzi* were compared on a basis of morphology, biometry, behavior, ultrastructure, virulence, histotropism, drug sensitivity, infectivity to vectors, and antigenic and enzymatic composition. These criteria have been used both to identify *T. cruzi* insinuating its possible infectivity to man and to show the diversity of the *T. cruzi*-like organisms. The classification of *T. cruzi*-like organisms will have to develop along the same line as in protozoan taxonomy in general, using a wide range of biochemical, physical, and nutritional characteristics in the form of numerical taxonomy.

Domestic and sylvatic animals which include dogs, cats, guinea pigs, opossums, foxes, ferrets, squirrels, armadillos, anteaters, porcupines, rats, and mice are the reservoirs of *T. cruzi*. The marsupials of the genus *Didelphis* are regarded as playing an important role in establishing a link between the sylvatic and domestic cycles. In these animals the parasitemia is frequent and probably lifelong, and transmits the infection through domiciliary triatomes directly to man or through domestic animals such as the cat and the dog. Once established, the transmission from man to man is probably the most common cycle of infection (Fife 1978). A high incidence of 9 to 28% of infection has been recorded in dogs and cats (literature quoted by Zeledòn 1974). In northeast Brazil, it was found that *T. cruzi* infection was present in about 18% of domestic cats and dogs and these species were important reservoirs of *T. cruzi* in an endemic area where *P. megistus* is the only domiciliary triatome vector (Mott *et al.* 1978). In the southeastern states of the USA 24 out of 365 dogs were found to be serologically positive for *T. cruzi* (Tomlinson *et al.* 1981). In man, only 1% of all infections cause enough clinical signs to attract the attention of the physician. A comparable situation may exist in dogs and cats and it is only when clinical signs are severe, which may occur months or years after infection, that the disease is detected. It has been stated in a review of the role of domestic species that infections in large domestic animals seldom, if ever, occur (Minter 1976). However, lambs, kids, and calves may be infected experimentally (Diamond and Rubin 1958). The pig has also been shown to be susceptible to experimental infection and may serve as a reservoir host (Marsden *et al.* 1970).

INFECTION

Infectivity

Infectivity, defined as the ability of trypanosomes to invade and multiply in a host, is variable depending on the species and strain of trypanosomes. A species of trypanosome is, first of all, either infective or noninfective for a particular species of host. If it is infective, there is then variability of the relative ease with which the organism establishes itself in the host. Infectivity within a species of trypanosomes varies with strains, and is also dependent on the heterogeneity of susceptibilities of individuals within a species of host. It is measured by the numbers of organisms required to establish an infection and is, therefore, a quantifiable attribute of trypanosomal populations. Infectivity can be modified for a species of animal by serial passage of trypanosomes in the species of host.

All species of Salivarian trypanosomes have a wide range of domestic and wild mammalian hosts. Of the domestic animals, *T. brucei*, *T. evansi*, and *T. congolense* infect cattle, sheep, goats, horses, donkeys, camels, pigs, dogs, and cats. In addition to these hosts, *T. evansi* also infects water buffalo. *Trypanosoma vivax* also infects all those animal species infected with the other tsetse-fly-transmitted species with the exception of the dog, cat, and pig. *Trypanosoma equiperdum* is restricted to horses and donkeys. *Trypanosoma simiae* infects pigs, camels, sheep, and goats, but in the last two species the infectivity is variable; it is not infective for cattle. The other species, *T. suis* causing trypanosomiasis in pigs, is not infective for other species of animals. *Trypanosoma cruzi* is made up of numerous subpopulations or strains which vary in the infectivity for man and animals. Natural infections do not occur in most domestic species with the exception of dogs, cats, and rarely pigs. Experimental infections, however, have been established in calves, lambs, and kids.

Literature

Infectivity is the first criteria used to describe the interaction between pathogenic trypanosomes and their hosts. It has generally been accepted that all domestic animals with the exception of poultry are susceptible to infections with pathogenic African trypanosomes. Recently, however, it has been shown that chickens are susceptible to infections by *T. brucei* and *T. rhodesiense*, but the parasitemias were low and detectable only by subinoculation into mice (Minter-Goedbloed 1981). An absolute resistance of a host to a species of trypanosome is easily demonstrable, but a description of varying degrees of infectivity for a susceptible host requires quantitation using standardized laboratory materials and methods (Mshelbwala and Ormerod 1973; Phillips 1960a, b; Phillips and Bertram 1967).

The biological behavior, including infectivity, of tsetse-transmitted trypanosomes isolated from nature depend in part on the species of tsetse fly and host from which it is isolated; it is further affected by manipulations in the laboratory. Because of this extensive heterogeneity in character and activity of trypanosome populations, standardization of nomenclature and many of the basic techniques is essential. A system of nomenclature has been proposed which identifies the origin and subsequent animal passages used in the maintenance of trypanosomes in the laboratory (Lumsden and Herbert 1975; Lumsden 1977). The preservation of unchanged trypanosomes in the laboratory while they are under study is the key to the research of trypanosome behavior. The maintenance of viable trypanosomes *in vitro* for short periods of time depends on the obligatory composition of physiological solutions (Raether and Seidenath 1972, 1973, 1974; Taylor *et al.* 1974). The storage of trypanosomes in ice showed a reduced virulence of *T. gambiense* and *T. rhodesiense*, which survived for 7 days and remained infective for 3 to 4 days. On the other hand *T. congolense* survived for 4 days but remained infective for 2 days, while *T. vivax* only survived for 1 day. Dilution of the inoculant had an effect on the survival (Princewill 1980).

Most studies also require storage of trypanosomes in a stable state for long periods of time. This is achieved by cryopreservation based on the general principles applied for freezing of protozoa, and the frozen material is called stabilate (Dalgliesh 1972; Lumsden 1972a, b). The ultrastructural alterations, infectivity, and motility of *T. brucei* caused by cryopreservation after 10% glycerin has been added were compared and it was found that morphological changes were observed in 50% of the deep-frozen trypanosomes; significant loss of motility and infectivity was observed to go hand in hand with these morphological changes (Schupp *et al.* 1980). Having these methods for handling of live trypanosomes enables determination of the infectivity of suspensions. Lumsden *et al.* (1963, 1968) and Lumsden (1972a) published the pioneering work on the quantitative definition of the infectivity of trypanosomes. He introduced the use of ID_{63} and, although the method was criticized by Overdulve and Antonisse (1970), it formed a basis for quantitative study of trypanosome infectivity. However, a better method has been available based on the use of ID_{50} as determined by the mathematical model proposed by Shortley and Wilkins (1965). This method has some very important advantages which include demonstration whether the test population of animals is homogeneous in its susceptibility and, if it is not, determines the ID_{50} for each of the heterogeneous subgroups. The application of this model to the study of infectivity of hemoprotozoa was reviewed by Losos *et al.* (1982).

Laboratory investigation of the infectivity and other aspects of trypanosomiasis caused by *T. vivax* has been limited because of the resistance of laboratory rodents to infection. A technique of injecting large quantities of bovine serum together with the infecting trypanosomes caused infections in rodents, and after numerous subpassages by this method *T. vivax* became adapted and did not require further injection of serum (Desowitz and Watson 1951, 1952; Desowitz 1963). More recently a strain of *T. vivax* from West Africa has been found to be infective and transmissible through rats without the injections of bovine sera (De Gee *et al.* 1976; Leeflang *et al.* 1976a, b).

Parasitemia and tissue tropism

Various species of pathogenic trypanosome cause infections in the mammalian host which differ in their distributions in the tissues and in their levels of parasitemia. Tissue tropism and numbers of organisms circulating in the blood depend on the subgenera, species, and strain of trypanosomes, and on the species of host infected. Infections by all species begin with the injection or penetration of trypanosomes into the subcutaneous or submucosal connective tissue. At this site, multiplication may occur and may be associated with a local inflammatory reaction. In man infected with *T. rhodesiense* and *T. cruzi*, a characteristic local lesion develops. Similar lesions have not been reported in natural infections of domestic animals. However, experimental infections with *T. brucei* in laboratory animals and with *T. congolense* in cattle can cause local inflammation associated with multiplication of organisms. There is also evidence from studies in laboratory animals infected with *T. brucei* that the local response varies with the species of animal. In domestic animals, although multiplication of tsetse-transmitted species of trypanosomes may occur at the site of the bite, the inflammatory reaction is not clinically detected under field conditions. Inflammation of the external genital organs is usually observed in the initial stages of *T. equiperdum* infections in horses and is associated with tissue multiplication of trypanosomes.

From the site of the infection, the trypanosomes enter the blood, either directly or through the lymphatics, and are disseminated throughout the body by the circulating blood. During this first wave of parasitemia some species leave the blood and localize in various tissues and organs. Although parasitemia occurs throughout the course of infection in all forms of trypanosomiasis, its level varies with different species and strains of trypanosome and with various species of host. With those trypanosomes which localize in solid tissue (the *brucei*-like organisms) the parasitemia is usually lower than with those species which remain in the circulation. In most infections, parasitemia is usually higher during the early rather than in the chronic stages.

Considerable importance has been attached to detection of trypanosomes in the blood and levels of parasitemia in the diagnosis and study of the pathogenesis of trypanosomiasis. High parasitemia is often associated with acute severe disease, while low levels are usually observed in chronic syndromes characterized by mild clinical signs or in asymptomatic responses seen in the carrier state. The virulence of a strain is thus often reflected in the level of parasitemia it causes. However, because infections caused by various species of pathogenic trypanosomes differ in their distributions, the role of parasitemia in the development of disease varies and may not be reflected in the levels which occur. Circulating trypanosomes are either the main population causing infection, or are merely a fraction of the total, a subpopulation which may or may not be representative of the numbers and behavior of the whole population.

Following the development of parasitemia, localization occurs in solid tissues with many species of trypanosomes. Most of the Salivarian species, *T. brucei*, the related trypanosomes affecting man, *T. evansi* and *T. equiperdum* are widely disseminated throughout various organs and tissues, localizing intracellularly in their connective tissue stroma. Although there are proposals to the contrary, there is no clear evidence for the existence of morphologically distinct tissue forms other than the blood form trypomastigotes. A cycle of development of the vertebrate host which involves morphological transformation has not been found. Specific organ or tissue tropism has also not been demonstrated for either the various species or strains of *brucei*-like trypanosomes, but the involvement of certain organs, e.g. brain, heart, and eye results in the most noticeable clinical signs. There is evidence that tissue tropism may be dependent to some degree on duration of infection and also on the species of host. Invasion of the central nervous system in cattle and camels occurs during the latter stages of infection. In laboratory animals, the central nervous system is rarely affected in the rat and neither heart nor brain is affected in the rabbit, but massive localization occurs in the subcutaneous and submucosal tissues of the head. *Trypanosoma congolense*, after its initial multiplication at the site of the bite by the vector, localizes in the capillaries by attaching itself to the endothelial cells. The most noticeable accumulation of trypanosomes occurs in the microvasculature of the brain and heart. The last member of the Salivarian group, *T. vivax*, is also capable of leaving the circulation and invading solid tissue, particularly the heart. However, there is evidence that its invasive capabilities are not comparable to those of the *brucei*-like organisms, and the majority of the trypanosome population is found in the circulatory blood.

Trypanosoma cruzi differs from the other pathogenic trypanosomes by dividing, not in blood or tissue fluid, but in various cells with a well-developed and varied tissue tropism observed with different strains, as well as having cyclic development in cells which involves morphological transformation and multiplication. These qualitative and quantitative differences and similarities between the parasitemias and tissue distributions caused by various pathogenic trypanosomes reflect the distinct and common host–parasite relationship of various species which are responsible for the similarities and differences in the clinical signs and pathogenesis.

Literature

The local skin reaction at the site of the tsetse-fly bite have been studied in man and laboratory animals infected with *T. brucei* and *T. rhodesiense,* and differences between various species of host were observed in the extent of inflammation and multiplication (Fairbain and Godfrey 1957; Fantham 1911; Gordon *et al.* 1956; Gordon and Willett 1958; Willett and Gordon 1957). There were no reports of local skin reactions in domestic animals under even severe field challenge, suggesting that they are not common or difficult to detect clinically. In experimental *T. congolense* infection of cattle, nodules developed at the site of the tsetse-fly bite and the organisms multiplied and subsequently appeared in the local drainage lymph node (Roberts *et al.* 1969; Luckins and Gray 1978, 1979a). Tsetse flies infected with *T. congolense* or *T. vivax* caused local skin reactions in goats which were detected with *T. congolense* 7 days after infection, became maximum 3 days later, and were characterized by an initial neutrophil infiltration followed by accumulation of lymphocytes, macrophages, and plasma cells. Moderate numbers of trypanosomes were observed in tissues at the height of the inflammatory actions. *Trypanosoma vivax* injected by tsetse fly also produced a skin nodule 7 days after infection and contained large numbers of lymphocytes and macrophages and only a few neutrophils, with small numbers of trypanosomes being associated with the lesions. It was concluded that the skin reactions caused by *T. congolense, T. vivax,* and *T. brucei* were different in their histological appearance, severity, and time of response (Emery *et al.* 1980; Emery and Moloo 1981).

Infections of rabbits, calves, and sheep caused by tsetse flies infected with *T. congolense* resulted in local skin reaction developing after 6 to 10 days at the site of the bite. Substantial numbers of trypanosomes were located in the deep dermis between 7 and 12 days after the infection and were then observed in the local drainage lymph nodes. In the calves, a few trypanosomes persisted at the site of the bite up to day 30. The local multiplication of trypanosomes was accompanied by inflammatory exudate and necrosis of dermis in the vicinity of blood vessels (Gray and Luckins 1980). Infective *T. congolense* forms from cultures also caused similar local skin reactions in rabbits (Luckins *et al.* 1981). In calves and sheep infected experimentally with *T. congolense* the migration of *T. equiperdum* after intradermal infection of dogs revealed that afferent lymph contained trypanosomes 5 to 27 minutes after inoculation. Lymph nodes draining the site and blood were positive as early as 5 minutes after injection (Theis and Bolton 1980). Attention has been drawn to the sequence of events which occur at this site of first contact between the invading organisms and host because of the importance of the mechanism which governs whether infections are established or eliminated, and as with other aspects of pathogenesis it may vary significantly with the species of trypanosome.

The time to the development of parasitemia after infection, known as the prepatent period, and the levels and fluctuations of parasitemia have been studied throughout the course of various forms of trypanosomiases in domestic and laboratory animals. The usefulness of a quantitative description of parasitemia depends on the precision of the sampling schedule and the accuracy of the enumeration techniques which are used. The precision of one as compared to multiple samples taken within 24 hours was determined in *T. vivax* infection in goats (Losos *et al.* 1982). A number of enumeration methods have been used which vary in their level of accuracy. A rapid approximate method of estimating parasitemia was devised by matching density of organisms observed in a microscope field of a wet mount with a precalculated count (Herbert and Lumsden 1976). Low numbers of trypanosomes have been counted by a drop method which examined a relatively large volume of blood. Direct counts in a hemocytometer were compared to the indirect estimations obtained by relating to the density of trypanosomes to white blood cells (Creemers 1972a, b). To facilitate counting, lysis of red blood cells by ammonium chloride and concentration of the trypanosomes have been used (Hoff 1974). The enumeration of trypanosomes in blood was aided by the selected lysis of erythrocytes and leukocytes by aerolysin, a toxin produced by the bacterium *Aeromonas hydrophila* (Pearson *et al.* 1982). The use of electronic particle counters required the separation of trypanosomes from blood (Martin *et al.* 1972). Cytofluorometric methods were promising but required some improvement to enable rapid and accurate counting of trypanosomes at low levels (Jackson *et al.* 1977; Mills and Valli 1978). Another way of describing the parasite load of a parasitemia is by the volume of the trypanosomes making up the infecting population, and has been undertaken in *T. vivax* and *T. congolense* infections of cattle (Maxie *et al.* 1978).

High levels of parasitemia have often been associated with acute severe syndromes of trypanosomiasis both in domestic and laboratory animals. Two morphologically different subpopulations of *T. congolense* have been observed to cause different levels of parasitemia which resulted in two syndromes of varying severity (Godfrey 1960, 1961). The levels of *T. vivax* infection in East Africa are lower than in West

Africa and are also related to milder forms of the disease. Low levels of parasitemia also characterize the mild or asymptomatic form of trypanosomiasis in trypano-tolerant breeds of cattle (Murray and Morrison 1979a). The relationship between levels of parasitemia and the severity of diseases in cattle caused by single and multiple infections with *T. brucei, T. congolense,* and *T. vivax* have been confirmed (Losos 1979; Murray and Morrison 1979a).

These observations in cattle have been supported by results in laboratory animals, with more severe syndromes developing in those strains of mice which had higher parasitemia (Morrison *et al.* 1978; Raether 1971). Comparison of a susceptible and a resistant strain of mice to *T. congolense* showed that initially both strains caused similar levels of anemia, parasitemia, biochemical derangement, and immunosuppression. The remarkable difference after 8 days of infection was the sustained high levels of parasitemia in the susceptible strain of mice and a marked decrease, a reduction of 10^3 trypanosomes per ml, occurred in the resistant strain (Whitelaw *et al.* 1980). Inbred strains of mice showed marked differences in susceptibility to infections with *T. congolense,* as judged by survival and levels of parasitemia, and the genetic basis of susceptibility was likely to be under complex control (Morrison and Murray 1979b). It has also been shown that virulence of *T. brucei* for mice was associated with high levels of parasitemia, and was dependent on a particular antigenic type (McNeillage and Herbert 1968; Clayton 1978). However, it was also shown that infectivity and virulence of *T. brucei* for mice did not appear to be related to the variable antigenic type because two populations of trypanosomes of the same antigenic type, one subjected to many passages through animals, and another, isolated closer to the original stock, produced two syndromes of different severity (Barry 1979). In acute fatal *T. brucei* infection in mice, the inability of the host to achieve effective levels of circulating antibody was the result of continued rapid multiplication of trypanosomes and not due to any significant degree of immunosuppression; in chronic forms of the disease a slower replication rate allowed the antibody to reach levels which permitted effective opsonization (MacAskill *et al.* 1981).

The suppression of IgM responses induced by different strains of trypanosomes could be related to the virulence as expressed in two strains of mice which differed considerably in their ability to survive infection dependent on their ability to mount an IgM response (Selkirk and Sacks 1980; Sacks and Askonas 1980; Sacks *et al.* 1980). The infectivity of *T. congolense* in mice was altered – as evidenced by the prolonged survival time – by preincubation with bovine antilymphocyte sera, suggesting cross-reactivity between the antibodies and trypanosomal antigens (Weiland *et al.* 1981). Administration of immunostimulants, such as *Corynebacterium parvum,* bacillus-Calmette-Guérin, or *Bordetella pertussis,* increased the survival time in mice with a reduction in parasitemia and its onset (Murray and Morrison 1979b). Virulence has been associated with the following species of tsetse fly: *T. simiae* were isolated in Kenya from *G. brevipalpis,*

G. austeni, and *G. pallipides*. All strains from *G. brevipalpis* were very virulent for pigs and on subpassage retained their virulence. Strains in *G. pallipides* caused a chronic infection, often self-limiting, and strains from *G. austeni* were intermediate between the other two strains in their virulence (Janssen and Wijers 1974). The factors, both of the trypanosomes and the host, which affect virulence have been reviewed by Herbert and Parratt (1979).

Fluctuations of numbers of trypanosomes observed in the blood are characteristic of most forms of trypanosomiasis, and the periodic peaks of parasitemia suggest rapid changes in the circulating populations. Obvious cyclic waves of parasitemia were observed to occur about every 6 days in *T. vivax* but not *T. congolense* infections (Maxie *et al.* 1979). During the first peak, the generation time was approximately 8 hours which is equal to the optimal growth rate reported for *T. brucei* in culture (Hirumi *et al.* 1977). Circadian rhythm has been reported with *T. congolense* infection of cattle and rats, and in the first species it was associated with morning and afternoon temperature changes (Hornby and Bailey 1931; Hawking 1978a). Circadian and other rhythms in parasitic infections, including pathogenic and nonpathogenic trypanosomes, were reviewed by Hawking (1975). Because it is now generally accepted that many infections by pathogenic Salivarian trypanosomes result in invasions of solid tissues or other tissue localizations, changes in the levels of parasitemia have to be regarded as involving a number of factors affecting the population kinetics such as multiplication in the blood, elimination by the host's defense mechanisms of circulating trypanosomes, and the migration of organisms between blood and solid tissues.

In the literature before 1930, species of pathogenic trypanosomes were differentiated by their ability to invade solid tissues (reviewed by Hornby 1952, and Losos and Ikede 1972). Since 1930, and until fairly recently, this feature of Salivarian trypanosomes has not been generally emphasized and infections have been thought to be limited primarily to the blood. It has now been clearly re-established that *T. brucei*, *T. rhodesiense*, *T. gambiense*, and *T. evansi* invade and localize in solid tissues (Goodwin 1970; Losos and Ikede 1970; Morales and Carreno 1976; Yutuc and Sher 1949), and their penetrating ability has been related to their vigorous twisting forward motility (Evans and Ellis 1975). Their cyclic or otherwise behavior in the solid tissues has not been established. Most of the tissue forms observed have been the blood form trypomastigotes, although a few amastigote forms have also been found (Losos and Ikede 1972; Peruzzi 1928). Whether these were part of a tissue life cycle or merely degenerative forms has not been established. Soltys and Woo (1969, 1970) claimed that these amastigote tissue forms were infective. Large numbers of what was thought to be amastigote forms were also observed in the choroid plexus, but the supporting illustration was unconvincing since in routine histological preparations trypomastigotes in blood look like amastigote forms (Ormerod and Vankatesan 1971a, b). Ormerod (1979) reviewed the life cycle in the mammalian host of the species in the subgenus

Trypanozoon. This included consideration of the variability of the morphology of blood trypomastigotes, including the slender, intermediate, and stumpy forms, and their relationship to the variable genetic constitution, sexual dimorphism, and degeneration. He concluded that these forms appeared to present the successive development of three stages of a life cycle. The literature on the development of these species in solid tissues was reviewed, pointing out the attitudes and conclusions of various groups of workers, and a number of hypotheses to explain the diversity of structural forms observed in both blood and tissue was presented. Unfortunately, the reexamination of all of these data still fails to resolve how complex is the life cycle in the mammalian host and whether the forms which have been described are regenerative or degenerative.

Also in the older literature, *T. congolense* was regarded as localizing in small blood vessels (Hornby 1952). Now it is known that these organisms attach themselves to the endothelial cells by their flagella (Banks 1978; Bungener and Muller 1976). The mechanism *T. congolense*, an intravascular parasite binding to the endothelium wall and erythrocytes of infected hosts, was proposed to be due to the surface of *T. congolense* containing a protein-associated site which binds to sialic acid of the host cell (Banks 1979). Injury induced by the lysis of trypanosomes by antibody–complement interaction damaged the endothelial cells, resulting in increased vascular permeability at the site of *T. congolense* attachment in the microcirculation (Banks 1980). The populations which are found in the microvasculature were up to a thousandfold higher than those found in the circulating blood (Banks 1978). There was also conclusive evidence that once there, this species does not leave the circulatory system, and this is based on histological examination of tissues and lymph from infected domestic and laboratory animals (Losos *et al.* 1973a; Ssenyonga 1974; Ssenyonga and Adam 1975; Tizard *et al.* 1978e). Comparative study of the distribution of *T. brucei* and *T. congolense* in tissues of mice and rats showed *T. brucei* in the connective tissues and body fluids, while *T. congolense* was found in capillaries and not in either fluids of the body cavities or lymph, and an extensive mononuclear cell infiltration in the interstitial tissues was not observed (Ssenyonga 1980a). This attachment is disrupted by the action of the trypanocidal drug diamidine aceturate and trypanosomes are liberated into the circulating blood (Maxie *et al.* 1976). Various species of trypanosomes attach to the cells of the tsetse flies during their cyclic development and this has been considered as an indispensable property in their ability to cause infections in the invertebrate host. A similar situation exists in the case of *T. congolense* in the mammalian host.

Hornby (1952) regarded *T. vivax* as a species capable of invading solid tissues. Work undertaken in West Africa to verify this did not confirm his observations (Losos and Ikede 1972). However, recent reports have shown conclusively that *T. vivax* invaded solid tissues, particularly the heart, and caused an inflammatory response (Bungener and Mehlitz 1977; van den Ingh and de Neijs-Bakker

1979). The *T. vivax* infections of tissues appeared to differ from *T. brucei* in that they were not generalized throughout the body of the host. The tissue localization of *T. cruzi* depends on the cell tropism of different strains. It has been proposed that originally in the evolution of the host–parasite relationship this trypanosome invaded the cells of the reticuloendothelial system and only subsequently adapted itself to other tissues and organs such as muscle, liver, brain, peripheral nerves, ovary, and testes. Once in the cell, the blood trypomastigote underwent a life cycle involving transformation to epimastigotes and amastigotes which multiplied in a pseudocyst structure. The rupture of the pseudocyst resulted in further dissemination of infection. Entry into the cell was dependent in part on the active motility and action of the flagellum, and with some types of cells such as the macrophage, on the presence of a protease-sensitive component of the host cell plasma membrane (Noguiera and Cohn 1976, 1977; Sooksri and Inoki 1972). Strains of *T. cruzi* have remarkably well-developed cell tropisms, probably due to differences in the membrane composition of host cells and in the receptors on the trypanosomes. It has also been proposed that contact between cells of various tissues and trypanosomes was not random but dependent on some form of attracting mechanism (Dvorak and Howe 1976; Melo and Brener 1978).

The numbers of Salivarian trypanosomes in tissues varies with the severity of the clinical syndrome. Massive numbers occur in acute diseases caused by *brucei*-like organisms in dogs, sheep, goats, and some laboratory species. In the rat, the early tissue localization is overshadowed by the massive intravascular population. *Trypanosoma cruzi* is also found in large numbers in the acute diseases of man and dog. In chronic diseases and in asymptomatic carriers all species of pathogenic trypanosomes were difficult to find in tissues. A similar situation with regard to the association of tissue parasitosis and severity of the syndrome was also seen in *T. congolense* infections. The relationships between numbers of trypanosomes in the tissues and those circulating in the blood have not been established for most species. There has been little information published on this correlation. Hanson and Robertson (1974) noted a positive relationship between numbers of *T. cruzi* in tissues and the blood trypomastigotes in acute experimental disease in mice, while in *T. congolense* infection of cattle, both acute and chronic, no correlation was observed between size of population localized in the capillaries of the brain and heart, and those in the general circulation. The localization of *T. congolense* in the widened capillaries of the cerebral cortex was observed but few trypanosomes were found in the microcirculation of the muscle and liver. These changes were observed in the 6-month-old calves and not in the neonatal calves. The effects of the various drugs on this localization of *T. congolense* showed that Berenil and dexamethasone had a significant effect on the trypanosome count in the peripheral circulation and that epinephrine caused a fleeting increase in parasitemia. While Hetastarch, dectran and cyclophosphamide have no effect, Berenil cleared the capillaries of the trypanosomes within 30 minutes (Mills *et al.* 1980). Because of the localization of *T. congolense* in the peripheral circulation its isolation from the infected animal is more difficult than with other species of trypanosomes. The yield is increased by placing the rat in an environment of 37 °C for 1 hour prior to sacrifice and by replacing of the blood removed by lactated Ringer's solution with 5% glucose (Rosen *et al.* 1979).

CLINICAL SIGNS

Infections by pathogenic trypanosomes cause diseases which vary in severity depending on the virulence of the organisms and susceptibility of the host. Strains in each species of trypanosomes are capable of evoking a range of responses including acute, chronic, and asymptomatic carrier syndromes. There are very marked differences between species and breeds of animals in their susceptibility to the development of clinical disease. Also, even under identical conditions of challenge, remarkable differences in individual animal susceptibility are observed in uniform groups of animals. The acute disease usually occurs shortly after infection, lasts for days or a few weeks, and terminates in either death or development of a chronic form of the disease. Chronic syndromes, with or without the initial acute phase, last for months, in some cases years, and terminate in either death, elimination of infection, or carrier state. Many chronic forms of trypanosomiasis are characterized by periodic exacerbation of clinical signs throughout the course of infection and at such times the animal may die. Asymptomatic carriers are either a sequel to chronic forms of the disease or develop without prior signs of disease.

The type of clinical signs which develop depend on host–parasite interaction involving the behavior of the organisms in the host and the response they stimulate. Most forms of trypanosomiasis do not have pathognomonic clinical signs, which are useful in diagnosis. The similarities and differences between symptoms in the various diseases caused by the different species of trypanosomes are related to common and distinct characteristics of the different infections. Similar clinical manifestations result from the common features of the infections caused by different species and the relatively limited range of responses, both local and systemic, which the host is able to generate. Distribution of the organisms in the tissues of the host is responsible for the most obvious clinical differences. An important form of animal trypanosomiasis, which is observed in herds resident in enzootic areas infested by tsetse flies, is caused by concomitant infections by more than one species of trypanosomes, and the diseases are more severe than those caused by a simple species.

Diseases caused by *Nannomonas*

There are two species, *T. congolense* and *T. simiae*, in the subgenus *Nannomonas*. The first affects all species of domestic mammals, and the second infects primarily pigs but also possibly camels, sheep, and goats. Animal species vary in their susceptibility to the development of disease caused by *T. congolense*, and the most severe syndrome is observed in dogs with death often occurring within 2 weeks after infection. The syndromes in cattle are more severe in East than West Africa. In cattle, sheep, goats, and horses the acute syndrome caused by *T. congolense* lasts 4 to 6 weeks with intermittent pyrexia, increased respiratory and heart rate, depression, pale mucous membranes, subcutaneous edema of the jaw, and prominent jugular pulse. In horses, the edema may be more generalized and affect the ventral abdominal wall and legs. Fever is usually first observed with the initial wave of parasitemia, and thereafter elevation of temperature is often associated with an increase in the number of trypanosomes in the blood. The appetite is depressed and there is rapid loss of weight. Death is associated with severe anemia and circulatory collapse. During the terminal stages the animal becomes recumbent for 1 to 3 days, lies quietly, and does not show any central nervous system involvement. The chronic syndromes may last for months, resulting in extreme emaciation and severe anemia.

Trypanosoma simiae causes a very acute disease, probably the most fulminating form of trypanosomiasis, in pigs with death occurring virtually within hours after trypanosomes first appear in the blood. The increasing parasitemia is accompanied by fever, increased respiration, dullness, stiff and unsteady gait, and hyperemia of the skin.

Literature

Clinical signs of various forms of trypanosomiasis of domestic animals have been presented by Stephen (1970). A somewhat more complex description of the course of infection in cattle than the one presented by Stephen (1970) and found in more recent publications (Krampitz 1970; Maxie *et al.* 1979; Valli *et al.* 1978a; Wellde *et al.* 1974) was proposed by Fiennes (1950, 1970) and Fiennes *et al.* (1946) and was based on the occurrence of the so-called 'crises' which were exacerbations of clinical signs associated with the destruction of large numbers of trypanosomes and red blood cells in the circulation at specific periods during infection. In recent studies, the development of anemia and disease was progressive without occurrence of these 'crises' and anemia occurred with the first wave of parasitemia (Maxie *et al.* 1979). In calves, enlargement of lymph and hemolymph nodes was observed (Valli *et al.* 1978a), but not in older cattle (Maxie *et al.* 1979; Wellde *et al.* 1974). Very few reports are available on the clinical signs in the other species: horses (Kimberling and Ewing 1973; Stephen 1962a), goats and sheep (Edwards *et al.* 1956a, b) and camels (Uilenberg 1964). *Trypanosoma congolense* caused three syndromes of disease in goats. The first two syndromes, acute and subacute, were either fatal or resulted in a self-cure while the chronic syndrome was inevitably fatal (Griffin and Allonby 1979d). A complete review of the disease caused by *T. simiae* in natural outbreaks and experimental infection was presented by Stephen (1966a).

Diseases caused by *Duttonella*

Trypanosoma vivax infections occur in cattle, sheep, goats, horses, and camels, but not in dogs and pigs. The severity of the disease in cattle differs, with its geographic distribution being more severe in West than in East Africa. However, in East Africa acute outbreaks occur in enzootic areas and are characterized by a fulminating septicemic-like syndrome with extensive hemorrhages on mucous membranes, bloody nasal discharge, and blood in the feces. In the more commonly observed less severe, but still acute, syndromes the hemorrhages are only occasionally observed. The high peaks of parasitemia are associated with elevation of temperature and death often occurs during these periods. The lymph nodes are enlarged, the mucous membranes are pale, and there is rapid loss of weight and appetite. The chronic syndromes are characterized by a series of peaks of parasitemia but at lower levels than in the acute syndromes. Extreme emaciation and subcutaneous edema of the throat are observed. Death in both acute and chronic syndromes is often sudden and not preceded by recumbency. In sheep and goats the disease is similar to those in cattle. In horses the disease is considered to be milder, but a severe acute syndrome may be produced experimentally. In addition to those signs seen in cattle there is more extensive edema of legs and ventral abdomen with the occurrence of urticaria-like plaques.

Literature

In West Africa, mortality was reported as high as 100% in an infected group, but the severity of the syndrome and time to death varied greatly between individual animals (Unsworth 1953; Maxie *et al.* 1979). The fulminating syndrome has been reported in East Africa (Hudson 1944; Boyt and MacKenzie 1970). Acute fatal hemorrhagic disease in exotic dairy cattle reported from Kenya caused by *T. vivax* was characterized by abortion, bloody diarrhea, and death (Mwongela *et al.* 1981). The fever was well correlated to elevation of parasitemia, the respiratory and heart rates were increased, and the lymph nodes obviously enlarged (Maxie *et al.* 1979; van den Ingh *et al.* 1976b). In South America the disease in cattle was predominantly chronic with death being only occasionally observed (Shaw and Lainson 1972). In the chronic syndromes of cattle there was progressive emaciation, anemia, and variable enlargement of lymph nodes. In the horse, a relatively mild chronic form of the disease was observed (Stephen and Mackenzie 1959).

Diseases caused by *Trypanozoon*

The subgenus *Trypanozoon* has five species which are pathogenic to man, cattle, sheep, goats, horses, donkeys, dogs, cats, pigs, camels, and water buffalo. There are considerable differences in the severity of the syndromes produced in the various species of host. The most acute natural syndromes are observed in horses and dogs while relatively mild chronic forms of the disease are seen in cattle.

The acute syndrome lasts for up to 3 months and is characterized by prominent enlargement of lymph nodes, subcutaneous edema, urticarial plaques, fever, anemia, and occasionally ophthalmitis. The elevation of temperature may or may not be correlated to the increase of the numbers of circulating trypanosomes. The ophthalmitis and urticarial plaques are temporary but recurrent. The anemia varies considerably and is generally not as severe as in the other forms of trypanosomiasis. In the chronic syndromes most of the clinical signs are less distinctive, with emaciation, anemia, and recurrent pyrexia being observed. However, there is often obvious central nervous system involvement characterized by weakness, hyperexcitability, and incoordination, usually progressing to terminal paresis and paralysis. In cattle, *T. brucei* usually causes a mild or asymptomatic response. However, there is evidence that prolonged infections may terminate in central nervous system involvement and death. Acute syndromes have also been produced experimentally. On this basis, *T. brucei* should be regarded as being potentially pathogenic for cattle. Its effect may be overlooked because of the low parasitemia, particularly in mixed infection where it is overshadowed by the higher parasitemia caused by other species.

Trypanosoma evansi causes syndromes which closely resemble those caused by *T. brucei*. In cattle and buffalo, the diseases are usually less severe than those observed in camels, dogs, horses, and donkeys. In camels, acute syndromes of 2 to 3 months' duration are common and chronic forms may last for up to 3 years. In carnivore and equines, the acute disease may be as short as 2 to 3 weeks, the chronic syndromes lasting up to 4 months. The disease in horses in South America, known as *mal de caderas* and *murrina*, is characterized by signs of a gradual development of central nervous system involvement.

Trypanosoma equiperdum causes three types of syndrome: asymptomatic, edematous, and neurologic. The asymptomatic condition is afebrile without parasitemia and the diagnosis can be made only serologically. The edematous form is characterized by recurrent edema of the external genitalia which may extend along the abdominal wall. The lymph nodes are enlarged and transient urticarial skin plaques may develop. There is an accompanying pyrexia and loss of weight and appetite. This form of disease progresses to the neurologic syndrome characterized by short periods of hypoaesthesis, incoordination, and finally paralysis. During this stage the animals are extremely emaciated.

Literature

In the older literature reference has been made to *T. brucei* causing severe disease in cattle. However, this was thought by some to be due to mixed infections with other species of trypanosomes. The question of the pathogenicity of *T. brucei* for cattle has not been settled, although more evidence has been gathered that it was a significant pathogen of cattle. The low pathogenicity of *T. brucei* for cattle has been pointed out and supported by reference to the older literature (Killick-Kendrick 1971) and by experimental work (MacKenzie and Boyt 1973). *Trypanosoma rhodesiense* has also been shown to be nonpathogenic for cattle (Wilde and French 1945). However, in more recent studies experimental infections in mature cattle and calves caused severe clinical signs and lesions including brain involvement (Ikede and Losos 1972c; Moulton and Sollod 1976). The differences in pathogenicity for cattle were probably due to differing strains. Also in sheep and goats, the two species for which there are no detailed reports of natural diseases, a severe syndrome has been produced experimentally with the neurologic signs occurring in 9 of the 11 animals studied (Ikede and Losos 1975a). The development of central nervous system signs was associated with the chronic stages in horses (Neitz and McCully 1971) and donkeys (Ikede *et al.* 1977a). Acute neurologic syndromes have been reported in the dog (Ikede and Losos 1972b).

The diseases caused by *T. evansi* in domestic animals has been reviewed recently (Losos 1980). The previous most complete description of the clinical signs were in a textbook by Innes and Saunders (1962). The last two authors pointed out the scarcity of information on the disease from South America. An account of the course of diseases in cattle and buffalo calves has been presented by Verma and Gautam (1978). More recently two studies of the clinical pathology were reported. Plasma monoamine oxidase levels in acute and chronic trypanosomiasis in camels caused by *T. evansi* were found to be significantly lower than in normal animals (Raisinghani *et al.* 1980). Increased levels of sorbitol dehydrogenase, glutamic pyruvic transaminase, and glutamic oxaloacetic transaminase, and decreased levels of alkaline phosphatase were recorded in serum in *T. evansi* infections in camels and were associated with cellular destruction and lysis of trypanosomes (Boid *et al.* 1980b). On *T. equiperdum* there was a report published recently on immunologic responses, clinical signs, and chemotherapy (Barrowman 1976a, b).

Diseases caused by *Pyenomonas*

Trypanosoma suis infection in the pig causes the rarest and the most undefined form of trypanosomiasis. There are but a few reports of the disease it produces which appears to resemble, to a certain extent, chronic syndromes caused by *T. brucei*. It was last reported in Burundi in 1954.

Literature

The last report was by Peel and Chardome (1954) and the available information on *T. suis* was reviewed by Stephen (1966a).

Diseases caused by *Trypanosoma cruzi*

There appear to be few descriptions published of the natural disease in dogs which is characterized by signs of cardiac malfunction including tachycardia, weak pulse, enlarged liver and spleen, distended abdomen, pale mucous membranes, and lethargy. There is an accompanying loss of weight, enlargement of lymph nodes, diarrhea, and anorexia. Central nervous system involvement with ataxia, weakness, and chorea is also observed. Cases are reported where apparently normal animals die suddenly and, on postmortem examination, the cause is an acute heart failure due to myocarditis.

Literature

Reports on *T. cruzi* causing natural diseases in nine dogs were by Williams *et al.* (1977) and by Goble (1952) on experimental infections. More recent publications include Lopes *et al.* (1980) and Andrade *et al.* (1980, 1981).

Diseases in wild animals

Wild animals, although infected with one or more species of pathogenic trypanosomes, are regarded as being resistant to the development of clinical diseases. This is supported by the presence of large herds of wild animals with a high incidence of infection in tsetse-fly-infested areas of Africa. However, this does not mean that diseases and deaths do not occur in these species. Based on experimental work on *T. brucei* and *T. rhodesiense* infections in a variety of species of African wild animals, a surprising number of species are susceptible to infections which terminate in death. In the field, factors such as the effect of continuous exposure of a wild animal population to challenge by trypanosomes in a particular locality, and the selection of certain species by tsetse flies as the preferential food host may determine the susceptibility of various wild species to trypanosomes. *Trypanosoma evansi* spreading to new areas causes severe diseases and deaths in local wild animal populations.

Literature

Microscopic lesions, suggestive of *T. brucei* and aggregates of *T. congolense* organisms, have been observed in some of the naturally infected animals (Losos and Gwamaka 1973). *Trypanosoma brucei* infections have been associated with natural disease of a zebra and lion (McCulloch 1967; Sachs *et al.* 1967). Ashcroft *et al.* (1959) reviewed the previous results published on experimental infections and summarized their own experimental work of 18 years on *T. brucei*. He concluded that of the 20 species, 9 were susceptible to the development of disease and died, 7 were infected but not diseased, 3 were difficult to infect and 1 was completely resistant. Numerous species have been shown to be susceptible to *T. evansi* infections which caused severe disease and death, and the subject has been reviewed by Hoare (1972) and Morales *et al.* (1976).

Diseases in laboratory and animal models

Mice, rats, rabbits, and a variety of other less common laboratory animals are used extensively in the studies of behavior of pathogenic trypanosomes in the development of the diseases. In rats and mice infected with various tsetse-transmitted varieties acute diseases are not characterized by any remarkable clinical signs. The chronic forms of infection occasionally cause central nervous system involvement and are particularly useful in the development of chemotherapy against human trypanosomiasis. In the rabbit, species in the subgenus *Trypanozoon* cause characteristic skin inflammation of the head and genitalia. Experimental *T. cruzi* infection in laboratory rodents cause a variety of syndromes which vary with the strains in severity and tissue tropism.

The literature, which includes some clinical aspects of trypanosomiases in laboratory animals, is presented in the section on the pathology of trypanosomiases in laboratory animals.

PATHOLOGY

The similarities and differences between the clinical syndromes caused by the different species of trypanosomes are reflected in the variability of the pathogenesis of the disease. An important factor of all forms of trypanosomiasis is the occurrence – at times dominance of some field situations – of infections which do not cause disease. Therefore, in trypanosomiasis a simple direct relationship of all infections causing disease does not exist. To understand the development of clinical disease it is necessary to take into account not only qualitative, but also quantitative features of both the infecting trypanosome populations and the resulting host responses.

The basic mechanisms by which trypanosomes injure tissues are probably multifactorial for any species of trypanosome and involve utilization and excretion of metabolites, excretion of toxic substances, mechanical disruption of host's tissue, and immunologically mediated injury. These mechanisms, singularly or in combination, are potentially harmful. However, the actual tissue damage is dependent, in addition to these inherent noxious properties of the infecting trypanosome organism, on the level of infection and the capability of the infected tissues to tolerate levels of parasitemia without significant impairment of function.

Lesions found in various forms of trypanosomiasis can be regarded as being either primary, i.e. caused by the direct effect of the injurious mechanisms usually on the infected target organs, or secondary, resulting from the subsequent malfunction of organs and tissues affected by the primary lesions. Because of the limited responses of the host tissues to injury some lesions, e.g. anemia, may have a different underlying causative mechanism in various forms of trypanosomiasis. The description which follows will include gross and microscopic tissue changes for each subgenera and at times for each species, a discussion of the possible mechanisms of injury, and the pathogenesis of lesions.

Pathogenesis of diseases caused by *Nannomonas*

Primary lesions caused by *T. congolense* are in the blood, blood vessels, and in the lymphoid system. Secondary lesions occur in various other tissues and organs as a result of the circulatory system malfunction. With the first wave of parasitemia, the packed cell volume (PCV), white blood cells (WBC), and thrombocyte levels are decreased. Depending on the severity of the syndromes, these levels either continue to drop until the animal dies or plateau out in the chronic form of the disease at subnormal levels. At postmortem examination there are no pathognomonic lesions. In the acute syndrome the carcass is pale and there is variable atrophy of adipose and skeletal muscle tissue. Extensive edema affects the loose connective tissue stroma throughout the carcass, but it is most pronounced in the mesentery, abomasal mucosa, and perirenal fat. In the chronic syndrome there is extensive emaciation with generalized edema, with the carcass having the appearance of nonspecific cachexia. The spleen is enlarged, meaty, and the white pulp is prominent in both acute and chronic syndromes. The lymph nodes are wet, and are either enlarged or normal size depending on the duration and severity of the infection. The hemolymph node size is variable, but at times they are large and palpable through the skin. The thymus is markedly atrophied. The heart, liver, and kidneys are enlarged, but this is not readily discernible without weighing the organs. There are usually no hemorrhages on the serosal and mucosal surfaces. On microscopical examination, trypanosomes are found localized in the small blood vessels of all organs and tissues, but are found in particularly large numbers in the brain and heart. This localization is accompanied by widespread dilatation of the microvascular system and hypertrophy of the endothelial cells.

Aggregates of mononuclear cells, predominantly macrophages, are found in the blood vessels. The perivascular connective tissue is edematous and there are occasionally few mononuclear cells in some organs, e.g. heart and kidneys. However, these are not comparable to the extensive mononuclear inflammatory reactions which characterize lesions caused by those species of trypanosome which invade solid tissues. The glomeruli are enlarged and hypercellular, with dilatation of the capillaries and thickening of the basement membrane. Depending on the severity of the terminal anemia, central lobular ischemic necrosis may be seen in the liver. In the acute syndrome, there is an obvious depletion of small lymphocytes from the cortical areas of the lymph nodes and the white pulp of the spleen. In the more protracted infection, depending on the severity of the disease, there is considerable variability in the amount of depletion, hypertrophy, and hyperplasia of various cellular components of the lymphoid system.

Although a number of proposals have been put forward as to the mechanisms by which *T. congolense* causes tissue damage and the sequence of development of lesions, the pathogenesis has not been clearly established. A biologically active extract, with hemolytic and inflammatory properties, has been identified from the trypanosomes. Immunologically mediated cytotoxicity, related to antigen–antibody complexes on host cells and activation of complement, may also be involved in the destruction of the blood cells and in causing vascular changes affecting permeability. The principal target tissue for colonization by *T. congolense* is the microvasculature, causing dilatation and structural changes in the vessel walls which are indicative of circulatory malfunction. Atrophy and hyperplasia of various lymphoid tissues indicates the variable effect of the severity and duration of infections of different syndromes. The absence of obvious necrosis and inflammation suggests that the underlying cellular changes are degenerative in both the primary and secondary lesions associated with circulatory system malfunction.

The fulminating septicemic syndrome caused by *T. simiae* in pigs is associated with large numbers of intravascular trypanosomes and thrombosis, resulting in tissue necrosis and hemorrhages.

Literature

A number of in-depth studies have been undertaken on the clinical pathology, hemodynamics, and lesions in solid tissues of cattle infected with various strains of *T. congolense*. The initial hemolytic anemia was macrocytic and normochronic with the bone marrow being responsive, particularly in young animals (Losos *et al.* 1973a, b; Maxie *et al.* 1976, 1979; Valli *et al.* 1978b; Wellde *et al.* 1974). The half-life of erythrocytes was greatly reduced as a result of *T. congolense* infection of calves due to hemolysis (Preston *et al.* 1979). Although the anemia caused by *T. congolense* was normochronic and macrocytic in the acute phase, it became normocytic in chronic infections. The anemia was hemolytic and responsive with the half-life of red blood cells halved in the acute phase with an increase in plasma volume. The red blood cell destruction occurred in the liver as the major site (Valli *et al.* 1978a, b).

Anemia was milder in the neonatal calves than in 6-month-old calves. Differences were also observed in the leukocytosis between the two age groups, but the plasma iron turnover rates were not different (Valli and Mills 1980). Accompanying the anemia there was leukopenia and thrombocytopenia (Wellde *et al.* 1978). The role of hemodilution in the development of anemia has not been totally resolved; some of the results were contradictory and probably affected by the variations and inadequacies of the techniques used (Dargie *et al.* 1979a; Mamo and Holmes 1975; Maxie and Valli 1979; Tartour and Idris 1973; Valli *et al.* 1978b).

Significant decreases of total serum proteins and albumin levels were also reported, but whether this was due to dilution or the increased rate of catabolism has not been determined (Tabel 1979; Tabel *et al.* 1980). The responses of N'Dama and Zebu cattle to *T. congolense* were compared and the peak of parasitemia was significantly lower, occurred later, and was of shorter duration in the N'Dama breed. Animals in both breeds become anemic, the severity of which being related to the level and duration of parasitemia which was not pronounced in the Zebu. Hemodilution was not a feature of the anemia. It was concluded that the resistance of the N'Dama cattle to the development of clinical diseases lies in the control of parasitemia rather than more efficient erythropoietic response (Dargie *et al.* 1979a). The red blood cell destruction rate was determined in two breeds of goats infected with *T. congolense* and *H. contortus*. Both breeds had more rapid cell loss with the dual infection than with the single infection, and the *T. congolense* rendered goats more susceptible to *Haemonchus contortus* infestation (Griffin *et al.* 1981a). It is important to note in hematological studies that variation in the hematological parameters was observed between samples from ear and jugular vein in cattle with natural infection with *T. congolense* and *T. vivax* with the ear blood being more sensitive for the detection of parasitemia (Greig *et al.* 1979).

The anemia in infected cattle has been associated with antigen–antibody complexes and complement on the surface of the erythrocytes (Kobayashi and Tizard 1976). This observation, however, had not been verified by using the direct Coomb's test against various classes of antibody (Tabel *et al.* 1981). These results were inconclusive and it was proposed that agglutination was due to coating of erythrocytes by materials released from disintegrating trypanosomes. A lysate of trypanosomes was found to have hemolytic activity *in vitro* in its free fatty acid component (Tizard and Holmes 1976, 1977; Tizard *et al.* 1978a, b, c). The subject has been reviewed recently (Tizard *et al.* 1978d, 1979). Circulating free fatty acids were significantly altered in trypanosome infections and thought to be a possible factor in the disturbance of the clotting mechanism (Roberts and Clarkson 1977).

Phagocytosis of erythrocytes and leukocytes, because of trypanosome material on their surface, was postulated to contribute to the decreased levels (MacKenzie and Cruickshank 1973; MacKenzie *et al.* 1978). In the circulating blood, phagocytosis of trypanosomes by macrophages could also be an important mechanism in eliminating the *in situ* organisms attached to the endothelial cells (Young *et al.* 1975). Another cause of the low levels of blood cells was proposed to be a granulcycle–macrophage maturation inhibitory factor in the plasma (Kaaya *et al.* 1979). Sera from calves infected with either *T. congolense* or *T. vivax* inhibited bovine granulocyte–macrophage colony formation *in vitro*, but not erythroid colony formation, indicating the presence of an inhibitory factor (Kaaya *et al.* 1980) which was related to the degree of parasitemia (Kaaya *et al.* 1979). Myeloid and erythroid cultures from calves infected with *T. congolense* showed a decrease in the number of myeloid colonies in 6-month-old calves as compared to neonatal calves, but there was no difference between the infected and noninfected groups with regard to the numbers of erythroid colonies (Lawson *et al.* 1980). The ineffective thrombopoiesis was observed in calves infected with *T. congolense*, indicating that in chronic forms of this form of trypanosomiasis there was a partial compensated consumption coagulopathy (Forsberg *et al.* 1979). The coagulation parameter partial thromboplastin time in goats, sheep, and horses infected with *T. brucei* and *T. congolense* was abnormally prolonged and could be used to monitor infection and recovery (Essien and Ikede 1976). Thrombocytopenia accompanied partial coagulation disturbances with increased turnover of fibrinogen and prolongation of thromboplastin times and was associated with increases in the parasitemia (Forsberg *et al.* 1979; Wellde *et al.* 1978). Also, inadequate maturation of megakaryocytes has been observed as a contributory factor (Valli *et al.* 1979) to the thrombocytopenia.

There were no changes in the electrolytes and osmolality in sera from neonatal and 6-month-old calves infected with *T. congolense*. Decrease in total serum protein occurred in 6-month-old calves caused by a decrease in albumin and beta$_2$-globulin fractions. The total serum protein in neonatal calves was constant, but the decrease in albumin was compensated by increases in the alpha- and gamma-globulin fractions. Total serum lipids and cholesterol were decreased and triglyceride levels and erythrocide phospholipid levels were significantly elevated in both age groups. Adrenal and hepatic functions were not affected in the infected groups while thyroid function tests showed that T_3 was significantly elevated in 6-month-old calves and T_4 was significantly decreased in neonatal calves (Valli *et al.* 1980).

The absence of inflammatory, necrotic, and extensive degenerative lesions, making the gross and microscopic difficult to define, has led to quantitative and ultrastructural histologic studies to demonstrate the tissue changes (Losos and Mwambu 1979; Mwambu and Losos 1979; Valli *et al.* 1979). It was reported that *T. congolense* caused hemosiderosis, cellular infiltration in the kidney, changes in the walls of the arteries in the lung, scattered local perivascular and meningeal infiltrations, and glial nodules in the central nervous system (Kaliner 1974). However, the presence of a few mononuclear cells in some tissues was not interpreted as an overt inflammatory reaction, but was more likely to be a cellular response to the degenerative tissue changes associated with the tissue edema. The widespread dilatation of capillary beds in tissue was probably the most significant lesion causing severe circulatory impairment by pooling of a large volume of blood in microvasculature. Calves infected with *T. congolense* had generalized microvascular dilatation which was most prominent in the liver and mesentery. There was an increase in the cellularity in the lung, with alveolar thickening and accumulation of hemosiderin containing cells. Accumulation of lymphocytes were found at the corticomedullary junction of the kidneys with well-developed membranoproliferative glomerulonephritis. Reticuloendothelial changes consisted of marrow hyperplasia with an erythroid shift, moderate hemosiderosis, and moderate dysthrombopoiesis, while in other lymphoid organs there was marked thymic (cortical) atrophy, hypersplenism, and enlarged nodes with reduced cellular density, paracortical atrophy, and medullary sclerosis (Valli and Forsberg 1979). *Trypanosoma congolense* infection in goats also caused degeneration of the testes (Kaaya and Oduor-Okela 1980).

How the trypanosomes attached to the endothelial cell caused structural and functional alteration has not been determined, but the release of biologically active substances from disintegrating intravascular trypanosomes, which were inflammatory and activate complement-releasing pharmacologically active agents, could play a role in the increased vascular permeability (Nielsen *et al.* 1978a, b, c, d, 1979; Tizard and Holmes 1976, 1977). The activation of complement was also proposed as a mechanism responsible for a disruption of lymphoid tissue (Nielsen *et al.* 1979). The variable lesions, including atrophy and hyperplasia of lymphoid tissue cells, were associated with the different stages of infection (Morrison and Murray 1979a). Observations on lesions in lymphoid tissue in rats corroborated observations in cattle, showing obvious differences in the responses between *T. congolense* and *T. brucei* infections (Brown and Losos 1977).

There are two recent reports of diseases caused by *T. simiae* in pigs. Large numbers of trypanosomes in small blood vessels were associated with thrombosis and ischemic tissue necrosis (van Dijk *et al.* 1973; Isoun 1968).

Pathogenesis of diseases caused by *Duttonella*

Primary lesions caused by *T. vivax* occur in the blood, blood vessels, lymphoid system, and, to a limited degree, in some of the solid tissue, particularly the heart. With the first wave of parasitemia the PCV, WBC, and thrombocytes decrease in levels. The PCV may continue to drop gradually until the death of the animal or level off with the development of a chronic syndrome. There is also an initial drop in WBC counts which may return to normal levels early in the infection. The number of thrombocytes decline rapidly and progressively in the acute syndromes.

Secondary lesions are observed in tissues and organs as a result of anemia and intravascular thrombosis. In the acute syndrome of cattle, sheep, and goats, extensive subcutaneous mucosal and serosal hemorrhages characterize the disease. The lesions are associated with obvious disturbances of the blood-clotting mechanisms as exemplified by the hemorrhagic diathesis and bleeding tendency following any cutaneous injury such as caused by needle puncture or biting flies. In the chronic syndrome, the hemorrhages are much less obvious and the postmortem findings are of a chronic wasting disease, with cachexia and subcutaneous edema not accompanied by any pathognomonic lesions. There is experimental evidence that intermittent intravascular coagulation occurs throughout the course of infection and is associated with the peaks of parasitemia. In acute and chronic syndromes, there may be an increase in pericardial fluid with fibrinous or fibrous tags on the serosal surface. The liver, kidneys, spleen and lymph nodes are enlarged. The splenic red pulp is usually friable and the white pulp is prominent.

Microscopic lesions in acute syndromes have, as a main feature, large numbers of trypanosomes in large blood vessels associated with fibrinous thrombi, occasionally undergoing organization. Ischemic necrosis due to infarction is most often observed in the lung and spleen. The pericarditis is characterized by an extensive mononuclear cell infiltration of the epicardium, and to a lesser degree the myocardium, and is associated with extravascular infiltration of trypanosomes. The lymphoid tissues of lymph nodes and spleen are hyperplastic with phagocytosis of trypanosomiasis by macrophages.

Literature

The pathogenesis, involving anemia, disseminated intravascular coagulation, and to some degree, inflammation of solid tissues associated with extravascular localization of trypanosomes, has been studied in cattle, sheep, and goats. The behavior and the pathogenesis of three mouse-infective *T. vivax* strains isolated in West Africa were reviewed (Zwart 1979) and the transmission and maintenance of two stocks of *T. vivax* by tsetse fly and by syringe passage were studied in cattle, goats, rabbits, rats, and mice (Moloo 1982). During the initial stages of infection with *T. vivax* in cattle trypanosomes were detected in lymph nodes. Lymph nodes and spleen showed proliferative response between days 10 and 17 of infection, characterized by an increase in size of germinal centers and proliferating lymphocytes in the medullary cords, in the paracortex of lymph nodes and in the white pulp of the spleen which was accompanied by an increase in the plasma cells. During the remainder of infection there was a gradual reduction in the activity of the lymphoid organs. It was concluded that an intact, orderly immune response occurred to the infection and questioned the relative importance of immunodepression in bovine trypanosomiasis (Masake and Morrison 1981). The subsequent anemia was hemolytic with extensive hemosiderosis in various tissues (Maxie *et al.* 1976, 1979; van den Ingh *et al.* 1976a, b; Veenendaal *et al.* 1976). Splenectomy reduced the incubation period of *T. vivax* in sheep but did not affect the duration and mortality observed in the disease. The anemia was hemolytic with the spleen as the major site of the red blood cell destruction in the mild forms of anemia, and the liver as the major site in severely anemic animals. Bone marrow erythroid hyperplasia was observed early in the infection but became normal in the later stages (Anosa and Isoun 1980a). *Trypanosoma vivax* infection of sheep and goats caused increased blood and plasma volumes, decreased red blood cell volume, increased serum proteins and gamma globulins, and decreased serum albumin, indicating anemia attributable partly to hemadilution and decreased volume of red blood cells (Anosa and Isoun 1976). Free plasma amino acid profiles in *T. vivax*-infected sheep was studied (Isoun *et al.* 1978). In cattle, the total serum proteins decrease (Tabel and Losos 1980).

Whether hemodilution plays a significant role in the pathogenesis of the anemia has not been clearly established, but plasma volume changes have been reported (Clarkson *et al.* 1975; Anosa and Isoun 1976). The acute syndrome, with extensive hemorrhages and thrombosis, has been produced experimentally in cattle, sheep, and goats with both the West and East African strains of *T. vivax* (Boyt and MacKenzie 1970; van den Ingh *et al.* 1976a, b). The organs affected were kidneys, lungs, liver, lymph nodes, and adrenal glands (Masake 1980). The thrombosis causing tissue infarction was observed to occur early and late in a relatively mild form of the disease and was associated with peaks of parasitemia. Thrombosis was also shown to occur in rats infected with a rodent-adapted strain of *T. vivax* (Isoun 1975).

In addition to the infarction observed in the acute forms of the disease, a pericarditis and a myocarditis, associated with the invasion of trypanosomes of solid tissues, was reported. This particular lesion resembled the inflammatory reaction seen in *T. brucei* infections (van den Ingh and deNeijs-Bakker 1979). Infection in goats and cattle caused marked lymph node enlargement associated with an increase in number and size of the lymphatic follicles accompanied by germinal center formation. Lesions were also observed in the heart, with myocardial fiber degeneration and occasional necrosis, and mononuclear cell infiltration accompanied by extravascular trypanosomes. Inflammatory lesions were also observed in the testes and pituitary (Masake 1980). These observations changed the conclusion reached earlier that *T. vivax* was a strict plasma parasite (Losos and Ikede 1972) and confirmed those of Hornby (1952) that *T. vivax* does in fact invade solid tissue. However, the question still remained of the importance of this lesion in the pathogenesis. Based on the fact that only pericarditis has been reported and other sites did not appear to be common, the tissue distribution was not as extensive as seen in *T. brucei* infections. The effect of *T. vivax* on the male genital organs and the invasion of the fetus by trypanosomes have been considered as indicating reproductive disturbances in this form of trypanosomiasis (Isoun and Anosa 1974; Ikede and Losos 1972d). Testicular degeneration in *T. vivax* infection of sheep and goats was associated with pyrexia with fibrin thrombi in testicular vessels also a possible secondary mechanism which occasionally resulted in infarction (Anosa and Isoun 1980b).

The mechanism of injury in *T. vivax* infections has been related to the release of pharmacologically active substances such as serotonin and kinins by immunological responses, high parasitemia, and thrombocytopenia; their actions on the circulatory and gastrointestinal systems have been proposed (Veenendaal *et al.* 1976). The recent adaptation of a West African strain of *T. vivax* to the rodent has enabled the development of a model which could be used for more extensive studies of the pathogenesis of diseases caused by *T. vivax*. The isolation and propagation of this strain in rats and the pathogenesis of *T. vivax* in cattle and goats, have been recently reviewed (Zwart 1979).

Pathogenesis of diseases caused by *Trypanozoon*

There is considerable similarity between the lesions and the pathogenesis of the diseases caused by *T. brucei*, *T. evansi*, and *T. equiperdum* affecting animals, and *T. rhodesiense* and *T. gambiense* causing disease in man. The characteristic lesion is an extensive inflammation of the primary tissues affected, which are the connective tissues of the stroma of various tissues and organs, the blood, and the lymphoid system. The dominant lesions are found in the solid tissues and the draining lymph nodes, while in many of the syndromes changes in the blood appear to be of secondary importance. Varying degrees of anemia occur in all syndromes and are accompanied by either leukopenia or leukocytosis and thrombocytopenia. In the acute syndromes, which are common in natural infections of dogs and horses, large populations of trypanosomes localize in the connective tissues accompanied by extensive mononuclear cell infiltration and exudation of inflammatory fluid containing these cells into the body cavities, especially the pericardium. The widespread distribution of trypanosomes in tissue causes a variety of lesions in the acute syndrome, including subcutaneous edema of the head, limbs, and genitalia, urticarial plaques, keratitis, and ophthalmitis, extensive enlargement of lymph nodes and spleen, and accumulation of turbid inflammatory exudates in the pericardium, pleural, and abdominal cavities.

This is accompanied by rapid loss of weight and varying degrees of anemia. Some of the lesions observed in the acute syndrome, e.g. the urticarial plaques and ophthalmitis, are transitory and may be recurrent. The lymph nodes and spleen are enlarged and there is usually evidence of pericarditis with the presence of fibrinous or fibrous tags. In the chronic syndromes the tissue inflammation is less severe, but there is more extensive emaciation and often cachexia. In some of the mild chronic forms, lesions may not be detectable on gross postmortem examinations.

Microscopically, the inflammatory exudate consists of lymphocytes, macrophage, and plasma cells associated with the presence of trypanosomes in the tissues. Tissue tropism is observed with *T. equiperdum* which localizes in the genitalia. Whether different tissue tropism occurs with the other species and strains has not been demonstrated.

It appears rather that widespread localization occurs with most strains and that invasion of some tissues, such as the brain, occurs in the late stages of the infections.

Based on this mononuclear inflammation, delayed hypersensitivity reaction is an obvious possible mechanism of injury. However, degenerating trypanosomes also release components which cause tissue inflammation directly. Other immunologically mediated cytotoxic reactions associated with antigen–antibody complexes have been incriminated in the destruction of erythrocytes and thrombocytes, disturbances in the coagulation mechanism, and development of proliferative glomerulonephritis. The release of pharmacologically active substances, particularly kinins, during infection have also been considered to play a role in the pathogenesis. The decrease in the tissue metabolism, as seen with the reduction of the tissue trytophan level in the brain due to its utilization by trypanosomes, has been proposed as the basis for functional disturbances.

Literature

The study of the pathogenesis of the diseases caused by trypanosomes in the subgenus *Trypanozoon* have included investigations of the pathology of acute syndromes in sheep, goats, cattle, and horses, as well as various other aspects of pathogenesis in laboratory animals. The detailed study of the pathology in small ruminants have included descriptions of the lesions in the eyes, heart, reproductive organs, and endocrine system (Ikede 1974, 1979; Ikede and Losos 1972a, 1975b, c; Losos and Ikede 1970). Lesions similar to those observed in sheep and goats have also been observed in acute cases in cattle (Ikede and Losos 1972b). In sheep infected with *T. brucei,* initial lymphoid stimulation was overshadowed by intense proliferation of reticuloendothelial cells which subsequently decreased, and there was a recurrence of proliferation of lymphoid cells resulting in an increase of primary follicles with formation of germinal centers and production of plasma cell precursors. Both reticuloendothelial and lymphoid components exhibited marked cellular necrosis which increased throughout the course of infection (Barrowman and Roos 1979). Infection of dwarf goats with *T. vivax, T. congolense,* and *T. brucei* resulted in diseases which with *T. brucei* infection was characterized by mononuclear cell infiltration in the brain and heart, as well as in other tissues and organs; *T. congolense* and *T. vivax* produced very little histological alteration (Bungener and Mehlitz 1976). Lesions comparable to those seen in ruminants occurred in experimental acute and chronic infections in donkeys and horses (Ikede *et al.* 1977a; McCully and Neitz 1971). A meningoencephalitis caused by *T. evansi* in horses was reported, closely resembling human African trypanosomiasis (Seiler *et al.* 1981).

The central nervous system involvement in dourine was shown to be associated with the ability of *T. equiperdum* to cross the blood–brain barrier (Barrowman 1976a, b). The downer mare syndrome was reported to be associated with dourine of horses (Collins 1980). The involvement of the brain in a natural case of *T. brucei* was observed in a dog (Ikede and Losos 1972c). The disease in dogs caused by *T. brucei* infection was characterized by widespread invasion of trypanosomes in various tissues and organs which was associated with mononuclear cell infiltration, severe cellular degeneration, and focal necrosis, with the most consistent lesions occurring in the heart, eyes, and central nervous system (Morrison *et al.* 1981), while in the lymphoid organs there was, during the initial stages, an extensive generation of large numbers of immunoglobulin-producing cells and, in the latter stages, a marked decrease of cellular reactivity, with disorganization and depletion of the lymphoid system (Morrison and Murray 1979a). The pathogenesis of sleeping sickness in man has been recently reviewed and it has been concluded that the mechanisms have not been clarified (Greenwood and Whittle 1980).

Although *T. brucei* and *T. equiperdum* cause acute syndromes, the most common disease in cattle, buffalo, and camels was the chronic form, which was often asymptomatic (Ikede and Losos 1972c; Verma and Gautam 1977). A chronic syndrome in cattle was described by Moulton and Sollod (1976) and confirmed further the conclusion that *T. brucei* could be pathogenic to cattle. Because these infections were characterized by invasion of tissues by trypanosomes and by either low or absent parasitemia, the detection of trypanosomes was difficult. The localization of trypanosomes in genital and endocrine organs, together with the virtual absence of blood infections, could result in insipid syndromes which would be difficult to diagnose. Infections in rams resulted in a nonsuppurative granulomatous periorchitis associated with extravascular localizations of trypanosomes in areas of inflammation and focal necrosis (Ikede 1979). This situation could be important in cattle because of the high incidence of *T. brucei* infections.

The most extensive studies in the pathogenesis of trypanosomiasis caused by Salivarian species have been in laboratory infection of rats, mice, and rabbits by *brucei*-like organisms pathogenic to man and animals. In mice and rats, the commonest syndrome investigated has been an acute disease characterized by massive parasitemia and death within a few days; it is not the ideal model for animal trypanosomiases which are predominantly chronic diseases. The more chronic syndromes in these two laboratory species were characterized by anemia associated with extensive erythrophagocytosis in the spleen, emaciation, enlargement of spleen and lymph nodes, and an increase in pericardial fluid (Murray *et al.* 1974; Brown and Losos 1977). The lymph nodes were stimulated during the first stages of the disease and later became depleted of various lymphoid cells (Morrison *et al.* 1978). The changes in the spleen in *T. brucei* infections of deer mice were characterized by extensive infiltration of plasma cells (Moulton 1980).

In the acute and most chronic syndromes, central nervous system infections do not occur. However, on occasion *T. brucei*, *T. equiperdum*, and *T. gambiense* have been reported to cause brain lesions in a percentage of infected animals. There was a need to develop a model which consistently produced brain lesions and in this way resembled more closely the natural infections of man and animals. A useful model has been reported to develop in mice with extensive encephalitis and meningitis 6 to 9 weeks after infection with *T. rhodesiense* (Fink and Schmidt 1979). Another model with these attributes was produced in deer mice infected with *T. brucei* and *T. equiperdum* (Moulton *et al.* 1974; Stevens and Moulton 1977a, b). Although brain lesions developed regularly in these infections, there was considerable variation between animals as to the severity, distribution, and type of lesions which occurred. Another useful model has been caused in the rabbit by most of the *brucei*-like species, resulting in a disease characterized by low parasitemia and an exudative dermatitis affecting the face, ears, and scrotum. Many lesions in this species were comparable to those observed in domestic animals and have been described in detail (van den Ingh 1977; van den Ingh and van Dijk 1975; van den Ingh *et al.* 1977). Ocular lesions caused by *T. brucei* in rabbits had numerous trypanosomes in the aqueous and vitreous humor, cornea, sclera, iris, and ciliary processes (Ssenyonga 1980b).

One of the leading articles on the pathogenesis of trypanosomiasis using the rabbit model was published by Goodwin (1970). His observations center around the localization of *T. brucei* in connective tissue, and on the accompanying changes occurring in fibroblasts, collogen, interstitial fluid, and blood vessels which described the cellular injury and inflammatory reaction (Goodwin 1971; Goodwin and Guy 1973; Goodwin *et al.* 1973). One particular observation, which may be important as to why this tissue was preferentially colonized, was the detection of some of the antibodies in these tissue fluids about 5 days after their titers were high in the blood. This delay would enable the trypanosomes to escape temporarily from the serological defenses and, through exponential growth within this period, permit sequented trypanosomes to multiply to large numbers.

Immunologically mediated cellular injury has been incriminated in various forms of trypanosomiasis. A review of the immunology and pathogenesis of trypanosomiasis focused on some of the newer ideas of the role of immunological responses in pathogenesis (Henson and Noel 1979) and was presented as a composite view encompassing the same pathogenesis of all forms of trypanosomes (Urquhart 1980). A symposium on the pathogenesis including human trypanosomiasis was held in 1980. Although many workers have tried to establish the exact mechanisms of pathogenesis, the mechanisms have not yet been defined. A mouse model for chronic trypanosomiasis, in which the immunopathological and chemotherapeutic studies were undertaken with the focus on the two target organs, the heart and the brain, was described by Poltera (1980) and Poltera *et al.* (1980a, b). The isolation and characterization of a strain of *T. rhodesiense* which causes a chronic course of the infection in mice was also reported (Campbell *et al.* 1979). It has been demonstrated that *T. brucei* and *T. rhodesiense* caused a cell-mediated hypersensitivity to live organisms and could be related to the extensive mononuclear cell inflammatory reaction accompanying the invasion of connective tissues by trypanosomes (Tizard and Soltys 1971). Another immunologically induced lesion was the deposition of antigen–antibody complexes in the glomeruli, described in *T. equiperdum* infection of deer mice (Moulton *et al.* 1974), in *T. brucei* in rabbits (Facer *et al.* 1978) and in *T. rhodesiense* in monkeys and rats (Lindsley *et al.* 1978; Nagle *et al.* 1974).

Variable severity of glomerulonephritis was observed in rats infected with different strains of *T. rhodesiense*, secondary to the presence of immune complexes, as indicated by granular immune deposits in the glomeruli (Lindsley *et al.* 1980). Deposits of IgG, IgM, and C3 were found in renal glomeruli associated with hypercellularity and proteinuria, as evidenced by an increase in tubular hyaline droplets (Nagle *et al.* 1980). Extensive granular deposits of C3, IgG1, and IgG3, together with small quantities of IgG2a, IgG2b, and IgM, but with no evidence of trypanosomal antigen, were detected in deposits on the glomeruli of mice with chronic *T. gambiense* infections (van Marck *et al.* 1981). In *T. brucei*-infected mice, small amounts of trypanosomal antigen were found in animals which were vaccinated with purified variable antigen (van Marck and Vervoort 1980). The occurrence of immune complexes in cerebrospinal fluid in African trypanosomiasis in man is an indicator of continued central nervous system disease and may be useful in monitoring patient care (Lambert *et al.* 1981). The importance of this renal lesion in the pathogenesis was not clear in view of the often widespread severe inflammation occurring in other tissues. Autoantibodies to kidneys, liver, brain, and heart have also been observed in rabbits infected with what was thought to be *T. congolense*, but the description of the lesions indicated a *brucei*-like organism (Mansfield and Kreier 1972). Antibodies to liver, Wasserman antigens, and components of the fibrin–fibrinogen system have also been reported (MacKenzie and Boreham 1974; Boreham and Facer 1974b). What role these antibodies against tissues play in the pathogenesis has not been determined.

A number of mechanisms have been proposed as causing the anemia. The anemia was observed to be more severe in the Zebu breed than in the N'Dama, and due to the increased rate of red blood cell destruction, but with no hemodilution occurring, this greater resistance of N'Dama to *T. brucei* was not attributed to a more efficient erythropoiesis response (Dargie *et al.* 1979b). Anemia caused by *T. brucei* in rats and mice was macrocytic with normoblastic hyperplasia of bone marrow and spleen; the circulating half-life of red blood cells was reduced. These changes together with hemosiderosis and marked splenic erythrophagocytosis indicate a hemolytic anemia (Jennings *et al.* 1974). The parasitemia, plasma volumes, leukocyte, and bone marrow cell counts were investigated in *T. brucei* infection in splenectomized and intact mice (Anosa 1980). Hemolysis was associated with the presence of trypanosome antigens and antibodies combined with complement on erythrocytes (Woo and Kobayashi 1975). However, antibodies on red blood cells were only rarely demonstrated during the late stages of infections in mice (Ikede *et al.* 1977b). Hemolytic factors have been found in *T. brucei* autolysate (Tizard *et al.* 1978c), and associated with the protein component of the trypanosome suspension (Huan *et al.* 1975). Splenomegaly, a constant feature of most trypanosomiases, might also contribute to the anemia by nonspecific increase of erythrocyte destruction, although splenectomy did not alleviate the anemia which indicated that erythrocytes were being destroyed in other tissues (Anosa *et al.* 1977). The anemia and the role of the spleen in its pathogenesis was investigated in rabbits infected with *T. brucei,* with splenectomy delaying the onset of anemia and lessening its severity (Jenkins *et al.* 1980; McCrorie *et al.* 1980).

Disturbances in the blood coagulation mechanisms have been studied in the pathogenesis. It has been proposed that the thrombocytopenia observed in infections was due to immune complexes by trypanosome antigens and antibodies and was not associated with a consumptive coagulopathy as proposed by some (Robins-Browne *et al.* 1975). Platelet injury also occurred without involvement of an immunological response and was caused by whole trypanosomes and their soluble extracts (Davis *et al.* 1974). Rats infected with *T. brucei* developed anemia, thrombocytopenia, and hypocomplementemia associated with elevated titers of cold-active hemagglutinin, antibody to fibrinogen–fibrin related products, and immunoconglutinin. It was proposed that microthrombosis resulted in immunologic interactions of complex-coated blood cells with immunoconglutinin (Rickman and Cox 1980; Rickman *et al.* 1981b). Other studies on the blood coagulation system in rabbits infected with *T. brucei* have shown an increase in fibrinogen and fibrinogen–fibrin degradation products considered to result from an increased fibrinolytic activity associated with the formation of microthrombi in the circulation (Boreham and Facer 1974a). These degradation products were found in the urine, suggesting either an increased permeability of glomeruli or local fibrinogenolysis in kidney tubules (Boreham and Facer 1977). Fibrinogen and nacroglobulins in plasma were thought to cause erythrocyte aggregation, sludging, and microthrombi (Facer 1976). Associated with the extensive inflammatory reaction in tissues has been the release of pharmacologically active substances, such as the kallikreins found in plasma and urine and thought to result from immune complexes activating the kallikrein–kinin system by the Hageman factor, which in turn was involved in the coagulation, fibrinolysis, and complement systems (Boreham 1977, 1979; Wright and Boreham 1977). The increased viscosity and hypertension associated with the plasma kinins was considered to cause local and general circulatory malfunction (Boreham and Wright 1976). Changes in the vascular smooth muscle contractility were also observed with *T. brucei* infections in rats (Greer *et al.* 1979).

Another approach to the study of pathogenesis has been by determining changes in the metabolism of tissues in the host infected with trypanosomes. An increase in oxygen metabolism occurred in the liver, heart, and brain slices from *T. rhodesiense*-infected rodents (Lincicombe and Bruce 1965; Lee and Aboko-Cole 1972; Lee *et al.* 1972). Also, malfunction of the liver, as determined by biochemical and ultrastructural abnormalities, which included glycogen deposition and alteration in the enzyme functions, was related to the terminal hypoglycemia observed in rodent trypanosomiasis (Marciacq and Seed 1970; Lumsden *et al.* 1972; Ashman and Seed 1973). Hypertriglyceridemia was observed in rabbits infected with *T. brucei* and resulted from a defect in the triglyceride degradation (Rouzer and Cerami 1980). Mice infected with *T. brucei* had reduced hepatic mixed function oxidase activity, which could also be decreased by the use of Suramin and Melarsoprol B which indicated that in trypanosomiasis its chemotherapy significantly impaired the capacity of the liver to metabolize foreign compounds (Shertzer *et al.* 1981). A decrease in tryptophan levels and accumulation metabolites produced by trypanosomes in tissues has been associated with alteration of brain function (Stibbs and Seed 1975a, b, c; Newport *et al.* 1977). Serum lipid and cholesterol values increased three- to fourfold towards the terminal stages of *T. gambiense* infection in rabbits. Electrophoresis of serum lipids showed increased beta- and pre-beta-lipoprotein and the appearance of a chylomicron band, while serum protein bound iodine values were decreased (Diehl and Risby 1974). Phospholipase A_1 was also found in tissue fluid in *T. brucei*-infected rabbits at higher levels than observed in the blood and was thought to be of trypanosomal origin (Hambrey *et al.* 1980).

Pathogenesis of diseases caused by *Schizotrypanum*

Trypanosoma cruzi causes an acute syndrome in young dogs comparable in various features of its pathogenesis to the acute syndrome in man. Chronic natural disease has not been described although it is likely to occur, but may be difficult to diagnose. In the acute syndrome, high levels of tissue infections are observed and cardiac lesions are the most important finding. The heart is dilated, particularly the right atrium and ventricle, and discolored by yellow, gray, or white areas under the epicardium and endocardium, which at times affect the entire thickness of the heart wall. Accompanying these mycordial lesions there is pulmonary edema, enlargement and congestion of the liver, and enlargement of the spleen and lymph nodes. On microscopic examination the myocardial lesion is characterized by a granulomatous myocarditis with varying degrees of myocardial fiber degeneration, necrosis, and fibrosis. The severity of the lesions is associated with the numbers of trypanosomes in the tissue. Occasionally, large numbers of amastigotes are found extracellularly and are accompanied by an acute, purulent, necrotizing local lesion. The granulomatous lesions are found in other organs, such as the gastrointestinal tract and brain, where the amastigote forms are found in the macrophages.

The main mechanism of tissue injury is currently thought to be mediated by immunological responses. In the past, toxins were considered to be involved, but this was not verified. Although intracellular pseudocysts cause structural changes in the cell organelles which may reflect functional disturbances, it is the extracellular trypanosomes in the interstitial tissue which stimulate the inflammatory reaction. These trypanosomes cause a delayed hypersensitivity reaction which may be involved in destroying intact and parasitized connective tissue and myocardial cells. Antibodies to plasma membrane of muscle and endothelial cells have also been incriminated as another form of immunologic injury.

Literature

The pathogenesis of Chagas' disease in man and experimental animals has been reviewed by Koberle (1968, 1974) and Tafuri (1979) who described the lesions in acute and chronic syndromes. The occurrence of natural acute syndromes in dogs in the USA, including description of clinical signs, pathology, and pathogenesis, has been reported by Tippit (1978) and Williams and colleagues (1977). Naturally occurring *T. cruzi* infection in a dog associated with myocarditis was reported in Louisiana (Snider *et al.* 1980). Nine dogs experimentally infected with *T. cruzi* developed an acute disease within 15 to 25 days, followed by a chronic asymptomatic period that varied from 8 months to 3 years. The electrocardiogram (ECG) changes were minimal, but the animals showed a mild focal chronic myocarditis with a few microscopic foci of fibrosis. In the atrioventricular node, focal or diffuse fibrosis, scleroatrophy, and fatty replacement were present in various parts of the conducting system. Comparable lesions in the conducting system may be responsible for ECG changes in human patients who were otherwise asymptomatic (Andrade *et al.* 1981). Infected striped skunks (*Mephitis mephitis*) caused moderately severe chronic granulomatous myocarditis with typical amastigotes in the myocardial fibers (Davis *et al.* 1980).

Surprisingly, there appear to be no other descriptions in either recent or older literature of natural diseases in dogs and cats in enzootic areas of South and Central America. Dogs have been used in experimental studies of Chagas' disease and their susceptibility to various strains of *T. cruzi*, immunology, and pathology, including citation of older literature, have been presented by Goble (1952, 1970). Experimental infection with culture forms of *T. cruzi* of farm animals, pigs, lambs, goats, and calves, with a North American strain of *T. cruzi* isolated from a raccoon was reported (Diamond and Rubin 1958). The available published information on *T. cruzi* infection in farm animals is fragmentary and the author reviews the older literature on the subject on the attempts at experimental infections in pigs, lambs, and goats. The results were not consistent; pigs were found to be parasitemic up to day 57 of infection and, in one, animal tissue forms were observed on day 27. Lambs and kids infected showed positive parasitemia by culture method on days 85 and 38 respectively. One calf was found to be parasitemic up to day 21 after infection. Out of the total of 20 animals used in these experiments, only in 2 were tissue forms observed. All infections were not accompanied by clinical signs and there was an absence of pathological alterations at low levels of parasitemia. The conclusion was reached that farm animals in contact with reduviid vectors could become infective with *T. cruzi* (Diamond and Rubin 1958).

Most studies of the mechanisms of tissue injury, as observed in the development of lesions and tissue tropisms in the acute and chronic syndromes in man, have been made in laboratory animals. Tafuri (1979) reviewed the role played by the characteristics of the parasites, such as polymorphism of the blood forms in their infectivity and virulence, the tissue tropism of various strains, the penetration of the cells by different forms, and the rate of degeneration of tissue forms resulting in the release of antigens and as inflammatory mediators. The host-dependent factors, such as sex, age, genetic constitution, and species are also known to affect the susceptibility to infections and their outcome.

The first step in the pathogenic process was the attraction of the trypanosome to a certain cell type and was thought to be due to something present in target cells or organs which made them physiologically attractive and stimulated growth (Dvorak and Howe 1976; Shoemaker and Hoffman 1974). The actual invasion of the cells involves both the active penetration of the trypanosome and the phagocytic capabilities of the different host cells (Alexander 1975; Kipnis *et al.* 1979). The alteration of the surface composition, either the glycoprotein or the plasma membrane of host cells, inhibits their infection by *T. cruzi*, suggesting that membranes of these cells do not play a merely passive role in the infection of cells (Henriquez *et al.* 1981). Once in the cell, a life cycle occurred involving morphological changes and multiplication with the final formation of a pseudocyst. The interaction of *T. cruzi* with lysosomes in macrophages was followed 24 hours later by multiplication in the cytoplasm, not the vacuoles but free in the cytoplasm (Milder and Kloetzel 1980). Overt cellular injury has not been associated with the process of penetration of cells and the growth of pseudocysts and the extrusion of the various stages of trypanosomes into the interstitial tissue. This resulted in the extensive granulomous inflammatory reaction and the occasional purulent focus associated with cellular necrosis. The macrophages in the inflammatory exudate destroy the ingested trypanosomes (Scorza and Scorza 1972). The fate of trypanosomes phagocytosed by macrophages depended on whether they had been activated and on the life-cycle stage of trypanosomes which had been phagocytosed. Macrophages activated by either previous exposure to trypanosome antigens or nonspecifically, destroyed the trypanosomes in phagocytic vacuoles, while normal macrophages could permit their multiplication

(Kress *et al.* 1975, 1977). Animals in which macrophages had been activated were more resistant to challenge by *T. cruzi*, while blockage of the reticuloendothelial system decreased resistance (Kierszenbaum 1979). The induced delayed hypersensitivity reaction by trypanosomes has been proposed as a method by which host cells are injured. Sensitized lymphocytes destroyed *in vitro* parasitized fibroblasts and myocardial cells, and nonparasitized myocardial cells (Kuhn and Murnane 1977; Santos-Buch and Teixeira 1974; Teixeira and Santos-Buch 1975). Delayed hypersensitivity to heart antigens was also observed in man infected with *T. cruzi* both with and without evidence of cardiomyopathy (Mosca and Plaja 1981). Another immunologically mediated injurious mechanism was related to the presence of antibodies against plasma membranes of muscle and endothelial cells and considered to cause morphological changes in these cells not associated with the interstitial inflammatory exudate (Cossio *et al.* 1974; Laguens *et al.* 1975). The subject of immunologically mediated cellular injury has been reviewed by Teixeira (1976).

IMMUNOLOGY

In practical terms, immunologic responses of domestic animals to pathogenic trypanosomes are important in the diagnosis, resistance to infections and diseases, susceptibility to secondary infections by other microorganisms, and development of lesions. The host's immunologic responses, both qualitative and quantitative, are dependent to a degree on the species of trypanosomes causing infection and on the species of host. This variability is further affected by the severity of the syndromes produced and the complexity of some of the diseases caused by multiple infections of the tsetse-transmitted species. There is not sufficient published information to describe accurately the responses in each of the various diseases and syndromes. Only a general discussion is possible of the basic interactions between the host and parasite affecting the immunological responses. Much of the available information is based on infections in man and laboratory animals, particularly on those types of trypanosomes easily handled in the laboratory. Only limited studies have been made in domestic animals.

The immunologic responses in trypanosomiasis depend on their complex antigenic composition. The antigens are divided into two types; one type is known as homogenate internal or common antigens and is derived from the disintegrated whole organism, while the other is called released, surface, or variant antigens found on the surface of trypanosomes. The common antigens originate from various components of the disrupted nucleus and cytoplasm and are not protective but responsible for the serological cross-reactions between species. The variant antigens, because of their heterogenicity in infecting populations of trypanosomes are enabled to survive and multiply in spite of the protective antibodies they stimulate. At any time during infection, one or more variant antigens making up the major part of the population determine the specific antibody response. The subsequent elimination of these dominant antigenic types of trypanosomes is followed by the growth of others against which antibodies had not been produced during the previous period of infection. This change of dominant antigenic types occurs every 2 to 4 days and many, probably an indefinable number, of different types develop. However, there is some organization which tends to limit diversity. Infections caused by one strain tend to be characterized by a few dominant antigenic variants which usually occur in the same sequence in different animals. A further restriction to antigenic variability is imposed by passage through tsetse flies in which the dominant antigen occurring in the course of infection by a strain revert to common basic antigenic types seen in metacyclics.

In the next section, resistance to infection and development of disease and susceptibility to secondary infection of animals with trypanosomiasis are described. The serological diagnosis and the role of immunologically mediated tissue injury have been presented in the section on diagnosis and pathogenesis. Resistance to trypanosomiasis involves insusceptibility to infection and ability to withstand infection without development of overt clinical disease. The defense mechanisms against trypanosome infections are either innate or acquired. Innate resistance is best shown as it occurs in absolute terms in those host species which totally repel infections to some subgenera of trypanosomes without prior exposure. It is independent of the challenging dose of organisms of the breed of a particular species of host, e.g. resistance of dogs to *T. vivax* infections. Partial innate resistance undoubtedly also exists and probably plays a role in the interspecies variation in susceptibilities observed in various species of domestic animals. Innate defence mechanisms are difficult to identify. In some cases they are known to be associated with certain natural antibodies, but in others they are probably related to a combination of physiological factors in the constitution of the resistant host. Acquired resistance, on the other hand, results from prior contact between trypanosomes and the host, and involves protective immunologic responses. This acquired insusceptibility is at best partial, usually limited to challenge by the specific variant antigenic types which had initiated the original immunologic response. The ability of a host to tolerate infections without developing disease also depends on the pathogenicity of the invading trypanosomes, as well as the defence mechanism of the host. It appears that suppressing the trypanosome population to low levels results in reduction of the severity of the syndromes. This resistance to disease is dependent on both the innate resistance of the individual animal and species and may be related to the efficiency of the defence mechanism, particularly the immunologic protective responses which come into play during infection.

Variability in the susceptibility occurs at three levels, being most obvious between species, less pronounced between breeds, and least discernible between individuals within a breed. Because acquired, this resistance is variable and partial; it is difficult to assess, requiring quantitative evaluation of the host responses to infection. In most cases the infected host is in a precarious balance which may be readily upset, resulting in overt clinical signs by unfavorable conditions, such as poor husbandry practices, concurrent infections, and severity of trypanosomal challenge.

Partial resistance to the development of disease by natural challenge, trypanotolerance, occurs in a number of breeds of cattle commonly referred to as the dwarf and shorthorn breeds, indigenous to tsetse-fly-infested areas of West and Central Africa. In comparison to other breeds, such as the Zebu and imported varieties, these indigenous trypanotolerant breeds show a remarkable ability to withstand challenge by pathogenic trypanosomes. The responses are often mild or asymptomatic, permitting relatively normal productivity in spite of the infection. This inherent ability is dependent on continuous exposure to a challenge limited by the confines of a permanent habitat of these cattle and is overcome by a challenge outside this habitat and adverse conditions, such as husbandry, affecting the host. Certain breeds of sheep also show trypanotolerance. These breeds of cattle and sheep are potentially useful in limiting losses from trypanosomiasis, but because trypanotolerance is partial and may break down, it necessitates close monitoring of the health of the animals under challenge.

Increased resistance to trypanosomiasis, both to the incidence of infection and severity of syndromes, appears to occur in cattle following one or more prophylactic or therapeutic treatments with trypanocides. It is thought to result from the stimulation of defense mechanisms, probably immunologic, which become more efficient following repeated challenge and treatment. Calves appear to be more tolerant than adult cattle and this may also be related to the responsiveness of the immune system. The full exploitation of the infection and treatment method in a field situation has to be accompanied by the judicious use of various trypanocides to prevent the development of resistant strains. The successful use of trypanotolerant cattle and of the infection and treatment method in increasing the resistance to trypanosomiasis hinges on the constant close veterinary supervision of the animals under challenge.

An opposite effect to the stimulation of immunity following infection and treatment is the increased susceptibility to secondary infections by other microorganisms observed in infected untreated animals. The underlying mechanism is thought to be immunosuppression, probably involving unresponsiveness of lymphoid tissue caused by suppressive and deleting mechanisms. This immunosuppression also affects the responsiveness to bacterial and viral vaccines, but is rapidly alleviated following treatment with trypanocides.

Literature

A general introductory review on the immunologic responses in infection and resistance in animals was published by Weitz (1970) and a useful summary, emphasizing immunology of trypanosomiasis of veterinary importance, was presented by Clarkson (1976b). Much of the information available, and particularly those studies which provided the basic concepts of immunology in trypanosomiases, has come from work on *T. brucei* and other species in the subgenus *Trypanozoon* because they are readily maintained and easily handled in the laboratory. Much of this information appears to be applicable to the complex situations in the field. A great deal of attention has been given to the antigens, especially the variant antigens, because of their fundamental role in the ability of the trypanosomes to persist in the host in spite of the immunologic defense mechanisms, and they have been the subject of a number of general comprehensive reviews (Doyle 1977; Gray and Luckins 1976; Seed 1974; Vickerman 1974, 1978), including the chemical composition of the variant antigens (Cross 1978). The relation of antigenic variation to pathogenicity was also discussed in papers in a symposium (Losos and Chouinard 1979).

The Salivarian trypanosomes have a unique capacity for antigenic variation at the cell surface and serve as mechanisms for evasion of the host's response. The chemical and immunological characterization and uniqueness of soluble surface coat glycoprotein from *T. rhodesiense* identified them as variant specific surface coat antigens responsible for antigenic variability (Olenick 1981). The variation is mediated through expression of an extensive repertoire of variant surface glycoproteins, and different amino acid sequences are responsible for the antigenic diversity. All variants of *T. brucei* contained an immunologically cross-reacting glycosyl side chain at the C-terminus (Cross *et al.* 1980). Two conformationally distinct regions were obtained by cryptic cleavage of variant surface glycoproteins of *T. brucei*, the N-terminal fragment and C-terminal fragments; the distinction between them may be significant in relation to their organization and function (Johnson and Cross 1979). The N-terminal half of the protein makes up the outer layer of the surface coat, whereas the C-terminal is associated with the cell membrane and carries a carbohydrate side chain. One trypanosome clone can make up at least 100 different variant surface glycoproteins (Borst *et al.* 1981). The amino acid sequence of the variant surface glycoprotein of *T. brucei* showed extensive variation between the N-terminal amino acid sequences and the common antigenic determinant in the C-terminal portion (Matthyssens *et al.* 1981). Variant specific glycoproteins of *T. equiperdum* were also shown to have cross-reacting determinants located in the C-terminal part of the molecule (Labastie *et al.* 1981). Oligosaccharide residues have importance in the antigenic structure of variable surface glycoproteins containing cross-reacting antigenic determinants (Barbet *et al.* 1981).

The redistribution of surface variable antigen and its movement to the flagellar pocket region which occurred on application of homologous antiserum in indirect immunofluorescence tests was unlikely to be relevant to antigenic variation *in vivo* (Barry 1979). An optimal scheme was developed which separated mechanically more than

90% of the coat protein from *T. congolense* (Reinwald *et al.* 1979). The purification and partial chemical characterization of early bloodstream variants of T. congolense were investigated (Onodera *et al.* 1981; Rosen *et al.* 1981). Variant specific antigen was detected in the plasma of rats and mice infected with *T. brucei* and its quantity correlated with the numbers of parasites in the blood. No parasite antigen other than the variant specific antigen were detected in the plasma of the infected host (Diffley *et al.* 1980). Radioimmunoassay of variant surface glycoproteins of *T. brucei* grown in rats and in culture had amounts of glycoproteins which were similar (McGuire *et al.* 1980). Immunoelectrophoretic study was undertaken on antigens of *T. evansi* (Purohit and Jatkar 1979).

Monoclonal antibodies were used immunochemically to characterize variant specific surface coat glycoprotein from *T. rhodesiense* (Lyon *et al.* 1981). Monoclonal antibodies are ideal probes for studying the localization of antigenic sites on antigen molecules and for studying antigen synthesis, glycocylation, and architecture in relation to the cell surface. Two-dimensional gel maps show that only major differences in the protein profiles of the nonnuclear materials from different clones of trypanosomes were attributable to the variable surface antigens (Pearson *et al.* 1981). Studies of the relationship of glycoprotein structure to antigenic specificity, the genetic basis for antigenic diversity, the control of the expression of alternative antigens, and the role of immune responses in the instigation of variation will be undertaken in the future using recombinant DNA techniques and the *in vitro* cultivation of both metacyclic and bloodstream forms (Cross 1979).

Borst and co-workers stated that the DNA recombinant methods involved isolation of recombinant plasmids containing DNA complementary to the messenger RNAs (mRNAs). Four different variant surface glycoproteins of *T. brucei* had no homology of the mRNAs detectable by hybridization and the expression of variant surface glycoprotein genes was not controlled at the translation level. The variant specific glycoprotein genes have evolved by gene duplication and/or divergence. The process of gene duplication and deletion leads to continuing further evolution of the variant surface glycoprotein repertoire at constant genome size. It was concluded that the whole repertoire of variant surface glycoprotein genes was present in each variant, but the activation of a gene leads to the appearance of an additional copy of that gene and the simplest explanation was that the variant surface glycoprotein gene activation was accompanied by duplication of this gene and its transposition to the expression site (Borst *et al.* 1980a, b, 1981). The genetic basis of antigenic variation of *T. brucei* was investigated by analyzing the structure of the genome involved in the gene cooling (Williams *et al.* 1980, 1981). The structural analysis of variant and invariant genes was investigated in *T. brucei.* Regulation of the variant antigen gene expression was at the level of transcription and the variant antigen genomic sequences differed in their arrangement between the variants (Agabian *et al.* 1980). Gene duplication and transpositions linked to genetic variation in *T. brucei* was investigated (Pays *et al.* 1981). The cloning and characterization of

DNA sequences complementary to messenger RNA coating for the synthesis of two surface antigens of *T. brucei* was studied (Pays *et al.* 1980). The immunological purification and partial characterization of variant-specific surface antigen messenger RNA of *T. brucei* was also studied (Lheureux *et al.* 1979). An immunochemical method for purification of mRNA encoding trypanosome variable surface antigens was developed (Shapiro and Young 1981). The mRNA was purified and characterized for a specific surface antigen of *T. gambiense* (Merritt 1980). The nucleotide sequence data in *T. brucei* have also been investigated (Boothroyd *et al.* 1980). The role of polysomes in the synthesis and processing of variant surface antigen has been studied and has been used in recombinant DNA research (Cordingley and Turner 1980a.). The biosynthesis of variant surface glycoprotein of *T. brucei* has been studied (Rovis and Dube 1981). The inhibition of glycosylation of the major variable surface coat glycoprotein was investigated (Strickler and Patton 1980).

The antigenic variation of Salivarian trypanosomes was reviewed by Gray and Luckins (1976) who emphasized the importance of this characteristic in the host–parasite interactions which result in persistence of infection and in the possible development of new methods in its control by vaccination. The basic concepts of behavior of trypanosomes with regard to their antigenic variability and their organization into the dominant and basic types were developed in cattle infected with *T. brucei* (Gray, 1965, 1966). Additional investigations showed stability of the antigenic variants which characterized a strain causing an infection over a period of 5 years in the field (Gray 1970). On the basis of their dominant antigens, strains isolated from within one area were less variable than those obtained from different localities (Paris and Wilson 1976). In cattle infected with *T. brucei*, trypanosomes with antigenic compositions similar to that of the infecting population reappeared 3 weeks after the initial infection (Nantulya *et al.* 1979). In *T. congolense* infections of cattle, dominant antigenic variants also developed according to a set sequence and reverted to a basic type on passage through the tsetse fly (Wilson and Cunningham 1970, 1971, 1972). Metacyclic populations of different antigenic types were obtained from isolates from different areas, and a concurrent infection of tsetse flies with a mixture of different isolates resulted in a population of metacyclic trypanosomes which contained the characteristic variable antigens of each isolate (Nantulya *et al.* 1980). In further surveys of tsetse flies in different areas to establish whether serological classification of strains was possible (Dar *et al.* 1973a, b), large and probably unmanageable numbers of antigenic types of *T. brucei* (Goedbloed *et al.* 1973), *T. congolense* (Wilson *et al.* 1973), and *T. vivax* (Dar *et al.* 1973b) were observed. Cross-reaction occurred between strains from these various areas and there was evidence that the metacyclics in a fly may be made up of more than one antigenic type. Further investigations on the antigenic relationship of four isolates of *T. congolense* from different regions of Africa indicated that at least three different strains were present (Luckins and Gray 1979b).

On the basis of these observations, neither serotyping nor prospects of inducing effective protection by immunization against a limited number of antigens appeared to be practical. The antigenic behavior of *T. vivax* in calves and sheep was similar to that reported for *T. brucei* with new dominant types appearing at 2- to 3-day intervals (Jones and Clarkson 1972, 1974). Absence of a surface coat on the metacyclic *T. vivax* suggested that the mechanism of antigenic variation is different from that observed in metacyclic forms of *T. brucei* and *T. congolense* (Tetley *et al.* 1981). *Trypanosoma vivax* organisms isolated from the blood of cattle do not have bovine serum proteins on their surface (Tabel and Losos 1980). Similar results were observed with *T. vivax* infection in mice (De Gee and Rovis 1981). The sequence of antigenic variants was compared in mice and goats infected with *T. vivax* and significant differences were observed in the antigenic composition, both during the initial and relapse populations, suggesting a selective growth of different variable antigens in different hosts (De Gee *et al.* 1979, 1981).

In laboratory animals, the heterogeneity of antigenic types in a population of trypanosomes causing infection was demonstrated. Transmission through tsetse flies resulted in reversion of different antigenic variants of *T. brucei* in mice to a common antigenic type, but the first parasitemia after transmission was antigenically heterogeneous (Hudson *et al.* 1980). The variable antigen type ingested by the tsetse fly influenced the antigenic composition of the first parasitemia in tsetse-transmitted infection in mice (Hajduk and Vickerman 1981). Further heterogeneity was observed in tissue cultures. Metacyclic trypanosomes in head salivary gland trypanosome cultures initiated with cloned bloodstream forms were also heterogeneous with respect to their variable antigenic type, and early parasitemia in immunosuppressed mice infected and metacyclics produced in culture also resulted in a range of variable antigenic types (Gardiner *et al.* 1980a, b). Antigenic variation was observed to occur in clones of *T. brucei* grown in tissue culture (Doyle *et al.* 1980). Multiple variable antigen types were observed in a metacyclic population of *T. brucei* derived from a clone (Barry *et al.* 1979a, b). The loss of variable antigens occurred *in vitro* with *T. brucei* during transformation of the bloodstream to procyclic forms (Barry and Vickerman 1979). Whether the dominant antigenic variants in a population arise in an ordered sequence or randomly was investigated by the use of a coefficient of concordance applied to data available in the literature, and a definite tendency towards a reproducible order of occurrence of variants and further analysis indicated that random generation and selection by growth rate alone could not produce the degree of variant orderliness. However, larger numbers of animals and direct investigation of variant growth rate and competitive interactions are necessary before the random generation-selection hypothesis can be proven or disproven (Kosinski 1980). In mice infected with *T. brucei* new variant antigenic types different for each parent variant antigenic type were expressed according to a statistically defined order of priority, and some variants were able to change to others only by passing through intermediate types (Miller and Turner 1981).

A review of the immunity to *T. cruzi* was recently published by Brener (1980). The article deals with the antigenic composition of the trypanosomes, natural immunity, humoral and cellular immunity effects of immunosuppressors, immunodepression, evasion of immune responses by *T. cruzi* autoimmune reactions, and vaccination. Hudson (1981) presented a brief review on the immunal biology of *T. cruzi* and the prospects of using monoclonal antibodies by genetic engineering in immunal diagnosis and the production of protecting antigens. A method was described to obtain a glycoprotein fraction containing a surface determinant common to trypomastigotes and amastigotes of different *T. cruzi* strains (Repka *et al.* 1980). A surface glycoprotein was observed in trypomastigotes but not in the metacyclic and epimastigote forms, and was thought to be responsible for the antiphagocytic factor (Noguiera *et al.* 1981). The antigenic composition of *T. cruzi* culture forms was identified to have a specific component characterized by its unique antigenicity and immunogenicity (Afchain *et al.* 1979).

In the serological responses of cattle to various species of trypanosome the levels of various classes of antibodies were reviewed by Tabel (1979). Natural mixed infections with *T. congolense, T. vivax,* and *T. brucei* caused an increase in the IgG (Desowitz 1959; Luckins 1972) and especially in IgM (Bideau *et al.* 1966; Gidel and Leporte 1962; Luckins 1972), with similar observations being made in experimental infection (Luckins and Mehlitz 1976). The serum levels of IgM and IgG to *T. vivax, T. congolense,* and *T. brucei* infection in sheep were determined and a significant rise in levels occurred in all sheep within 2 weeks of infection, with the exception that IgG levels failed to rise in sheep dying of acute *T. congolense* infection (MacKenzie *et al.* 1979). However, other studies on experimental infection with *T. congolense* in cattle reported levels of IgG_1, IgG_2, and IgM to be either elevated, normal, or depressed, depending on the duration of infection (Kobayashi and Tizard 1976; Luckins 1976; Nielsen *et al.* 1978 a, b, c, d). Antibody titers were slightly lower in primary and secondary responses of cattle infected with *T. congolense* and inoculated with antigens, and required more time to reach the peak titers (Sollod and Frank 1979). Similar variability in the IgG_1 and IgG_2 levels, but relatively constant levels of IgM, were observed in *T. vivax* infection (Clarkson 1976c; Luckins 1976). It was reported that infections of calves by *T. vivax* were characterized by a marked rise in the IgM concentration commencing about 10 days after infection, and by a rise in IgG concentration commencing about 65 days after infection. Successful treatment resulted in a fall of IgM (Clarkson *et al.* 1975).

Significant differences in antibody levels were found to occur between individual animals within a relatively uniform group of cattle (Tabel 1979). Severe hypocomplementemia occurred in experimental *T. vivax* and *T. congolense* infections in cattle (Nielsen *et al.* 1978b, d; Nielsen and Sheppard 1977). In experimental *T. brucei* infections, the IgG and IgM were also elevated (Moulton and Sollod 1976). These various serological responses have not been related to protection; only extensive studies correlating resistance to natural and experimental challenge would be likely to show a relationship between antibody responses and resistance to infection (Weitz 1970). Camels experimentally infected with *T. evansi* had a decrease of albumin level and an overall increase in gamma-globulin levels with no changes observed in alpha and beta globulins, while in naturally infected camels in addition to these changes beta-globulin levels were also lower. In both experimentally and naturally infected camels IgM levels increased and remained high despite treatment (Boid *et al.* 1980a).

The role played by cellular immunity in trypanosomiasis has not been investigated extensively either in domestic or laboratory animals. Recent studies have shown that the proliferative response of bovine leukocytes was significantly decreased in infected cattle (Masake *et al.* 1981). Transformation *in vitro* of leukocytes to trypanosomal antigens from infected and immunized cattle was assayed and the kinetics of mitosis paralleled the development of delayed-skin reaction (Emery *et al.* 1980). In *T. brucei* and *T. congolense* infections of calves there was a slight increase in the number of circulating T- and B- and null cells (Ahmed *et al.* 1981). *Trypanosoma vivax* infection in goats caused suppression of the T- as well as the B-lymphocyte function (van Dam *et al.* 1981). The T-lymphocyte proliferation was assayed in *T. brucei* infection in mice (Gasbarre *et al.* 1980) and a suppression of the T-lymphocyte proliferative response to *T. brucei* resulted from an effect of trypanosomes on both the T-lymphocyte and macrophage populations (Gasbarre *et al.* 1981). It is likely that there will be considerable variability in the cellular immune responses, depending on the species of host and trypanosomes involved and the course of the clinical syndrome.

The effectors of resistance, both innate and acquired, have been investigated in laboratory animals in infections by pathogenic and nonpathogenic trypanosomes. Innate resistance was reviewed by Terry (1976) and he dealt with the insusceptibility of the cotton rat to *T. vivax*, the mouse to *T. lewisi* infection, and man to *T. brucei*. The nature of the trypanocidal mechanism associated with this form of resistance was not determined but appeared to involve, in some cases, plasma proteins, referred to as 'natural' antibodies, and, in others, factors related to the constitution and metabolism of the host. Because of the difficulty in determining specific factors responsible for such resistance – and once identified they could prove impossible to induce – much more attention has been drawn to the acquired resistance which could readily be manipulated experimentally. Here again the majority of the work has been on *T. brucei* and related species, and the protective trypanocidal immunologic mechanisms in experimental animals have been reviewed by Murray and Urquhart (1977). These involved antibodies in different classes of immunoglobulins specific for the variant antigens which induced cytotoxicity, sensitized lymphocytes, macrophages, and cell-mediated responses. One or more of these mechanisms probably also occur in natural infections in domestic animals, but the predominant trypanocidal factor may differ with the various syndromes caused by different species of trypanosome.

More recently it has been shown that elevated levels of IgM and IgG immunoglobulins in cattle infected with *T. brucei* were specific for the trypanosome, and IgM antibodies appeared to be more efficient in killing trypanosomes than IgG_1 antibodies during the first peak, the reverse being true during the second peak of infection (Musoke *et al.* 1981). Clearance of trypanosomes is accomplished by antibody-mediated hepatic phagocytosis which in passively immunized animals is dependent on opsonization involving C3 with no evidence of intravascular lysis or activation of macrophages being involved in the immune clearance (MacAskill *et al.* 1980). In *T. brucei*-infected mice, the complement has no essential role in the mechanisms of control of successive variant populations of trypanosomes in the blood, and variant specific IgM antibodies acting as agglutinins of trypanosomes probably controlled the blood infections (Shirazi *et al.* 1980). *Trypanosoma brucei* and *T. congolense* can either inactivate or eliminate potentially trypanolytic surface immune complexes containing antibodies to variant-specific antigens (Balber *et al.* 1979). The mechanisms in innate and acquired immunity in *T. cruzi* infections have been reviewed by Teixeira (1977). The innate insusceptibility was complement dependent in birds, involved macrophages in lower vertebrates, and was not well developed in mammals. In relation to acquired immunity, *T. cruzi* stimulated immunologic responses involving antibodies, complement, and macrophages which destroyed trypanosomes. Because this trypanosomal infection was predominantly localized in tissues, lymphocytes and macrophages in the cellular inflammatory responses appeared to have a dominant role in acquired immunity.

Recent investigations have shown that in *T. cruzi* infection in mice the protective antibodies were preferentially located in the IgG_2b subclass, while the IgM and IgG_1 fractions had little if any protection (Takehara *et al.* 1981). The defensive role of humoral immunity was emphasized in the protection of congenitally athymic mice against *T. cruzi* by passive antibody transfer. The antibody caused mobility of surface antigens of live blood forms of *T. cruzi*. (Kierszenbaum 1980). When the organisms were exposed to human or animal antisera the aggregation of surface antigens occurred to form an anterior or a posterior cap (Schmunis *et al.* 1980). Amastigotes of *T. cruzi* were more actively phagocytosed than other forms in the presence of a specific serum (Villalta *et al.* 1981). The passive transfer of lymphocytes from lymph nodes and spleen are effective in protection against *T. cruzi* (Burgess and Hanson 1979). The main antibody-dependent cellular cytotoxicity activity in man was detected in the granulocyte-rich fraction (Madeira *et al.* 1979). The bloodstream forms of *T. cruzi* were destroyed by human lymphoid cells, neutrophils, and eosinophils in the presence of specific antibodies (Kierszenbaum 1979). Further work indicated that the destruction by eosinophils was due to the discharge of basic granule components which were directly toxic to the trypanosomes (Kierszenbaum *et al.* 1981).

The occurrence of acquired immunity to various forms of natural trypanosomiasis, although only partial, had led to immunization against *brucei*-like trypanosomes, *T. congolense* and *T. cruzi* of laboratory animals and, to some extent, of domestic animals. Vaccination against Salivarian species has been reviewed by Murray and Urquhart (1977) and Stercorarian species by Teixeira (1977) and Hanson (1976). The prospect for vaccination against African trypanosomes is discussed in a brief review (Murray *et al.* 1980) and included discussion of immunological prevention against tsetse flies, immunostimulants, trypanotolerance, and infection and treatment methods, with the optimistic conclusion that, while vaccine against trypanosomiasis is not an immediate prospect, there are several promising avenues for immunological exploration. With the Salivarian species, three techniques have been used: injection of dead trypanosomes or their components, live irradiated trypanosomes, and the infection and treatment method. The use of the first two methods resulted in incomplete immunity at best, against homologous challenge only. Irradiated *T. rhodesiense*, but not *T. congolense*, protected cattle against challenge by the same pathogenic strains (Duxbury *et al.* 1972; Wellde *et al.* 1973). At present, the most potentially useful method applicable to wide field use, once it is properly assessed, is the infection and treatment procedure. Discussions of the effectiveness of this method have been presented (Gray 1967; Williamson 1970, 1976; Whiteside 1962a, b). Some of the more recent investigations have not added further support to the usefulness of this method (Wilson *et al.* 1975a, b, 1976) and have shown that multiple experimental infection and treatment methods merely increased the prepatent period and survival time after challenge and did not prevent infection (Scott *et al.* 1978). However, under field conditions the infection and treatment method would probably involve exposure to a greater variety of trypanosomes which could result in more effective immunity. The critical factors which affect the successful application of this method depend on the prevention of development of resistant strains to the trypanocides and on evaluation of the efficiency under various degrees of trypanosome challenge.

Increased resistance to trypanosomiasis has also been demonstrated in calves, as compared to adult cattle, and in certain trypanotolerant breeds indigenous to tsetse-fly areas of West and Central Africa. With regard to calf susceptibility to infection, much attention was given to this in the early literature (reviewed by Fiennes 1970) and has been supported by a more recent study of Wellde *et al.* (1979). Substantial age resistance to *T. congolense* was observed in that young animals underwent a relatively severe disease process, but all survived, while animals over 2 years of age invariably succumbed to infection. Resistance to challenge by the same strain was observed in both the young and older animals which recovered from infection after Berenil treatment (Wellde *et al.* 1981). However, young sheep and goats are found to be more susceptible to *T. congolense* than adults, as indicated by clinical effects and mortality (Griffin *et al.* 1981b).

The survival of trypanotolerant breeds, particularly the N'Dama breed, in the tsetse-fly-infested zones had drawn attention to the possibility of their greater use to overcome the restrictions imposed by trypanosomiasis on cattle production in Africa. Their productivity and their present and future economic importance in livestock development have been the subject of a study in 1977 by FAO, and UNDP. Already with the first investigation of these breeds, it was evident that the resistance was partial and precarious, dependent on a number of factors such as continuous exposure to restricted challenge, and on husbandry conditions (Chandler 1952, 1958; Roberts and Gray 1973a, b; Murray *et al.* 1979; Stephen 1966b). Various breeds of goats and sheep, indigenous and exotic to East Africa, were shown to have marked differences in trypanotolerance, which was high in indigenous, medium in crossbreeds, and low in exotic breeds (Griffin and Allonby 1979c). The wider acceptance and more effective use of all these methods of increasing resistance to trypanosomiasis whether breed, age, or drug related, will depend on the full recognition of their limitations and their judicious use in livestock production in Africa.

Of considerable importance in the discussion of resistance, whether in the field or laboratory, is the variability which may be observed between individual animals even under uniform challenge. This diversity of resistance appeared in many reports in trypanotolerant breeds (Maxie *et al.* 1979; Toure 1977; Toure *et al.* 1978). Although this variability makes the assessment of resistance difficult for any particular group of animals, it does provide the possibility of studying syndromes of varying severity under ideally uniform experimental conditions within. It also suggests that selection within a breed for resistance may be possible.

Immunosuppression occurs in various forms of trypanosomiasis of livestock and man. Under field conditions it is manifested by secondary infection which may mask the underlying trypanosomiasis. Experimental infections resulting in an acute syndrome in cattle were associated with acute septicemic and enteric forms of salmonellosis and subcutaneous tissue abscesses (Maxie *et al.* 1979). Another indication of immunologic malfunction was the lowered serological response to bacterial and viral vaccines in infected cattle (Scott *et al.* 1977; Rurangirwa *et al.* 1978; Whitelaw *et al.* 1979) which could be prevented by administering a trypanocide at the time of vaccination (Rurangirwa *et al.* 1979). The underlying mechanisms have been investigated in laboratory models and found to be due to such mechanisms as depression of various lymphocyte responses related to reduction of complement levels and involvement of suppressor cells (Albright *et al.* 1977; Eardley and Jayawardena 1977; Corsini *et al.* 1977; Pearson *et al.* 1978; Nielsen *et al.* 1978c).

In more recent studies it has been shown that goats infected with *T. congolense* had a significant, but not complete, suppression of antibody response to *Brucella melitensis* which was most marked with the onset of parasitemia which increased immediately after treatment with a trypanocidal drug (Griffin *et al.* 1980). Immunoconglutinin responses in calves experimentally infected with *T. congolense* were depressed as trypanosome infections inhibited the immunoconglutinin response to *B. abortus* (Tizard *et al.* 1979). There was no effect on cell-mediated effector mechanisms. A comparable degree of immuno-depression did not occur in *T. congolense*-infected cattle as observed in small laboratory animals (Sollod and Frank 1979).

Suppression of both IgM and IgG responses in mice infected with *T. congolense* was attributed to polyclonal activation and subsequent depletion or exhaustion of B-cells because of blastogenic stimulus due to the saturated fatty acids in trypanosomes (Assoku *et al.* 1979). The spleen was the primary site of immune depression with other lymphoid organs being little affected (Kar *et al.* 1981). In mice infected with *T. brucei* the immunosuppressive effect was related to a membrane fraction of the parasite (Clayton *et al.* 1979). In mice infected with *T. brucei, T. gambiense,* and *T. equiperdum* the immune depression was not the result of clonal exhaustion as measured by IgM levels, but was closely associated with the presence of living trypanosomes in chronic infections (Baltz *et al.* 1981). A soluble immunosuppressive substance was also extracted from the spleen of deer mice infected with *T. brucei* which blocked germinal center formation and prevented plasma cell differentiation in the spleen (Moulton and Coleman 1979). Immunosuppression was virtually complete in acute infection and associated with failure to control the first relapse variant; the suppression in chronic infection was less severe and subsequent variant populations were successfully controlled. The severity of the trypanosome-induced suppression of the antiparasite response, particularly IgM response, determined the course of the trypanosome infection (Sacks and Askonas 1980; Sacks *et al.* 1980). Vaccination against either louping-ill virus or lymphocytic choriomeningitis virus of groups of trypanosome-infected mice showed that T-cell responses are only diminished and the major immunosuppressive effect of trypanosomes is brought about by B-cell unresponsiveness (Reid *et al.* 1979). Immunosuppression and the suppressor cell activity relationship in *T. rhodesiense*-infected mice was investigated and it was shown that the suppressor cell population is restricted to the spleen; loss of immunocompetence in the lymph node may be due to factors other than suppressor cell activity (Wellhausen and Mansfield 1980). Macrophages were also shown to be the key cells as mediators of an immune dysfunction caused by *T. brucei* in mice (Grosskinsky and Askonas 1981).

It has yet also to be resolved how these immunologic malfunctions affect the sequential production of antibodies to the various dominant variant antigens throughout infection and the effect general debility, seen in chronic trypanosomiasis, has in susceptibility to secondary infection.

DIAGNOSIS

Parasitological methods

Procedures used for the detection of Salivarian trypanosomal infections and diagnosis of disease in the field depend on available laboratory facilities, the local epidemiological situation, and whether a single animal or herd is involved. Additional considerations in selecting diagnostic methods have also been given to the species of host and to the suspected species of trypanosome, e.g. with cattle and camels infected with trypanosomes in subgeneras *Trypanozoon* more complicated laboratory procedures have to be used. In epizootic tsetse-infested areas, the possibility of multiple infections must be kept in mind. The identification of the species of trypanosomes has a bearing on the type and level of trypanocide which has to be used and on the prognosis.

In general, because of the absence of pathognomonic signs, clinical examination is of little help in the diagnosis of trypanosomiasis with the possible exception of the more acute syndromes caused by the subgenus *Trypanozoon*. In horse, dogs, cats, camels, cattle, and small ruminants, *brucei* and *T. evansi* cause acute diseases characterized by enlargement of lymph nodes, subcutaneous edema, ophthalmitis, and central nervous system involvement. In addition, in dourine the external genitalia are affected. One important clinical feature of many forms of trypanosomiasis, particularly the chronic debilitating syndromes, is the secondary infection by other microorganisms which complicate and mask the underlying trypanosomiasis.

Definitive diagnosis of trypanosomiasis depends on the demonstration of trypanosomes. Serological tests indicate exposure to trypanosomal antigens which may result from a current or past infection. Therefore, depending on the particular epidemiological situation involved, either immunological or parasitological examinations, or both, are used. Routine parasitological examinations are on the blood, and less frequently on lymph node aspirates, cerebrospinal fluid, inflammatory exudes from eye and genital system, and edema fluid in skin plaques. Repeated examination, over a time, of fluids in wet mounts and stained preparation may be necessary because of the rapidly fluctuating levels of parasitemia in most forms of trypanosomiasis. The sensitivity of the direct parasitological examinations depends on the volumes of blood or tissue fluids examined. A common practical method is the standard hematocrit technique which concentrates the trypanosomes in the buffy coat. Another method with those species infective for laboratory rodents involves the subinoculation of relatively large volumes of blood or other tissue fluids into the peritoneal cavity of rodents. This is a particularly useful technique with species in the subgenus *Trypanozoon*, but the infectivity of other species varies to some extent with the different species in this subgenus and, to a lesser degree, with strains.

Trypanosoma congolense is less infective and *T. vivax* is generally considered to be not infective for rodents.

The detection of *T. cruzi* in blood depends on levels of parasitemia which are related to the acuteness of the disease. In dogs and cats, the parasitemia is usually low because of the predominantly chronic form and carrier state in these species. Subinoculation of laboratory rodents and culture methods are generally not regarded as reliable. The most sensitive method is xenodiagnosis using a species of triatomine bugs which, in a particular area, are known to be the principal vector. Because there are other species in the subgenus *Schizotrypanum* infecting wild and domestic animals which are morphologically indistinguishable from *T. cruzi*, identification of *cruzi*-like infections as *T. cruzi* can often only be made with certainty when several criteria are evaluated, including the local epidemiological situation of disease in man, morphology, serology, and biological behavior on subinfection of laboratory animals, cultures, and triatomine bugs.

Literature

The diagnostic methods in Salivarian trypanosome infections have been reviewed by Killick-Kendrick (1968) and Molyneux (1975). Various parasitological techniques, including microscopic examinations and animal subinoculations, have been evaluated in laboratory infections and under natural conditions. In West Africa, using six common methods, it was shown that in the field any one technique by itself was unsatisfactory and a combination of either the hematocrit concentration or thick smear techniques, together with thin smear was recommended; examination of lymph node aspirates did not increase the sensitivity (Leeflang *et al.* 1978). In East Africa, infections in cattle were more often detected in the peripheral than in jugular blood, and lymph node smears were essential in diagnosis of *T. vivax* (Robson and Ashkar 1972a, b; Rickman and Robson 1972). Other workers did not observe an increased efficiency in detecting infections by examination of lymph nodes of sheep and goats (Zwart *et al.* 1973). With trypanosomes infective for rodents, the subinoculation technique is particularly useful in diagnosis of very low parasitemia, as occurred in such infections as *T. evansi* in camels (Godfrey and Killick-Kendrick 1962; Pegram and Scott 1976). In these cases a single microscopic examination missed 80% of infections (Bennett 1933). Among the species in the subgenera *Trypanozoon* the infectivity to rodents varied, with *T. brucei* and *T. rhodesiense* being more infective than *T. gambiense* and *T. equiperdum*. The latter two species could infect rabbits by intratesticular inoculation (Heisch *et al.* 1970; Molyneux 1973). Even within those species regarded as infective, strains are present which are either noninfective or have low infectivity, a situation also often observed with trypanosomes exposed to trypanocides. With the other Salivarian species, *T. congolense* is less infective, while *T. vivax* is the least infective for rodents. Recently, *T. vivax* in West Africa was reported to be infective during the first 4 weeks of natural infections of cattle (Leeflang *et al.* 1976b).

The other common methods used to detect low numbers of trypanosomes in the blood involve either concentration or separation of trypanosomes from relatively large volumes of blood. The microhematocrit techniques, based on the method of Devignat and Dresse (1955), have been modified and adopted for routine use in the field (Woo 1969a, 1970; Murray *et al.* 1977). The reliability of the microhematocrit centrifugation technique in *T. vivax* infections was indicated by the fact that 62.5 to 75% of positive samples were not detected by the wet or thin film alone under field conditions (Toro *et al.* 1981). It is more sensitive with *T. vivax* and *brucei*-like species than with *T. congolense*, which has a specific gravity closer to that of erythrocytes, is less mobile, and adheres to erythrocytes (Woo and Rogers 1974). Separation of low numbers of trypanosomes by anion-exchange, followed by either centrifugation or filtration, is useful in research and has been adapted for field use (Godfrey and Lanham 1971; Lanham *et al.* 1972; Lumsden *et al.* 1977, 1979). In the field diagnosis of human sleeping sickness, miniature anion-exchange centrifugation was more sensitive than the microhematocrit and the thick blood film methods (Lumsden *et al.* 1977, 1979).

Differentiation of morphologically indistinguishable species and strains which are particularly important in distinguishing biological behavior, e.g. infectivity for man, have been attempted with some encouraging success by characterization of some of their intrinsic biochemical compositions (reviewed by Godfrey 1977). These methods provide objective reliable markers useful in studies of epidemiology and pathogenesis. Although the majority of this work has been on *T. brucei* and trypanosomes infecting man, initial work on *T. vivax* has shown three distinct isoenzyme patterns of different subpopulations, and two of the characteristic isoenzymes were stable, persisting in a field infection for a year (Kilgour *et al.* 1975; Kilgour and Godfrey 1977). *Trypanosoma gambiense* was shown to have one isoenzyme pattern different from *T. brucei*, and *T. rhodesiense* has three patterns which appeared related to different serological types (Godfrey and Kilgour 1976). These techniques have been used to determine the *T. gambiense* carrier status of pigs and dogs in Liberia, with the conclusion that pigs were a likely reservoir host (Gibson *et al.* 1978). Godfrey (1977) has also indicated that these techniques were promising in identifying *T. cruzi* subpopulations with different biological behavior.

The importance of detecting animal infection with *brucei*-like organisms infective for man has led to the wide use of the blood incubation infectivity test (BIIT) which is based on the infectivity of trypanosomes after incubation with human blood, serum, or plasma for rats. The characteristic of human serum resistance and isoenzyme patterns of *T. brucei* and *T. gambiense* did not change when being maintained in the new host and remained constant for an extended period of time (Schutt and Mehlitz 1981). The mechanism by which three carbohydrates alter trypanocidal activity of normal human serum on *T. brucei* was investigated and it was shown that the inhibitory effect of metabolizable carbohydrates on the trypanocidal activity is exerted at the point where the carbohydrate molecule interacts with its transport carrier site on the membrane of the trypanosomes (D'hondt and Kondo 1980). This test was recently reintroduced by Rickman and Robson (1970a, b, 1972) and has gained practical application but needs more rigid standardization of materials and methods to avoid the inconstant (equivocal) results reported by various authors (reports reviewed by Hawking 1979). A further complication in interpretation has been the observation that both negative and positive results in BIIT tests can be obtained with each of the clones of *T. brucei* and *T. rhodesiense* and were related to the development of specific antigenic types (Rickman 1977a, b; van Meirvenne *et al*. 1973, 1976). This variation in the susceptibility of successive variant antigen types to normal human sera would exert a natural selective pressure in favor of development of serum-resistant variant antigen types during metacyclic formation (Rickman and Kolala 1981). If these types of *T. brucei* resistant to human serum were in fact infective for man, it would have a very important bearing on the whole epidemiology of human sleeping sickness. Also, significant trypanolytic activity of sera from some African game animals was shown to *T. brucei* and *T. rhodesiense* and variable antigen types were found to vary widely in their sensitivity to different sera (Rickman *et al*. 1981a).

The subject of the effect of human blood components on various species of tsetse-transmitted trypanosomes has been reviewed by Hawking (1979). This review included the older literature up to 1935 when considerable interest was shown in this activity, and analyzed the observations and conclusions reported since the subject was reexamined by Rickman and Robson (1970a, b, 1972). Based on his own observation on the resistance and susceptibility of *T. brucei, T. rhodesiense, T. gambiense, T. evansi, T. congolense*, and *T. vivax*, Hawking concluded that in *brucei*-like organisms there are subpopulations which are either highly resistant, subresistant, or sensitive (Hawking 1973, 1976a, b, 1977, 1978b). These subpopulations in turn are composed of individual trypanosomes which are heterogeneous in their susceptibility to human sera. Therefore, the differences between BIIT negative, equivocal, and positive results depended on how many of the trypanosomes survived exposure to human serum. These results demonstrate a quantitative rather than a qualitative feature of subpopulations and must be evaluated statistically. In addition, the ability of trypanosome populations to resist the effect of human sera was changeable by exposure to human sera *in vivo* and *in vitro*, and by passage through different species of animals. Broader investigations of the susceptibility of *T. congolense, T. vivax*, and *T. evansi* to human sera has shown a wide range of sensitivity, giving rise to the possibility that even these three species may cause occasional infections in man (Hawking 1978b). This elegant concept of host specificity being a quantitative rather than a qualitative feature of trypanosome population would explain the diversity of infectivity of various trypanosomes for different species of hosts, which characterizes the trypanosomiasis in the field.

Serological methods

Serological tests in Salivarian trypanosomiasis are divided into two categories – those which use antigens extracted from lysed trypanosomes and others which use living organisms. Tests using trypanosome extracts include complement fixation (CF), precipitation, passive hemagglutination and fluorescent antibody tests, while live trypanosomes are used in immune adherence, neutralization cytotic, and respiratory tests. Tests based on trypanosome extracts enable better standardization of materials and methods and have a wider application in the field. Serological tests are used to detect antibody responses which are common to infections caused by the three subgenera and also those which are subgenus specific. Further refinement of some of the tests enables detection of different variant specific antigens. For field diagnosis, large survey tests which detect responses common to all subgenera are useful, but for the differentiation of infections caused by the three subgenera, there is yet no reliable standardized field test.

The usefulness of serological tests in the diagnosis of trypanosomiasis depends on the same criteria as for parasitological methods, namely, whether diagnosis is to be made on a single animal or on a herd basis, and in or outside epizootic areas. Because these tests detect immunologic responses after contact between trypanosomes and the host, they are necessarily correlated at the time of testing to patent or latent infection, e.g. after treatment, serological responses persist for a variable period of time. A number of factors influence the type and level of the serological responses and include species of host and trypanosomes, duration of infection, and severity of the disease. Therefore, serodiagnosis is usually undertaken to supplement parasitological examinations and by itself is useful in screening to determine the incidence of exposure of animals to trypanosomiasis. Serological tests are also more useful with those species, *T. equiperdum* and *T. evansi*, which are mechanically transmitted. The sensitivity of the CF test enabled the eradication of dourine from most parts of the world; with *T. evansi* the passive hemagglutination reaction is used. Fluorescent antibody tests are the most promising tests with all forms of trypanosomiasis which can be used under field conditions.

Because of the predominantly latent nature of *T. cruzi* infection in dogs, cats, and wild animal reservoirs, detection of parasitemia is often difficult. A similar situation exists in Chagas' disease of man for which a number of serological tests have been developed. Complement fixation, hemagglutination, and direct and indirect immunofluorescent tests have been used in surveys of cats and dogs. Cross-reactions with nonpathogenic trypanosomes, such as *T. rangeli* and with *Leishmania* may occur.

Literature

The majority of the serodiagnostic procedures with Salivarian and Stercorarian trypanosomes have been investigated in laboratory animals and man. The basic techniques in African trypanosomiasis were summarized by Weitz (1970) and their application in the field by Molyneux (1973). Some of these tests have been used in domestic animals. The indirect fluorescent antibody (IFA) test incorporating antigens from *T. brucei, T. congolense,* and *T. vivax* was found useful in screening large numbers of cattle (Toure *et al.* 1975; Wilson 1969). The IFA test was shown to be highly efficient in experimental *T. vivax* of South American origin for detecting serological response throughout infection (Platt and Adams 1976). This test has also been used with varying success to differentiate serological responses to the three species, and was found to be more specific than the CF reaction (Lotzsch and Deindl 1974; Mehlitz 1975; Mehlitz and Deindl 1972; Politzar 1974; Schindler 1972). Modification of the CF test by incorporation of either fluorescence or peroxidase was useful, with the additional advantage that the latter technique was more sensitive and specific. The conjugate can be used independent of the species of animal and is therefore useful in surveys (Horchner *et al.* 1979; Perié *et al.* 1975). The immunoperoxidase test, the immunofluorescent test, and the immunoperoxidase CF test were compared in the serological diagnosis and differentiation of *T. brucei, T. congolense,* and *T. vivax*. The latter was more specific and sensitive and had the advantage that it was independent of the species of animal examined (Horchner *et al.* 1979). Both the IFA and CF tests were useful in demonstrating a fall in serological responses following successful chemotherapy (Staak and Kelley 1979; Staak and Lohding 1979; Wilson 1971).

The enzyme-linked immunosorbent assay (ELISA) test was compared with the IFA test in cattle and shown to be more sensitive under certain situations, but it did not differentiate between *T. brucei, T. congolense,* and *T. vivax* (Luckins 1977; Luckins and Mehlitz 1978). In the epizootiological study of trypanosomiasis in trypanotolerant and susceptible cattle serological tests, the ELISA test and the titers under continuous tsetse challenge did not correlate with the direct detection of trypanosomes (Bernard *et al.* 1980). Antigens from culture forms of *T. brucei* were used to determine ELISA antibodies of cattle to *T. brucei, T. vivax,* and *T. congolense* by the micro test which was found to be as sensitive as the tests carried out with antigens of bloodstream forms of *T. brucei* (Silayo *et al.* 1980). In dogs infected with *T. brucei,* the IFA, CF, direct agglutination, and indirect hemagglutination tests yielded comparable results (Schindler and Sachs 1970). Both IFA and the indirect hemagglutination tests detected antibodies in sheep to *T. congolense* and *T. vivax* (Clarkson *et al.* 1971a, b; Kobayashi *et al.* 1976a, b).

A number of biochemical tests which depend on elevation of immunoglobulin levels have been used in the past to diagnose *T. evansi* infection, particularly in camels. Of these, the formal gel and the modified mercuric chloride precipitation tests appeared to be best but still had a poor correlation to patent parasitemia. The IFA and the ELISA tests were more sensitive than the biochemical tests (Luckins *et al.* 1979). Also, in camels the indirect hemagglutination test has been recommended for field diagnosis (Jatkar and Singh 1971; Jatkar *et al.* 1977). In buffalo and cattle, the passive hemagglutination test was found to be more sensitive and reliable than the gel diffusion and IFA tests (Verma and Gautam 1977).

An extensive amount of literature is available on the serological diagnosis of Chagas' disease in man and laboratory animals, and review articles were cited in the section on immunology. Their application to diagnosis in dogs and cats has not been evaluated, but they have been used in serological surveys.

CHEMOTHERAPY AND CHEMOPROPHYLAXIS

Trypanocides used in treatment and protection are the most common single method employed for the control of animal trypanosomiases. Effective application of chemotherapy and chemoprophylaxis in the field depends on several factors which include the species of trypanosome causing infection, severity of the challenge, species of animal, and lastly the occurrence of resistant strains. The complexity of the epizootiological situation also affects this method of control which is especially difficult when applied on a large scale for protection of livestock constantly under challenge, as occurs in tsetse-fly-infested areas of Africa. Outside enzootic areas, chemotherapy is relatively simple. The species of trypanosome determines the type of curative compound used. The trypanocides are divided into two types – those effective against *brucei*-like species, and others against *T. congolense* and *T. vivax*. The dosage used, within the recommended safety limits, depends on the species of trypanosome, local and systemic tolerance of the drug by the species of animal, and the possibility of occurrence of partial resistance in the infecting trypanosomes. Prophylactic and curative regimes, involving different doses and schedules of treatment, used in areas of continuous challenge, depend on the risk of infection, also called the severity of challenge. High challenge requires more frequent use of drugs at higher dosage levels.

The one factor which further complicates the use of trypanocides more than any other in the enzootic areas is the rapid development of drug resistance in the trypansome populations. The induction of resistance depends on the compound being less apt to occur with the rapidly excreted curative drugs rather than with the long-lasting prophylactics which have declining levels over long periods of time. Cross-resistance is a further complication and usually occurs between those compounds which are related in their chemical structure. Because all of the available compounds have been used extensively for over 20 years, resistance to some is widely spread, but fortunately against a few drugs it is still relatively rare and difficult to induce. The number of drugs available for field use is limited and requires the most judicious use to prevent the development of resistant strains. This depends to a great extent on the application of the 'sanative' method which involves the use, interchangeably, of compounds which are active against resistant strains produced by others. The 'sanative' drugs recommended are Berenil and Ethidium used to supplement each other, or other curative or prophylactic drugs, with which they do not have either reciprocal or one-sided cross-resistance. A 'sanative' drug is used interchangeably with the other drugs, either curative or prophylactic, at a prescribed schedule when breakthrough infections are likely to occur, or when actual resistant strains are observed. In practice, the most effective and most efficient economic method is established through constant monitoring of the incidence of infection, and accordingly either changing the type of drug used or adjusting the dosage and frequency of treatment.

In addition to the practical division of trypanocides used in livestock into those active against the two groups of trypanosomes, *brucei*-like on the one hand and *T. congolense* and *T. vivax* on the other, these compounds can also be classified according to their chemical structure. However, in both classifications the classes overlap, with some compounds having either an effect on both types of trypanosomes or common features in their chemical structure. Chemical relationships are particularly important from the standpoint of development of cross-resistance between various trypanocides. The currently used trypanocides are divided according to their chemical composition into acid naphthylamine, phenanthridine, quinaldine, and diamidine groups. Usually each compound within a group is used separately, but occasionally trypanocides from two groups are combined and administered as a complex.

In the naphthylamine group there is only one compound, Suramin (Antrypol*), (Naganol†), principally a product against human trypanosomiasis, which is used as a curative and a prophylactic agent of 1 to 4 months' duration against *T. brucei, T. evansi,* and *T. equiperdum* in horses, donkeys, and camels at 10 mg/kg IV (intravascular) given for two or three treatments at weekly intervals. The effectiveness is variable and the compound has more recently been replaced by others.

In the phenanthridine group, there are three compounds in current use. Homidium bromide (Ethidium bromide‡) and its derivative soluble in cold water, homidium chloride (Novidium§), are curative drugs against *T. congolense* and *T. vivax* in cattle, sheep, goats, and

* Imperial Chemical (Pharmaceutical) Ltd.
† Bayer.
‡ Boots Pure Drug Co.
§ May and Baker Ltd.

horses, at doses of 1.0 mg/kg IM (intramuscular). Prothidium bromide (Prothidium*) is used as both a curative and a prophylactic agent in cattle, sheep, goats, horses, and donkeys infected with *T. congolense* and *T. vivax* at 0.2 to 0.4 and 2.0 mg/kg respectively. It has also been used in dogs and donkeys against *T. evansi* at curative doses of 1 to 2 mg/kg, and for prophylaxis at 2.0 mg/kg. The last derivative to be developed in this group isometamidium (Samorin†), is now used more extensively than the others at a curative level of 0.5 to 2.0 mg/kg, also at the higher levels as a prophylactic against *T. vivax* and *T. congolense* in cattle, sheep, goats, and horses and against *T. evansi* in donkeys and dogs. The prophylactic effect of these phenanthridine compounds lasts from 3 to 6 months depending on the severity of the challenge. All members of this group cause an inflammatory tissue reaction at the site of injection characterized by swelling skin necrosis, which is especially severe with higher doses and when the drug is administered subcutaneously rather than intramuscularly. These lesions may be severe enough to cause lameness and affect the quality of the carcass. The local inflammation is reduced by incorporating the drug in an oil/grease base. Other methods used to eliminate these undesirable effects including dividing the dose and injecting it into several sites, and injecting the dewlap where the skin lesion is less important. Although liver damage may be produced by these trypanocides, it occurs at doses considerably higher than the therapeutic levels recommended. Whether systemic toxicity occurs following frequent repeated uses is not established, and it probably depends to some extent on the species and on the general health of the animals.

In the quinaldine group, quinapyramine dimethylsulfate (Antrycide sulfate‡) has been widely used as a curative agent against *T. congolense* and *T. vivax* in cattle at 4.4 mg/kg SC and against *T. evansi* and *T. equiperdum* in horses and camels at 3 to 5 mg/kg. Quinapyramine chloride (not available commercially) is also a prophylactic compound against *T. simiae* at doses of 50 mg/kg SC (subcutaneous). The prophylactive derivative of this quinapyramine compound, Antrycide prosalt,‡ is a mixture of chloride and dimethylsulfate and has activity up to 3 months against *T. vivax, T. congolense,* and *T. brucei,* and against *T. evansi* at doses of 7.4 mg/kg in cattle, horses, and camels. It is curative against *T. simiae* and can be used prophylactically against *T. equiperdum*. These two compounds produce a local encapsulated inflammatory reaction which may appear as a subcutaneous swelling. Transient systemic reaction characterized by tremors, salivation and sweating, and recumbency, occasionally resulting in death, may occur, especially in debilitated animals.

Diminazene aceturate (Berenil§), the only member of the diamidine group used routinely in small animal trypanosomiases, is the

* Boots Pure Drug Co.
† May and Baker Ltd.
‡ Imperial Chemical (Pharmaceutical) Ltd.
§ Farbwerke Hoechst AG.

commonest drug currently used against tsetse transmitted species, and qualifies as a wide-spectrum trypanocide. It is effective in cattle, sheep, horses, and dogs against *T. congolense* and *T. vivax* at 3 to 5 mg/kg and at 5 to 7 mg/kg levels against *T. brucei*. Higher doses of 10 mg/kg have been used against *T. evansi* infections in cattle. The drug is contraindicated in camels, and low tolerance has been observed in dogs. In these species it causes vascular injury manifested in extensive brain damage. It is used primarily as a curative drug and as a 'sanative' drug in replacing other trypanocides.

Trypanocidal complexes have been tried, usually under experimental conditions, using Suramin in combination with either Antrycide, Ethidium, Prothidium, or Berenil. The Antrycide–Suramin complex has been shown to be active as a curative and prophylactic agent against *T. evansi* in horses at various doses, and protective against *T. simiae* at 40 mg/kg. The complexes involving members of the phenonthridive group usually have a markedly increased trypanocidal effect, but cause a severe reaction at site of infection which makes them unacceptable for general field use.

Cross-resistance appears largely to be due to structural relationship between various trypanocides. Cross-resistance to high curative doses occurs among members of the phenanthridine group and, to a lesser extent, between phenanthridine trypanocides and Antrycide. Strains of trypanosomes resistant to Antrycide usually show partial resistance to curative doses of the three phenanthridine compounds. Cross-resistance is thought not to occur between Berenil and the phenanthridine group but one-sided resistance, partially resistant to Berenil, occurs in Antrycide-resistant strains. Based on this pattern of cross-resistance, Berenil is the drug of choice in the 'sanative' method involving any of the other commonly used compounds.

The widespread use of these compounds, particularly Berenil, over the last 20 years has altered the pattern and incidence of resistance and cross-resistance. The continued effective use of this limited number of available trypanocides now depends on their judicious use under close veterinary supervision to eliminate and prevent the further development of resistant strains. With the effectiveness of all trypanocides being reduced through the development of resistant strains, there is an urgent need for new drugs.

Literature

The most comprehensive review on the development, history of field use, and mode of action of human and animal trypanocides was published by Williamson (1970). This excellent presentation is primarily on the tsetse-fly-transmitted species but also includes reference to *T. evansi* and *T. equiperdum*. Unfortunately, many of the articles cited in the text are not listed in the bibliography. However, most of these citations are to be found in an earlier review article by the same author (Williamson 1962). Other reviews dealing with animal trypanocides are also available (Davey 1957; Hawking 1966) and include an analysis of the observations made in the initial extensive field trials undertaken in East Africa (Whiteside 1958a, b, 1962a, b). A monograph on the therapy of African trypanosomiasis which includes an exhaustive literature citation for various species of livestock has recently been published by Ruchel (1975). The present status of chemotherapy and chemoprophylaxis of African trypanosomiasis in animals was reviewed by Leach and Roberts (1981) with the following conclusion. The effectiveness of drugs favorable for use in African trypanosomiasis has been reduced by development of drug resistance. However, chemotherapy and chemoprophylaxis of animal trypanosomiasis could be effective and economically justified. Most of the currently available drugs can be used in a limited clearly defined situation, but cannot be used with the confidence with which they were employed in the 1960s. Therefore, the continued use of drugs requires greater expenditures on the surveillance and testing for resistance. Little research has been undertaken on the development of new drugs because of the tremendous cost and the relatively small markets. The author expresses the pessimistic view that control of trypanosomiasis by immunological methods is not likely to be achieved in the immediate future. The present state of chemotherapy and chemoprophylaxis of human trypanosomiasis caused by *T. cruzi* in the Western Hemisphere was reviewed by Brener (1979), who concluded that the pharmaceutical industry appeared not to consider Chagas' disease a rewarding market. There was a lack of a specific drug suitable for mass treatment and for safely treating individual patients.

In these reviews, summaries, and other published articles, there is considerable diversity as to the type of trypanocides, dose, and schedule of treatment which have been used for the various forms of trypanosomiasis of livestock. This reflects the complexity of chemotherapy and prophylaxis which, in the field, is affected by many factors pertaining to the species of animal and trypanosome, degree of challenge, occurrence of either complete or partial resistance, cross-resistance, and differences caused by geographical distribution. The majority of the literature published on the chemotherapy and chemoprophylaxis against Salivarian species in livestock is related to the initial experimental trials of field applications of newly developed trypanocides. Since then, trypanocides have been used extensively for a long time. Berenil, the newest compound, has now been in use for over 20 years. The effectiveness of the compounds has changed over time because of the development of resistance and cross-resistance and the changing epizootiology of trypanosomiases by altered distributions of tsetse flies and different methods of animal husbandry. Unfortunately, very little published information is available on either a local or regional basis on the efficacy of present-day methods of chemotherapy and prophylaxis. However, there are reports of rapid development of resistance following wide field application of most of the trypanocides. For the last 20 years, no new trypanocides have been developed for field use and this alarming situation was discussed in a number of recent articles on the chemotherapy of protozoa and the prohibitive costs of development of new drugs (Goodwin 1978; Hutner 1977).

The oldest drug used in animals, but now with decreasing frequency, was Suramin for the *brucei*-like infections in horses, donkeys, and camels. Its early use was in therapy and gave some protection at the 4 to 10 mg/kg level (Knowles 1927; Bennett 1933). Resistance developed quickly and has been demonstrated more recently in camels (Leach 1961) and Antrycide has now replaced this drug. Another use of Suramin was in complexes with other trypanocides, and the literature is presented in those sections dealing with compounds. Recent work has shown that after a single intravenous injection of Suramin the rate of removal of the drug from plasma into other tissues of the rat was independent of the initial concentration. Trypanosomes take up small amounts of the drug and do not concentrate the drug within the cell. Once within the cell, Suramin progressively inhibited respiration and glycolysis, but even in the highest dose levels tolerated by the rat the trypanosomes continued to increase in the bloodstream for at least 6 hours. In the final stages sufficient Suramin is released from the secondary lysosomes leading to disorganization of the metabolic function and death of the organism (Fairlamb and Bowman 1980a, c). Suramin has been reported to inhibit phosphorylation–dephosphorylation reactions in *T. gambiense* (Walter 1980).

The phenanthridine compounds have been used for about 30 years. Ethidium was used widely in East and West Africa for the first 5 years following its first field application, with the number of doses increasing tenfold from the few thousand used initially (Ford *et al.* 1953a, b; Unsworth 1954a, b; Wilde and Robson 1953). Although it was primarily a curative compound, some protection has been observed (Desowitz 1957; Leach *et al.* 1955; Whiteside 1960). More recently its prophylactic effect was observed on cattle for a period of up to 10 months with decreased incidence of infection and increased productivity (Mwambu 1971). The next derivative in this group, Prothidium, was developed as a prophylactic drug and was shown to be effective for up to 4 months in East and West Africa (Lyttle 1960; Marshall 1958; Whiteside *et al.* 1960). Shorter periods were associated with severe challenge (Robson 1961).

The last compound in this group to be developed for both curative and prophylactic use was Isometamidium (Marshall 1958; Kirby 1961; Robson 1962). The duration of protection could be increased by using higher doses of 4 to 5 mg/kg (Smith and Brown 1960; Stephen 1960). Concentrations of Isometamidium in goat tissues were examined following either a single intravenous or intramuscular dose of 0.5 mg/kg. Appreciable amounts of the drug were observed in the liver and kidneys 12 weeks after injection. Intramuscular injection resulted in a lower and less sustained concentration of drugs in tissue. The drug was not observed in adipose tissue, spleen, or skeletal muscle (Braide and Eghianruwa 1980). Isometamidium dextran complex was prepared by adding a 4% solution of dextran sulfate to an equal volume of 4% solution of Isometamidium chloride. Treatment with 1 or 2 mg/kg subcutaneously protected the animals for 90 days. At the injection site, a firm subcutaneous nodule formed (Aliu and Sannusi 1979). The toxicity and activity against *T. vivax* and *T. congolense* in rats and mice of Isometamidium dextran complex showed a reduction in the local and systemic toxicity with the complex and increased therapeutic index by four times (Aliu and Chineme 1980). During the early stages of its use it was thought to be effective against strains resistant to all other trypanocides. However, in subsequent extensive field trials it did not live up to these expectations and cross-resistance was observed (Jones-Davies and Folkes 1967). It is now considered that cross-resistance may occur between Prothidium and all other compounds except Berenil. The first experimental phenanthridine compounds which led to the development of the three currently in use caused liver damage. The three derivatives now in use cause liver lesions only at doses substantially higher than therapeutic levels. However, Isometamidium at high therapeutic doses of 4 mg/kg has caused systemic toxic effects with staggering, recumbency, and occasional death (Robson 1962).

Antrycide has been used extensively as a curative drug for all forms of tsetse-transmitted trypanosomiases, as well as against *T. evansi* and *T. equiperdum* (Curd and Davey 1950; Evans 1956; Leach 1961). The prophylactic derivative has also been used (Marshall 1958; Whiteside *et al.* 1960; Deom 1960). Systemic toxicity due to its curare-like properties has been reported at 5 mg/kg (Unsworth and Chandler 1952; Davey 1957).

The newest compound, Berenil, has in many parts of Africa replaced Ethidium and Antrycide as the curative trypanocide of choice. The activity of this compound in the field was presented by Fussganger and Bauer (1958). Intravenous injection of Berenil was followed in 5 minutes by an increase in the jugular blood parasite count of *T. congolense*-infected cattle. The peak parasitemia, reached at 8 minutes after injection, was 15 times greater than the pretreatment parasitemia (Maxie and Losos 1977). It has a high therapeutic index and a broad spectrum of activity, and widespread resistance has as yet not been reported. Although it was considered to be rapidly excreted and therefore strictly curative in nature, some prophylactic activity has been reported (van Hoeve and Cunningham 1964). Recent investigations in experimental animals have shown that Berenil at low concentrations that occur in tissue may exert some antihistaminic activity or antiinflammatory effect in addition to its trypanocidal action (Arowolu and Adepolu 1981). On exposure of *T. evansi* to Berenil a dyskinetoplastic form developed which caused a chronic infection (Gobel and Dennig 1981). Also, loss of kinetoplast occurred in a strain of *T. equiperdum* by successive treatments of infected rats with Berenil (Riou and Benard 1980). Because of the short-lasting curative action, it has been used as a means of judging severity of challenge by the so-called Berenil index which is defined as the average time required between Berenil treatment to eliminate infections in animals under constant challenge (Boyt *et al.* 1963). In most livestock neither local nor systemic toxicity was regarded as a problem except in the case of dogs and camels. At high therapeutic levels extensive hemorrhagic malacia of central nervous tissue associated with underlying vascular lesions was observed in dogs (Losos and Crockett 1969; Schmidt *et al.* 1978). In camels, Berenil is contraindicated and caused death at therapeutic levels (Leach 1961; Abdel-Latif 1963a) with lesions which were comparable to those observed in dogs (R. Heinnonen, personal communication). The first formulation combining Suramin and Pentamidine for human use led to the incorporation of the animal trypanocides into complexes to reduce systemic toxicity and increase their curative and prophylactic properties. The method of combining these compounds into complexes was described by Williamson and Desowitz (1956).

The results of the initial trials showed that the trypanocidal properties were markedly increased, e.g. with Ethidium and Prothidium at higher doses the protection was extended up to 10 months (Desowitz 1957; Smith 1959; Robson and Cawdery 1958; Robson 1958a, b; Stephen and Williamson 1958; Stephen 1962b). Although the systemic toxicity was also reduced, the local inflammatory reaction at the site of injection was too severe for wide application of these complexes in the field (Wilson 1959; Williamson and Stephen 1961). The Antrycide complex has been recommended as a curative and prophylactic drug against *T. simiae,* because it is resistant to all other trypanocides in common use (Stephen 1966b; Stephen and Gray 1960).

The treatment against *T. evansi* requires some special consideration because the variable efficacy of different trypanocides has been reported and appears to be dependent on the animal species and geographic distribution. Cattle and buffalo have been treated successfully with 10 mg/kg of Berenil (Verma *et al.* 1973, 1976; Razzaque and Mishra 1977). It is not effective in dogs at 3.5 mg/kg (Bansal and Pathak 1968), but higher doses of 6 to 7 mg/kg were found to be curative in dogs and horses (Abdel-Latif, 1963a, b). Antrycide has been widely used as a curative and prophylactic drug in cattle and horses (Ray *et al.* 1953; Fernandez *et al.* 1965) and is also effective in buffalo and caraboa (Castillo 1962). Isometamidium was effective at doses 1 to 2 mg/kg in treatment of dogs and horses (Chand and Singh 1970; Srivastava and Malhotra 1967), while in camels it only suppressed the infection but was not curative (Balis and Richard 1977). There was also mention of Isometamidium being effective in cattle. (Raghaven and Khan 1970). The Suramin and Antrycide complex gave considerably longer protection in horses from 6 to 23 months as compared to the 2 to 3 months obtained with Antrycide Prosalt (Gill 1972; Gill and Malhotra 1971). Antrypol, at a 5 gm dose, antrycide methyl sulfate at 1.5 gm, Nagonal at 5 gm, and Berenil at 2 gm were found equally trypanocidal in action in 40 naturally infected camels with *T. evansi* (Raisinghani and Lodha 1980a). Six camels were experimentally infected with *T. evansi* and treated 3 months after infection with Berenil. Death was reported at 3.75 mg/kg but was thought not to be associated with drug toxicity. The drug was found to be effective at 2.5 and 1.25 mg/kg. However, the claim of nontoxic response is questionable (Raisinghani and Lodha

1980b). Samorin (Isometamidium chloride) was effective against *T. evansi* in mice after a single intraperitoneal injection of 1 to 2 mg/kg but doses of 40 mg/kg were toxic, resulting in death (Homeida *et al.* 1980).

With the extensive use of trypanocides in Africa to maintain livestock in tsetse-fly belts, the development of resistant strains and the increase in tolerance of livestock to trypanosomiasis because of the prolonged exposure to challenge permitted by the protective trypanocides has been discussed by Williamson (1970). The detection of resistant strains was usually undertaken in sheep and goats because small laboratory animals were often not susceptible to subinoculation of these resistant strains (Williamson and Stephen 1960). It was also shown that drug resistance is stable and transmissible by passage through tsetse flies (Gray and Roberts 1971). Following infection and treatment, the breakthrough infections had lower subsequent pathogenicity in the treated animals, but not necessarily on subpassage to other animals. In tsetse-transmitted varieties of trypanosomiases resistant strains develop in conjunction with increased tolerance of cattle, a situation which could be exploited more effectively through more judicial use of trypanocides.

Recent advances in the study of trypanosomal metabolism have encouraged the development of new chemotherapeutic agents specifically designed to exploit known biochemical differences between trypanosomes and their mammalian hosts. A semi-automated microtesting for quantitation of antitrypanosomal activity in *in vitro* utilized bloodstream forms of *T. rhodesiense* and the inhibition of the uptake of radiolabeled thymidine and L-leucine by parasite served as the indicators of antitrypanosomal activity (Desjardins *et al.* 1980). Twenty-four of 27 compounds of 2-acetyl-pyridine thiosemicarbazones and analogs exhibited antitrypanosomal activity comparable to that found with Ethidium bromide (Casero *et al.* 1980). Treatment with a single dose of salicylhydroxamic acid was shown to be effective against infections caused by monomorphic but not pleomorphic members of the *Trypanozoon*, with a reoccurrence of parasitemia in the pleomorphic infections (Evans and Brightman 1980). The trypanocidal effect of salicylhydroxamic and glycerol was found to be associated with a synergistic factor which affected both the speed and completeness of destruction of *T. brucei* (Amole and Clarkson 1981). Low-molecular-weight interferon inducers did not affect *T. equiperdum* infections in mice (Gláz 1978). Antitumor antibiotic beta gleomycin was found to be effective against *T. brucei* in mice (Nathan *et al.* 1981). An experimental infection with *T. cruzi* treated with a nitrofuranic drug and cortico-steroids showed an almost complete elimination of inflammation when cortico-steroid was added. Treatment with corticoids enabled some of the animals to reach the chronic phase. It was concluded that the combination of a nitrofuranic drug with corticoids resulted in parasite destruction and inhibited the inflammatory response (Andrade *et al.* 1980). The effects of allopurinol on four different strains of *T. cruzi* with varied parasitemia patterns and mortality rates showed differences in drug response which appeared to be related to the biological characteristics of the host–parasite interaction (Avila *et al.* 1981).

BIBLIOGRAPHY

Abdel-Latif, K., 1958. The incidence of diseases caused by intercorpuscular blood parasites in camels in Egypt, *Vet. Med. J. Gizam*, **4**(4): 43–54.

Abdel-Latif, K., 1963a. Berenil in the treatment of trypanosomiasis 'El-Debab'. II. A study on the efficacy of Berenil in the treatment of camels and donkeys affected with 'El-Debab', *J. Arab Vet. Med. Ass.*, **23**(3): 204–13.

Abdel-Latif, K., 1963b. Berenil in treatment of trypanosomiasis 'El-Debab'. III. A study on the efficacy of Berenil in the treatment of dogs experimentally infected with 'El-Debab', *J. Arab Vet. Med. Ass.*, **23**: 293–300.

Abdel-Latif, K., 1963c. On the possibility of the congenital transmission of *Trypanosoma* of El-Debab, *J. Arab Vet. Med. Ass.*, **28**: 287–92.

Adekolu-John, E. O., 1978. The significance of migrant Fulani for human trypanosomiasis in Kainji lake areas of Nigeria, *Trop. geogr. Med.*, **30**: 285–93.

Afchain, D., Le Ray, D., Fruit, J. and Capron, A., 1979. Antigenic make-up of *Trypanosoma cruzi* culture forms: identification of a specific component, *J. Parasitol.*, **65**(4): 507–14.

Agabian, N., Thomashow, L., Milhausen, M. and Stuart, K., 1980. Structural analysis of variant and invariant genes in trypanosomes, *Am. J. Trop. Med. Hyg.*, **29**(Suppl. 5): 1043–9.

Ahmed, J. S., Salker, R., Zweygarth, E., Rehbein, G. and Horchner, F., 1981. Influence of *Trypanosoma* infection on the formation of E, EA, and EAC rosettes with peripheral blood lymphocytes from calves, *Z. Tropenmed. Parasit.*, **32**: 55–7.

Albright, J. F., Albright, J. W. and Dusanic, D. G., 1977. Trypanosome-induced splenomegaly and suppression of mouse spleen cell response to antigen and mitogens, *J. Reticuloendothel. Soc.*, **21**(1): 21–31.

Alexander, J., 1975. Effect of the antiphagocytic agent Cytochalasin B on macrophage invasion by *Leishmania mexicana* promastigotes and *Trypanosoma cruzi* epimastigotes, *J. Protozool.*, **22**(2): 237–40.

Aliu, Y. O., 1975. Dry season Fulani transhumance and cattle trypanosomiasis: the nature of the relationship, *Niger. J. Anim. Prod.*, **2**(2): 204–11.

Aliu, Y. O. and Chineme, C. M., 1980. Isometamidium–dextran complex: toxicity and activity against *Trypanosoma vivax* and

Trypanosoma congolense in rats and mice, *Toxicol. Appl. Pharmacol.*, **53**: 196–203.

Aliu, Y. O. and Sannusi, A., 1979. Isometamidium–dextrose complex: therapeutic activity against *Trypanosoma vivax* infection in Zebu cattle, *J. vet. Pharmacol. Therap.*, **2**: 265–74.

Amole, B. O. and Clarkson, A. B. Jr., 1981. *Trypanosoma brucei*: host–parasite interaction in parasite destruction by salicylhydroxamic acid and glycerol in mice, *Exp. Parasitol.*, **51**: 133–40.

Anderson, E., Saxe, L. H. and Beams, H. W., 1956. Electron microscope observations of *Trypanosoma equiperdum*, *J. Parasitol.*, **42**: 11–16.

Andrade, S. G., Andrade, Z. A. and Sadigursky, M., 1980. Combined treatment with a nitrofuranic and a corticoid in experimental Chagas' disease in the dog, *Am. J. Trop. Med. Hyg.*, **29**(5): 766–73.

Andrade, Z. A., Andrade, S. G., Sadigursky, M. and Maguire, J. G., 1981. Experimental Chagas' disease in dogs. A pathologic and ECG study of the chronic indeterminate phase of the infection, *Arch. Pathol. Lab. Med.*, **105**: 460–4.

Anosa, V. O., 1980. Studies on the parasitemia, plasma volumes, leucocyte and bone marrow cell counts, and the moribund state in *Trypanosoma brucei* infection of splenectomised and intact mice, *Zbl. Vet. Med.*, **B27**: 169–80.

Anosa, V. O. and Isoun, T. T., 1976. Serum proteins, blood plasma volumes in experimental *Trypanosoma vivax* infections of sheep and goats, *Trop. Anim. Hlth Prod.*, **8**: 14–19.

Anosa, V. O. and Isoun, T. T., 1980a. Haematological studies on *Trypanosoma vivax* infection of goats and intact and splenectomized sheep, *J. Comp. Path.*, **90**: 155–68.

Anosa, V. O. and Isoun, T. T., 1980b. Further observations on the testicular pathology in *Trypanosoma vivax* infection of sheep and goats, *Res. vet. Sci.*, **28**: 151–60.

Anosa, V., Jennings, F. W. and Urquhart, G. M., 1977. The effect of splenectomy on anaemia in *Trypanosoma brucei* infection of mice, *J. Comp. Path.*, **87**: 569–79.

Apted, F. I. C., 1980. Present status of chemotherapy and chemoprophylaxis of human trypanosomiasis in the Eastern hemisphere, *Pharmac. Ther.*, **11**: 391–413.

Arowolu, R. O. and Adepolu, F. O., 1981. The interaction of Berenil with histamine on isolated mammalian tissues, *R. Soc. trop. Med. Hyg.*, **75**(2): 302.

Ashcroft, M. T., 1957. The polymorphism of *Trypanosoma brucei* and *Trypanosoma rhodesiense*, its relation to relapses and remission of infections in white rats, and the effect of cortisone, *Ann. trop. Med. Parasit.*, **51**: 301–12.

Ashcroft, M. T., Burtt, E. and Fairbairn, H., 1959. The experimental infection of some African wild animals with *Trypanosoma rhodesiense*, *T. brucei*, and *T. congolense*, *Ann. trop. Med. Parasit.*, **53**: 147–61.

Ashman, P. U. and Seed, J. R., 1973. Biochemical studies in the vole, *Microtus montanus*. II. The effects of a *Trypanosoma brucei gambiense* infection on the diurnal variation of hepatic glucose-6-phosphatase and liver glycogen, *Comp. Biochem. Physiol.*, **45B**: 379–92.

Assoku, R. K. G., Hazlett, C. A. and Tizard, I., 1979. Immunosuppression in experimental African trypanosomiasis. Polyclonal B-cell activation and mitogenicity of trypanosome-derived saturated fatty acids, *Int. Arch. Allergy app. Immun.*, **59**: 298–307.

Avila, J. L., Avila, A. and Munoz, E., 1981. Effect of Allopurinol on different strains of *Trypanosoma cruzi, Am. J. Trop. Med. Hyg.*, **30**(4): 769–74.

Avila, J. L., Casanova, M. A., Avila, A. and Bretana, A., 1979. Acid and neutral hydrolases in *Trypanosoma cruzi.* Characterization and assay, *J. Protozool.*, **26**(2): 304–11.

Awkati, A. J. and Al-Khatib, G. M., 1972. Trypanosomiasis in domestic animals of Iraq, *J. Egypt. Vet. Med. Assoc.*, **32**: 203–6.

Bacchi, C. J., 1981. Content, synthesis, and function of polyamines in trypanosomatids: relationship to chemotherapy, *J. Protozool.*, **28**(1): 20–7.

Bacchi, C. J., Vergara, C., Garofalo, J., Lipschik, G. Y. and Hutner, S. H., 1979. Synthesis and content of polyamines in bloodstream *Trypanosoma brucei, J. Protozool.*, **26**(3): 484–8.

Baker, J. R., 1970. Techniques for detection of trypanosome infections. In *The African Trypanosomiases*, ed. H. W. Mulligan. George Allen & Unwin (London), pp. 67–88.

Balber, A. E., 1972. *Trypanosoma brucei*: fluxes of the morphological variants in intact and x-irradiated mice, *Exp. Parasitol.*, **31**: 307–19.

Balber, A. E., Bangs, J. D., Jones, S. M. and Proia, R. L., 1979. Inactivation or elimination of potentially trypanolytic complement-activating immune complexes by pathogenic trypanosomes, *Infect. Immun.*, **24**(2): 617–27.

Balis, J. and Richard, D., 1977. Trypanocide action of Isometamidium chloride hydrochlorate on *Trypanosoma evansi* and an attempt to control trypanosomiasis in dromedary, *Rev. Elev. Méd. vét. Pays trop.*, **30**: 369–72.

Baltz, T., Baltz, D., Giroud, C. and Pautrizel, R., 1981. Immune depression and macroglobulinemia in experimental subchronic trypanosomiasis, *Infect. Immun.*, **32**(3): 979–84.

Banks, K. L., 1978. Binding of *Trypanosoma congolense* to the walls of small blood vessels, *J. Protozool.*, **25**(2): 241–45.

Banks, K. L. 1979. *In vitro* binding of *Trypanosoma congolense* to erythrocytes, *J. Protozool.*, **26**(1): 103–8.

Banks, K. L., 1980. Injury induced by *Trypanosoma congolense* adhesion to cell membranes, *J. Parasitol.*, **66**(1): 34–7.

Bansal, S. R. and Pathak, R. C., 1968. Therapeutic efficacy of Berenil in experimental trypanosomiasis (Surra), *Indian J. Anim. Hlth*, **7**: 283–8.

Barbet, A. F., Musoke, A. J., Shapiro, S. Z., Mpimbaza, G. and McGuire, T. C., 1981. Identification of the fragment containing cross-reacting antigenic determinants in the variable surface glycoprotein of *Trypanosoma brucei*, *Parasitology*, **83**: 623–37.

Barrois, M., Riou, G. and Galibert, F., 1981. Complete nucleotide sequence of minicircle kinetoplast DNA from *Trypanosoma equiperdum*, *Proc. Natl. Acad. Sci. USA*, **78**(6): 3323–7.

Barrowman, P. R., 1976a. Observations on the transmission, immunology, clinical signs and chemotherapy of dourine (*Trypanosoma equiperdum* infection) in horses, with special reference to cerebro-spinal fluid, *Onderstepoort J. vet. Res.*, **43**(2): 55–66.

Barrowman, P. R., 1976b. Experimental intraspinal *Trypanosoma equiperdum* infection in a horse, *Onderstepoort J. vet. Res.*, **43**(4): 201–2.

Barrowman, P. R. and Roos, J. A., 1979. Lymph node pathology in *Trypanosoma brucei*-infected sheep, *Onderstepoort J. vet. Res.*, **46**: 9–17.

Barrowman, P. R. and van Vuuren, M., 1976. The prevalence of dourine in southern Africa, *J. S. Afr. vet. med. Ass.*, **47**(2): 83–5.

Barry, J. D., 1979. Capping of variable antigen on *Trypanosoma brucei*, and its immunological and biological significance, *J. Cell Sci.*, **37**: 287–302.

Barry, J. D., Hajduk, S. L., Vickerman, K. and Le Ray, D., 1979a. Detection of multiple variable antigen types in metacyclic populations of *Trypanosoma brucei*, *Trans. R. Soc. trop. Med. Hyg.*, **73**(2): 205–8.

Barry, J. D., Le Ray, D. and Herbert, W. J., 1979b. Infectivity and virulence of *Trypanosoma* (*Trypanozoon*) *brucei* for mice. IV. Dissociation of virulence and variable antigen type in relation to pleomorphism, *J. Comp. Path.*, **89**: 465–70.

Barry, J. D. and Vickerman, K., 1979. *Trypanosoma brucei*: loss of variable antigens during transformation from bloodstream to procyclic forms *in vitro*, *Exp. Parasitol.*, **48**: 313–24.

Bennett, S. C. J., 1933. The control of camel trypanosomiasis, *J. Comp. Path.*, **46**: 67–77, 174–85.

Berens, R. L., Marr, J. J. and Brun, R., 1980. Pyrazolopyrimidine metabolism in African trypanosomes: metabolic similarities to *Trypanosoma cruzi* and *Leishmania* spp., *Mol. Biochem. Parasitol.*, **1**: 69–73.

Bernard, S., Haase, M. and Guidot, G., 1980. Trypanosomiasis of cattle in Upper Volta, epizootiological investigations and a contribution to the problem of trypano-tolerance. II. Enzyme linked immunosorbent assay and indirect immunofluorescence for examination of antibodies against trypanosomes in trypanotolerant and trypanosensitive breeds, *Berl. Münch. Tierarztl. Wschr.*, **93**: 482–5.

Bideau, J., Gidel, R. and Moity, J., 1966. Note préliminaire sur l'étude immunoelectrophorétique de serum de bovins trypanosomés, *Bull. Soc. Path. exot.*, **59**: 817–25.

Bienen, E. J., Hammadi, E. and Hill, G. C., 1980. Initiation of trypanosome transformation from bloodstream trypomastigotes to procyclic trypomastigotes, *J. Parasitol.*, **66**(4): 680–2.

Bienen, E. J., Hammadi, E. and Hill, G. C., 1981. *Trypanosoma brucei*: biochemical and morphological changes during *in vitro* transformation of bloodstream- to procyclic-trypomastigotes, *Exp. Parasitol.*, **51**: 408–17.

Bittencourt, A., 1976. Congenital Chagas' disease, *Am. J. Dis. Child.*, **130**: 97–103.

Boehringer, E. G., 1977. Infestación natural del vacuno por *Trypanosoma equinum* (Vogues 1901), *Rev. Invast. Ganad.*, **11**: 63–8.

Boid, R., Luckins, A. G., Rae, P. F., Gray, A. R., Mahmoud, M. M. and Malik, K. H., 1980a. Serum immunoglobulin levels and electrophoretic patterns of serum proteins in camels infected with *Trypanosoma evansi*, *Vet. Parasitol.*, **6**: 333–45.

Boid, R., Mahmoud, M. M. and Gray, A. R., 1980b. Changes in the levels of some serum enzymes in dromedary camels infected with *Trypanosoma evansi*, *Res. vet. Sci.*, **28**: 336–40.

Boothroyd, J. C., Cross, G. A. M., Hoeijmakers, J. H. J. and Borst, P., 1980. A variant surface glycoprotein of *Trypanosoma brucei* synthesized with a C-terminal hydrophobic 'tail' absent from purified glycoprotein, *Nature*: **288**: 624–6.

Boreham, P. F. L., 1977. Kallikrein – its release and possible significance in trypanosomiasis, *Ann. Soc. belge Méd. trop.*, **57**(4–5): 249–52.

Boreham, P. F. L., 1979. Pharmacologically active substances in *Trypanosoma brucei* infections. In *Pathogenicity of Trypanosomes*, eds G. J. Losos, A. Chouinard. IDRC (Ottawa), **132e**, pp. 114–19.

Boreham, P. F. L. and Facer, C. A., 1974a. Fibrinogen and fibrinogen/fibrin degradation products in experimental African trypanosomiasis, *Int. J. Parasitol.*, **4**: 143–51.

Boreham, P. F. L. and Facer, C. A., 1974b. Autoimmunity in trypanosome infections. II. Anti-fibrin/fibrinogen (anti-F) autoantibody in *Trypanosoma* (*Trypanozoon*) *brucei* infections of the rabbit, *Int. J. Parasitol.*, **4**: 601–7.

Boreham, P. F. L. and Facer, C. A., 1977. Fibrinogen and fibrinogen/fibrin degradation products in the urine of rabbits infected with *Trypanosoma* (*Trypanozoon*) *brucei*, *Z. Parasitenkd.*, **52**: 257–65.

Boreham, P. F. L. and Wright, I. G., 1976. Hypotension in rabbits infected with *Trypanosoma brucei*, *Br. J. Pharmac.*, **58**: 137–9.

Borst, P., Arnberg, A. C., Bernards, A., Cross, G. A. M., Frasch, A. C. C., Hoeijmakers, J. H. J. and van der Ploeg, L. H. T., 1980b. DNA rearrangements involving the genes for variant antigens in *Trypanosoma brucei*, *Cold Spring Harbor Symposia on Quantitative Biology*, **45**: 935–43.

Borst, P., Fase-Fowler, F. and Gibson, W. C., 1981. Quantitation of genetic differences between *Trypanosoma brucei gambiense, rhodesiense* and *brucei* by restriction enzyme analysis of kinetoplast DNA, *Mol. Biochem. Parasitol.*, **3**: 117–31.

Borst, P., Frasch, A. C. C., Bernards, A., Hoeijmakers, J. H. J., van der Ploeg, L. H. T. and Cross, G. A. M., 1980a. The genes for variant antigens in trypanosomes, *Am. J. trop. Med. Hyg.*, **29**(Suppl. 5): 1033–6.

Bowman, I. B. R. and Flynn, I. W., 1976. Oxidative metabolism of trypanosomes. In *Biology of the Kinetoplastida*, eds W. H. R. Lumsden, D. A. Evans. Academic Press (New York), vol. 1, pp. 435–76.

Boyt, W. P., Lovemore, D. F., Pilson, R. D. and Smith, I. D., 1963. *A Preliminary Report on the Maintenance of Cattle by Various Drugs in a mixed* Glossina morsitans *and* Glossina pallidipes *Fly-belt*. ISCTR, Publ. 88, vol. XI, pp. 71–9.

Boyt, W. P. and MacKenzie, P. K. I., 1970. A preliminary note on a virulent strain of *Trypanosoma vivax* in Rhodesia, *Rhod. vet. J.*, **1**: 57–62.

Braide, V. B. and Eghianruwa, K. I., 1980. Isometamidium residues in goat tissues after parenteral administration, *Res. vet. Sci.*, **29**: 111–13.

Brener, Z., 1973. Biology of *Trypanosoma cruzi, Ann. Rev. Microbiol.*, **27**: 347–82.

Brener, Z., 1976. Summarization. In *New Approaches in American Trypanosomiasis Research*, Proc. Int. Symp. Pan Am. Hlth Org., Sci. Publ. No. 318, pp. 403–10.

Brener, Z., 1979. Present status of chemotherapy and chemoprophylaxis of human trypanosomiasis in the western hemisphere, *Pharmac. Ther.*, **7**: 71–90.

Brener, Z., 1980. Immunity to *Trypanosoma cruzi*. In *Advances in Parasitology*, eds W. H. R. Lumsden, R. Muller, J. R. Baker. Academic Press (London), vol. 18, pp. 247–92.

Brohn, F. H. and Clarkson, A. B. Jr., 1980. *Trypanosoma brucei brucei*: patterns of glycolysis at 37 °C *in vitro, Mol. Biochem. Parasitol.*, **1**: 291–305.

Brown, L. A. and Losos, G. J., 1977. A comparative study of the responses of the thymus, spleen, lymph nodes and bone marrow of the albino rat to infection with *Trypanosoma congolense* and *Trypanosoma brucei, Res. vet. Sci.*, **23**: 196–203.

Brown, R. C., Evans, D. A. and Vickerman, K., 1973. Changes in oxidative metabolism and ultrastructure accompanying differentiation of the mitochondrion in *Trypanosoma brucei, Parasitology*, **3**: 691–704.

Brun, R., 1980. Hydroxyurea – effect on growth, structure and (^{3}H) thymidine uptake of *Trypanosoma brucei* procyclic culture forms, *J. Protozool.*, **27**(1): 122–8.

Brun, R., Jenni, M., Schonenberger, M. and Schell, K-F., 1981. *In vitro* cultivation of bloodstream forms of *Trypanosoma brucei,*

T. rhodesiense and *T. gambiense*, *J. Protozool.*, **28**(4): 470–9.

Brun, R. and Schonenberger, M., 1981. Stimulating effect of citrate and Cis-Aconitate on the transformation of *Trypanosoma brucei* bloodstream forms to procyclic forms *in vitro*, *Z. Parasitenkd.*, **66**: 17–24.

Bungener, W. and Mehlitz, D., 1976. Experimental *Trypanosoma* infections in Cameroon Dwarf goats: histopathological observations, *Z. Tropenmed. Parasit.*, **27**: 405–10.

Bungener, W. and Mehlitz, D., 1977. Extravascular localization of *Trypanosoma vivax* in cattle, *Z. Tropenmed. Parasit.*, **28**: 8–10.

Bungener, W. and Muller, G., 1976. Adherence phenomena in *Trypanosoma congolense*, *Z. Tropenmed. Parasit.*, **27**: 370–1.

Burger, J. F. and Thompson, F. C., 1981. The *Tabanus striatus* complex (*Diptera: tabanidae*): a revision of some oriental horse fly vectors of surra, *Proc. Entomol. Soc. Washington*, **83**(2): 339–58.

Burgess, D. E. and Hanson, W. L., 1979. Adoptive transfer of protection against *Trypanosoma cruzi* with lymphocytes and macrophages, *Infect. Immun.*, **25**(3): 838–43.

Burridge, M. J., Reid, H. W., Pullan, N. B., Sutherst, R. W. and Wain, E. B., 1970. Survey for trypanosome infections in domestic cattle and wild animals in areas of East Africa. II. Salivarian trypanosome infections in wild animals in Busoga District, Uganda, *Br. vet. J.*, **126**: 627–33.

Buyst, H., 1976. The treatment of congenital trypanosomiasis, *Trans. R. Soc. trop. Med. Hyg.*, **70**(2): 163–4.

Campbell, G. H., Esser, K. M., Wellde, B. T. and Diggs, C. L., 1979. Isolation and characterization of a new serodeme of *Trypanosoma rhodesiense*, *Am. J. Trop. Med. Hyg.*, **28**(6): 974–83.

Caporale, V. P., Battelli, G. and Semproni, G., 1980. Epidemiology of dourine in the equine population of the Abruzzi region, *Z. Vet. Med.*, **B27**: 489–98.

Carneiro, M. and Caldas, R. A., 1982. Evidence for three respiratory terminals in *Trypanosoma cruzi* epimastigotes, *Acta trop.*, **39**: 41–9.

Casero, R. A. Jr., Klayman, D. L., Childs, G. E., Scovill, J. P. and Desjardins, R. E., 1980. Activity of 2-acetylpyridine thiosemicarbazones against *Trypanosoma rhodesiense in vitro*, *Antimicrob. Agents Chemother.*, **18**(2): 317–22.

Castillo, A. M., 1962. Studies on Surra. II. Treatment with antrycide salts, *Philipp. J. Anim. Husb.*, **20**: 97–104.

Chand, K. and Singh, R. P., 1970. Therapeutic effect of Samorin in donkeys and dogs experimentally infected with *Trypanosoma evansi*, *Indian J. vet. Res.*, **47**: 475–9.

Chandler, R. L., 1952. Comparative tolerance of West African N'Dama cattle to trypanosomiasis, *Ann. trop. Med. Parasit.*, **46**: 127–34.

Chandler, R. L., 1958. Studies on the tolerance of N'Dama cattle to trypanosomiasis, *J. Comp. Path.*, **68**: 253–60.

Chaudhuri, R. P., Kumar, P. and Khan, M. H., 1965. Role of

stable-fly, *Stomoxys calcitrans*, in the transmission of surra in India, *Indian J. vet. Sci.*, **36**: 18–28.

Ciba Foundation, 1970. *Trypanosomiasis and Leishmaniasis with Special Reference to Chagas' Disease* (Ciba Foundation Symposium 20, new series). Associated Scientific Publishers (Amsterdam).

Clarkson, A. B. Jr., Grady, R. W., Grossman, S. A., McAllum, R. J. and Brohn, F. H., 1981. *Trypanosoma brucei brucei*: a systematic screening for alternatives to the salicylhydroxamic acid-glycerol combination, *Mol. Biochem. Parasitol.*, **3**: 271–91.

Clarkson, M. J., 1976a. Trypanosomiasis of domesticated animals of South America, *Trans. R. Soc. trop. Med. Hyg.*, **70**(2): 125–216.

Clarkson, M. J., 1976b. Trypanosomes, *Vet. Parasitol.*, **2**: 9–29.

Clarkson, M. J., 1976c. Immunoglobulin M in trypanosomiasis. In *Pathophysiology of Parasitic Infection*, ed. E. J. L. Soulsby. Academic Press (London), pp. 171–82.

Clarkson, M. J., Cottrell, B. A. and Enayat, M. S., 1971a. The indirect haemagglutination test in the study of *Trypanosoma vivax* infections of sheep, *Ann. Trop. Med. Parasitol.*, **65**(3): 335–40.

Clarkson, M. J., McCabe, W. and Colina, H. S., 1971b. Bovine trypanosomiasis in Venezuela, *Trans. R. Soc. trop. Med. Hyg.*, **65**: 275–6.

Clarkson, M. J., Penhale, W. J. and McKenna, R. B., 1975. Progressive serum protein changes in experimental infections of calves with *Trypanosoma vivax*, *J. Comp. Path.*, **85**: 397–410.

Clayton, C. E., 1978. *Trypanosoma brucei*: influence of host strain and parasite antigenic type on infections in mice, *Exp. Parasitol.*, **44**: 202–8.

Clayton, C. E., Sacks, D. L., Ogilvie, B. M. and Askonas, B. A., 1979. Membrane fractions of trypanosomes mimic the immunosuppressive and mitogenic effects of living parasites on the host, *Parasite Immunol.*, **1**: 241–9.

Collins, T. T., 1980. Dourine and the Downer mare (letter), *J. S. Afr. vet. Med. Ass.*, **51**: 201.

Cordingley, J. S. and Turner, M. J., 1980a. Isolation and characterization of polysomes from *Trypanosoma brucei*, *Parasitology*, **81**: 537–51.

Cordingley, J. S. and Turner, M. J., 1980b. 6.5 S RNA; preliminary characterisation of unusual small RNAs in *Trypanosoma brucei*, *Mol. Biochem. Parasitol.*, **1**: 91–6.

Corsini, A. C., Clayton, C., Askonas, B. A. and Ogilvie, B. M., 1977. Suppressor cells and loss of B-cell potential in mice infected with *Trypanosoma brucei*, *Clin. Exp. Immunol.*, **29**: 122–31.

Cossio, P. M., Laguens, R. P., Diez, C., Szarfman, A., Segal, A. and Arana, R. M., 1974. Chagasic cardiopathy. Antibodies reacting with plasma membrane of striated muscle and endothelial cells, *Circulation*, **50**: 1252–9.

Creemers, P. C., 1972a. Counting methods for low concentrations of trypanosomes in the blood. I. Drop method, *Exp. Parasitol.*, **32**(3): 343–7.

Creemers, P. C., 1972b. Counting methods for low concentrations of trypanosomes in blood. II. Accuracy of the indirect method, *Exp. Parasitol.*, **32**: 348–58.

Cross, G. A. M., 1978. Antigenic variation in trypanosomes, *Proc. R. Soc. Lond.*, **B202**: 55–72.

Cross, G. A. M., 1979. Immunochemical aspects of antigenic variation on trypanosomes. The third Fleming lecture, *J. Gen. Microbiol.*, **113**: 1–11.

Cross, G. A. M., Holder, A. A., Allen, G. and Boothroyd, J. C., 1980. An introduction to antigenic variation in trypanosomes, *Am. J. Trop. Med. Hyg.*, **29**(5) suppl.: 1027–32.

Cross, G. A. M. and Manning, J. C., 1973. Cultivation of *Trypanosoma brucei* spp. in semi-defined and defined media, *Parasitology*, **67**: 315–31.

Cunningham, I., 1973. Quantitative studies on trypanosomes in tsetse tissue culture, *Exp. Parasitol.*, **33**: 34–45.

Cunningham, I., 1977. New culture medium for maintenance of tsetse tissues and growth of Trypanosomatids, *J. Protozool.*, **24**(2): 325–9.

Cunningham, I. and Honigberg, B. M., 1977. Infectivity reacquisition by *Trypanosoma brucei brucei* cultivated with tsetse salivary glands, *Science*, **197**: 1279–82.

Cunningham, I., Honigberg, B. M. and Taylor, A. M., 1981. Infectivity of monomorphic and pleomorphic *Trypanosoma brucei* stocks cultivated at 28 °C with various tsetse-fly tissues, *J. Parasitol.*, **67**(3): 391–7.

Cunningham, I. and Taylor, A. M., 1979. Infectivity of *Trypanosoma brucei* cultivation at 28 °C with tsetse-fly salivary glands, *J. Protozool.*, **26**(3): 428–32.

Curd, F. H. S. and Davey, D. G., 1950. 'Antrycide' – a new trypanocidal drug, *Br. J. Pharmac. Chemother.*, **5**: 25–32.

D'Alesandro, P. A., 1976. Biology of *Trypanosoma* (*Herpetosoma*) *rangeli* Tejera, 1920. In *Biology of the Kinetoplastida*, eds W. H. R. Lumsden, D. A. Evans. Academic Press (London), vol. 1, pp. 328–93.

D'Alesandro, P. A., 1979. Rodent trypanosomiasis. In *Pathogenicity of Trypanosomes*, eds G. J. Losos, A. Chouinard. IDRC (Ottawa), **132e**, pp. 63–70.

Dalgliesh, R. J., 1972. Theoretical and practical aspects of freezing parasitic protozoa, *Aust. vet. J.*, **48**: 233–9.

Dar, F. K., Paris, J. and Wilson, A. J., 1973b. Serologic studies on trypanosomiasis in East Africa. IV. Comparison of antigenic types of *Trypanosoma vivax* group organisms, *Ann. trop. Med. Parasit.*, **67**(3): 319–29.

Dar, F. K., Wilson, A. J., Goedbloed, E., Ligthart, G. S. and Minter, D. M., 1973a. Serological studies on trypanosomiasis in East Africa. I. Introduction and techniques, *Ann. trop. Med. Parasit.*, **67**(1): 21–9.

Dargie, J. D., 1979. Effects of *Trypanosoma congolense* and *Trypanosoma brucei* on the circulatory volumes of cattle. In *Pathogenicity of Trypanosomes*, eds G. J. Losos, A. Chouinard. IDRC (Ottawa), **132e**, pp. 140–4.

Dargie, J. D., Murray, P. K., Murray, M., Grimshaw, W. and McIntyre, W. I. M., 1979a. Bovine trypanosomiasis: red cell kinetics of Ndama and Zebu cattle infected with *Trypanosoma congolense*, *Parasitology*, **78**: 271–86.

Dargie, J. D., Murray, P. K., Murray, M. and McIntyre, W. I. M., 1979b. The blood volumes and erythrokinetics of Ndama and Zebu cattle experimentally infected with *Trypanosoma brucei*, *Res. vet. Sci.*, **26**: 245–7.

Davey, D. G., 1957. The chemotherapy of animal trypanosomiasis with particular reference to the trypanosomal diseases of domestic animals in Africa, *Vet. Revs.*, **3**: 15–36.

Davis, C. E., Robbins, R. S., Weller, R. D. and Braude, A. I., 1974. Thrombocytopenia in experimental trypanosomiasis, *J. Clin. Invest.*, **53**: 1359–67.

Davis, D. S., Russell, L. H., Adams, L. G., Yaeger, R. G. and Robinson, R. M., 1980. An experimental infection of *Trypanosoma cruzi* in striped skunks (*Mephitis mephitis*), *J. Wildl. Dis.*, **16**(3): 403–6.

De Gee, A. L. W., Ige, K. and Leeflang, P., 1976. Studies on *Trypanosoma vivax*: transmission of mouse infective *Trypanosoma vivax* by tsetse flies, *Int. J. Parasitol.*, **6**: 419–21.

De Gee, A. L. W. and Rovis, L., 1981. *Trypanosoma vivax*: absence of host protein on the surface coat, *Exp. Parasitol.*, **51**: 124–32.

De Gee, A. L. W., Shah, S. D. and Doyle, J. J., 1979. *Trypanosoma vivax*: sequence of antigenic variance in mice and goats, *Exp. Parasi*[tol.,] **48**: 352–8.

De Gee, A. L. W., Shah, S. D. and Doyle, J. J., 1981. *Trypanosoma vivax*: host influence on appearance of variable antigen types, *Exp. Parasitol.* **51**: 392–9.

de Jesus, Z., 1951. Studies on the control of Surra. V. Experiments on Surra transmission, *Nat. appl. Sci. Bull. Univ. Philipp.*, **11**: 191–207.

de Jesus, Z., 1962. Resistance of *Trypanosoma evansi* determined by its relative viability in surra blood and meat, *Philipp. J. Vet. Med.*, **1**: 3–9.

Deom, J., 1960. *Outline Report on the Evolution of Trypanosomiasis in the Belgian Congo. Excerpts from 1959 and 1958 Annual Reports of the Ruanda-Urundi Veterinary Services*. ISCTR, vol. VIII, 15 pp.

Desjardins, R. E., Casero, R. A. Jr, Willett, G. P., Childs, G. E. and Canfield, C. J., 1980. *Trypanosoma rhodesiense*: semi-automated microtesting for quantitation of antitrypanosomal activity *in vitro*, *Exp. Parasitol.*, **50**: 260–71.

Desowitz, R. S., 1957. Suramin complexes. II. Prophylactic activity against *Trypanosoma vivax* in cattle, *Ann. trop. Med. Parasitol.*, **51**: 457–63.

Desowitz, R. S., 1959. Studies on immunity and host–parasite relationships. I. The immunological response of resistant and susceptible breeds of cattle to trypanosomal challenge, *Ann. trop. Med. Parasitol.*, **53**: 293–313.

Desowitz, R. S., 1963. Adaptation of trypanosomes to abnormal hosts, *Ann. N.Y. Acad. Sci.*, **113**: 74–87.

Desowitz, R. S., 1970. African trypanosomes. In *Immunity to Parasitic Animals*, eds G. A. Jackson, R. Herman, I. Singer. Appleton-Century-Crofts (New York), vol. 2, pp. 551–96.

Desowitz, R. S. and Watson, H. J. C., 1951. Studies on *Trypanosoma vivax*. I. Susceptibility of white rats to infection, *Ann. trop. Med. Parasitol.*, **45**: 207–19.

Desowitz, R. S. and Watson, H. J. C., 1952. Studies on *Trypanosoma vivax*. III. Observations on the maintenance of a strain in white rats, *Ann. trop. Med. Parasitol.*, **46**: 92–100.

Devignat, R. and Dresse, A., 1955. Micro-technique simple et rapide de concentration du sang en trypanosomes, *Ann. Soc. Belge. Méd. Trop. Parasitol. Mycol. Hum. Anim.*, **35**: 315–21.

D'hondt, J. and Kondo, M., 1980. Carbohydrate alters the trypanocidal activity of normal human serum with *Trypanosoma brucei*, *Mol. Biochem. Parasitol.*, **2**: 113–21.

Diamond, L. S. and Rubin, R., 1958. Experimental infection of certain farm mammals with a North American strain of *Trypanosoma cruzi* from the raccoon, *Exp. Parasitol.*, **7**: 383–90.

Diehl, E. J. and Risby, E. L., 1974. Serum changes in rabbits experimentally infected with *Trypanosoma gambiense*, *Am. J. Trop. Med. Hyg.*, **23**(6): 1019–22.

Diffley, P., Strickler, J. E., Patton, C. L. and Waksman, H., 1980. Detection and quantification of variant specific antigen in the plasma of rats and mice infected with *Trypanosoma brucei brucei*, *J. Parasitol.*, **66**(2): 185–91.

Dixon, J. B., Cull, R. S., Dunbar, I. F., Greenhill, R. J., Grimshaw, C. G., Hill, M. A., Landeg, F. J. and Miller, W. M., 1971. Non-cyclical transmission of trypanosomiasis in Uganda. II. Experimental assessment of the survival time of *Trypanosoma brucei* in *Stomoxys calcitrans*, *Vet. Rec.*, **89**: 233–5.

Doyle, J. J., 1977. Antigenic variation in the Salivarian trypanosomes. In *Immunity to Blood Parasites of Animals and Man*, eds L. H. Miller, J. A. Pino, J. J. McKelvey Jr. Plenum Press (New York), pp. 31–64.

Doyle, J. J., Hirumi, H., Hirumi, K., Lupton, E. N. and Cross, G. A. M., 1980. Antigenic variation in clones of animal-infective *Trypanosoma brucei* derived and maintained *in vitro*, *Parasitology*, **80**: 359–69.

Dräger, N. and Mehlitz, D., 1978. Investigations on the prevalence of trypanosome carriers and the antibody response in wildlife in northern Botswana, *Z. Tropenmed. Parasit.*, **29**: 223–33.

Duxbury, R. E., Anderson, J. S., Wellde, B. T., Sadun, E. H. and Muriithi, I. E., 1972. *Trypanosoma congolense*: immunization of mice, dogs and cattle with gamma-irradiated parasites, *Exp. Parasitol.*, **32**(3): 527–33.

Dvorak, J. A. and Howe, C. L., 1976. The attraction of *Trypanosoma cruzi* to vertebrate cells *in vitro, J. Protozool.*, **23**(4): 534–7.

Eardley, D. D. and Jayawardena, A. N., 1977. Suppressor cells in mice infected with *Trypanosoma brucei, J. Immun.*, **119**(3): 1029–33.

Edwards, E. E., Judd, J. M. and Squire, F. A., 1956a. Observations on trypanosomiasis in domestic animals in West Africa. I. The daily index of infection and the weekly haematological values in goats and sheep infected with *Trypanosoma vivax, T. congolense,* and *T. brucei, Ann. trop. Med. Parasit.*, **50**: 223–41.

Edwards, E. E., Judd, J. M. and Squire, F. A., 1956b. Observations on trypanosomiasis in domestic animals in West Africa. II. The effect on erythrocyte sedimentation rate, plasma protein, bilirubin, blood sugar, red cell osmotic fragility, body weight and temperature in goats and sheep infected with *Trypanosoma vivax, T. congolense* and *T. brucei, Ann. trop. Med. Parasit.*, **50**: 242–51.

Ellis, D. S., Evans, D. A., Ormerod, W. E., Holland, M. F. and Stamford, S., 1980. Preliminary observations on the infectivity of slender forms of *Trypanosoma brucei rhodesiense* to *Glossina morsitans morsitans, Trans. R. Soc. trop. Med. Hyg.*, **74**(1): 131–2.

Emery, D. L., Barry, J. D. and Moloo, S. K., 1980. Appearance of *Trypanosoma* (*Duttonella*) *vivax* in lymph following challenge of goats with infected *Glossina morsitans morsitans, Acta trop.*, **37**: 375–9.

Emery, D. L. and Moloo, S. K., 1981. The dynamics of the cellular reactions elicited in the skin of goats by *Glossina morsitans morsitans* infected with *Trypanosoma* (*Nannomonas*) *congolense* or *T.* (*Duttonella*) *vivax, Acta trop.*, **38**: 15–28.

Essien, E. M. and Ikede, B. O., 1976. Coagulation defect in experimental trypanosomial infection, *Haemostasis*, **5**: 341–7.

Esuoroso, W., 1974. The epizootiology, prevalence and economic aspects of bovine trypanosomiasis in Nigeria, *Proc. Ann. Meet. USAHA*, **77**: 160–75.

Evans, D. A., 1979. Cyclical transmission of *Trypanosoma brucei rhodesiense* and *Trypanosoma congolense* by tsetse-flies infected with culture-form procyclic trypanosomes, *J. Protozool.*, **26**(3): 425–7.

Evans, D. A. and Brightman, C. A., 1980. Pleomorphism and the problem of recrudescent parasitaemia following treatment with salicylhydroxamic acid (SHAM) in African trypanosomiasis, *Trans. R. Soc. trop. Med. Hyg.*, **74**(5): 601–4.

Evans, D. A. and Ellis, D. S., 1975. Penetration of mid-gut cells of *Glossina morsitans morsitans* by *Trypanosoma brucei rhodesiense, Nature*, **258**: 231–3.

Evans, J. T. R., 1956. Control of animal trypanosomiasis in Sudan. Conference on the use of drugs for the control of animal trypanosomiasis. TFTC (cc). Colonial Office (London), No. 50., 17 pp.

Facer, C. A., 1976. Blood hyperviscosity during *Trypanosoma (Trypanozoon) brucei* infections of rabbits, *J. Comp. Path.*, **86**: 393–407.

Facer, C. A., Molland, E. A., Gray, A. B. and Jenkins, G. C., 1978. *Trypanosoma brucei*: renal pathology in rabbits, *Exp. Parasitol.*, **44**: 249–61.

Fairbain, H. and Godfrey, D. G., 1957. The local reaction in man at site of infection with *Trypanosoma rhodesiense, Am. trop. Med. Parasit.*, **51**: 464–70.

Fairlamb, A. H. and Bowman, I. B. R., 1980a. An improved method for the estimation of suramin in plasma and *Trypanosoma* samples, *Mol. Biochem. Parasitol.*, **1**: 307–13.

Fairlamb, A. H. and Bowman, I. B. R., 1980b. *Trypanosoma brucei*: maintenance of concentrated suspensions of bloodstream trypomastigotes *in vitro* using continuous dialysis for measurement of endocytosis, *Exp. Parasitol.*, **49**: 366–80.

Fairlamb, A. H. and Bowman, I. B. R., 1980c. Uptake of the trypanocidal drug suramin by bloodstream forms of *Trypanosoma brucei* and its effect on respiration and growth rate *in vivo, Mol. Biochem. Parasitol.*, **1**: 315–33.

Falk, E., Akinrimisi, E. O. and Onoagbe, I., 1980. Malete dehydrogenase in African trypanosomes. I. Preliminary studies with *T. brucei, Int. J. Biochem.*, **12**: 647–50.

Fantham, H. G., 1911. The life-history of *Trypanosoma gambiense* and *Trypanosoma rhodesiense* as seen in rats and guinea pigs, *Proc. R. Soc. Lond.*, **83**: 212–34.

FAO/UNDP, 1977. *Expert Consultation on the Economics of Trypanosomiases*. FAO (Rome), W/L 5740.

Fernandez, D. B., Dumog, P. U. and Rico, F., 1965. Observations on an outbreak of Surra among cattle, *Philipp. J. Anim. Ind.*, **21**: 221–4.

Fiennes, R. N. T-W., 1950. The cattle trypanosomiases. Some considerations of pathology and immunity, *Ann. trop. Med. Parasit.*, **44**: 42–54.

Fiennes, R. N. T-W., 1970. Pathogenesis and pathology of animal trypanosomiases. In *The African Trypanosomiases*, ed. H. W. Mulligan. George Allen & Unwin (London), pp. 729–50.

Fiennes, R. N. T-W., Jones, E. R. and Laws, S. G., 1946. The course and pathology of *Trypanosoma congolense* (Broden) disease of cattle, *J. Comp. Path.*, **56**: 1–27.

Fife, E. H. Jr., 1978. *Trypanosoma (Schizotrypanum) cruzi*. In *Parasite Protozoa*, ed. J. P. Kreier. Academic Press (New York), vol. IV, pp. 135–73.

Finelle, P., 1974. African animal trypanosomiasis economic problems, *Wld Anim. Rev.*, **10**: 15–18.

Finelle, P., 1976. *Geographic Distribution and Incidence of Animal Trypanosomiasis*. Joint WHO/FAO Exp. Comm., AGA: Tryp/WP/76.30, 1–13.

Fink, E. and Schmidt, H., 1979. Meningoencephalitis in chronic

Trypanosoma brucei rhodesiense infection of the white mouse, *Z. Tropenmed. Parasit.*, **30**: 206–11.

Flynn, I. W. and Bowman, I. B. R., 1980. Purification and characterization of pyruvate kinase from *Trypanosoma brucei, Arch. Biochem. Biophys.*, **200**(2): 401–9.

Ford, E. J. H., Karib, A. A. and Wilmshurst, E. C., 1953a. Studies on Ethidium bromide. I. The treatment of early *Trypanosoma vivax* infection in cattle, *Vet. Rec.*, **65**: 589–90.

Ford, E. J. H. Karib, A. A. and Wilmshurst, E. C., 1953b. Studies on Ethidium bromide. II. The treatment of *Trypanosoma congolense* infections in cattle, *Vet. Rec.*, **65**: 907–8.

Ford, J., 1971. *The Role of Trypanosomiases in African Ecology. A Study of the Tsetse Fly Problem.* Clarendon Press (Oxford).

Forsberg, C. M., Valli, V. E. O., Gentry, P. W. and Donworth, R. M., 1979. The pathogenesis of *Trypanosoma congolense* infection in calves. IV. The kinetics of blood coagulation, *Vet. Pathol.*, **16**: 229–42.

Fussganger, R. and Bauer, F., 1958. Berenil ein neues chemotherapeuticum in der Veterinarmedizin, *Med. Chem.*, **6**: 504–31.

Gardiner, P. R., Jones, T. W., and Cunningham, I., 1980b. Antigenic analysis by immunofluorescence of *in vitro*-produced metacyclics of *Trypanosoma brucei* and their infections in mice, *J. Protozool.*, **27**(3): 316–20.

Gardiner, P. R., Lamont, L. C., Jones, T. W. and Cunningham, I., 1980a. The separation and structure of infective trypanosomes from cultures of *Trypanosoma brucei* grown in association with tsetse-fly salivary glands, *J. Protozool.*, **27**(2): 182–5.

Gasbarre, L. C., Hug, K. and Louis, J. A., 1980. Murine T-lymphocyte specificity for African trypanosomes. I. Induction of a T-lymphocyte-dependent proliferative response to *Trypanosoma brucei, Clin. Exp. Immunol.*, **41**: 97–106.

Gasbarre, L. C., Hug, K. and Louis, J., 1981. Murine T lymphocyte specificity for African trypanosomes. II. Suppression of the T-lymphocyte proliferative response to *Trypanosoma brucei* by systemic trypanosome infection, *Clin. Exp. Immunol.*, **45**: 165–72.

Gbenle, G. O. and Akinrimisi, E. O., 1981. Isolation of partial characterization of a calcium-dependent endoribonuclease of *Trypanosoma brucei* cytoplasm, *Biochem. Int.*, **2**(2): 219–28.

Geigy, R., Mwambu, P. M. and Kauffman, M., 1971. Sleeping sickness survey in Musoma district, Tanzania. IV. Examination of wild mammals as a potential reservoir for *Trypanosoma rhodesiense, Acta trop.*, **28**: 211–20.

Ghiotto, V., Brun, R., Jenni, L. and Hecker, H., 1979. *Trypanosoma brucei*: morphometric changes and loss of infectivity during transformation of bloodstream forms to procyclic culture forms *in vitro, Exp. Parasitol.*, **48**: 447–56.

Gibson, W. C., Marshall, T. F. de C. and Godfrey, D. G., 1980. Numerical analysis of enzyme polymorphism – a new approach to the epidemiology and taxonomy of trypanosomes from the subgenus *Trypanozoon*. In *Advances in Parasitology*, eds W. H. R. Lumsden, R. Muller, J. R. Baker. Academic Press (London), vol. 18, pp. 175–239.

Gibson, W., Mehlitz, W., Lanham, S. M. and Godfrey, D. G., 1978. The identification of *Trypanosoma brucei gambiense* in Liberian pigs and dogs by isoenzymes and by resistance to human plasma, *Z. Tropenmed. Parasit.*, **29**: 335–45.

Gidel, R. and Leporte, F., 1962. Etude électrophorétique quantitative en gélose des protéines seriques de bovins, *Rev. Elev. Méd. vét. Pays trop.*, **15**: 279.

Gill, B. S., 1972. Studies on Surra. IX. Prophylactic activity of quinapyramine, Suramin, and MSb. against *Trypanosoma evansi* infection in equines, *Indian J. Anim. Sci.*, **42**: 385–8.

Gill, B. S. and Malhotra, M. N., 1971. Chemoprophylaxis of *Trypanosoma evansi* infections in ponies, *Trop. Anim. Hlth Prod.*, **3**: 199–202.

Gláz, E.T., 1978. Effect of low molecular weight interferon inducers on *Trypanosoma equiperdum* infection of mice, *Ann. trop. Med. Parasit.*, **73**(1): 83–4.

Gobel, E. and Dennig, H. K., 1981. *Trypanosoma evansi*: micromorphological and biological behaviour before and after Berenil-exposition, *Berl. Münch. Tierarztl. Wschr.*, **94**: 241–6..

Goble, F. C., 1952. Observations on experimental Chagas' disease in dogs, *Am. J. Trop. Med. Hyg.*, **1**: 189–204.

Goble, F. C., 1970. South American trypanosomes. In *Immunity to Parasitic Animals*, eds G. A. Jackson, R. Herman, I. Singer. Appleton-Century-Crofts (New York), pp. 597–689.

Godfrey, D. G., 1960. Types of *Trypanosoma congolense*. I. Morphological differences, *Ann. trop. Med. Parasit.*, **54**: 428–38.

Godfrey, D. G., 1961. Types of *Trypanosoma congolense*. II. Differences in the courses of infection, *Ann. trop. Med. Parasit.*, **55**: 154–66.

Godfrey, D. G., 1977. Problems in distinguishing between the morphologically similar trypanosomes of mammals, *Protozoology*, **3**: 33–49.

Godfrey, D. G. and Kilgour, V., 1976. Enzyme electrophoresis in characterizing the causative organism of Gambian trypanosomiasis, *Trans. R. Soc. trop. Med. Hyg.*, **70**(3): 219–24.

Godfrey, D. G. and Killick-Kendrick, R., 1962. *Trypanosoma evansi* of camels in Nigeria: a high incidence demonstrated by the inoculation of blood into rats, *Ann. trop. Med. Parasit.*, **56**(1): 14–19.

Godfrey, D. G., Killick-Kendrick, R. and Ferguson, W., 1965. Bovine trypanosomiasis in Nigeria. IV. Observations on cattle trekked along a trade-cattle route through areas infested with tsetse-fly, *Ann. trop. Med. Parasit.*, **59**(3): 255–69.

Godfrey, D. G. and Lanham, S. M., 1971. Diagnosis of Gambian trypanosomiasis in man by isolating trypanosomes from blood passed through DEAE-Cellulose, *Bull. Wld Hlth Org.*, **45**: 13–19.

Goedbloed, E., Ligthart, F. K., Minter, D. M., Wilson, A. J., Dar, F. K. and Paris, J., 1973. Serological studies of trypanosomiasis in East Africa. II. Comparison of antigenic types of *Trypanosoma brucei* subgroup organisms isolated from wild tsetse flies, *Ann. trop. Med. Parasit.*, **67**(1): 31–43.

Goodwin, L. G., 1970. The pathology of African trypanosomiasis, *Trans. R. Soc. trop. Med. Hyg.*, **64**: 797–817.

Goodwin, L. G., 1971. Pathological effects of *Trypanosoma brucei* on small blood vessels in rabbit ear-chambers, *Trans. R. Soc. trop. Med. Hyg.*, **65**(1): 82–8.

Goodwin, L. G., 1978. Pharmacy and World Organization special programme, *Pharmaceut. J.*, **221**: 365–6.

Goodwin, L. G. and Guy, M. W., 1973. Tissue fluids in rabbits infected with *Trypanosoma* (*Trypanozoon*) *brucei*, *Parasitology*, **66**: 499–513.

Goodwin, L. G., Guy, M. W. and Brooker, B. E., 1973. Connective tissue changes in rabbits infected with *Trypanosoma* (*Trypanozoon*) *brucei*, *Parasitology*, **67**: 115–22.

Gordon, R. M., Crew, W. and Willett, K. C., 1956. Studies on the deposition, migration and development of the blood forms of trypanosomes belonging to the *Trypanosoma brucei* group. I. An account of the process of feeding adopted by the tsetse-fly when obtaining a blood-meal from the mammalian host, with special reference to the ejection of saliva and the relationship of the feeding process to deposition of the metacyclic trypanosomes, *Ann. trop. Med. Parasit.*, **50**: 426–37.

Gordon, R. M. and Willett, K. C., 1958. Studies on the deposition, migration, and development of the blood forms of trypanosomes belonging to the *Trypanosoma brucei* group. III. The development of *Trypanosoma rhodesiense* from the metacyclic forms, as observed in mammalian tissue and in culture, *Ann. trop. Med. Parasit.*, **52**: 346–65.

Gray, A. R., 1965. Antigenic variation in a strain of *Trypanosoma brucei* transmitted by *Glossina morsitans* and *G. palpalis*, *J. Gen. Microbiol.*, **44**: 195–214.

Gray, A. R., 1966. The antigenic relationship of strains of *Trypanosoma brucei* isolated in Nigeria, *J. Gen. Microbiol.*, **44**: 263–71.

Gray, A. R., 1967. Some principles on immunology of trypanosomiasis, *Bull. Wld Hlth Org.*, **37**: 177–93.

Gray, A. R., 1970. A study of the antigenic relationships of isolates of *Trypanosoma brucei* collected from a herd of cattle kept in one locality for five years, *J. Gen. Microbiol.*, **62**: 301–13.

Gray, A. R. and Luckins, A. G., 1976. Antigenic variation in Salivarian trypanosomes. In *Biology of the Kinetoplastida*, eds W. H. R. Lumsden, D. A. Evans. Academic Press (London), pp. 493–542.

Gray, A. R. and Luckins, A. G., 1980. The initial stage of infection with cyclically transmitted *Trypanosoma congolense* in rabbits,

calves and sheep, *J. Comp. Path.*, **90**: 499–512.
Gray, A. R. and Roberts, C. J., 1971. The cyclical transmission of strains of *Trypanosoma congolense* and *Trypanosoma vivax* resistant to normal therapeutic doses of trypanocidal drugs, *Parasitology*, **63**: 67–89.
Gray, M. A., Brown, C. G. D., Luckins, A. G. and Gray, A. R., 1979. Maintenance of infectivity of *Trypanosoma congolense in vitro* with explants of infected skin at 37 °C, *Trans. R. Soc. trop. Med. Hyg.*, **73**(4): 406–8.
Gray, M. A., Cunningham, I., Gardiner, P. R., Taylor, A. M. and Luckins, A. G., 1981. Cultivation of infective forms of *Trypanosoma congolense* from trypanosomes in the proboscis of *Glossina morsitans*, *Parasitology*, **82**: 81–95.
Greenwood, B. M. and Whittle, H. C., 1980. The pathogenesis of sleeping sickness, *Trans. R. Soc. trop. Med. Hyg.*, **74**(6): 716–25.
Greer, C. A., Cain, G. D. and Schottelius, B. A., 1979. Changes in vascular smooth muscle contractility associated with *Trypanosoma brucei* infections in rats, *J. Parasitol.*, **65**(5): 825–7.
Greig, W. A., Murray, M., Murray, P. K. and McIntyre, W. M., 1979. Factors affecting blood sampling for anaemia and parasitaemia in bovine trypanosomiasis, *Br. vet. J.*, **135**: 130–41.
Griffin, L. and Allonby, E. W., 1979a. Studies on the epidemiology of trypanosomiasis of sheep and goats in Kenya, *Trop. Anim. Hlth Prod.*, **11**: 133–42.
Griffin, L. and Allonby, E. W., 1979b. The economic effects of trypanosomiasis in sheep and goats at a range research station in Kenya, *Trop. Anim. Hlth Prod.*, **11**: 127–132.
Griffin, L. and Allonby, E. W., 1979c. Trypanotolerance in breeds of sheep and goats with an experimental infection of *Trypanosoma congolense*, *Vet. Parasitol.*, **5**: 97–105.
Griffin, L. and Allonby, E. W., 1979d. Disease syndromes in sheep and goats naturally infected with *Trypanosoma congolense*, *J. Comp. Path.*, **89**: 457–64.
Griffin, L., Allonby, E. W. and Preston, J. M., 1981b. The interaction of *Trypanosoma congolense* and *Haemonchus contortus* infections in two breeds of goat. 1. Parasitology, *J. Comp. Path.*, **91**: 85–95.
Griffin, L., Aucutt, M., Allonby, E. W., Preston, J. and Castelino, J., 1981a. The interaction of *Trypanosoma congolense* and *Haemonchus contortus* infections in 2 breeds of goat. 2. Haematology, *J. Comp. Path.*, **91**: 97–103.
Griffin, L., Waghela, S. and Allonby, E. W., 1980. The immunosuppressive effects of experimental *T. congolense* infections in goats, *Vet. Parasitol.*, **7**: 11–18.
Grosskinsky, C. M. and Askonas, B. A., 1981. Macrophages as primary target cells and mediators of immune dysfunction in African trypanosomiasis, *Infect. Immun.*, **33**(1): 149–55.
Gruvel, J. and Balis, J., 1965. *Trypanosoma evansi* infection of camels in the Chad Republic, principal vectors, *Rev. Elev. Méd. vét. Pays trop.*, **18**: 435–9.

Gutteridge, W. E., 1981. *Trypanosoma cruzi*: recent biochemical advances, *Trans. R. Soc. trop. Med. Hyg.*, **75**(4): 484–92.
Gutteridge, W. E. and Rogerson, G. W., 1979. Biochemical aspects of the biology of *Trypanosoma cruzi*. In *Biology of the Kinetoplastida*, eds W. H. R. Lumsden, D. A. Evans. Academic Press (London), vol. 2, pp. 620–82.

Haase, M., Bernard, S. and Guidot, G., 1980. Trypanosomiasis of cattle in Upper Volta – epizootiological investigations and a contribution to the problem of trypanotolerance. I. Studies concerning the incidence of trypanosomiasis and the application of trypanocide medicine, *Berl. Münch. Tierarztl. Wschr.*, **93**(20): 400–2.
Hadaway, A. B., 1977. The role of laboratory testing of insecticides for tsetse fly control. The relevance of laboratory studies to tsetse control, *Trans. R. Soc. trop. Med Hyg.*, **71**: 6–7.
Hajduk, S. and Vickerman, K., 1981. Antigenic differentiation of *Trypanosoma brucei*: studies on metacyclic and first parasitemia populations, *Trans. R. Soc. trop. Med. Hyg.*, **75**(1): 145–6.
Hambrey, P. N., Tizard, I. R. and Mellors, A., 1980. Accumulation of phospholipase A_1 in tissue fluid of rabbits infected with *Trypanosoma brucei*, *Z. Tropenmed. Parasit.*, **31**: 439–43.
Hammond, D. J. and Bowman, I. B. R., 1980a. *Trypanosoma brucei*: the effect of glycerol on the anaerobic metabolism glucose, *Mol. Biochem. Parasitol.*, **2**: 63–75.
Hammond, D. J. and Bowman, I. B. R., 1980b. Studies on glycerol kinase and its role in ATP synthesis in *Trypanosoma brucei*, *Mol. Biochem. Parasitol.*, **2**: 77–91.
Hanson, W. L., 1976. Immunology of American trypanosomiasis (Chagas' disease). In *Immunology of Parasitic Infections*, eds S. Cohen, E. Sadun. Blackwell Scientific Publications (London), pp. 222–34.
Hanson, W. L., 1977. Experiments on immunoprophylaxis against Chagas' disease. In *Immunity to Blood Parasites of Animals and Man*, eds L. H. Miller, J. A. Pino, J. J. McKelvey Jr. Plenum Press (New York), pp. 281–3.
Hanson, W. L. and Robertson, E. L., 1974. Density of parasites in various organs and the relation to numbers of trypomastigotes in the blood during acute infections of *Trypanosoma cruzi* in mice, *J. Protozool.*, **21**: 512–17.
Hawking, F., 1966. Chemotherapy of trypanosomiasis. In *Experimental Chemotherapy*, eds R. J. Schnitzer, F. Hawking. Academic Press (New York), vol. IV, pp. 398–417.
Hawking, F., 1973. The differentiation of *Trypanosoma rhodesiense* from *Trypanosoma brucei* by means of human serum, *Trans. R. Soc. trop. Med. Hyg.*, **67**(4): 517–27.
Hawking, F., 1975. Circadian and other rhythms of parasites, *Adv. Parasitol.*, **13**: 123–82.

Hawking, F., 1976a. The resistance to human plasma of *Trypanosoma brucei, T. rhodesiense* and *T. gambiense*. I. Analysis of the composition of trypanosome strains, *Trans. R. Soc. trop. Med. Hyg.*, **70**(5/6): 504–12.

Hawking, F., 1976b. The resistance to human plasma of *Trypanosoma brucei, T. rhodesiense* and *T. gambiense*. II. Survey of strains from East Africa and Nigeria, *Trans. R. Soc. trop. Med. Hyg.*, **70**: 513–20.

Hawking, F., 1977. The resistance to human plasma of *Trypanosoma brucei, T. rhodesiense* and *T. gambiense*. III. Clones of two plasma-resistant strains, *Trans. R. Soc. trop. Med. Hyg.*, **71**(5): 427–30.

Hawking, F., 1978a. Circadian rhythms of *Trypanosoma congolense* in laboratory rodents, *Trans. R. Soc. trop. Med. Hyg.*, **72**(6): 592–5.

Hawking, F., 1978b. The resistance of *Trypanosoma congolense, T. vivax* and *T. evansi* to human plasma, *Trans. R. Soc. trop. Med. Hyg.*, **72**(4): 405–7.

Hawking, F., 1979. The action of human serum upon *Trypanosoma brucei*, *Protozool. Abstr.*, **3**(7): 199–206.

Hecker, H., Burri, P. H. and Bohringer, S., 1973. Quantitative ultrastructural differences in the mitochondrium of pleomorphic bloodforms of *Trypanosoma brucei*, *Experientia*, **29**: 901–3.

Hecker, H., Burri, P. H., Steiger, R. and Geigy, R., 1972. Morphometric data on the ultrastructure of the pleomorphic bloodforms of *Trypanosoma brucei*, Plimmer and Bradford, 1899, *Acta trop.*, **29**(2): 182–98.

Heisch, R. B., Killick-Kendrick, R., Guy, M. W. and Dorrell, J., 1970. The development of trypanosomes. *Leishmaniae* and ascitic tumour cells in the testicles of laboratory animals, *Trans. R. Soc. trop. Med. Hyg.*, **64**(5): 679–82.

Henriquez, D., Piras, R. and Piras, M. M., 1981. The effect of surface membrane modifications of fibroblastic cells on the entry process of *Trypanosoma cruzi* trypomastigotes, *Mol. Biochem. Parasitol.*, **2**: 359–66.

Henson, J. B. and Noel, J. C., 1979. Immunology and pathogenesis of African animal trypanosomiasis, *Adv. Vet. Sci. Comp. Med.*, **23**: 161–82.

Herbert, W. J. and Lumsden, W. H. R., 1976. *Trypanosoma brucei*: a rapid 'matching' method for estimating the host's parasitemia, *Exp. Parasitol.*, **40**: 427–31.

Herbert, W. J. and Parratt, D., 1979. Virulence of trypanosomes in vertebrate host. In *Biology of Kinetoplastida*, eds W. H. R. Lumsden, D. A. Evans. Academic Press (London), vol. 2, pp. 481–522.

Hill, G. C., Shimer, S. P., Caughey, B. and Sauer, L. S., 1978. Growth of infective forms of *Trypanosoma rhodesiense in vitro*, the causative agent of African trypanosomiasis, *Science*, **202**: 763–5.

Hirumi, H., 1979. Cultivation of salivarian trypanosomes: application to *in vitro* studies of African trypanosomiases. In *Practical Tissue*

Culture Applications, eds K. Maramorosch, H. Hirumi. Academic Press (New York), pp. 309–30.

Hirumi, H., Doyle, J. J. and Hirumi, K., 1977. African trypanosomes: cultivation of animal-infective *Trypanosoma brucei in vitro*, *Science*, **196**: 992–4.

Hirumi, H., Hirumi, K., Doyle, J. J. and Cross, G. A. M., 1980. *In vitro* cloning of animal-infective bloodstream forms of *Trypanosoma brucei*, *Parasitology*, **80**: 371–82.

Hoare, C. A., 1949. Akinetoplastic strains of *Trypanosoma evansi* and the status of allied trypanosomes in America, *Revta. Soc. mex. Hist. nat.*, **10**(1–4): 81–90.

Hoare, C. A., 1957. The spread of African trypanosomes beyond their natural range, *Z. Tropenmed. Parasit.*, **8**: 157–61.

Hoare, C. A., 1965. Vampire bats as vectors and hosts of equine and bovine trypanosomes, *Parasitology*, **22**: 204–16.

Hoare, C. A., 1972. *The Trypanosomes of Mammals. A Zoological Monograph*. Blackwell Scientific Publication (Oxford).

Hoff, R., 1974. A method for counting and concentrating living *Trypanosoma cruzi* in blood lysed with ammonium chloride, *J. Parasitol.*, **60**(3): 527–8.

Homeida, A. M., El Amin, E. A., Adam, S. E. and Mahmoud, M. M., 1980. The effect of Samorin (isometamidium chloride) on *Trypanosoma evansi* infection in mice, *Br. J. exp. Path.*, **61**: 380–9.

Horchner, F., Bofenschen, F. and Zander, B., 1979. Serological differentiation between *Trypanosoma brucei-*, *T. congolense-* and *T. vivax*-infection, *Z. Tropenmed. Parasit.*, **30**: 265–73.

Hornby, H. E., 1952. *Animal Trypanosomiasis in East Africa, 1949*. HMSO (London).

Hornby, H. E. and Bailey, H. W., 1931. Diurnal variation in the concentration of *Trypanosoma congolense* in blood vessels of the ox's ear, *Trans. R. Soc. trop. Med. Hyg.*, **26**: 557–64.

Huan, C. N., Webb, L., Lambert, P. H. and Miescher, P. A., 1975. Pathogenesis of the anemia in African trypanosomiasis: characterization and purification of a hemolytic factor, *Schweiz med. Wschr.*, **105**(47): 1582–3.

Hudson, J. R., 1944. Acute and subacute trypanosomiasis in cattle caused by *Trypanosoma vivax*, *J. Comp. Path. Therapeu.*, **54**: 108–19.

Hudson, K. M., Taylor, A. E. R. and Elce, B. J., 1980. Antigenic changes in *Trypanosoma brucei* on transmission by tsetse-fly, *Parasite Immunol.*, **2**: 57–69.

Hudson, L., 1981. Immunobiology of *Trypanosoma cruzi* infection and Chagas' disease, *Trans. R. Soc. trop. Med. Hyg.*, **75**(4): 475–8.

Hutner, S. H., 1977. Essay and reviews of recent symposia on protozoan chemotherapy, *J. Protozool.*, **24**(3): 475–8.

Ikede, B. O., 1974. Ocular lesions in sheep infected with *Trypanosoma brucei*, *J. Comp. Path.*, **84**: 203–13.

Ikede, B. O., 1979. Genital lesions in experimental chronic

Trypanosoma brucei infection in rams, *Res. vet. Sci.*, **26**: 145–51.
Ikede, B. O., Akpokodje, J. U., Hill, D. H. and Adjidagba, P. O. A., 1977a. Clinical, haematological and pathological studies in donkeys experimentally infected with *Trypanosoma brucei*, *Trop. Anim. Hlth Prod.*, **9**: 93–8.
Ikede, B. O. and Losos, G. J., 1972a. Pathology of the disease in sheep produced experimentally by *Trypanosoma brucei*, *Vet. Path.*, **9**: 278–89.
Ikede, B. O. and Losos, G. J., 1972b. Spontaneous canine trypanosomiasis caused by *T. brucei*: meningo-encephalomyelitis with extravascular localization of trypanosomes in the brain, *Bull. epiz. Dis. Afr.*, **20**: 221–8.
Ikede, B. O. and Losos, G. J., 1972c. Pathological changes in cattle infected with *Trypanosoma brucei*, *Vet. Path.*, **9**: 272–7.
Ikede, B. O. and Losos, G. J., 1972d. Hereditary transmission of *Trypanosoma vivax* in sheep, *Br. vet. J.*, **128**: i–ii.
Ikede, B. O. and Losos, G. J., 1975a. Pathogenesis of *Trypanosoma brucei* infection in sheep. I. Clinical signs, *J. Comp. Path.*, **85**: 23–31.
Ikede, B. O. and Losos, G. J., 1975b. Pathogenesis of *Trypanosoma brucei* infection in sheep. II. Cerebrospinal fluid changes, *J. Comp. Path.*, **85**: 33–6.
Ikede, B. O. and Losos, G. J., 1975c. Pathogenesis of *Trypanosoma brucei* infection in sheep. III. Hypophysial and other endocrine lesions, *J. Comp. Path.*, **85**: 37–44.
Ikede, B. O., Lule, M. and Terry, R. J., 1977b. Anaemia in trypanosomiasis: mechanisms of erythrocyte destruction in mice infected with *Trypanosoma congolense* or *T. brucei*, *Acta trop.*, **34**: 53–60.
Innes, J. R. M. and Saunders, L. Z., 1962. *Comparative Neuropathology*. Academic Press (New York).
Isoun, M. J. and Isoun, T. T., 1974a. The effect of HEPES buffered media on the *in vitro* cultivation of *Trypanosoma vivax* and *T. brucei*, *Z. Tropenmed. Parasit.*, **25**(3): 283–7.
Isoun, M. J. and Isoun, T. T., 1981. Oxygen uptake by *Trypanosoma brucei* and three strains of *T. vivax*, *Vet. Parasitol.*, **8**: 127–31.
Isoun, T. T., 1968. The pathology of *Trypanosoma simiae* infection in pigs, *Ann. trop. Med. Parasit.*, **62**: 188–92.
Isoun, T. T., 1975. The histopathology of experimental disease produced in mice infected with *Trypanosoma vivax*, *Acta trop.*, **32**(3): 267–72.
Isoun, T. T. and Anosa, V. D., 1974. Lesions in the reproductive organs of sheep and goats experimentally infected with *Trypanosoma vivax*, *Z. Tropenmed. Parasit.*, **25**: 469–76.
Isoun, T. T. and Isoun, M. J., 1974b. *In vitro* cultivation of *Trypanosoma vivax* isolated from cattle, *Nature*, **251**(5475): 513–14.
Isoun, T. T., Isoun, M. J. and Anosa, V. D., 1978. Free plasma amino acid profiles of normal and *Trypanosoma vivax* infected sheep, *Z. Tropenmed. Parasit.*, **29**(3): 330–4.

Ito, Y., Furuya, M., Oka, M., Osaki, H. and Aikawa, M., 1981. Transmission and scanning electron microscopic studies of the micronemata of *Trypanosoma gambiense*, *J. Protozool.*, **28**(3): 313–16.

Jackson, P. R., Winkler, D. G., Kimzey, S. L. and Fisher, F. M. Jr., 1977. Cytofluorograf detection of *Plasmodium yoelii*, *Trypanosoma gambiense*, and *Trypanosoma equiperdum* by laser excited fluorescence of stained rodent blood, *J. Parasitol.*, **63**(4): 593–8.

James, D. M. and Born, G. V. R., 1980. Uptake of purine bases and nucleosides in African trypanosomes, *Parasitology*, **81**: 383–93.

Janssen, J. A. H. A. and Wijers, D. J. B., 1974. *Trypanosoma simiae* at the Kenya coast. A correlation between virulence and the transmitting species of *Glossina*, *Ann. trop. Med. Parasit.*, **68**(1): 5–19.

Jatkar, P. R., Rao, P. V. and Singh, M., 1977. Diagnosis of surra; capillary agglutination test, *Indian vet. J.*, **54**: 795–7.

Jaktar, P. R. and Singh, M., 1971. Diagnosis of surra in camels by passive agglutination test, *Br. vet. J.*, **127**: 283–8.

Jenkins, G. C., McCrorie, P., Forsberg, C. M. and Brown, J. L., 1980. Studies on the anaemia in rabbits infected with *Trypanosoma brucei brucei*, *J. Comp. Path.*, **90**: 107–21.

Jenni, L. and Brun, R., 1981. *In vitro* cultivation of pleomorphic *Trypanosoma brucei* stocks: a possible source of variable antigens for immunization studies, *Trans. R. Soc. trop. Med. Hyg.*, **75**(1): 150–1.

Jennings, F. W., Murray, P. K., Murray, M. and Urquhart, G. M., 1974. Anaemia in trypanosomiasis: studies in rats and mice infected with *Trypanosoma brucei*, *Res. vet. Sci.*, **16**: 70–6.

Johnson, J. G. and Cross, G. A. M., 1979. Selective cleavage of variant surface glycoproteins from *Trypanosoma brucei*, *Biochem. J.*, **178**: 689–97.

Jones, T. W. and Clarkson, M. J., 1972. The effect of syringe and cyclical passage on antigenic variants of *Trypanosoma vivax*, *Ann. trop. Med. Parasit.*, **66**(33): 303–12.

Jones, T. W. and Clarkson, M. J., 1974. The timing of antigenic variation in *Trypanosoma vivax*, *Ann. trop. Med. Parasit.*, **68**(4): 485–6.

Jones, T. W., Cunningham, I., Taylor, A. M. and Gray, A. R., 1981. The use of culture-derived metacyclic trypanosomes in studies on the serological relationships of stocks of *Trypanosoma brucei gambiense*, *Trans. R. Soc. trop. Med. Hyg.*, **75**(4): 560–5.

Jones-Davies, W. J. and Folkes, W. J., 1967. *Some Observations on Cross-resistance to Samorin and Berenil of Homidium-resistant Field Strains of* Trypanosoma congolense *in Northern Nigerian Cattle.* ISCTR, vol. XV, 34 pp.

Jordan, A. M., 1961. An assessment of the economic importance of tsetse species of southern Nigeria and southern Cameroons based on their trypanosome infection rates and ecology, *Bull. Ent. Res.*, **5**: 431–41.

Jordan, A. M., 1965. Bovine trypanosomiasis in Nigeria. V. The tsetse-fly challenge to a herd of cattle trekked along a trade-cattle route, *Ann. trop. Med. Parasit.*, **59**(3): 270–6.

Jordan, A. M., 1976. Tsetse control – present and future, *Trans. R. Soc. trop. Med. Hyg.*, **70**: 128–9.

Jordan, A. M., 1978. Principles of the eradication or control of tsetse flies, *Nature, Lond.*, **273**(5664): 607–9.

Kaaya, G. P. and Oduor-Okela, D., 1980. The effects of *Trypanosoma congolense* infection on the testis and epidemys of the goat, *Bull. Anim. Hlth Prod. Afr.*, **28**: 1–5.

Kaaya, G. P., Tizard, I. R., Maxie, M. G. and Vallie, V. E. O., 1980. Inhibition of leukopoiesis by sera from *Trypanosoma congolense* infected calves: partial characterization of the inhibitory factor, *Z. Tropenmed. Parasit.*, **31**: 232–8.

Kaaya, G. P., Valli, V. E. O., Maxie, M. G. and Losos, G. J., 1979. Inhibition of bone marrow granulocyte/macrophage colony formation *in vitro* by serum collected from cattle infected with *Trypanosoma vivax* and *Trypanosoma congolense*, *Z. Tropenmed. Parasit.*, **30**: 230–5.

Kaliner, G., 1974. *Trypanosoma congolense*. II. Histopathologic findings in experimentally infected cattle, *Exp. Parasitol.*, **36**: 20–6.

Kar, S. K., Roelants, G. E., Mayor-Withey, K. S. and Pearson, T. W., 1981. Immunodepression in trypanosome-infected mice. VI. Comparison of immune responses of different lymphoid organs, *Eur. J. Immunol.*, **11**: 100–5.

Kierszenbaum, F., 1979. Antibody-dependent killing of bloodstream forms of *Trypanosoma cruzi* by human peripheral blood leukocytes, *Am. J. Trop. Med. Hyg.*, **28**(6): 965–8.

Kierszenbaum, F., 1980. Protection of congenitally athymic mice against *Trypanosoma cruzi* infection by passive antibody transfer, *J. Parasitol.*, **66**(4): 673–5.

Kierszenbaum, F., Ackerman, S. J. and Gleich, G. J., 1981. Destruction of bloodstream forms of *Trypanosoma cruzi* by eosinophil granule major basic protein, *Am. J. Trop. Med. Hyg.*, **30**: 775–9.

Kilgour, V., 1980a. *Trypanosoma*: intricacies of biochemistry, morphology, and environment, *Int. J. Biochem.*, **12**: 325–32.

Kilgour, V., 1980b. The electrophoretic mobilities and activities of eleven enzymes of bloodstream and culture forms of *Trypanosoma brucei* compared, *Mol. Biochem. Parasitol.*, **2**: 51–62.

Kilgour, V. and Godfrey, D. G., 1977. The persistence in the field of two characteristic isoenzyme patterns in Nigerian *Trypanosoma vivax*, *Ann. Trop. Med. Parasitol.*, **71**(3): 387–9.

Kilgour, V. and Godfrey, D. G., 1978. The influence of lorry transport on the *Trypanosoma vivax* infection rate in Nigerian trade cattle, *Trop. Anim. Hlth Prod.*, **10**: 145–8.

Kilgour, V., Godfrey, D. G. and Na'Isa, B. K., 1975. Isoenzymes of two aminotransferases among *Trypanosoma vivax* in Nigerian cattle, *Ann. trop. Med. Parasit.*, **69**(3): 329–35.

Killick-Kendrick, R., 1964. The apparent loss of the kinetoplast of *Trypanosoma evansi* after treatment of an experimentally infected horse with Berenil, *Ann. trop. Med. Parasit.*, **58**(4): 481–90.

Killick-Kendrick, R., 1968. The diagnosis of trypanosomiasis of livestock; a review of current techniques, *Vet. Bull.*, **38**(4): 191–6.

Killick-Kendrick, R., 1971. The low pathogenicity of *Trypanosoma brucei* to cattle, *Trans. R. Soc. trop. Med. Hyg.*, **65**(1): 104.

Killick-Kendrick, R. and Godfrey, D. G., 1963. Bovine trypanosomiasis in Nigeria. II. The incidence among some migrating cattle, with observations on the examination of wet blood preparations as a method of survey, *Ann. trop. Med. Parasit.*, **57**(1): 117–26.

Kimberling, C. V. and Ewing, J. R., 1973. A case history of *Trypanosoma congolense* infection in two horses, *Bull. epiz. Dis. Afr.*, **21**: 249–51.

Kipnis, T. L., Calich, V. L. G. and Dias da Silva, W., 1979. Active entry of bloodstream forms of *Trypanosoma cruzi* into macrophages, *Parasitology*, **78**: 89–98.

Kirby, W. W., 1961. Prophylaxis under continuous exposure to the risk of natural infection with trypanosomiasis by tsetse-flies. A comparative trial of metamidium chloride, antrycide pro-salt and antrycide methylsulphate, *Vet. Rec.*, **73**: 411.

Knowles, R. H., 1927. Trypanosomiasis of camels in the Anglo-Egyptian Sudan: diagnosis, chemotherapy, immunity, *J. Comp. Path.*, **40**: 59–71.

Kobayashi, A., Soltys, M. A. and Woo, P. T. K., 1976b. Comparative studies on the laboratory diagnosis of experimental *Trypanosoma congolense* infection in sheep, *Ann. trop. Med. Parasit.*, **70**: 53–8.

Kobayashi, A. and Tizard, I. R., 1976. The response to *Trypanosoma congolense* infection in calves: determination of immunoglobulins IgG1, IgG2, IgM and C3 levels and the complement fixing antibody titres during the course of infection, *Z. Tropenmed. Parasit.*, **27**: 411–17.

Kobayashi, A., Tizard, I. R. and Woo, P. T. K., 1976a. Studies on the anemia in experimental African trypanosomiasis. II. The pathogenesis of the anemia in calves infected with *Trypanosoma congolense*, *Am. J. Trop. Med. Hyg.*, **25**(3): 401–6.

Koberle, F., 1968. Chagas' disease and Chagas' syndromes: the pathology of American trypanosomiasis, *Adv. Parasitol.*, **6**: 63–116.

Koberle, F., 1974. Pathogenesis of Chagas' disease. In *Trypanosomiasis and Leishmaniasis with Special Reference to Chagas' Disease*. Ciba Foundation Symposium 20 (new series), Associated Scientific Publishers (Amsterdam), pp. 135–58.

Kosinski, R. J., 1980. Antigenic variation in trypanosomes: a computer analysis of variant order, *Parasitology*, **80**: 343–57.

Kramer, J., 1966. Incidence of trypanosomes in West African dwarf sheep and goats in Nsukka, eastern Nigeria, *Bull. epiz. Dis. Afr.*, **14**: 423–8.

Krampitz, H. E., 1970. Studies on experimental infections of East African zebu cattle with strains of *Trypanosoma congolense* isolated from tsetse flies, *Z. Tropenmed. Parasit.*, **21**(1): 3–20.

Kress, Y., Bloom, B. R., Wittner, M., Rowan, A. and Tanowitz, H., 1975. Resistance of *Trypanosoma cruzi* to killing by macrophages, *Nature*, **257**(5525): 394–6.

Kress, Y., Tanowitz, H., Bloom, B. and Wittner, M., 1977. *Trypanosoma cruzi*: infection of normal and activated mouse macrophages, *Exp. Parasitol.*, **41**: 385–96.

Kreutzer, R. D. and Sousa, O. E., 1981. Biochemical characterization of *Trypanosoma* spp. by isozyme electrophoresis, *Am. J. Trop. Med. Hyg.*, **30**(2): 308–17.

Kuhn, R. E. and Murnane, J. E., 1977. *Trypanosoma cruzi*: immune destruction of parasitized mouse fibroblast *in vitro*, *Exp. Parasitol.*, **41**: 66–73.

Labastie, M. C., Baltz, T., Richet, C., Giroud, Ch., Duvillier, G., Pautrizel, R. and Degand, P., 1981. Variant specific glycoproteins of *Trypanosoma equiperdum*: cross reacting determinants and chemical studies, *Biochem. Biophys. Res. Comm.*, **99**(2): 729–36.

Laguens, R. P., Cossio, P. M., Diez, C., Segal, A., Vasquez, C., Kreutzer, E., Khoury, E. and Arana, R. M., 1975. Immunopathologic and morphologic studies of skeletal muscle in Chagas' disease, *Am. J. Path.*, **80**: 153–62.

Laird, M., (ed.), 1977. *Tsetse: The Future for Biological Methods in Integrated Control*. IDRC (Ottawa), **077e**.

Lambert, P. H., Berney, M. and Kazyumba, G., 1981. Immune complexes in serum and in cerebrospinal fluid in African trypanosomiasis. Correlation with polyclonal B cell activation and with intracerebral immunoglobulin synthesis, *J. Clin. Invest.*, **67**: 77–85.

Langley, P. A., 1977. Tsetse physiology. The relevance of laboratory studies to tsetse control, *Trans. R. Soc. trop. Med. Hyg.*, **71**: 5–6.

Lanham, S. M., Williams, J. E. and Godfrey, D. G., 1972. Detection of low concentrations of trypanosomes in blood by column-separation and membrane-filtration, *Trans. R. Soc. trop. Med. Hyg.*, **66**(4): 624–7.

Lawson, B. M., Valli, V. E. O., Mills, J. N. and Forsberg, C. M., 1980. The quantitation of *Trypanosoma congolense* in calves. IV. *In vitro* culture of myeloid and erythroid marrow cells, *Z. Tropenmed. Parasitol.*, **31**: 425–34.

Leach, T. M., 1961. Observations on the treatment of *Trypanosoma evansi* infection in camels, *J. Comp. Path.*, **71**: 109–17.

Leach, T. M., 1973. African trypanosomiases, *Adv. vet. Sci.*, **17**: 119–62.

Leach, T. M., El Karib, A. A., Ford, E. J. H. and Wilmshurst, E. C.,

1955. Studies on ethidium bromide. VI. The prophylactic properties of the drug, *J. Comp. Path.*, **65**: 130–42.

Leach, T. M. and Roberts, C. J., 1981. Present status of chemotherapy and chemoprophylaxis of animal trypanosomiasis in the eastern hemisphere, *Pharmac. Ther.*, **13**: 91–147.

Lee, C. M. and Aboko-Cole, G. F., 1972. Comparative metabolic activity of brain slices of rats infected with pathogenic and a non-pathogenic trypanosome evidenced by cell population and respiratory activity, *Z. Parasitenkd.*, **39**: 149–60.

Lee, C. M., Linicombe, D. R., Bruce, J. I., Akinyemi, J., Llano, C. and Mendes, T., 1972. *Trypanosoma rhodesiense*: oxygen uptake by mouse brain slices, *Exp. Parasitol.*, **32**: 282–8.

Leeflang, P., 1975. The predominance of *Trypanosoma vivax* infections of cattle at a distance from savannah tsetse concentration, *Trop. Anim. Hlth Prod.*, **7**: 201–4.

Leeflang, P., Buys, J. and Blotkamp, C., 1976a. Studies on *Trypanosoma vivax*: infectivity and serial maintenance of natural bovine isolates in mice, *Int. J. Parasitol.*, **6**: 413–17.

Leeflang, P., Buys, J. and Blotkamp, C., 1978. Studies on *Trypanosoma vivax*: comparison of parasitological diagnostic methods, *Int. J. Parasitol.*, **8**: 15–18.

Leeflang, P., Ige, K. and Olatunde, D. S., 1976b. Studies on *Trypanosoma vivax*: the infectivity of cyclically and mechanically transmitted ruminant infections for mice and rats, *Int. J. Parasitol.*, **6**: 453–6.

Letch, C. A. and Gibson, W., 1981. *Trypanosoma brucei*: the peptidases of bloodstream trypanosomes, *Exp. Parasitol.*, **52**: 86–90.

Lheureux, M., Lheureux, M., Vervoort, T., van Meirvenne, N. and Steinert, M., 1979. Immunological purification and partial characterization of variant-specific surface antigen messenger RNA of *Trypanosoma brucei brucei*, *Nucleic Acids Res.*, **7**(3): 595–609.

Lincicombe, D. A. and Bruce, J. I., 1965. Oxygen uptake of liver and heart slices of *Trypanosoma rhodesiense*-infected mice, *Exp. Parasitol.*, **17**: 332–9.

Lindsley, H. B., Nagle, R. B. and Stechschulte, D. J., 1978. Proliferative glomerulonephritis hypocomplementemia, and nucleic acid antibodies in rats infected with *Trypanosoma rhodesiense*, *Am. J. Trop. Med. Hyg.*, **27**(5): 864–72.

Lindsley, H. B., Nagle, R. B., Werner, P. A. and Stechschulte, D. J., 1980. Variable severity of glomerulonephritis in inbred rats infected with *Trypanosoma rhodesiense*. Correlation with immunoglobulin class-specific antibody responses to trypanosomal antigens and total IgM levels, *Am. J. Trop. Med. Hyg.*, **29**(3): 343–57.

Lopes, E. R., Chapadeiro, E., Macedo, V., Pires, L. L., Prata, A. R., Tafuri, W. L. and Tanus, R., 1980. Chagas' disease in dogs. Anatomo-pathological study of naturally infected animals, *Re. Inst. Med. Trop. Sao Paulo*, **22**: 135–43.

Losos, G. J., 1979. Infections caused by pathogenic African

trypanosomes. In *Pathogenicity of Trypanosomes*, eds G. J. Losos, A. Chouinard, IDRC (Ottawa), **132e**, pp. 59–62.

Losos, G. J., 1980. Diseases caused by *Trypanosoma evansi*, a review. In *Veterinary Research Communications*. Elsevier (Amsterdam), **4**:165–81.

Losos, G. J., 1981. Diseases caused by *Trypanosoma evansi*. A review, *Vet. Sci. Comm.*, **4**: 165–81.

Losos, G. J. and Chouinard, A., (eds), 1979. *Pathogenicity of Trypanosomes.* IDRC (Ottawa), **132e**.

Losos, G. J. and Crockett, E., 1969. Toxicity of Berenil in the dog, *Vet. Rec.*, **85**: 196.

Losos, G. J. and Gwamaka, G., 1973. Histological examination of wild animals naturally infected with pathogenic African trypanosomes, *Acta trop.*, **30**(1–2): 57–63.

Losos, G. J. and Ikede, B. O., 1970. Pathology of experimental trypanosomiasis in the albino rat, rabbit, goat, and sheep – A preliminary report, *Can. J. comp. Med.*, **34**(3): 209–12.

Losos, G. J. and Ikede, B. O., 1972. Review of pathology of diseases in domestic and laboratory animals caused by *Trypanosoma congolense, T. vivax, T. brucei, T. rhodesiense* and *T. gambiense, Vet. Pathol.*, **9**(Suppl.): 1–71.

Losos, G. J., Maxie, M. G. and Tabel, H., in preparation. Experimental bovine trypanosomiasis (*Trypanosoma vivax* and *Trypanosoma congolense*). IV. Pathology.

Losos, G. J. and Mwambu, P. M., 1979. Organ and tissue weights in diseases caused by *T. vivax* and *T. congolense*. In *Pathogenicity of Trypanosomes*, eds G. J. Losos, A. Chouinard. IDRC (Ottawa), **132e**, p. 178.

Losos, G. J., McMillan, I., Minder, Ch. E. and Soulsby, K., 1982. Quantitative methods in the study of the pathogenesis of haemoprotozoal diseases. In *Parasitology*, **84**: 537–65.

Losos, G. J., Paris, J., Wilson, A. J. and Dar, F. K., 1973a. Distribution of *Trypanosoma congolense* in tissues of cattle, *Trans. R. Soc. trop. Med. Hyg.*, **67**: 278.

Losos, G. J., Paris, J., Wilson, A. J. and Dar, F. K., 1973b. Pathology of the disease in cattle caused by *Trypanosoma congolense, Bull. epiz. Dis. Afr.*, **21**: 239–48.

Lotzsch, R. and Deindl, G., 1974. *Trypanosoma congolense*. III. Serological responses of experimentally infected cattle, *Exp. Parasitol.*, **36**: 27–33.

Luckins, A. G., 1972. Studies on bovine trypanosomiasis. Serum immunoglobulin levels in zebu cattle exposed to natural infection in East Africa, *Br. vet. J.*, **128**: 523–8.

Luckins, A. G., 1976. The immune response of zebu cattle to infection with *Trypanosoma congolense* and *T. vivax, Ann. trop. Med. Parasit.*, **70**(2): 133–45.

Luckins, A. G., 1977. Detection of antibodies in trypanosome-infected cattle by means of a microplate enzyme-linked immunosorbent assay, *Trop. Anim. Hlth Prod.*, **9**: 53–62.

Luckins, A. G., Boid, R., Rae, P., Mahmoud, M. M., El Malik, K. H. and Gray, A. R., 1979. Serodiagnosis of infection with *Trypanosoma evansi* in camels in the Sudan, *Trop. Anim. Hlth Prod.*, **11**: 1–12.

Luckins, A. G. and Gray, A. R., 1978. An extravascular site of development of *Trypanosoma congolense*, *Nature*, **272**(5654): 613–4.

Luckins, A. G. and Gray, A. R., 1979a. Trypanosomes in the lymph nodes of cattle and sheep infected with *Trypanosoma congolense*, *Res. vet. Sci.*, **27**: 129–31.

Luckins, A. G. and Gray, A. R., 1979b. Observations on the antigenicity and serological relationships of stocks of *Trypanosoma congolense* from East and West Africa, *Parasitology*, **79**: 337–47.

Luckins, A. G. and Mehlitz, D., 1976. Observations on serum immunoglobulin levels in cattle infected with *Trypanosoma brucei*, *T. vivax*, and *T. congolense*, *Ann. trop. Med. Parasit.*, **70**(4): 479–80.

Luckins, A. G. and Mehlitz, D., 1978. Evaluation of an indirect fluorescent antibody test, enzyme-linked immunosorbent assay and quantification of immunoglobulins in the diagnosis of bovine trypanosomiasis, *Trop. Anim. Hlth Prod.*, **10**: 149–59.

Luckins, A. G., Rae, P. and Gray, M. A., 1981. Development of local skin reactions in rabbits infected with metacyclic forms of *Trypanosoma congolense* cultured *in vitro*, *Ann. trop. Med. Parasit.*, **75**(5): 563–4.

Lumsden, R. D., Marciacq, Y. and Seed, J. R., 1972. *Trypanosoma gambiense*: cytopathologic changes in guinea pig hepatocytes, *Exp. Parasitol.*, **32**(3): 369–89.

Lumsden, W. H. R., 1962. Trypanosomiasis in African wild life, *Proc. 1st Conf. on Wildlife Disease, New York*, pp. 68–88.

Lumsden, W. H. R., 1972a. Infectivity of Salivarian trypanosomes to the mammalian host, *Acta trop.*, **29**(4): 300–20.

Lumsden, W. H. R., 1972b. Principles of viable preservation of parasitic protozoa, *Int. J. Parasit.*, **2**: 327–32.

Lumsden, W. H. R., 1977. Problems in characterization and nomenclature of trypanosome populations. *Ann. Soc. Belge Méd. trop.*, **57**(4–5): 361–8.

Lumsden, W. H. R., Cunningham, M. P., Webber, W. A. F., van Hoeve, K. and Walker, P. J., 1963. A method for the measurement of the infectivity of trypanosome suspensions, *Exp. Parasitol.*, **14**(3): 269–79.

Lumsden, W. H. R. and Evans, D. A. (eds), 1976. *Biology of Kinetoplastida*. Academic Press (London, New York, San Francisco), vol. 2.

Lumsden, W. H. R., Gitatha, S. K. and Lutz, W., 1968. Factors influencing the infectivity of a *Trypanosoma brucei* stabilate for mice, *J. Protozool.*, **15**(1): 129–31.

Lumsden, W. H. R. and Herbert, W. J., 1975. Pedigrees of the Edinburgh *Trypanosoma* (*Trypanozoon*) antigenic types (ETat), *Trans. R. Soc. trop. Med. Hyg.*, **69**(2): 205–8.

Lumsden, W. H. R., Kimber, C. D., Evans, D. A. and Doig, S. J.,

1979. *Trypanosoma brucei*: miniature anion-exchange centrifugation technique for detection of low parasitemias: adaptation for field use, *Trans. R. Soc. trop. Med. Hyg.*, **73**(3): 312–17.

Lumsden, W. H. R., Kimber, C. D. and Strange, M., 1977. *Trypanosoma brucei*: detection of low parasitemias in mice by a miniature anion-exchanger/centrifugation technique, *Trans. R. Soc. trop. Med. Hyg.*, **71**(5): 421–4.

Lyon, J. A., Pratt, J. M., Travis, R. W., Doctor, B. P. and Olenick, J. G., 1981. Use of monoclonal antibody to immunochemically characterize variant-specific surface coat glycoprotein from *Trypanosoma rhodesiense, J. Immunol.*, **126**(1): 134–7.

Lyttle, C. N., 1960. Field trials of Prothidium as a prophylactic in cattle trypanosomiasis, *J. Comp. Path.*, **70**: 18–35.

MacAskill, J. A., Holmes, P. H., Jennings, F. W. and Urquhart, G. M., 1981. Immunological clearance of ^{75}Se-labelled *Trypanosoma brucei* in mice. III. Studies in animals with acute infections, *Immunology*, **43**: 691–8.

MacAskill, J. A., Holmes, P. H., Whitelaw, D. D., McConnell, I., Jennings, F. W. and Urquhart, G. M., 1980. Immunological clearance of ^{75}Se-labelled *Trypanosoma brucei* in mice. II. Mechanisms in immune animals, *Immunology*, **40**: 629–35.

MacKenzie, A. R. and Boreham, P. F. L., 1974. Autoimmunity in trypanosome infections. I. Tissue autoantibodies in *Trypanosoma (Trypanozoon) brucei* infections of the rabbit, *Immunology*, **26**: 1225–38.

MacKenzie, P. K. I. and Boyt, W. P., 1973. The pathogenicity of local strains of *Trypanosoma brucei* for bovines in Rhodesia, *Rhod. vet. J.*, **4**(2): 23–8.

MacKenzie, P. K. I., Boyt, W. P. and Nesham, V. W., 1979. Serum immunoglobulin levels in sheep during the course of naturally acquired and experimentally induced trypanosomiasis, *Br. vet. J.*, **135**: 178–84.

MacKenzie, P. K. I., Boyt, W. P., Nesham, V. W. and Pirie, E., 1978. The aetiology and significance of phagocytosis of erythrocytes in sheep infected with *Trypanosoma congolense* (Broden, 1904), *Res. vet. Sci.*, **24**: 4–7.

MacKenzie, P. K. I. and Cruickshank, J. G., 1973. Phagocytosis of erythrocytes and leucocytes in sheep infected with *Trypanosoma congolense*, *Res. vet. Sci.*, **15**: 256–62.

MacLennan, K. J. R., 1970. The epizootiology of trypanosomiasis in livestock in West Africa. In *The African Trypanosomiases*, ed. H. W. Mulligan. George Allen & Unwin (London), pp. 751–67.

MacLennan, K. J. R., 1980. Tsetse-transmitted trypanosomiasis in relation to the rural economy in Africa. Part 1. Tsetse infestation, *Wld Anim. Rev.*, **36**: 2–17.

Madeira, E. D., de Andrade, A. F. B., Bunn-Moreno, M. M. and Barcinski, M., 1979. Antibody-dependent cellular cytotoxicity of

Trypanosoma cruzi: characterization of the effector cell from normal human blood, *Infect. Immun.*, **25**(1): 34–8.
Mahmoud, M. M. and Gray, A. R., 1980. Trypanosomiasis due to *Trypanosoma evansi* (Steel, 1885) Balbiani, 1888. A review of recent research, *Trop. Anim. Hlth Prod.*, **12**: 35–47.
Mamo, E. and Holmes, P. H., 1975. The erythrokinetics of zebu cattle chronically infected with *Trypanosoma congolense*, *Res. vet. Sci.*, **18**: 105–6.
Mancini, P. E. and Patton, C. L., 1981. Cyclic 3′,5′-adenosine monophosphate levels during the development cycle of *Trypanosoma brucei brucei* in the rat, *Mol. Biochem. Parasitol.*, **3**: 19–31.
Mandal, A. K., Rao, A. M. and Nandi, N. C., 1977. Outbreak of surra in bovines from Krishna district, Andhra Pradesh, *Indian J. Anim. Hlth*, **16**: 100.
Mansfield, J. M. and Kreier, J. P., 1972. Autoimmunity in experimental *Trypanosoma congolense* infections of rabbits, *Infect. Immun.*, **5**(5): 648–56.
Marciacq, Y. and Seed, J. R., 1970. Reduced levels of glycogen and glucose-6-phosphatase in livers of guinea pigs infected with *Trypanosoma gambiense*, *J. Infect. Dis.*, **121**(6): 653–5.
Marsden, P. D., Blackie, E. J., Rosenberg, M. E., Ridley, D. S. and Hagstrom, J. W. C., 1970. Experimental *Trypanosoma cruzi* infections in domestic pigs (*Sus scrofa domestica*), *Trans. R. Soc. trop. Med. Hyg.*, **64**(1): 156–8.
Marshall, R. S., 1958. *Animal Trypanosomiasis: Control Measures by Means of Drugs*. ISCTR, CCTA Pub. No. 41, vol. VI, pp. 13–24.
Martin, L. K., Sadun, E. H. and Ingram, G. D., 1972. Experimental infections with African trypanosomes. I. Quantitation of *Trypanosoma rhodesiense* by electronic particle counting, *Am. J. Trop. Med. Hyg.*, **21**(6): 880–4.
Masake, R. A., 1980. The pathogenesis of infection with *Trypanosoma vivax* in goats and cattle, *Vet. Rec.*, **107**: 551–7.
Masake, R. A. and Morrison, W. I., 1981. Evaluation of the structural and functional changes in the lymphoid organs of Boran cattle infected with *Trypanosoma vivax*, *Am. J. Vet. Res.*, **42**(10): 1738–46.
Masake, R. A., Pearson, T. W., Wells, P. and Roelants, G. E., 1981. The *in vitro* response to mitogens of leucocytes from cattle infected with *Trypanosoma congolense*, *Clin. Exp. Immunol.*,**43**: 583–9.
Mattern, P., Klein, F., Pautrizel, R. and Jongepier-Geerdes, Y. E. J. M., 1980. Anti-immunoglobulins and heterophil agglutinins in experimental trypanosomiasis, *Infect. Immun.*, **28**: 812–17.
Matthyssens, G., Michiels, F., Hamers, R., Pays, E. and Steinert, M., 1981. Two variant surface glycoproteins of *Trypanosoma brucei* have a conserved C. terminus, *Nature*, **293**(5829): 230–3.
Maxie, M. G. and Losos, G. J., 1977. Release of *Trypanosoma congolense* from the microcirculation of cattle by Berenil, *Vet. Parasitol.*, **3**: 277–81.

Maxie, M. G., Losos, G. J. and Tabel, H., 1976. A comparative study of the haematological aspects of the diseases caused by *Trypanosoma vivax* and *Trypanosoma congolense* in cattle. In *Pathophysiology of Parasitic Infections*, ed. E. J. L. Soulsby. Academic Press (New York), pp. 183–98.

Maxie, M. G., Losos, G. J. and Tabel, H., 1979. Experimental bovine trypanosomiasis (*Trypanosoma vivax* and *T. congolense*). I. Symptomatology and clinical pathology, *Z. Tropenmed. Parasit.*, **30**: 274–82.

Maxie, M. G., Tabel, H. and Losos, G. J., 1978. Determination of volumes of *Trypanosoma vivax* and *T. congolense* separated from cattle blood, *Z. Tropenmed. Parasit.*, **29**: 234–8.

Maxie, M. G. and Valli, V. E. O., 1979. Hemodilution in bovine trypanosomiasis. In *Pathogenicity of Trypanosomes*, eds G. J. Losos, A. Chouinard. IDRC 132e (Ottawa), pp. 145–50.

McCrorie, P., Jenkins, G. C., Brown, J. L. and Ramsey, C. E., 1980. Studies on the anaemia in rabbits infected with *Trypanosoma brucei brucei*. 2. Haematological studies on the role of the spleen, *J. Comp. Path.*, **90**: 123–37.

McCulloch, B., 1967. Trypanosomes of the *brucei* subgroup as a probable cause of disease in wild zebra (*Equus burchelli*), *Ann. trop. Med. Parasit.*, **61**: 261–4.

McCully, R. M. and Neitz, W. O., 1971. Clinicopathological study on experimental *Trypanosoma brucei* infections in horses. Part 2. Histopathological findings in the nervous system and other organs of treated and untreated horses reacting to Nagana, *Onderstepoort J. vet. Res.*, **38**(3): 141–76.

McGuire, T. C., Barbet, A. F., Hirumi, H., Meshnick, S. and Doyle, J. J., 1980. *Trypanosoma brucei*: radioimmunoassay of variant surface glycoproteins from organisms grown *in vitro* and *in vivo*, *Exp. Parasitol.*, **50**: 233–9.

McNeillage, G. J. C. and Herbert, W. J., 1968. Infectivity and virulence of *Trypanosoma* (*Trypanozoon*) *brucei* for mice. II. Comparison of closely related trypanosome antigenic types, *J. Comp. Path.*, **78**: 345–9.

Mehlitz, D., 1975. Serological studies on subgenus differentiation and persistence of antibodies following infections with trypanosomes, *Z. Tropenmed. Parasit.*, **26**: 265–75.

Mehlitz, D., 1979. Trypanosome infections in domestic animals in Liberia, *Z. Tropenmed. Parasit.*, **30**: 212–19.

Mehlitz, D. and Deindl, G., 1972. Serological studies on cattle experimentally infected with African trypanosomes. Preliminary communication, *Z. Tropenmed. Parasit.*, **23**: 411–17.

Melo, R. C. and Brener, Z., 1978. Tissue tropism of different *Trypanosoma cruzi* strains, *J. Parasitol.*, **64**(3): 475–82.

Merritt, S. C., 1980. Purification and cell-free translation of mRNA coding for a variant specific antigen from *Trypanosoma brucei gambiense*, *Mol. Biochem. Parasitol.*, **1**: 151–66.

Milder, R. and Kloetzel, J., 1980. The development of *Trypanosoma cruzi* in macrophages *in vitro*. Interaction with lysosomes and host cell fate, *Parasitology*, **80**: 139–45.

Miles, M. A., 1979. Transmission cycles and the heterogeneity of *Trypanosoma cruzi*. In *Biology of the Kinetoplastida*, eds W. H. R. Lumsden, D. A. Evans. Academic Press (London), vol. 2, pp. 118–212.

Miller, E. N. and Turner, M. J., 1981. Analysis of antigenic types appearing in first relapse populations of clones of *Trypanosoma brucei*, *Parasitology*, **82**: 63–80.

Miller, P. G. and Klein, R. A., 1980. Effects of oligomycin on glucose utilization and calcium transport in African trypanosomes, *J. Gen. Microbiol.*, **116**: 391–6.

Mills, J. N. and Valli, V. E. O., 1978. A cytofluorometric method of counting trypanosomes, *Z. Tropenmed. Parasit.*, **29**: 95–100.

Mills, J. N., Valli, V. E., Boo, K. S. and Forsberg, C. M., 1980. The quantitation of *Trypanosoma congolense* in calves. III. A quantitative comparison of trypanosomes in jugular vein and microvasculature and tests of dispersing agents, *Z. Tropenmed. Parasit.*, **31**: 299–312.

Minter, D. M., 1976. Effects on transmission of the presence of domestic animals in infested households. In *New Approaches in American Trypanosomiasis Research*, Proc. Int. Symp., Pan. Am. Hlth Org., Sci. Publ. No. 318, pp. 330–7.

Minter-Goedbloed, E., 1981. The susceptibility of chickens to *Trypanosoma brucei* subspecies, *Trans. R. Soc. trop. Med. Hyg.*, **75**(3): 345–53.

Moloo, S. K., 1982. Studies on transmission of two East African stocks of *Trypanosoma vivax* to cattle, goats, rabbits, rats and mice, *Acta trop.*, **39**: 51–9.

Moloo, S. K. and Kutuza, S. B., 1974. Sleeping sickness survey in Musoma district, Tanzania: further study on the vector role of *Glossina*, *Trans. R. Soc. trop. Med. Hyg.*, **68**(5): 403–9.

Moloo, S. K., Losos, G. J. and Kutuza, S. B., 1973. Transmission of *Trypanosoma brucei* to cats and dogs by feeding of infected goats, *Ann. trop. Med. Parasit.*, **67**(3): 331–4.

Moloo, S. K., Steiger, R. F., Brun, R. and Boreham, P. F. L., 1971. Sleeping sickness survey in Musoma district, Tanzania. II. The role of *Glossina* in the transmission of sleeping sickness, *Acta trop.*, **28**: 189–205.

Molyneux, D. H., 1973. Isolation of *Trypanosoma* (*Trypanozoon*) *brucei gambiense* in rabbits by intratesticular inoculation technique, *Ann. trop. Med. Parasit.*, **67**(4): 391–7.

Molyneux, D. H., 1975. Diagnostic methods in animal trypanosomiasis, *Vet. Parasitol.*, **1**: 5–17.

Morales, G. A. and Carreno, F., 1976. The Proechimys rat: a potential laboratory host and model for the study of *Trypanosoma evansi*, *Trop. Anim. Hlth Prod.*, **8**: 122–4.

Morales, G. A., Wells, E. A. and Angel, D., 1976. The capybara (*Hydrochoerus hydrochaeris*) as a reservoir host for *Trypanosoma evansi*, *J. Wildl. Dis.*, **12**: 572–4.

Morel, C. and Simpson, L., 1980. Characterization of pathogenic trypanosomatidae by restriction endonuclease fingerprinting of kinetoplast DNA minicircles, *Am. J. Trop. Med. Hyg.*, **29**(5) Suppl.: 1070–4.

Morrison, W. I. and Murray, M., 1979a. Lymphoid changes in African trypanosomiasis. In *Pathogenicity of Trypanosomes*, eds G. J. Losos, A. Chouinard. IDRC (Ottawa), **132e**, pp. 154–160.

Morrison, W. I. and Murray, M., 1979b. *Trypanosoma congolense*: inheritance of susceptibility to infection in inbred strains of mice, *Exp. Parasitol.*, **48**: 364–74.

Morrison, W. I., Murray, M., Sayer, P. D. and Preston, J. M., 1981. The pathogenesis of experimentally induced *Trypanosoma brucei* infection in the dog. I. Tissue and organ damage. II. Changes in the lymphoid organs. *Am. J. Pathol.*, **102**: 168–94.

Morrison, W. I., Roelants, G. E., Mayor-Withey, K. S. and Murray, M., 1978. Susceptibility of inbred strains of mice to *Trypanosoma congolense*: correlation with changes in spleen lymphocyte populations, *Clin. Exp. Immunol.*, **32**: 25–40.

Mosca, W. and Plaja, J., 1981. Delayed hypersensitivity to heart antigens in Chagas' disease as measured by *in vitro* lymphocyte stimulation, *J. Clin. Microbiol.*, **14**(1): 1–5.

Mott, K. E., Mota, E. A., Sherlock, I., Hoff, R., Muniz, T. M., Oliveira, T. S. and Draper, C. C., 1978. *Trypanosoma cruzi* infection in dogs and cats and household seroactivity to *T. cruzi* in a rural community in northeast Brazil, *Am. J. Trop. Med. Hyg.*, **27**(6): 1123–7.

Moulton, J. E., 1980. Experimental *Trypanosoma brucei* infection in deer mice: splenic changes, *Vet. Pathol.*, **17**: 218–25.

Moulton, J. E. and Coleman, J. L., 1979. A soluble immunosuppressor substance in spleen in deer mice infected with *Trypanosoma brucei*, *Am. J. vet. Res.*, **40**(8): 1131–3.

Moulton, J. E., Coleman, J. L. and Thompson, P. S., 1974. Pathogenesis of *Trypanosoma equiperdum* in deer mice (*Peromyscus maniculatus*), *Am. J. vet. Res.*, **35**(7): 961–76.

Moulton, J. E. and Sollod, A. E., 1976. Clinical, serologic, and pathologic changes in calves with experimentally induced *Trypanosoma brucei* infection, *Am. J. vet. Res.*, **37**(7): 791–801.

Mshelbwala, A. S. and Ormerod, W. E., 1973. Measurement of the infectivity of *Trypanosoma cruzi* in faeces of *Rhodnius* by comparison of dose–response curves, *J. Gen. Microbiol.*, **75**: 339–50.

Muhlpfordt, H., 1975. An electron microscopic study on a strain of *Trypanosoma vivax* maintained in cattle, *Z. Tropenmed. Parasit.*, **26**(1): 1–8.

Mulligan, H. W., 1970. *The African Trypanosomiases*. George Allen & Unwin (London).

Murray, M., Berry, J. D., Morrison, W. I., Williams, R. O., Hirumi, H. and Rovis, L., 1980. A review of the prospects for vaccination in African trypanosomiasis. Part II, *Wld Anim. Rev.*, **33**: 14–18.

Murray, M. and Morrison, W. I., 1979a. Parasitemia and host susceptibility to African trypanosomiasis. In *Pathogenicity of Trypanosomes*, eds G. J. Losos, A. Chouinard, IDRC (Ottawa), **132e**, pp. 71–81.

Murray, M. and Morrison, W. I., 1979b. Non-specific induction of increased resistance in mice to *Trypanosoma congolense* and *Trypanosoma brucei* by immunostimulants, *Parasitology*, **79**: 349–66.

Murray, M., Morrison, W. I., Murray, P. K., Clifford, D. J. and Trail, J. C. M., 1979. Trypanotolerance – a review, *Wld Anim. Rev.*, **31**: 2–12.

Murray, M., Murray, P. K., Jennings, F. W., Fisher, E. W. and Urquhart, G. M., 1974. The pathology of *Trypanosoma brucei* infection in the rat, *Res. vet. Sci.*, **16**: 77–84.

Murray, M., Murray, P. K. and McIntyre, W. I. M., 1977. An improved parasitological technique for the diagnosis of African trypanosomiasis, *Trans. R. Soc. trop. Med. Hyg.*, **71**(4): 325–6.

Murray, M. and Urquhart, G. M., 1977. Immunoprophylaxis against African trypanosomiasis. In *Immunity to Blood Parasites of Animals and Man*, eds L. H. Miller, J. A. Pino, J. J. McKelvey Jr. Plenum Press (New York), pp. 209–41.

Musoke, A. J., Nantulya, V. M., Barbet, A. F., Kironde, F. and McGuire, T. C., 1981. Bovine immune response to African trypanosomes: specific antibodies to variable surface glyco-proteins of *Trypanosoma brucei, Parasite Immunol.*, **3**: 97–106.

Mwambu, P. M., 1971. The effect of a block-treatment regimen, using Ethidium, on cattle trypanosomiasis in an endemic area, *E. Afr. Agric. For. J.*, **36**(4): 414–18.

Mwambu, P. M. and Losos, G. J., 1979. Ultrastructural changes in blood vessels of tissues of cattle experimentally infected with *Trypanosoma congolense* and *Trypanosoma vivax*: a preliminary report. In *Pathogenicity of Trypanosomes*, eds G. J. Losos, A. Chouinard. IDRC (Ottawa), **132e**, pp. 184–5.

Mwambu, P. M. and Mayende, J. S. P., 1971. Sleeping sickness survey in Musoma district, Tanzania. III. Survey of cattle for evidence of *Trypanosoma rhodesiense* infections, *Acta trop.*,**28**: 206–10.

Mwongela, G. N., Kovatch, R. M. and Fazil, M. A., 1981. Acute *Trypanosoma vivax* infection in dairy cattle in coast province, Kenya, *Trop. Anim. Hlth Prod.*, **13**: 63–9.

Nagle, R. B., Dong, S., Guillot, J. M., McDaniel, K. M. and Lindsley, H. B., 1980. Pathology of experimental African trypanosomiasis in rabbits infected with *Trypanosoma rhodesiense, Am. J. Trop. Med. Hyg.*, **29**(6): 1187–95.

Nagle, R. B., Ward, P. A., Lindsley, H. B., Sadun, E. H., Johnson, A. J., Berkaw, R. E. and Hildebrandt, P. K., 1974. Experimental infections with African trypanosomes. VI. Glomerulonephritis involving the alternate pathway of complement activation, *Am. J. Trop. Med. Hyg.*, **23**(1): 15–26.

Nantulya, V. M., Doyle, J. J. and Jenni, L., 1978. Studies on *Trypanosoma* (*Nannomonas*) *congolense*. I. On the morphological appearance of the parasite in the mouse, *Acta trop.*, **35**: 329–37.
Nantulya, V. M., Doyle, J. J. and Jenni, L., 1980. Studies on *Trypanosoma* (*Nannomonas*) *congolense*. III. Antigenic variation in three cyclically transmitted stocks, *Parasitology*, **80**: 123–31.
Nantulya, V. M., Musoke, A. J., Barbet, A. F. and Roelants, G. E., 1979. Evidence for reappearance of *Trypanosoma brucei* variable antigen types in relapse populations, *J. Parasitol.*, **65**(5): 673–9.
Nathan, H. C., Bacchi, C. J., Sakai, T. T., Rescigno, D., Stumpf, D. and Hutner, S. H., 1981. Bleomycin-induced life prolongation of mice infected with *Trypanosoma brucei brucei* EATRO 110, *Trans. R. Soc. trop. Med. Hyg.*, **75**(3): 394–8.
Neitz, W. O. and McCully, R. M., 1971. Clinicopathological study on experimental *Trypanosoma brucei* infections in horses. Part 1. Development of clinically recognizable nervous symptoms in Nagana-infected horses treated with subcurative doses of Antrypol and Berenil, *Onderstepoort J. vet. Res.*, **38**(3): 127–40.
Newport, G. R., Page, C. R. III, Ashman, P. U., Stibbs, H. H. and Seed, J. R., 1977. Alteration of free serum amino acids in voles infected with *Trypanosoma brucei gambiense*, *J. Parasitol.*, **63**(1): 15–24.
Newton, B. A., 1968. Biochemical peculiarities of trypanosomatid flagellates, *Am. Rev. Microbiol.*, **22**: 109–30.
Newton, B. A. and Burnett, J. K., 1972. DNS of *Kinetoplastidae*: a comparative study. In *Comparative Biochemistry of Parasites*, ed. H. van den Bossche. Academic Press (New York), pp. 185–98.
Nielsen, K. and Sheppard, J., 1977. Activation of complement by trypanosomes, *Experientia*, **33**(6): 769–71.
Nielsen, K., Sheppard, J., Holmes, W. and Tizard, T., 1978a. Experimental bovine trypanosomiasis. Changes in the catabolism of serum immunoglobulins and complement components in infected cattle, *Immunology*, **35**: 811–16.
Nielsen, K., Sheppard, J., Holmes, W. and Tizard, I., 1978b. Experimental bovine trypanosomiasis. Changes in serum complement and complement levels in infected cattle, *Immunology*, **35**: 817–26.
Nielsen, K., Sheppard, J., Holmes, W. and Tizard, I., 1978c. Increased susceptibility of *Trypanosoma lewisi* infected or decomplemented rats to *Salmonella typhimurium*, *Experientia*, **34**: 118–9.
Nielsen, K., Sheppard, J., Holmes, W. and Tizard, I., 1978d. Direct activation of complement by trypanosomes, *J. Parasitol.*, **64**(3): 544–6.
Nielsen, K., Sheppard, J. and Tizard, I., 1979. Complement in experimental trypanosomiasis. In *Pathogenicity of Trypanosomes*, eds G. J. Losos, A. Chouinard. IDRC (Ottawa), **132e**, pp. 94–102.
Njogu, R. M., Whittaker, C. J. and Hill, G. C., 1980. Evidence for a branched electron transport chain in *Trypanosoma brucei*, *Mol. Biochem. Parasitol.*, **1**: 13–29.

Noguiera, N., Chaplan, S., Tydings, J. D., Unkeless, J. and Cohn, Z., 1981. *Trypanosoma cruzi*. Surface antigens of blood and culture forms, *J. Exp. Med.*, **153**: 629–39.

Noguiera, N. and Cohn, Z., 1976. *Trypanosoma cruzi*: mechanism of entry and intracellular fate in mammalian cells, *J. Exp. Med.*, **143**: 1402–20.

Noguiera, N. and Cohn, Z., 1977. *Trypanosoma cruzi* uptake and intracellular fate in normal and activated cells, *Am. J. Trop. Med. Hyg.*, **26**(6): 194–203.

Nwagwu, M. and Opperdoes, F. R., 1982. Regulation of glycolysis in *Trypanosoma brucei*: hexokinase and phosphofructokinase activity, *Acta trop.*, **39**: 61–72.

Nyindo, M., Chimtawi, M. and Owor, J., 1980. Fine structure of metacyclic forms of *Trypanosoma brucei* grown in continuous culture, *Am. J. Trop. Med. Hyg.*, **29**(5): 774–8.

Nyindo, M., Chimtawi, M., Owor, J., Kaminjolo, J. S., Patel, N. and Darji, N., 1978. Sleeping sickness: *in vitro* cultivation of *Trypanosoma brucei* from the salivary glands of *Glossina morsitans*, *J. Parasitol.*, **64**(6): 1039–43.

O'Daly, J. A., 1975. A new liquid medium for *Trypanosoma (Schizotrypanum) cruzi*, *J. Protozool.*, **22**(2): 265–70.

Oduro, K. K., Bowman, I. B. R. and Flynn, I. W., 1980a. *Trypanosoma brucei*: preparation and some properties of a multienzyme complex catalysing part of the glycolytic pathway, *Exp. Parasitol.*, **50**: 240–50.

Oduro, K. K., Flynn, I. W. and Bowman, I. B. R., 1980b. *Trypanosoma brucei*: activities and subcellular distribution of glycolytic enzymes from differently disrupted cells, *Exp. Parasitol.*, **50**: 123–35.

Ogwu, D. and Nuru, S., 1981. Transplacental transmission of trypanosomes in animals and man. A review, *Vet. Bull.*, **51**(6): 381–4.

Okiwelu, S. N., 1977. Host preference and trypanosome infection rates of *Glossina morsitans morsitans* Westwood in the Republic of Zambia, *Ann. trop. Med. Parasit.*, **71**(1): 101–7.

Olenick, J. G., Travis, R. W. and Garson, S., 1981. *Trypanosoma rhodesiense*: chemical and immunological characterization of variant-specific surface coat glycoproteins, *Mol. Biochem. Parasitol.*, **3**: 227–38.

Onodera, M., Rosen, N. L., Lifter, J., Hotez, P. J., Bogucki, M. S., Davis, G., Patton, C. L., Konigsberg, W. H. and Richards, F. F., 1981. *Trypanosoma congolense*: surface glyco-proteins of two early bloodstream variants. II. Purification and partial chemical characterization, *Exp. Parasitol.*, **52**: 427–39.

Opperdoes, F. R., 1981. A rapid method for the isolation of intact glycosomes from *Trypanosoma brucei* by Percoll-gradient centrifugation in a vertical rotor, *Mol. Biochem. Parasitol.*, **3**: 181–6.

Ormerod, W. E., 1958. A comparative study of cytoplasmic inclusions (volutin granules) in different species of trypanosomes, *J. gen. Microbiol.*, **19**: 271–88.

Ormerod, W. E., 1976. Ecological effect of control of African trypanosomiasis, *Science*, **191**: 815–21.

Ormerod, W. E., 1979. Development of *Trypanosoma brucei* in mammalian host. In *Biology of the Kinetoplastida*, eds W. H. R. Lumsden, D. A. Evans. Academic Press (London), vol. 2, pp. 339–84.

Ormerod, W. E. and Page, M. J., 1967. Lipid staining of type II. granules in trypanosomes, *Trans. R. Soc. trop. Med. Hyg.*, **61**: 12.

Ormerod, W. E. and Venkatesan, S., 1971a. An amastigote phase of the sleeping sickness trypanosome, *Trans. R. Soc. trop. Med. Hyg.*, **65**(6): 736–41.

Ormerod, W. E. and Venkatesan, S., 1971b. The occult visceral phase of mammalian trypanosomes with special reference to the life cycle of *Trypanosoma* (*Trypanozoon*) *brucei*, *Trans. R. Soc. trop. Med. Hyg.*, **65**(6): 722–35.

Ormerod, W. E., Venkatesan, S. and Carpenter, R. G., 1974. The effect of immune inhibition on pleomorphism in *Trypanosoma brucei rhodesiense*, *Parasitology*, **68**: 355–67.

Overdulve, J. P. and Antonisse, H. W., 1970. Measurement of the effect of low temperature on protozoa by titration. I. A mathematical model for titration, using prepatent period or survival time; with a discussion of method of ID_{63}, *Exp. Parasitol.*, **27**: 310–22.

Pan American Health Organization, 1976. *New Approaches in American Trypanosomiasis Research*, Proc. Int. Symp., Scientific Publ. No. 318. WHO (Washington, DC).

Paris, J. and Wilson, A. J., 1976. A study of the antigenic relationships of isolates of *Trypanosoma brucei* from three areas of East Africa, *Ann. trop. Med. Parasit.*, **70**(1): 45–51.

Pays, E., Delronche, M., Lheureux, M., Vervoort, T., Bloch, J., Gannon, F. and Steinert, M., 1980. Cloning and characterization of DNA sequences complementary to messenger ribonucleic acids coding for synthesis of two surface antigens of *Trypanosoma brucei*, *Nuclei Acids Res.*, **8**(24): 5965–81.

Pays, E., van Meirvenne, N., Le Ray, D. and Steinert, M., 1981. Gene duplication and transposition linked to antigenic variation in *Trypanosoma brucei*, *Proc. Natl Acad. Sci., USA*, **78**(5): 2673–7.

Pearson, T. W., Kar, S. K., McGuire, T. C. and Lundin, L. B., 1981. Trypanosome variable surface antigens: studies using two-dimensional gel electrophoresis and monoclonal antibodies, *J. Immunol.*, **126**(3): 823–8.

Pearson, T. W., Roelants, G. E., Lundin, L. B. and Mayor-Withey, K. S., 1978. Immune depression in trypanosome-infected mice. I. Depressed T lymphocyte responses, *Eur. J. Immunol.*, **8**: 723–7.

Pearson, T. W., Saya, L. E., Howard, S. P. and Buckley, J. T., 1982.

The use of aerolysin toxin as an aid for visualization of low numbers of African trypanosomes in whole blood, *Acta trop.*, **39**: 73–7.

Peel, E. and Chardome, M., 1954. *Trypanosoma suis* – Ochmann 1905 – trypanosome monomorphe pathogène de mammifères, évaluant dans les glandes salivaires de *Glossina brevipalpis*, Newst., Mosso (Urundi), *Ann. Soc. Belge Méd. trop.*, **34**: 277–95.

Pegram, R. G. and Scott, J. M., 1976. The prevalence and diagnosis of *Trypanosoma evansi* infection in camels in southern Ethiopia, *Trop. Anim. Hlth Prod.*, **8**: 20–7.

Perié, N. M., Tinnemans-Anggawidjaja, T. and Zwart, D., 1975. A refinement of the immunofluorescent complex fixation test for trypanosome infections, *2. Tropenmed. Parasit.*, **25**: 399–404.

Peruzzi, M., 1928. Pathologic-anatomical and serological observations in trypanosomiases, *Final Report, League of Nations, Int. Comm. Human Trypanosomiasis*, **3**: 245–328.

Phillips, N. R., 1960a. Experimental studies on the quantitative transmission of *Trypanosoma cruzi*: consideration regarding the standardization of materials, *Ann. trop. Med. Parasit.*, **54**: 60–71.

Phillips, N. R., 1960b. Experimental studies on the quantitative transmission of *Trypanosoma cruzi*: aspects of the rearing, maintenance and testing of vector material, and of the origin and course of infection in the vector, *Ann. trop. Med. Parasit.*, **54**: 397–414.

Phillips, N. R. and Bertram, D. S., 1967. Laboratory studies of *Trypanosoma cruzi* infections, *J. Med. Ent.*, **4**: 168–74.

Platt, K. B. and Adams, L. G., 1976. Evaluation of the indirect fluorescent antibody test for detecting *Trypanosoma vivax* in South American cattle, *Res. vet. Sci.*, **21**: 53–8.

Politzar, H., 1974. Serological studies on cattle experimentally infected with several species of African trypanosomes, *Z. Tropenmed. Parasit.*, **25**: 22–7.

Poltera, A. A., 1980. Immunopathological and chemotherapeutic studies in experimental trypanosomiasis with special reference to the heart and brain, *Trans. R. Soc. trop. Med. Hyg.*, **74**(6): 706–15.

Poltera, A. A., Hochmann, A. and Lambert, P. H., 1980a. A model for cardiopathy induced by *Trypanosoma brucei brucei* in mice. A histologic and immunopathologic study, *Am. J. Pathol.*, **99**(2): 325–51.

Poltera, A. A., Hochmann, A., Rudin, W. and Lambert, P. H., 1980b. *Trypanosoma brucei brucei*: a model for cerebral trypanosomiasis in mice – an immunological, histological and electromicroscopic study, *Clin. Exp. Immunol.*, **40**: 496–507.

Preston, J. M., Wellde, B. T. and Kovatch, R. M., 1979. *Trypanosoma congolense*: calf erythrocyte survival, *Exp. Parasitol.*, **48**: 118–25.

Princewill, T. J., 1980. Effect of storage on ice on pathogenicity of salivarian trypanosomes, *Bull. Anim. Hlth Prod. Afr.*, **28**: 115–29.

Purohit, S. K. and Jatkar, P. R., 1979. Antigenic analysis of *Trypanosoma evansi*, *Indian vet. J.*, **56**: 91–4.

Raether, W., 1971. Experimental infections of *Mastomys natalensis* (Smith 1834) with trypanosome species of the *Lewisi-Congolense* and *Brucei-evansi* group, *Z. Tropenmed. Parasit.*, **22**(4): 351–9.

Raether, W. and Seidenath, H., 1972. Infectivity of various protozoan species after extended storage in liquid nitrogen, *Z. Tropenmed. Parasit.*, **23**: 428–31.

Raether, W. and Seidenath, H., 1974. Influence of different physiologic solutions on the motility and infectivity of trypanosomes (*T. rhodesiense*) from fresh blood, *Z. Tropenmed. Parasit.*, **24**: 285–95.

Rather, W. and Seidenath, H., 1974. Influence of different physiologic solutions on the motility and infectivity of trypanosomes after deep-freezing in liquid nitrogen (*T. rhodesiense, T. brucei*), *Z. Tropenmed. Parasit.*, **25**: 28–41.

Raghaven, R. S. and Khan, N. A., 1970. Bovine trypanosomiasis – control with Samorin, *Indian vet. J.*, **47**: 187–8.

Raisinghani, P. M., Bhatia, J. S., Dwaraknath, P. K. and Lodha, K. R., 1980. Plasma monamine oxidase (MOA) levels in trypanosomiasis in the camel, *Indian vet. J.*, **57**: 780–2.

Raisinghani, P. M. and Lodha, K. R., 1980a. Prognostic values of some haematological and biochemical parameters of camels affected with surra following the treatment with Antrypol, antrycide methyl sulphate, Naganol and Berenil, *Indian vet. J.*, **57**: 579–84.

Raisinghani, P. M. and Lodha, K. R., 1980b. Chemotherapeutic levels of Berenil (Hoechst) in experimental surra in camel, *Indian vet. J.*, **57**: 891–5.

Rangel, H. A., Araujo, P. M. F., Camargo, I. J. B., Bonfitto, M., Repka, D., Sakurada, J. K. and Atta, A. M., 1981. Detection of a proteinase common to epimastigote, trypomastigote and amastigote of different strains of *Trypanosoma cruzi*, *Z. Tropenmed. Parasit.*, **32**: 87–92.

Ray, H. N., Short, G. N., Shivnani, G. A. and Hawkins, P. A., 1953. Therapy and prophylaxis of Indian equine and bovine trypanosomiasis by antrycide formulation, *Indian vet. J.*, **29**: 627–35.

Razzaque, A. and Mishra, S. S., 1977. Comparative efficacy of Berenil, Antrycide, Prosalt, and Acriflavin in the treatment of experimental surra in buffalo-calves, *Bull. Anim. Hlth Prod.*, **25**: 409–14.

Reid, H. W., Burridge, M. J., Pullan, N. B., Sutherst, R. W. and Wain, E. B., 1970a. Survey for trypanosome infections in domestic cattle and wild animals in areas of East Africa. I. Introduction, *Br. vet. J.*, **126**: 622–6.

Reid, H. W., Burridge, M. J., Pullan, N. B., Sutherst, R. W. and Wain, E. B., 1970b. Survey for trypanosome infections in domestic cattle and wild animals in areas of East Africa. IV. Stercorarian trypanosome infections in cattle and wild animals in East Africa, *Br. vet. J.*, **126**: 642–7.

Reid, H. W., Holmes, P. H. and Skinner, H. H., 1979. Immunosuppression in experimental trypanosomiasis: effects of *Trypanosoma brucei* on immunization against louping-ill virus and lymphocytic choriomeningitis virus, *J. Comp. Path.*, **89**: 581–5.

Reinwald, E., Rautenberg, P. and Risse, H-J., 1979. *Trypanosoma congolense*: mechanical removal of the surface coat *in vitro*, *Exp. Parasitol.*, **48**: 384–97.

Repka, D., Camargo, I. J. B., Sanatana, E. M., Cunha, W. M., de Souza, O. C., Sakurada, J. K. and Rangel, H. A., 1980. Surface antigenic determinant of epimastigote forms common to *Trypanosoma cruzi*, *Z. Tropenmed. Parasit.*, **31**: 239–46.

Rickman, L. R., 1977a. Variation in the test responses of clone-derived *Trypanosoma* (*Trypanozoon*) *brucei brucei* and *T.* (*T*) *B. rhodesiense* relapse antigenic variants, examined by a modified blood incubation infectivity test and its possible significance in Rhodesian sleeping sickness transmission, *Med. J. Zambia*, **11**(2): 31–7.

Rickman, L. R., 1977b. Variation in the sensitivity to normal human serum of clone-derived antigenic variants of *Trypanosoma* (*Trypanozoon*) *brucei* complex trypanosomes, *Med. J. Zambia*, **11**(2): 41–2.

Rickman, L. and Kolala, F., 1980. The sequential testing of successive variable antigen types produced in clone induced *Trypanosoma brucei* species infections serially syringe-passaged in white rats. *Proc. 16th Meet. int. Scient. Comm. Trypanosom.* (*Yaoundé*). OAU/STRC publ.

Rickman, L., Kolala, F. and Mwanza, S., 1981a. Variation in the sensitivity of successive variable antigen types in a *Trypanosoma* (*Trypanozoon*) *brucei* subspecies clone to some African game animal sera, *Acta trop.*, **38**: 115–24.

Rickman, L. R. and Robson, J., 1970a. The blood incubation infectivity test: a simple test which may serve to distinguish *Trypanosoma brucei* from *T. rhodesiense*, *Bull. Wld Hlth Org.*, **42**: 650–1.

Rickman, L. R. and Robson, J., 1970b. The testing of proven *Trypanosoma brucei* and *T. rhodesiense* strains by the blood incubation infectivity test. *Bull. Wld Hlth Org.*, **42**: 911–16.

Rickman, L. R. and Robson, J., 1972. Some supplementary observations on the blood incubation infectivity test, *Bull. Wld Hlth Org.*, **46**: 403–4.

Rickman, W. J. and Cox, H. W., 1980. Immunologic reactions associated with anemia, thrombocytopenia, and coagulopathy in experimental African trypanosomiasis, *J. Parasitol.*, **66**(1): 28–33.

Rickman, W. J., Cox, H. W. and Thoongsuwan, S., 1981b. Interactions of immunoconglutinin and immune complexes in cold autohemagglutination associated with African trypanosomiasis, *J. Parasitol.*, **67**(2): 159–63.

Riordan, K., 1977. Long term variations in trypanosome infection rates in highly infected tsetse flies on a cattle route in southwestern Nigeria, *Ann. trop. Med. Parasit.*, **71**(1): 11–20.

Riou, G. and Barrois, M., 1979. Restriction cleavage map of kinetoplast DNA minicircles from *Trypanosoma equiperdum*, *Biochem. Biophys. Res. Comm.*, **90**(2): 405–9.

Riou, G. and Barrois, M., 1981. The kinetoplast DNA of *Trypanosoma gambiense*: comparison with the kDNA of *Trypanosoma equiperdum*, *Biochimie*, **63**(10): 755–65.

Riou, G. and Benard, J., 1980. Berenil induces the complete loss of kinetoplast DNA sequences, *Biochem. Biophys. Res. Comm.*, **96**(1): 350–4.

Riou, G. F. and Saucier, J. M., 1979. Characterization of the molecular components in kinetoplast-mitochondrial DNA of *Trypanosoma equiperdum*. Comparative study of the dyskinetoplastic and wild strains, *J. Cell. Biol.*, **82**: 248–63.

Roberts, C. J. and Clarkson, M. J., 1977. Free fatty acids, lysophosphatidylcholine and pathogenesis of trypanosomiasis, *Lancet* (i): 952–3.

Roberts, C. J. and Gray, A. R., 1973a. Studies on trypanosome-resistant cattle. I. The breeding and growth performance of N'Dama, Muturu, and Zebu cattle maintained under the same conditions of husbandry, *Trop. Anim. Hlth Prod.*, **5**: 211–19.

Roberts, C. J. and Gray, A. R., 1973b. Studies on trypanosome-resistant cattle. II. The effect of trypanosomiasis on N'Dama, Muturu, and Zebu cattle. *Trop. Anim. Hlth Prod.*, **5**: 220–33.

Roberts, C. J., Gray. A. R. and Gray. M. A., 1969. Local skin reactions in cattle at the site of infection with *Trypanosoma congolense* by *Glossina morsitans* and *tachinoides*, *Trans. R. Soc. trop. Med. Hyg.*, **63**: 620–4.

Robins-Browne, R. M., Schneider, J. and Metz, J., 1975. Thrombocytopenia in trypanosomiasis, *Am. J. trop. Med. Hyg.*, **24**(2): 226–31.

Robson, J., 1958a. A field trial of prophylactic drugs against trypanosomiasis in zebu cattle, *Vet. Rec.*, **70**(46): 925–7.

Robson, J., 1958b. *Observations on the Use of Prothidium in Tanganyika Territory*. ISCTR, CCTA Publ. No. 41, vol. VII, pp. 55–8.

Robson, J., 1961. Prophylaxis against trypanosomiasis in zebu cattle. II. The duration of prophylaxis conferred by preparations of prothidium compared with antrycide prosalt, *Vet. Rec.*, **73**(26): 641–5.

Robson, J., 1962. Prophylaxis against trypanosomiasis in zebu cattle. IV. A field trial of metamidium and isometamidium, *Vet. Rec.*, **74**(34): 913–17.

Robson, J. and Ashkar, T. S., 1972a. The efficiency of different diagnostic methods in animal trypanosomiasis; based on surveys carried out in Nyanza province, Kenya, *Bull. epiz. Dis. Afr.*, **20**: 303–6.

Robson, J. and Ashkar, T. S., 1972b. Trypanosomiasis in domestic livestock in the Lambwe Valley area and a field evaluation of various diagnostic techniques, *Bull. Wld Hlth Org.*, **47**: 727–34.

Robson, J. and Cawdery, M. J. H., 1958. Prophylaxis against

trypanosomiasis in zebu cattle. A comparison of prothidium, the suraminates of ethidium and RD 2902 and antrycide prosalt, *Vet. Rec.*, **70**: 870–6.

Rosen, N. L., Onodera, M., Hotez, P. J., Bogucki, M. S., Elce, B., Patton, C., Konigsberg, W. H., Cross, G. A. M. and Richards, F. F., 1981. *Trypanosoma congolense*: surface glyco-proteins of two early bloodstream variants. I. Production of a relapsing infection in rodents, *Exp. Parasitol.*, **52**: 210–18.

Rosen, N. L., Onodera, M., Patton, C. L., Lipman, M. B. and Richards, F. F., 1979. *Trypanosoma congolense*: isolation and purification, *Exp. Parasitol.*, **47**: 378–83.

Rouzer, C. A. and Cerami, A., 1980. Hypertriglyceridemia associated with *Trypanosoma brucei brucei* infection in rabbits: role of defective tryglyceride removal, *Mol. Biochem. Parasitol.*, 210–18.

Rovis, L. and Baekkeskov, S., 1980. Subcellular fractionation of *Trypanosoma brucei*. Isolation and characterization of plasma membranes, *Parasitology*, **80**: 507–24.

Rovis, L. and Dube, D. K., 1981. Studies on the biosynthesis of the variant surface glycoprotein of *Trypanosoma brucei*: sequence of glycosylation, *Mol. Biochem. Parasitol.*, **4**: 77–93.

Ruchel, H., 1975. Chemoprophylaxis of bovine trypanosomiasis. Thesis Vet. Institute. Univ. Göttingen, pp. 1–248.

Rurangirwa, F. R., Tabel, F. R., Losos, G. J., Masiga, W. N., Mwambu, P., 1978. Immunosuppressive effect of *Trypanosoma congolense* and *Trypanosoma vivax* on the secondary immune response of cattle to *Mycoplasma mycoides* subs. *mycoides*, *Res. vet. Sci.*, **25**: 395–7.

Rurangirwa, F. R., Tabel, H., Losos, G. J. and Tizard, I. R., 1979. Suppression of antibody response to *Leptospira biflexa* and *Brucella abortus* and recovery from immunosuppression after Berenil treatment, *Infect. Immun.*, **26**: 822–6.

Sachs, R., Schaller, G. B. and Baker, J. R., 1967. Isolation of trypanosomes of the *Trypanosoma brucei* group from a lion, *Acta trop.*, **24**: 109–12.

Sacks, D. L. and Askonas, B. A., 1980. Trypanosome-induced suppression of anti-parasite responses during experimental African trypanosomiasis, *Eur. J. Immunol.*, **10**: 971–4.

Sacks, D. L., Selkirk, M., Ogilvie, B. M. and Askonas, B. A., 1980. Intrinsic immunosuppressive activity of different trypanosome strains varies with parasite virulence, *Nature*, **283**: 476–8.

Santos-Buch, C. A. and Teixeira, A. R. L., 1974. The immunology of experimental Chagas' disease. III. Rejection of allogenic heart cells *in vitro*, *J. exp. Med.*, **140**: 38–53.

Schindler, R., 1972. Studies of the applicability of serological methods to the differential diagnosis of cattle trypanosomiasis in Africa. *Z. Tropenmed. Parasit.*, **23**: 78–88.

Schindler, R. and Sachs, R., 1970. Serological studies on dogs infected with *Trypanosoma brucei*. *Z. Tropenmed. Parasit.*, **21**(4): 339–46.

Schmidt, H., Kaduk, B., Fink, E., 1978. Pathomorphology of side-effects of trypanocide diamidines. *Vet. Pathol.*, **15**: 574.

Schmunis, G. A., Szarfman, A., de Souza, W. and Langembach, T., 1980. *Trypanosoma cruzi*: antibody-induced mobility of surface antigens, *Exp. Parasitol.*, **50**: 90–102.

Schneider, I., 1979. Tsetse fly tissue culture and its application to the propagation of African trypanosomes *in vitro*. In *Practical Tissue Culture Applications*, eds K. Maramorsch, H. Hirumi. Academic Press (London), pp. 373–86.

Schupp, E., Michel, R., Raether, W., Niemitz, H. and Uphoff, M., 1980. Ultrastructural alterations, infectivity, and motility of *Trypanosoma brucei* before and after cryopreservation in nitrogen, *Z. Parasitenkd.*, **62**: 213–30.

Schutt, I. D. and Mehlitz, D., 1981. On the persistence of human serum resistance and isoenzyme patterns of *Trypanozoon* in experimentally infected pigs, *Acta trop.*, **38**: 367–73.

Scorza, C. and Scorza, J. V., 1972. The role of inflammatory macrophages in experimental acute Chagasic myocarditis, *J. Reticuloendothel. Soc.*, **11**: 604–16.

Scott, J. M., Holmes, P. H., Jennings, F. W. and Urquhart, G. M., 1978. Attempted protection of zebu cattle against trypanosomiasis using a multi-stabilate vaccine, *Res. vet. Sci.*, **25**: 115–17.

Scott, J. M., Pegram, R. G., Holmes, P. H., Pay, T. W. F., Knight, P. A., Jennings, F. W. and Urquhart, G. M., 1977. Immunosuppression in bovine trypanosomiasis field studies using foot-and-mouth disease vaccine and clostrodial vaccine, *Trop. Anim. Hlth Prod.*, **9**: 159–65.

Seed, J. R., 1974. Antigens and antigenic variability of the African trypanosomes, *J. Protozool.*, **21**(5): 639–45.

Seiler, R. J., Omar, S. and Jackson, A. R., 1981. Meningoencephalitis in naturally occurring *Trypanosoma evansi* infection (surra) of horses, *Vet. Pathol.*, **18**: 120–2.

Selkirk, M. E. and Sacks, D. L., 1980. Trypanotolerance in inbred mice: an immunological basis for variation in susceptibility to infection with *Trypanosoma brucei*, *Z. Tropenmed. Parasit.*, **31**: 435–8.

Shapiro, S. Z. and Young, J. R., 1981. An immunochemical method for mRNA purification. Application to messenger RNA encoding trypanosome variable surface antigen, *J. Biol. Chem.*, **256**(4): 1495–8.

Shaw, J. J. and Lainson, R., 1972. *Trypanosoma vivax* in Brazil, *Ann. trop. Med. Parasit.*, **66**: 25–32.

Shertzer, H. G., Hall, J. E. and Seed, J. R., 1981. Hepatic mixed-function oxidase activity in mice infected with *Trypanosoma brucei gambiense* or treated with trypanocides, *Mol. Biochem. Parasitol.*, **3**: 199–204.

Shirazi, M. F., Holman, M., Hudson, K. M., Klaus, G. G. B., Terry, R. J., 1980. Complement (C3) levels and the effect of C3 depletion in infections of *Trypanosoma brucei* in mice, *Parasite Immunol.*, **2**: 155–61.

Shoemaker, J. P. and Hoffman, R. V., 1974. *Trypanosoma cruzi*: possible stimulatory factor(s) in brown adipose tissue of mice, *Exp. Parasitol.*, **35**: 272–4.

Shortley, G. and Wilkins, J. R., 1965. Independent-action and birth-death models in experimental microbiology, *Bact. Rev.*, **29**: 102–41.

Silayo, R. S., Gray, A. R. and Luckins, A. G., 1980. Use of antigens of cultured *Trypanosoma brucei* in tests for bovine trypanosomiasis, *Trop. Anim. Hlth Prod.*, **12**: 127–31.

Simpson, A. M. and Simpson, L., 1980. Kinetoplast DNA and RNA of *Trypanosoma brucei*, *Mol. Biochem. Parasitol.*, **2**: 93–108.

Smith, I. M., 1959. Chemoprophylaxis against bovine trypanosomiasis. I. Duration of protection from prothidium, ethidium and R.D. 2902 suraminates, in an area of high tsetse density, *J. Comp. Path.*, **69**: 105–15.

Smith, I. M. and Brown, K. N., 1960. Chemoprophylaxis against bovine trypanosomiasis. II. Duration of protection afforded by metamidium, prothidium and antrycide prosalt in an area of high tsetse density, *J. Comp. Path.*, **70**: 161–75.

Snider, T. G., Yaeger, R. G. and Dellucky, J., 1980. Myocarditis caused by *Trypanosoma cruzi* in a native Louisana dog, *J. Am. vet. Med. Ass.*, **177**(3): 247–9.

Sollod, A. E. and Frank, G. H., 1979. Bovine trypanosomiasis: effect on the immune response of the infected host, *Am. J. vet. Res.*, **40**(5): 658–64.

Soltys, M. A., Thomason, S. M. R. and Woo, P. T. K., 1973. Experimental transmission of *Trypanosoma brucei* and *Trypanosoma congolense* in rats and guinea pigs through skin and intact mucous membranes, *Ann. trop. Med. Parasit.*, **67**(4): 399–402.

Soltys, M. A. and Woo, P., 1969. Multiplication of *Trypanosoma brucei* and *T. congolense* in vertebrate hosts, *Trans. R. Soc. trop. Med. Hyg.*, **63**(4): 490–4.

Soltys, M. A. and Woo, P., 1970. Further studies on tissue forms of *Trypanosoma brucei* in a vertebrate host, *Trans. R. Soc. trop. Med. Hyg.*, **64**(5): 692–4.

Sooksri, V. and Inoki, S., 1972. Electron microscopic studies on penetration and development of *Trypanosoma cruzi* in HELA cells, *Biken J.*, **15**: 179–91.

Srivastava, R. V. N. and Malhotra, M. N., 1967. Efficacy of MelW-trimelarsan-melarsonyl potassium and samorinisometamidium chloride against *Trypanosoma evansi* infection in experimental dogs, *Indian J. Anim. Hlth*, **7**: 291–7.

Ssenyonga, G. S. Z., 1974. The distribution of *Trypanosoma brucei* and *T. congolense* in tissue of mice, *Parasitology*, **69**: 25.

Ssenyonga, G. S. Z., 1980a. A comparative study on the distribution of *Trypanosoma brucei* and *T. congolense* in tissues of mice and rats, *Bull. Anim. Hlth Prod. Afr.*, **28**: 312–26.
Ssenyonga, G. S. Z., 1980b. Ocular lesions associated with *Trypanosoma* (*Trypanozoon*) *brucei* infection in the rabbits, *Bull. Anim. Hlth Prod. Afr.*, **28**: 342–6.
Ssenyonga, G. S. Z., and Adam, K. M. G., 1975. The number and morphology of trypanosomes in the blood and lymph of rats infected with *Trypanosoma brucei* and *T. congolense*, *Parasitology*, **70**: 255–61.
Staak, C. and Kelley, S., 1979. The complement fixation test and African trypanosomiasis. II. The complement fixation test as an aid for assessing therapy, *Z. Tropenmed. Parasit.*, **30**: 283–6.
Staak, C. and Lohding, A., 1979. The complement fixation test and African trypanosomiasis. I. Experimental infection and re-infection in cattle before and after treatment, *Z. Tropenmed. Parasit.*, **30**: 13–18.
Stanghellini, A. and Duvallet, G., 1981. The epidemiology of human trypanosomiasis due to *Trypanosoma gambiense* in a focus of the Ivory Coast. 1. The distribution of the disease in the population, *Z. Tropenmed. Parasit.*, **32**(3): 141–4.
Steiger, R. F., 1973. On the ultrastructure of *Trypanosoma* (*Trypanozoon*) *brucei* in the course of its life cycle and some related aspects, *Acta trop.*, **30**(1–2): 64–168.
Steiger, R. F., Opperdoes, F. R. and Bontemps, J., 1980. Subcellular fractionation of *Trypanosoma brucei* bloodstream forms with special reference to hydrolases, *Eur. J. Biochem.*, **105**: 163–75.
Steiger, R. F., Steiger, E., Trager, W. and Schneider, I., 1977. *Trypanosoma congolense*: partial cyclic development in a *Glossina* cell system and oxygen consumption, *J. Parasitol.*, **63**(5): 861–7.
Stephen, L. E., 1958. Suramin complexes. IV. Ethidium bromide complex: a large scale laboratory trial of its prophylactic activity in cattle, *Ann. trop. Med. Parasit.*, **52**: 417–26.
Stephen, L. E., 1960. The prophylactic and therapeutic activity of metamidium and its suramine salt against trypanosomiasis in cattle, *Vet. Rec.*, **72**(5): 80–4.
Stephen, L. E., 1962a. Experimental *Trypanosoma congolense* infection in a horse, *Vet. Rec.*, **74**(31): 853–5.
Stephen, L. E., 1962b. Suramin complexes. X. Comparison of the prophylactic activity of prothidium–suramin complex and prothidium bromide in West African zebu cattle, *Ann. trop. Med. Parasit.*, **56**: 406–14.
Stephen, L. E., 1963. The chemotherapy and chemoprophylaxis of *Trypanosoma simiae* infections, *Vet. Bull.*, **33**: 599–604.
Stephen, L. E., 1966a. *Pig Trypanosomiasis in Tropical Africa*. Commonwealth Bureau of Animal Health Review Series No. 8 (Weybridge), pp. 1–16.
Stephen, L. E., 1966b. Observations on the resistance of West African N'Dama and zebu cattle to trypanosomiasis following a challenge

by wild *Glossina morsitans* from an early age, *Ann. trop. Med. Parasit.*, **60**(2): 230–46.

Stephen, L. E., 1970. Clinical manifestations of trypanosomiases in livestock and other domestic animals. In *The African Trypanosomiases*, ed. H. W. Mulligan. George Allen & Unwin (London), pp. 774–94.

Stephen, L. E. and Gray, A. R., 1960. Suramin complexes. VI. The prophylactic activity of antrycide–suramin complex and antrycide chloride against *Trypanosoma simiae* in pigs, *Ann. trop. Med. Parasit.*, **54**: 493–507.

Stephen, L. E. and Mackenzie, C. P., 1959. Experimental *Trypanosoma vivax* infection in the horse, *Vet. Rec.*, **71**(26): 527–31.

Stephen, L. E. and Williamson, J., 1958. Suramine complexes. V. Ethidium complex: attempts to overcome the injection-site reaction in cattle, *Ann. trop. Med. Parasit.*, **52**: 427–42.

Stevens, D. R. and Moulton, J. E., 1977a. Meningoencephalitis in *Trypanosoma equiperdum* infection of deer mice (*Peromyscus maniculatus*), *J. Comp. Path.*, **87**: 109–18.

Stevens, D. R. and Moulton, J. E., 1977b. Experimental meningoencephalitis in *Trypanosoma brucei* infection of deer mice (*Peromyscus maniculatus*). A light immunofluorescent, and electron microscopic study, *Acta neuropath.* (*Berl.*), **38**: 173–80.

Stibbs, H. H. and Seed, J. R., 1975a. Further studies on the metabolism of tryptophan in *Trypanosoma brucei gambiense*: cofactors, inhibitors and end-products, *Experientia*, **29**: 274–8.

Stibbs, H. H. and Seed, J. R., 1975b. Effect of *Trypanosoma brucei gambiense* infection on incorporation of ^{14}C-tryptophan by *Microtus montanus*, *J. Parasitol.*, **61**(1): 143–4.

Stibbs, H. H. and Seed, J. R., 1975c. Short-term metabolism of (^{14}C) tryptophan in rats infected with *Trypanosoma brucei gambiense*, *J. Infect. Dis.*, **131**(4): 459–62.

Strickler, J. E. and Patton, C. L., 1980. *Trypanosoma brucei brucei*: inhibition of glycosylation of the major variable surface coat glycoprotein by tunicamycin, *Proc. Natl Acad. Sci. USA*, **77**(3): 1529–33.

Stuart, K., 1980. Cultivation of dyskinetoplastic *Trypanosoma brucei*, *J. Parasitol.*, **66**(6): 1060–1.

Stuart, K. and Gelvin, S. R., 1980. Kinetoplast DNA of normal and mutant *Trypanosoma brucei*, *Am. J. Trop. Med. Hyg.*, **29**(5)Suppl.: 1075–84.

Tabel, H., 1979. Serum protein changes in bovine trypanosomiasis: a review. In *Pathogenicity of Trypanosomes*, eds G. J. Losos, A. Chouinard. IDRC 132e (Ottawa), pp. 151–3.

Tabel, H. and Losos, G. J., 1980. Absence of host proteins from the surface of *Trypanosoma vivax* of cattle, *Vet. Parasitol.*, **7**: 297–303.

Tabel, H., Losos, G. J. and Maxie, M. G., 1980. Experimental bovine trypanosomiasis (*T. vivax* and *T. congolense*). II. Serum levels of

total protein, albumin, hemolytic complement and complement component C3, *Z. Tropenmed. Parasit.*, **31**(1): 99–104.
Tabel, H., Losos, G. J. and Maxie, M. G., 1981. Experimental bovine trypanosomiasis (*Trypanosoma vivax, Trypanosoma congolense*). III. Serum levels of immunoglobulins, heterophile antibodies and antibodies to *Trypanosoma vivax, Z. Tropenmed. Parasit.*, **32**: 149–53.
Tafuri, W. L., 1979. Pathogenesis of *Trypanosoma cruzi* infections. In *Biology of Kinetoplastida,* eds W. H. R. Lumsden, D. A. Evans. Academic Press (London), vol. 2, pp. 547–652.
Takehara, H. A., Perini, A., da Silva, M. H. and Mota, I., 1981. *Trypanosoma cruzi*: role of different antibody classes in protection against infection in the mouse, *Exp. Parasitol.*, **52**: 137–46.
Tanner, M., Jenni, L., Hecker, H. and Brun, R. 1980. Characterization of *Trypanosoma brucei* isolated from lymph nodes of rats, *Parasitology*, **80**: 383–91.
Tartour, G. and Idris, O. F., 1973. Iron metabolism in *Trypanosoma congolense* infection in zebu cattle: serum iron and serum iron-binding capacity, *Res. vet. Sci.*, **15**: 24–32.
Taylor, A. E. R. and Baker, J. R., 1968. *Cultivation of Parasites* in vitro. Blackwell Scientific Publications (Oxford).
Taylor, A. E. R., Lanham, S. M. and Williams, J. E., 1974. Influence of methods of preparation on the infectivity, agglutination, activity, and ultrastructure of bloodstream trypanosomes, *Exp. Parasitol.*, **35**: 196–208.
Teixeira, A. R. L., 1976. Autoimmune mechanisms in Chagas' disease. In *New Approaches in Trypanosomiasis Research*, Proc. Int. Symp., Pan Am. Hlth Org. No. 318, pp. 98–108.
Teixeira, A. R. L., 1977. Immunoprophylaxis against Chagas' disease. In *Immunity to Blood Parasites of Animals and Man*, eds L. H. Miller, T. A., Pino, J. J. McKelvey Jr. Plenum Press (New York), pp. 243–83.
Teixeira, A. R. L. and Santos-Buch, C. A., 1975. The immunology of experimental Chagas' disease. II. Delayed hypersensitivity to *Trypanosoma cruzi* antigens, *Immunology*, **28**: 401–10.
Terry, R. J., 1976. Innate resistance to trypanosome infections. In *Biology of the Kinetoplastida*, eds W. H. R. Lumsden, D. A. Evans. Academic Press (London), vol. 1, pp. 477–92.
Tetley, L., Vickerman, K. and Moloo, S. K., 1981. Absence of a surface coat from metacyclic *Trypanosoma vivax*: possible implications for vaccination against *vivax* trypanosomiasis, *Trans. R. Soc. trop. Med. Hyg.*, **75**(3): 409–14.
Theis, J. H. and Bolton, V., 1980. *Trypanosoma equiperdum*: movement from the dermis, *Exp. Parasitol.*, **50**: 317–30.
Tippit, T. S., 1978. Canine trypanosomiasis (Chagas' disease), *SWest. Vet.*, **31**: 97–104.
Tizard, I. R., Hay, J. and Wilkie, B. N., 1978e. The absence of *Trypanosoma congolense* from the lymph of an infected sheep, *Res. vet. Sci.*, **25**: 131–2.

Tizard, I. R. and Holmes, W. L., 1976. The generation of toxic activity from *Trypanosoma congolense, Experientia*, **32**(12): 1533–4.

Tizard, I. R. and Holmes, W. L., 1977. The release of soluble vaso-active material from *Trypanosoma congolense* in intraperitoneal diffusion chambers, *Trans. R. Soc. trop. Med. Hyg.*, **71**(1): 52–5.

Tizard, I. R., Holmes, W. L. and Nielsen, K., 1978a. Mechanism of the anemia in trypanosomiasis: studies on the role of the hemolytic fatty acids derived from *Trypanosoma congolense, Z. Tropenmed. Parasit.*, **29**: 108–14.

Tizard, I. R., Mellors, A., Holmes, W. L. and Nielsen, K., 1978b. The generation of phospholipase A hemolytic fatty acids by autolysing suspensions of *Trypanosoma congolense, Z. Tropenmed. Parasit.*, **29**: 127–33.

Tizard, I. R., Neilsen, K. H., Mellors, A. and Assoku, R. K. G., 1979. Biologically active lipids generated by autolysis of *T. congolense*. In *Pathogenicity of Trypanosomes*, eds G. J. Losos, A. Chouinard. IDRC 132e (Ottawa), pp. 103–10.

Tizard, I. R., Nielsen, K. H., Seed, J. R. and Hall, J. E., 1978d. Biologically active products from African trypanosomes, *Microbiol. Rev.*, **42**(4): 661–81.

Tizard, I. R., Sheppard, J. and Nielsen, K., 1978c. The characterization of a second class of haemolysins from *Trypanosoma brucei, Trans. R. Soc. trop. Med. Hyg.*, **72**(2): 198–200.

Tizard, I. R. and Soltys, M. A., 1971. Cell-mediated hypersensitivity in rabbits infected with *Trypanosoma brucei* and *Trypanosoma rhodesiense, Infect. Immun.*, **4**(6): 674–7.

Tobie, E. J., 1964. Cultivation of mammalian trypanosomes, *J. Protozool.*, **11**: 418–23.

Tomlinson, M. J., Chapman, W. L., Hanson, W. L. and Gosser, H. S., 1981. Occurrence of antibody to *Trypanosoma cruzi* in dogs in the southeastern United States, *Am. J. vet. Res.*, **42**(8): 1444–6.

Toro, M., Leon, E. and Lopez, R., 1981. Hematocrit centrifugation technique for the diagnosis of bovine trypanosomiasis, *Vet. Parasitol.*, **8**: 23–9.

Toure, S. M., 1977. Trypanotolerance. Review on actual knowledge, *Rev. Elev. Méd. vét. Pays trop.*, **30**(2): 157–74.

Toure, S. M., Gueye, A., Seye, M., Ba, M. A., Mane, A. *et al.*, 1978. Experiment on comparative pathology of zebu and N'Dama cattle naturally infected by pathogenic trypanosomes, *Rev. Elev. Méd. vét. Pays trop.*, **31**(3): 293–313.

Toure, S. M., Seydi, M., Seye, M. and Kebe, B., 1975. Value of the indirect fluorescence antibody test in the diagnosis and the epizootiological survey on bovine trypanosomiases, *Rev. Elev. Méd. vét Pays trop.*, **28**(4): 463–72.

Trager, W., 1959. Tsetse-fly tissue culture and development of trypanosomes to the infective stage, *Ann. trop. Med. Parasit.*, **53**: 473–91.

Trager, W., 1975. On the cultivation of *Trypanosoma vivax*: a tale of two visits in Nigeria, *J. Parasitol.*, **61**(1): 3–11.

Trager, W. and Krassner, S. M., 1967. Growth of parasitic protozoa in tissue cultures. In *Research in Protozoology*, ed. Tze-Tuan Chen. Pergamon Press (New York), vol. 2, pp. 357–82.

Uilenberg, G., 1964. A case of *Trypanosoma congolense* infection in the camel (*Camelus dromedarius*), *Tijdschr. Diergeneesk*, **84**: 610–11.

Unsworth, K., 1953. Studies on *Trypanosoma vivax*. VIII. Observations on the incidence and pathogenicity of *T. vivax* in zebu cattle in Nigeria, *Ann. trop. Med. Parasit.*, **47**: 361–6.

Unsworth, K., 1954a. The curative effect of ethidium bromide against *Trypanosoma vivax* infections of zebu cattle in West Africa, with observations on the toxicity of the drug, *Ann. trop. Med. Parasit.*, **48**: 229–36.

Unsworth, K., 1954b. Further observations on the curative effect of ethidium bromide against *Trypanosoma vivax* infections in zebu cattle in West Africa, *Ann. trop. Med. Parasit.*, **48**: 237–41.

Unsworth, K. and Chandler, R. L., 1952. Field trials with prophylactic antrycide in West Africa, *Ann. trop. Med. Parasit.*, **46**: 240–49.

Urquhart, G. M., 1980. The pathogenesis and immunology of African trypanosomiasis in domestic animals, *Trans. R. Soc. trop. Med. Hyg.*, **74**(6): 726–9.

Valli, V. E. O. and Forsberg, C. M., 1979. The pathogenesis of *Trypanosoma congolense* infection in calves. V. Quantitative histological changes, *Vet. Pathol.*, **16**: 334–68.

Valli, V. E. O., Forsberg, C. M. and McSherry, B. J., 1978b. The pathogenesis of *Trypanosoma congolensis* infection in calves. III. The neutropenia and myeloid response, *Vet. Pathol.*, **16**: 96–107.

Valli, V. E. O., Forsberg, C. M. and McSherry, B. J., 1978b. The pathogenesis of *Trypanosoma congolense* infection in calves. II. Anemia and erythroid response, *Vet. Pathol.*, **15**: 732–45.

Valli, V. E. O., Forsberg, C. M. and Robinson, G. A., 1978a. The pathogenesis of *Trypanosoma congolense* infection in calves. I. Clinical observations and gross pathological changes, *Vet. Pathol.*, **15**: 608–20.

Valli, V. E. O. and Mills, J. N., 1980. The quantitation of *Trypanosoma congolense* in calves. I. Hematological changes, *Z. Tropenmed. Parasit.*, **31**: 215–31.

Valli, V. E. O., Mills, J. N., Lumsden, J. H., Rattray, J. B. and Forsberg, C. M., 1980. The quantitation of *Trypanosoma congolense* in calves. II. Biochemical changes, *Z. Tropenmed. Parasit.*, **31**: 288–98.

van Dam, R. H., van Kooten, P. J. S., Bosman-Kooyman, C. A. M., Nieuwenhuijs, J., Perie, N. M. and Zwart, D., 1981. Trypanosome mediated suppression of humoral and cell-mediated immunity in goats. *Vet. Parasitol.*, **8**: 1–11.

van den Ingh, T. S. G. A. M., 1977. Pathomorphological changes in *Trypanosoma brucei brucei* infection in the rabbit, *Zbl. Vet. Med.*, **B24**: 773–86.

van den Ingh, T. S. G. A. M. and de Neijs-Bakker, M. H., 1979. Pancarditis in *Trypanosoma vivax* in cattle, *Z. Tropenmed. Parasit.*, **31**: 239–43.

van den Ingh, T. S. G. A. M., Schotman, A. J. H., van Duin, C. T. M., Busser, F. J. M., ten Hoedt, E. and de Neys, M. H. H., 1977. Clinicopathological changes during *Trypanosoma brucei brucei* infection in the rabbit, *Zbl. Vet. Med.*, **B24**: 787–97.

van den Ingh, T. S. G. A. M. and van Dijk, J. E., 1975. Pathology of chronic *Trypanosoma brucei* infection in the rabbit, *Zbl. Vet. Med.*, **B22**: 729–36.

van den Ingh, T. S. G. A. M., Zwart, D., Schotman, A. J. H., van Miert, A. S. J. P. A. M. and Venendaal, H. G., 1976a. The pathology and pathogenesis of *Trypanosoma vivax* infection in the goat, *Res. vet. Sci.*, **21**: 264–70.

van den Ingh, T. S. G. A. M., Zwart, D., van Miert, A. S. J. P. A. M. and Schotman, A. J. H., 1976b. Clinico-pathological and pathomorphological observations in *Trypanosoma vivax* infection in cattle, *Vet. Parasitol.*, **2**: 237–50.

van Dijk, J. E., Zwart, D. and Leeflang, P., 1973. A contribution to the pathology of *Trypanosoma simiae* infection in pigs, *Zbl. Vet. Med.*, **B20**: 374–91.

van Hoeve, K. and Cunningham, M. P., 1964. Prophylactic activity of Berenil against trypanosomes in treated cattle, *Vet. Rec.*, **76**: 260.

van Marck, E. A., Beckers, A., Deelder, A. M., Jacob, W., Wery, M. and Gigase, P. L., 1981. Renal disease in chronic experimental *Trypanosoma gambiense* infections, *Am. J. Trop. Med. Hyg.*, **30**(4): 780–9.

van Marck, E. A. E. and Vervoort, T., 1980. *Trypanosoma brucei*: detection of antigen deposits in glomeruli of mice vaccinated with purified variable antigen, *Trans. R. Soc. trop. Med. Hyg.*, **74**(5): 666–7.

van Meirvenne, N., Janssens, P. G. and Magnus, E., 1973. Further studies on the lytic and neutralizing action of human serum on *Trypanosoma brucei, Ann. Soc. belge Méd trop.*, **53**: 49–56.

van Meirvenne, N., Magnus, E. and Janssens, P. G., 1976. The effect of normal human serum on trypanosomes of distinct antigenic type (ETat 1 to 12) isolated from strain of *Trypanosoma brucei rhodesiense, Ann. Soc. belge Méd. trop.*, **56**: 55–63.

Veenendaal, G. H., van Miert, A. S. J. P. A. M., van den Ingh, T. S. G. A. M., Schotman, A. J. H. and Zwart, D., 1976. A comparison of the role of kinins and serotin in endotoxin induced fever and *Trypanosoma vivax* infections in the goat, *Res. vet. Sci.*, **21**: 271– 9.

Verma, B. B. and Gautam, O. P., 1977. Serological diagnosis of experimental bovine surra (*Trypanosoma evansi* infection) – a comparison of passive haemagglutination, gel diffusion and indirect fluorescent antibody test, *Indian vet. J.*, **54**: 809–13.

Verma, B. B. and Gautam, O. P., 1978. Studies on experimental surra (*Trypanosoma evansi* infection) in buffalo and cow calves, *Indian vet. J.*, **55**: 648–53.

Verma, B. B., Gautam, O. P. and Malik, P. D., 1973. Diminazine aceturate in the treatment of experimental *Trypanosoma evansi* infection in buffalo calves, *Vet. Rec.*, **93**: 465–7.

Verma, B. B., Gautam, O. P. and Malik, P. D., 1976. *Trypanosoma evansi*: therapeutic efficacy of Diminazine aceturate in crossbred calves, *Bos taurus* and *B. indicus*, *Exp. Parasitol.*, **40**: 406–10.

Vickerman, K., 1962. The mechanism of cyclic development in trypanosomes of the *Trypanosoma brucei* subgroup: an hypothesis based on ultrastructural observations, *Trans. R. Soc. trop. Med. Hyg.*, **56**: 487–95.

Vickerman, K., 1969. The fine structure of *Trypanosoma congolense* in its bloodstream phase, *J. Protozool.*, **16**: 54–69.

Vickerman, K., 1970. Ultrastructure of *Trypanosoma* and relation to function. In *The African Trypanosomiases*, ed. H. W. Mulligan. George Allen & Unwin (London), pp. 60–6.

Vickerman, K., 1974. Antigenic variation in African trypanosomes. In *Parasites in the Immunized Host: Mechanisms of Survival*. Ciba Foundation Symp. 25 (new series), Associated Scientific Publishers (Amsterdam), pp. 53–70.

Vickerman, K., 1978. Antigenic variation in trypanosomes, *Nature*, **273**: 613–17.

Villalta, F., Oda, L. M., Angluster, J., Alviano, C. S. and Leon, W., 1981. Phagocytosis of the three developmental forms of *Trypanosoma cruzi*: effect of specific sera, *Acta trop.*, **38**: 375–81.

Visser, N. and Opperdoes, F. R., 1980. Glycolysis in *Trypanosoma brucei*, *Eur. J. Biochem.*, **103**: 623–32.

von Brand, T., 1967. Metabolism of *Trypanosoma cruzi*. A review of recent developments. In: *Medicina Tropical*, ed. A. Aselmi. pp. 261–75.

von Brand, T. (ed.), 1973. *Biochemistry of Parasites*. Academic Press (New York).

Voorheis, H. P., 1980. Fatty acid uptake by bloodstream forms of *Trypanosoma brucei* and other species of the kinetoplastida, *Mol. Biochem. Parasitol.*, **1**: 177–86.

Voorheis, H. P. and Martin, B. R., 1980. 'Swell dialysis' demonstrates that adenylate cyclase in *Trypanosoma brucei* is regulated by calcium ions, *Eur. J. Biochem.*, **113**: 223–7.

Voorheis, H. P. and Martin, B. R, 1981. Characteristics of the calcium-mediated mechanism activating adenylate cyclase in *Trypanosoma brucei*, *Eur. J. Biochem.*, **116**: 471–7.

Wain, E. B., Sutherst, R. W., Burridge, M. J., Pullan, N. B. and Reid, H. W., 1970. Survey for trypanosome infections in domestic cattle and wild animals in areas of East Africa. III. Salivarian trypanosome infections in cattle in relation to the *Glossina* distribution in Busoga district, Uganda, *Br. vet. J.*, **126**: 634–41.

Walter, R. D., 1980. Effect of suramin on phosphorylation–dephosphorylation reactions in *Trypanosoma gambiense, Mol. Biochem. Parasitol.*, **1**: 139–42.

Weiland, G., Gurster, F., Schmid, D. O. and Cwik, S., 1981. Investigations on the influence of bovine sera on infectivity and pathogenicity of *Trypanosoma congolense* in mice, *Berl. Münch. Tierarztl. Wschr.*, **94**(8): 150–3.

Weitz, B. G. F., 1970. Infection and resistance. In *The African Trypanosomiases*, ed. H. W. Mulligan. George Allen & Unwin (London), pp. 97–124.

Wellde, B. T., Bhogal, M. S., Hockmeyer, W. T. and Kovatch, R. M., 1979. Immunity in the bovine to *Trypanosoma congolense* induced by self-cure or chemotherapy. In *Pathogenicity of Trypanosomes*, eds G. J. Losos, A. Chouinard. IDRC (Ottawa), **132e**, pp. 82–6.

Wellde, B. T., Chumo, D. A, Kovatch, R. M. and Wykoff, D. E., 1978. *Trypanosoma congolense*: thrombocytopenia in experimentally infected cattle, *Exp. Parasitol.*, **45**: 26–33.

Wellde, B. T., Duxbury, R. T., Sadun, E. H., Langbehn, H. R., Lotzsch, R., Deindl, G. and Warui, G., 1973. Experimental infections with African trypanosomes. IV. Immunization of cattle with gamma-irradiated *Trypanosoma rhodesiense, Exp. Parasitol.*, **34**: 62–8.

Wellde, B. T., Hockmeyer, W. T., Kovatch, R. M., Bhogal, M. S. and Diggs, C. L., 1981. *Trypanosoma congolense*: natural and acquired resistance in the bovine, *Exp. Parasitol.*, **52**: 219–32.

Wellde, B. T., Lotzsch, R., Deindl, G., Sadun, E., Williams, J. and Warui, G., 1974. *Trypanosoma congolense*. I. Clinical observations of experimentally infected cattle, *Exp. Parasitol.*, **36**: 6–19.

Wellhausen, S. R. and Mansfield, J. M., 1980. Lymphocyte function in experimental African trypanosomiasis. III. Loss of lymph node cell responsiveness, *J. Immunol.*, **124**(3): 1183–6.

Wells, E. A., 1972. The importance of mechanical transmissions in the epidemiology of Nagana: a review, *Trop. Anim. Hlth Prod.*, **4**: 74–88.

Wells, E. A., Betancourt, A., and Page, W. A., 1970. The epidemiology of bovine trypanosomiasis in Colombia, *Trop. Anim. Hlth Prod.*, **2**: 111–25.

Wells, E. A., Betancourt, A. and Ramirez, L. E., 1977. Serological evidence for the geographical distribution of *Trypanosoma vivax* in the New World, *Trans. R. Soc. trop. Med. Hyg.*, **71**: 448–9.

Wenyon, C. M., 1926. *Protozoology*. Baillière, Tindall and Cox (London), vol. 1.

Whitelaw, D. D., MacAskill, J. A., Holmes, P. H., Jennings, F. W. and Urquhart, G. M., 1980. Genetic resistance to *Trypanosoma congolense* infections in mice, *Infect. Immun.*, **27**(3): 707–13.

Whitelaw, D. D., Scott, J. M., Reid, H. W., Holmes, P. H., Jennings,

F. W. and Urquhart, G. M., 1979. Immunosuppression in bovine trypanosomiasis: studies with louping-ill vaccine, *Res. vet. Sci.*, **26**: 102–7.

Whiteside, E. F., 1958a. The control of animal trypanosomiasis in Kenya. In *Symposium on Animal Trypanosomiasis*. Int. Afr. Advisory Comm. Epiz. Dis., Luanda, Publ. No. 45, CCTA, pp. 81–116.

Whiteside, E. F., 1958b. *The Maintenance of Cattle in Tsetse-infested Country*. ISCTR, CCTA Publ. No. 41, vol. VII, pp. 83–90.

Whiteside, E. F., 1960. *Recent Work in Kenya on the Control of Drug-resistant Cattle Trypanosomiasis*. ISCTR, vol. VIII, 22 pp.

Whiteside, E. F., 1962a. Interaction between drugs, trypanosomes and cattle in the field. In *Drugs, Parasites and Hosts*, eds L. G. Goodwin, R. H. Ninimo-Smith, F. and A. Churchill (UK), pp. 117–132.

Whiteside, E. F., 1962b. The control of cattle trypanosomiasis with drugs in Kenya: methods and costs, *E. Afric. Agric. For. J.*, **26**: 67–73.

Whiteside, E. F., Bax, P. L. N. and Fairclough, R., 1960. *Annual Report for 1959 of the Zoological Section, Dept. Vet. Services, Kenya*, ISCTR (VIII), 8, pp. 7–13.

Wijers, D. J. B., 1959. Polymorphism in *Trypanosoma gambiense* and *Trypanosoma rhodesiense* and the significance of the intermediate forms, *Ann. trop. Med. Parasit.*, **53**: 59–68.

Wijers, D. J. B. and Willett, K. C., 1960. Factors that may influence the infection rate of *Glossina palpalis* with *Trypanosoma gambiense*. II. The number of morphology of the trypanosomes present in the blood of the host at the time of the infected feed, *Ann. trop. Med. Parasit.*, **54**: 341–50.

Wilde, J. K. H. and French, M. H., 1945. An experimental study of *Trypanosoma* infections in zebu cattle, *J. Comp. Path.*, **55**: 206–28.

Wilde, J. K. H. and Robson, J., 1953. The effect against *Trypanosoma congolense* in zebu cattle of three new phenanthridine compounds, *Vet. Rec.*, **65**: 49–51.

Willett, K. C., 1970. Epizootiology of trypanosomiasis in livestock in East and Central Africa. In *The African Trypanosomes*, ed. H. W. Mulligan. George Allen & Unwin (London), pp. 766–73.

Willett, K. C. and Gordon, R. M., 1957. Studies on the deposition, migration, and development of blood forms of trypanosomes belonging to the *Trypanosoma brucei* group. II. An account of the migration of trypanosomes from the site of their deposition in the rodent host to their appearance in the general circulation with some observations on their probable routes of migration in human host, *Ann. trop. Med. Parasit.*, **57**: 471–92.

Williams, G. D., Adams, L. G., Yaeger, R. G., McGrath, R. K., Read, W. K. and Bilderbach, W. R., 1977. Naturally occurring trypanosomiasis (Chagas' disease) in dogs, *J. Am. vet. Med. Ass.*, **171**(2): 171–7.

Williams, R. O., Majiwa, P. A. and Young, J. R., 1979. Genomic rearrangements correlated with antigenic variation in *Trypanosome brucei*, *Nature*, **282**: 847–9.

Williams, R. O., Young, J. R., Majiwa, P. A., Doyle, J. J. and Shapiro, S. Z., 1980. Analyses of variable antigen gene rearrangements in *Trypanosoma brucei, Am. J. Trop. Med. Hyg.*, **29**(5): 1037–42.

Williams, R. O., Young, J. R., Majiwa, P. A. O., Doyle, J. J. and Shapiro, S. Z., 1981. Contextural genomic rearrangements of variable-antigen genes in *Trypanosoma brucei, Cold Spring Harbor Symp. on Quantitative Biology*, **45**: 945–9.

Williamson, J., 1962. Chemotherapy and chemoprophylaxis of African trypanosomiasis, *Exp. Parasitol.*, **12**: 274–322.

Williamson, J., 1970. Review of chemotherapeutic and chemoprophylactic agents. In *The African Trypanosomes*, ed. H. W. Mulligan. George Allen & Unwin (London), pp. 125–221.

Williamson, J., 1976. Chemotherapy of African trypanosomiasis, *Trop. Dis. Bull.*, **73**: 531–42.

Williamson, J. and Desowitz, R. S., 1956. Prophylactic activity of suramin complexes in animal trypanosomiasis, *Nature, Lond.*, **177**: 1074–5.

Williamson, J. and Stephen, L. E., 1960. A test for drug-resistant trypanosomes in experimental tsetse-fly challenge of cattle, *Ann. trop. Med. Parasit.*, **54**: 366–70.

Williamson, J. and Stephen, L. E., 1961. Suramin complexes. VIII. Further attempts to overcome the ethidium complex injection site reaction, *Ann. trop. Med. Parasit.*, **55**: 97–106.

Wilson, A. J., 1959. Studies on toxicity of ethidium bromide for English cattle, *Br. vet. J.*, **110**: 233–7.

Wilson, A. J., 1969. Value of the indirect fluorescent antibody test as a serological aid to diagnosis of *Glossina*-transmitted bovine trypanosomiasis, *Trop. Anim. Hlth Prod.*, **1**: 89–95.

Wilson, A. J., 1971. Immunological aspects of bovine trypanosomiasis. III. Patterns in the development of immunity, *Trop. Anim. Hlth Prod.*, **3**: 14–22.

Wilson, A. J. and Cunningham, M. P., 1970. Immunological aspects of bovine trypanosomiasis. II. Antigenic variation in a strain of *Trypanosoma congolense* transmitted by *Glossina morsitans, Trans. R. Soc. trop. Med. Hyg.*, **64**(6): 818–21.

Wilson, A. J. and Cunningham, M. P., 1971. Immunological aspects of bovine trypanosomiasis. IV. Patterns in the production of common antibodies, *Trop. Anim. Hlth Prod.*, **3**: 133–9.

Wilson, A. J. and Cunningham, M. P., 1972. Immunological aspects of bovine trypanosomiasis. I. The immune response of cattle to infection with *Trypanosoma congolense* and the antigenic variation of the infecting organism, *Exp. Parasitol.*, **32**: 165–73.

Wilson, A. J., Dar, F. K. and Paris, J., 1973. Serological studies on trypanosomiasis in East Africa. III. Comparison of antigenic types of *Trypanosoma congolense* organisms isolated from wild flies, *Ann. trop. Med. Parasit.*, **67**(3): 313–17.

Wilson, A. J., Dar, F. K. and Paris, J., 1975b. Maintenance of a herd of breeding cattle in an area of high trypanosome challenge, *Trop. Anim. Hlth Prod.*, **7**: 63–71.

Wilson, A. J., Le Roux, J. H., Paris, J., Davidson, C. R. and Gray, A. R., 1975a. Observations on a herd of beef cattle maintained in a tsetse (*Glossina*) area. I. Assessment of chemotherapy as a method for control of trypanosomiasis, *Trop. Anim. Hlth Prod.*, **7**: 187–99.

Wilson, A. J., Paris, J., Luckins, A. G., Dar, F. K. and Gray, A. R., 1976. Observations on a herd of beef cattle maintained in a tsetse (*Glossina*) area. II. Assessment on the development of immunity in association with trypanocidal drug treatment, *Trop. Anim. Hlth Prod.*, **8**: 1–11.

Wilson, S. G., Morris, K. R. S., Lewis, E. A. and Krog, E., 1963. The effects of trypanosomiasis on rural economy: with special reference to the Sudan, Bechuanaland, and West Africa, *Bull. Wld Hlth Org.*, **28**: 595–613.

Woo, P. T. K., 1969a. The haematocrit centrifuge for the detection of trypanosomes in blood, *Can. J. Zool.*, **47**: 921–3.

Woo, P. T. K., 1969b. The development of *Trypanosoma canadensis* of *Rana pipiens* in *Placobdella* sp., *Can. J. Zool.*, **47**: 1257–9.

Woo, P. T. K., 1970. The haematocrit centrifuge technique for the diagnosis of African trypanosomiasis, *Acta trop.*, **27**(4): 384–6.

Woo, P. T. K. and Kobayashi, A. 1975. Studies on the anaemia in experimental African trypanosomiasis. I. A preliminary communication on the mechanism of the anaemia, *Ann. Soc. belge Méd. trop.*, **55**(1): 37–45.

Woo, P. T. K. and Rogers, D. J., 1974. A statistical study of the sensitivity of haematocrit centrifuge technique in the detection of trypanosomes in the blood, *Trans. R. Soc. trop. Med. Hyg.*, **68**(4): 319–26.

Wright, I. G. and Boreham, P. F. L., 1977. Studies on urinary kallikrein in *Trypanosoma brucei* infections of the rabbit, *Biochem. Pharmac.*, **26**: 417–23.

Yesufu, H. M. and Mshelbwala, A. S., 1973. Trypanosomiasis survey in cattle and tsetse flies along a trade cattle route in southwestern Nigeria, *Ann. trop. Med. Parasit.*, **67**(3): 307–12.

Young, A. S., Kanhai, G. K. and Stagg, D. A., 1975. Phagocytosis of *Trypanosoma (Nannomonas) congolense* by circulating macrophages in African buffalo (*Syncerus caffer*), *Res. vet. Sci.*, **19**: 108–10.

Yutuc, L. M., 1949. Observations on the prevalence of tabanid flies and surra-transmission experiments, *Philipp. J. Sci.*, **78**: 379–88.

Yutuc, L. M. and Sher, H., 1949. Observations on the distribution of *Trypanosoma evansi* in the bodies of rats and guinea pigs during different stages of infection, *Philipp. J. Sci.*, **78**: 155–65.

Zeledòn, R., 1974. Epidemiology, modes of transmission and reservoir hosts of Chagas' disease. In *Trypanosomiasis and Leishmaniasis with Special Reference to Chagas' Disease*. Ciba Foundation Symp. 20

(new series), Associated Scientific Publishers (New York), pp. 51–85.

Zwart, D., 1979. A review of studies on three mouse-infective *T. vivax* strains, *Vet. Sci. Comm.*, **3**: 187–206.

Zwart, D., Perie, N. M., Keppler, A. and Goedbloed, E., 1973. A comparison of methods for the diagnosis of trypanosomiasis in East African domestic ruminants, *Trop. Anim. Hlth Prod.*, **5**: 79–87.

Chapter

4

Leishmaniasis

CONTENTS

INTRODUCTION

Leishmaniasis is primarily a disease of man and dog is caused by several species of protozoa in the genus *Leishmania*. Leishmanial infections without clinical signs are common in a wide variety of wild animals which act as reservoir hosts. Leishmaniasis is a zoonosis transmitted by sandflies, and is of veterinary importance because of its very wide distribution in the dog and in the wild animal populations.

The subject of *Leishmania* and leishmaniasis is very complex, and continues to increase in complexity with the addition of more information on the parasites, vectors, and hosts which are involved. Descriptions of human leishmanial infections and clinical syndromes are based on clinical and epidemiological criteria. The various leishmanial species involved are morphologically identical and closely related antigenically. Classification of organisms into species and subspecies is confusing and based on a variety of local names.

The majority of information which is available is based on studies in man and laboratory models. Relatively little attention has been given to the diseases in dogs and other naturally infected animals. In this chapter, for convenience of description the diseases and infections are divided into visceral and cutaneous forms caused by species found in the Old and New Worlds. Visceral forms in man and dog are caused by *L. donovani* and *L. infantum* in the Old and *L. chagasi* in the New World. In man, the cutaneous leishmaniasis of the Old World is caused by *L. major* and *L. tropica* which induce two clinical syndromes differing in the incubation period, severity of lesions, and duration of infections. In the New World two main types of cutaneous forms are also found and are caused by *L. mexicana* and *L. braziliensis*. In the dog a comparable variety of cutaneous syndromes has not been described.

Literature

The literature on leishmaniasis is very extensive, but there is remarkably little information on natural disease in dogs and wild animals. Information available on various aspects of the host–parasite interaction involved in the pathogenesis is based on observations made on man and in laboratory animal models.

Literature which has been cited in this chapter includes primarily review articles on human leishmaniasis and those publications which deal specifically with infections and diseases in dogs. Comprehensive general reviews on leishmaniasis were presented by Bray (1974a), Cahill and Cox (1975), Manson-Bahr (1971, 1977), and Zuckerman and Lainson (1977). Other articles have dealt with specific aspects of leishmaniasis and are cited in the appropriate sections.

ETIOLOGY

Human leishmaniasis is caused by at least 14 different species and subspecies in the genus *Leishmania*. Classification is difficult and is based on morphology, behavior in the vertebrate and invertebrate host, *in vitro* growth, serology, epidemiology, and antigenic and biochemical criteria. Differences in the host–parasite relationship exist which cause either visceral or cutaneous forms of infections.

The life cycle of leishmania involves the vertebrate host and the phlebotomine vector. In the mammalian host, leishmania are obligate intracellular parasites which exist in the amastigote form in macrophages. The morphology of various species of leishmania does not vary. The amastigote is an oval, rounded body measuring 2 to 3 nm and with Giemsa's or Wright's stains the organisms appear as a mass of red-staining granules surrounded by blue cytoplasm. Multiplication is by binary fission, ultimately destroying the host cell. In the insect vector they are motile extracellular promastigotes. These forms are pear-shaped or slender spindle-shaped bodies, 15 to 25 nm in length and 1 to 4 nm in width, and have a flagellum.

In culture systems, leishmania grow either in the promastigote or amastigote forms. Some isolates do not grow easily in culture and no one single method suffices. Their ability to grow depends to a large degree on the species. There is some relationship between the rate of growth *in vitro* and the multiplication *in vivo*. One method involves 16 cultures of amastigotes in macrophages which are readily infected by promastigotes as well as amastigotes. A number of complex or relatively simple media are also used and include diphasic, semi-solid or liquid media which contain agar, certain nutrients, and blood. Isolates from the mammalian host grow on a biphasic medium of agar and blood incubated between 21 and 26 °C. Growth is observed in 7 to 10 days but may take considerably longer, and cultures have to be maintained for 4 to 6 weeks. The amastigotes transform into replicating motile promastigotes in about 24 hours. Strains maintained as promastigotes by serial passage *in vitro* progressively lose their invasiveness for the laboratory hosts.

Literature

Leishmania have been placed in the order Kinetoplastida, suborder Trypanosomatina, family Trypanosomatidae, and genus *Leishmania* (Levine *et al.* 1980). Gardener (1977) published a review which dealt with the taxonomy of the genus *Leishmania* including nomenclature and classification, and pointed out that a major problem in human leishmaniasis is the speciation of each etiological agent. Leishmanial species have been identified by the geographical distribution, epidemiology, and by laboratory investigations including characteristics in culture, serological tests, response in various experimental hosts, and the behavior in the phlebotomine host. Further examinations, using modern technologies have been employed to verify classifications made on the basis of conventional biological criteria and included nuclear and kinetoplast deoxyribonucleic acid buoyant densities, isoenzymes, antigenic compositions of amastigotes and promastigotes, and exometabolites secreted by the parasites (Zuckerman and Lainson 1977). Reclassification of leishmania on the basis of the developmental patterns in the sandfly was proposed by Lainson and Shaw (1979). The leishmania were divided into three major types depending on the development and migration of the organisms within the gut. For example, leishmania from warm-blooded vertebrates developed in the anterior portion and from cold-blooded animals in the posterior part of the insect gut. A list of the animal species and the localization of the related leishmania in the gut of the fly was presented.

EPIZOOTIOLOGY

General

Leishmania have a wide distribution in tropical and subtropical countries, extending through Central and South America, the Mediterranean countries, Africa, central Asia, India, and China. The climate ranges from humid rain forests of South and Central America to the dry savannahs of Africa and deserts of the Middle East. Leishmaniasis in man is considered among the protozoal diseases and of secondary importance only to malaria, with treatment and control being considerably more difficult. The distribution is determined by reservoir hosts from which vectors transmit the infection.

All forms of visceral and cutaneous leishmaniasis of man are zoonotic diseases, with species and subspecies of leishmania being transmitted from a variety of wild and, more rarely, domestic animals. The species of animal reservoir vary according to the type of syndrome as well as its geographic distribution. The importance of various reservoir species depends on the distribution, contact with sandfly vector, and the levels of infection being sufficiently high to be readily transmitted. Leishmania are a primary parasite of lizards, marsupials, rodents, carnivores, edentates, insectivores, and only secondarily of man and dogs severe disease develops, characterized either by skin lesions or or more of the wild species from which they are transmitted to dogs and man. Some species of leishmania are strictly host-specific, while others lack host-specificity. Infections in these natural mammalian hosts are usually benign without apparent clinical disease. In man and dog severe disease develops, characterized either by skin lesions or generalized visceral involvement. Man is a relatively poor source of infection for the sandfly, and man-to-man transmission is not considered to be of importance.

Among domestic animals, the dog is the reservoir for South American and Mediterranean visceral leishmaniasis. In endemic foci, incidence of infections in dogs varies considerably from one region to another and may be far more common in dogs than in man with an infection rate varying from 10 to 35% in the dogs surveyed. In spite of this prevalence the importance of canine leishmaniasis has received remarkably little attention. The cutaneous and mucocutaneous leishmaniases of South America is not associated with infections in domestic species. A cutaneous form of leishmania has been described in horses and donkeys in South America, and reference to leishmanial infections in calves has been made in the early literature.

Literature

The complex epidemiology and epizootiology of leishmaniasis in South America has been extensively reviewed by Adler (1964), Bray (1974b), Lainson and Shaw (1978, 1979) and Lainson (1982).

Hoare (1955) and Cahill and Cox (1975) briefly reviewed the epizootiological role of animal reservoirs in human leishmaniasis. Animal reservoirs were presented according to the various regions and countries by Garnham (1965). Bray (1974c) listed the species of leishmania found in various species of wild animals. The species of infected host differed with particular species of leishmania and with its geographical distribution. Manson-Bahr (1977) also listed the reservoir host including domestic and wild carnivora and various species of rodents. Tables of the recorded mammalian hosts found in South America were given for the different species causing visceral and cutaneous leishmaniasis (Lainson and Shaw 1978, 1979; Lainson 1982). A historical account of investigations which incriminated wild and domestic animals as reservoirs was presented by Lainson (1982). Lainson and Shaw (1979) concluded that, although surveys of American leishmaniasis were undertaken in domestic animals, infections other than in the dog were very rarely reported. Earlier, Adler (1964) cited early literature on infection in domestic animals and included reports by Mazza (1927) on a few infected dogs in the Argentine, infection in a cat in Brazil (Mello 1940), and a case of cutaneous leishmaniasis in a donkey (Alencar 1959). The incidences of leishmaniasis in various species of domestic animals have not been either adequately investigated or documented.

An important addition to the knowledge of leishmaniasis in domestic animals other than the dog has been made recently by Bonfante-Garrido *et al.* (1981). The authors stated that equine infections could be relatively common in some endemic areas of South America and summarized the three reports available on cutaneous syndromes. In one report cited, Mazza (1927) described a leishmanial ulcer on the inner corner of the right eye of a horse. Alencar (1959) reported one case of leishmaniasis in a donkey, and Pons (1968) described the lesions in two of six donkeys examined. Bonfante-Garrido *et al.* (1981) initially found eight donkeys in Venezuela with ulcerative lesions on the scrotum, penis, and legs, and on smear examination from these lesions all animals were found to be infected with leishmania. Further investigation in the same location of 116 donkeys showed that 28 animals had one or more ulcerative lesions, 13 of which were scrotal and others being on the legs and neck. Of the animals with lesions, 17 were positive for leishmania. This article has brought attention to the possibility that other domestic animals could be infected and develop skin lesions which up to this time have not been recognized as caused by leishmanial infections.

Both invertebrate and vertebrate hosts were of equal importance in maintaining leishmania parasites in enzootic foci. Although various strains of leishmania have been isolated from vertebrates in different parts of the world, the relationship between these strains and those causing human infections has not been established (Cahill and Cox 1975). Grouping of leishmania, primarily on the visceral or cutaneous classifications, was not warranted. The organisms did not always maintain their cutaneous or visceral tropisms which varied with strains in the species (Lainson and Shaw 1979). However, convention has made it necessary to make this distinction.

Visceral leishmaniasis is widely spread throughout the world but varies in its local epidemiology. *Leishmania donovani*, causing a syndrome in man known as kala-azar, has been a parasite found in rodents, canids, and man, which represent three different types of reservoirs resulting in three different endemic situations. Generally the rodent reservoir served as a source of sporadic infection in Africa south of the Sahara, but outbreaks of infection occurred when susceptible human populations moved into these endemic areas (Hoare 1955; Manson-Bahr 1977). In Kenya, the relationship between the incidence of visceral leishmaniasis in man and contact with domestic animals has been considered. Although infections in these animals were not determined, a relationship was postulated but not shown to exist between the development of visceral leishmaniasis and the close contact with calves, goats, sheep, chickens, dogs, and cats (Southgate and Oriedo 1962). Canine reservoirs of the disease, including wild jackals, foxes and dogs, was found in the Mediterranean countries, the Middle East, southern USSR, and northern China. In these regions, infections were not spread from man to man. In India, the epidemiological situation was different in that the kala-azar syndrome was spread only from human reservoirs and was transmitted predominantly by one species of sandfly (Manson-Bahr 1977).

The visceral leishmaniasis in children, caused by *L. infantum*, has been associated with the canine reservoir and found in the Mediterranean countries, North Africa, central Asia and the Far East. The reservoir hosts were the fox, dog, jackal, wolf, and porcupine (Zuckerman and Lainson 1977). Although canids were the principal host of this species, other animals including rats have also been recognized as reservoirs (Lainson 1982).

In South America, *L. chagasi* has been responsible for visceral leishmaniasis with foxes, dogs, and cats with these species serving as reservoir hosts. A sylvatic cycle, involving rodents and wild canids, was the source of infection for dogs which in turn served as an important reservoir for man. The canine visceral leishmaniasis was regarded as prevalent and could result in epizootics in man (Lainson and Shaw 1979).

The cutaneous form of leishmaniasis is common in both man and dogs. Man has been regarded as an accidental host and as not playing a significant role as a reservoir host. The cutaneous syndromes in the Old World have been divided into two different types, the wet rural form caused by *L. major* and the dry urban variety caused by *L. tropica*. These species have been isolated from a variety of rodents which play important roles as reservoirs. *Leishmania tropica* infections in dogs and occasionally also in cats have been the source of infection. In rural areas, *L. major* has been transmitted from rodents. In the New World, *L. mexicana* causes cutaneous leishmania in man, with the small forest rodents serving as reservoir. Small insignficant leishmanial lesions were present on the tail, ears, and limbs of these animals (Manson-Bahr 1977). Lainson and Shaw (1979) presented in detail the ecology of different subspecies of leishmania in the groups of *L. braziliensis* and *L. mexicana*, and the variety of rodents and marsupials which served as reservoirs. Dogs were an important reservoir host in some forms of cutaneous leishmaniasis. Experimental infection in dogs induced by inoculating material into the skin of the nose or ears caused small localized lesions.

Surveys in dogs

There have been reports on surveys undertaken in dogs on the prevalence of leishmanial infections as determined by either serological tests, isolation of organisms, demonstration of organisms in tissues, or a combination of their methods from various regions and countries. Standardization of methods for the investigation of leishmaniasis in dogs was discussed and included sampling procedures, serological techniques, as well as parasitological examinations (Lanotte *et al.* 1977). Garnham (1971a, b) reviewed the literature on the incidence of visceral and cutaneous infection found and referred to articles which gave the incidence rate in dogs in various parts of the world. Infection rates in dogs were found to be as high as 50% in some localities.

In the recent literature, additional information has been presented from various countries on the incidences of infection in dogs. In Kenya, dogs were considered an important reservoir for visceral leishmaniasis (Ngoka and Mutinga 1977). Surveys of wild and domestic animals in Kenya were undertaken by Ngoka and Mutinga (1978). Mutinga *et al.* (1980) briefly reviewed reports from eastern Africa on the presence of leishmaniasis in dogs. In a survey of an area where human leishmaniasis was enzootic, 2 of 288 dogs were found to be infected and the organisms were characterized enzymatically and serologically to be comparable to the strains observed in man. In comparison, 25% of the dogs were said to harbor a Mediterranean form of visceral leishmaniasis (Hoare 1962). The occurrence of canine leishmaniasis in Senegal was reported by Ranque *et al.* (1970).

Rifaat and Hassan (1967) summarized the earlier surveys of canine leishmaniasis in Africa and the Middle East. In the United Arab Republic a survey was undertaken using the formol-gel test and examinations of spleen, liver, and skin by smears and culture techniques. In the 340 dogs examined 7 were positive by the formol-gel test. There were no positive cases by direct smear examination, and only a proportion of the dogs found positive by the formol-gel test were positive by the culture technique. In Tunisia, 1219 dogs were examined serologically and 5.6% were found to be positive (Dedet *et al.* 1973). Sukkar *et al.* (1981) summarized information on the isolation of leishmania from dogs in Iraq and reported on one case. In India, serological surveys using fluorescent antibodies were also useful in the diagnosis of cutaneous leishmaniasis in the dog (Mishra and Lodha 1975). The amastigotes of *L. donovani* were found in smears of spleen and livers of jackal (*Canis* (*Thos*) *aureos*) (Maruashvili and Bardzhadze 1980).

Pozio *et al.* (1981b) summarized some of the more recent incidences published in Italy and compared their survey results. They found an incidence of 24% as compared to the reports of others who used serological techniques and found incidences of 10.2% (Bucci *et al.* 1975) and 7.6% (Colella *et al.* 1979). Out of 171 dogs surveyed by Pozio *et al.* (1981b) 41 were positive by the fluorescent antibody (FA) test, 17 of these showed signs of the disease, and only 12 were positive by microscopic examination of lymph nodes. Examination of these animals 1 year later revealed that 88% of the dogs with clinical signs had died and 36 of the asymptomatic infected dogs either developed clinical signs and recovered, or died. In other earlier surveys, approximately 2 of 97 dogs were found to be positive for leishmania by direct examinations of organisms (Tasselli and Colella 1960). Seven cases were observed on examination of 102 dogs at postmortem for the presence of leishmania in various tissues (Colella and Casamassima 1975). Using a technique of injecting spleen homogenates into hamsters, isolates were also made from the black rat (*Rattus rattus*) and fox (Bettini *et al.* 1980; Pozio *et al.* 1981a), who also presented a list of references reporting isolation of leishmania from wild rodents and carnivora in a region of Italy.

Surveys of canine leishmaniasis in southern France involved 4270 animals and the incidences varied in different regions from 0.23 to 3.1% (Lanotte *et al.* 1978; Dunan 1978). In earlier work, the distribution of canine leishmaniasis in France was reported and discussed as to its possible danger to children (Guilhon 1950, 1965). Positive cases were observed in packs of hounds (Houin *et al.* 1977). Foxes were surveyed as possible reservoir hosts in southern France and two animals were found to be infected (Rioux *et al.* 1968).

In an early report from China, out of 1430 dogs 44 had alopecia and seborrhea, and leishmania were demonstrated in a high percentage of these animals, both by examination of skin biopsy and of the bone marrow (Ho *et al.* 1947).

In Panama, 333 dogs were surveyed between 1965 and 1973 for cutaneous leishmaniasis and 11 cases were found. Infections were associated with ulcerative skin lesions characterized by depigmentation and inflammation and found primarily on the base of the ear and on the nostrils. These lesions persisted for up to 45 months. The organism did not disseminate from the local lesions to the viscera or other areas of the skin. The organism was categorized as *L. braziliensis.* A summary of earlier reports of canine cutaneous leishmaniasis in South America was also presented (Herrer and Christensen 1976).

In North America, the majority of cases reported in the USA were found in dogs imported from Greece and South America (George *et al.* 1976). One cases of endemic leishmaniasis was found in several animals in a kennel of foxhounds in Oklahoma (Anderson *et al.* 1980).

Transmission

Transmission is by sandflies of the genera *Phlebotomus* in the Old World and *Lutzomyia* in the New World. Sandflies are active primarily at night and inhabit shady, highly humid environments. Although they are weak fliers, they may be carried long distances by wind. The species involved vary with the geographical area, depending on suitable climatic conditions which govern the existence and predominance of a particular species. The vectors are most numerous at breeding and resting sites of optimal humidity and temperature. Certain species are closely associated with specific locations such as rodent burrows.

The vector feeds by piercing the skin and creating a pool of blood. Ingested amastigotes develop into motile promastigotes in the anterior portion of the gut during the first 72 hours. They multiply by binary fission and then move to the salivary glands within a period of about 10 days. The length of life cycle in the vector depends both on the species of fly and of the organism, as well as on the environment which may be from 1 to 2 months in the summer but longer in winter. The transmission takes place when the organisms are injected through the proboscis into the skin of the new host.

Literature

Bray (1974c) presented a brief review of the zoonosis of leishmaniasis, giving an overview of the various aspects of transmission. Lainson and Shaw (1979) reviewed the infection of the vector by different species of leishmania. Killick-Kendrick (1979) discussed the biology of leishmania in the vector, particularly its development in the various parts and the efficiency of transmission.

In both visceral and cutaneous leishmaniasis, the ingested parasites were in the macrophages of the dermis. The numbers of organisms available to the fly varied greatly with different regions of the skin. The site of predisposition for the bite of the sandfly contained the highest numbers. In dogs with visceral leishmaniasis the skin was heavily infected for a long period of time, resulting in alopecia which enabled widespread feeding by the fly, thereby resulting in efficient transmission. In cutaneous leishmaniasis the organisms were confined to specific sites which were usually the areas of exposed skin where sandflies tended always to bite (Bray 1974a). The transmission of American cutaneous leishmaniasis to a number of wild, domesticated, and laboratory animals was reported, including passage between dogs to dog and cat (Medina 1966).

It was pointed out that remarkably little has been documented of the detailed biology of various species of leishmania in the invertebrate host with the complete cycles in the vector seldom being described. The basic sequence of events in the transmission involved multiplication in the gut and migration – first to the pharynx, then to the proboscis, and finally to the mouthparts (Killick-Kendrick 1979). The time needed for localization in the anterior parts of the alimentary tract and for the invasion of the biting mouthparts varied with different species of leishmania. Transmission was considered to be relatively efficient. Although the organisms were localized in the pharynx and hypopharynx, their presence in this location did not assure easy transmission because the excretion of saliva did not flush the organism into the site of bite in the host (Bray 1974a).

INFECTION

In man, infections do not necessarily induce lesions or disease, and in endemic areas of leishmaniasis high incidences of serologically positive and asymptomatic carriers exist. In reservoir animals, the host–parasite relationship is well established and there are usually no overt lesions or clinical signs. In these asymptomatic forms, the parasites localize in normal skin. Because man and dog are unnatural hosts the host–parasite interaction results in development of either cutaneous or visceral lesions.

Once inoculated into the skin of the host, the fate of the organism depends on a number of factors such as temperature at the site of the bite, susceptibility of the host, and numbers of organisms injected. Infection may become either localized in a small area of skin or spread throughout the entire reticuloendothelial system. Temperature of tissues plays a role in the localization. Some organisms thrive at the low temperatures of bare skin where the fly is able to bite and will not survive at the higher temperatures, either in other areas of the skin or in internal viscera. In the skin, infections may be associated with lesions, but also occur in normal skin. The viscerotropic and dermatropic characteristics of a leishmania isolate are not always retained during transmission between wild animals and man. Some organisms which cause cutaneous leishmaniasis in man are isolated from viscera of reservoir hosts. In the visceral forms, amastigotes can be widely distributed throughout apparently normal skin.

Literature

After dermal inoculation by the vector, the promastigotes were phagocytosed by macrophages in a local mononuclear cell inflammatory reaction. Within the macrophage, the organism developed into amastigotes which divided by binary fission. Infection was spread by infected macrophages, dividing or rupturing of infected cells with phagocytosis of amastigotes by other macrophages, and migration throughout various tissues of the host. The fate of leishmania in activated macrophages depended on its ability to survive therein. Species which were infective for a specific host have resisted the microbicidal activity of macrophages (Mauel *et al.* 1974). In a natural host, the balance was established with only moderate numbers developing under the control of an immune system, being overcome by the delayed hypersensitivity type of response (Lainson 1982). Cutaneous infections were often self-limiting resulting in immunity. In the cutaneous forms in man, caused by *L. tropica* and *L. mexicana*, lesions were restricted to one area of the skin by cell mediated immunity. In *L. braziliensis* infections, development of cell-mediated immunity was delayed, enabling a wider spread of infections to other areas of skin and mucocutaneous junctions (Manson-Bahr 1977).

Visceral leishmaniasis developed after an initial multiplication at the site of injection and subsequent infection of the reticuloendothelial cells, spleen, bone marrow, lymph glands, and other organs. Delay in the development of cellular immune response in visceral forms enabled widespread dissemination of infection throughout the entire reticuloendothelial system. The cellular inflammatory reaction in visceral form was comparable to that observed in cutaneous lesions and involved proliferation of macrophages and secondary infiltration by lymphocytes and plasma cells. In visceral leishmaniasis of dogs and rodents, infected macrophages were always distributed throughout the dermis, while in man the infection of the dermis was variable (Adler 1964). In dogs and foxes infected, there was a massive invasion of the skin by *L. infantum* and *L. chagasi* (Lainson and Shaw 1979). The survival and the elimination of leishmania in the macrophages was reviewed by Mauel *et al.* (1974).

In laboratory animal models, tissue tropism of isolates often reflected predisposition observed in natural infections. Strains isolated from cutaneous human or rodent lesions localized in the skin and caused lesions, while strains from visceral leishmaniasis infected the viscera and did not spread to the skin. However, there were exceptions, and some strains which caused cutaneous lesions in man caused visceral infections in laboratory animals; conversely, some strains causing cutaneous lesions in man have been isolated from visceral organs of reservoir animals (Zuckerman and Lainson 1977).

Experimental infections were induced in dogs at the susceptible site, which was the dorsal aspect of the nose, by cultures of South American strain freshly isolated from lesions in man as well as lesions in dogs (Herrer and Battistini 1951). In experimental infection, *L. donovani* was transmitted from dog to dog by sandflies, and after an incubation period of 15 months visceral leishmaniasis developed (Rioux *et al.* 1979). The visceral disease in foxes was comparable to that of the dog (Rioux *et al.* 1968, 1971).

A variety of species of animals have been used extensively as experimental models. Experimental infections with *L. donovani* have been established in mice, rats, guinea pigs, rabbits, gerbils, hamsters, jackals, dogs, and monkeys; with *L. tropica* in mice, rats, guinea pigs, and monkeys; and with *L. braziliensis* in mice, hamsters, cotton rats, opossum, bats, several forest rodents, and monkeys. The clinical patterns of animal syndromes generally parallel those described for visceral and cutaneous leishmaniasis observed in man (Cahill and Cox 1975). Some laboratory models have been used extensively in the study of leishmaniasis. Selection of the host depended on the purpose of infection; for example, hamsters have been used for the isolation and growth of the organisms and guinea pigs have been used to study cell-mediated immunity. Various mouse models of inbred strains were used to study susceptibility and development of cell-mediated immunity (Zuckerman and Lainson 1977). In many investigations of pathogenesis hamsters have been the species of choice because they are very susceptible, with a mortality occurring 3 to 6 months after infection. Infected cutaneous tissue suspensions were inoculated intradermally into the nose and feet, and intraperitoneally when visceral infections were suspected. Animals were maintained at 23 to 26 °C because higher temperatures inhibited development of the cutaneous lesions. A variety of lesions developed over several months which included either asymptomatic localized infections, cutaneous nodules or ulcers, or large nonvascular tumor-like growths which grew quickly and metastasized (Lainson 1982).

CLINICAL SIGNS

A considerable amount of information is available on the various clinical syndromes occurring in man, but remarkably little information is published on the natural diseases of dogs. Clinical leishmaniasis is a spectrum of diseases with the host's immune mechanism determining the type of syndrome which develops. Syndromes range from mild self-limiting local skin lesions to systemic fatal diseases.

Visceral leishmaniasis starts as a cutaneous lesion and the infection spreads through the various organs, particularly the spleen, liver, and bone marrow. In man, the clinical picture in visceral leishmaniasis is similar in all regions but the duration of the disease differs. There are other distinct features which differentiate the disease in India from that observed in the Mediterranean region. In India, the disease is found in adults but not in dogs, while in the Mediterranean the infantile syndrome is seen in children and in dogs. There is a good association between the incidence of the infantile visceral leishmaniasis and the occurrence of disease in dogs. In these geographic regions up to 20% of dogs are infected. Clinical manifestations of American visceral leishmaniasis syndromes are also similar.

Cutaneous leishmaniasis is made up of a spectrum of syndromes. In the Old World, the syndrome is divided into the dry or urban form caused by *L. tropica* and occurring in the Mediterranean countries, Asia, and northern Africa, with the dog acting as the reservoir host. *Leishmania major* causes the wet or rural form and occurs in Asia and Africa, with reservoir hosts being gerbils and other rodents. Variation in the immunological responses, particularly in cell-mediated responses, determines the clinical differences of these syndromes. Cutaneous leishmania in the Western Hemisphere is classified into two major groups: *L. mexicana* and *L. braziliensis* complexes, each containing a number of different isolates regarded as being different subspecies. *Leishmania mexicana* has a number of subspecies and has a natural reservoir in forest rodents and other animals where it is found either in dermal nodules, plaques, ulcers, or noninfected skin. *Leishmania braziliensis* complex has a wide range of wild sylvatic animals and some organisms have the dog as reservoir host. The organisms can be isolated from inconspicuous skin lesions, normal skin, and occasionally from viscera. Syndromes caused by *L. tropica* or *L. mexicana* are often self-limiting diseases while mucocutaneous lesions caused by *L. braziliensis* may be persistent and progressive and complicated by secondary bacterial infections. Severe cutaneous syndromes are associated with alterations in the immune response, especially cell-mediated reactions. Severe lesions occur when it is largely lacking and when there is an allergic state in which antibody production and cell-mediated reaction are overdeveloped causing hypersensitivity. At one end of the spectrum, severe diffuse cutaneous leishmaniasis is characterized by massive invasion of skin, mucous membranes, and drainage lymph nodes, while at the other pole there is localized skin lesion with few parasites.

Literature

Zuckerman and Lainson (1977) presented in detail the classification and characteristics of the various forms of leishmaniasis in man in the Eastern Hemisphere. Some workers have thought that the visceral form of leishmaniasis was introduced to South America by the early settlers (Garnham 1971b). An epidemiological and clinical relationship between Mediterranean visceral leishmaniasis in man and dogs was noted by various workers (Berberian 1959; Hoare 1955).

In dogs, comprehensive studies of the clinical syndrome, either visceral or cutaneous, have not been presented. Most of the information in the more current literature has been limited to the examination of individual cases either naturally or experimentally infected. The cutaneous forms are confined to small focal lesions in the skin. Generalized skin involvement is more often observed in the visceral syndromes. Adler and Theodor (1932) reviewed the earlier literature on the visceral leishmaniasis in the dog and reported that the main signs consisted of emaciation, anemia, keratitis, scaling of skin, and alopecia. It was also found that some heavily infected dogs did not have any clinical signs. Frequently there was also a discrepancy between the intensity of infection and the clinical condition in dogs. Skin infections associated with the visceral form could be readily differentiated from those induced by cutaneous variety of leishmaniasis (Adler and Theodor 1932; Di Domizio 1955). The infection in the peripheral skin could be more extensive than that found in the internal organs. Organisms were found in the eyes and in the eyelids, resulting in discharge and corneal opacity (Adler and Tchernomoretz 1946). Symptomology of the visceral syndromes in dogs in the Mediterranean basin was variable. Common signs were seborrhea, partial alopecia, ulceration, and emaciation, but some animals were asymptomatic (Adler 1964). In a case report of a dog with visceral leishmaniasis caused by *L. donovani*, infection was found to be confined to the eyes and adjacent tissues and was manifested by severe bilateral endophthalmitis and blepharitis (McConnell *et al.* 1970). In another case reported of generalized visceral leishmaniasis in the dog, there was hypergammaglobulinemia and bilateral ophthalmitis (Giles *et al.* 1975). In the clinical course of natural cutaneous and visceral forms of canine leishmaniasis in Uzbekistan, skin lesions were a primary manifestation of disease. In the cutaneous form, the lesions were localized and terminated by healing or ran a chronic intermittent course (Isaev 1966). The disease in dogs caused by *L. chagasi* was usually fatal and the clinical signs observed were extreme weakness, wasting, diarrhea, edema of the feet, ulceration, alopecia of skin, and eye inflammation leading to blindness (Lainson and Shaw 1979). The variability of the disease syndrome was stressed in four different experimental cases (Sanchis *et al.* 1976).

There have been numerous clinical reports of occurrences of single cases, primarily of the visceral form, from various parts of the world: Mozambique (Tendeiro *et al.* 1968), Iran (Rafyi *et al.* 1968), Algeria (Donatien and Lestoquand 1938), Italy (Muscarella *et al.* 1981), Madagascar (Buck *et al.* 1951). In North America, a number of cases have been reported in dogs imported from Greece and Spain (Thorson *et al.* 1955; Gleiser *et al.* 1957; Corbeil *et al.* 1976; George *et al.* 1976; Tryphonas *et al.* 1977; Theran and Ling 1967). Visceral leishmaniasis has also been found in a fennec fox (*Fennecus zerda*) which was imported into the USA from northern Africa (Conroy *et al.* 1970).

PATHOLOGY

The basic lesion of cutaneous and visceral leishmaniasis consists of injection by macrophages of the organism which is accompanied by lymphocyte and plasma cell infiltrations. This lesion is considered to indicate the induction of a cell-mediated immunological response. Tissue tropisms vary with strains and species of organism, resulting in lesions of different degrees of severity ranging from a well-defined local skin granulatomous lesion to widespread infections and hyperplasia of the reticuloendothelial systems throughout various tissues and organs.

Literature

Grossly visible visceral lesions in dogs were similar to those observed in man and include emaciation, anemia, splenomegaly, hepatomegaly, lymphadenopathy, and ophthalmitis (George *et al.* 1976). Histologically, the lesion is characterized by the accumulation of infected macrophages accompanied by a lymphocytic and plasma cell response (Adler and Theodor 1934; Conroy *et al.* 1970; Gleiser *et al.* 1957). In addition to other lesions, kidney involvement has been observed consisting primarily of fibrous tissue reaction and lymphocytosis (Millin *et al.* 1975; Lainson *et al.* 1969). In natural infection with *L. donovani*, glomerulomesangial thickening diagnosed as proliferative glomerulonephritis was reported (Rojas Ayala 1973). Experimental infection of dogs with a strain of *L. donovani* resulted in histiocytic granulomas with very few leishmania in the liver and skin. Tumor-like histiocytic infiltrates were found in the heart, lungs, liver, kidneys, pancreas and muscles, with the development of amyloidosis which was regarded as an atypical course of *L. donovani* infection in dogs (Bungener and Mehlitz 1977). Elevation in proteins, globulins, and lipoproteins were also observed (Groulade and Groulade 1959; Kammerman and Buhlmann 1965). In dogs the cutaneous leishmaniasis caused lesions on the nose, ears, extremities, and other hairless parts, apparently where the phlebotomus flies fed. In the dermis, histological reaction consisted of macrophages, lymphocytes and plasma cells (Mishra and Lodha 1977). Skin lesions have also been described in dogs and donkeys in Venezuela by Pons (1968). The histologic appearance of localized and diffuse cutaneous lesions was different. In diffuse skin leishmaniasis, granulomatous formations were made up exclusively of macrophages filled with parasites, while in localized lesions epitheloid or tuberculoid nodules were surrounded by exclusive infiltrations of lymphoid cells. In some intermediate syndromes a combination of both types of cellular responses were observed. These characteristic histological responses were considered to reflect host defenses with extensive proliferation of organisms and widespread lesions indicating ineffectual defenses. It was concluded that pathogenicity and virulence were not directly related to some inherent feature of a particular isolate (Convit and Pinardi 1974; Giles *et al.* 1975; Conroy *et al.* 1970). In the

New and Old World lesions in rodents commonly occurred at the base of the tail, on the ears, and in dogs on the nose and face, but some reservoir hosts were infected without development of lesions (Manson-Bahr 1977).

IMMUNOLOGY

The importance of cell-mediated immunity dominates immunological responses of the mammalian host to leishmanial infections. It is responsible for the destruction of the organisms and controls the severity of the lesions and induction of protection. Humoral antibodies accompanying cellular immunity occur in all forms of cutaneous leishmaniasis except in the syndromes characterized by the diffuse cutaneous lesions. In man and dogs, large numbers of serological tests are used, but the results vary with the strain of leishmania causing infection and with the clinical syndromes.

Literature

Immunology of leishmaniasis in man was reviewed (Heyneman 1971; Zuckerman 1975; Zuckerman and Lainson 1977). Stauber (1970) discussed the innate and acquired immunity to both cutaneous and visceral leishmaniasis in man. The cell-mediated and humoral responses to protozoan infections were related to the protective immunity by Mauel and Behin (1974).

Resistance was dependent on cell-mediated immunity. Leishmanial antigens sensitized lymphocytes which in turn activated macrophages against the homologous antigens and against nonspecific heterologous antigen. These sensitized lymphocytes were cytotoxic to the infected macrophages and parasiticidal to the organisms. Infected macrophages were observed to be surrounded lymphocytes and plasma cells. Cell-mediated immunity has been assayed in *in vivo* and *in vitro* systems by lymphoblastoid transformation, macrophage migration inhibition, production of biologically active substances, and adapted transfer of delayed hypersensitivity (Zuckerman and Lainson 1977). The immunity associated with this cellular response was unique in the protozoal infections because it was complete and long-lasting and was not dependent on low levels of persistent infection (Manson-Bahr 1977).

In man, hyperglobulinemia was observed in visceral leishmaniasis but not in mucocutaneous forms. The rise in immunoglobulins was due almost entirely to IgG which was reflected in the nonspecific formol-gel test. The serum proteins and globulins in dogs changed (Vitu *et al.* 1973). There was an increase in various globulin levels, particularly of IgG and IgA (Corbeil *et al.* 1976).

The antigenic composition of leishmania is complex with common antigens being responsible for cross-reactivity among various species of leishmania and between leishmania and trypanosomes, limiting the reliability because of specificity of many of the immunological tests. A number of serological tests including hemagglutination, complement fixation (CF), immobilization, passive cutaneous anaphylactic, precipitin, indirect hemagglutination, FA, and the Noguchi–Adler tests have been used in man but their application to dogs has not been determined. The nonspecific tests which have been used depend on the extreme hyperglobulinemia. Antibodies are not reliable indicators of immunity and serological studies are of limited value. Most serological tests are of limited value, for example the CF test was useful only with active form of visceral form, but cross-reactions occurred with cases of trypanosomiasis. Results of the indirect hemagglutination test varied with various clinical syndromes and was impractical for diagnosis. Fluorescent antibodies appeared early in systemic infection before the development of overt clinical signs and lasted for 2 or 3 years after recovery. The Adler test has been used exclusively to demonstrate antigenic differentiation of leishmanial species but required careful standardization. It consisted of agglutination and replacement of motile flagellates by amoeboid forms of organisms in the promastigotes cultured in the presence of immune sera (Zuckerman and Lainson 1977). Electrophoresis and chromatography provided characteristic specific patterns of proteins, particularly of enzymes, and could prove to be a reliable method of identifying leishmania (Bray 1976; Zuckerman and Lainson 1977).

Leishmanial antigen was used successfully by Rioux and Golvan (1969) in testing dogs and foxes for antibodies to *L. infantum*. Complement fixation with antigens prepared from *Mycobacterium butyricum* have been used in the diagnosis of human and canine kala-azar (Nussenzweig 1956; Pellegrino *et al*. 1958).

DIAGNOSIS

Diagnosis of leishmaniasis in man and dogs is made on microscopic demonstration of organisms, culture of tissue explants, infection of laboratory rodents, testing for delayed hypersensitivity, and the nonspecific test to demonstrate the extensive rise of serum globulins. Serological tests are useful in epidemiological studies rather than for diagnosis of cases but have to be interpreted carefully. Nonspecific tests such as the aldehyde test, the antimony test, and the precipitation test are nonspecific and cannot be regarded as definitive. Because low levels of infection characterize cutaneous forms and infections in reservoir hosts, examination of tissue smears is not efficient and has to be verified. Cultures and injection of susceptible laboratory animals are much more sensitive. In the visceral form in man, the method of choice is the culture bone marrow aspirates. From visceral syndromes tissue samples are examined from the spleen, bone marrow, liver, and lymph nodes. Aspirates from lymph nodes are routinely examined in dogs. In man the leishmanin skin test is used in the diagnosis of all forms of leishmaniasis. Levels of infections vary, and in man amastigotes are relatively more abundant in the Old World than in New World varieties of cutaneous leishmaniasis. Hamsters are also used to isolate the organisms and have to be kept under observation for 9 to 12 months after infection.

Literature

In man and dogs the demonstration of leishmania for diagnostic purposes has often been difficult and, under some field conditions, impossible. Culture of organisms require specialized laboratory procedures which are often unavailable. Because of the difficulty of demonstrating the organisms, the leishmanin intradermal test has been extensively used in man as an epidemiological tool for studying the incidence, geographical distribution, and the diagnosis of leishmaniasis. The antigen consisted of a phenol-killed suspension of cultured leptomonads and the response was a delayed hypersensitivity reaction resulting in an area of induration greater than 5 mm in diameter in 24 to 48 hours. The test was positive at different times with the various forms of the disease, being most useful with the cutaneous as opposed to the visceral varieties. The reaction was nonspecific for various species of leishmania and other flagellates including *Trypanosoma cruzi*. The false-positive rate was 1 to 5%. False negatives were encountered due to age or complication by other infections. The cutaneous forms were positive 8 to 10 days after infection, and in the visceral type were positive in subclinical infections early in the course and after 2 to 3 months following spontaneous or chemical cure (Cahill and Cox 1975).

The immunodiagnosis of leishmaniasis in man was reviewed by Bray (1976). The antigen was derived from flagellated promastigotes grown in culture. Antibodies were detected by the FA, precipitation, and indirect hemagglutination tests in those syndromes where the organisms had spread from the original site of infection.

A summary was presented of the techniques which were used in the diagnosis of canine leishmaniasis, and the methods involved aspiration of lymph nodes, CF, and immunofluorescent tests (Lanotte *et al.* 1975). The reliability of various serological tests has not been established, and it was pointed out that there has been a great need for reliable serodiagnostic methods for surveying dogs (Bray 1976). A relatively good correlation was observed between immunofluorescent techniques and parasitological examinations (Lanotte *et al.* 1975). Lymph node biopsy was found to be useful (Ranque *et al.* 1948).

Hamsters have been the laboratory animals of choice for the isolation of leishmania. Materials from cutaneous form of leishmania were inoculated into the nose or feet. In suspected visceral cases inoculations were intraperitoneal. Well-established laboratory species induced well-defined proliferative lesions known as histiocytoma at the site of the injection, with the histiocytes containing large numbers of amastigotes. With recent isolates comparable lesions were not formed and were characterized by vascular components with comparatively few amastigotes. The extent of metastasia and the severity of lesions in the hamster depended on the species, subspecies, and strain of leishmania. Some species were unable to cause infection. It has been recommended that the hamsters are kept under observation for at least 1 year and a more detailed examination of tissues should be undertaken at postmortem (Lainson 1982).

CHEMOTHERAPY

Most forms of cutaneous leishmaniasis do not require therapy because they are self-healing. A variety of agents have been used in the treatment of mucocutaneous and visceral leishmaniasis of man, which include pentavalent antimony preparations, aromatic diamidines, and amphotericin B. The antifolic drugs, pyrimethamine and cycloguanil pamoate, are useful in the treatment of American cutaneous leishmaniasis. Current therapy of various forms of leishmaniasis in dogs is inadequate and management of secondary infections is critical.

Literature

Current approaches in the chemotherapy of leishmaniasis in man were reviewed by Newton (1974). The main chemotherapeutic agents consisted of a number of antimonials and aromatic diamidines (Zuckerman and Lainson 1977). Drug resistance of leishmania was reviewed by Peters (1974). In man, the treatment varies depending on the type of infection, the geographical origin of the disease, and the extent and duration of illness. Pentavalent antimony (urea stibamine and/or sodium antimony gluconates) were the basic drugs used in mucocutaneous infections. Control of secondary bacterial infections was essential in all forms of leishmaniasis (Cahill and Cox 1975).

Fifteen cases of canine leishmaniasis were treated with pentasodium antimony, methylglucamine, and cycloguamil pamoate and this therapy was only partially successful with only temporary improvement in skin lesions. The therapy was complicated by local and systemic toxic responses (Nicoletti and Fruin 1974). A case of visceral leishmaniasis in a dog was treated with *N*-methylglucoamine antimoniate and with supportive therapy, with clinical recovery after two treatments (Persechino and Agresti 1973). With antimony compounds and aromatic diamidines, it was found that although the visceral infections were cleared the infection in the skin and lymph nodes persisted (Adler and Tchernomoretz 1946). Organisms were found to persist for long periods after treatment after symptoms had disappeared (Bray 1974a; Poul and Pallas 1962).

CONTROL

Control of human leishmaniasis depends on the particular syndrome and epizootiological situation, and measures are directed towards the organism, the vector, and the reservoir host. Opportunity and feasibility for control of each of these components, singly or together, varies in different parts of the world. Control must be adapted to local situations in each endemic area once baseline data of the various components is available. Although the weakest link is the relatively fragile vector, the extensive technology required for its control is frequently unavailable. Insecticides may be used effectively in urban conditions. Control is also possible through destruction of the wild rodent reservoirs and dogs. In some epizootiological situations, control is based on diagnosis and therapy of human infections and avoidance of endemic sites.

Literature

Many review articles discuss some component of the control of leishmaniasis. Inoculation with living promastigotes of *L. tropica major* has been practised extensively with great success in the control of the cutaneous form of leishmaniasis in the Middle East. Similar treatment against American cutaneous leishmaniasis and kala-azar has not been undertaken (Manson-Bahr 1977). These measures have not been tried in dogs.

BIBLIOGRAPHY

Adler, S., 1964. Leishmania, *Adv. Parasitol.*, **2**: 35–96.

Adler, S. and Tchernomoretz, I., 1946. Failure to cure natural canine visceral leishmaniasis, *Ann. trop. Med. Parasit.*, **40**: 320–4.

Adler, S. and Theodor, O., 1932. Investigations on Mediterranean kala-azar. VI. Canine visceral leishmaniasis. *Proc. R. Soc. Lond.*, **110**: 402–12.

Adler, S. and Theodor, O., 1934. Investigations on Mediterranean kala-azar. VII. Further observations on canine visceral leishmaniasis, *Proc. R. Soc. Lond.*, **116**: 494–504.

Alencar, J. E., 1959. Um caso de leishmaniose tegumentarem *Equus asinus*. In *XIV Congresso Brasileiro de Higiene* (*Niteroi*), pp. 18–21.

Anderson, D. C., Buckner, R. G., Glenn, B. L. and MacVean, D. W., 1980. Endemic canine leishmaniasis, *Vet. Pathol.*, **17**: 94–6.

Berberian, D. A., 1959. Relationship of Mediterranean kala-azar to canine kala-azar, *Trans R. Soc. trop. Med. Hyg.*, **53**: 364–5.

Bettini, S., Pozio, E. and Gradoni, L., 1980. Leishmaniasis in Tuscany (Italy): (11) *Leishmania* from wild Rodentia and Carnivora in a human and canine leishmaniasis focus, *Trans. R. Soc. trop. Med. Hyg.*, **74**(1): 77–83.

Bonfante-Garrido, R., Melendez, E. C., Torres, R. A., Morillo, N. C., Arredondo, C. C. and Urdeneta, I., 1981. Enzootic equine cutaneous leishmaniasis in Venezuela, *Trans. R. Soc. trop. Med. Hyg.*, **75**(3): 471.

Bray, R. S., 1974a. Leishmania, *Ann. Rev. Microbiol.*, **28**: 189–217.

Bray, R. S., 1974b. Epidemiology of leishmaniasis: some reflections on causation. In *Trypanosomiasis and Leishmaniasis with Special Reference to Chagas' Disease*, Ciba Foundation Symposium 20 (new series). Elsevier, Excerpta Medica, North Holland, Associated Scientific Publishers (Amsterdam, London, New York), pp. 87–101.

Bray, R. S., 1974c. Zoonoses in leishmaniasis. In *Parasitic Zoonoses. Clinical and Experimental Studies*, ed. E. J. L. Soulsby. Academic Press (London), pp. 65–77.

Bray, R. S., 1976. Immunodiagnosis of leishmaniasis. In *Immunology of Parasitic Infections*, eds S. Cohen, E. Sadun. Blackwell Scientific Publications (Oxford), pp. 65–75.

Bucci, A., Puccini, V., Casaglia, O. and Colella, G., 1975. Epizoologia della leishmaniosi in provincia di Foggia: la leishmaniosi del cane, *Parassitologia*, **17**: 25–37.

Buck, G., Courdurier, J., Dorel, R. and Quesnel, J. J., 1951. Premier cas de leishmaniose canine à Madagascar, *Bull. Soc. Path. Exot.*, **44**: 428–30.

Bungener, W. and Mehlitz, D., 1977. Atypical course of *Leishmania donovani* infections in dogs. Histopathological findings, *Z. Tropenmed. Parasit.*, **28**: 175–80.

Cahill, K. M. and Cox, K. B., 1975. Leishmaniasis. In *Diseases Transmitted from Animals to Man*, eds W. T. Hubbert, W. F. McCulloch, P. R. Schnurrenberger. Charles C. Thomas (Springfield, Ill.), pp. 777–8.

Colella, G., Bucci, A., Puccini, C., Casaglia, O., La Salandra, M., Rendine, C., Sebastiani, A. and Proietti, A. M., 1979. Epizoology of leishmaniasis in the province of Matera (Italy): spreading of dog leishmaniasis and collecting of phlebotomines, *Clin. Vet.*, **102**: 35–41.

Colella, G. and Casamassima, E., 1975. La leishmaniosi del cane in provincia di Matera, *Vet. Italiana*, **26**(9–12): 393–402.

Conroy, J. D., Levine, N. D. and Small, E., 1970. Visceral leishmaniosis in a fennec fox (*Fennecus zerda*), *Path. Vet.*, **7**: 163–70.

Convit, J. and Pinardi, M. E., 1974. Cutaneous leishmaniasis. The clinical and immunopathological spectrum in South America. In *Trypanosomiasis and Leishmaniasis with Special Reference to Chagas' Disease*, Ciba Foundation Symposium 20 (new series). Elsevier,

Excerpta Medica, North Holland, Associated Scientific Publishers (Amsterdam, London, New York), pp. 159–68.
Corbeil, L. B., Wright-George, J., Shively, J. N., Duncan, J. R., LaMotte, G. B. and Schultz, R. D., 1976. Canine visceral leishmaniasis with amyloidosis: and immunopathological case study, *Clin. Immunol. Immunopathol.*, **6**: 165–73.

Dedet, J., Ben Osman, F., Croset, C. H. and Rioux, J.-A., 1973. Leishmaniasis in Tunisia. Sero-immunological survey about the frequency of infestation, *Ann. Parasitol. (Paris)*, **48**(5): 653–60.
Di Domizio, G., 1955. Casi mortali di leishmaniosi visceraie canina autoctona in Bologna – contributo allo studio anatomopatologico e parassitologico, *Zooprofilassi*, **10**(7): 399–414.
Donatien, A. and Lestoquand, F., 1938. Sur l'évolution de la leishmaniose générale du chien, *Arch. Inst. Pasteur d'Algerie*, **16**: 191–202.
Dunan, S., 1978. Interpretation of biological results in leishmaniasis in man and the dog, *Rec. Méd. vét.*, **154**(3): 251–61.

Gardener, P. J., 1977. Taxonomy of the genus *Leishmania*: a review of nomenclature and classification, *Trop. Dis. Bull.*, **74**(12): 1069–88.
Garnham, P. C. C., 1965. The leishmanias, with special reference to the role of animal reservoirs, *Am. Zoologist.*, **5**: 141–51.
Garnham, P. C. C., 1971a. The genus *Leishmania*, *Bull. Wld Hlth Org.*, **44**: 477–89.
Garnham, P. C. C., 1971b. American leishmaniasis, *Bull. Wld Hlth Org.*, **44**: 521–7.
George, J. W., Nielsen, S. W., Shively, J. N., Hopek, S. and Mroz, S., 1976. Canine leishmaniasis with amyloidosis, *Vet. Pathol.*, **13**: 365–73.
Giles, R. C. Jr, Hildebrandt, P. K., Becker, R. L. and Montgomery, C. A. Jr, 1975. Visceral leishmaniasis in a dog with bilateral endophthalmitis, *J. Am. Anim. Hosp. Ass.*, **11**: 155–9.
Gleiser, C. A., Thiel, J. and Cashell, I. G., 1957. Visceral leishmaniasis in a dog imported into the United States, *Am. J. Trop. Med. Hyg.*, **6**: 227–31.
Gradoni, L., Pozio, E., Bettini, S. and Gramiccia, M., 1980. Leishmaniasis in Tuscany (Italy). III. The prevalence of canine leishmaniasis in two foci of Grosseto Province, *Trans. R. Soc. trop. Med. Hyg.*, **74**(3): 421–2.
Groulade, P. and Groulade, J., 1959. Leishmaniose canine hématologie et micro-electrophorèse sur papier, *Bull. Soc. Path. Exot.*, **32**: 343–52.
Guilhon, J., 1950. Répartition geographique de la leishmaniose canine en France, *Bull. Acad. Vet. France*, **23**: 69–74.
Guilhon, M. J., 1965. Extension de la leishmaniose canine, en France, et son possible danger pour les enfants, *Acad. Nat. Méd. Bull.*, **149**: 638–43.

Herrer, A. and Battistini, M. G., 1951. Estudios sobre leishmaniasis tegumentaria en el Peru. I. Infecion experimental de perros con cepas de leishmanias proce dentes de casos de Uta, *Revta. de Med. Exp. (Lima)*, **8**: 12–28.

Herrer, A. and Christensen, H. A., 1976. Natural cutaneous leishmaniasis among dogs in Panama, *Am. J. trop. Med. Hyg.*, **25**(1): 59–63.

Heyneman, D., 1971. Immunology of leishmaniasis, *Bull. Wld Hlth Org.*, **44**: 499–514.

Ho, E. A., Hsu, T-H. H. and Soong, T-H., 1947. Canine visceral leishmaniasis in villages west of Lanchow, China, *Trans. R. Soc. trop. Med. Hyg.*, **40**(6): 889–94.

Hoare, C. A., 1955. The epidemiological role of animal reservoirs in human leishmaniasis and trypanosomiasis, *Vet. Rev. Annot.*, **1**: 62–8.

Hoare, C. A., 1962. Reservoir hosts and natural foci of human protozoa infections, *Acta trop.*, **19**: 281.

Houin, R., Jolivet, G., Combescot, C., Deniau, M., Puel, F., Barbier, D., Romano, P. and Kerbœuf, D., 1977. Etude préliminaire d'un foyer de leishmaniose canine dans la région de Tours. In *Ecologie des Leishmanioses*. Editions du centre National de la Recherche scientifique (Paris), vol. 239, pp. 109–22.

Isaev, L. M., 1966. The pathogenesis and clinical course of canine leishmaniasis in Uzbekistan, *Medskaya Parazit.*, **35**: 250–62.

Kammermann, B. and Buhlmann, L., 1965. Zu einem Fall von leishmaniase beim hund, *Schweizer Archiv fur Tierheilkunde*, **107**(7): 371–85.

Killick-Kendrick, R., 1979. Biology of *Leishmania* in phlobotomine sandflies. In *Biology of the Kinetoplastida*, eds W. H. R. Lumsden, D. A. Evans. Academic Press (London), vol. 2, pp. 395–460.

Lainson, R., 1982. Leishmanial parasites of mammals in relation to human disease, *Symp. Zool. Soc. Lond.*, **50**: 137–79.

Lainson, R. and Shaw, J. J., 1978. Epidemiology and ecology of leishmaniasis in Latin-America, *Nature*, **273**(22): 595–600.

Lainson, R. and Shaw, J. J., 1979. The role of animals in the epidemiology of South American leishmaniasis. In *Biology of the Kinetoplastida*, eds W. H. R. Lumsden, D. A. Evans. Academic Press (London), vol. 2, pp. 1–99.

Lainson, R., Shaw, J. J. and Lins, Z. C., 1969. Leishmaniasis in Brazil: IV. The fox, *Cerdocyon thous* (L) as a reservoir of *Leishmania donovani* in Para State, Brazil, *Trans. R. Soc. trop. Med. Hyg.*, **63**(6): 741–5.

Lanotte, G., Rioux, J. A., Croset, H. and Vollhardt, Y., 1975. Ecology of leishmaniasis in the South of France. 8. Complement to the immunofluorescent technique applied to epidemiology: geometric and arithmetic mean titers in a canine leishmaniasis survey, *Ann. Parasitol.*, **50**(1): 1–5.

Lanotte, G., Rioux, J. A., Croset, H. and Vollhardt, Y., 1977. Dépistage de la leishmaniose canine stratégie d'enquête utilisée dans le foyer des cevennes méridionales. In *Ecologie des Leishmanioses*. Editions du centre National de la Recherche scientifique (Paris), vol. 239, pp. 117–28.

Lanotte, G., Rioux, J. A., Croset, H. and Vollhardt, Y., 1978. Ecology of leishmaniasis in the South of France. 9. Sampling methods in the study of the canine enzootic, *Ann. Parasitol. (Paris)*, **53**(1): 33–45.

Lanotte, G., Rioux, J. A., Croset, H., Vollhardt, Y. and Martini-Dumas, A., 1974. Ecology of leishmaniasis in the South of France. 7. Research of canine reservoir by the mean of serological reactions, *Ann. Parasitol. (Paris)*, **49**(1): 41–62.

Levine, N. D., Corliss, J. O., Cox, F. F. *et al.*, 1980. A newly revised classification of the protozoa, *J. Protozool.*, **27**: 37–58.

Manson-Bahr, P. E. C., 1971. Leishmaniasis, *Int. Rev. Trop. Med.*, **4**: 123–140.

Manson-Bahr, P. E. C., 1977. Leishmaniasis. In *Infectious Diseases: A Modern Treatise of Infectious Processes*, ed. P. D. Hoeprich. Harper and Row (Hagerstown, Md.), pp. 1088–99.

Maruashvili, G. M. and Bardzhadze, B. G., 1980. New natural reservoir of *Leishmania donovani* in Georgia, *Med. Parazitol.*, **49**: 77–8.

Mauel, J. and Behin, R., 1974. Cell-mediated and humoral immunity to protozoan infections (with special reference to leishmaniasis), *Tranplant Rev.*, **19**: 121–46.

Mauel, J., Behin, R., Biroum-Noerjasin and Doyle, J. J., 1974. Survival and death of *Leishmania* in macrophages. In *Parasites in the Immunized Host: Mechanisms of Survival*, Ciba Foundation Symposium 25 (new series). Elsevier, Excerpta Medica, North Holland, Associated Scientific Publishers (Amsterdam, London, New York), pp. 225–37.

Mazza, S., 1927. Leishmaniasis curanea en el caballo y nueva observacion de la misma en el petro, *Bol. Inst. Clin. Quirurgico (Buenos Aires)*, **3**: 462–4.

McConnell, E. E., Chaffee, E. F., Cashell, I. G. and Garner, F. M., 1970. Visceral leishmaniasis with ocular involvement in a dog, *J. Am. vet. med. Ass.*, **156**(2): 197–203.

Medina, R., 1966. Leishmaniasis experimental en animales silvestres, *Dermatologica Venezuelana*, **5**: 91–119.

Mello, S. B., 1940. Natural infection of a cat with *Leishmania sp.*, *Rev. Bras. Med.*, **54**: 189.

Millin, J., Fine, J. M., Groulade, J. and Groulade, P., 1975.

Leishmaniasis and dysglobulinaemia in a dog, *Rev. Méd. vét.*, **126**(12): 1655–64.
Mishra, A. K. and Lodha, K. R., 1975. Serodiagnostic tests in *Leishmania tropica* (Wright, 1903) Luhe, 1906 infection in dogs, *Indian vet. J.*, **52**: 395–7.
Mishra, A. K. and Lodha, K. R., 1977. Histopathological study: cutaneous leishmaniasis in dogs, *Indian vet. J.*, **54**: 475–6.
Muscarella, A., Galofaro, V. and Macri, B., 1981. A study of a case of canine leishmaniasis, *Arch. Vet. Ital.*, **32**(1–2): 15–23.
Mutinga, M. J., Ngoka, J. M., Schnur, L. F. and Chance, M. L., 1980. The isolation and identification of leishmanial parasites from domestic dogs in the Machakos District of Kenya, and the possible role of dogs as reservoirs of kala-azar in East Africa, *Ann. trop. Med. Parasit.*, **74**(2): 139–44.

Newton, B. A., 1974. The chemotherapy of trypanosomiasis and leishmaniasis: towards a more rational approach. In *Trypanosomiasis and Leishmaniasis with Special Reference to Chagas' Disease*, Ciba Foundation Symposium 20 (new series). Elsevier, Excerpta Medica, North Holland, Associated Scientific Publishers (Amsterdam, London, New York), pp. 309–28.
Ngoka, J. M. and Mutinga, M. J., 1977. The dog a reservoir of visceral leishmaniasis in Kenya, *Trans. R. Soc. trop. Med. Hyg.*, **71**(5): 447–8.
Ngoka, J. M. and Mutinga, M. J., 1978. Visceral leishmaniasis animal reservoirs in Kenya, *E. Afr. med. J.*, **55**(7): 332–6.
Nicoletti, P. and Fruin, J., 1974. Treatment of canine cutaneous leishmaniasis, *Trop. Anim. Hlth Prod.*, **6**: 85–8.
Nussenzweig, V., 1956. *Hospital* (*Rio de J.*), **2**: 217.

Pellegrino, J., Brener, Z. and Soutos, M. M., 1958. Complement fixation test in Kalazai using *Mycobacterium butyricum* antigen (m), *J. Parasitol.*, **44**: 645.
Persechino, A. and Agresti, A., 1973. Su di un caso di leishmaniosi canina osservato nell cita' di Napoli, *Acta Med. Vet.*, **19**(3–4): 233–43.
Peters, W., 1974. Drug resistance in trypanosomiasis and leishmaniasis. In *Trypanosomiasis and Leishmaniasis with Special Reference to Chagas' Disease*, Ciba Foundation Symposium 20 (new series). Elsevier, Excerpta Medica, North Holland, Associated Scientific Publishers (Amsterdam, London, New York), pp. 309–28.
Pons, A. R., 1968. Leishmaniasis tegumentaria Americana en el asentamiento campesino de Zipa-Yare, *Su importancia en la Reforma Agraria, Kasmera*, **3**: 5–59.
Poul, J. and Pallas, P., 1962. Persistance de *Leishmania donovani* dans l'organisme du chien après la guérison clinique et sérologique de

la leishmaniose générale, *Arch. Inst. Pasteure d'Algérie*, **40**: 25–32.

Pozio, E., Gradoni, L., Bettina, S. and Gramiccia, M., 1981a. Leishmaniasis in Tuscany (Italy): V. Further isolation of *Leishmania* from *Rattus rattus* in the province of Grosetto, *Ann. trop. Med. Parasit.*, **75**: 393–5.

Pozio, E., Gradoni, L., Bettini, S. and Gramiccia, M., 1981b. Leishmaniasis in Tuscany (Italy): VI. Canine leishmaniasis in the focus of Monte Argentario (Grosseto), *Acta trop.*, **38**: 383–93.

Rafyi, A., Niak, A. L., Naghshineh, R. and Aboutorabian, H., 1968. Canine visceral leishmaniasis in Iran, *Vet. Rec.*, **83**: 269–78.

Ranque, J., Ranque, M., Cabassu, J. and Cabassu, H., 1948. Le diagnostic précoce de la leishmaniose canine par la ponction ganglionnaire. Réflexions àpropos de soixante examens positifs obtenus en dix mois dans la région marseillaise, *Bull. Acad. Nat. Med.*, **132**: 339–40.

Ranque, P., Bussiéras, J., Chevalier, J.-L., Quillici, M. and Mattei, X., 1970. Importance actuelle de la leishmaniose canine au Sénégal. Intérêt du diagnostic immunologique. Incidence possible en pathologie humaine, *Acad. Nat. Méd. Bull.*, **154**: 510–12.

Rifaat, M. A. and Hassan, Z. A., 1967. Canine leishmaniasis in the U.A.R., *J. Trop. Med. Hyg.*, **70**: 209–14.

Rioux, J. A., Albert, J.-L., Houin, R., Dedet, J.-P. and Lanotte, G., 1968. Ecologie des leishmanioses dans le sud de la France. 2. Les réservoirs selvatique. Infestation spontanée du renard (*Vulpes vulpes* L.), *Ann. Parasitol. (Paris)*, **43**(4): 421–8.

Rioux, J. A. and Golvan, Y. J., 1969. Epidémiologie des leishmanioses dans le sud de la France, *Monogr. Inst. Nat. Santé Rech. Méd.*, No. 37 (Paris), 220 pp.

Rioux, J. A., Killick-Kendrick, R., Leaney, A. J., Young, C. J., Turner, D. P., Lanotte, G. and Bailly, M., 1979. Ecology of leishmaniasis in the south of France. 11. Canine leishmaniasis: successful experimental transmission from dog to dog by the bite of *Phlebotomus ariasi* Tonnoir, 1921, *Ann. Parasitol. (Paris)*, **54**(4): 401–7.

Rioux, J. A., Lanotte, G., Destombes, P., Vollhardt, Y., Croset, H. and Martini-Dumas, A., 1971. Leishmaniose expérimentale du renard *Vulpes vulpes* (L), *Rec. Méd. Vét.*, **147**: 489–98.

Rojos Ayala, M. A., 1973. Alteracoes renais no calazar canino espontaneo, *Revta. Soc. Brasil. Med. Trop.*, **7**(6): 353–8.

Sanchis, R., Vitu, C. and Giauffret, A., 1976. Laboratory tests in dog's leishmaniasis. II. Evaluation of biological tests in experimental disease, *Rev. Méd. vet.*, **127**(8–9): 1191–1202.

Sheriff, D., 1957. Canine visceral leishmaniasis in foxhounds near Baghdad, *Trans. R. Soc. trop. Med. Hyg.*, **51**(5): 467.

Southgate, B. A. and Oriedo, B. V. E., 1962. Studies in the

epidemiology of East African leishmaniasis. I. The circumstantial epidemiology of kala-azar in the Kitui district of Kenya, *Trans. R. Soc. trop. Med. Hyg.*, **56**(1): 30–47.

Stauber, L. A., 1970. Leishmanias. In *Immunity to Parasitic Animals*, eds G. J. Jackson, R. Herman, I. Singer. Appleton-Century-Crofts (New York), vol. 2, pp. 739–69.

Sukkar, F., Al-Mahdawi, S. K., Al-Doori, N. A. and Kadhum, J. A., 1981. Isolation of *Leishmania* from the spleen of a dog in Iraq, *Trans. R. Soc. trop. Med. Hyg.*, **75**(6): 859–60.

Tasselli, E. and Colella, G., 1960. Presence of canine leishmaniosis in the province of Matera, *Vet. Ital.*, **11**: 293–7.

Tendeiro, J., Petisca, J. L. de N. and Serra, J. L., 1968. Observacoes sobre leishmaniose canina em Mocambique, *Revta. de Ciencias Veterinarias (Lourenco Marques)*, VI ser. A, pp. 95–110.

Theran, P. and Ling, G. V., 1967. Case records of the Angell Memorial Hospital, *J. Am. vet. med. Ass.*, **150**(1): 82–8.

Thorson, R. E., Bailey, W. S., Hoerlein, B. F. and Seibold, H. R., 1955. A report of a case of imported visceral leishmaniasis of a dog in the United States, *Am. J. Trop. Med.*, **4**: 18–21.

Tryphonas, L., Zawidska, Z., Bernard, M. A. and Janzen, E. A., 1977. Visceral leishmaniasis in a dog: clinical hematological and pathological observations, *Can. J. comp. Med.*, **41**: 1–12.

Vitu, C., Sanchis, R. and Giauffret, A., 1973. Evolution des protéines sériques dans la leishmaniose canine, *Comptes Rendus des Seances de la Soc. de Biologie*, **167**(3–4): 513–18.

Zuckerman, A., 1975. Parasitological review. Current status of the immunology of blood and tissue protozoa. 1. *Leishmania, Exp. Parasitol.*, **38**: 370–400.

Zuckerman, A. and Lainson, R., 1977. Leishmania. In *Protozoa of Veterinary and Medical Interest*, ed. J. P. Kreier. Academic Press (New York), pp. 57–133.

PART
II

VIRAL DISEASES

Chapter

5

African horse sickness

CONTENTS

INTRODUCTION

African horse sickness (AHS) is an acute or subacute arboviral disease of horses and related species, characterized by fever, hemorrhages and edema of the subcutaneous tissues, lungs, and internal cavities. It is enzootic in Africa, where it is geographically well defined. The disease spread during the 1930s, causing extensive losses through epizootics outside the traditional enzootic areas of sub-Saharan Africa.

Literature

The historical incidence and geographical distribution of AHS in South Africa were reviewed by Henning (1956). African horse sickness was discussed at conferences on emerging diseases held under the auspices of the OIE–FAO in Ankara, Turkey, in 1961 (Anon. 1961a). A special conference on African swine fever and AHS was held in Paris in 1961 (Anon. 1961c). Summaries of the reports on AHS presented at the Third International Conference on Equine Infectious Diseases were published in 1972 (Anon. 1972).

ETIOLOGY

African horse sickness virus belongs to the orbivirus group of the family Reoviridae. It contains double-stranded ribonucleic acid (RNA), is icosahedral in shape, measures between 40 and 80 nm, has 32 capsomeres, and is closely related to bluetongue (BT) virus.

African horse sickness virus retains its infectivity under various laboratory conditions and is relatively stable under adverse conditions such as putrefaction, desiccation, and temperature variation.

The virus can be readily passaged by intracerebral inoculation of mice. The adaptation and propagation of the virus in chicken embryos is more readily attained with the neurotropic strain than with the viscerotropic virus isolated from horses. Chicken embryo fibroblast cells also support the growth of low-passage mouse-brain-adapted virus, but cytopathic effects do not develop. The virus can be propagated in mosquito cells and in a variety of kidney cell lines originating from various species. The virus has been adapted to monkey kidney stable (MKS) cell and VERO cell lines. The MKS cell cultures are used for serological and diagnostic tests, the study of infections in cells, and the development of live and inactivated vaccines. Viral growth is characterized by the occurrence of an eclipse phase lasting 8 hours, followed by the release of a new virus and the appearance of cytopathic effects. The cytopathic effects, consisting of degenerative and necrotic changes, are observed 36 hours after infection, and are completed by the fourth day. Plaquing techniques can be employed for the quantification and cloning of different strains.

Literature

The physicochemical properties of AHS virus have been studied. African horse sickness virus has a double-stranded RNA genome, is icosahedral in shape, measures 55 nm in diameter, and consists of 32 capsomeres (Oellermann *et al.* 1970). The size of the particles from seven different strains of AHS virus was examined and found to vary between 40 and 80 nm (Bakaya and Gurturk 1962). During an investigation of the particle size distribution of a neurotropic strain of AHS virus, it was determined that the infective particles had two sedimentation constants (Polson and Madsen 1954). Electron-microscopic examination of AHS virus established that the virus was a member of the orbivirus genus of the family Reoviridae (Bremer 1976) and that it was morphologically similar to BT virus (Oellermann *et al.* 1970). Gel electrophoretic patterns of the polypeptides and the RNA also demonstrated that there was a close relationship between AHS and BT viruses (Bremer 1976).

The physicochemical properties of AHS virus were studied using highly susceptible hosts and various tissue culture systems. Mouse-adapted AHS virus was found to resist the action of ether, chloroform, trypsin, and sodium deoxycholate (Tewari *et al.* 1972). The stability of neurotropic AHS virus was influenced by the media in which the virus was suspended (Polson *et al.* 1953). The sensitivity of the virus to beta propiolactone and pH was determined in studies undertaken to establish the experimental conditions necessary for the production of inactivated vaccines. The virus was inactivated within 15 minutes at pHs below 5.6 and above 10.9 (Parker 1975). The infectivity of both neurotropic and viscerotropic AHS virus decreased markedly when the virus, suspended in tissue culture medium or in phosphate buffered saline, was stored at temperatures between −20 and −30 °C. It was established that various salts contained in the solutions were responsible for the inactivation of the virus. The infectivity was protected by the addition of sugars. The AHS virus was stable at −70 °C (Ozawa 1968; Ozawa and Bahrami 1966).

Virulent viscerotropic AHS virus was initially isolated from horses by the intracerebral inoculation of mice, and serial mouse-brain passage resulted in neurotropic adaptation of the virus. The growth of neurotropic and viscerotropic strains of AHS virus was studied in chicken embryos. In this system, virus titers were high and comparable to those obtained in mouse brains. The neurotropic strains retained their affinity for brain tissue after six consecutive passages in embryonated eggs (Goldsmit 1967). In other studies, it was found that different neurotropic strains of AHS virus required different incubation temperatures for optimal growth in developing chick embryos. These strains also differed in their ability to maintain neurotropism on serial egg passage (Prasad and Gulrajani 1975).

African horse sickness virus was first propagated in tissue culture by Mirchamsy and Taslimi (1962, 1963). They cultivated low-passage mouse-brain-adapted virus in hamster kidney cells and observed a progressive cytopathic effect from the second transfer onwards. Chicken embryo fibroblasts were also used for primary isolation of the virus, but no specific cytopathic effect developed (Eramus 1963a, 1964). The ability of the virus to propagate in MKS cell cultures led many laboratories to abandon the use of mice as a source of virus (Hazrati and Ozawa 1965a). Two strains of AHS virus already adapted either to mouse brain or to MKS cell culture were also readily grown in a mosquito cell line. Cytopathic effects were not evident in the infected mosquito cells, but the virus was detected in the cytoplasm and around the nuclei of infected cells by the fluorescent antibody (FA) technique and acridine orange staining (Mirchamsy *et al.* 1960; Tessler 1972; Davies and Lund 1974). In a study of the growth pattern of AHS virus in fetal camel kidney cells, the maximum virus yield was obtained 48 hours after infection. Various cytopathic and histochemical changes were observed in the infected cells (Farid *et al.* 1974). The interference demonstrated between different antigenic types of AHS virus in tissue culture was either partial or complete, depending on the time between infection with the interfering virus and inoculation of the challenge virus (Ozawa 1966).

The AHS virus was adapted to hamster kidney cells, and the interaction between the virus and the cells in a single growth cycle was described (Mirchamsy and Taslimi 1963). Attenuated neurotropic strains and virulent field strains both caused distinct cytopathic changes in MKS cell cultures. After passage, the incubation period became shorter and cytopathic changes were observed 2 to 3 days after infection. Plaques ranging from 1 to 3 mm in diameter formed after 10 days of incubation (Ozawa and Hazrati 1964). The effect of a number of variables on plaque formation by AHS virus on different cell lines was determined (Oellermann 1970). Virus particles were occasionally detected in the cytoplasm during the advanced stage of infection (Ozawa *et al.* 1967). The presence of intranuclear and intracytoplasmic structureless inclusions in MKS cells was demonstrated by electron microscopy. Enzyme digestion showed that these inclusions were proteinaceous (Breese and Ozawa 1969; Breese *et al.* 1969). Single-passage growth patterns of AHS virus in two different MKS cell lines (MS and VERO) were compared by titrating the extracellular virus in cultures infected at high multiplicity. The FA and acridine orange staining techniques both showed that large antigenic bodies containing RNA were present in the cytoplasm of the VERO but not the MS cells (Ozawa 1967). The MS and VERO cell cultures also differed with respect to the distribution and appearance of viral antigens in the cytoplasm (Ozawa 1968). In other studies using the direct FA technique, the virus was detected in or around the nucleus of MS cells 8 hours after infection and was observed in the cytoplasm at 24 and 48 hours (Mirchamsy and Taslimi 1964a). Actinomycin D inhibited the yield of virus in monkey kidney cells and it was suggested that the virus contained deoxyribonucleic acid (DNA) or was an RNA virus whose replication was dependent on DNA (Mirchamsy and Taslimi 1966, 1967c).

EPIZOOTIOLOGY

Geographical distribution and incidence

African horse sickness is enzootic and widely distributed throughout the continent of Africa, where it has a rhythmic seasonal incidence, occurring during the summer and being prevalent in warm, wet regions. In dry tropical climates, the dissemination of the disease is favored by hot and humid conditions. Enzootic conditions exist in regions of Africa with a Sahelian climate which favors the breeding of horses. The spread of the AHS virus is due to the introduction of equidae, to the dissemination of insect vectors, and to the nomadic conditions of livestock-rearing in many endemically infected countries. The climatic conditions which affect the vectors play a major role in the spread of the virus outside the established enzootic areas. With the onset of winter, the epizootics subside in most of the affected countries.

Until the 1960s, AHS was most common in eastern, western, and southern Africa. As early as the 1930s, however, the disease spread out of the regions south of the Sahara to Egypt, Israel, and Lebanon. The next extensive outbreak occurred between 1959 and 1960 in Afghanistan, Pakistan, India, Iran, Iraq, Jordan, Syria, Turkey, Lebanon, and Cyprus. Between 1965 and 1966, the virus was evident in Morocco, Libya, Algeria, Tunisia, and Spain.

Literature

The most recent and comprehensive reviews of the epizootiology of AHS were presented by Bourdin (1973), Bourdin and Laurent (1974), and Mirchamsy and Hazrati (1973). Bourdin (1973) reviewed the geographical distribution of AHS in the past and present and discussed the incidence of the disease in relation to climatic conditions and topography. In a review of the 1960 epizootic which occurred in the Middle East and southwest Asia, Howell (1960) presented a most comprehensive picture of the sequence of events in the spread of the disease. In addition, there have been a number of international conferences at which the AHS situation was updated on a country-by-country basis (Anon. 1961a, b, c, d). Further research was inspired by the devastating spread of this virus outside the African continent (Howell and Erasmus 1963).

The history of AHS in Egypt, from the first outbreak in 1928, was reported (Anon. 1961a). African horse sickness was also recognized in Yemen (1930) and Israel (1944) and later reappeared in Egypt (1958). During 1959 and 1960, other countries in the Persian Gulf area were affected, and outbreaks were simultaneously reported in Afghanistan, Pakistan, India, and most of the Middle Eastern countries. This region lost over 300 000 animals between 1959 and 1961 (Mirchamsy and Hazrati 1973). At an international meeting on emerging diseases held in 1961, the position of AHS in Pakistan, Iraq, Nigeria, the Sudan, Israel,

Iran, Lebanon, and Jordan was discussed, and various control measures, including mass immunization of all equines, were recommended (Anon. 1961a). The status of the disease in Afghanistan, Cyprus, Greece, India, Iran, Iraq, Israel, Jordan, Lebanon, Saudi Arabia, Pakistan, Senegal, Turkey, Syria, and the USSR was described in a summary of the proceedings of an international conference on AHS. In a number of these countries, the disease first became apparent around 1960 (Anon. 1961b). The AHS situation from 1959 to 1963 was summarized in a table listing the numbers of outbreaks and affected animals in various African, Middle Eastern, and southwest Asian countries (Eichhorn 1963). The involvement of a very large area and the dissemination of the virus over great distances are consequences of the movement of large numbers of nomadic people which inhabit these regions (Howell 1960).

Subsequently, investigations were undertaken to define the incidence and epizootiology of AHS on a country-by-country basis. Two cases of type 9 virus infection were observed in Chad (Doutre and Leclercq 1962). A serological survey of horses for type 9 virus was undertaken in Chad, the Central African Republic, and Cameroon, and it was concluded that this strain was widespread but less virulent (Maurice and Provost 1967). A number of reports have been published on AHS in Nigeria. African horse sickness was first isolated and identified in Nigeria by Kemp *et al.* (1971). A clinical case was described, and a small-scale survey indicated widespread incidence of AHS antibody at low levels in horses, donkeys, and dogs in Nigeria (Alhaji *et al.* 1974). An outbreak of a frequently fatal disease caused by type 9 AHS virus, affecting only imported horses, occurred in Nigeria in 1974 (Best *et al.* 1975). African horse sickness was considered an important disease of equines, particularly in the highly susceptible animals introduced into the country (Abegunde 1975). In a serological survey of horses in Nigeria, approximately 81% of the sera were positive for precipitating antibodies to AHS virus (Nawathe *et al.* 1981) A recent survey for complement-fixing and neutralizing antibodies to AHS virus carried out sera collected from indigenous Nigerian horses demonstrated that most types of AHS virus had been present in Nigeria in the past and that type 9 was the current predominant serotype. Inapparent infections might occur in enzootic areas; hence, wild and domestic equidae with subclinical cases of AHS were potential reservoirs of the virus (Parker *et al.* 1977). In Cyprus, a serological study of native horses revealed that there was a 95% incidence of neutralizing antibodies only in animals at least 11 years of age. These results indicated that the virus did not persist on the island after the 1960–61 epizootic (Parker 1974). The disease was observed in Libya (Michamsy and Hazrati 1973), Morocco (Anon. 1969; Laaberki 1969), and Algeria (Anon. 1966) in 1965 and reached Tunisia (El Fourgi 1967) in 1966. The occurrence and eradication of AHS in Spain in 1966 were described in detail (Montilla and Marti 1967, 1968).

Transmission

Hematophagous arthropods have been incriminated as possible vectors of AHS virus by circumstantial epizootiological evidence as well as by experimental transmission. *Culicoides* and mosquitoes are mainly suspected. The infection is transmitted mechanically and biologically when these vectors feed on viremic animals. Because the disease is probably transmitted by *Culicoides* and by other biting arthropods, it has the potential to spread widely throughout the world, and the possibility of transmission is increased by livestock trade and travel between different parts of the world. Transmission by wind-borne insects is also a possibility. The disease is not contagious on contact, but can be transmitted experimentally by a variety of routes.

A most important factor in the epizootiology of AHS is the reservoir host. The existence of reservoirs of infection is suggested by the fact that the disease passes from one season to another in a particular area. Serological investigations have not clearly identified the reservoir hosts or vectors which maintain the virus during the winter and interepizootic periods.

Literature

The information on the transmission of AHS by arthropods was summarized by Mirchamsy and Hazrati (1973). The transmission of AHS virus by various arthropods was suspected on the basis of circumstantial evidence, but was not verified extensively by experimental work. The available evidence indicated that the virus could be transmitted mechanically as well as biologically to highly susceptible equine populations by nocturnal biting insects (Mirchamsy and Hazrati 1973). Numerous arthropod species have been incriminated in the mechanical transmission of AHS, but only a few species have been shown to be important in the biological transmission (Bourdin 1973). The virus was shown to be transmitted primarily by *Culicoides* species. Although the mosquitoes of the genus *Aedes* harbored the virus for 1 week following experimental infection, they could not transmit the disease, while *Anopheles stephensis, Culex pipiens,* and *Aedes aegypti* mosquitoes were able to transmit the virus (Mirchamsy and Hazrati 1973).

In other investigations, it was shown that *Culicoides variipennis* midges fed on infected chick embryos were able to transmit the virus to uninfected embryonated eggs, indicating that this insect is a biological vector of AHS virus in the laboratory (Boorman *et al.* 1975). Type 9 AHS virus multiplied in *C. nubeculosus* as well as in *C. variipennis* after intrathoracic inoculation and was transmitted by the latter species after 4 days of incubation (Mellor *et al.* 1975). This strain of AHS virus multiplied to a high titer in *C. puncticollis* after intrathoracic inoculation and persisted for at least 10 days. However, the virus failed to multiply in this insect following oral ingestion and was not detected beyond the fourth postinfection day (Mellor *et al.* 1981).

African horse sickness virus was transmitted experimentally to a horse by the bites of *A. aegypti* which had been infected orally (Ozawa *et al.* 1966; Anon. 1967). *Anopheles stephensi* and *Culex pipiens* fed 15 to 22 days previously on infected blood also transmitted the disease (Ozawa and Nakata 1965). Under experimental conditions, less than 3% of *Aedes aegypti* mosquitoes were infected by feeding. However, intrathoracic injection of the virus caused high infection rates. It was concluded that this species was unlikely to be an effective vector of AHS virus (Braverman and Boorman 1978). In other studies, *A. aegypti, C. pipiens fatigans* and *Culicoides* species fed on infected horses were found to be negative when subsequently tested for infectivity by intracerebral inoculation of mice (Wetzel *et al.* 1970).

It was shown that AHS could be transmitted by other biting vectors. African horse sickness virus was isolated from *Hyalomma dromedarii* in Egypt by Samia Khidr (1980). Recent work on infected ticks demonstrated that the virus was not transmitted from engorged females to eggs, but could be transmitted from larvae to nymphs and from nymphs to adults. There was a progressive increase in the amount of virus present at each stage (Awad *et al.* 1981).

Recovered horses did not maintain the virus for long periods of time, and the viral titers existing in the presence of neutralizing antibody were considered too low for efficient vectorial transmission (Mirchamsy and Hazrati 1973). It was proposed that the virus might be present in indigenous wild and domestic equines of Africa. In enzootic situations, the disease tended to occur in a subclinical form, and animals with such infections were considered a possible source of virus for susceptible horses (Bourdin 1973; Pilo-Moron *et al.* 1969). In a review of the epizootiology of the disease, McIntosh (1958) discussed the possibility that nonequine species maintained the virus in enzootic regions. In subsequent studies, neutralizing and complement-fixing antibodies were detected in the sera of zebra and elephants (Davies and Otieno 1977). Analyses of outbreaks of African horse sickness showed that movement of infected *Culicoides* midges on the wind was most likely responsible for the spread of the disease over the sea from Morocco to Spain in 1966, from Turkey to Cyprus in 1960, and from Senegal to the Cape Verde Islands in 1943. The risk of spread to countries outside the endemic areas should be assessed by reference to possible wind dispersal of infected midges (Sellers *et al.* 1977).

INFECTION

African horse sickness is primarily a disease of equines. Horses are most susceptible, mules and donkeys are more resistant, and zebras are highly resistant. It is known from the early work in South Africa that different strains of AHS virus vary considerably in their virulence for susceptible equines. This variation is also observed in experimental murine infections. African horse sickness virus slowly loses its virulence for horses on passage through mice, whereas attenuation occurs rapidly on passage through tissue culture. Dogs are the only species of domestic animal known to be susceptible to infection by the ingestion of infected meat.

African horse sickness virus can be readily transmitted experimentally by a variety of parenteral routes. Viremia develops during the febrile stage; the virus is closely associated with the red blood cells and may be found in the blood for up to 90 days after the onset of fever. The virus is viscerotropic; the highest titers are found in the spleen, while lower concentrations are present in other internal organs. African horse sickness virus is also present in tissue fluids, urine, milk, and fetal tissue.

Suckling mice can be experimentally infected by the intracerebral and intraperitoneal inoculation of blood and tissue from infected horses. This system has been used for primary isolation of the virus. The viscerotropic virus is converted into a neurotropic form by serial intracranial passage through mice, and the resultant attenuation of the virulence for horses is achieved without any loss of antigenic properties. The viscerotropic virus isolated from natural infections in horses grows in embryonated chicken eggs, and serial passage through this system also produces attenuation.

Literature

Experimentally, AHS virus is infective for horses by a variety of parenteral routes, including intratracheal inoculation. The disease could be transmitted by ingestion only when very large quantities of infective material were administered. The high infectivity of the virus inoculated by the intravenous route was demonstrated by the fact that as little as 0.0001 ml of infected blood may cause the disease (Mirchamsy and Hazrati 1973). In the horse, there was a short period of viremia which began with the onset of the febrile reaction. A low level of viremia was observed in equine species less susceptible than the horse (Bourdin 1973). The demonstration of infective AHS virus in the presence of high concentrations of specific neutralizing antibody (McIntosh 1953) suggested that the virus was located on or in the erythrocyte membrane, where it was protected from the circulating antibody. Ozawa *et al.* (1972, 1973) titrated the virus in plasma, buffy coat, and erythrocyte fractions of infected blood and found that infectivity was highest in the erythrocyte fraction, thus indicating that the virus was closely associated with the red blood cells. In an attempt to develop a simple method for recovering AHS virus from infected horse blood, Ozawa *et al.* (1972, 1973) subjected washed erythrocytes to a variety of treatments, including trypsinization, ultrasonication, and hemolysis by the addition of distilled water. The virus was most readily recovered when washed erythrocytes were hemolyzed by ultrasonication. The effect of low temperature on the preservation of infectivity was also investigated (Ozawa *et al.* 1972, 1973). Specimens of various internal organs and skeletal muscle collected from infected horses at postmortem were examined for the presence of AHS virus by means of the FA test; only the spleen was shown to contain virus (Tessler 1970). Although some of the early work showed that the virus could be isolated from a convalescent horse up to the ninetieth postinfection day, more recent work indicated that the virus could not be isolated from recovered animals (Maurer and McCully 1963).

Mules were less susceptible than horses. The Egyptian donkey (*Equus asinus africanum domesticus*) was much less susceptible than the mule but more susceptible than the South African donkey (*E. asinus asinus*), which was rarely affected (McIntosh 1958; Maurer and McCully 1963). The susceptibility of zebra to AHS virus infections was shown by Erasmus *et al.* (1978). In these experiments, zebra did not develop clinical illness following infection. However, the viremia lasted for 8 to 11 days, and there were indications that the virus could persist in very low titers in the tissues despite the presence of a neutralizing antibody (Erasmus *et al.* 1978).

During the early investigations of the disease, it was found that dogs were susceptible to AHS virus (Henning 1956). There have been three reports of outbreaks of AHS among dogs which ate raw meat from diseased horses. Some of these animals became ill and died with symptoms and lesions typical of AHS. Although dogs could be infected intravenously or by the ingestion of contaminated meat, vectorial transmission was considered unlikely under natural conditions (Mirchamsy and Hazrati 1973). Recently, AHS virus type 9 was isolated from the blood of 6 of 111 street dogs examined in Egypt. These animals were thought to have become infected by feeding on contaminated meat. Horses experimentally infected with the canine isolates developed clinical symptoms and pathological lesions characteristic of AHS. It was proposed that dogs might play a role in the epizootiology of AHS (Salama *et al.* 1981). The susceptibility of other domestic species has not been established, although some of the early work suggested that this was possible.

Alexander (1935) performed the classical work on the neurotropic fixation on AHS virus in various species of animals. Neurotropic variants were produced by serial intracerebral passage of viscerotropic strains through 2-month-old mice. The virus was recovered from the brain, spinal cord, and peripheral nerves and was only rarely isolated from the liver, kidney, and spleen; infectivity was never found in the blood. Thus, the neurotropism of the mouse-adapted virus was relatively strict (Alexander 1935). During the first two intracerebral passages, the mortality was not high and the incubation period varied between 9 and 26 days. With successive passages, the viscerotropic properties were lost, the incubation period gradually shortened, and the mortality generally reached 100% within 3 to 5 days. Infections could also be induced in mice by intranasal instillation of a mouse-adapted neurotropic strain of AHS virus. The suckling mouse proved to be the animal of choice for primary isolation, neurotropic fixation, and attenuation of AHS virus because it is highly susceptible and produced high virus titers (Mirchamsy and Hazrati 1973).

Guinea pigs were another species of laboratory animal which could be used in the study of AHS virus, but they were only susceptible to mouse-adapted neurotropic virus. The virus multiplied in the brain and then spread peripherally in the nervous tissue. However, the concentrations of the virus were up to 100 times lower than those found in mouse brains. Once the virus became adapted to the guinea pig, additional passages were not difficult and intracerebrally passaged virus increased in virulence for this host. Guinea pigs could also be infected by the intraperitoneal and intranasal routes of inoculation; however, these methods are less efficient than intracerebral injection. The intranasal route of infection was the most sensitive method of demonstrating the infectivity of mouse-adapted strains of AHS virus in guinea pigs (Mirchamsy and Hazrati 1973). The guinea pig was also valuable for the selection of viral strains of high antigenic potency because there was a good correlation between the antigenicity of the virus in guinea pigs and that in horses (Erasmus 1963b). The pathogenicity of AHS virus isolated from India was investigated in guinea pigs and mice (Datt *et al.* 1972b).

A limited amount of work was conducted on viscerotropic virus infections in ferrets and neurotropic infections in rats (Mirchamsy and Hazrati 1973).

CLINICAL SIGNS

Four clinical forms of AHS have been defined: the febrile form, the pulmonary form, the cardiac form, and the mixed form. Clinically the disease is characterized by hyperthermia, dyspnea, edema of the supraorbital fossae, subcutaneous edema of the head and neck, pulmonary edema, cardiac involvement, accumulation of pericardial and pleural fluids, and hemorrhage of the internal organs. The mortality in epizootics varies from 25 to 95%.

Literature

The literature on the clinical signs and pathogenesis of AHS was reviewed by Mirchamsy and Hazrati (1973), Henning (1956), and Maurer and McCully (1963). Mild febrile, acute pulmonary, subacute cardiac, and mixed forms of AHS were distinguished on the basis of their clinical characteristics. The classification of AHS into four different clinical syndromes was useful since it indicated the course and prognosis of the disease. The gross lesions observed in many studies of AHS indicated that, in the majority of cases, the syndromes were mixed to a certain extent, and the relative severity of involvement of the heart and lungs determined whether the syndrome was predominantly of the pulmonary or cardiac form. The localized distribution of the subcutaneous edema suggested the involvement of an inflammatory process which arose from localized damage caused by the virus. Increased vascular permeability was thought to be responsible for the subcutaneous inflammatory edema (Maurer and McCully 1963).

In experimental cases, the incubation period was usually between 5 and 7 days. Fever occurred in all forms of the disease and developed gradually or rapidly, depending on the virulence of the virus. Death resulted from pulmonary or cardiac failure (Henning 1956).

The febrile form of the disease, called AHS fever, was very mild and frequently subclinical. It was characterized by an elevation of body temperature, anorexia, slight dyspnea, increased pulse rate, and inflammation of the conjunctiva (Maurer and McCully 1963). The pulmonary form was acute and found in severe outbreaks. The most characteristic symptoms were severe dyspnea, coughing, and discharge of a large amount of frothy fluid from the nostrils. The onset was sudden, depression occurred, and the animal died within a few hours. During the terminal stages, the horse virtually drowned in its own fluids (Henning 1956). The subacute cardiac form was characterized by swelling of the head and neck, with marked edema of the supraorbital fossae being a classical lesion. With the progression of the edema, signs comparable to those seen in the pulmonary form developed. In the mixed form, the clinical signs were a combination of those observed in the pulmonary and cardiac syndromes. Both pulmonary edema and cardiac failure contributed to hypoxia and death (Maurer and McCully 1963).

There were a few other reports on the clinical symptoms observed during outbreaks in different countries. Draft horses imported into Nigeria died of AHS within 2 months of importation (Akinboade *et al.* 1980). The clinical and serological observations made during one of the first outbreaks of AHS in India were reported (Gorhe *et al.* 1962; Shah 1964; Parnaik *et al.* 1965).

An outbreak of AHS was observed in a pack of foxhounds fed infected meat. The syndromes ranged in severity from peracute to mild. The main symptoms in acute fatal cases were dyspnea, retching, marked congestion of the visible mucous membranes, facial edema, and high temperature. Hemorrhages were observed on the mucous membranes of the mouth. Death occurred 12 to 24 hours after the first symptoms were observed (Haig *et al.* 1956; Piercy 1951).

PATHOLOGY

In the acute pulmonary form of the disease, the characteristic lesions are edema of the lungs and hydrothorax. The interlobular and subpleural connective tissues are infiltrated with a yellow gelatinous fluid, the lung oozes a clear, yellow fluid, and froth is present in the bronchi. The local drainage lymph nodes are swollen, soft, and wet. Hemorrhages may be found on the mucosal surface of the intestine. In the cardiac form, there are hemorrhages on the endocardium and gross evidence of myocardial degeneration, necrosis, and hydropericardium. Edematous fluid is found subcutaneously throughout the fascia and intramuscular tissue, but the lungs are only slightly affected by congestion and edema. The underlying histological lesions have not been described in detail but appear to be vascular, affecting primarily pulmonary and cardiac blood vessels.

Literature

The gross and microscopic lesions of AHS were described by Henning (1956) and Maurer and McCully (1963). The latter two authors presented a detailed account of the observations made on 14 cases. The fundamental lesions consisted of generalized hemorrhages, edema, myocarditis with focal necrosis, and extensive hemorrhage in the epicardium and endocardium. The primary edema of the lungs and other tissues was considered to be of inflammatory origin. The degenerative and necrotic changes observed in the heart were associated with the infiltration of inflammatory cells and fibrosis. In the lymph nodes, there were reactive changes associated with the draining of the edematous tissues. In the gastrointestinal tract, hemorrhages or excoriations were found on the ventral surface of the tongue. One of the most constant features was the extensive congestion and hemorrhage of the glanular portion of the stomach, with edematous thickening of the wall and occasional erosions. The lesions found throughout the body were associated with impaired circulation due to cardiac and pulmonary lesions (Maurer and McCully 1963). Eosinophilic cytoplasmic inclusion bodies were observed in the urinary tubule epithelial cells of experimentally infected horses (Amjadi and Ahourai 1971).

In acutely infected dogs, the main lesions were pulmonary edema, hydrothorax, splenomegaly, extensive extravasation of blood, and enteritis (Haig *et al.* 1956).

IMMUNOLOGY

A plurality of antigenically different strains of AHS virus exists. The differences in the antigenic structures are considered quantitative rather than qualitative. Field observations made early in the study of AHS have established that horses thought to be completely resistant to natural infection in one area could succumb to the disease when transferred to another enzootic area. Antigenic variation also occurs during serial passage of the virus from horse to horse, and a horse immunized against a particular strain may become infected with homologous strains from a different passage level.

Animals develop strong natural immunity in those regions of the world where the disease has been enzootic. Recovered equines are immune to homologous challenge, and because of the antigenic relationship between strains, immunity engendered by one strain confers partial protection against infection by a heterologous strain. In South Africa, immunity is observed in 'salted' horses which have recovered from clinical AHS or have survived symptom-free for many years in localities where the disease was frequently observed. Foals from immune dams do not have neutralizing antibodies at birth. Passive protection is transferred through the antibodies in the colostrum and persists for approximately 5 or 6 months. Subsequent injection either of pantropic or attenuated neurotropic virus does not induce the high antibody titers associated with active immunity. Passive immunity can also be established by the transfer of hyperimmune serum from one animal to another.

Complement fixation (CF) and neutralization tests in animals and tissue culture systems are used to detect antibodies, and the latter test is used to distinguish different antigenic types.

Literature

McIntosh (1958) reviewed the work on the antigenic plurality of AHS virus strains and their role in the induction of immunity. Intracerebral neutralization tests in mice were used to group 42 mouse-adapted strains of virus into 7 antigenic types. All strains of AHS virus are antigenically related, and horses immune to one strain possess some degree of immunity to all other strains (McIntosh 1958). The antigenic plurality of naturally occurring strains of AHS virus was further investigated using neutralization tests, and an additional two antigenic types, represented by widely distributed strains of low virulence, were identified (Howell and Erasmus 1963). The immunologic specificity of hyperimmune sera and sera from naturally infected and vaccinated horses for eight antigenic types of AHS virus was demonstrated by the hemagglutination inhibition test (Pavri and Anderson 1963a). The identification of AHS virus strains isolated from Morocco, Tunisia, and Algeria was accomplished by demonstrating their pathogenicity for laboratory animals and horses and their ability to fix the complement in the CF test. The serum neutralization test was used to define the antigenic types (Hazrati 1967). The preparation and characterization of a soluble precipitating antigen from AHS virus grown in tissue culture were described (Hazrati and Ozawa 1968; Hazrati and Dayhim 1971; Hazrati and Mirchamsy 1973).

In serological studies of horses, complement-fixing antibodies usually appeared first followed by neutralizing antibodies (Ozawa *et al.* 1973). The CF and mouse neutralization tests were employed extensively in the serological work on AHS virus (Pavri 1961). The CF test was not type-specific, while the neutralization test could be used to define antigenic differences. The value of the CF test was primarily in making a diagnosis (Howell 1962; McIntosh, 1956). The CF and FA tests readily detected recently infected horses because these animals contained high levels of group-specific antibodies, but the CF test does not necessarily detect antibodies for a long period of time after infection. The test was less sensitive than the neutralization test in enzootic and epizootic situations (Parker 1976). Plaque techniques for the titration and purification of AHS virus and for neutralization tests were developed in MKS cells. Factors affecting plaque formation were investigated, and the structures of plaques produced by different strains of AHS virus were compared (Hopkins *et al.* 1966).

Other serological tests have been used. In an immunodiffusion test, there were serological cross-reactions between AHS and BT viruses, indicating that they were closely related (Ozawa and Hafez 1972). The agar double-diffusion precipitation test was standardized for use in the study of precipitation reactions between AHS antigen–antibody systems and the precipitating viral antigens were characterized (Hazrati and Dayhim 1971; Hazrati *et al.* 1968). The conglutinating complement-absorption test could be used to detect high antibody titers in horses following vaccination. However, the reliability of the test was affected by small variations in procedure (Prasad and Gulrajani 1970). Hemagglutination and hemagglutination-inhibition techniques were used but required further development (Maurice and Provost 1966; Pavri 1961). Recently, Tokuhisa *et al.* (1982) have shown that, using concentrated cell culture fluids of AHS virus, agglutinate erythrocytes from cattle, horses, sheep, goats, guinea pigs, rabbits, and poultry at 4 °C, room temperature, and 37 °C, the titers observed were dependent on pH and NaCl molarity of the diluent, optimal titers being obtained at pH 7.5 and 0.6 M NaCl. The hemagglutination-inhibiting antibodies to two AHS viruses were proven to be type specific.

Dogs infected with neurotropic and viscerotropic AHS viruses were studied serologically. Complement-fixing and virus-neutralizing antibodies were detected in the sera of dogs exposed to a neurotropic strain of AHS virus by a variety of routes. Dogs fed meat contaminated with viscerotropic virus also developed antibodies and transitory viremia. All of the dogs used in these studies remained clinically healthy (Dardiri and Ozawa 1969).

DIAGNOSIS

The diagnosis of the disease in enzootic areas may be more difficult because of the prevalence of the milder forms. In these regions, however, the clinical signs in acute cases are generally so characteristic that it is considered unnecessary to isolate and identify the virus. Clinical findings such as dyspnea, edema of the supraorbital fossae, subcutaneous edema of the head and neck, pulmonary and cardiac involvement, excess pericardial and pleural fluids, and gastritis provide sufficient evidence for field diagnosis. In epizootic situations, the clinical signs are pathognomonic and infections are confirmed either by demonstrating the virus or by serological methods. The virus is isolated by the intracerebral inoculation of mice with defibrinated horse blood collected at the peak of fever. Neutralization tests may be conducted on intracerebrally infected mice.

Literature

The pertinent literature has been presented in the etiology and immunology sections. No specific techniques appear to have been adopted for the purpose of rapid and efficient diagnosis.

CONTROL

The control measures taken against AHS depend on whether a country is endemically infected or disease-free. The relatively recent spread of the disease outside the African continent has focused attention on the need for international efforts to curtail and prevent further spread of the infection.

Literature

The control measures instituted during outbreaks of AHS in countries previously free of the disease consisted of quarantine, destruction of clinical cases, spraying of stables with insecticides, and massive vaccination campaigns undertaken with the assistance of international organizations. The establishment of large buffer zones of immunized animals between infected and free zones was recommended. The international technical assistance provided during the epizootics which started in Egypt in 1958 has been described (Reid 1961). An international plan to prevent the spread of AHS involved the establishment of immune buffer zones around infected areas, disinfestation procedures at international airports and seaports, extensive production of vaccines, and internationally coordinated vaccination campaigns (Anon. 1961a). Social, economic, and geographical factors greatly hindered the efforts of veterinary services to contain the disease by imposing various control measures (Howell 1960).

VACCINATION

The horse sickness neurotropic mouse brain vaccine and the neurotropic tissue culture vaccine have been used extensively for the last 40 years. The mouse brain polyvalent vaccine is produced by using up to eight strains of neurotropic virus propagated intracerebrally in mice. Vaccinated horses have a mild fever after 5 to 13 days. The vaccine provides protection in 21 days; full immunity is reached after 6 months and lasts for up to 5 to 8 years. Foals from immune mothers are effectively vaccinated only after 7 months of age. Strains attenuated in mice are potentially neurotropic for horses, but clinical evidence of central nervous system infection in vaccinated horses is usually found only in the most susceptible animals on primary vaccination.

The widespread outbreak of AHS in 1959 and 1960 in the Middle East and Asia stimulated the development of polyvalent and monovalent tissue culture vaccines using primarily kidney cell culture systems. The vaccines do not induce adverse clinical signs and a period of 5 to 6 months is necessary to produce maximum protection.

Because there is always the possibility that the attenuated vaccine virus might become virulent during serial passage through horses, live vaccines are not used outside enzootic regions. Although inactivated vaccines have been developed and employed against homologous challenge with limited success, this method of vaccination has not been used extensively.

Literature

McIntosh (1958) reviewed the history of immunization against AHS in South Africa. The development of a polyvalent attenuated-virus vaccine was attributed to the work of Alexander *et al.* (1936) and McIntosh (1958). The intracerebral passage of the virus in mice resulted in a decrease in virulence, but the strains retained their antigenic and immunizing properties, becoming sufficiently attenuated by approximately 100 cerebral passages. The number of passages required for attenuation differed with different strains. The guinea pig was found to be a good experimental host for testing the degree of attenuation of mouse-passaged strains before their inclusion in a polyvalent vaccine (Howell and Erasmus 1963). A vaccine using a neurotropic strain adapted to the central nervous system of the guinea pig was also described (Cilli 1961). In enzootic areas, annual immunization was practiced in the belief that repeated administration of a polyvalent vaccine would provoke a broad-spectrum antibody response which would protect the animals against homologous as well as heterologous strains. However, the occurrence of minor epizootics caused by viral strains homologous with the antigenic types incorporated in the polyvalent vaccine indicated that the vaccine did not induce true polyvalent immunity. It was found that certain components of the vaccine were poorly antigenic and could not stimulate antibody formation (Howell and Erasmus 1963). Although polyvalent neurotropic vaccine prepared in mice using eight strains induced immunity up to 8 years, annual vaccination was recommended to produce the widest possible polyvalent immunity (McIntosh 1953). Although polyvalent vaccines were more effective, monovalent types were also used. A strain isolated in India was safely attenuated at the sixtieth and seventieth passage levels and used in a monovalent vaccine (Datt *et al.* 1972a; Kumar *et al.* 1972). A monovalent vaccine was prepared against an Iranian strain (Hazrati and Ozawa 1965b).

Initially, it was thought that these neurotropic vaccine strains did not have any affinity for the central nervous system of horses. With wide use of the vaccine, however, there were field reports of postvaccinal blindness in mules and madness in horses. Subsequently, vaccine strains were isolated from the brain of equines in Israel, India, and Iran, and it was suggested that these viruses could multiply in the brain and induce blindness, neurologic disorders, and fatal encephalitis (Howell and Erasmus 1963; Mirchamsy and Hazrati, 1973). The virus obtained from immunized horses undergoing breakdown reactions was not infective for mice by intracerebral injection but could be isolated in the horse, dog, and ferret (Howell 1963; McIntosh 1953). Adverse reactions to the South African polyvalent mouse-adapted vaccine occurred in horses in India. The virus was isolated from two animals which died 32 and 47 days after immunization with a polyvalent vaccine, and one of the isolated vaccine strains was associated with the development of encephalitis (Pavri and Anderson 1963b). The clinical signs which developed following the administration of the polyvalent vaccine resembled the relatively mild symptoms seen in natural cases. On one farm mild, transient, neurological signs were observed in foals and yearlings 3 to 7 weeks after vaccination, and most of the animals were viremic for 14 to 23 days (Shah *et al.* 1964).

Egg-adapted virus at various passage levels became attenuated without losing its antigenicity when injected into horses. The potential for vaccine production was poor due to the low concentration of the virus and low antibody titers (Mirchamsy and Hazrati 1973). In one study, it was shown that neurotropic vaccine strains propagated in chicken embryos and in mouse brains were of comparable efficiency: there was no difference in the levels of neutralizing antibody induced by these vaccinal strains or in the animals' ability to resist challenge 4.5 months after vaccination (Goldsmit 1968).

A tissue culture-adapted neurotropic virus vaccine developed by Mirchamsy and Taslimi (1964b, c) was used in the Middle East, Tunisia, Algeria, Morocco, and Spain. Because of the difficulties of producing the vaccine in mice and the exigencies of the widespread 1960 epizootic of AHS, research efforts were directed toward producing vaccines in tissue culture. A polyvalent live attenuated tissue culture vaccine was prepared using seven neurotropic viruses and the type 9 virus isolated in Iran after from 5 to 20 passages in MKS cells or in baby hamster kidney cells. During the 1959–61 epizootic of AHS in the Middle East and Asia, the causal virus, classified as type 9, was antigenically different from the six to seven known attenuated neurotropic strains used in the polyvalent live vaccine, but the vaccine was shown to confer satisfactory immunity against this heterologous type (Davies 1976; Goldsmit 1968). Monovalent and polyvalent tissue culture vaccines were produced using MKS cells and baby hamster kidney (BHK) cells. Protective antibodies were induced in vaccinated horses and no adverse postvaccination reactions developed (Ozawa *et al.* 1965). Monovalent and polyvalent vaccines prepared in MKS cell lines were tested for thermal stability. Loss of activity was related to the time of storage and the temperature, with lyophilization enabling storage for 12 to 18 months (Mirchamsy and Taslimi 1967b). The attenuation of a virulent strain of AHS was also carried out in BHK cells. Horses immunized with this vaccine virus at the tenth and twentieth passage levels did not develop clinical reactions and were resistant to challenge 12 weeks after vaccination (Erasmus 1965). The virus was irreversibly attenuated by seven passages in mosquito cell lines and three or seven passages in BHK cell lines (Mirchamsy *et al.* 1972a). Horses initially immunized with a polyvalent cell culture vaccine and revaccinated 2 years later showed a fourfold rise in neutralizing antibodies (Mirchamsy and Taslimi 1967d). In order to obtain strains of virus which were avirulent for mice, a wild strain and a neurotropic strain were serially passaged in MKS lines at decreasing temperatures. A relationship was observed between the neurovirulence of the AHS virus for mice and its immunogenicity for horses (Mirchamsy and Taslimi 1967a).

An inactivated monovalent tissue culture vaccine was shown to be effective when used with adjuvants and when given in multiple injections (Mirchamsy *et al.* 1970). A vaccine produced from a neurotropic or virulent strain of type 9 virus was grown in MKS cell lines and inactivated with beta-propiolactone or formaldehyde. The immunogenicity of the vaccine was increased by the addition of aluminum hydroxide as an adjuvant. Neutralizing antibodies developed within 4 weeks and protected against homologous virulent virus challenge. Two injections administered 4 weeks apart resulted in high neutralizing antibody titers which persisted for 6 months (Mirchamsy and Taslimi 1968). Mirchamsy *et al.* (1972b) evaluated the use of formalin-inactivated AHS vaccines mixed with a variety of adjuvants in foals. Following the original work on the development of an inactivated vaccine used in conjunction with adjuvants, further work was undertaken on two inactivated cell culture vaccines and four different adjuvants. The adjuvants induced local skin reactions which, in the case of aluminum hydroxide, persisted for a few days, whereas with the saponin and Freund's incomplete vaccines, the reactions lasted for weeks (Mirchamsy *et al.* 1973). Other work showed that formalized vaccine, prepared either from viscerotropic or neurotropic type 9 virus cultivated in MKS cell cultures, induced immunity which protected animals from challenge 5 weeks after vaccination (Ozawa and Bahrami 1966). The inactivated vaccines was administered in Iran, and two strains of type 9 virus were used in the production of live and inactivated vaccines (Kaveh 1968). The production and control of the inactivated vaccine were described by Stellmann *et al.* (1969).

BIBLIOGRAPHY

Abegunde, A., 1975. Epizootiology of African horse sickness: the situation in Nigeria, *Bull. Off. int. Epiz.*, **83**(11–12): 1091–5.

Akinboade, O. A., Awani, O., Best, O. and Cole T., 1980. The reaction of imported British Shire horses to African horse sickness: a case report, *Vet. Quarterly*, **2**(3): 179–80.

Alexander, R. A., 1935. Studies on the neurotropic virus of horsesickness. I. Neurotropic fixation, *Onderstepoort J. vet. Sci. Anim. Ind.*, **4**(2): 291–322.

Alexander, R. A., Neitz, W. O. and Du Toit, P. J., 1936. Horsesickness: immunization of horses and mules in the field during the season 1934–1935 with a description of the technique of preparation of polyvalent mouse neurotropic vaccine, *Onderstepoort J. vet. Sci. Anim. Ind.*, **7**: 17–30.

Alhaji, I., Humburg, M. and Kemp, G. E., 1974. African horse sickness in Nigeria – a case report, *Bull. Anim. Hlth Prod. Afr.*, **22**: 311–14.

Amjadi, A. R. and Ahourai, P., 1971. Observation of inclusion bodies in renal epithelial cells of experimentally infected horses with African horse-sickness virus, *Arch. Inst. Razi*, **23**: 125–8.

Anon., 1961a. F.A.O.–O.I.E. Meeting on Emerging Diseases (Ankara, 19–24 June 1961), *Bull. Off. int. Epiz.*, **55**: 1223–59.

Anon., 1961b. Summary of the proceedings of the conference on African horse sickness. Present situation, *Bull. Off. int. Epiz.*, **55**: 330–40.

Anon., 1961c. Special conference on African swine fever and African horse sickness. Paris 17–20th January 1961, *Bull. Off. int. Epiz.*, **55**: 361–537.

Anon., 1961d. African horse sickness in Turkey, *Bull. Off. int. Epiz.*, **55**: 292–7.

Anon., 1966. Note on an outbreak of African horse sickness in Algeria, *Bull. Off. int. Epiz.*, **66**: 675–80.

Anon., 1967. Transmission of African horse sickness by *Aedes aegypti* Linnaeus in Iran, *Vet. Rec.*, **80**(2): 39.

Anon., 1969. Report on African horse sickness in Morocco, *Bull. Off. int. Epiz.*, **72**: 1123–31.

Anon., 1972. Summaries of the reports on African horse sickness. 3rd Int. Conf. on Equine Infectious Diseases, July 17–21, 1972, *Bull. Off. int. Epiz.*, **77**: 1601–20.

Awad, F. I., Amin, M. M., Salama, S. A. and Samia Khidr, 1981. The role played by *Hyalomma dromedarii* in the transmission of African horse sickness virus in Egypt, *Bull. Anim. Hlth Prod. Afr.*, **29**: 337–40.

Bakaya, H. and Gurturk, S., 1962. Morphological study of the virus of African horse sickness, *Dtsch. Tierarztl. Wschr.*, **69**: 451–2.

Best, J. R., Abegunde, A. and Taylor, W. P., 1975. An outbreak of African horse sickness in Nigeria, *Vet. Rec.*, **97**: 394.

Boorman, J., Mellor, P. S., Penn, M. and Jennings, M., 1975. The growth of African horse sickness virus in embryonated hen eggs and the transmission of virus by *Culicoides variipennis* Coquillett (Diptera, Ceratopogonidae), *Arch. Virol.*, **47**: 343–9.

Bourdin, P., 1973. Ecology of African horsesickness. In *Equine Infectious Diseases*, eds J. T. Bryans, H. Gerber. Karger (Basle), vol. III, pp. 12–30.

Bourdin, P. and Laurent, A., 1974. Note sur l'écologie de la peste équine africaine, *Rev. Elev. Méd. vét. Pays trop.*, **27**(2): 163–8.

Braverman, Y. and Boorman, J., 1978. Rates of infection in, and transmission of, African horse-sickness virus by *Aedes aegypti* mosquitoes, *Acta virol.*, **22**: 329–32.

Breese, S. S. Jr and Ozawa, Y., 1969. Intracellular inclusions resulting from infection with African horsesickness virus, *J. Virol.*, **4**(1): 109–12.

Breese, S. S. Jr, Ozawa, Y. and Dardiri, J. H., 1969. Electron microscopic characterization of African horse-sickness virus, *J. J. Am. vet. med. Ass.*, **155**(2): 391–400.

Bremer, C. W., 1976. A gel electrophoretic study of the protein and nucleic acid components of African horsesickness virus, *Onderstepoort J. vet. Res.*, **43**(4): 193–200.

Cilli, V., 1961. Study of two neurotropic strains of African horse sickness virus isolated in Eritrea, *Vet. Ital.*, **12**: 623–8.

Dardiri, J. H. and Ozawa, Y., 1969. Immune and serologic response of dogs to neurotropic and viscerotropic African horse-sickness viruses, *J. Am. vet. med. Ass.*, **155**(2): 400–7.

Datt, N. S., Sehgal, C. L., Sharma, G. L. and Kumar, S., 1972a. Studies on African horsesickness virus type IX ('Jaipur' strain): immunological studies with mouse-adapted virus, *Indian J. Anim. Sci.*, **42**(6): 442–5.

Datt, N. S., Sehgal, C. L., Sharma, G. L., Pandey, M. C. and Kumar, S., 1972b. Studies on African horsesickness virus type IX ('Jaipur' strain): host-range pathogenicity including adaptation to guinea-pigs and mice, *Indian J. Anim. Sci.*, **42**(6): 438–41.

Davies, F. G., 1976. AHS vaccine, *Vet. Rec.*, **98**: 36.

Davies F. G. and Lund, L. J., 1974. The application of fluorescent antibody techniques to the virus of African horse sickness, *Res. Vet. Sci.*, **17**: 128–30.

Davies, F. G. and Otieno, S., 1977. Elephants and zebras as possible reservoir hosts for African horse sickness virus, *Vet. Rec.*, **100**: 291–2.

Doutre, M. P. and Leclercq, A., 1962. Existence of African horse sickness virus type 9 in Chad, *Rev. Elev. Méd. vét. Pays trop.*, **15**(3): 241–5.

Eichhorn, E. A., 1963. Report on SAT 1, African horse sickness and African swine fever, *Proc. 17th Wld Vet. Congr.*, **3**: 73–84.

El Fourgi, M., 1967. Note on African horse sickness in Tunisia, *Bull. Off. int. Epiz.*, **68**: 715–17.

Erasmus, B. J., 1963a. Cultivation of horsesickness virus in tissue culture, *Nature*, **200**: 716.

Erasmus, B. J., 1963b. Preliminary observations on the value of the guinea-pig in determining the innocuity and antigenicity of neurotropic attenuated horsesickness strains, *Onderstepoort J. vet. Res.*, **30**(1): 11–21.

Erasmus, B. J., 1964. Some observations on the propagation of horse sickness virus in tissue culture, *Bull. Off. int. Epiz.*, **62**: 923–8.

Erasmus, B. J., 1965. The attenuation of viscerotropic horsesickness virus in tissue culture, *Bull. Off. int. Epiz.*, **64**: 697–702.

Erasmus, B. J., Young, E., Pieterse, L. M. and Boshoff, S. T., 1978. The susceptibility of zebra and elephants to African horsesickness virus. In *Equine Infectious Diseases*, eds J. T. Bryans, H. Gerber. Veterinary Publications (Princeton, New Jersey, USA), vol. III, pp. 409–13.

Farid, A., Tantawi, H. H., Shalaby, M. A., Sallama, S. and Abdel Ghani, M., 1974. Growth, histopathological and histochemical changes in foetal camel kidney cells infected with African horse sickness virus, *J. Egyptian vet. Med. Assoc.*, **34**: 438–47.

Goldsmit, L., 1967. Growth characteristics of six neurotropic and one viscerotropic African horsesickness virus strains in fertilized eggs, *Am. J. vet. Res.*, **28**(122): 19–24.

Goldsmit, L., 1968. Immunization of horses against African horse-sickness with attenuated neurotropic viral strains propagated in chicken embryos, *Am. J. vet. Res.*, **29**(1): 133–41.

Gorhe, D. S., Parnaik, D. T., Nisal, M. B. and Khot, J. B., 1962. Observations on South African horse sickness in Maharashtra, *Indian vet. J.*, **39**: 260–4.

Haig, D. A., McIntosh, B. M., Cumming, R. B. and Hempstead, J. F. D., 1956. An outbreak of horsesickness, complicated by distemper in a pack of foxhounds, *J. S. Afr. vet. med. Ass.*, **27**(4): 245–9.

Hazrati, A., 1967. Identification and typing of horsesickness virus strains isolated in the recent epizootic of the disease in Morocco, Tunisia, and Algeria, *Arch. Inst. Razi*, **19**: 131–43.

Hazrati, A. and Dayhim, F., 1971. The study of African horsesickness virus by the agar double-diffusion precipitation test. II. Characterization of the precipitating antigen, *Arch. Inst. Razi*, **23**: 33–43.

Hazrati, A., Mastan, B. and Bahrami, S., 1968. The study of African horsesickness virus by the agar double-diffusion precipitation test. 1. Standardization of the technique, *Arch. Inst. Razi*, **20**: 49–66.

Hazrati, A. and Mirchamsy, H., 1973. Preparation and characterization of a soluble precipitating antigen from African horsesickness virus propagated in cell cultures, *Proc. 3rd Int. Conf. Equine Infectious Diseases*, Paris, 1972. Karger (Basle), pp. 38–44.

Hazrati, A. and Ozawa, Y., 1965a. Serologic studies of African horsesickness virus with emphasis on neutralization test in tissue culture, *Can. J. comp. Med.*, **29**: 173–8.

Hazrati, A. and Ozawa, Y., 1965b. Monovalent live-virus horse-sickness vaccine, *Bull. Off. int. Epiz.*, **64**: 683–95.

Hazrati, A. and Ozawa, Y., 1968. Quantitative studies on the neutralization reaction between African horse sickness virus and antiserum, *Arch. ges. Virusforsch.*, **25**: 83–92.

Henning, M. W., 1956. African horsesickness, Perdesiekte, Pestis equorum. In *Animal Diseases in South Africa. Being an Account of the Infectious Diseases of Domestic Animals*. 3rd Central News Agency Ltd (South Africa), pp. 785–808.

Hopkins, I. G., Hazrati, A. and Ozawa, Y., 1966. Development of plaque techniques for titration and neutralization tests with African horse-sickness virus, *Am. J. vet. Res.*, **27**(116): 96–105.

Howell, P. G., 1960. The 1960 epizootic of African horsesickness in the Middle East and S.W. Asia, *J. S. Afr. vet. med. Ass.*, **31**(3): 329–34.

Howell, P. G., 1962. The isolation and identification of further antigenic types of African horsesickness virus, *Onderstepoort J. vet. Res.*, **29**(2): 139–49.

Howell, P. G., 1963. Observations on the occurrence of African horsesickness amongst immunised horses, *Onderstepoort J. vet. Res.*, **30**(1): 3–10.

Howell, P. G. and Erasmus, B. J., 1963. Recent contributions to the study of the virus of African horse sickness, *Bull. Off. int. Epiz.*, **60**: 883–7.

Kaveh, M., 1968. African horse sickness: recent developments in North Africa and Europe. Research on vaccines at the Razi Institute (Iran), *Bull. Off. int. Epiz.*, **69**(1–2): 263–9.

Kemp, G. E., Humburg, J. M. and Alhaji, I., 1971. Isolation and identification of African horse-sickness virus in Nigeria, *Vet. Rec.*, **4**: 127–8.

Kumar, S., Datt, N. S., Sharma, R. N., Mathur, B. B. L. and Sharma, G. L., 1972. Studies on African horsesickness virus type IX ('Jaipur' strain): development of modified mouse strain vaccine, *Indian J. Anim. Sci.*, **42**: 446–9.

Laaberki, A., 1969. The development of an outbreak of African horse sickness in Morocco (February 1966–December 1966), *Bull. Off. int. Epiz.*, **71**(7–8): 921–36.

Maurer, F. D. and McCully, R. M., 1963. African horsesickness – with emphasis on pathology, *Am. J. vet. Res.*, **24**(99): 235–66.
Maurice, Y. and Provost, A., 1966. Hemagglutination and hemagglutination inhibition tests with horse sickness virus. Limits of their interpretation, *Rev. Elev. Méd. vét. Pays trop.*, **19**(4): 439–50.
Maurice, Y. and Provost, A., 1967. Horse sickness caused by type 9 virus in central Africa. Serological survey, *Rev. Elev. Méd. vét. Pays trop.*, **20**(1): 21–5.
McIntosh, B. M., 1953. The isolation of virus in mice from cases of horse-sickness in immunized horses, *Onderstepoort J. vet. Res.*, **26**: 183–95.
McIntosh, B. M., 1956. Complement fixation with horse sickness viruses, *Onderstepoort J. vet. Res.*, **27**(2): 165–9.
McIntosh, B. M., 1958. Immunological types of horse sickness virus and their significance in immunization, *Onderstepoort J. vet. Res.*, **27**(4): 465–538.
Mellor, P. S., Boorman, J. and Jennings, M., 1975. The multiplication of African horse-sickness virus in two species of *Culicoides* (Diptera, Ceratopogonidae), *Arch. Virol.*, **47**: 351–56.
Mellor, P. S., Jennings, D. M., Braverman, Y. and Boorman, J., 1981. Infection of Israeli *Culicoides* with African horse sickness, bluetongue, and Akabane viruses, *Acta virol.*, **25**: 401–7.
Mirchamsy, H. and Hazrati, A., 1973. A review on aetiology and pathogeny of African horsesickness, *Arch. Inst. Razi*, **25**: 23–46.
Mirchamsy, H., Hazrati, A., Bahrami, S. and Shafyi, A., 1960. Growth and persistent infection of African horse-sickness virus in a mosquito cell line, *Am. J. vet. Res.*, **31**(10): 1755–61.
Mirchamsy, H., Hazrati, A., Bahrami, S., Shafyi, A. and Mahinpoor, M., 1972a. Comparative attenuation of African horse sickness virus in mosquito (*Aedes albopictus*) and in hamster kidney (BHK-21) cell lines, *Bull. Off. int. Epiz.*, **77**(11–12): 1614.
Mirchamsy, H., Hazrati, A., Bahrami, S., Shafyi, A. and Nazari, P., 1972b. Development of new African horse sickness cell culture killed vaccines, *Bull. Off. int. Epiz.*, **77**(11–12): 1617–18.
Mirchamsy, H., Hazrati, A., Bahrami, S., Shafyi, A. and Nazari, P., 1973. Development of new African horsesickness cell culture killed vaccines, *Proc. 3rd Int. Conf. Equine Infectious Diseases*, Paris 1972. Karger (Basle), pp. 81–7.
Mirchamsy, H. and Taslimi, H., 1962. Adaptation de virus de la peste equine à la culture cellules, *C.R. Acad. Sci. (Paris)*, **25**: 424.
Mirchamsy, H. and Taslimi, H., 1963. Adaptation of horse sickness virus to tissue culture, *Nature*, **198**: 704–6.
Mirchamsy, H. and Taslimi, H., 1964a. Visualization of horse sickness

virus by the fluorescent antibody technique, *Immunology*, **7**: 213–16.

Mirchamsy, H. and Taslimi, H., 1964b. Attempts to vaccinate foals with living tissue culture adapted horse sickness virus, *Bull. Off. int. Epiz.*, **62**: 911–21.

Mirchamsy, H. and Taslimi, H., 1964c. Immunization against African horse sickness with tissue-culture-adapted neurotropic viruses, *Br. vet. J.*, **120**: 481–6.

Mirchamsy, H. and Taslimi, H., 1966. The nucleic acid of African horse sickness virus, *J. Hyg. Camb.*, **64**: 255–9.

Mirchamsy, H. and Taslimi, H., 1967a. Some properties of avirulent cold variants of African horse sickness virus, *Res. vet. Sci.*, **8**: 195–200.

Mirchamsy, H. and Taslimi, H., 1967b. Thermal stability of African horse sickness virus, *Arch. ges. Virusforsch.*, **20**: 275–7.

Mirchamsy, H. and Taslimi, H., 1967c. Cytochemical studies with African horse sickness virus by fluorescent microscopy, *Arch. Inst. Razi*, **19**: 67–9.

Mirchamsy, H. and Taslimi, H., 1967d. Serological responses of horses immunized with live attenuated African horse sickness vaccine, *J. Comp. Pth.*, **77**: 431–8.

Mirchamsy, H. and Taslimi, H., 1968. Inactivated African horse sickness virus cell culture vaccine, *Immunology*, **14**: 81–8.

Mirchamsy, H., Taslimi, H. and Bahrami, S., 1970. Recent advances in immunization of horses against African horsesickness, *Arch. Inst. Razi*, **22**: 11–18.

Montilla, R. D. and Marti, P., 1967. Epizootiology of African horse sickness in Spain, *Bull. Off. int. Epiz.*, **68**: 705–14.

Montilla, R. D. and Marti, P. P., 1968. African horse sickness, *Bull. Off. int. Epiz.*, **70**: 647–62.

Nawathe, D. R., Synge, E., Okoh, A. E. J. and Abegunde, A., 1981. Persistence of African horse sickness in Nigeria, *Trop. Anim. Hlth Prod.*, **13**: 167–8.

Oellermann, R. A., 1970. Plaque formation by African horsesickness virus and characterization of its RNA, *Onderstepoort J. vet. Res.*, **37**(2): 137–43.

Oellermann, R. A., Els, H. J. and Erasmus, B. J., 1970. Characterization of African horsesickness virus, *Arch. ges. Virusforsch.*, **29**: 163–74.

Ozawa, Y., 1966. Interference between African horsesickness viruses in tissue culture, *Am. J. vet. Res.*, **27**(116): 106–9.

Ozawa, Y., 1967. Studies on the replication of African horse-sickness virus in two different cell line cultures, *Arch. ges. Virusforsch.*, **21**: 155–69.

Ozawa, Y., 1968. Studies on the properties of African horse-sickness virus, *Jap. J. Med. Sci. Biol.*, **21**: 27–39.

Ozawa, Y. and Bahrami, S., 1966. African horse-sickness killed-virus tissue culture vaccine, *Can. J. comp. Med. vet. Sci.*, **30**: 311–14.

Ozawa, Y. and Hafez, S. M., 1972. Serological relationship between African horse sickness and bluetongue viruses, *Bull. Off. int. Epiz.*, **77**(11–12): 1612–13.

Ozawa, Y. and Hazrati, A., 1964. Growth of African horse-sickness virus in monkey kidney cell cultures, *Am. J. vet. Res.*, **25**(105): 505–11.

Ozawa, Y., Hazrati, A. and Erol, N., 1965. African horse-sickness live-virus tissue culture vaccine, *Am. J. vet. Res.*, **26**(110): 154–68.

Ozawa, Y., Hopkins, I. G., Hazrati, A., Modjitabai, A. and Kaveh, P., 1967. Cytology of monkey kidney cells infected with African horse-sickness virus, *Arch. Inst. Razi*, **19**: 51–6.

Ozawa, Y. and Nakata, G., 1965. Experimental transmission of African horse-sickness by means of mosquitoes, *Am. J. vet. Res.*, **26**(112): 744–8.

Ozawa, Y., Nakata, G., Shad-del, F. and Navai, S., 1966. Transmission of African horse-sickness by a species of mosquito, *Aedes aegypti* Linnaeus, *Am. J. vet. Res.*, **27**(118): 695–7.

Ozawa, Y., Salama, S. A. and Dardiri, A. H., 1972. Methods for recovering African horse sickness virus from blood of horses, *Bull. Off. int. Epiz.*, **77**(11–12): 1615.

Ozawa, Y., Salama, S. A. and Dardiri, A. H., 1973. Methods for recovering African horse sickness virus from horse blood. In *Proc. 3rd Int. Conf. Equine Infectious Diseases*, Paris 1972. Karger (Basle), pp. 58–68.

Parker, J., 1974. African horse sickness virus antibodies in Cyprus – 1971–72, *Vet. Rec.*, **94**: 370–3.

Parker, J., 1975. Inactivation of African horse-sickness virus by betapropiolactone and by pH, *Arch. Virol.*, **47**: 357–65.

Parker, J., 1976. African horse sickness, *Vet. Rec.*, **98**: 204.

Parker, J., Armstrong, R. M., Abegunde, A. and Taylor, W. P., 1977. African horse sickness virus antibodies in northern Nigeria 1974–1975, *Res. vet. Sci.*, **26**: 274–80.

Parnaik, D. T., Gorhe, D. S. and Khot, J. B., 1965. Observation on South African horsesickness in Maharashtra, *Indian J. vet. Sci.*, **35**(2): 94–101.

Pavri, K. M., 1961. Haemagglutination and haemagglutination-inhibition with African horse-sickness virus, *Nature*, **189**: 249.

Pavri, K. M. and Anderson, C. R., 1963a. Haemagglutination-inhibition tests with different types of African horse-sickness virus, *Indian J. vet. Sci.*, **33**: 113–17.

Pavri, K. M. and Anderson, C. R., 1963b. Isolation of a vaccine strain of African horse-sickness virus from brains of two horses given polyvalent vaccine, *Indian J. vet. Sci.*, **33**: 215–19.

Piercy, S. E., 1951. Some observations on African horsesickness including an account of an outbreak amongst dogs, *E. Afr. Agric. J.*, **17**: 62–4.

Pilo-Moron, E., Vincent, J., Ait Mesbah, O. and Forthomme, G., 1969. Origine de la peste équine en Afrique du Nord: résultats d'une enquête sur les ânes du Sahara algérien, *Arch. Inst. Pasteur Algérie*, **47**: 105–18.

Polson, A. and Madsen, T., 1954. Particle size distribution of African horsesickness virus, *Biochim. Biophys. Acta*, **14**: 366–73.

Polson, A., von Rooy, P. J., Lawrence, S. M. and Dent, J., 1953. The stability of neurotropic African horsesickness virus in solutions of different chemical composition, *Onderstepoort J. vet. Res.*, **26**(2): 197–206.

Prasad, S. and Gulrajani, T. S., 1970. A note on the application of the conglutinating complement-absorption test in African horsesickness antigen–antibody system, *Indian J. Anim. Sci.*, **40**: 145–8.

Prasad, S. and Gulrajani, T. S., 1975. Studies on African horse-sickness virus. 1. Adaptation of neurotropic strains of virus in developing chick embryo, *Indian J. Anim. Sci.*, **45**: 479–83.

Reid, N. R., 1961. African horse sickness. The 1959–60 epizootic of African horse sickness in the Near East region and India, and a note on technical assistance provided by the Food and Agriculture Organization of the United Nations, *Br. vet. J.*, **118**: 137–42.

Salama, S. A., Dardiri, A. H., Awad, F. I., Soliman, A. M. and Amin, M. M., 1981. Isolation and identification of African horse sickness virus from naturally infected dogs in Upper Egypt, *Can. J. comp. Med.*, **45**: 392–6.

Samia Khidr, 1980. Studies on African horse-sickness disease. Thesis presented to Faculty of Vet. Med., Cairo University.

Sellers, R. F., Pedgley, D. E. and Tucker, M. R., 1977. Possible spread of African horse sickness on the wind, *J. Hyg. Camb.*, **79**: 279–98.

Shah, K. V., 1964. Investigation of African horse-sickness in India. I. Study of the natural disease and the virus, *Indian J. vet. Sci.*, **34**(1): 1–14.

Shah, K. V., Chinoy, D. N. and Gokhale, T. B., 1964. Investigation of African horse-sickness in India. II. Reactions in non-immune horses after vaccination with the polyvalent African horse-sickness vaccine, *Indian J. vet. Sci.*, **34**(2): 75–83.

Stellmann, C., Mirchamsy, H., Giraud, M., Favre, H., Santucci, J. and Gilbert, H., 1969. Production and control of inactivated vaccines against African horse sickness, *Bull. Off. int. Epiz.*, **71**(7–8): 1031–57.

Tessler, J., 1970. Immunofluorescent study of African horse-sickness virus in tissues, *Am. Soc. Microb. Bact. Proc.*, p. 179.

Tessler, J., 1972. Detection of African horsesickness viral antigens in tissues by immunofluorescence, *Can. J. comp. Med.*, **36**(2): 167–9.

Tewari, S. C., Datt, N. S. and Kumar, S., 1972. Studies on physico-chemical properties of African horsesickness virus, *Indian J. Anim. Sci.*, **42**(7): 536–8.

Tokuhisa, S., Inaba, Y. and Sato, K., 1982. Factors associated with improved haemagglutination by African horse sickness virus, *Vet. Microbiol.*, **7**: 177–81.

Wetzel, H., Nevill, E. M. and Erasmus, B. J., 1970. Studies on the transmission of African horsesickness, *Onderstepoort J. vet. Res.*, **37**(3): 165–8.

Chapter

6

African swine fever

CONTENTS

INTRODUCTION

African swine fever (ASF) is an acute contagious viral disease of domestic pigs caused by an as yet unclassified virus originating from the wild species of the Suidae family in Africa. The disease emerged in East Africa between 1900 and 1910 in domestic pigs originally imported from Europe, and has since then occurred sporadically in various countries throughout the continent. It spread to southwestern Europe in 1957, the West Indies in 1971, and South America in 1978, and at present it constitutes a very major threat to the swine production industry throughout the world.

Literature

Before the spread of ASF from the continent of Africa, the majority of research was undertaken in East, Central, and South Africa. Based on these investigations, a number of reviews were published which together gave a comprehensive description of ASF (DeTray 1963; Hess 1971; Neitz 1963; Scott 1965a, b, c). In addition, there have been periodic brief reports on work being undertaken (DeTray 1957a, 1960) and summaries of conferences (Anon. 1961a, b). Since the outbreak of the disease on the Iberian Peninsula, more intensive and coordinated research programs were undertaken on classical swine fever (hog cholera, HC) and ASF in laboratories in Europe, under the auspices of the Office International des Epizooties (OIE) and the European Economic Community, and resulted in the publication of a monograph on the properties and differential diagnosis of these two diseases, including detailed descriptions of the clinical signs, lesions, and materials and methods of various serological tests (Anon. 1971). In 1976 a symposium was held on these two diseases and the proceedings were published (Anon. 1977). A bibliography has been compiled up to 1978 by the United States Department of Agriculture* (Anon. 1978). More recently, the reports on consultations and symposia on ASF have been published by international organizations (FAO 1979; Anon. 1979, 1980). In 1981, Hess critically reassessed the available knowledge of the various aspects of ASF and the advances made by the current research programs.

Particular attention should be drawn to some of the earliest reports on the disease in Africa, for example that of Montgomery (1921), which presented outstanding accounts of the investigations on ASF.

ETIOLOGY

African swine fever virus (ASFV) is a cytoplasmic deoxyribovirus with a diameter between 175 and 215 μm and an icosahedral shape. It infects and replicates in the cells of the reticuloendothelial system causing deoxyribonucleic acid (DNA)-containing inclusions. The virus is remarkably resistant under laboratory and natural conditions to various physical and chemical stresses, remaining infective for long periods of

* Available from the Director, Emergency Programs, Veterinary Services, Federal Building, Hyattsville, Maryland 20782, USA.

time in adverse environment. It can be readily isolated and grown in porcine-buffy-coat and bone-marrow cell cultures in which it causes adsorption of red blood cells (hemadsorption) to the cell surface and a cytopathic effect (CPE). By prolonged maintenance and serial passage many strains can be adapted to established continuous cell culture systems originating from pigs and other species. Maintenance and passage in cell culture systems, embryonated eggs, and rabbits modifies the virus, resulting in decreased infectivity and pathogenicity, causing a lowered incidence of disease and production of a carrier state.

Literature

The classification, nomenclature, morphology, and chemical composition of ASFV were reviewed by Hess (1971). Its morphology in electron-microscopic studies was similar to a number of other viruses which were listed by Breese and DeBoer (1966), and these similarities and differences were discussed by Hess (1971). On the basis of these compiled characteristics, it has been concluded that ASFV could not be included in any of the recognized families of viruses (Lucas and Carnero 1968); in 1978 it was listed as an unclassified virus in the *Manual of Standardized Methods for Veterinary Mycobiology* (Cottral 1978) although in 1976 Fenner proposed that the tentative classification of ASFV should be an Iridiovirus.

The size and morphology of the replicating virus in tissue cultures as observed by electron microscopy was first described by Breese and DeBoer (1966) and Haag *et al.* (1966). The internal composition of the viral structure was described by Almeida *et al.* (1967) and Moura Nunes *et al.* (1975), and of the nonhemadsorbing variant by Els and Pini (1977). The replication of the viral DNA and synthesis of antigens in the cytoplasm of the host cell was demonstrated by autoradiography and immunofluorescence (Vigário *et al.* 1967). The morphology of ASFV in the tissue of infected pigs was similar to that observed in tissue cultures but the level of infection was lower (Garcia-Gancedo *et al.* 1974). The sedimentation coefficient of the infective unit of ASF in tissue culture harvest fluids was measured in a preparative ultracentrifuge and ranged from 3000 to 8000 Svedberg units representing many classes of infective particles, and many types of virus-containing units were observed by electron microscopy (Trautman *et al.* 1980).

The porcine-buffy-coat and bone-marrow cell cultures were developed by Malmquist and Hay (1960) and constituted a major advancement in the research on ASFV. In these systems, the virus caused intercytoplasmic inclusions, usually one per cell, about 12 hours after infection, coinciding with the first cellular degenerative changes which progressed to cell lysis (Moulton and Coggins 1968a). These inclusions stained red, like the nuclear chromatin, and appeared as complete, incomplete, or crescent forms in single cells and as large amorphic inclusions in the multinucleated giant cells. In pig kidney cultures the inclusions were round, oval, or elongated, and were occasionally multiple. Their DNA composition was demonstrated directly by Feulgen and acridine orange staining techniques (Haag and Larenaudie 1965; Plowright *et al.* 1966), and indirectly by using inhibitors of DNA synthesis and the incorporation of thiamidine in the inclusions (Haag *et al.* 1965; Moreno *et al.* 1978; Moulton and Coggins 1968a; Plowright *et al.* 1966). The infective DNA has also been extracted from the ASFV (Adldinger *et al.* 1966).

The development of suitable isolation and purification techniques of the virus has enabled further characterization of the protein composition (Black and Brown 1976), and determination of the molecular weight of the DNA component (Enjuanes *et al.* 1976b). The kinetics of protein synthesis in ASF infected cells, the localization of protein within the cells, and the classification of early and late proteins as well as the viral structural polypeptides, with their localization within the virion and their antigenic role in the induction of natural infections, were investigated (Tabarés *et al.* 1980a, b). The synthesis of DNA in cells infected with ASF fever occurs in the nucleus (Tabarés and Sanchez Botija 1979). The ribonucleic acid (RNA) synthesis by ASF virions was also investigated recently (Salas *et al.* 1981). The ASFV had a DNA-dependent RNA polymerase activity which did not require the addition of exogenous DNA (Kuznar *et al.* 1980). The nucleoside triphosphate phosphohydrolase activities were investigated in ASFV (Kuznar *et al.* 1981). The virus was observed to replicate in the cytoplasm, moving to the cytoplasmic membrane, and emerging as a budding process during which it acquired an outer coat composed of material from the plasma membrane (Breese and DeBoer 1966).

The porcine-buffy-coat and bone-marrow cell cultures have been widely adopted for the isolation, identification, and titration of ASFV (Malmquist and Hay 1960; Hess and DeTray 1960, 1961). The materials and methods of these culture systems have also been presented in detail in the review by DeTray (1963). The replication of the virus in these systems took place in the monocyte–macrophage series with the monocyte being the most susceptible (Wardley and Wilkinson 1977), and by immunofluorescent techniques appeared as fine stipplings evenly distributed in the cytoplasm of the VERO cells and in monocytes (Pan *et al.* 1980). Macrophages from species other than the pig were not infected (Enjuanes *et al.* 1977). Lymphocytes (Wardley *et al.* 1979) and endothelial cells (Wilkinson and Wardley 1978) were also infected in primary cultures. Both virulent and attenuated strains infected and multiplied in macrophages but the latter had a higher infectivity (Wardley *et al.* 1979). An important property of the infected cells was the adsorption of red blood cells to their surfaces, and this had been used in the identification and titration of ASFV. However, not all ASFV isolates cause hemadsorption. Nonhemadsorbing strains have been isolated from the natural field infections (Pini 1977) and segregated by dilution techniques from the hemadsorbing component, suggesting heterogeneity in the viral population making up a strain (Coggins 1968a). These nonhemadsorbing isolates have been associated with reduced pathogenicity, but not in all cases (Pini 1977). Also, some attenuated strains could not be detected by the hemadsorption test in experimentally infected pigs (Sanchez Botija 1963b). Comparison of the virulence of two nonhemadsorbing ASFV isolates and two hemadsorbing viruses showed that one nonhemadsorbing virus induced a milder form of the disease than the other three. This was not a constant phenomena, and it was concluded that hemadsorption could not be used as a marker of virulence (Thomson *et al.* 1979).

The buffy-coat cultures were found to be too fragile for repeated manipulations, and other culture systems, using a number of established continuous cell lines originating from pigs and other species, were developed and have been used as assay tools and methods by which the viral pathogenicity was modified. All of these techniques involved adaptation of the virus by prolonged incubation and serial passage (Hess *et al.* 1965; Malmquist 1962; Haag and Larenaudie 1965). The growth curve of various strains of ASFV have been investigated in their different culture systems (Enjuanes *et al.* 1976b; Coggins 1966; Malmquist 1962; Plowright *et al.* 1966). Other methods have also been developed for titration of the virus and included standard plaque formation (Greig 1975; Parker and Plowright 1968), immunofluorescent (Tessler *et al.* 1974) and immunoperoxidase plaque methods (Pan *et al.* 1978). The propagation of the virus in embryonated chicken eggs and laboratory rodents has been reviewed by DeTray (1963). African swine fever virus has been attenuated by serial passage through porcine-buffy-coat and bone-marrow cell culture systems (Coggins *et al.* 1966; Manso Ribeiro *et al.* 1963; Sanchez Botija 1963c; Malmquist 1962).

The virus remained viable over a wide range of physicochemical conditions used to determine the intrinsic properties of the virus, its inactivation for the purposes of immunization, and relation to its transmission. A systematic quantitative study of the effect of pH and heat on ASFV showed that storage for long periods at −20 °C was deleterious but not at +4 or −70 °C (Plowright and Parker 1967). The early qualitative studies on survival of the virus were reviewed by Neitz (1963) and the more recent quantitative information by Hess (1971), who pointed out that the variability in the stability of the virus could be caused by differences in the composition of the medium.

EPIZOOTIOLOGY

In Africa ASF was first reported in Kenya, and since then sporadic outbreaks of the disease have occurred in Tanzania, Zambia, Zimbabwe, Angola, Mozambique, Malawi, South Africa, Zaïre, South West Africa, Senegal, Benin, and Algeria. The distribution and incidence in most of these countries are dependent on the prevalence of carriers, either wild or domestic pigs, the extent of the swine industry, type of husbandry practiced, and the efficacy of the recommended control practices. All regions which have wild pigs are regarded as potential enzootic areas. The reservoirs are warthogs, bush pigs, and giant forest hogs. The warthogs are the most important source of the virus, but not all populations carry ASFV and there are regional differences in the incidence of infection.

In 1957, ASFV spread to the Iberian Peninsula, probably by importation of infected pork, and subsequently became established as an enzootic disease in Portugal and Spain, while in France and Italy it was eradicated. In 1971, an outbreak occurred in Cuba; the disease was subsequently eradicated but it reappeared again in 1979. Until 1978 the only outbreak which occurred outside the Iberian Peninsula and Africa was in France in 1974. In March 1978, the disease occurred in Malta and Sardinia, was subsequently reported in Brazil in May, and was confirmed in the Dominican Republic and Haiti in July.

Two types of enzootics, old and new, characterize the epizootiology of ASF. The old enzootic situation is found in Africa and is related to the transmission from the wild species to domestic pigs. The new enzootics involve spread of the virus by chronically diseased and asymptomatic carrier domestic pigs. The outbreaks of ASF in the old enzootic areas are characterized by an acute disease syndrome with morbidity and mortality of nearly 100%, with the few survivors developing a chronic form of the disease which eventually terminates in death. Occasionally an animal may become infected, not develop clinical signs, and become a carrier. Many outbreaks of the disease in Africa are of this type, but within these countries, where communal free-ranging practices are maintained, a new enzootic situation has been established and the disease has changed to a less acute form, with a more frequent occurrence of chronic syndromes and asymptomatic carriers. A similar situation now also exists in Portugal and Spain where the disease continues to change to a less severe form. In these two countries the epizootiology is complicated by the use of a partially attenuated live viral vaccine which causes a reaction in a relatively high percentage of the vaccinated animals and establishes carriers.

Among the warthogs, ASFV is apparently transmitted primarily by the argasid tick, *Ornithodorus moubata porcinus*, a multihost tick in which the virus multiplies and is transmitted transovarially and sexually. The spread to domestic pigs from warthogs is associated by contact such as occurs under free-ranging husbandry practices. It was originally thought to be caused by ingestion of fomites, but subsequent experimental work showed that domestic pigs could not be infected by close contact with warthogs. It is now postulated that transmission by the vector tick is the most likely method. The acute disease in domestic pigs is highly contagious because of the high levels of viremia resulting in excretion of large amounts of virus in feces and urine. Chronically diseased animals are also viremic and may transmit the virus in the same way, but the asymptomatic carrier animals have lower levels of infection and are less infective. It is not clear how important is direct contact between asymptomatic carriers and susceptible pigs, in comparison to the possible transmission by the tick, *O. erraticus*, and to a lesser degree by the louse, *Hematopinus suis*. An important method of spread is by pork in uncooked swill and this has been responsible for most of the initial outbreaks in Portugal and Spain. Another consideration in the transmission is the particular resistance of the virus to various chemical and physical environmental factors. Contaminated premises may be infective for up to 3 months, and the virus withstands putrefaction in some tissues for several weeks and in chilled and frozen pork for up to 6 months. Under laboratory conditions it remains viable at 5 °C for years. These factors necessitate particularly stringent precautions and measures to prevent the spread of the virus.

Literature

The worldwide outbreaks of ASF are monitored by the OIE and are reported in the OIE information notes, monthly epizootic circulars, statistics in the *FAO–WHO–OIE Animal Health Year Book*, and the Inter-African Bureau for Animal Resources (IBAR) bulletins. The position of ASF epizootiology in Latin America was reviewed and the disease introduction into Brazil, the Dominican Republic, and Haiti, where it was discovered in 1978, was discussed (Peritz 1980). There were additional reports and discussions on the spread to other countries outside Africa (Bool 1967; Carnero *et al.* 1975, 1979; Doyle 1961; Gasse 1963; Polo Jover and Sanchez Botija 1961; Ribeiro *et al.* 1975; Pereira Henriques *et al.* 1976; Spuhler 1967; Terpstra 1961).

The epizootiology of ASF was divided into the old and new epizootic cycles which differed in the reservoir host, main mode of transmission, and the severity of the diseases (Scott 1965a, c). It was noted that in South Africa outbreaks appeared to have a cyclic pattern, occurring at about 12-year intervals and lasting for 12 to 13 years (Pini 1977). Because of the relatively limited swine industry in many countries in Africa, the past epizootic usually involved transmission from wild pigs, the incidence being related to the distribution and prevalence of the main reservoir, the warthog (Anon. 1962). In Angola and South Africa, the carrier domestic pigs have also been shown to be important in some of the outbreaks (Leite Velho 1956; Pini and Hurter 1975). The reservoir species of wild pigs were the warthog (*Phaeochoerus aethiopicus*), bush pig (*Potomochoerus porcus*), and the giant forest hog (*Hylochoerus minertzhageni*), with the incidence in warthogs being tenfold higher than in other wild pigs (DeTray 1957b, 1963; DeTray *et al.* 1961). Already, during the first outbreaks in Kenya, warthogs had been incriminated by farmers as the source of ASFV (Steyn 1932) and the presence of warthogs not infected with ASFV in some regions of Africa has been associated with absence of the disease (Mansvelt 1963; Scott and Hill 1966; Taylor *et al.* 1977). The giant forest hog, because of its habitat in remote bush areas, probably plays the least important role in the epizootiology (Heuschele and Coggins 1965b; Mansvelt 1963; Scott and Hill 1966; Taylor *et al.* 1977). The hippopotamus (*Hippopotamus amphibius*), because of its joint feeding habitat with warthogs and close relation to the Suidae family, has been investigated as another possible carrier species. Although two apparent isolations were made, later more extensive surveys proved negative (Stone and Heuschele 1965). In the enzootic areas, the incidence in warthog populations varied from 20 to 70%, with the highest rate being observed in animals 4 to 10 months of age (DeTray 1957b; DeTray *et al.* 1961; Plowright *et al.* 1969a).

Based on experimental observations, transmission among warthogs by contact was thought to be unlikely, and transfer by ingestion, across the placenta, and by biting vectors was proposed (DeTray 1963; Hammond and DeTray 1955; Heuschele *et al.* 1965; Heuschele and Coggins 1969). The latter method was highly probable since parenteral administration by various routes of even relatively low doses readily established infections. Further more definitive investigations showed that neither ingestion nor transplacental transfer were likely and that the tick, *O. dorus moubata porcinus,* was the vector (Heuschele and Coggins 1965a; Plowright *et al.* 1969a). The prevalence of ticks and their infection rates varied in different enzootic regions, with infections being highest in the adult stages. The virus was maintained in the tick populations by sexual – primarily male to female – and transovarian transmission, and multiplied in various tissues of the newly infected tick (Greig 1972b; Plowright *et al.* 1969b, 1970a, b, 1974). These findings have changed the basic concepts of the epizootiology of ASF in Africa and indicate the possible importance of arthropod vectors in the spread of the virus in other regions. A tick species indigenous to the USA, *O. coriaceus,* did not show transovarial transmission of ASF in adult females. However, nymphs maintained the virus for 77 to 118 days through the molting stage and transmitted the strain to susceptible animals (Groocock *et al.* 1980). Feral pigs from Florida were susceptible to AFSV by intranasal and oral inoculation, causing high mortality and a typical postmortem picture associated with the acute syndrome (McVicar *et al.* 1981).

Although transmission from warthogs to pigs had dominated the epizootiology of ASF in Africa, a few enzootics within the domestic pig population developed in South Africa, but these were quickly brought under control (De Kock *et al.* 1940; Pini and Hurter 1975). In Angola, a new type of enzootic was established because of free-ranging swine production practices and delay in controlling the spread of ASFV within the domestic pig population, and was characterized by increased numbers of chronic cases and asymptomatic carriers (Mendes and Daskalos 1955). This was attributed to decreased pathogenicity of the virus as a result of its association with domestic pigs (Leite Velho 1956, 1958), a situation which also characterizes the epizootiology of ASF in Europe (DeTray 1957a; Sanchez Botija 1962, 1963a). The clinical and pathological observations were compared between the more virulent Lisbon 60 strain of ASFV and those isolates made from Brazil and the Dominican Republic. The two latter strains had a longer clinical course and a lower mortality associated with a more pronounced leukopenia (Mebus and Dardiri 1979).

This concept of reduced virulence because of the transmission between domestic pigs has been questioned by Hess (1971) who pointed out that it has not been verified experimentally and that, in fact, DeTray (1963) reported increased virulence, as seen by the decreased incubation period of from 5 to 15 days to 4 to 5 days after 45 pig passages of the Hinde strain. However, this does not invalidate the hypothesis of the cause of the reduced virulence as observed in the field because DeTray presumably passaged a virus causing acute syndromes, while in a natural situation the virus associated with chronic and carrier states would be responsible for maintaining the enzootics. Therefore, the virus associated with chronic diseases would be transmitted and could be partly attenuated.

In an outbreak the acute disease is contagious because of the high levels of virus excreted in feces and urine. Transmission was shown to occur by ingestion and nuzzling but was not considered to be airborne (Montgomery 1921; Steyn 1932). However, recent experimental work has shown that airborne spread is possible (Wilkinson and Donaldson 1977). The survivors of the acute syndrome developed chronic disease and virus continued to be excreted, but only some of the animals showing inapparent infection remained as carriers and had intermittent viremia (De Kock *et al.* 1940; DeTray 1957a). The importance of direct contact with asymptomatic carriers in transmission has not been established, although there is circumstantial evidence that they have been responsible for outbreaks (De Kock *et al.* 1940). It now appears that transmission from a carrier by an arthropod vector could be important. It has been shown in Europe that the tick, *O. erraticus*, found in premises after an outbreak of ASF retained the virus for a year and could transmit the infection (Sanchez Botija 1962, 1963b). The louse (*Hematopinus suis*) has also been reported to be infected and able to transmit ASFV (Sanchez Botija and Badiola 1966). Therefore vector transmission, particularly by the ticks, has to be considered as an important means of transmission (Plowright *et al.* 1969a, b).

Many of the outbreaks have been associated with the spread of ASFV through infected pork fed in uncooked swill which was considered to be responsible for 84% of the outbreaks in Spain (Anon. 1961a). The virus has shown a remarkable ability to survive in the environment and tissues. Contaminated sties have been reported to remain infective for about 5 days (Montgomery 1921) and 3 months (Sanchez Botija 1962). The carcasses of pigs dying of ASF were infective for at least 17 hours and putrefying blood for 16 days when stored at room temperature (Montgomery 1921). De Kock *et al.* (1940) reported that 10 weeks was required to render the virus noninfective from putrefaction, and blood stored in a cold room remained infective for 5 to 6 years (De Kock *et al.* 1940; Kovalenko *et al.* 1965). Hams prepared commercially had contained virus for up to 6 months (Sanchez Botija 1962) and chilled meat had viable virus after 15 weeks (Kovalenko *et al.* 1964). Virus in tissues irradiated at a 50 kGy dose inactivated the virus and such material could be used as a source of positive controls in fluorescent antibody (FA) tests for up to 18 months when stored at −70 °C (McVicar *et al.* 1982). These reports indicate that ASFV is extremely stable under a variety of environmental conditions. The time periods reported should be regarded as merely indications of its durability and should not be considered as definitive time frames. A great deal of more systematic quantitative investigations are required to determine the length of time ASFV can survive in the environment.

INFECTION

The process of infection by ASFV includes the entry, growth, dissemination throughout tissues, and excretion, and forms the basis of the pathogenesis of the disease and the transmission of the virus. The routes of infections vary somewhat with the epizootiological situation. The parenteral route by bite of the vector tick is probably the main method of spread of infection among warthogs and from warthogs to pigs, and it may also be important in transmission from carrier pigs. The virus is maintained in a resident tick population for long periods of time after an outbreak of the disease on the premises. This conclusion that arthropod vectors are important is further supported by the experimental work which shows, first of all that in contact transmission from warthogs does not occur, and secondly that experimental parenteral infections are relatively easy and require relatively small doses of virus. The difficulty of transmitting ASFV to pigs by contact with warthogs and with some asymptomatic carrier pigs is probably because of the low and transient levels of viremia which cause the excretion of the virus at subinfective levels. However, the carrier state observed in the chronic disease may have higher infective levels of virus in the excretions. Transmission from acute cases to stall-mates and by feeding of uncooked infected pork is thought to occur through the upper respiratory and upper gastrointestinal routes. This has been verified experimentally, and it has also been shown that primary infection can occur through the lungs and lower gastrointestinal tissues.

At the site of infection the virus multiplies in the local reticuloendothelial tissue component and in the drainage lymph node. The subsequent viremia disseminates the virus throughout other tissues and high titers are observed in those organs which have a large reticuloendothelial tissue component. The virus initially infects reticular cells and macrophages, then lymphoid cells, and then endothelial cells during the later stages of the disease. The excretion of the virus is dependent on the presence of viremia.

Literature

Titers of the virus in tissues during its spread have been determined after intranasal (Heuschele 1967; Plowright *et al.* 1968), oral (Colgrove *et al.* 1969), airborne (Wilkinson and Donaldson 1977), and in contact infections (Greig and Plowright 1970). The Malta isolate was compared with other isolates as to clinical signs, pathology, and viremia. The clinical syndromes and severity of postmortem examinations were less severe with the Malta strain, and the virus titers in blood and tissues were similar with the African virus isolate (Wilkinson *et al.* 1981). Pigs recovered from acute infection with Brazilian or the Dominican Republic isolates of ASF were clinically normal. These animals were observed not to shed the virus or to shed it at low titers which were not infective to contact pigs; however, tissues from these pigs were infective when fed to susceptible pigs (Mebus and Dardiri 1980). The distribution and levels of virus in tissues have also been investigated in warthogs (Plowright *et al.* 1969a). The microtechnique for the titration of ASFV was less sensitive than the conventional tube assay (Wardley and Wilkinson 1980c).

After intranasal infection the virus was first detected at 24 hours in tonsils, mandibular lymph nodes, and in circulating leukocytes which were thought to disseminate the virus into other tissues, particularly those which contained a large reticuloendothelial component and showed infection on the third day (Heuschele 1967). Further studies on the dissemination of the virus after intranasal infection showed that the viral growth was already established within 16 to 24 hours in the retropharyngeal lymph nodes and spread to other tissues within 72 hours by its association with erythrocytes (Plowright *et al.* 1968). The sources of this circulating virus were the lymph nodes with contributions made by liver, lung, and bone marrow. The oral route of the infection of newborn pigs resulted in the initial infection of the tonsils and mandibular lymph nodes, with evidence that some cases of primary infection become established through either the lungs or the mesenteric lymph nodes (Colgrove *et al.* 1969). Viremia in these young pigs was already detected at 8 hours after infection and increased to higher levels by 15 to 24 hours, being caused by the virus growing in the spleen, liver, lymph nodes, and lungs. After in contact exposure, primary infections occurred in the pharyngeal tonsils at 24 hours, but there was also evidence, in some cases, that viral invasion occurred through the nasal, bronchial, and gastric mucosa (Greig 1972a). The excretion of the virus was first observed in the nasal and pharyngeal secretions and 1 and 2 days before the onset of fever (Greig and Plowright 1970). The failure of infected pigs to transmit the virus through direct contact during the first 12 to 24 hours of fever was thought to be due to low titers in the excretions. Fecal and urinary excretions were less important in the transmission during the early stages, but became more significant during the protracted course of the disease. A recent publication has shown that ASF can be transmitted by the airborne virus, contrary to the conclusions reached by Montgomery (1921) and Wilkinson and Donaldson (1977). By this route, the site of primary infection is the lower respiratory tract and the virus is carried in a fine aerosol. Airborne transmission is apparently only over short distances but could be important in intensive swine production facilities.

In warthogs the virus was found primarily in external and internal lymph nodes (Plowright *et al.* 1969a). The spleen had a much lower incidence of infection and viremia was not observed in any of the infected animals. In warthogs and possibly in some carrier pigs, the virus localized predominantly in tissue, especially the lymph nodes, and viremia occurred only intermittently.

CLINICAL SIGNS

African swine fever is described to occur in peracute, acute, subacute, chronic, and asymptomatic carrier forms and this is based on the length of incubation period, severity of symptoms, and duration of disease. This classification represents the range of syndromes which may occur in outbreaks under different epizootiological conditions. In epizootics caused by transmission from warthogs, the peracute and acute syndromes predominate while outbreaks in enzootic areas related to transmission from pigs have less severe symptoms.

In the acute syndromes, including the peracute, acute, and subacute forms, the symptoms are most pronounced in those cases which are last to die. Thus, in the peracute disease there are virtually no signs other than the development of high temperature followed within 48 hours by death. This form is often observed in the first stage of an acute outbreak with death occurring in a few pigs before any disease is detected. This is followed in 5 to 6 days by death in other pigs which developed the acute form. In cases where the outbreak is due to uncooked swill, the initial incidence is more explosive with peracute and acute syndromes occurring initially in large numbers of pigs. In the acute form, the incubation period is 2 to 5 days in the experimental and 5 to 9 days in natural disease. This is followed by high temperatures from 40 to 42 °C. During the initial 2 to 3 days of pyrexia, there are no apparent symptoms and the animals continue to eat. Then the pigs become depressed, do not eat, lie huddled, and are reluctant to move, showing lameness and stiffness of the hindquarters. The other signs include hyperemia of the skin which may progress to cyanosis, subcutaneous hemorrhages which may form hematomas on the ears and haunches, and localized skin necrosis. Further evidence of a generalized hemorrhagic disorder is evidenced by epistaxis, dysentery, and vomiting of blood. In the terminal stages, the animals become recumbent and either comatose or show convulsions and muscle tremors, dying within 24 hours. In the subacute syndrome, the incubation period is longer, 8 to 15 days, the clinical signs are usually more pronounced than in the acute form, and the pigs live for 12 to 15 days.

The chronic syndrome usually follows a period during which symptoms of acute disease are manifested and may last for several months. The temperature returns to normal and the appetite returns. There is subsequent progressive emaciation, intermittent fever, dyspnea and cough, lameness accompanied by soft swelling of joints, and inadvertently the animal dies, usually due to pulmonary involvement. The ASFV is present throughout the course of chronic syndromes. Inapparent infections which are not accompanied by any overt clinical disease characterize the asymptomatic carrier state.

Literature

The acute syndromes were described in detail by the early workers in Africa (De Kock *et al.* 1940; Montgomery 1921; Steyn 1932) and have been summarized in the more recent reviews, particularly by Neitz (1963). The more chronic forms of the disease have been described, although not in detail, from the enzootic regions outside Africa: from Spain (Polo Jover and Sanchez Botija 1961), Portugal (Manso Ribeiro *et al.* 1963), Cuba (Rodriguez *et al.* 1972), and in association with the use of the partially attenuated strains of vaccines (Manso Ribeiro *et al.* 1963; Sanchez Botija 1963c). The postvaccine reaction, in addition to the prominent pulmonary involvement, included locomotor disturbance, abortion, impaired milk production, and development of tumor-like lesions, resembling myxoma, in the skin. Other clinical signs which occur irregularly but were considered to characterize ASF symptomatology were summarized in the report of the Commission of European Communities (Anon. 1971).

PATHOLOGY

The cellular changes which underlie the development of lesions occur in the lymphoid tissues and blood vessels, and consist of hypertrophy, hyperplasia, and necrosis of various cellular components of the reticuloendothelial system. Reticular cells, macrophages, endothelial cells, and lymphocytes are affected, with hyperplasia being dominant in the more chronic syndromes and necrosis characterizing the acute forms. The resulting lesions affect the whole lymphoid system, including lymphoid organs, circulating lymphocytes, and its peripheral component made up of the migrating mononuclear cells in the connective tissue stroma of various solid tissues. The endothelial cells are affected predominantly in the small arteries and capillaries.

The resulting gross lesions in the various organs and tissues are caused by the changes occurring in their circulatory and lymphoid tissue components which in turn are responsible for the secondary lesions in the parenchymous tissues. The lymph nodes are enlarged and very hemorrhagic, appearing often as hematoma-like lesions. Microscopically, there is extensive necrosis of various types of cells resulting in widespread cellular depletion. These changes are of particular diagnostic importance in the gastrohepatic nodes and spleen. The spleen is also enlarged and there is marked congestion. The circulating lymphocytes are depleted, and inclusions may be observed in association with this leukopenia. There is mononuclear cell infiltration of stroma of various tissues, including the walls of the blood vessels in the brain, liver, heart, and lungs, resulting in encephalitis, hepatitis, myocarditis, and interstitial pneumonia. Accompanying these cellular changes in solid tissues there are lesions in the blood vessels, which in the acute stage consist of degeneration and necrosis of the endothelium and thrombosis, causing interstitial edema, extensive hemorrhage, and varying degrees of infarction. The combination of the lesions in the lymphoid and vascular system causes the widespread hemorrhages, which occasionally result in hematomas of serosal surfaces, subcutaneous tissues, and muscle facial sheaths. Particularly severe hemorrhages are observed in the epicardium, endocardium, and kidney cortex. Edema accompanies the vascular lesions and affects the lungs, gall bladder, and subcutaneous tissue and results in accumulation of serohemorrhagic fluid in the pericardial, pleural, and peritoneal cavities. Accompanying these lesions there is injury to the parenchymous tissues with cellular degeneration occurring in the brain, liver, and gastrointestinal tract. In the latter tissue, there is congestion and necrosis of the mucosa, with ulceration, fibrin, and blood present in the lumen. In the more chronic cases, a necrotizing pleuropneumonia, fibrinous pericarditis, and arthritis are present. Extensive myxomatous thickening and focal necrosis of skin also are observed in the more severe acute cases.

The frequency and severity of various lesions observed in an outbreak are dependent to a large degree on the epizootiological situation which governs the acuteness of the syndromes. The disease continues to evolve within an enzootic area and the predominance of many of the characteristic lesions changes with time.

Literature

The pathogenesis of ASF has been summarized in the review articles cited in the previous sections with an additional brief review, more specifically on pathogenesis, presented by Coggins (1974). Because of the close similarity between ASF and HC, both on clinical and pathological observations, more detailed comparisons were studied and it was shown that, although the primary lesions in both diseases were found in the lymphoid tissues and in the walls of blood vessels, a more severe karyorrhexis occurred in AFS (Maurer *et al.* 1958). Comparing acute and chronic lesions of AFS, the former was characterized by inflammation of the spleen, lymph nodes, tonsils, kidneys, skin, eyes, liver, brain, gastrointestinal tract, and early interstitial pneumonia, while the chronic cases, in addition to the above lesions, also had pericarditis, well-developed interstitial pneumonia, and hyperplasia of lymph nodes (Moulton and Coggins 1968b). The proliferation of cells in lympho-endothelial-reticular systems in acute ASF and the accompanying changes in the liver have been described (Konno *et al.* 1971a, b, 1972). The leukopenia was shown to occur 4 days after exposure, resulting from an increase in juvenile neutrophils and decrease of lymphocytes; the other cellular blood components were within normal ranges (DeTray and Scott 1957). The macroscopic lesions in the pigs infected with more virulent Lisbon 60 isolates were typical for the AFS syndrome and characterized by enlarged reddish-black friable spleen and enlarged reddish-black visceral lymph nodes. Microscopically, these lesions were associated with extensive necrosis of reticular cells. These lesions were less severe with the less virulent isolates from Brazil and the Dominican Republic, particularly in those animals which had a longer course of illness. Because the low mortality decreased the classical lesions of AFS, its initial diagnosis could be overlooked. Also, the development of antibody would be likely to interfere with the direct immunofluorescent antibody and hemadsorption diagnostic tests and the disease could become widely spread because clinically recovered animals or meat products can be a source of the virus (Mebus and Dardiri 1979).

The injurious mechanisms causing cell necrosis have not been determined, but it has been proposed that, on the basis of symptoms and lesions, an allergic reaction could be involved and ASF was classified as an immunopathological disease (Korn 1964). Immunofluorescent studies on the chronic pneumonia have shown immunoglobulins and complement found in association with ASFV antigens in and on macrophages; these antigen–antibody complexes were proposed as the possible mechanism causing necrosis (Pan *et al.* 1974a, b). Immune deposits consisting of AFS antigen, immunoglobulin G, and native C3 were found in glomeruli of surviving pigs after 2 weeks of infection. Leukocyte-bound immunoglobulin E was demonstrated and was associated with secondary platelet aggregation and vaso-active amine release (Slauson and Sanchez-Vizcaino 1981). Infected tissue culture cells were lysed by the classical complement pathway and not the alternative pathway, a system unique among reported virus infections (Norley and Wardley 1982).

IMMUNOLOGY

The role of immunological responses in resistance to infection and to development of disease is not completely established. Pigs recovered from natural and artificial ASFV infections are usually refractory to challenge with homologous but not heterologous strains. The protection produced by partially attenuated strains passaged in tissue cultures depends on the virulence of the virus and its ability to cause an apparent clinical response. Antibodies are detected by precipitin, fluorescent, and complement-fixing reactions, but are not associated with immunity to challenge. Neutralizing antibodies may occur, as evidenced by the *in vivo* challenge experiments, but have not been detected *in vitro*. It is also possible that the resistance to reinfection is due to some inhibitory factor which is associated with the persistent viral infections characterizing the resistant states of pigs recovering from challenge by virulent or attenuated virus. On the basis of cross-immunity experiments undertaken in the early investigations on ASF, immunologically distinct strains are demonstrated. Further support for the presence of isolate or strain specific antigens are provided by the *in vitro* hemadsorption inhibition reaction which enables serological typing of ASF. However, strains cannot be differentiated by precipitin, fluorescent, and complement-fixation (CF) reactions.

Laboratory and field vaccination trials with attenuated ASF have been attempted. Although results in laboratories indicated high levels of protection with acceptable level of morbidity and mortality from the vaccine in view of the losses from natural disease, field trials caused severe postinfection in 10 to 50% of vaccinated pigs, as well as widespread dissemination of the attenuated virus.

Literature

Hess (1971) referred to the 'obscure immunology' of ASF to describe the present state of knowledge. Yet because of the impending danger of worldwide dissemination of ASF and its devastating effect on swine production in epizootic and enzootic areas, improved diagnostic and protective methods involving adequately defined immunologic mechanisms are absolutely essential. Already during the early investigations in Africa on ASF, the few pigs which recovered from infection were shown to be refractory to subsequent reinfections. This resistance was incomplete, being at best limited to the challenge by the homologous strain (Montgomery 1921; Steyn 1932). With the development of the attenuated strains which caused either chronic or inapparent clinical responses, more intensive studies of immunological studies were undertaken. The resistance to reinfection was related to the virulence of the virus and required the development of clinical response, e.g. fever (Malmquist 1963; Sanchez Botija 1963c).

Natural and experimental infections with attenuated virus caused serological responses which were demonstrated by precipitin, immunofluorescent, and complement-fixing antibodies (Boulanger *et al.* 1966; Coggins and Heuschele 1966; Cowan 1961; Korn 1963; Malmquist 1963). Relatively high levels of these antibodies developed in those animals which had been vaccinated with attenuated virus and subsequently challenged with the homologous virulent virus. However, these antibodies were not associated with protection and were thought to be related to several antigens associated with ASFV infected cells and not necessarily with the virus itself (Malmquist 1963). The interaction of viral antigens with ferritin-conjugated antibody was studied by electron microscopy (Breese *et al.* 1967). All of these serological reactions were not strain-specific and appeared to be immunologically different, as shown by *in vivo* cross-resistance studies.

Antigenic differences were detected by the hemadsorption-inhibition test (Carnero *et al.* 1967; Coggins 1968b; Malmquist 1963; Vigário *et al.* 1970, 1974), and to some degree the isoelectric precipitation technique which separated the antigenic viral fractions (Stone and Hess 1965). Another method used for the study of antigenic components of ASFV-infected cells was the crossed immunoelectrophoresis (Dalsgaard *et al.* 1977). In spite of the serological responses to various antigens and evidence of partial immunity *in vivo*, neutralizing antibodies have not been detected *in vitro* (DeBoer 1967; DeBoer *et al.* 1969). Attempts to protect against ASF by vaccination with inactivated virus by physical and chemical means, using many of the techniques successful with HC, have failed (Hess 1971). Further work with noninfective antigens has shown that precipitin and complement-fixing, but not neutralizing, antibodies were produced and there was no resistance to challenge (Stone and Hess 1967). On the basis of the serological reactions and in spite of the extensive cellular necrosis in lymphoid tissues in ASF, the humoral responses appeared to be intact.

In chronic diseases, hyperglobulinemia was even demonstrated (Pan *et al.* 1970, 1974a, b). It was also shown that the delayed hypersensitivity was not impaired following infection with attenuated virus and subsequent challenge with the homologous virulent strain (Shimizu *et al.* 1977). The lymphopenia and the decreased percentage of circulating T-lymphocytes were observed as early as 7 days after pigs were inoculated and this was accompanied by depressed lymphocyte function, indicating a depression of cellular immunity (Sanchez-Vizcaino *et al.* 1981). The cytolytic effect of the virus caused a proportionately greater drop in B- rather than T-lymphocytes. Sensitized lymphocytes were observed to appear 10 days after infection in the circulating leukocytes (Wardley and Wilkinson 1980a, b). Various serological reactions have been modified and adapted for the diagnosis of the ASF and the literature is cited in that section.

Due to the critical epizootic situation in the Iberian Peninsula, large field vaccination trials were undertaken using a partially attenuated virus strain. Although laboratory results indicated acceptable levels of protection and incidence of postvaccination reactions, the subsequent field trials resulted in a much greater incidence of deleterious reaction which included death of 10 to 50% over prolonged periods of time and established an enzootic ASF situation in these regions (Manso Ribeiro *et al.* 1963; Sanchez Botija 1963c).

DIAGNOSIS

Control of ASF depends on rapid diagnosis, which consists of making a provisional diagnosis on epizootiological, clinical, and pathological bases and a definitive diagnosis demonstrating the ASFV. In view of the continued spread of ASF throughout the world and the establishment of new enzootic areas outside Africa, the danger of spread to

ASF-free regions has increased greatly. Therefore, the onus is on rapid and accurate diagnosis, especially on the initial recognition of outbreaks of diseases in pigs which have a high probability of being ASF. On the basis of this stage of diagnosis the first phase of control measures can be implemented. The epizootiology of ASF varies with different regions and affects the severity of the syndromes and their clinical, pathological, and serological responses. Therefore, a tentative diagnosis must include taking into consideration the local and regional epizootiological situation, history, morbidity, clinical signs, mortality, and lesions. Definitive diagnosis depends on the demonstration of the virus and, in certain situations, also on the presence of ASF specific antibodies. Because of this variability of the various features of ASF in different epizootiological situations, the diagnosis, both tentative and definitive, usually requires the use of several diagnostic procedures.

The local and regional epizootiology of ASF is of primary importance since it indicates the possibility of an outbreak occurring, and the course and severity of the disease. Epizootics in ASF-free regions are usually characterized in the initial stages by acute syndromes, as are warthog to pig transmissions in enzootic areas, while pig-to-pig spread causes development of more chronic forms, especially where disease has been established for some time with a high incidence of carrier animals. Because international movement of animals and control of disease are under the control of national governments, the distribution of ASF is best considered on a country basis. In countries free from ASF, diagnosis takes into consideration the proximity of enzootic areas, international movement of animals (both legal and illegal), and the possible access to pork products from international air- and seaports. Many outbreaks have occurred in the vicinity of airports and have been associated with the feeding of uncooked swill originating probably from international flights.

In epizootics of acute disease, with morbidity and mortality approaching 100%, the syndrome is septicemic, dominated by tissue hemorrhages and necrosis of lymphoid organs. A differential diagnosis has to be made from a number of acute bacterial septicemic viremias including salmonellosis and erysipelas. The chronic forms of ASF result in intestinal, pneumonic, arthritic, and cutaneous lesions which are observed in many of the common bacterial diseases of swine. In HC enzootic areas, ASF cannot be differentiated on a clinical and pathological basis. Therefore, the provisional diagnosis of ASF in many enzootic situations is difficult, requiring rapid confirmation by definitive diagnosis demonstrating the virus.

Definitive diagnosis depends primarily on the demonstration of the virus and the presence of specific humoral antibodies. A number of methods are available and their efficacy depends on the levels of virus and antibody which vary with the stage and the severity of the diseases, whether acute, chronic, or asymptomatic. Therefore, several laboratory techniques are used in each suspected outbreak of ASF. Virus in tissues of pigs is detected by direct FA techniques, and by cell cultural methods. Smears of leukocytes and infected tissues, particularly lymphoid and frozen section techniques, are used to demonstrate and identify the virus. In acute forms of the disease the viral titers are high and ASFV can be readily detected in smears of buffy-coat and lymphoid organs, and in frozen sections by direct FA techniques. Although the virus is present in the circulatory leukocytes during the clinical course of the disease, it appears only for a relatively short time period. African swine fever virus is isolated from tissues in cultures of buffy-coat cells or other continuous cell lines not requiring a period during which the virus has to be adapted, and is identified by hemadsorption and by direct FA techniques. Demonstration of the virus is relatively more difficult in chronic cases having low titers, and often is not identifiable on primary isolation by the hemadsorption method. In these cases, precipitin CF, and FA tests are utilized. The most efficient and sensitive serological tests developed to date are the immunoelectroosmophoresis and the enzyme-linked immunosorbent assay (ELISA) tests.

Literature

The diagnosis of ASF has been discussed in all the reviews (DeTray 1963; Hess 1971; Neitz 1963; Scott 1965a, c). In addition, a detailed presentation of the clinical, pathological, and immunological methods was given in a monograph compiled by the Commission of the European Communities (Anon. 1977) with special emphasis on the differential diagnosis from HC. Diagnostic procedures have also been reported from various countries and related to the local epizootiological situation: Portugal (Manso Ribeiro 1970), Cuba (Rodriguez *et al.* 1972), Spain (Sanchez Botija and Ordas 1969), and Angola (Leite Velho 1956).

The original technique demonstrating hemadsorption described by Malmquist and Hay (1960) was modified by Hess and DeTray (1961) using leukocyte culture from defibrinated blood. This method has also been described in detail by DeTray (1963). The question has been raised as to the specificity of this test for other viruses isolated from pigs with which nonspecific hemadsorption was reported (Drager *et al.* 1965). A further complication to identifying ASFV through hemadsorption has been the presence of nonhemadsorbing strains mixed with hemadsorbing varieties in a single isolate (Coggins 1968a, b). The test has limited value in chronic and inapparent carrier animals from which isolates cause cytopathic effect but require serial passage before hemadsorption is observed (Sanchez Botija *et al.* 1971). Therefore, the usefulness of this test in the diagnosis is limited with the changing epizootiology occurring outside Africa. Because of this shortcoming, alternate techniques were developed using FA techniques to demonstrate the virus in primary isolations in leukocyte and other cell line cultures (Bool *et al.* 1969; Carnero *et al.* 1968; Heuschele and Hess 1973; Sanchez Botija 1971). In acute cases, ASFV has also been demonstrated in tissues by FA techniques and other serological tests (Boulanger *et al.* 1966, 1967a, b, c). The virus has also been detected in circulating leukocytes by the FA test (Colgrove 1968, 1969).

Serological responses in the CF (Cowan 1961, 1963) and agar-gel diffusion precipitation tests (Coggins and Heuschele 1966) were demonstrated by detecting chronic and carrier cases. Modification of the precipitation reaction by immunoelectroosmophoresis increased the sensitivity and decreased the time to run the test (Pan *et al.* 1972). For further application to field use, the reverse single radial immunodiffusion test was recommended (Pan *et al.* 1974b). The radioimmunoassay detected antibodies 3 to 4 days after infection while immunoelectroosmophoresis and the reverse single radial immunodiffusion test did not detect antibodies until 10 days after infection. The hemadsorption assay was more sensitive than the radioimmunoassay for the detection of antigens in tissues (Wardley and Wilkinson 1980a). The micro agar-gel precipitation test was found to be more economical, although not as simple as the reverse single radial immunodiffusion test which also, at times, gave equivocal results (Simpson and Drager 1979). The ELISA test was considered to be more sensitive than the other currently used serological tests, and in addition to its specificity and sensitivity it is rapid, inexpensive, and can be undertaken with modest laboratory equipment, enabling it to be used as a practical diagnostic test (Hamdy and Dardiri 1979, 1980). Therefore, the ELISA was recommended as an efficient method of testing large numbers of sera in epizootic situations. The ELISA-positive sera which were negative with the indirect immunofluorescent test in about 7% of sera tested had a nonspecific reaction associated with poor serum quality due to contamination (Hamdy *et al.* 1981).

PREVENTION, CONTROL, AND ERADICATION

Methods used to prevent, control, and eradicate ASF vary with the regional epizootiological situation and depend on whether the outbreak occurs in enzootic or ASF-free areas and if wild species of pigs are involved. The efficacy of the various measures depends on the ability of individual countries to implement the internationally recognized regulations. The continued spread of ASFV, since its original escape from Africa in 1959, underlines the difficulty of implementing these regulations.

Effective preventative measures in those regions of Africa inhabited by the wild species in the genus *Suis* depend on the complete isolation of domestic pigs from contact with warthogs and the arthropod vector. In those regions of Africa and Europe where the disease has become enzootic in the pig population, the spread of the virus can be limited by rigid restrictions on the movement of pigs and pork products, and in particular on the feeding of uncooked swill. Strict regulations on the disinfections of premises should also be applied. Outbreaks in disease-free countries have been often associated with the feeding of uncooked swill originating from international air or sea transport. Therefore, preventative mesures are dependent on, first of all, prohibiting the importation of pigs and pork products from enzootic areas, cooking all swills of animal origin, and the destruction of waste foods from national transport at ports of entry. Although, to date, transmission of ASFV has not been associated with the introduction of wild pig species into zoological gardens or with the importation of biological materials, such as sera and ticks of porcine origin, these sources should be regarded as being potentially dangerous.

The control of an outbreak in an enzootic area depends on the rapid diagnosis, quarantine, slaughter, disposal of carcasses, and disinfection of premises. One major weakness has been the prevention of disposal of infected animals or their products before the full regulations come into effect. The difficulty of implementing these classical measures, because of administrative and financial reasons in some regions, especially those in which communal free-ranging husbandry is practiced, has necessitated attempts to control ASF through vaccination with an attenuated virus. This was considered possible in Europe because of the occurrence of a single antigenic type, unlike the enzootic situation in Africa where a number of different types are found. The method is not without serious disadvantages which include heavy loss from post-vaccine reaction resulting in chronic forms of disease and the creation of a permanent carrier status in the pig population, with as yet unpredictable and undetermined pathogenicity on continued pig-to-pig transmission. Therefore, the use of this method, in face of the need to prevent heavy losses through either eradication methods or allowing the uninhibited spread of the disease, has to be judged against the long-term effect it has on the swine production industry in a particular country.

Literature

Prevention, control, and eradication has been the subject of many international meetings dealing with the spread of ASFV outside Africa, which have been published in summaries and in full text in the *Bulletin of Epizootiologic Diseases of Africa*. The full text of international regulations and recommendations was published in 1961 and included those for horse sickness (Anon. 1961a, b) and in 1977 included classical swine fever (Anon. 1977). The historical account of the outbreaks in Kenya and their successful control was presented by Dorman (1965). The most comprehensive discussion of prevention, control, and eradication was published by Scott (1965b). The use of live attenuated virus vaccines has been described in Spain (Sanchez Botija 1963c) and in Portugal (Manso Ribeiro *et al.* 1963).

BIBLIOGRAPHY

Adldinger, H. K., Stone, S. S., Hess, W. R. and Bachrach, H. L., 1966. Extraction of infectious deoxyribonucleic acid from African swine fever virus, *Virology*, **30**: 750–2.

Almeida, J. D., Waterson, A. P. and Plowright, W., 1967. The morphological characteristics of African swine fever virus and its resemblance to *Tipula* iridescent virus, *Arch. Virusforsch.*, **20**: 392–6.

Anon., 1961a. Summary of the Proceedings of the Conference on African Swine Fever (ASF), *Bull. Off. int. Epiz.*, **55**: 223–9.

Anon., 1961b. Report of the FAO/OIE emergency meeting on African horse sickness and African swine fever, held in Paris, France, 17–20 Jan., *Bull. Off. int. Epiz.*, **55**: 75–537.

Anon., 1962. The geographical distribution of wart-hog and domestic pigs in Africa, *Bull. epiz. Dis. Afr.*, **10**: 91–2.

Anon., 1971. *Properties of the Virus of Classical Swine Fever and Differential Diagnosis of Classical and African Swine Fever.* Directorate-general for Agriculture, Commission of the European Communities.

Anon., 1977. Agricultural Research Seminar on Hog Cholera/Classical Swine Fever and African Swine Fever. Tierarztliche Hochschule Hannover, 6–11 Sept. 1976, Luxemburg. Director-General XIII.

Anon., 1978. *Bibliography on African Swine Fever.* Emergency Programs Veterinary Services, United States Department of Agriculture.

Anon., 1979. *Proceedings 83rd Annual Meeting of United States Animal Health Association.*

Anon., 1980. *Proc. 2nd Int. Symp. Vet. Lab. Diagnost.*, 24, 25, 26 June 1980, Lucerne (Switzerland).

Black, D. N. and Brown, F., 1976. Purification and physicochemical characteristics of African swine fever virus, *J. gen. Virol.*, **32**: 509–18.

Bool, P. H., 1967. Afrikaanse vorkenpest. African swine fever, *Tijdschr. Diergeneesk.*, **92**(25): 1731–6.

Bool, P. H., Ordas, A. and Botija, C. S., 1969. Diagnosis of African swine fever by immunofluorescence, *Bull. Off. int. Epiz.*, **72**: 819–39.

Boulanger, P., Bannister, G. L., Gray, D. P., Ruckerbauer, G. M. and Willis, N. G., 1967a. African swine fever. II. Detection of virus in swine tissues by means of the modified direct complement-fixation test, *Can. J. comp. Med.*, **31**: 7–11.

Boulanger, P., Bannister, G. L., Gray, D. P., Ruckerbauer, G. M. and Willis, N. G., 1967b. African swine fever. III. The use of agar double-diffusion precipitation test for the detection of the virus in swine tissues, *Can. J. comp. Med.*, **31**: 12–15.

Boulanger, P., Bannister, G. L., Greig, A. S., Gray, D. P. and Ruckerbauer, G. M., 1966. Diagnosis of African swine fever by

immunofluorescence and other serological methods, *Bull. Off. int. Epiz.*, **66**: 723–39.
Boulanger, P., Bannister, G. L., Greig, A. S., Gray, D. P., Ruckerbauer, G. M. and Willis, N. G., 1967c. African swine fever. IV. Demonstration of the viral antigen by means of immunofluorescence, *Can. J. comp. Med.* **31**: 16–23.
Breese, S. S. Jr and DeBoer, C. J., 1966. Electron microscope observations of African swine fever in tissue culture cells, *Virology*, **28**: 420–8.
Breese, S. S. Jr, Stone, S. S., DeBoer, C. J. and Hess, W. R., 1967. Electron microscopy of the interaction of African swine fever virus with ferritin-conjugated antibody, *Virology*, **31**: 508–13.

Carnero, R., Costes, C. and Picard, M., 1975. African swine fever: a clinical and laboratory study of the epizootical wave in January–March 1974, *Proc. 20th World Vet. Congr. Thessaloniki*, No. 3: 2201–3.
Carnero, R., Costes, C. and Picard, M., 1979. Peste porcine africaine. II. La maladie – sa prophylaxie, *Bull. Acad. Vét. France*, **52**: 391–400.
Carnero, R., Larenaudie, B., Ruiz Gonzalvo, F. and Haag, J., 1967. Peste porcine Africaine. Etudes sur la réaction d'hémadsorption et son inhibition par des anticorps spécifiques, *Rec. Méd. vét.*, **143**: 49–59.
Carnero, R., Lucas, A., Ruiz Gonzalvo, F. and Larenaudie, B., 1968. African swine fever. Use of immunofluorescence to study the virus in tissue culture, *Rec. Méd. vét.*, **144**: 937–49.
Coggins, L., 1966. Growth and certain stability characteristics of African swine fever virus, *Am. J. vet. Res.*, **27**(120): 1351–8.
Coggins, L., 1968a. Segregation of a nonhemadsorbing African swine fever virus in tissue culture, *Cornell Vet.*, **58**: 12–20.
Coggins, L., 1968b. A modified hemadsorption–inhibition test for African swine fever virus, *Bull. epiz. Dis. Afr.*, **16**: 61–4.
Coggins, L. P., 1974. African swine fever virus. Pathogenesis, *Progr. Med. Virol.*, **18**: 48–63.
Coggins, L. and Heuschele, W. P., 1966. Use of agar diffusion precipitation test in the diagnosis of African swine fever, *Am. J. vet. Res.*, **27**(117): 485–8.
Coggins, L., Moulton, J. E. and Colgrove, G. S., 1966. Studies with Hinde attenuated African swine fever virus, *Cornell Vet.*, **58**: 525–40.
Colgrove, G. S., 1968. Immunofluorescence and inclusion bodies in circulating leukocytes of pigs infected with African swine fever virus, *Bull. epiz. Dis. Afr.*, **16**: 341–3.
Colgrove, G. S., 1969. Diagnosis of African swine fever by fluorescent antibody staining of blood films and buffy coat smears, *Bull. epiz. Dis. Afr.*, **17**: 39–44.
Colgrove, G. S., Haelterman, E. O., Coggins, L., 1969. Pathogenesis

of African swine fever in young pigs, *Am. J. vet. Res.*, **30**: 1343–59.

Cottral, G. E. (ed.), 1978. *Manual of Standardized Methods for Veterinary Microbiology*. Cornell University Press (Ithaca, NY).

Cowan, K. M., 1961. Immunological studies on African swine fever virus. I. Elimination of the precomplementary activity of swine serum with formalin, *J. Immunol.*, **86**: 465–70.

Cowan, K. M., 1963. Immunologic studies on African swine fever virus. II. Enhancing effect of normal bovine serum on the complement-fixation reaction, *Am. J. vet. Res.*, **24**: 756–61.

Dalsgaard, K., Overby, E. and Sanchez Botija, C., 1977. Crossed immunoelectrophoretic characterization of virus-specified antigens in cells infected with African swine fever (ASF) virus, *J. gen. Virol.*, **36**(1): 203–6.

DeBoer, C. J., 1967. Studies to determine neutralizing antibody in sera from animals recovered from African swine fever and laboratory animals inoculated with African virus with adjuvants, *Arch. Virusforsch.*, **20**: 164–79.

DeBoer, C. J., Hess, W. R. and Dardiri, A. H., 1969. Studies to determine the presence of neutralizing antibody in sera and kidneys from swine recovered from African swine fever, *Arch. ges. Virusforsch.*, **27**: 44–54.

De Kock, G., Robinson, E. M., and Keppel, J. J. G., 1940. Swine fever in South Africa, *Onderstepoort J. Sci. Anim. Indust.*, **14**: 31–93.

DeTray, D. E., 1957a. African swine fever – a review, *Bull. epiz. Dis. Afr.*, **5**: 475–8.

DeTray, D. E., 1957b. African swine fever in warthogs (*Phacochoerus aethiopicus*), *J. Am. vet. med. Ass.*, **130**: 537–40.

DeTray, D. E., 1960. African swine fever – an interim report, *Bull. epiz. Dis. Afr.*, **8**: 217–23.

DeTray, D. E., 1963. African swine fever, *Adv. Vet. Sci.*, **8**: 299–333.

DeTray, D. E. and Scott, G. R., 1957. Blood changes in swine with African swine fever, *Am. J. vet. Res.*, **18**: 484–90.

DeTray, D. E., Zaphiro, D. and Hay, D., 1961. The incidence of African swine fever in warthogs in Kenya – a preliminary report, *J. Am. vet. med. Ass.* **138**: 78–80.

Dorman, A. E., 1965. The control of African swine fever in Kenya, *Bull. Off. int. Epiz.*, **63**: 807–23.

Doyle, T. M., 1961. African pig disease, *Br. vet. J.*, **117**: 229–38.

Drager, K. S., Kamphans, S. and Weigand, D., 1965. Zur Frage der Spezifität des Hamadsorptionstestes bei der afrikanischen Schweinepest, *Tierarztl. Umschau.*, **20**: 1–4.

Els, H. J. and Pini, A., 1977. Negative staining of a non-hemadsorbing strain of African swine fever virus, *Onderstepoort J. Vet. Res.*, **44**(1): 39–46.

Enjuanes, L., Carrascosa, A. L., Moreno, M. A. and Vinuela, E.,

1976a. Titration of African swine fever (ASF) virus, *J. gen. Virol.*, **32**(3): 471–7.
Enjuanes, L., Carrascosa, A. L. and Vinuela, E., 1976b. Isolation and properties of the DNA of African swine fever (ASF) virus, *J. gen. Virol.*, **32**: 479–92.
Enjuanes, L., Cubero, I. and Vinuela, E., 1977. Sensitivity of macrophages from different species to African swine fever (ASF) virus, *J. gen. Virol.*, **34**: 455–63.

FAO, 1979. *Report of the Technical Consultation on African Swine Fever.* Consultation convened by FAO in collaboration with the Ministry of Agricultural Development of Panama.
Fenner, F., 1976. Classification and nomenclature of viruses. Second report of the International Committee on Taxonomy of Viruses, *Intervirology*, **6**: 1–12.

Garcia-Gancedo, A., Ronda-Lain, E. and Rubio-Huertos, M., 1974. Ultrastructure of spleen and liver of swine infected with African swine fever, *Microbiol. Espanola.*, **27**: 177–89.
Gasse, H., 1963. Prévention de l'introduction éventuelle en France de la peste porcine Africaine, *Bull. Off. int. Epiz.*, **59**(11–12): 1867–72.
Greig, A., 1972a. Pathogenesis of African swine fever in pigs naturally exposed to the disease, *J. Comp. Path.*, **82**: 73–9.
Greig, A., 1972b. The localization of African swine fever virus in the tick *Ornithodorus moubata porcinus, Arch. ges. Virusforsch.*, **39**: 240–7.
Greig, A., 1975. The use of microtitration technique for the routine assay of African swine fever virus, *Arch. Virol.*, **47**: 287–9.
Greig, A. and Plowright, W., 1970. The excretion of two virulent strains of African swine fever virus by domestic pigs, *J. Hyg., Camb.*, **68**: 673–82.
Groocock, C. M., Hess, W. R. and Gladney, W. J., 1980. Experimental transmission of African swine fever virus by *Ornithodorus coriaceus*, an argasid tick indigenous to the United States, *Am. J. vet. Res.*, **41**(4): 591–4.

Haag, J. and Larenaudie, B., 1965. Peste porcine Africaine. L'effet cytopathogène du virus en culture leucocytaire, *Bull. Off. int. Epiz.*, **63**: 191–8.
Haag, J., Larenaudie, B. and Ruiz-Gonzalvo, F., 1965. Peste porcine Africaine. Action de la 5-iodo-2'désoxyuridine sur la culture du virus *in vitro, Bull. Off. int. Epiz.*, **63**(5–6): 717–22.
Haag, J., Lucas, A., Larenaudie, B., Ruiz-Gonzalvo, F. and Carnero, R., 1966. Peste porcine Africaine. Recherches sur taille et la morphologie du virus, *Rec. Méd. vét.*, **142**: 801–8.
Hamdy, F. M., Colgrove, G. S., de Rodriguez, E. M., Snyder, M. L.

and Stewart, W. C., 1981. Field evaluation of enzyme-linked immunosorbent assay for detection of antibody to African swine fever virus, *Am. J. vet. Res.*, **42**(8): 1441–3.

Hamdy, F. M. and Dardiri, A. H., 1979. Enzyme-linked immunosorbent assay for the diagnosis of African swine fever, *Vet. Rec.*, **105**: 445–6.

Hamdy, F. and Dardiri, A., 1980. Detection of antibody to African swine fever virus by enzyme-linked immunosorbent assay, *Proc. 2nd Int. Symp. Vet. Lab. Diagnost.*, Lucerne (Switzerland), pp. 240–3.

Hammond, R. A. and DeTray, D. E., 1955. A recent case of African swine fever in Kenya, East Africa, *J. Am. vet. med. Ass.*, **126**: 389–91.

Hess, W. R., 1971. African swine fever virus, *Virology Monographs*, **9**: 1–33.

Hess, W. R., 1981. African swine fever: a reassessment, *Ad. Vet. Sci. Comp. Med.*, **25**: 39–69.

Hess, W. R., Cox, B. F., Heuschele, W. P. and Stone, S. S., 1965. Propagation and modification of African swine fever virus in cell cultures, *Am. J. vet. Res.*, **26**: 141–6.

Hess, W. R. and DeTray, D. E., 1960. The use of leukocyte cultures for diagnosing African swine fever (ASF), *Bull. epiz. Dis. Afr.*, **8**: 317–20.

Hess, W. R. and DeTray, D. E., 1961. The use of leukocyte cultures for diagnosing African swine fever (ASF), *Bull. Off. int. Epiz.*, **55**: 201–4.

Heuschele, W. P., 1967. Studies on the pathogenesis of African swine fever. I. Quantitative studies on the sequential development of virus in pig tissues, *Arch. ges. Virusforsch.*, **21**: 349–56.

Heuschele, W. P. and Coggins, L., 1965a. Studies on the transmission of African swine fever virus by arthropods, *Proc. 69th Ann. Meet. US Livestock Sanit. Ass.*, 1965, pp. 94–100.

Heuschele, W. P. and Coggins, L., 1965b. Isolation of African swine fever virus from a giant forest hog, *Bull. epiz. Dis. Afr.*, **13**: 255–6.

Heuschele, W. P. and Coggins, L., 1969. Epizootiology of African swine fever virus in warthogs, *Bull. epiz. Dis. Afr.*, **17**: 179–83.

Heuschele, W. P. and Hess, W. R., 1973. Diagnosis of African swine fever by immunofluorescence, *Trop. Anim. Hlth Prod.*, **5**: 181–6.

Heuschele, W. P., Stone, S. S. and Coggins, L., 1965. Observations on the epizootiology of African swine fever, *Bull. epiz. Dis. Afr.*, **13**: 157–60.

Konno, S., Taylor, W. D. and Dardiri, A. H., 1971a. Acute African swine fever. Proliferative phase in lymphoreticular tissue and the reticuloendothelial system, *Cornell Vet.*, **16**: 71–84.

Konno, S., Taylor, W. D., Hess, W. R. and Heuschele, W. P., 1971b. Liver pathology in African swine fever, *Cornell Vet.*, **61**: 125–50.

Konno, S., Taylor, W. D., Hess, W. R. and Heuschele, W. P., 1972. Spleen pathology in African swine fever, *Cornell Vet.*, **62**(3): 486–506.

Korn, G., 1963. Uber die afrikanische Schweinepest und die Spezifität des Hamadsorptionstestes zu ihrer Diagnose, *Mschr. Tierheilk.*, **15**: 225–32.

Korn, G., 1964. The pathogenesis of swine fever as an immunopathological process in the allergic sense (with evidence of similar relationships in African swine fever, equine infectious anaemia and bovine mucosal disease), *Zbl. Vet. Med.*, **B11**: 379–92.

Kovalenko, Y. R., Sidorov, M. A. and Burba, L. G., 1964. Viability of African swine fever virus in environment, *Vestnik Sel, skokhoz, Nauki*, **9**: 62–5.

Kovalenko, Y. R., Sidorov, M. A. and Burba, L. G., 1965. Experimental investigations on African swine fever, *Bull. Off. int. Epiz.*, **63**: 169–89.

Kuznar, J., Salas, M. L. and Vinuela, E., 1980. DNA-dependent RNA polymerase in African swine fever virus, *Virology*, **101**: 169–75.

Kuznar, J., Salas, M. L. and Vinuela, E., 1981. Nucleoside triphosphate phosphohydrolase activities in African swine fever virus, *Arch. Virol.*, **69**: 307–10.

Leite Velho, E., 1956. Observations sur la peste porcine en Angola, *Bull. Off. int. Epiz.*, **46**: 335–40.

Leite Velho, E., 1958. La peste porcine africaine, *Bull. Off. int. Epiz.*, **48**: 395–402.

Lucas, A. and Carnero, R., 1968. Situation du virus de la peste porcine africaine dans la systématique virale, *C.R. Acad. Sci. (Paris)*, **266**: 1800–1.

Malmquist, W. A., 1962. Propagation, modification, and hemadsorption of African swine fever virus in cell cultures, *Am. J. vet. Res.*, **23**: 241–7.

Malmquist, W. A., 1963. Serologic and immunologic studies with African swine fever virus, *Am. J. vet. Res.*, **24**: 450–9.

Malmquist, W. A. and Hay, D., 1960. Hemadsorption and cytopathic effect produced by African swine fever virus in swine bone marrow and buffy coat cultures, *Am. J. vet. Res.*, **21**: 104–8.

Manso Ribeiro, J., 1970. Diagnosis of African swine fever, *Bull. Off. int. Epiz.*, **73**(11–12): 1045–55.

Manso Ribeiro, J., Nunes Petisa, J. L., Lopez Frazao, F. and Sobral, M., 1963. Vaccination against African swine fever, *Bull. Off. int. Epiz.*, **60**: 921–37.

Mansvelt, P. R., 1963. The incidence and control of African swine fever in the Republic of South Africa, *Bull. Off. int. Epiz.*, **60**: 889–94.

Maurer, F. D., Griesemer, R. A. and Jones, T. C., 1958. The pathology of African swine fever – a comparison with hog cholera, *Am. J. vet. Res.*, **19**(72): 517–39.

McVicar, J. W., Mebus, C. A., Becker, H. N., Belden, R. C. and Gibbs, E. P. J., 1981. Induced African swine fever in feral pigs, *J. Am. vet. med. Ass.*, **179**(5): 441–6.

McVicar, J. W., Mebus, C. A., Brynjolfsson, A. and Walker, J. S., 1982. Inactivation of African swine fever virus in tissues by gamma radiation, *Am. J. vet. Res.*, **43**(2): 318–19.

Mebus, C. A. and Dardiri, A. H., 1979. Additional characteristics of disease caused by the African swine fever viruses isolated from Brazil and the Dominican Republic, *Proc. 83rd Ann. Meet. US Anim. Hlth Ass.*, **83**: 227–39.

Mebus, C. A. and Dardiri, A. H., 1980. Western hemisphere isolates of African swine fever virus: asymptomatic carriers and resistance to challenge inoculation, *Am. J. vet. Res.*, **41**(11): 1867–9.

Mendes, A. M. and Daskalos, de O. A. M., 1955. Studies on the lapinization of swine fever virus in Angola, *Bull. epiz. Dis. Afr.*, **3**: 9–14.

Montgomery, R. E., 1921. On a form of swine fever occurring in British East Africa (Kenya Colony), *J. Comp. Path.*, **34**: 159–91, 243–62.

Moreno, M. A., Carrascosa, A. L., Ortin, J. and Venuela, E., 1978. Inhibition of African swine fever (ASF) virus replication by phosphonoacetic acid, *J. gen. Virol.*, **39**: 253–8.

Moulton, J. and Coggins, L., 1968a. Synthesis and cytopathogenesis of African swine fever virus in porcine cell cultures, *Am. J. vet. Res.*, **29**(2): 219–32.

Moulton, J. and Coggins, L., 1968b. Comparison of lesions in acute and chronic African swine fever, *Cornell Vet.*, **58**: 364–88.

Moura Nunes, J. F., Vigario, J. D. and Terrinha, A. M., 1975. Ultrastructural study of African swine fever virus replication in cultures of swine bone marrow cells, *Arch. Virol.*, **49**: 59–66.

Neitz, W. O., 1963. African swine fever. In *Emerging Diseases of Animals*. FAO Agricultural Studies (Rome), vol. 61, pp. 1–70.

Norley, S. G. and Wardley, R. C., 1982. Complement-mediated lysis of African swine fever virus-infected cells. *Immunology*, **46**: 75–82.

Pan, I. C., De Boer, C. J. and Hess, W. R., 1972. African swine fever: application of immunoelectroosmophoresis for the detection of antibody, *Can. J. comp. Med.*, **36**(3): 309–16.

Pan, I. C., De Boer, C. J. and Heuschele, W. P., 1970. Hypergammaglobulinemia in swine infected with African swine fever virus (34794), *Proc. Soc. Exp. Biol. Med.*, **134**: 367–71.

Pan, I. C., Shimizu, M. and Hess, W. R., 1978. African swine fever:

microplaque assay by an immunoperoxidase method, *Am. J. vet. Res.*, **39**(3): 491–7.

Pan, I. C., Shimizu, M. and Hess, W. R., 1980. Replication of African swine fever virus in cell cultures, *Am. J. vet. Res.*, **41**(9): 1357–67.

Pan, I. C., Trautman, R., DeBoer, C. J. and Hess, W. R., 1974a. African swine fever: hypergammaglobulinemia and the iodine agglutination test, *Am. J. vet. Res.*, **35**(5): 629–31.

Pan, I. C., Trautman, R., Hess, W. R., DeBoer, C. J. and Tessler, J., 1974b. African swine fever: detection of antibody by reverse single radial immunodiffusion, *Am. J. vet. Res.*, **35**(3): 351–4.

Parker, J. and Plowright, W., 1968. Plaque formation by African swine fever virus, *Nature*, **219**: 524–5.

Pereira Henriques, R., Nunes Petisca, J. L. and Costa Durao, J., 1976. Situation actuelle des pestes porcines au Portugal, *Bull. Off. int. Epiz.*, **85**(3–4): 461–6.

Peritz, F. J., 1980. African swine fever in Latin America, *Wld Anim. Rev.*, **36**: 29–33.

Pini, A., 1977. African swine fever: some observations and considerations, *S. Afr. J. Sci.*, **73**: 133–4.

Pini, A. and Hurter, L. R., 1975. African swine fever: an epizootiological review with special reference to the South African situation, *J. S. Afr. vet. med. Ass.*, **46**: 227–32.

Plowright, W., Brown, F. and Parker, J., 1966. Evidence for the type of nucleic acid in African swine fever virus, *Arch. ges. Virusforsch.*, **19**: 289–304.

Plowright, W. and Parker, J., 1967. The stability of African swine fever virus with particular reference to heat and pH inactivation, *Arch. ges. Virusforsch.*, **21**: 383–402.

Plowright, W., Parker, J. and Pierce, M. A., 1969a. The epizootiology of African swine fever in Africa, *Vet. Rec.*, **85:** 668–74.

Plowright, W., Parker, J. and Pierce, M. A., 1969b. African swine fever virus in ticks (*Ornithodorus moubata*, Murray) collected from animal burrows in Tanzania, *Nature, Lond.*, **221**: 1071–3.

Plowright, W., Parker, J. and Staple, R. F., 1968. The growth of a virulent strain of African swine fever virus in domestic pigs, *J. Hyg. Camb.* **66**: 117- 34.

Plowright, W., Perry, C. T. and Greig, A., 1974. Sexual transmission of African swine fever virus in the tick, *Ornithodorus moubata porcinus*, Walton, *Res. vet. Sci.*, **17**: 106–13.

Plowright, W., Perry, C. T. and Peirce, M. A., 1970a. Transovarial infection with African swine fever in the argasid tick, *Ornithodoros moubata porcinus*, *Res. vet. Sci.*, **11**: 582–4.

Plowright, W., Perry, C. T., Peirce, M. A. and Parker, J., 1970b. Experimental infection of the argasid tick, *Ornithodorus moubata porcinus*, with African swine fever virus, *Arch. ges. Virusforsch.*, **31**: 33–50.

Polo Jover, F. and Sanchez Botija, C., 1961. African swine fever in Spain, *Bull. Off. int. Epiz.*, **55**: 107–47.

Ribeiro, A. M. R., Vigario, J. D. and Lage, M. D., 1975. African swine fever in Portugal, *Proc. 20th Wld Vet. Congr. Thessaloniki*, No. 3: 2190–4.

Rodriguez, O. N., Fernandes, A., Chamizo, E. and del Pozo, E., 1972. Observaciones clínicas y morfológicas en el brote de fiebre porcina africana en Cuba, *Revta. cuban. Cienc. vet.*, **3**(1): 1–18.

Salas, M. L., Kuznar, J. and Vinuela, E., 1981. Polyadenylation, methylation, and capping of the RNA synthesized *in vitro* by African swine fever virus, *Virology*, **113**: 484–91.

Sanchez Botija, C., 1962. Estudios sobre la peste porcine African en Espàna, *Bull. epiz. Dis. Afr.*, **58**: 707–27.

Sanchez Botija, C., 1963a. La peste suina Africana, *Zooprofilassi*, **18**: 587–607.

Sanchez Botija, C., 1963b. Reservorios del virus de la peste porcina Africana. Investigación del virus de la P.P.A. en los artrópodos mediante la prueba de la hemoadsorción, *Bull. Off. int. Epiz.*, **60**: 895–9.

Sanchez Botija, C., 1963c. Modificación del virus peste porcina Africana en cultivos celulares. Contribución al conocimiento de la acción patógena y del poder de protección de las estirpes atenuadas, *Bull. Off. int. Epiz.*, **60**: 901–19.

Sanchez Botija, 1971. Diagnostic de la peste porcine Africaine par l'immunofluorescence, *Bull. Off. int. Epiz.*, **73**: (11–12): 1025–36.

Sanchez Botija, C. and Badiola, C., 1966. Presencia del virus de la peste porcine Africana en el *Haematopinus suis*, *Bull. Off. int. Epiz.*, **66**: 699–705.

Sanchez Botija, C., Garcio-Gonzales, J. and Ordas, A., 1971. Indirect immunofluorescence to detect antibodies to African swine fever. Its diagnostic value, *Zooprofilassi*, **26**: 111–28.

Sanchez Botija, C. and Ordas, A., 1969. Diagnóstico differencial de rutina de la peste porcine Clasica y de la peste porcine Africana por immunofluorescencia y hemoadsorción asociadas, *Bull. Off. int. Epiz.*, **72**: 763–84.

Sanchez-Vizcaino, J. M., Slauson, D. O., Ruiz-Gonzalvo, F. and Valero, F., 1981. Lymphocyte function and cell-mediated immunity in pigs with experimentally induced African swine fever, *Am. J. vet. Res.*, **42**: (8): 1335–41.

Scott, G. R., 1965a. The virus of African swine fever and its transmission, *Bull. Off. int. Epiz.*, **63**(5–6): 645–77.

Scott, G. R., 1965b. II. Prevention, control, and eradication of African swine fever, *Bull. Off. int. Epiz.*, **63**(5–6): 751–64.

Scott, G. R., 1965c. African swine fever, *Vet. Rec.*, **77**: 1421–7.

Scott, G. R. and Hill, D. H., 1966. Failure to detect African swine fever virus in Nigerian dwarf pigs, *Bull. epiz. Dis. Afr.*, **14**: 55–7.

Shimizu, M., Pan, I. C. and Hess, W. R., 1977. Cellular immunity demonstrated in pigs infected with African swine fever virus, *Am.*

J. vet. Res., **38**(1): 27–31.

Simpson, V. R. and Drager, N., 1979. African swine fever antibody detection in warthogs, *Vet. Rec.*, **105**: 61.

Slauson, D. O. and Sanchez-Vizcaino, J. M., 1981. Leukocyte-dependent platelet vasoactive amine release and immune complex deposition in African swine fever, *Vet. Pathol.*, **18**: 813–26.

Spuhler, V., 1967. Uber die africanische Schweinepest, *Schweizer Arch. Tierheilk.*, **109**(5): 273–80.

Steyn, D. G., 1932. East African virus disease in pigs, *18th Rep. Dir. vet. Ser. Anim. Indust., S. Afr.*, **1**: 99–109.

Stone, S. S. and Hess, W. R., 1965. Separation of virus and soluble noninfectious antigens in African swine fever virus by isoelectric precipitation, *Virology*, **26**: 622–9.

Stone, S. S. and Hess, W. R., 1967. Antibody responses to inactivated preparation of African swine fever virus in pigs, *Am. J. vet. Res.*, **28**: 475–81.

Stone, S. S. and Heuschele, W. P., 1965. The role of the hippopotamus in the epizootiology of African swine fever: (A survey of the incidence of African swine fever virus in hippopotami in Queen Elizabeth National Park, Uganda), *Bull. epiz. Dis. Afr.*, **13**: 23–8.

Tabarés, E., Marcotegui, M. A., Fernandez, M. and Sanchez Botija C., 1980a. Proteins specified by African swine fever virus. I. Analysis of viral structural proteins and antigenic properties, *Arch. Virol.*, **66**: 107–17.

Tabarés, E., Martinez, J., Ruiz Gonzalvo, F. and Sanchez Botija, C., 1980b. Proteins specified by African swine fever virus. II. Analysis of proteins in infected cells and antigenic properties, *Arch. Virol.*, **66**: 119–32.

Tabarés, E. and Sanchez Botija, C., 1979. Synthesis of DNA in cells infected with African swine fever, *Arch. Virol.*, **61**: 49–59.

Taylor, W. P., Best, J. R. and Colquhoun, I. R., 1977. Absence of African swine fever from Nigerian warthogs, *Bull. Anim. Hlth Prod.*, **25**: 196–7.

Terpstra, J. I., 1961. African swine fever, *Tijdschr. Diergeneesk.*, **20**: 1324–31.

Tessler, J., Hess, W. R., Pan, I. C. and Trautman, R., 1974. Immunofluorescence plaque assay for African swine fever virus, *Can. J. comp. Med.*, **38**: 443–7.

Thomson, G. R., Gainaru, M. D. and van Dellen, A. F., 1979. African swine fever: pathogenicity and immunogenicity of two non-hemadsorbing viruses, *Onderstepoort J. vet. Res.*, **46**: 149–54.

Trautman, R., Pan, I. C. and Hess, W. R., 1980. Sedimentation coefficient of African swine fever virus, *Am. J. vet. Res.*, **41**(11): 1874–8.

Vigário, J. D., Relvas, M. E., Ferraz, F. P., Ribeiro, J. M. and Pereira, C. G., 1967. Identification and localization of genetic material of African swine fever virus by autoradiography, *Virology*, **33**: 173–5.

Vigário, J. D., Terrinha, A. M., Bastos, A. L., Moura-Nunes, J. F., Marques, D. and Silva, J. F., 1970. Serological behaviour of isolated swine fever virus. Brief report, *Arch. ges. Virusforsch.*, **31**: 387–9.

Vigário, J. D., Terrinha, A. M. and Moura-Nunes, J. F., 1974. Antigenic relationships among strains of African swine fever virus, *Arch. ges. Virusforsch.*, **45**: 272–7.

Wardley, R. C., Hamilton, F. and Wilkinson, P. J., 1979. The replication of virulent and attenuated strains of African swine fever virus in porcine macrophages, *Arch. Virol.*, **61**: 217–25.

Wardley, R. C. and Wilkinson, P. J., 1977. The growth of virulent African swine fever virus in pig monocytes and macrophages, *J. gen Virol.*, **38**: 183–6.

Wardley, R. C. and Wilkinson, P. J.,1980a. Detection of African swine fever virus antigen and antibody by radioimmunoassay, *Vet. Microbiol.*, **5**: 169–76.

Wardley, R. C. and Wilkinson, P. J., 1980b. Lymphocyte responses to African swine fever virus infection, *Res. vet. Sci.*, **28**: 185–9.

Wardley, R. C. and Wilkinson, P. J., 1980c. A microtechnique for the titration for African swine fever virus. Brief report, *Arch. Virol.*, **64**: 93–5.

Wilkinson, P. J. and Donaldson, A. I., 1977. Transmission studies with African swine fever virus. The early distribution of virus in pigs infected by airborne virus, *J. Comp. Path.*, **87**: 497–501.

Wilkinson, P. J. and Wardley, R. C., 1978. The replication of African swine fever virus in pig endothelial cells, *Br. vet. J.*, **134**: 280–2.

Wilkinson, P. J., Wardley, R. C. and Williams, S. M., 1981. African swine fever virus (Malta/78) in pigs, *J. Comp. Path.*, **91**: 277–84.

Chapter

7

Bluetongue

CONTENTS

INTRODUCTION

Bluetongue (BT) is an arboviral disease of sheep and cattle which occasionally affects other ruminants. It is characterized by inflammation of the mucous membranes of the digestive and respiratory tracts, necrosis of skeletal muscles, placentitis, abortion, and fetal malformation. Emaciation and weakness follow the acute disease, resulting in protracted convalescence and serious loss of productivity. There is currently considerable interest in BT virus because of the apparent spread of the disease outside the African continent. It is likely that, in those countries outside Africa where the virus is currently identified and is of concern because of restrictions imposed by the international movement of livestock, infection has already occurred at some distant port.

Ibaraki and epizootic hemorrhagic disease (EHD) of deer viruses are antigenically related to members of the BT complex and cause diseases which are clinically similar to BT. Ibaraki virus was originally isolated in Japan in 1959. It affects cattle but not sheep and causes an acute febrile disease characterized by fever, stomatitis, and deglutitive difficulty. Epizootic hemorrhagic disease of deer occurs in North America and primarily affects deer, to some degree cattle, but not sheep.

Literature

The history of BT in Africa and the geographic distribution of the disease were described by Henning (1956) and Neitz (1966). Major reviews were published by Howell (1963, 1966) and particular aspects of the disease were discussed by Owen (1965). An early description of BT in sheep, a syndrome referred to as 'soremuzzle', was provided by Hardy and Price (1952). The isolation of BT virus from cattle in the USA was by Bowne *et al.* (1966). An early report on the occurrence of BT in the USA was presented by McGowan (1953). Comprehensive reviews were published by Howell and Verwoerd (1971) and Bowne (1971). The papers presented at a symposium on BT were published in 1975 (Symposium on bluetongue 1975; Anon. 1974). The latest reviews on BT, Ibaraki disease, and EHD were presented by Sellers (1981), and by Jones *et al.* (1981).

ETIOLOGY

Bluetongue is a virus of the *Orbivirus* genus in the family Reoviridae. The BT virus complex consists of many serologically related species and serotypes. The serological specificity is defined by the neutralization test. The virus is 65 to 80 nm in diameter, the genome is a double-stranded ribonucleic acid (RNA) comprised of 10 segments, and the capsid has 32 capsomeres. Bluetongue virus is resistant to adverse conditions and retains its viability even in decomposed blood for considerable periods of time, but it is inactivated by postmortem changes occurring in muscle at a pH below 6. It is stable at 4 and

−70 °C, but loses infectivity when frozen at −20 °C. The stability is dependent to a certain degree on the medium. Although the composition of the virus is stable in some tissues and biological fluids, it is extremely unstable in media which do not contain protein.

Bluetongue virus from natural infections can be isolated in embryonated chicken eggs and with some difficulty in tissue cultures. However, an egg-adapted virus can be grown in a variety of tissue cultures, including lamb and bovine kidney cells, causing a cytopathic effect which is the basis of plaque assay techniques. Intravascular inoculation is the most effective method of infecting embryonated chicken eggs, which are used to isolate the virus from blood and semen samples and various cell cultures. Suckling mice are also susceptible to intracerebral infection. The incubation temperature influences the efficiency of isolation and the multiplication of virus and is optimal at 33.6 °C. There is a linear relationship between the virus titer inoculated and the survival time of the embryo.

Bluetongue and related viruses in the *Orbivirus* genus are placed in a serological subgroup based on the results of complement fixation (CF) tests, but at times the agar-gel immune diffusion and fluorescent antibody (FA) tests are used for classification purposes. Bluetongue viruses are members of the subgroup which had identical serological reactions in subgroup reactive tests. The subgroups contained different antigenic types as determined by the neutralization test.

Literature

Various arboviruses, including BT and EHD disease of deer, were classified on the basis of stability to solvents, lability at pH 3.0, and serological and morphological relationships (Borden *et al.* 1971). Bluetongue and African horse sickness viruses (AHSVs) were similar with respect to structure, chemical composition, and biological properties and could be distinguished mainly on serological grounds and by differences in host specificity. The double-stranded RNAs from these two viruses were tested for hybridization with messenger RNA derived from BT virus- and reovirus-infected cells. A small amount of hybridization between BT and AHSVs was obtained (Verwoerd and Huismans 1969).

The physicochemical and morphological relationships of various arthropod-borne viruses to BT virus have been investigated, and a new taxonomic group was proposed with bluetongue virus as the prototype (Murphy *et al.* 1971). Foster (1976) summarized the morphology, stability, and molecular synthesis of BT virus. Two distinct morphological types of BT virus particles were isolated from tissue culture; both were infectious and contained a double-stranded RNA genome (Bowne and Ritchie 1970; Martin and Zweerink, 1972; Verwoerd, 1969). In tissue culture, the nonenveloped virus was 100 nm in diameter, and there was evidence that the particle had an icosahedral shape (Owen and Munz 1966). The capsid of the virion consisted of a single layer of 32 capsomeres (Els and Verwoerd 1969). Like BT virus, Ibaraki virus contained double-stranded RNA, was 55 nm in diameter, lacked an envelope, and had a capsid composed of 32 capsomeres (Ito *et al.* 1973; Inaba 1975).

Oligonucleotide fingerprinting was used to characterize BT virus isolates. The results indicated that viruses represented naturally occurring reassortant viruses (Sugiyama *et al.* 1981). Bluetongue virus type 20, an Australian isolate, contained unique sequences in its genome as determined by oligonucleotide mapping. Using an RNA–RNA reassociation assay, no significant homology could be demonstrated between the genome segments of BT virus type 20 and selected viruses of the BT and Eubenangee serogroups (Gorman *et al.* 1981). Protein synthesis in BT virus-infected cells was investigated (Huismans 1979), and the activation and characterization of a BT virus-associated transcriptase was studied (van Dijk and Huismans 1980). Bluetongue virus was found to be an exceptionally good inducer of interferon in animals and cell cultures derived from many species (Jameson and Grossberg 1981).

The resistance of BT virus of pH, temperature, and chemicals has been investigated in infected biological material and premises. The persistence of BT virus in the muscle of ovine and bovine carcasses was dependent on postmortem pH changes and on the stage of the disease at which the animal was slaughtered. Inactivation occurred below a pH of 6.3. The virus could survive for a period of 30 days at 4 °C in mutton when the pH did not fall below 6.3 (Owen 1964). The thermal stability of BT virus under various conditions was studied. At pH 7.0 it was stable for 3 years at room temperature (Svehag 1963). The thermal stability of the virus could be improved by the addition of protein to the medium (Howell *et al.* 1967). The temperature-sensitive mutants of BT virus were characterized in terms of early or late physiological functions affected and on the ability to synthesize RNA (Shipham and de la Rey 1979). Virucidal chemical agents commonly used for disinfectant purposes were sufficiently effective to inactivate BT virus even when a considerable quantity of extraneous material was present (McCrory *et al.* 1959). The resistance of the virus to various chemical agents is also influenced by protein composition which is present in the medium (Howell and Verwoerd 1971).

Considerable work has been undertaken on culture systems for isolation and growth of various isolates. The intravenous inoculation of embryonating chicken eggs for the isolation and identification of BT virus was found to be an improvement over the yolk-sac route of inoculation. The difference between the LD_{50} titers of the virus in the eggs inoculated by the intravenous and yolk-sac routes was 3 logs. The mortality of the embryo after intravenous inoculation was 100% in the first egg passage. Ten days were required for the isolation and typing of the virus when the intravenous route was used. With the yolk-sac method of inoculation, mortality did not reach 100% until the sixth or seventh passage and the time required for typing of the virus was 7 to 8 weeks (Goldsmit and Barzilai 1968). Intravascular inoculation of embryonating chicken eggs enabled a direct assay for BT virus that was as sensitive as the inoculation of susceptible sheep (Foster and Luedke 1968; Foster *et al.* 1972).

The cultivation of the virus in lamb kidney cells was first described by Haig *et al.* (1956). Subsequently, a number of systems were employed for isolating the virus and studying its development in tissue culture. Embryonating chicken eggs and VERO cell cultures were used for the isolation of the virus from semen samples (Breckon *et al.* 1980). The cytopathogenic effects of the virus on various tissues of newborn lambs in primary explant cultures following inoculation *in vitro* were investigated. In cultures inoculated after the production of good cellular outgrowth, a complete cytopathogenic effect occurred within 6 days of infection. No significant differences were observed in the susceptibility of the different tissue explants to BT virus. However, there was some indication that fibroblast-like cells were more susceptible than epithelial-like cells (Fernandes 1959).

The growth and replication of BT virus in tissue culture was investigated using the FA titration and microscopic techniques. The virus was adsorbed and the cell was penetrated by means of pinocytosis within the first 5 to 10 minutes (Howell and Verwoerd 1971). Using acridine orange and fluorescent-tagged antibody procedures, it was demonstrated that mature particles were formed in the cytoplasm of infected cells (Livingston and Moore 1962). Two types of intracytoplasmic inclusion bodies were demonstrated in cultured cells infected with BT virus. Type I inclusion bodies arose from the perinuclear space within the nuclear envelope and were not associated with viral synthesis. Type II inclusion bodies appeared to originate in the nucleus, were associated with viral synthesis, and fluoresced in response to specific BT virus conjugate when they migrated to the cytoplasm (Bowne and Jochim 1967).

The formation of antigens stained with FA was related to the production of infective particles in cultured baby hamster kidney (BHK) cells (Ohder *et al.* 1970). In cells infected with BT virus, the first cytopathic effect was usually observed after an incubation period of about 40 to 70 hours, but evidence of cellular destruction might be seen as early as 24 hours. Initially, the cytopathic effects were limited to a few cells which became swollen and detached from the glass. The process of cellular destruction spread rapidly and eventually affected all cells in the culture (Howell and Verwoerd 1971). The cytopathic effects caused by three strains of BT virus consisted of shrinkage of cells and increased granularity. Although these changes were not specific, the presence of the virus was confirmed by the FA technique (Girard *et al.* 1967). Plaque formation by BT virus in a line of mouse fibroblast cells was described. The cytopathic changes were related to the increase in the titer of the virus. The growth pattern was consistent for a particular isolate, but the rate of multiplication and yield of virus varied between different strains. Antigenically different strains varied with respect to plaque morphology and size. In addition, environmental factors appeared to influence the development and size of plaques (Howell *et al.* 1967). Ibaraki and BT viruses shared a number of biological properties, including the ability to multiply in embryonated eggs, tissue cultures, and the brains of mice (Inaba 1975). Ibaraki virus was isolated in bovine cell cultures and became less virulent for calves upon serial passage. The bovine cell culture system was less sensitive than calf inoculation for the primary detection of the virus (Omori *et al.* 1969b). This virus induced cytopathogenic effects in primary cultures of sheep and BHK and chick embryo cells (Inaba 1975).

EPIZOOTIOLOGY

Geographical distribution and incidence

Bluetongue probably originated in southern Africa and spread to various regions of the world, most likely primarily by shipment of livestock, and possibly on some occasions by movement of the vector. The disease was first recognized in South Africa between 1870 and 1880. It subsequently spread to East, West, and North Africa, the Mediterranean countries, North and South America, the Caribbean, Asia, and Australia. The disease was reported in Cyprus, the eastern Mediterranean and the USA between 1940 and 1950, and it was recognized in Europe, Pakistan, and Japan between 1950 and 1960. Due to its rapid and continuous dissemination throughout the world, BT has become an important disease which causes considerable economic loss to the sheep-raising and cattle industries from loss of exports. Major economic losses result from the high morbidity and mortality in ewes and lambs. In surviving animals, there is a prolonged convalescent period, unthriftiness, and damage to the wool. Losses are also caused by embargoes on the movement of animals and semen and by the serological testing necessary in the international livestock trade.

Ibaraki disease has been reported only in cattle in southeast Asia, while EHD of deer has been observed primarily in North America.

In enzootic areas, outbreaks of BT and related diseases occur annually during the summer months, and the extent of the epizootics varies from one year to another. These diseases disappear with the onset of winter.

Serological surveys have shown that the BT complex has a worldwide distribution. However, in a discussion of epizootiology, important distinctions have to be made between the occurrence of the disease, inapparent infections, and the presence of antibodies which, depending on the serological test used, may cross-react with other viruses. The disease entity was originally defined in and confined to Africa. Because BT virus varies considerably in its virulence for sheep and other ruminants, mild and inapparent infections occur. The infections may remain undetected unless a particular strain of virus is sufficiently virulent to cause disease. The virus may circulate in the local breeds without causing clinical syndromes.

Literature

The history of the isolation and spread of BT virus in South Africa was reviewed by Henning (1956) and Neitz (1966). Bluetongue infections have been recognized as causing significant economic losses. Direct losses are due to high mortality and morbidity, and indirect losses are a consequence of protracted convalescence which results in a marked loss of condition, retarded wool growth, damage to the musculature, susceptibility to secondary infections, and reduced breeding efficiency (Erasmus 1975a).

A survey of the species composition and prevalence of the *Culicoides* midge populations in BT-enzootic areas of Kenya was conducted to determine some of the epizootiological factors involved in the dissemination of the disease. Bluetongue virus was isolated from several *Culicoides* species known to feed on cattle and sheep, and a high proportion of wild and domestic bovids were seropositive for the virus (Walker and Davies 1971). When the sera of cattle, sheep, goats, and 11 wild bovid species from different locations in Kenya were screened for antibody to BT virus by indirect immunofluorescence, it was found that the distribution of clinical disease was more restricted than the distribution of antibody. *Culicoides pallidipennis*, the most widespread species, was the presumptive vector of BT in Kenya (Davies and Walker 1974). Nineteen different serological types of BT antibodies were found in a group of sentinel cattle in Kenya. These animals were continuously challenged by the 19 strains each year (Davies 1978). A survey in Botswana demonstrated precipitating antibodies to BT virus in the sera of cattle, camels, sheep, goats, and seven species of game animals. In sheep, the incidence was approximately 40%, while in the other three species it was 80 to 90% (Simpson 1979). Serological studies of domestic and wild animals in Nigeria showed that the incidence of antibodies to BT and related viruses was high in cattle and sheep. Antibodies were not detected in the sera of swine, chickens, shrews, rodents, or wild birds (Moore and Kemp 1974). Using the agar-gel diffusion test, it was determined that about 30 to 50% of the cattle, sheep, and goats in northern Nigeria were seropositive for BT (Taylor and McCausland 1976). The agar-gel precipitation technique showed that the incidence of BT virus antibodies in the sera of camels, cattle, goats, and sheep in the Sudan was approximately 5 to 28% (Eisa *et al.* 1979). There was a report on the epizootics of BT which occurred in Egypt in 1969 and 1970 (Soliman *et al.* 1972). Serological tests for BT were performed in Egypt, and antibodies were detected in sheep, water buffalo, cattle, goats, and camels. The incidence of BT precipitating antibodies in ovine sera collected from disease-free and enzootic areas was about 9 and 37% respectively (Hafez and Ozawa 1973).

It was postulated that the disease spread outside the African continent by the movement of infected animals into regions where the insect vectors and prevailing climatic conditions were favorable for the persistence and dissemination of the virus. It was probable that the virus was more widespread than was generally accepted, but because the infections did not induce clinical signs or lesions, it was not recognized. The lack of gross clinical symptoms was possibly due to the high natural resistance of the indigenous breeds of sheep and other ruminants and/or the presence of strains of virus of low virulence (Howell 1963).

The disease was first diagnosed outside the African continent in Cyprus and then in the eastern Mediterranean countries. The disease has been observed on the island since 1924, although the virus was not isolated and identified until 1949. After an analysis of the primary outbreaks, it was concluded that the epizootic cycle could arise from changes in the virus on the island or from the introduction of new antigenic types from abroad (Sellers 1975). The possible origin of the BT virus responsible for outbreaks in Cyprus in 1977 was thought to be wind-borne midges from remote enzootic regions (Sellers *et al.* 1979). In this epizootic, 13.1% of 27 837 sheep were affected (Polydorou 1978).

Verge and Paraf (1957) reviewed the epizootiology of the disease in the Iberian Peninsula. The occurrence of BT in Spain was described by Lopez (1957), who reported that there was a wide variation in the morbidity and mortality observed in different locations in Spain during the 1956 epizootic. The overall morbidity and mortality rates were approximately 3 and 1.5% respectively (Lopez and Sanchez Botija 1958). During the 1956 epizootic in Portugal, the incidence of morbidity was approximately 11% and that of mortality was about 6% (Manso-Ribeiro *et al.* 1957). The possible sources of the latter epizootic were examined. The introduction of the disease through the importation of wild or domestic ruminants was considered unlikely, and the possibility of wind-borne spread of *Culicoides* midges from North Africa was discussed (Sellers *et al.* 1978).

The virus has been reported from other Mediterranean countries. In Iraq, the incidence of BT was approximately 6% in sheep, 24% in goats, and 8% in cattle (Hafez 1978). A serological survey showed that sheep, cattle, goats, camels, and pigs in Iran had an infection rate between 0.6 and 13.6%, but serum samples from water buffalo were negative (Afshar and Kayvanfar 1974). A strain of BT virus was identified in Israel in 1952 (Komarov and Haig 1952). During an epizootic of BT in Israel in 1964, the general rate of morbidity was approximately 21% and the mortality was 31.4% (Dafni 1966).

The epizootiology of bluetongue in the USA was reviewed, with particular emphasis on entomological factors (Jones *et al.* 1981). The findings of surveys performed in the USA between 1968 and 1978 on sera obtained from cattle and other ruminants were summarized by Metcalf *et al.* (1981). In a survey conducted during 1978 and 1979, serological and viral identification techniques were used to study the epizootiology of BT in four western states. Four of the 20 known serotypes of BT were isolated from sheep, cattle, and goats, and herds and flocks with multiple serotype infections were reported. On most ranches where the virus was recovered from sheep and cattle, multiple serotype infections occurred in cattle only, indicating that cattle might be the reservoir. Viral isolates were made from cattle and sheep which had no demonstrable evidence of agar-gel precipitating antibodies

(Osburn *et al.* 1981). The presence of BT in sheep in California was confirmed in 1952 (McKercher *et al.* 1953). Initially, the disease was enzootic in the Southwest and then spread to other regions (Bowne *et al.* 1964). The earlier work on the identification and epizootiology of BT in sheep in the USA was reported (McCrory *et al.* 1957; Price and Hardy 1954; McKercher *et al.* 1957b; Anon. 1958), and the incidence and distribution of the virus during the period from 1948 to 1966 were described (Kennedy 1968; Anon. 1965). The epizootiology of the disease in the USA was reviewed up to 1973 (Hourrigan and Klingsporn, 1975b). The geographical distribution of various serotypes of BT virus detected in the USA between 1953 and 1977 was summarized (Barber 1979). A serological survey of cattle, goats, sheep, and wildlife in the USA in 1978 indicated that the overall incidence of BT was 2% (Klingsporn 1978). Approximately 3% of the caprine sera and 30% of the bovine sera collected in Louisiana from 1979 to 1981 were positive for BT viral antibodies by an immunodiffusion test (Fulton *et al.* 1981, 1982). In a serological survey of cattle slaughtered in the USA during the winter of 1977–78, the prevalence of BT viral antibodies ranged from 0 to 79%, with a national prevalence of approximately 18% (Metcalf *et al.* 1979, 1980, 1981). In South Carolina, serologically positive dairy cattle were not found to have associated reproductive problems (Barnes *et al.* 1982).

Serological studies indicated that the distribution of BT virus in wild ruminants in North America paralleled that of the disease in livestock (Trainer and Jochim 1969). Epizootic hemorrhagic disease of deer was reported in the USA in 1955 (Sellers 1981). Sera obtained from mule deer in New Mexico were found to be positive for antibodies to BT and EHD (Couvillion *et al.* 1980). In India, an outbreak of BT occurred in sheep in 1967 (Bhambani and Singh 1968). Using the micro-agar-gel precipitation test, Sodhi *et al.* (1981) determined that the incidence of BT in sheep and goats in Punjab, India, was approximately 1 and 7% respectively. In a similar survey, it was demonstrated that dairy cattle in the same region had an average infection rate of about 7% and that buffalo were seronegative (Sharma *et al.* 1981).

There are a number of reports on the current status of BT infection in Australia. The first isolation of BT virus in this country was from *Culicoides* midges collected in 1975; positive identification of the virus was made in 1977. However, clinical disease was not associated with the evidence of BT infection in any livestock species in Australia. The virus was designated a new serotype and was experimentally shown to be moderately pathogenic for sheep (Anon. 1979; Snowdon and Gee 1978). A survey conducted during 1978 and 1979 to determine the extent of BT infection among cattle and sheep in Western Australia revealed that only bovine sera contained group- and serotype-specific BT virus antibodies (Coackley *et al.* 1980). More recently, two additional BT virus isolations were made in Australia, and none of the three Australian isolates caused disease in sheep or cattle under natural conditions (Della-Porta *et al.* 1981b). Serological surveys of cattle, buffalo, sheep, and deer in Papua New Guinea disclosed that the incidence of group antibodies to BT virus ranged from 8% in deer to about 60% in cattle. The only evidence of disease was the slight nasal discharge exhibited by some cattle (van Kammen and Cybinski 1981).

Ibaraki virus caused an epizootic in cattle in Japan during 1959 and 1960. Approximately 44 000 cattle were affected; the mortality was about 10% and severe clinical signs were observed in 20 to 30% of the animals. Although Ibaraki disease clinically resembled BT, the two viruses were serologically distinguishable (Inaba *et al.* 1966).

Transmission

The primary vectors of BT are midges of the genus *Culicoides*. Transmission is therefore dependent on the climatic and environmental conditions which govern the distribution and prevalence of these insects. It has been shown that lice, other biting insects, and ticks may also act as vectors. The virus undergoes a cycle of multiplication in the biting midges. The vector can transmit the infection among species and between species of ruminants as between sheep and cattle, and from vaccinated sheep to susceptible sheep. The seasonal incidence of the disease is associated with the prevalence of the vector. Although the virus may be shed in the urine and other excretions, BT is not contracted by direct contact. However, because the virus is present in semen, it can be transmitted to the female. In the pregnant animal, it is transmitted through the placenta to the fetus.

Literature

The general entomological aspects of the epizootiology of BT in the USA were reviewed by Jones *et al.* (1981). In a brief review of the epizootiology of the disease in Africa, they discussed the variety of environmental factors which influence the breeding of the insect vectors *C. pallidipennis* and *C. variipennis* and thus affect the incidence and distribution of the virus in both domestic and various wild species (Erasmus 1975b). The blood meals obtained from *Culicoides* collected in Kenya were analyzed, and it was found that *C. pallidipennis* fed primarily on cattle and to a lesser extent on sheep (Walker and Borham 1976). Bluetongue and related viruses were isolated from *Culicoides* species trapped near Ibadan, Nigeria (Lee *et al.* 1974). The isolation of BT virus from *Culicoides* collected in the Northern Territory of Australia was reported by St George *et al.* (1978). *Culicoides variipennis* was identified as the primary vector of BT in the USA (Jones *et al.* 1981).

Various species of *Culicoides* fed on viremic sheep were found to differ in their susceptibility to BT infection (Standfast *et al.* 1978). Under experimental conditions, the infection rate of *C. variipennis* was related to the titer of virus in the blood meal (Foster and Jones 1979a). *Culicoides variipennis* was susceptible to infection by both ingestion and inoculation, but *C. nubeculosus* could not be experimentally infected with BT virus by the oral route. However, some *C. nubeculosus* midges developed high titers of BT virus when simultaneously infected with the virus and the microfilariae of *Onchocerca cervicalis*, suggesting that penetration of the gut wall by the microfilariae enabled infection of the vector (Mellor and Boorman 1980). A 10 000-fold increase in viral titer developed 5 to 8 days after the intrathoracic inoculation of virus into the hemocoele of *C. variipennis* and was maintained for 26 days. The duration of incubation and the amount of inoculant influenced the viral titer (Jochim and Jones 1966). There was a great increase in titer in *C. variipennis* females by day 4 after oral infection. A second phase of multiplication resulted in a 100-fold increase in titer by day 14, and this maximum titer was maintained until day 35 (Foster and Jones 1979b). *Culicoides variipennis* midges incubated for 10 to 16 days after feeding on BT-infected sheep or cattle could transmit the virus from cattle to sheep, from sheep to cattle, from sheep to sheep, and from cattle to cattle (Luedke *et al.* 1967; Foster *et al.* 1963).

Various theories have been advanced to explain the overwintering mechanism of BT virus. In South Africa, the summer cycle between *Culicoides* and cattle might persist at a lower level throughout the winter since the temperatures were high enough for immature midges to continue developing and for adults to remain active (Nevill 1971). It was proposed that cattle acted as a reservoir of infection and were the host on which *Culicoides* midges preferentially fed. It was suggested that cattle run in close proximity to sheep could serve to protect them from natural infection by attracting the vector (du Toit 1962). Bluetongue and EHD viruses were both isolated from a diseased heifer and *C. variipennis* midges on a farm in Colorado (Foster *et al.* 1980). The sheep ked *Melophagus ovinus* was capable of transmitting BT virus, probably by mechanical means (Luedke *et al.* 1965).

INFECTION

Bluetongue virus infects sheep, goats, cattle, and wild ruminants. On the African continent, the susceptibility of sheep varies between breeds as well as among strains within the same breed. The European breeds appear to be more susceptible than the native African and Asiatic breeds. Although goats vary in their susceptibility to BT, they are more resistant than sheep and usually develop an asymptomatic infection. Cattle serve as a reservoir of the disease in nature and develop infections characterized by latency and periodic viremia. Some species of wild ruminants are also susceptible to BT, which may induce responses ranging from inapparent to acute. The marked variation in the susceptibility of individual animals and the wide range of virulence exhibited by antigenically different strains of BT virus are responsible for the unpredictable morbidity and mortality observed during an epizootic.

Relatively little is known about the pathogenesis of BT. After inoculation by the vector, the virus multiplies in the lymph nodes, draining the site of the injection. This is followed by a viremia and further dissemination of the virus throughout the body. The peak of viremia in sheep and cattle is associated with the peak fever and maximum leukopenia. Bluetongue virus has a particular affinity for red blood cells and can persist in them for weeks despite the presence of neutralizing antibodies. It also multiplies in lymphocytes, macrophages, and the endothelial linings of blood vessels. The infection of the endothelial cells results in the development of lesions characterized by fluid exudate and hemorrhages. The virus passes through the placenta and multiplies in the fetus and, depending on the stage of fetal development, causes death or various degrees of malformation of the central nervous system. In addition, it causes malfunction and anomalies of other virus tissues.

Literature

Intradermal inoculation of sheep was an effective method of inducing infection. Although sheep repeatedly given oral dosages of BT virus developed clinical reactions, the majority of these animals did not have significant levels of serum-neutralizing antibody (Jochim *et al.* 1965). West African dwarf sheep experimentally infected with EHD virus or BT virus did not develop clinical signs. However, viremia was detected in susceptible sheep exposed to BT virus but not in animals with EHD virus infection. Primary infection with either BT or EHD virus resulted in the production of complement-fixing antibodies against both homologous and heterologous virus (Tomori 1980).

Following infection, the virus underwent localized multiplication, probably in lymph nodes. During the viremic phase, the virus could be isolated from peripheral lymphocytes, but BT infectivity was predominantly associated with the red blood cells. Intracellular localization of the virus was indicated by the fact that the infectivity in the blood was neutralized after the erythrocytes were lysed and exposed to specific BT virus antibody. The virus was protected from circulating antibodies by its intraerythrocytic location. Bluetongue virus also replicated in bone-marrow stem cells, resulting in the release of infected erythrocytes into the bloodstream. Because of the long life span of red blood cells in the circulation, the viremia persisted for a long time (Alstad *et al.* 1977). The results of some early investigations indicated that the viremia in sheep did not persist for more than a few days after the peak of the febrile response, but occasionally the circulating virus was demonstrated for several weeks (Alexander 1959). In other studies, the virus was recovered from the peripheral circulation of convalescent sheep and cattle for a considerable length of time after the initial infection (Howell and Verwoerd 1971). In a study of various isolation methods used for monitoring viremia, it was found that sheep, chick embryo, and tissue culture systems were of comparable sensitivity (Thomas *et al.* 1975). Using embryonating chicken eggs, BT virus was detected in sheep blood 1 to 31 days after the animals had been inoculated. Peak viremia usually occurred 6 to 7 days after infection and was correlated with temperature elevation and leukopenia (Luedke 1969).

High concentrations of virus were present in the spleen, tonsils, and certain lymph nodes prior to the onset of viremia or the febrile reaction, thus implicating lymphoid tissue as the primary site of viral replication (Erasmus 1975a). Viral multiplication also took place in the cytoplasm of vascular endothelial cells (Hoff and Hoff 1976). Using various assay systems, it was determined that the virus was associated with the buffy coat and that the spleen and mesenteric lymph nodes were the best organs for virus isolation at postmortem (Pini *et al.* 1966). The pathogenesis of BT was studied by the titration of the virus in tissue samples taken from individual sheep killed at daily intervals over an 11-day period following infection. Four days after the animals had been subcutaneously inoculated in the ear, the virus was demonstrated in the lymph nodes of the cephalic region, the tonsils, and the spleen. Viremia occurred on the sixth day, and macroscopic lesions developed by the eighth day. The virus was not detected in tissue taken 6, 8, or 16 weeks after infection (Pini 1976).

Sheep infected at mid-gestation produced normal lambs which were viremic for 2 months after birth despite the ingestion of colostrum (Gibbs *et al.* 1979). Fetal and newborn lambs at different gestational and neonatal ages were experimentally infected with BT virus. The period during which the virus was recoverable depended on the age of the fetus at the time of exposure. Lambs inoculated at birth became persistently viremic, and it was suggested that such infections were a consequence of the physiological stress associated with birth (Osburn *et al.* 1975).

In goats, the viremia was comparable to that observed in sheep, but clinical signs did not develop. The susceptibility of goats to BT virus was variable, but generally this species was resistant to natural infections (Luedke and Anakwenze 1972).

Jochim and Bowne (1980) presented a review of BT virus infection in cattle. In infections caused by *C. variipennis* bites or by intradermal inoculation, the viremia started as early as the second day after the cattle were exposed, increased to a peak by the seventh day, and gradually decreased but was still detectable on the twenty-sixth day. The virus was also recovered from some animals tested on the fiftieth day. The viremia was observed at the same time that high levels of serum-neutralizing antibodies were found. The only clinical signs were loss of appetite, thickening of skin, and severe pityriasis (Luedke *et al.* 1969). In cattle, the viremia persisted for as long as 16 weeks. The annual recurrence of the viremia suggested that the animals were reinfected by different strains (du Toit 1962). Bluetongue infections in cattle were also associated with other clinical signs and sequelae, including mouth lesions and congenital deformities, but in most cases the disease was inapparent. In contrast to the peak incidence of BT observed in sheep during the summer and fall, the virus could be isolated from cattle throughout the year (Luedke *et al.* 1970).

Serial passage of the virus through calves caused viremia and antibody formation, but there was no enhancement of virulence for either calves or sheep (Gray *et al.* 1967). Infection of cows during the first 3 months of gestation, and less frequently between the third and sixth months, often resulted in the death of the fetus or the birth of weak calves which had various degrees of abnormalities. Calves that survived were apt to carry the infection but did not have circulating antibodies. Diagnosis of these persistent or latent infections was difficult because the virus could not be readily demonstrated. However, viremia could be induced in some latently infected cattle by the stimulatory action of the bite of *C. variipennis*. Cattle, therefore, could act as reservoirs of the virus without producing detectable antibody or virus titers (Jones *et al.* 1981). In other investigations, pregnant heifers at 60 and 120 days of gestation were experimentally infected with BT by the bites of *C. variipennis*. Viremia was detected in 60 and 33% of these animals on postinfection days 50 and 100 to 102 respectively. The virus was abortigenic and teratogenic, resulting in an overall reproductive failure of 30%. The calves born to infected heifers had demonstrable viremia at birth, but did not have detectable specific neutralizing or precipitating antibodies in the sera before the ingestion of colostrum, and some developed clinical signs during the first 6 months of life (Luedke *et al.* 1977a). Calves exposed to the virus *in utero* and reinfected at 6 months of age by *C. variipennis* had latent virus infection which continued as they matured. Some of these cattle did not develop detectable antibodies or clinical signs (Luedke *et al.* 1977b).

The virus has been isolated from a latently infected bull by the blood autograft technique in sheep. In these sheep, the washed bovine erythrocytes used as inocula caused a delayed but classical BT reaction, even after storage at 4 °C for up to 14 months (Luedke *et al.* 1980). Abnormalities and virus-like particles were seen in the semen of two latently infected bulls (Foster *et al.* 1979). Bluetongue virus could be isolated from the semen of experimentally infected bulls only by inoculating this material into sheep (Parsonson *et al.* 1981).

Strains of BT virus representing all of the antigenic types were successfully adapted to multiplication in the brains of suckling mice, but most strains required preliminary passage through embryonated eggs. Primary isolation of field strains of virus in suckling mice by intracerebral inoculation was unsuccessful. In 3- to 4-week old mice, viral multiplication occurred without evidence of clinical effect (Howell and Verwoerd 1971). The relationship between the age of the mouse and susceptibility to infection was affected by the passage level of the virus used. As the age of the mouse increased, there was a marked prolongation of survival time and a reduction of virus titer in the brain tissue (Svehag 1962). In mice, the immature cells of the subventricular zone were selectively infected by the virus, and the age dependency of the lesions was not determined by the immaturity of the immune system (Narayan *et al.* 1972). Successful infections of suckling hamsters with strains of mouse- and egg-adapted BT virus by the intracerebral route of inoculation was also reported (Howell and Verwoerd 1971).

Bluetongue infections were investigated in wild ruminants. Experimentally infected North American elk (*Cervus canadensis*) developed mild or inapparent clinical reactions. A pronounced viremia occurred, and antibody production persisted for 6 to 7 months postinoculation (Murray and Trainer 1970). Pregnant North American elk with experimental BT infection were asymptomatic and not viremic, but virus could be isolated from the spleen and bone marrow. The elk calves were latently infected, and the virus could be transmitted by biting gnats (Stott *et al.* 1982). Fatal and nonfatal infections were induced in white-tailed deer experimentally exposed to BT virus. The clinical syndromes observed in BT-infected sheep and deer were similar. However, the course of the disease was more acute in deer than sheep (Trainer *et al.* 1967; Vosdingh *et al.* 1968). Natural infection of captive Texas white-tailed deer resulted in the development of clinical signs and death (Stair *et al.* 1968). An outbreak of a hemorrhagic disease which occurred in six species of exotic ruminants in the San Diego Zoo in 1970–71 was caused by BT virus (Hoff *et al.* 1973).

White-tailed deer appeared to be the primary host of EHD, but mule, deer, and antelope were also susceptible (Trainer 1967). Epizootic hemorrhagic disease and BT were considered clinically and pathologically indistinguishable, and evidence of experimental or natural infection was recorded for 29 species of wild ruminants (Hoff and Hoff 1976).

Ibaraki virus could be transmitted serially in calves by the intravenous inoculation of blood obtained at the height of the febrile reaction. Sheep infected with this virus developed a low-grade viremia and a specific neutralizing antibody, but clinical manifestations of disease were absent (Inaba 1975).

CLINICAL SIGNS

Clinical syndromes are most common and most severe in sheep. Indigenous breeds in enzootic areas are less susceptible than imported exotic breeds, but there is considerable variation between individuals in any breed. Sheep approximately 1 year old are more susceptible: suckling lambs have some innate resistance. The mortality varies from 2 to 30%. Bluetongue infections in goats and cattle are milder; a transient fever and hyperemia may be the only evidence of disease. Occasionally, however, these animals develop clinical signs comparable to those observed in affected sheep.

Sheep with BT virus infection may develop acute, subacute, or mild syndromes depending on the strain of the virus and the breed susceptibility. In the acute form, the first clinical signs are fever, reddening of the buccal mucosa, and anorexia. Shortly thereafter, swelling and hyperemia of the lips, tongue, gums, and muzzle are evident. In some animals, the discoloration of the buccal and nasal mucosae intensifies to an almost purplish blue. There may be inflammation and excoriation of the mucous membrane of the gums, cheeks, and tongue. Swallowing becomes difficult when the tongue is very edematous and swollen and the mucosal erosions are pronounced. These lesions heal slowly under a diphtheritic membrane. A nasal discharge develops soon after the first rise in temperature and changes from serous to serosanguineous to mucopurulent as the disease progresses. The nostrils become encrusted with the mucopurulent nasal discharge, resulting in dyspnea and snorting. During the latter stages of the disease, some sheep develop inflamed and painful claws due to severe coronitis. Degenerative changes in the skeletal muscles cause stiffness and muscular weakness. An animal may stand with its back arched and its neck twisted. Thus, acutely affected animals suffer a rapid and severe loss of condition which is attributable to the presence of oral and muscular lesions; if recovery ensues, the debility persists for weeks. Animals with the subacute form of the disease do not have severe symptoms, but there is extreme emaciation, prolonged muscular weakness, occasional torticollis, and protracted convalescence. In the mild form, the only apparent clinical sign is a transient elevation of body temperature. Pregnant ewes infected with BT virus may abort or produce malformed or weak lambs.

In a small percentage of cattle, Ibaraki virus causes syndromes that are of comparable severity to BT infections in sheep, but most cattle exhibit mild signs or are asymptomatic.

Literature

The natural and experimental clinical syndromes have been described by Henning (1956), Neitz (1966), Howell and Verwoerd (1971), Bowne (1971), and Sellers (1981). The clinical and pathological aspects of BT in sheep and goats were reviewed by Erasmus (1975a). The natural syndromes are usually more severe than those induced experimentally. The fetal abnormalities and reproductive problems associated with BT virus infection were comprehensively discussed in a review of the disease in cattle (Hourrigan and Klingsporn 1975a).

Howell and Verwoerd (1971) presented the following description of the sequential development of clinical signs in sheep. After the experimental inoculation of sheep with BT virus-infected blood, incubation periods of 5 to 8 days were usually observed, but they could vary from 2 to 15 days. The first sign was an elevation in temperature which may persist for 6 to 8 days. There was no correlation between the intensity of the febrile reaction and the severity of the clinical signs that were exhibited during the early stages of the disease. Within 24 to 36 hours after the rise in temperature, hyperemia of the buccal and nasal mucosae developed, followed by salivation, frothing, and licking movements of the tongue. A catarrhal discharge leaked from the nostrils and eyes. After 48 hours, edema involved the lips, tongue, face, ears, and throat and extended down the ventral surface of the neck. The oral mucosa acquired a distinct purplish-blue cast as the hyperemia became more pronounced and petechial hemorrhages appeared. About 5 to 8 days after the initial rise in temperature, the mucous membranes of the mouth became extensively ulcerated and covered by necrotic exudate. With the formation of a diphtheritic membrane, a fetid odor was given off from the mouth. Respiration was impaired by the accumulation of dried mucopurulent exudate around the nostrils. At the end of the febrile period, the coronary bands reddened and the feet became warm and painful, causing lameness. Hyperemia of the skin often developed in various regions of the body. Rapid emaciation occurred as a result of inanition and specific muscular lesions. A sequela of the disease was breaking of the wool fibers and shedding of the fleece from various parts of the body about 3 to 4 weeks after the subsidence of the fever (Howell and Verwoerd 1971). In mild cases, the prognosis is favorable; recovery is generally rapid and uncomplicated. In severe cases, however, the prognosis should be more guarded since there may be severe debility and protracted convalescence (Henning 1956).

Sheep in enzootic areas were less severely affected than sheep introduced from BT-free areas. The appearance of clinical cases of BT in sub-Saharan Africa was related to the introduction of exotic breeds, particularly the highly susceptible Merino sheep (Owen 1965). In a recent outbreak of BT in the Sudan, the morbidity and mortality rates in adult sheep were estimated at 30 and 2% respectively; the corresponding rates in lambs were approximately 80 and 100% (Eisa *et al.* 1980). In Australia, the experimental infection of sheep with a new isolate, designated BT virus serotype 20 (BTV-20), produced mild to moderate clinical disease. When BTV-20 was injected into pregnant ewes, there was no evidence of abortion or transplacental transfer of the virus, although viremia was detected in these animals between days 3 and 11 postinoculation (Flanagan *et al.* 1982). Bluetongue virus serotype 20 was isolated from the blood of infected sheep and cattle but caused clinical syndromes only in the sheep (St George and McCaughan 1979). Losses in newborn lambs were reported in flocks in which ewes at 4 to 8 weeks of pregnancy were vaccinated against BT virus using a different serotype. Some lambs were stillborn or spastic or appeared dumb, whereas others were small and putrefied or deformed (Shultz and DeLay 1955).

Three serotypes of BT virus were recovered from goats in the USA. These isolates were associated with the development of a variety of clinical signs and sequelae, including weakness, pneumonia, keratoconjunctivitis, anemia, swollen joints, abortion, and fetal abnormalities (Inverso *et al.* 1980).

Cattle maintained under strict isolation conditions have not been observed to develop the severe clinical signs that have been reported in sheep (Bowne *et al.* 1968). Less than 5% of naturally infected adult cattle showed clinical symptoms. The primary problem caused by BT virus in enzootic areas was the decrease in calf production due to early fetal deaths and congenital defects (Jones *et al.* 1981). In cattle, the disease was characterized by fever, hyperemia of the mucous membranes, and ulcerations on the gingival and buccal mucosae and on the tongue. Lesions were also found on the teats of lactating cattle (Metcalf and Luedke 1978). The definitive diagnosis of BT in cattle was difficult, but the infection could be differentiated from some other symptomatically related viral diseases. One of the more extensive lesions was the massive necrosis of the dental pad. There was also inflammation in the coronary region, and severe damage to the coronet, sometimes resulted in the sloughing of the horny lamina. Pityriasis was a common clinical feature; the skin thickened, cracked, and scaled, especially on parts of the neck and perineal region. In severe cases, sloughing of the skin occurred (Reynolds 1971; Bowne 1973).

The clinical and pathological manifestations of BT and EHD in various wild artiodactyles were summarized in a review by Hoff and Hoff (1976). The experimental infection of pronghorn antelopes (*Antilocapra americana*) with BT virus caused clinical disease and death in animals which had no neutralizing antibodies to the virus, while antelopes with neutralizing antibodies did not become infected (Hoff and Trainer 1972). The occurrence of clinical BT disease in desert bighorn sheep was reported (Robinson *et al.* 1967).

Epizootic hemorrhagic disease of deer was characterized by depression, weakness, anorexia, pyrexia, edema, nasal exudation, and salivation. In addition, the buccal mucosa was ulcerated and hemorrhagic (Frank and Willis 1975).

Epizootiological, clinical, and pathological observations were made during outbreaks of Ibaraki disease in Japan (Omori *et al.* 1969a). The illness began with fever which lasted for 2 to 10 days and was accompanied by anorexia, lacrymation, foamy salivation, and ruminal stasis. This was followed by leukopenia and congestion and edema of the conjunctiva and oral and nasal mucous membranes. In more severe cases, the mucous membranes became cyanotic and small ulcers developed. Painful swelling of the joints and coronitis occurred. The most conspicuous clinical sign was difficulty in swallowing. This was observed in up to 30% of the affected animals and was associated with extensive lesions in the esophagus, pharynx, or tongue. The difficulty in swallowing led to dehydration, emaciation, and aspiration pneumonia. In mild cases, the animals recovered completely within 2 to 3 days (Inaba 1975).

PATHOLOGY

In sheep, the character of the lesions varies greatly depending on the strain of the virus, the severity of the disease, and the stage of the syndrome. Later stages of the disease are complicated by secondary infections. The changes which occur in the digestive, respiratory, and locomotory systems are indicative of an inflammatory process. The oral and nasal mucosae are primarily affected and become edematous, hyperemic, hemorrhagic, and ulcerated. The excoriations of the oral epithelium are covered with gray necrotic material. The tongue and mucous membranes of the mouth become swollen and are purple or dark blue in color. Aspiration pneumonia is a common sequela. Degeneration of the skeletal musculature is another important feature. There is infiltration of clear reddish fluid into the intermuscular fasciae, and hemorrhages and necrosis are evident. The lymph nodes draining the head are usually edematous and hemorrhagic. The hyperemia of the skin may be patchy, resulting in irregular crusty or exanthematous areas and a localized dermatitis. Generalized flushing of the skin may also occur, and excoriations develop on parts of the body that are subject to abrasion.

In pregnant animals, there is a hemorrhagic, necrotic placentitis. Depending on the stage of gestation, transplacental infection of the fetus may result in fetal death or an inflammatory reaction of the meninges and brain tissue, as well as developmental abnormalities.

The pathogenesis of BT has not yet been fully explained. Vascular degeneration constitutes the primary pathological change and is responsible for the secondary inflammatory exudation and the necrosis of the epithelium of the upper gastrointestinal, and respiratory tracts.

Literature

The macroscopic lesions were described in detail by Moulton (1961). Edema was subcutaneous, fascial, and intermuscular; it also occurred in the body cavities. This fluid was colorless or yellowish and occasionally bloodstained. The local drainage lymph nodes were enlarged, reddened, and edematous. Hemorrhage and necrosis in the myocardium and skeletal musculature appeared as diffuse opacities or grayish mottling or streaks. In the heart, the lesions were most prominent in the papillary muscle of the left ventricle. Hyperemia and petechiae were found throughout the gastrointestinal tract. Ulcers and erosions affected the buccal and nasal mucosae.

The general histological changes were described by Erasmus (1975a). Vascular injury was the principal factor in the pathogenesis of the lesions. The virus had an affinity for the endothelium and the cells surrounding the capillaries, arterioles, and venules. Large quantities of virus were observed in the small blood vessels underlying stratified squamous epithelium, particularly that of the oral mucosa, skin, and coronet of the hoof. In the endothelial cells, the virus caused cytoplasmic vesiculation, nuclear and cytoplasmic hypertrophy, pyknosis, and karyorrhexis. The necrosis and subsequent proliferative cellular changes in the endothelium induced vascular occlusion, stasis of inflammatory fluid, and exudation. This process resulted in the development of lesions in the overlying epithelium (Erasmus 1975a).

Lesions began as a swelling and ballooning of the cells of the striated epithelium, followed by pyknosis, cellular disintegration, and neutrophil infiltration. The necrosis extended downwards to involve all layers of the stratified epithelium (Howell and Verwoerd 1971). The severity of these secondary lesions was affected by mechanical abrasion and bacterial infection. It was suggested that the distribution of lesions was related to temperature gradients within the host. The most severe lesions developed in superficial tissues which had a temperature lower than that of the internal organs (Erasmus 1975a).

The most significant pathological changes occurred in the striated muscles. Thomas and Neitz (1947) divided the process involved in the formation of muscular lesions into five stages: altered staining reaction of affected fibers, swelling and distortion, disintegration and resorptions, hemorrhage, and regeneration. The plasma levels of glutamic oxalacetic transaminase, glutamic pyruvic transaminase, lactic dehydrogenase, and aldolase were elevated, probably as a result of the skeletal myopathy (Clark and Wagner 1967).

A number of studies were undertaken to determine the changes which occurred in the placentas and fetuses of sheep experimentally infected with BT virus. In one series of experiments, transplacental transmission of the virus occurred in 30% of the ewes inoculated during the fifth or sixth week of gestation. The results of these experiments suggested that placental lesions were a reflection of the direct effect of the virus on both the maternal and fetal vascular systems. The most common lesion was vasculitis of the arteries and arterioles in the endometrial stroma of the placentomes (Anderson and Jensen 1969). The skeletal abnormalities and encephalopathy seen in newborn lambs from a farm flock were attributed to BT virus (Griner *et al.* 1964), and cerebral malformations were observed in two fetuses from ewes in a BT-enzootic flock (Schmidt and Panciera 1973). Experimental BT infection caused cerebral anomalies in young fetal sheep, while a nonsuppurative meningoencephalitis developed in older fetuses. This change in the response of the nervous system occurred between the seventieth and ninetieth day of gestation and was correlated with the development of immunological responsiveness. Similarly, a focal necrotizing lesion was produced in young suckling mice, whereas a nonsuppurative meningoencephalitis was found in older animals. Thus, the lesions found in the central nervous systems of infected sheep and mice varied with the age of the animals and appeared to be influenced by the immunological maturity of the host (Richards and Cordy 1967). Ten to 15 days after ovine fetuses were inoculated with BT virus, there was a diffuse infiltration of macrophages into the interstitial tissue of the lung, and by day 20, nodules of macrophages were present. The only macroscopic lesions observed in these fetuses were enlarged lymph nodes and prominent lymphoid nodules in the spleen. The virus was recoverable from fetuses which had serum-neutralizing antibody (Enright and Osburn 1980).

There were outbreaks of hydranencephaly among newborn calves in California and Oregon in 1968. Evidence obtained from serological tests indicated that hydranencephaly developed as a result of fetal infection with BT virus (Richards *et al.* 1971; McKercher *et al.* 1970). The lesion was produced experimentally in two bovine fetuses which had been inoculated intramuscularly with attenuated BT virus on postconceptual days 126 and 138 respectively (Barnard and Pienaar 1976).

The attenuated vaccine virus also caused lesions in the central nervous system of ovine fetuses. Approximately 21% of the ewes vaccinated on day 40 of gestation gave birth to lambs with brain lesions, but these lesions were not observed after vaccination between days 19 and 29 of gestation. The lesions were characterized by either diffuse or focal necrotizing meningoencephalitis with vasculitis, hemorrhages, mineralization, and microcavitation of the cerebellar tissues. The administration of BT vaccine virus to ewes between days 35 and 42 of gestation produced the highest incidence of encephalopathy (Young and Cordy 1964). The morphologic characteristics of the hydranencephaly, porencephaly, and retinal dysplasia found in BT-infected ovine fetuses closely resembled those observed in infants with similar congenital malformations. Bluetongue vaccine virus infection in fetal lambs was thus proposed as an animal model of brain damage in man (Osburn and Silverstein 1972; Osburn *et al.* 1970). Virulent and vaccinal strains of BT virus differed in that the former caused generalized necrosis of ovine fetal hepatocytes and death of the fetus (Bwangamoi 1978).

In white-tailed deer which died of experimental BT infection, the predominant lesions were extensive thrombosis associated with hemorrhages, and degenerative and necrotic changes in a variety of tissues and organs. These lesions were those observed in BT-infected sheep and in deer with EHD (Karstad 1967; Karstad and Trainer 1967; Frank and Willis 1975).

In Ibaraki disease, lesions formed in the mucous membranes lining the upper portions of the respiratory tract and the gastrointestinal tract as far as the abomasum. The epithelial cells in these lesions exhibited vacuolation and nuclear disintegration. Lesions also developed in the blood vessels. In severe syndromes there was extensive degeneration and necrosis of the striated muscles of the pharynx, larynx, tongue, and esophagus. These lesions could also be observed in the skeletal muscles of the chest and limbs (Inaba 1975). Severe lesions in the esophageal and laryngopharyngeal musculature caused difficulty in swallowing, resulting in dehydration and emaciation, and occasionally in aspiration pneumonia. The pathologic changes which occurred in cattle with Ibaraki disease were comparable to those observed in sheep and cattle infected with BT virus (Omori *et al.* 1969a).

IMMUNOLOGY

There is a plurality of antigenically different strains of BT virus, and to date at least 20 antigenic types are known throughout the world. The distribution of the various antigenic strains among the host and vector populations is random, and specific antigenic types are related to particular geographic regions. Each strain has antigens common to all strains and a number of other antigens which are strain- or isolate-specific.

Because of the plurality of viral strains and the variation in susceptibility among the various breeds of sheep, the duration of immunity after infection has not been well defined. Sheep challenged by homologous virus following vaccination are immune for 12 months. Newborn lambs which ingest colostrum from immune dams acquire passive immunity which may persist for up to 68 days. The immunity of cattle following field challenge has not been determined, but the fact that they develop a milder form of the disease is indicative of a less efficient immunological response. The antibodies detected by various serological tests persist for different periods of time.

Neutralizing, fluorescent, hemagglutinating, complement-fixing, and agar-gel precipitating antibodies are used to obtain a complete picture of an animal's serological response and the antigenic composition of different strains. The applicability of the CF, FA, and agar-gel precipitin (AGP) tests depends on the duration of serum antibodies. The tests are group-specific and serve to detect antibodies to numerous strains. The AGP test is relatively simple, rapid, and economical. The agar-gel immunodiffusion tests are used commonly to screeen animals involved in international trade.

The serum virus neutralization test is commonly used to determine the distinct antigenic types of virus. This technique has been performed in a variety of systems, including intracerebrally inoculated suckling mice, embryonated eggs, and tissue culture. The results vary from laboratory to laboratory because there has been little uniformity in procedures. A number of variables, such as the serum and virus concentrations, strain of virus, route of infection, and methods of assessing end points, can affect the outcome of the test. The plaque assay is used routinely for the determination of viral titers and the detection of the neutralizing antibody.

The serotyping system for BT is in the World Reference Centre in South Africa.

Literature

Using serum virus neutralization tests, naturally occurring strains of BT virus were originally classified into 16 immunological groups (Howell 1970); 20 different antigenic types are currently recognized (Sellers 1981). Viruses isolated from cattle exposed to natural infections over two consecutive seasons were typed using the serum neutralization method; 11 established antigenic groups and several different new antigenic types were represented. No single antigenic type was found to occur in the same bovine for two consecutive seasons (Owen *et al.* 1965). Strains of BT virus in the USA were serologically characterized by means of the plaque reduction neutralization test. Four serotypes have been isolated from sheep and five from cattle. There was no cross-reaction between BT and EHD viruses (Barber and Jochim 1973; Thomas and Trainer, 1971).

Three different serotypes of BT virus were isolated from sentinel cattle in the Northern Territory of Australia and were not associated with natural clinical disease in sheep or cattle (Della-Porta *et al.* 1981a, b; St George, 1980). These isolates were further compared by cross-hybridization and cross-immune precipitation methods (Huismans and Bremer 1981). Two of the new serotypes of BT virus were mildly to moderately pathogenic in experimentally infected sheep (Squire *et al.* 1981).

The main differences between BT and EHD viruses were host specificity and antigenic composition. No cross-reaction occurred in a number of serological tests conducted on the sera of various ruminants. However, serological tests using mouse hyperimmune fluids demonstrated a minor antigenic component common to both viruses (Frank and Willis 1975). The number of serotypes of EHD virus was not known, although several were believed to exist. The antigenic relationship between EHD virus and BT virus has not been fully established (Hoff and Hoff 1976).

There was no evidence of a serological relationship between BT and Ibaraki viruses, but the information was incomplete (Inaba 1975). The antigenic relationship between Ibaraki, BT and EHD viruses was investigated. There was no relationship between the group- or serotype-specific antigens of Ibaraki and BT viruses. However, Ibaraki virus and EHD virus were related antigenically (Campbell *et al.* 1978).

Serological cross-reactions between the AHSV and the BT virus were demonstrated by an immunodiffusion technique. The AHSV possessed a group-specific complement-fixing antigen which did not react with the BT group-specific complement-fixing antibody (Ozawa and Hafez 1972, 1973).

The information obtained regarding the development and persistence of antibodies after infection varied with the experimental procedures and serological tests used. In a comparison of the plaque neutralization, CF, and AGP tests, the BT virus antibody was measured in the sera of cattle, sheep, and deer. Plaque neutralization titers began earlier than the other types, were much higher than the CF titers, and peaked 2 to 3 weeks after exposure (Thomas *et al.* 1976). The persistence of BT virus and complement-fixing antibodies was studied in experimentally infected calves. The duration of the immune response varied with the different strains used, and antibodies were found up to day 162 after infection and viremia was detected up to day 60. Antibodies were demonstrated at the time that virus isolations were made (Pearson *et al.* 1973). Antibodies passively transferred in the colostrum of BT-immune dams persisted in lamb sera for as long as 3 months (Livingston and Hardy 1964).

The need for an *in vitro* test to demonstrate the presence and incidence of antibodies to BT virus resulted in the development of the serum virus neutralization test. This technique involved the production of cytopathogenic effects by an egg-propagated strain of the virus in cultures of sheep kidney cells and the inhibition of these effects by serum from BT-immune sheep (Haig *et al.* 1956; Howell 1960). Embryonated chicken eggs and suckling mice were used to determine the sensitivity of quantal and graded responses to BT virus for the quantification of neutralizing antibody. The graded response was based on survival times and enabled the demonstration of antibody in highly dilute serum. The quantal response, which recorded the percentage death, was not sufficiently sensitive to detect low titers of antibody (Svehag 1966). The identification of strains was facilitated by the development of improved cell culture techniques which were considerably more economical in terms of time and materials than other serum virus neutralization tests in eggs, tubes, or petri dishes (Davies and Blackburn 1971; Howell *et al.* 1970). A rapid BT virus plaque neutralization test which required minimal antibody–virus contact time was considered to be effective for wide-scale screening or for the detection of dose–response lines (Thomas and Samagh 1979). The plaque inhibition method was simpler and required less time than the plaque neutralization technique (Stott *et al.* 1978). The neutralization of BT and EHD viruses was enhanced by the addition of rabbit anti-species gamma globulin to the virus–antibody mixtures in a plaque neutralization procedure (Jochim and Jones 1977). Comparisons of BT virus isolates by plaque neutralization and relatedness tests were reported. The relatedness of the viruses was studied by quantitatively measuring the cross-reaction. The cross-reactivity formed a spectrum from virtually no evidence of unrelatedness to clear antigenic differences (Thomas *et al.* 1979). Various factors affecting the BT virus neutralization antibody response and the virus–antibody reaction were studied. The conditions under which the virus was stable and the plaque neutralization test was optimally sensitive were defined. The antigen–antibody reaction was serotype-specific, and both IgM and IgG antibodies could neutralize the virus, although IgM reached maximum levels sooner than IgG (van der Walt 1979; Svehag 1960).

The CF test was used to detect the production of BT virus antibodies in sheep and cattle (Robertson *et al.* 1965). A number of methods using various sources of antigen were developed. Antigens prepared from infected mouse brains and chicken embryos gave inconsistent results in CF tests, while antigens prepared from lamb kidney cell cultures were satisfactory (Shone *et al.* 1956; Kipps 1956). Improvements were made in the modified direct CF test and in the preparation of antigen from infected mouse brain (Carrier and Boulanger 1975). Two CF methods for the detection of antibodies to BT were compared (Boulanger *et al.* 1967). Bluetongue virus group specificity, as measured by CF, was shown to be determined by a major polypeptide in the viral core, whereas a polypeptide in the capsid layer was the main determinant of serotype specificity (Huismans and Erasmus 1981). It was found that the precipitin test was more accurate than the CF test (Breckon *et al.* 1980).

Fluorescent antibody techniques were used in the identification of viral antigens in cultures and tissues. The results of experiments employing fluorescein-conjugated BT virus indicated that the reaction was group-specific rather than serotype-specific (Pini *et al.* 1966). The FA technique was used to detect BT virus in bovine fetal kidney cell cultures inoculated with tissues and blood from experimentally infected animals. Direct examination of infected tissues, either by impression smears or by frozen sections, was not a reliable method of demonstrating BT virus since there is no typical pattern in the distribution of virus in the organs. The viral antigen appeared as dust-like particles randomly distributed throughout the field (Ruckerbauer *et al.* 1967). An indirect fluorescent antibody (IFA) technique was used to detect BT virus in tissue smears from *Culiccides variipennis* (Jennings and Boorman 1980). Bluetongue and EHD viruses were identified and differentiated with an IFA test. A certain level of dilution was required to eliminate heterologous two-way cross-reactions. Cell cultures infected with these viruses had specific fluorescence as early as 12 hours after inoculation. The BT virus-infected cells had predominantly juxtanuclear spherical inclusions and granular materials in the cytoplasm, while the EHD virus-infected cells had fewer discrete inclusions and irregularly shaped aggregations of antigen around the nucleus (Jochim *et al.* 1975).

The more commonly used serological tests had certain limitations. For example, the modified CF test caused technical problems due to the many variables involved in the technique (Hubschle *et al.* 1981). Therefore a number of new tests were developed. Bluetongue virus hemagglutinated erythrocytes from a variety of animal species, and the reaction could be inhibited by specific antisera. The virulent strains readily agglutinated erythrocytes, while the avirulent type tested produced only a slight hemagglutination. It was recommended that the hemagglutination-inhibition test be used as a means of identifying various BT virus serotypes (Hubschle 1980). The hemagglutination and hemagglutination-inhibition tests were fast and easy to perform. The hemagglutination reaction was independent of variations in the pH, temperature, buffer system, and source of the test erythrocytes, and the hemagglutination-inhibition test was serotype-specific (van der Walt 1980). The hemagglutination titers of BT virus were increased by boosting the sodium chloride molarity of the diluent (Tokuhisa *et al.* 1981). The hemolysis-in-gel test was developed to detect and quantitate antibodies to BT virus. The test did not differentiate among antibodies to four serotypes of BT virus, but it did differentiate between anti-BT virus and anti-EHD virus (Jochim and Jones 1980). The enzyme-linked immunosorbent assay detected group-specific antibodies and was more sensitive than the modified CF test (Hubschle *et al.* 1981). This assay proved to be a rapid and sensitive method for the detection of antiviral IgG in the sera of sheep exposed to BT virus (Manning and Chen 1980).

VACCINATION

Both attenuated and inactivated vaccines have been developed. The monovalent live attenuated vaccine is effective, but in enzootic areas where several antigenic types of BT virus may be present simultaneously, a polyvalent vaccine is necessary. The use of polyvalent vaccines is complicated by interference between strains, differences in the immunizing potencies, and growth rates of the attenuated strains and pronounced differences in the response of individual animals to these vaccines. Live vaccines are not safe for pregnant animals because the fetus may be affected. The passage of attenuated vaccine virus through *Culicoides* may cause reversion to virulence. Therefore, vaccination with attenuated virus would be practical only in enzootic areas. In the USA, the only federally licensed vaccine available is a monovalent attenuated cell culture vaccine in sheep.

The inactivated vaccines are partially successful in enhancing the immune response to subsequent challenge with a virulent virus. These vaccines are advantageous in that there is no possibility of reversion to virulence or of fetal infection.

Literature

A method of immunization developed around 1900 in South Africa involved the simultaneous inoculation of immune serum and infective blood. The attenuation of a strain of virus was achieved after limited serial passage in sheep. This was referred to as Theiler's vaccine, and over a period of 40 years more than 50 millon doses were used. This vaccine was inadequate because of the plurality of virus strains occurring in nature. Although each strain produced a solid, durable immunity against homologous challenge, it induced a variable degree of protection against challenge by heterologous strains (Howell and Verwoerd 1971). Serial passage of BT virus through embryonated chicken eggs incubated at 33.5 °C resulted in a markedly attenuated strain (Henning 1956). The use of egg-attenuated BT virus in the production of polyvalent vaccine for sheep was discussed. The vaccine was found to be effective and the virus did not regain its virulence by serial passage (Alexander and Haig 1951; McKercher *et al.* 1957a). In field trials, the modified live virus vaccine induced satisfactory immunity in approximately 92% of the sheep challenged with virulent virus 6 weeks after vaccination. The only reaction observed was a moderate hyperemia of the muzzle and ears which occurred in approximately 10% of the animals (McGowan *et al.* 1956).

An experimental inactivated vaccine was produced in BHK cell cultures and inoculated as an emulsion in Freund's complete adjuvant (Barber *et al.* 1979). Sheep given either multiple injections of an inactivated vaccine or a single injection of the vaccine in adjuvant were protected against challenge with homologous virulent virus, even though viral neutralizing antibodies did not develop (Osburn *et al.* 1979).

A similar inactivated vaccine caused the development of both complement-fixing and agar-gel precipitating antibodies as well as a strong cell-mediated response. After vaccination, the sheep were more refractory to challenge at 6 weeks than at 4 weeks (Stott *et al.* 1979).

DIAGNOSIS

The diagnosis of BT is made on the basis of epizootiological circumstances, clinical signs, isolation and identification of the virus, and demonstration of group-specific antibodies. In sheep, the diagnosis is not difficult in acutely ill animals with obvious typical clinical signs such as lesions of the muzzle, eyes, and face. When uncharacteristic signs and secondary infections are present, clinical diagnosis is difficult. In cattle, the clinical picture is not as well defined and diagnosis cannot be made on the basis of the symptoms presented. The initial presumptive diagnosis has to be confirmed by virus isolation. The virus can be isolated from the blood during the early stages of the disease. The most sensitive and reliable methods of isolation involve injection of susceptible sheep and embryonated chicken eggs. Other systems used for the isolation of BT virus include susceptible tissue cell cultures and suckling mice, but these have not been routinely used because serial passage of the virus is required for adaptation to each system. However, more efficient tissue culture techniques may soon become available. Identification of the virus has been achieved by animal inoculation, antibody determination, and FA reactions in cultures and tissues. Diagnosis should be made on a herd basis by the collection of blood from several animals.

Literature

The diagnosis of BT has traditionally depended on the infection of susceptible sheep with suspected material from field cases. Propagation of the virus in embryonated chicken eggs was a more efficient laboratory method. However, isolation and serological problems resulted from the fastidiousness of some strains, the close association of the virus with erythrocytes, and the coexistence of the virus with specific circulating antibodies. Serological diagnosis was complicated by the difficulty of interpreting test results and the presence of virus without a detectable antibody response (Metcalf and Luedke 1974). The serological methods used for the diagnosis of BT included the modified direct CF test, the micro agar-gel precipitation test, the FA technique and the plaque reduction neutralization test. The antibodies in the sera of cattle, sheep, and deer could not be detected by the direct CF test until it was modified by the addition of 5% non-heat-inactivated normal bovine serum (Boulanger and Frank 1975). Immunofluorescence was used to demonstrate viral antigens in chicken embryos and in the labial mucosa of calves (at postinoculation day 4 or 7) which had not yet developed gross lesions. The viral antigens were observed in the vascular walls and in the perivascular tissues (Gleiser *et al.* 1969).

CONTROL

The control of enzootic BT requires consideration of the reservoirs of virus, the vectors, and the susceptible species of hosts. Because the virus has a wide host range and is biologically transmitted by insects, control measures are based primarily on the immunization of susceptible animals and on the prevention of contact with insect vectors. Although attenuated vaccines are of value, the existence of a variety of serotypes makes prophylactic immunization difficult.

The spread of BT virus beyond the African continent is probably due to the movement of livestock. There is also the danger of transmission by the importation of infected frozen semen. The control measures undertaken in the face of an outbreak in disease-free regions vary, depending on the epizootiological situation.

Literature

The control of BT virus was recently reviewed by Erasmus (1975c). Unless the epizootic situation is well defined, the control procedures have to be based on good general principles. Prophylaxis must be considered in relation to various aspects of the epizootiology of BT virus. Some of the important epizootiological factors are the variety of antigenic types and the complicated pattern of their occurrence within enzootic areas, the role of certain susceptible species as reservoirs, and the role of vectors (Howell 1966). In South Africa, *C. imicola* was found preferentially to feed on cattle; the maintenance of cattle near sheep led to a reduction in the incidence of BT in sheep. This 'decoy' approach was recommended as a practical means of protecting sheep from BT infection (Nevill 1978).

Geering (1975) expressed the opinion that once BT virus had been introduced into a country, there was little hope of its eradication. However, in the Iberian Peninsula, successful eradication of the disease was accomplished by quarantine, compulsory vaccination, and slaughter of infected animals. The contingency plans for the control of BT in an epizootic situation in Australia were discussed. The measures were based on current knowledge of the pathogenesis of BT and the biology of *Culicoides*. The steps to be undertaken include reduction of the number of viremic animals, reduction of the population density of *Culicoides*, and reduction of the numbers of susceptible hosts. Laboratory diagnosis of the virus was based on the detection of viremia in experimentally infected sheep which were examined for 4 to 6 weeks for the development of fever and clinical signs of BT. The diagnosis was confirmed by serological examination of paired sera from test sheep and demonstration of the virus (Geering 1975). The dangers of introducing BT virus into a BT-free area by the importation of infected semen were discussed (Grant *et al.* 1967).

BIBLIOGRAPHY

Afshar, A. and Kayvanfar, H., 1974. Occurrence of precipitating antibodies to bluetongue virus in sera of farm animals in Iran, *Vet. Rec.*, **94**: 233–5.

Alexander, R. A., 1959. Bluetongue as an international problem, *Bull. Off. int. Epiz.*, **51**: 432–9.

Alexander, R. A. and Haig, D. A., 1951. The use of egg attenuated bluetongue virus in the production of a polyvalent vaccine for sheep. A. Propagation of the virus in sheep, *Onderstepoort J. vet. Res.*, **25**(1): 3–15.

Alstad, A. D., Burger, D., Frank, F. W., McCain, C. S., Moll, T. and Stauber, E. S., 1977. Localization of bluetongue virus in red blood cells of experimentally infected sheep, *Proc. 20th Ann. Am. Assoc. Vet. Lab. Diagnost.*, pp. 273–90.

Anderson, C. K. and Jensen, R., 1969. Pathologic changes in placentas of ewes inoculated with bluetongue virus, *Am. J. vet. Res.*, **30**(6): 987–99.

Anon., 1958. Bluetongue in the United States in 1957, *J. Am. vet. med. Ass.*, **133**: 104–5.

Anon., 1965. Incidence of bluetongue reported in sheep in the U.S.A. during calendar year 1964, *Bull. Off. int. Epiz.*, **63**: 1344–5.

Anon., 1974. Bluetongue, *Bull. Off. int. Epiz.*, **81**(9–10): 867–77.

Anon., 1979. The present position of bluetongue virus in Australia, *Wld Anim. Rev.*, **32**: 49–50.

Barber, T. L., 1979. Temporal appearance, geographic distribution, and species of origin of bluetongue virus serotypes in the United States, *Am. J. vet. Res.*, **40**(1): 1654–6.

Barber, T. L. and Jochim, M. M., 1973. Serologic characterization of selected bluetongue virus strains from the United States, *Proc. 77th Ann. Meet. US Anim. Hlth Assoc.*, 14–19 Oct. 1973, pp. 352–9.

Barber, T. L., Stott, J. L., Osburn, B. I. and Sawyer, M., 1979. Development of an experimental inactivated bluetongue virus vaccine for sheep, *J. Am. vet. med. Ass.*, **175**: 611.

Barnard, B. J. H. and Pienaar, J. G., 1976. Bluetongue virus as a cause of hydranencephaly in cattle, *Onderstepoort J. vet. Res.*, **43**(3): 155–8.

Barnes, M. A., Wright, R. E., Bodine, A. B. and Alberty, C. F., 1982. Frequency of bluetongue and bovine parvovirus infection in cattle in South Carolina dairy herds, *Am. J. vet. Res.*, **43**(6): 1078–80.

Bhambani, B. D. and Singh, P. P., 1968. Bluetongue disease of sheep in India, *Indian vet. J.*, **45**: 370–1.

Borden, E. C., Shope, R. E. and Murphy, F. A., 1971. Physicochemical and morphological relationships of some arthropod-borne viruses to bluetongue virus – a new taxonomic group. Physicochemical and serological studies, *J. gen. Virol.*, **13**: 261–71.

Boulanger, P. and Frank, J. F., 1975. Serological methods in the diagnosis of bluetongue, *Aust. vet. J.*, **51**: 185–9.

Boulanger, P., Ruckerbauer, G. M., Bannister, G. L., Gray, D. P. and Girard, A., 1967. Studies on bluetongue. III. Comparison of two complement-fixation methods, *Can. J. comp. Med. Vet. Sci.*, **31**: 166–70.

Bowne, J. G., 1971. Bluetongue disease, *Adv. vet. Sci. comp. Med.*, **15**: 1–46.

Bowne, J. G., 1973. Is bluetongue an important disease in cattle? *J. Am. vet. med. Ass.*, **163**(7): 911–14.

Bowne, J. G. and Jochim, M. M., 1967. Cytopathologic changes and development of inclusion bodies in cultured cells infected with bluetongue virus, *Am. J. vet. Res.*, **28**(125): 1091–105.

Bowne, J. G., Luedke, A. J., Foster, N. M. and Jochim, M. M., 1966. Current aspects of bluetongue in cattle, *J. Am. vet. med. Ass.*, **148**(10): 1177–80.

Bowne, J. G., Luedke, A. J., Jochim, M. M. and Foster, N. M., 1964. Current status of bluetongue in sheep, *J. Am. vet. med. Ass.*, **144**(7): 759–64.

Bowne, J. G., Luedke, A. J., Jochim, M. M. and Metcalf, H. E., 1968. Bluetongue disease in cattle, *J. Am. vet. med. Ass.*, **153**(6): 662–8.

Bowne, J. G. and Ritchie, A. E., 1970. Some morphological features of bluetongue virus, *Virology*, **40**: 903–11.

Breckon, R. D., Luedke, A. J. and Walton, T. E., 1980. Bluetongue virus in bovine semen; viral isolation, *Am. J. vet. Res.*, **41**(3): 439–42.

Bwangamoi, O., 1978. Pathology of ovine foetus infection with bluetongue virus, *Bull. Anim. Hlth Prod. Afr.*, **26**: 79–97.

Campbell, C. H., Barber, T. L. and Jochim, M. M., 1978. Antigenic relationship of Ibaraki, bluetongue, and epizootic hemorrhagic disease viruses, *Vet. Microbiol.*, **3**: 15–22.

Carrier, S. P. and Boulanger, P., 1975. Improvements in the modified direct complement fixation test and its application in the detection of bluetongue antibodies in cattle and sheep sera, *Can. J. comp. Med. Vet. Sci.*, **39**: 231–3.

Clark, R. and Wagner, A. M., 1967. Plasma enzymes in bluetongue, *J. S. Afr. vet. med. Ass.*, **33**(3): 221–3.
Coackley, W., Smith, V. W. and Maker, D., 1980. A serological survey for bluetongue virus antibody in Western Australia, *Aust. vet. J.*, **56**: 487–91.
Couvillion, C. E., Jenney, E. W., Pearson, J. E. and Coker, M. E., 1980. Survey for antibodies to viruses of bovine virus diarrhea, bluetongue, and epizootic hemorrhagic disease in hunter-killed mule deer in New Mexico, *J. Am. vet. med. Ass.*, **177**(9): 790–1.

Dafni, I., 1966. Bluetongue in Israel in the years 1964 and 1965, *Bull. Off. int. Epiz.*, **66**: 319–27.
Davies, F. G., 1978. Bluetongue studies with sentinel cattle in Kenya, *J. Hyg., Camb.*, **30**: 197–204.
Davies, F. G. and Blackburn, N. K., 1971. The typing of bluetongue virus, *Res. vet. Sci.*, **12**: 181–3.
Davies, F. G. and Walker, A. R., 1974. The distribution in Kenya of bluetongue virus and antibody, and the *Culicoides* vector, *J. Hyg., Camb.*, **72**: 265–72.
Della-Porta, A. J., Herniman, K. A. J. and Sellers, R. F., 1981a. A serological comparison of the Australian isolate of bluetongue virus type 20 (CSIRO 19) with bluetongue group viruses, *Vet. Microbiol.*, **6**: 9–21.
Della-Porta, A. J., McPhee, D. A., Parsonson, I. M. and Snowdon, W. A., 1982. Classification of the arboviruses. Confusion in the use of terms bluetongue virus, bluetongue-like virus, bluetongue-related virus and the overall nomenclature, *Aust. vet. J.*, **58**: 164–5.
Della-Porta, A. J., McPhee, D. A., Wark, M. C., St George, T. D. and Cybinski, D. H., 1981b. Serological studies of two additional Australian bluetongue virus isolates CSIRO 154 and 156, *Vet. Microbiol.*, **6**: 233–45.
du Toit, R. M., 1962. Bluetongue – recent advances in research. The role played by bovines in the transmission of bluetongue in sheep, *J. S. Afr. vet. med. Ass.*, **33**(4): 483–90.

Eisa, M., Karrar, A. E. and Abd Elrahim, A. H., 1979. Incidence of bluetongue virus precipitating antibodies in sera of some domestic animals in the Sudan, *J. Hyg., Camb.*, **83**: 539–45.
Eisa, M., Osman, O. M., Karrar, A. E. and Abdel Rahim, A. A., 1980. An outbreak of bluetongue in sheep in the Sudan, *Vet. Rec.*, **106**: 481–2.
Els, H. J. and Verwoerd, D. W., 1969. Morphology of bluetongue virus, *Virology*, **38**: 213–19.
Enright, F. M. and Osburn, B. I., 1980. Ontogeny of host responses in ovine fetuses infected with bluetongue virus, *Am. J. vet. Res.*, **41**: 224–9.

Erasmus, B. J., 1975a. Bluetongue in sheep and goats, *Aust. vet. J.*, **51**(4): 165–70.
Erasmus, B. J., 1975b. The epizootiology of bluetongue: the African situation, *Aust. vet. J.*, **51**: 196–8.
Erasmus, B. J., 1975c. The control of bluetongue in an enzootic situation, *Aust. vet. J.*, **51**: 209–10.

Fernandes, M. V., 1959. Cytopathogenic effects of lamb tissues *in vitro*, *Texas Reports on Biology*, **17**: 94–105.
Flanagan, M., Wilson, A. J., Trueman, K. F. and Shepherd, M. A., 1982. Bluetongue virus serotype 20 infection in pregnant Merino sheep, *Aust. vet. J.*, **59**: 18–20.
Foster, N. M., 1976. Bluetongue virus characterization, *Proc. 79th Ann. Meet. US Anim. Hlth Ass.*, pp. 350–66.
Foster, N. M., Alders, M. A., Luedke, A. J. and Walton, T. E., 1979. Abnormalities, virus-like particles and infectivity in spermatozoa from bluetongue virus latently infected bulls, *Abstracts Ann. Meet. Am. Soc. Microbiol.*, p. 263.
Foster, N. M. and Jones, R. H., 1979a. Effect of normal and supranormal concentrations of bluetongue virus on the infection rate of the vector *Culicoides variipennis*, *Abstracts Ann. Meet. Am. Soc. Microbiol.*, p. 286.
Foster, N. M. and Jones, R. H., 1979b. Multiplication rate of bluetongue virus in the vector *Culicoides variipennis* (Diptera: Ceratopogonidae) infected orally, *J. Med. Entomol.*, **15**(3): 302–3.
Foster, N. M., Jones, R. H. and McCrory, B. R., 1963. Preliminary investigations on insect transmissions of bluetongue virus in sheep, *Am. J. vet. Res.*, **24**(103): 1195–200.
Foster, N. M. and Luedke, A. J., 1968. Direct assay for bluetongue virus by intravascular inoculation of embryonating chicken eggs, *Am. J. vet. Res.*, **29**: 749–53.
Foster, N. M., Luedke, A. J. and Metcalf, H. E., 1972. Bluetongue in sheep and cattle: efficacy of embryonating chicken eggs in viral isolations, *Am. J. vet. Res.*, **33**: 77–81.
Foster, N. M., Metcalf, H. E., Barber, T L., Jones, R. H. and Luedke, A. J., 1980. Bluetongue and epizootic hemorrhagic disease virus isolations from vertebrate and invertebrate hosts at a common geographic site, *J. Am. vet. med. Ass.*, **176**(2): 126–9.
Frank, J. F. and Willis, N. G., 1975. Bluetongue-like disease of deer, *Aust. vet. J.*, **51**: 174–7.
Fulton, R. W., Nicholson, S. S., Pearson, N. J., Potter, M. T., Archbald, L. F., Pearson, J. E. and Jochim, M. M., 1982. Bluetongue infections in Louisiana cattle, *Am. J. vet. Res.*, **43**(5): 887–91.
Fulton, R. W., Potter, M. T., Pearson, N. J. and Hagstad, H. V., 1981. Prevalence of bluetongue viral antibodies in Louisiana goats, *Am. J. vet. Res.*, **42**(1): 1985–6.

Geering, W. A., 1975. Control of bluetongue in an epizootic situation: Australian plans, *Aust. vet. J.*, **51**: 220–4.

Gibbs, E. P. J., Lawman, M. J. P. and Herniman, K. A. J., 1979. Preliminary observations on transplacental infection of bluetongue virus in sheep – a possible overwintering mechanism, *Res. vet. Sci.*, **27**(1): 118–20.

Girard, A., Ruckerbauer, G. M., Gray, D. P., Bannister, G. L. and Boulanger, P., 1967. Studies on bluetongue. IV. Studies of three strains in primary bovine foetal kidney cell cultures, *Can. J. comp. Med. Vet. Sci.*, **31**: 171–4.

Gleiser, C. A., Stair, E. L. and McGill, L. D., 1969. Diagnosis of bluetongue in cattle by intravascular inoculation of chicken embryos and immunofluorescence, *Am. J. vet. Res.*, **30**(6): 981–6.

Goldsmit, L. and Barzilai, E., 1968. An improved method for the isolation and identification of bluetongue virus by intravenous inoculation of embryonating chicken eggs, *J. Comp. Path.*, **78**: 477–87.

Gorman, B. M., Taylor, J., Walker, P. J., Davidson, W. L. and Brown, F., 1981. Comparison of bluetongue type 20 with certain viruses of the bluetongue and Eubenangee serological groups of orbiviruses, *J. gen. Virol.*, **57**: 251–61.

Grant, K. M., Clay, A. L. and Hale, K. B., 1967. Action taken in Queensland to prevent a possible introduction of bluetongue virus in cattle semen, *Aust. vet. J.*, **43**: 31–3.

Gray, D. P., Willis, N. G., Girard, A., Ruckerbauer, G. M., Boulanger, P. and Bannister, G. L., 1967. Studies on bluetongue. VI. Animal transmission studies, *Can. J. comp. Med. Vet. Sci.*, **31**: 182–8.

Griner, L. A., McCrory, B. R., Foster, N. M. and Meyer, H., 1964. Bluetongue associated with abnormalities in newborn lambs, *J. Am. vet. med. Ass.*, **145**(10): 1013–19.

Hafez, S. M., 1978. Serological survey of bluetongue in Iraq, *Bull. Off. int. Epiz.*, **89**(1–2): 13–22.

Hafez, S. M. and Ozawa, Y., 1973. Serological survey of bluetongue in Egypt, *Bull. epiz. Dis. Afr.*, **21**(3): 297–304.

Haig, D. A., McKercher, D. G. and Alexander, R. A., 1956. The cytopathogenic action of bluetongue virus on tissue cultures and its application to the detection of antibodies in the serum of sheep, *Onderstepoort J. vet. Res.*, **27**(2): 171–7.

Hardy, W. T. and Price, D. A., 1952. Soremuzzle of sheep, *J. Am. vet. med. Ass.*, **120**: 23–5.

Henning, M. W., 1956. Bluetongue, bloutong (catarrhal fever of sheep). In *Animal Diseases in South Africa. Being an Account of the Infectious Diseases of Domestic Animals*. Central News Agency (South Africa), pp. 809–27.

Hoff, G. L. and Hoff, D. M., 1976. Bluetongue and epizootic hemorrhagic disease: a review of these diseases in non-domestic

artiodactyles, *J. Zoo. Anim. Med.*, **7**(2): 26–30.
Hoff, G. L., Griner, L. A. and Trainer, D. O., 1973. Bluetongue virus in exotic ruminants, *J. Am. vet. med. Ass.*, **163**: 565–7.
Hoff, G. L. and Trainer, D. O., 1972. Bluetongue virus in pronghorn antelope, *Am. J. vet. Res.*, **33**(5): 1013–16.
Hourrigan, J. L. and Klingsporn, A. L., 1975a. Bluetongue: the disease in cattle, *Aust. vet. J.*, **51**(4): 170–4.
Hourrigan, J. L. and Klingsporn, A. L., 1975b. Epizootiology of bluetongue: the situation in the United States of America, *Aust. vet. J.*, **51**: 203–8.
Howell, P. G., 1960. A preliminary antigenic classification of strains of bluetongue virus, *Onderstepoort J. vet. Res.*, **28**(3): 357–64.
Howell, P. G., 1963. Bluetongue. In *Emerging Diseases of Animals*, No. 61. FAO/UN (Rome, Italy), pp. 111–53.
Howell, P. G., 1966. Some aspects of the epizootiology of bluetongue, *Bull. Off. int. Epiz.*, **66**: 341–52.
Howell, P. G., 1970. The antigenic classification and distribution of naturally occurring strains of bluetongue virus, *J. S. Afr. vet. med. Ass.*, **41**(3): 215–23.
Howell, P. G., Kumm, N. A. and Botha, M. J., 1970. The application of improved techniques to the identification of strains of bluetongue virus, *Onderstepoort J. vet. Res.*, **37**(1): 59–66.
Howell, P. G. and Verwoerd, D. W., 1971. Bluetongue virus, *Virology Monographs*, **9**: 37–74.
Howell, P. G., Verwoerd, D. W. and Oellermann, R. A., 1967. Plaque formation by bluetongue virus, *Onderstepoort J. vet. Res.*, **34**(2): 317–32.
Hubschle, O. J. B., 1980. Bluetongue virus hemagglutination and its inhibition by specific sera, *Arch. Virol.*, **64**: 133–40.
Hubschle, O. J. B., Lorenz, R. J. and Matheka, H. D., 1981. Enzyme-linked immunosorbent assay for detection of bluetongue virus antibodies, *Am. J. vet. Res.*, **42**(1): 61–5.
Huismans, H., 1979. Protein synthesis in bluetongue virus-infected cells, *Virology*, **92**: 385–96.
Huismans, H. and Bremer, C. W., 1981. A comparison of an Australian bluetongue virus isolate (CSIRO 19) with other bluetongue virus serotypes by cross-hybridization and cross-immune precipitation, *Onderstepoort J. vet. Res.*, **48**: 59–67.
Huismans, H. and Erasmus, B. J., 1981. Identification of the serotype-specific and group-specific antigens of bluetongue virus, *Onderstepoort J. vet. Res.*, **48**: 51–8.

Inaba, Y., 1975. Ibaraki disease and its relationship to bluetongue, *Aust. vet. J.*, **51**(4): 178–85.
Inaba, Y., Ishii, S. and Omori, T., 1966. Bluetongue-like disease in Japan, *Bull. Off. int. Epiz.*, **66**: 329–40.
Inverso, M., Lukas, G. N. and Weidenbach, S. J., 1980. Caprine bluetongue virus isolations, *Am. J. vet. Res.*, **41**(2): 277–8.

Ito, Y., Tanaka, Y., Inaba, Y. and Omori, T., 1973. Electron microscopy of Ibaraki virus, *Arch. ges. Virusforsch.*, **40**: 29–46.

Jameson, P. and Grossberg, S. E., 1981. Preparation and characterization of bluetongue virus. In *Methods in Enzymology*. Academic Press (New York), vol. 78, pp. 312–15.

Jennings, M. and Boorman, J., 1980. Use of the indirect fluorescent antibody technique for the detection of bluetongue virus antigen in tissue smears from *Culicoides variipennis* (Diptera, Ceratopogonidae), *Vet. Microbiol.*, **5**: 13–18.

Jochim, M. M., Barber, T. L. and Bando, B. M., 1975. Identification of bluetongue and epizootic hemorrhagic disease viruses by the indirect fluorescent antibody procedure, *Proc. 17th Ann. Meet. Am. Assoc. Vet. Lab. Diagnost.*, pp. 91–103.

Jochim, M. M. and Bowne, J. G., 1980. Bluetongue. In *Bovine Medicine and Surgery*, 2nd edn, ed. H. E. Amstutz. American Veterinary Publications, Vol. 1, pp. 176–82.

Jochim, M. M. and Jones, R. H., 1966. Multiplication of bluetongue virus in *Culicoides variipennis* following artificial infection, *Am. J. Epidem.*, **84**(2): 241–6.

Jochim, M. M. and Jones, S. C., 1977. Enhancement of bluetongue and epizootic hemorrhagic disease viral neutralization with anti-gamma globulin, *Proc. 20th Ann. Meet. Am. Assoc. Vet. Lab. Diagnost.*, pp. 255–72.

Jochim, M. M. and Jones, S. C., 1980. Evaluation of a hemolysis-in-gel test for detection and quantitation of antibodies to bluetongue virus, *Am. J. vet. Res.*, **41**(4): 595–9.

Jochim, M. M., Luedke, A. J. and Bowne, J. G., 1965. The clinical and immunogenic response of sheep to oral and intradermal administration of bluetongue virus, *Am. J. vet. Res.*, **26**(115): 1254–60.

Jones, R. H., Luedke, A. J., Walton, T. E. and Metcalf, H. E., 1981. Bluetongue in the United States. An entomological perspective toward control, *Wld Anim. Rev.*, **38**: 2–8.

Karstad, L., 1967. Comparative histopathology of experimental bluetongue disease and epizootic hemorrhagic disease of deer, *Bull. Wildl. Dis. Assoc.*, **3**: 119.

Karstad, L. and Trainer, D. O., 1967. Histopathology of experimental bluetongue disease of white-tailed deer, *Can. vet. J.*, **8**(11): 247–54.

Kennedy, P. C., 1968. Some aspects of bluetongue in the United States, *Aust. vet. J.*, **44**: 191–4.

Kipps, A., 1956. Complement fixation with antigens prepared from bluetongue virus-infected mouse brains, *J. Hyg., Camb.*, **54**: 79–88.

Klingsporn, A. L., 1978. Report of the Committee on disease of sheep and goats, *Proc. 82nd Ann. Meet. USA Anim. Hlth Assoc.*, 29–31

Oct., 1–3 Nov. 1978, pp. 409–11.

Komarov, A. and Haig, D. A., 1952. Identification of a strain of bluetongue virus isolated in Israel, *J. S. Afr. vet. med. Ass.*, **23**(2): 153–6.

Lee, V. H., Causey, O. R. and Moore, D. L., 1974. Bluetongue and related viruses in Ibadan, Nigeria: isolation and preliminary identification of viruses, *Am. J. vet. Res.*, **35**(8): 1105–8.

Livingston, C. W. and Hardy, W. T., 1964. Isolation of an antigenic variant of bluetongue virus, *Am. J. vet. Res.*, **25**(109): 1598–600.

Livingston, C. W. and Moore, R. W., 1962. Cytochemical changes of bluetongue virus in tissue cultures, *Am. J. vet. Res.*, **23**(95): 701–10.

Lopez, A. C., 1957. Rapport sur l'épizootie de fièvre catarrhal ovine 'langue bleue' en Espagne, *Bull. Off. int. Epiz.*, **48**: 605–11.

Lopez, A. C. and Sanchez Botija, C., 1958. Bluetongue in Spain, *Bull. Off. int. Epiz.*, **50**: 67–93.

Luedke, A. J., 1969. Bluetongue in sheep: viral assay and viremia, *Am. J. vet. Res.*, **30**(4): 499–509.

Luedke, A. J. and Anakwenze, E. I., 1972. Bluetongue virus in goats, *Am. J. vet. Res.*, **33**(9): 1739–45.

Luedke, A. J., Jochim, M. M. and Bowne, J. G., 1965. Preliminary bluetongue transmission with the sheep ked *Melophagus ovinus* (L), *Can. J. comp. Med. Vet. Sci.*, **29**: 229–31.

Luedke, A. J., Jochim, M. M., Bowne, J. G. and Jones, R. H., 1970. Observations on latent bluetongue virus infection in cattle, *J. Am. vet. med. Ass.*, **156**(12): 1871–9.

Luedke, A. J., Jochim, M. M. and Jones, R. H., 1969. Bluetongue in cattle: viremia, *Am. J. vet. Res.*, **30**(4): 511–16.

Luedke, A. J., Jochim, M. M. and Jones, R. H., 1977a. Bluetongue in cattle: effects of *Culicoides variipennis*-transmitted bluetongue virus on pregnant heifers and their calves, *Am. J. vet. Res.*, **38**(11): 1687–95.

Luedke, A. J., Jochim, M. M. and Jones, R. H., 1977b. Bluetongue in cattle: effects of vector-transmitted bluetongue virus on calves previously infected *in utero*, *Am. J. vet. Res.*, **38**(11): 1697–700.

Luedke, A. J., Jochim, M. M. and Jones, R. H., 1977c. Bluetongue in cattle: repeated exposure of two immunologically tolerant calves to bluetongue virus by vector bites, *Am. J. vet. Res.*, **38**(11): 1701–4.

Luedke, A. J., Jones, R. H. and Jochim, M. M., 1967. Transmission of bluetongue between sheep and cattle by *Culicoides variipennis*, *Am. J. vet. Res.*, **28**(123): 457–60.

Leudke, A. J., Jones, R. H. and Walton, T. E., 1977d. Overwintering mechanism for bluetongue virus: biological recovery of latent virus from a bovine by bites of *Culicoides variipennis*, *Am. J. trop. Med. Hyg.*, **26**(2): 313–25.

Luedke, A. J., Walton, T. E. and Breckon, R. D., 1980. Blood autograft in sheep for isolation of bluetongue virus from latently infected cattle, *Proc. 84th Ann. Meet. USA Hlth Assoc.*, 2–7 Nov. 1980, pp. 203–14.

Manning, J. S. and Chen, M. F., 1980. Bluetongue virus: detection of antiviral immunoglobulin G by means of enzyme-linked immunosorbent assay, *Curr. Microbiol.*, **4**: 381–5.

Manso-Ribeiro, J., Rosa-Azevedo, J. A., Noronha, F. O., Braço-Forte, M. C. Jr, Grave-Pereira, C. and Vasco-Fernandes. M., 1957. Bluetongue in Portugal, *Bull. Off. int. Epiz.*, **48**: 350–67.

Martin, S. A. and Zweerink, H. J., 1972. Isolation and characterization of two types of bluetongue virus particles, *Virology*, **50**: 495–506.

McCrory, B. R., Bay, R. C. and Foster, N. M., 1957. Observations on bluetongue in sheep, *Proc. 61st Ann. Meet. US Livestk sanit. Ass.*, St Louis, 1957, pp. 271–5.

McCrory, B. R., Foster, N. M. and Bay, R. C., 1959. Virucidal effect of some chemical agents on bluetongue virus, *Am. J. vet. Res.*, **20**: 665–9.

McGowan, B., 1953. An epidemic resembling soremuzzle or bluetongue in California sheep, *Cornell Vet.*, **43**: 213–16.

McGowan, B., McKercher, D. G. and Shultz, G., 1956. Studies on bluetongue. IV. Field trial of a modified live virus vaccine, *J. Am. vet. med. Ass.*, **128**: 454–6.

McKercher, D. G., McGowan, B., Cabasso, V. J. and Roberts, G. I., 1957a. Studies on bluetongue. III. The development of a modified live virus vaccine employing American strains of bluetongue virus, *Am. J. Vet. Res.*, **18**: 310–16.

McKercher, D. G., McGowan, B., Howarth, J. A. and Saito, J. K., 1953. A preliminary report on the isolation and identification of the bluetongue virus from sheep in California, *J. Am. vet. med. Ass.*, **122**: 300–1.

McKercher, D. G., McGowan, B. and McCrory, B. R., 1957b. Studies on bluetongue. V. Distribution of bluetongue in the United States as confirmed by diagnostic tests, *J. Am. vet. med. Ass.*, **130**: 86–9.

McKercher, D. G., Saito, J. K. and Singh, K. V., 1970. Serologic evidence of an etiologic role for bluetongue virus in hydranencephaly of calves, *J. Am. vet. med. Ass.*, **156**(8): 1044–7.

Mellor, P. S. and Boorman, J., 1980. Multiplication of bluetongue virus in *Culicoides nubeculosus* (Meigen) simultaneously infected with the virus and the microfilariae of *Onchocerca cervicalis* (Railliet and Henry), *Ann. trop. Med. Parasitol.*, **74**(4): 463–9.

Metcalf, H. E., Lomme, J. and Beal, V. C. Jr, 1980. Estimate of incidence and direct economic losses due to bluetongue in Mississippi cattle during 1979, *Proc. 84th Ann. Meet. US Anim. Hlth Assoc.*, pp. 186–202.

Metcalf, H. E. and Luedke, A. J., 1974. Bluetongue: problems in diagnosis and incidence measurement, *J. Am. vet. med. Ass.*, **165**: 737.

Metcalf, H. E. and Luedke, A. J., 1978. Bluetongue and related diseases. In *Veterinary Preventive Medicine and Epidemiology*. Work Conference, USDA, pp. 44–58.

Metcalf, H. E., Pearson, J. E. and Klingsporn, A. L., 1979. Bluetongue in cattle: a serological study in the United States, using slaughter cattle sera, *J. Am. vet. med. Ass.*, **175**(6): 612.

Metcalf, H. E., Pearson, J. E. and Klingsporn, A. L., 1981. Bluetongue in cattle: a serological survey of slaughter cattle in the United States, *Am. J. vet. Res.*, **42**(6): 1057–61.

Moore, D. L. and Kemp, G. E., 1974. Bluetongue and related viruses in Ibadan, Nigeria: serologic studies of domesticated and wild animals, *Am. J. vet. Res.*, **35**(8): 1115–20.

Moulton, J. E., 1961. Pathology of bluetongue in sheep, *J. Am. vet. med. Ass.*, **138**(9): 493–8.

Murphy, F. A., Borden, E. C., Shope, R. E. and Harrison, A., 1971. Physicochemical and morphological relationships of some arthropod-borne viruses to bluetongue virus – a new taxonomic group. Electron microscopic studies, *J. gen. Virol.*, **13**(2): 273–88.

Murray, J. O. and Trainer, D. O., 1970. Bluetongue virus in North American elk, *J. Wildl. Dis.*, **6**: 144–8.

Narayan, O., McFarland, H. F. and Johnson, R. T., 1972. Effects of viral infection on nervous system development, *Am. J. Path.*, **68**(1): 15–22.

Neitz, W. O., 1966. Bluetongue, *Bull. Off. int. Epiz.*, **65**(9–10): 1749–58.

Nevill, E. M., 1971. Cattle and *Culicoides* biting midges as possible overwintering hosts of bluetongue virus, *Onderstepoort J. vet. Res.*, **38**(2): 65–72.

Nevill, E. M., 1978. The use of cattle to protect sheep from bluetongue infection, *J. S. Afr. vet. med. Ass.*, **49**: 129–30.

Ohder, H., Lund, L. J. and Whiteland, A. P., 1970. Observations on the growth and development of bluetongue, Nairobi sheep disease and Rift Valley fever viruses by fluorescent antibody technique and titration in a tissue culture system, *Arch. ges. Virusforsch.*, **29**: 127–38.

Omori, T., Inaba, Y., Morimoto, T., Tanaka, Y., Ishitani, R., Kurogi, H., Munakata, K., Matsuda, K. and Matumoto, M., 1969a. Ibaraki virus, and agent of epizootic disease of cattle resembling bluetongue. I. Epidemiologic, clinical and pathologic observations and experimental transmission to calves, *Jap. J. Microbiol.*, **13**(2): 139–57.

Omori, T., Inaba, Y., Morimoto, T., Tanaka, Y., Kono, M., Kurogi, H. and Matumoto, M., 1969b. Ibaraki virus, an agent of epizootic disease of cattle resembling bluetongue. II. Isolation of the virus in bovine cell culture, *Jap. J. Microbiol.*, **13**(2): 159–68.

Osburn, B. I., McGowan. B., Heron, B., Loomis, E., Bushnell, R., Stott, J. and Utterback, W., 1981. Epizootiologic study of bluetongue: virologic and serologic results, *Am. J. vet. Res.*, **42**(5): 884–7.

Osburn, B. I., Sawyer, M., Stabenfeldt, G. H. and Trees, C., 1975. Persistent viremia in neonatal lambs infected with bluetongue virus at the height of physiological stress, *Fed. Proc.*, **34**(3): 836.

Osburn, B. I. and Silverstein, A. M., 1972. Animal model: bluetongue-vaccine-virus infection in fetal lambs, *Am. J. Path.*, **67**(1): 211–14.

Osburn, B. I., Silverstein, A. M. and Prendergast, R. A., 1970. Relation of age, immune competence and the pathology of fetal lambs infected with attenuated bluetongue virus vaccine, *Fed. Proc.*, **29**: 286.

Osburn, B. I., Stott, J. L., Barber, L. and Sawyer, M., 1979. Development of an inactivated bluetongue virus vaccine, *Fed. Proc.*, **38**:(3 pt 1): 1159.

Owen, N. C., 1964. Investigations into the pH stability of bluetongue virus and its survival in mutton and beef, *Onderstepoort J. vet. Res.*, **31**(2): 109–18.

Owen, N. C., 1965. Recent advances in the study of bluetongue, *Bull. Off. int. Epiz.*, **64**: 671–5.

Owen, N. C., du Toit, R. M. and Howell, P. G., 1965. Bluetongue in cattle: typing of viruses isolated from cattle exposed to natural infection, *Onderstepoort J. vet. Res.*, **32**: 3–6.

Owen, N. C. and Munz, E. K., 1966. Observations on a strain of bluetongue virus by electron microscopy, *Onderstepoort J. vet. Res.*, **33**(1): 9–14.

Ozawa, Y. and Hafez, S. M., 1972. Serological relationship between African horse sickness and bluetongue viruses, *Bull. Off. int. Epiz.* **77**(11/12): 1612–13.

Ozawa, Y. and Hafez, S. M., 1973. Antigenic relationship between African horsesickness and bluetongue viruses, *Proc. 3rd int. Conf. Equine Infect. Dis.*, Paris, 1972. Karger (Basle), pp. 31–7.

Parsonson, I. M., Della-Porta, A. J., McPhee, D. A., Cybinski, D. H., Squire, K. R. E., Standfast, H. A. and Uren, M. F., 1918. Isolation of bluetongue virus serotype 20 from the semen of an experimentally infected bull, *Aust. vet. J.*, **57**: 252–3.

Pearson, J. E., Carbrey, E. A. and Gustafson, G. A., 1973. Bluetongue virus in cattle: complement fixing antibody response and viremia in experimentally infected animals, *Proc. 77th Ann. Meet. US Anim. Hlth Assoc.*, St Louis, Missouri, 14–19 Oct. 1973, pp. 524–31.

Pini, A., 1976. A study on the pathogenesis of bluetongue: replication of the virus in the organs of infected sheep, *Onderstepoort J. vet. Res.*, **43**(4): 159–64.

Pini, A., Coackley, W. and Ohder, H., 1966. Concentration of

bluetongue virus in experimentally infected sheep and virus identification by immune fluorescence technique, *Arch. ges. Virusforsch.*, **18**: 385–90.
Polydorou, K., 1978. The 1977 outbreak of bluetongue in Cyprus, *Trop. Anim. Hlth Prod.*, **10**: 229–32.
Price, D. A. and Hardy, W. T., 1954. Isolation of the bluetongue virus from Texas sheep – *Culicoides* shown to be a vector, *J. Am. vet. med. Ass.*, **124**(925): 255–8.

Reynolds, G. E., 1971. Clinical aspects of bluetongue in Oregon cattle, *Proc. 75th Ann. Meet. US Anim. Hlth Assoc.*, Oklahoma, 24–29 Oct. 1971, pp. 74–9.
Richards, W. P. C. and Cordy, D. R., 1967. Bluetongue virus infection: pathologic response of nervous systems in sheep and mice, *Science*, **156**: 530–1.
Richards, W. P. C., Crenshaw, G. L. and Bushnell, R. B., 1971. Hydranencephaly of calves associated with natural bluetongue virus infection, *Cornell Vet.*, **61**: 336–48.
Robertson, A., Appel, M., Bannister, G. L., Ruckerbauer, G. M. and Boulanger, P., 1965. Studies on bluetongue. II. Complement-fixing activity of ovine and bovine sera, *Can. J. comp. Med. Vet. Sci.*, **29**: 113–17.
Robinson, R. M., Hailey, T. L., Livingston, C. W. and Thomas, J. W., 1967. Bluetongue in the desert bighorn sheep, *J. Wildl. Mgmt*, **31**: 165–8.
Ruckerbauer, G. M., Gray, D. P., Girard, A., Bannister, G. L. and Boulanger, P., 1967. Studies on bluetongue. V. Detection of the virus in infected materials by immunofluorescence. *Can. J. comp. Med. vet. Sci.*, **31**: 175–81.

St George, T. D., 1980. The isolation of two bluetongue viruses from healthy cattle in Australia, *Aust. vet. J.*, **56**: 562–3.
St George, T. D. and McCaughan, C. I., 1979. The transmission of the CSIRO 19 strain of bluetongue virus type 20 to sheep and cattle, *Aust. vet. J.*, **55**: 198–9.
St George, T. D., Standfast, H. A., Cybinski, D. H., Dyce, A. L., Muller, M. J., Doherty, R. L., Carley, J. G., Filippich, C. and Frazier, C. L., 1978. The isolation of a bluetongue virus from *Culicoides* collected in the Northern Territory of Australia, *Aust. vet. J.*, **54**: 153–4.
Schmidt, R. E. and Panciera, R. J., 1973. Cerebral malformation in fetal lambs from a bluetongue-enzootic flock, *J. Am. vet. med. Ass.*, **162**: 567–8.
Sellers, R. F., 1975. Bluetongue in Cyprus, *Aust. Vet. J.*, **51**: 198–203.
Sellers, R. F., 1981. Bluetongue and related diseases. In *Virus Diseases of Food Animals. A World Geography of Epidemiology and Control*, ed. E. P. J. Gibbs. Academic Press, Disease Monographs (London), vol. II, pp. 567–83.

Sellers, R. F., Gibbs, E. P. J., Herniman, K. A. J., Pedgley, D. E. and Tucker, M. R., 1979. Possible origin of the bluetongue epidemic in Cyprus, August 1977, *J. Hyg., Camb.*, **83**: 547–55.

Sellers, R. F., Pedgley, D. E. and Tucker, M. R., 1978. Possible windborne spread of bluetongue to Portugal, June-July 1956, *J. Hyg., Camb.*, **81**: 189–96.

Sharma, S. N., Oberoi, M. S., Sodhi, S. S. and Baxi, K. K., 1981. Bluetongue virus precipitating antibodies in dairy animals of Punjab, India, *Trop. Anim. Hlth Prod.*, **13**: 193.

Shipham, S. O. and de la Rey, M., 1979. Genetic and physiological characterization of temperature-sensitive mutants of bluetongue virus, *Onderstepoort J. vet. Res.*, **46**: 87–94.

Shone, D. K., Haig, D. A. and McKercher, D. G., 1956. The use of tissue culture propagated bluetongue virus for complement fixation studies on sheep sera, *Onderstepoort J. vet. Res.*, **27**(2): 179–82.

Shultz, G. and DeLay, P. D., 1955. Losses in newborn lambs associated with bluetongue vaccination of pregnant ewes, *J. Am. vet. med. Ass.*, **127**: 224–6.

Simpson, V. R., 1979. Bluetongue antibody in Botswana's domestic and game animals, *Trop. Anim. Hlth Prod.*, **11**: 43–9.

Snowdon, W. A. and Gee, R. W., 1978. Bluetongue virus infection in Australia, *Aust. vet. J.*, **54**: 505.

Sodhi, S. S., Oberoi, M. S., Sharma, S. N. and Baxi, K. K., 1981. Prevalence of bluetongue virus precipitating antibodies in sheep and goats of Punjab, India, *Zbl. Vet. Med.*, **B28**: 421–3.

Soliman, A. M., Hafez, S. M. and Ozawa, Y., 1972. Recent epizootics of bluetongue in Egypt, *Bull. epiz. Dis. Afr.*, **20**(2): 105–12.

Squire, K. R. E., Uren, M. F. and St George, T. D., 1981. The transmission of two new Australian serotypes of bluetongue virus to sheep, *Aust. vet. J.*, **57**: 301.

Stair, E. L., Robinson, R. M. and Jones, L. P., 1968. Spontaneous bluetongue in Texas white-tailed deer, *Path. vet.*, **5**: 164–73.

Standfast, H. A., St George, T. D., Cybinski, D. H., Dyce, A. L. and McCaughan, C. A., 1978. Experimental infection of *Culicoides* with a bluetongue virus isolated in Australia, *Aust. vet. J.*, **54**: 457–8.

Stott, J. L., Barber, T. L. and Osburn, B. I., 1978. Serotyping bluetongue virus: a comparison of plaque inhibition (disc) and plaque neutralization methods, *Proc. 21st Ann. Meet. Am. Assoc. vet. Lab. Diagnost.*, 29–31 Oct. 1978, pp. 399–410.

Stott, J. L., Lauerman, L. H. and Luedke, A. J., 1982. Bluetongue virus in pregnant elk and their calves, *Am. J. vet. Res.*, **43**(3): 423–8.

Stott, J. L., Osburn, B. I. and Barber, T. L., 1979. The current status of research on an experimental bluetongue virus vaccine, *Proc. 83rd Ann. Meet. US Anim. Hlth Assoc.*, 28–31 Oct., 1–2 Nov. 1979, pp. 55–62.

Sugiyama, K., Bishop, D. H. L. and Roy, P., 1981. Analyses of the genomes of bluetongue viruses recovered in the United States.

1. Oligonucleotide fingerprint studies that indicate the existence of naturally occurring reassortant BTV isolates, *Virology*, **114**: 210–17.
Svehag, S-E., 1960. Effect of different 'contact conditions' on the bluetongue virus–antibody reaction, *Fed. Proc.*, **19**(pt 1): 203.
Svehag, S-E., 1962. Quantitative studies of bluetongue virus in mice, *Arch. ges. Virusforsch.*, **12**: 363–86.
Svehag, S-E., 1963. Thermal inactivation of bluetongue virus, *Arch. ges. Virusforsch.*, **13**: 499–510.
Svehag, S-E., 1966. Quantal and graded dose-responses of bluetongue virus: a comparison of their sensitivity as assay methods for neutralizing antibody, *J. Hyg., Camb.*, **64**: 231–44.
Symposium on bluetongue, 1975. Contributions by various authors, *Aust. vet. J.*, **51**: 165–232.

Taylor, W. P. and McCausland, A., 1976. Studies with bluetongue virus in Nigeria, *Trop. Anim. Hlth Prod.*, **8**: 169–73.
Thomas, A. D. and Neitz, W. O., 1947. Further observations on the pathology of bluetongue in sheep, *Onderstepoort J. vet. Sci. Anim. Ind.*, **22**: 27–40.
Thomas, F. C., Girard, A., Boulanger, P. and Ruckerbauer, G., 1976. A comparison of some serological tests for bluetongue virus infection, *Can. J. comp. Med.*, **40**: 291–7.
Thomas, F. C., Morse, P. M. and Seawright, G. L., 1979. Comparisons of some bluetongue virus isolates by plaque neutralization and relatedness tests, *Arch. Virol.*, **62**: 189–99.
Thomas, F. C. and Samagh, B. S., 1979. A rapid plaque neutralization test for bluetongue virus, *Can. J. comp. Med.*, **43**: 234–6.
Thomas, F. C. and Trainer, D. O., 1971. Bluetongue virus: some relationships among North American isolates and further comparisons with EHD virus, *Can. J. comp. Med.*, **35**: 187–91.
Thomas, F. C., Willis, N. G., Ruckerbauer, G. M., Girard, A. and Boulanger, P., 1975. A comparison of methods for monitoring viremia in a bluetongue virus infected bovine, *Proc. 18th Ann. Meet. Am. Assoc. vet. Lab. Diagnost.*, Portland, Oregon, 2–4 Nov. 1975, pp. 175–86.
Tokuhisa, S., Inaba, Y., Miura, Y. and Sato, K., 1981. Salt-dependent hemagglutination with bluetongue virus. Brief report, *Arch. Virol.*, **70**: 75–8.
Tomori, O., 1980. Bluetongue and related viruses in Nigeria: experimental infections of West African dwarf sheep with Nigeria strains of the viruses of epizootic hemorrhagic disease of deer and bluetongue, *Vet. Microbiol.*, **5**: 177–85.
Trainer, D. O., 1967. Epizootiology of epizootic hemorrhagic disease, *Bull. Wildl. Dis. Assoc.*, **3**: 120.
Trainer, D. O. and Jochim, M. M., 1969. Serologic evidence of bluetongue in wild ruminants of North America, *Am. J. vet. Res.*, **30**(1): 2007–11.

Trainer, D. O., Vosdingh, R. A. and Easterday, B. C., 1967. Experimental bluetongue disease in white-tailed deer, *Bull. Wildl. Dis. Assoc.*, **3**: 120.

van der Walt, N. T., 1979. Factors affecting the bluetongue virus neutralizing antibody response and the reaction between virus and antibody, *Onderstepoort J. vet. Res.*, **46**: 111–16.

van der Walt, N. T., 1980. A haemagglutination and haemagglutination inhibition test for bluetongue virus, *Onderstepoort J. vet. Res.*, **47**: 113–17.

van Dijk, A. A. and Huismans. H., 1980. The *in vitro* activation and further characterization of the bluetongue virus-associated transcriptase, *Virology*, **104**: 347–56.

van Kammen, A. and Cybinski, D. H., 1981. A serological survey for antibodies to bluetongue virus in Papua New Guinea, *Aust. vet. J.*, **57**: 253–5.

Verge, J. and Paraf, A., 1957. Bluetongue, *Rec. Méd. Vét.*, **133**: 3–22.

Verwoerd, D. W., 1969. Purification and characterization of bluetongue virus, *Virology*, **38**: 203–12.

Verwoerd, D. W. and Huismans, H., 1969. On the relationship between bluetongue, African horsesickness and reoviruses: hybridization studies, *Onderstepoort J. vet. Res.*, **36**(2): 175–80.

Vosdingh, R. A., Trainer, D. O. and Easterday, B. C., 1968. Experimental bluetongue disease in white-tailed deer, *Can. J. comp. Med. Vet. Sci.*, **32**: 382–7.

Walker, A. R. and Boreham, P. F. L., 1976. Blood feeding of *Culicoides* (Diptera, Ceratopogonidae) in Kenya in relation to the epidemiology of bluetongue and ephemeral fever, *Bull. ent. Res.*, **66**: 181–8.

Walker, A. R. and Davies, F. G., 1971. A preliminary survey of the epidemiology of bluetongue in Kenya, *J. Hyg., Camb.*, **69**: 47–60.

Young, S. and Cordy, D. R., 1964. An ovine fetal encephalopathy caused by bluetongue vaccine virus, *J. Neuropathol. exp. Neurol.*, **23**: 635–59.

Chapter

8

Bovine ephemeral fever

CONTENTS

INTRODUCTION

Bovine ephemeral fever (BEF) is a noncontagious viral disease of cattle and water buffalo which is characterized by acute fever, stiffness, and lameness. Although there is high morbidity, the mortality rate is low and affected animals exhibit a rapid, spontaneous recovery. The virus is probably transmitted by insects; mosquitoes and *Culicoides* are the most likely vectors.

Literature

The most comprehensive review of BEF was published by Mackerras *et al*. (1940) and concerned studies conducted in Australia. St George (1981) presented the most recent review of the literature and included his personal observations. The disease has been studied in most detail in Africa, Japan, and Australia.

ETIOLOGY

Bovine ephemeral fever virus is classified as a rhabdovirus on the basis of its physical and biochemical properties. Its shape varies from rhabdoid to conical, depending on the stage of infection in tissue culture or experimental animals. Mammalian and insect tissue cultures are used to propagate BEF virus. Although the virus has been grown in a number of these systems, very few attempts have been made to use them for obtaining primary isolations.

Literature

Doherty (1978) briefly described the various characteristics of BEF virus, and Inaba (1973) reviewed the literature concerning this disease. Cone-shaped virus particles typical of rhabdoviruses were observed in cell cultures and in mouse brains infected with BEF virus (Murphy *et al*. 1972). The shape of BEF virus differed from the regular bullet-shaped morphology of some rhabdoviruses in that it was conical or slightly deviant from the rhabdoid morphology (Della-Porta and Brown 1979). In electron microscopic studies, the virus was shown to be cone-shaped and had a basal diameter of approximately 176 nm and a height of about 80 nm (Lecatsas 1969, 1970). The virus isolated from South Africa was cone-shaped, while the strains studied in Japan and Australia were bullet-shaped (Lecatsas *et al*. 1969a, b). Since both bullet- and cone-shaped forms were observed in later investigations of the South African and Japanese strains, it was suggested that the virus was pleomorphic and that its shape was dependent on the temperature and duration of infection in a culture system (Theodoridis and Lecatsas 1973). Cone-shaped particles (185 × 73 nm) were observed with light, immunofluorescent, and electron-microscopic techniques during the early stages of BEF virus infections in cell cultures and mice, and variation in shape occurred late in the infection. It was concluded that the morphological variation was not strain-related; the appearance of broad-based cones was more likely associated with varying growth rate (Murphy *et al.* 1972). Tanaka *et al.* (1972) found that BEF virus contained double-stranded ribonucleic acid and therefore proposed that this agent could not be classified in the rhabdovirus group, but these findings were challenged by those of Della-Porta and Brown (1979).

The sensitivity of BEF virus to changes in the temperature and pH was studied. The virus was inactivated within 10 minutes at 56 °C, within 18 hours at 37 °C, and within 120 hours at 25 °C. A slight loss of titer was observed after the virus had been stored at 4 °C for 30 days, but infectivity was lost progressively with storage at −35 °C. Bovine ephemeral fever virus was inactivated within 10 minutes at pH 2.5 and 12.0 and infectivity was lost in 60 and 90 minutes at pH 5.1 and 9.1 respectively (Heuschele 1970).

Although the virus grows readily in mammalian and insect tissue cultures, there has been little published work on the use of these systems to obtain primary isolates from natural cases and vectors. The infectivity of BEF virus for different *in vitro* culture systems varied with the strain (St George 1981). The virus propagated in hamster, bovine, and rat cell cultures (Matumoto *et al.* 1970). Bovine ephemeral fever virus was isolated from infected bovine blood titrated in VERO cell cultures. Cytopathic effects (CPEs) may accompany viral multiplication in tissue cultures. A strain of BEF was grown in bovine kidney, testis, and synovial cell monolayers and produced CPEs in 24 hours (Tzipori 1975c). Bovine ephemeral fever virus was grown in baby hamster kidney (BHK) 21 and VERO cell cultures. It was found that the replication of the virus was restricted to only a few types of primary cell cultures of rat origin (Gaffar Elamin and Spradbrow 1978b). The cytopathology observed in VERO cells involved an extended phase of cell rounding that was followed by extreme cytoplasmic vacuolation and condensation which terminated in lysis (Murphy *et al.* 1972). The virus propagated best in BHK21–W12 cells of hamster kidney origin and induced extensive cellular changes which decreased at lower temperatures (Matumoto *et al.* 1970). Later it was found the cells derived from a pig kidney cell line were more satisfactory for growing and assaying BEF virus than BHK21 and VERO cells (Della-Porta and Snowdon 1979), although plaque assays could be conducted in VERO cells (Heuschele 1970).

EPIZOOTIOLOGY

Geographic distribution

Bovine ephemeral fever occurs in Africa, Australia, and Asia, with extension into the subtropics and some temperate regions. In some regions, sporadic outbreaks occurred during the years between extensive epizootics.

Wild ruminants appear to act as a reservoir or amplifying hosts and are implicated in the interepizootic maintenance of the virus. In an epizootic, a few sporadic cases may precede the main outbreak by a week or more.

Literature

Henning (1956) reviewed the history of BEF in Africa and Asia. A more recent review of the epizootiology of BEF virus in Africa (particularly Zimbabwe, South Africa, and Kenya), Japan, and Australia was presented by St George (1981). The incidence of the disease in various countries was described by Burgess (1971). Bovine ephemeral fever was first reported in southeastern Africa during the mid nineteenth century and early twentieth century. The distribution of the disease has been relatively well established. However, the vectors have not been completely determined.

In Australia, there have been major epizootics (1936–37, 1955–56, and 1967–68) and numerous sporadic outbreaks during the interepizootic periods (Newton and Wheatley 1970). Snowdon (1971) presented evidence which supported the hypothesis that the virus persisted in areas of Australia during interepizootic periods. Because little or no clinical disease occurred during these intervals, Snowdon suggested that BEF virus might be of low pathogenicity and immunogenicity for cattle. Gee *et al.* (1969) and Murray (1970) described the 1967–68 Australian epizootic. St George *et al.* (1973) discussed the epizootic of BEF which occurred in 1972–73 in Australia. Parallelism could be discerned there in the patterns of spread of these epizootics, suggesting that critical factors such as wind movements, rainfall, distribution of susceptible cattle, and vector populations might have all been similar during these periods (Burgess 1971; Murray 1970; Newton and Wheatley 1970; Standfast *et al.* 1973).

The disease occurred in summer and autumn and spread according to wind patterns. The epizootics were generally associated with rain (St George 1981). St George *et al.* (1977) reviewed the epizootiology of BEF in Australia and Papua New Guinea from the discovery of the disease to the 1967–68 epizootic and provided a detailed description of the epizootiological situation since 1968. The sera of cattle and buffalo in sentinel herds located in many areas of Australia and Papua New Guinea were examined for antibodies to arboviruses. It was established that sporadic outbreaks and subclinical infections occurred between major epizootics of BEF in Australia, but the virus was not detected in Papua New Guinea. Individual sentinel cattle developed antibody to BEF before clinical signs were observed, but the majority of animals in these herds developed antibodies to the virus following the passage of the epizootic through the group. Bovine ephemeral fever antibodies were also detected in 11% of the domesticated and feral water buffalo. The sentinel herd system provided valuable information because some serum samples were collected in a methodical sequential fashion (St George *et al.* 1977; St George 1980). In Australia, antibodies to BEF virus were found in deer, but not in marsupials (St George, 1981). Uren *et al.* (1983) discussed the epizootiology of BEF in Australia from 1975 to 1981 and concluded that during these years the character and pattern of spread was different from previous epizootics characterized by explosive outbreaks. Recently, isolations of new rhabdoviruses related serologically to BEF have been made in Australia which will further complicate the epizootiology (Cybinski and Zakrzewski 1983; Gard *et al.* 1983).

Epizootiological studies were undertaken utilizing antibody tests to determine the incidence of BEF in Japan (Yamada 1964a, b, c, d). In the 1949–51 outbreak, 770 000 cases were reported and about 10 000 deaths occurred (Inaba 1973).

Henning (1956) discussed the distribution of BEF in southern Africa. In Kenya, epizootics of BEF were associated with rainfall, but the disease also occurred during dry periods (St George 1981). A pattern has been observed where there were years when epidemic disease occurs, between which there were years marked by sporadic outbreaks and subclinical infection. In a more recent study on the epizootiology of BEF in Kenya, antibodies to the disease were detected in cattle located in various ecological zones which included highland forest, grassland, desert, and semidesert regions. Antibodies were found in several species of game animals, particularly in the waterbuck (*Kobus ellipsiprymnus*) and buffalo (*Syncerus caffer*), where more than 50% of the serum samples were positive. The wildebeest (*Connochaetes taurinus*) and hartebeest (*Alcelaphus buselaphus*) also had sera positive for neutralizing antibodies, although the incidence did not exceed 9%. These findings indicate that the virus was cycling in the wild ruminant populations which served as reservoirs during the interepizootic periods (Davies *et al.* 1975). Bovine ephemeral fever virus was isolated in Nigeria (Kemp *et al.* 1973).

Transmission

There is circumstantial evidence that BEF is spread by insects. Biologically transmitted arboviruses multiply in the vector and are inoculated with the saliva when a blood meal is obtained whereas mechanically transmitted agents are transported directly from host to host. Bovine ephemeral fever virus can be experimentally grown in species of *Culicoides* and mosquitoes and has been isolated from wild-caught members of these groups. Thus, although vector transmission of BEF has not been demonstrated experimentally, the virus is probably biologically transferred. The methods of feeding used by *Culicoides* and mosquitoes significantly affect the pathogenesis and epidemiology of the disease.

Literature

Based on convincing circumstantial evidence, it has been assumed that BEF is transmitted by biting insects. Early attempts to use mosquitoes and stable flies for mechanical and biological transmission of BEF were unsuccessful, and it was concluded that the appropriate species had not been identified. The disease is probably transmitted via biological means since the virus was shown to be capable of propagating in mosquitoes (Burgess 1971). Mechanical dissemination of arboviruses by biting flies is possible when the host has high titers of circulating virus and the thermal stability of the agent is such that it can withstand exposure on the vector's mouthparts. The dynamics of transmission depend on the vector's abundance, distribution, host preferences, and susceptibility to infection (Standfast and Dyce 1972).

The potential insect vectors of arboviruses of cattle and buffalo in Australia were studied. On the bases of observed attack rates, general abundance, distribution, and host range, certain species of biting midges (Ceratopogonidae) and mosquitoes (Culicidae) were considered to be the most likely vectors of BEF (Standfast and Dyce 1972). During the 1967–68 epizootic of the disease in Australia, attempts were made to isolate the virus from mosquitoes and ceratopogonids collected near affected herds. Eight viruses were isolated, but no strain of BEF was found. The materials from these arthropod pools also failed to produce a febrile reaction or antibody response in cattle (Doherty *et al.* 1972). Five viruses, all unrelated to BEF virus, were isolated in South Africa from *Culicoides* biting midges collected near herds of cattle in which the disease had occurred. The cattle possessed antibodies to most of these isolates (Theodoridis *et al.* 1979). In Kenya, BEF virus was successfully isolated from a pool of *Culicoides,* while nine other *Culicoides* pools and five mosquito pools were negative (Davies and Walker 1974). In Australia, two isolations of BEF virus were made from pools of mosquitoes collected in areas where a clinical disease was reported (St George *et al.* 1976).

INFECTION

The most effective means of mechanically transmitting BEF to cattle is by intravenous injection of blood collected during the occurrence of fever. Experimental transmission was not achieved when blood or other body fluids were injected by other parenteral routes. The virus is associated with the leukocytes and platelet fraction of the blood; its presence and multiplication in various tissues and organs cannot be easily demonstrated. The virus remains infective in blood held for 2 days at room temperature. Bovine ephemeral fever virus is naturally infective for the Asian buffalo, in which it causes clinical signs. Sheep with experimental infections respond immunologically, but do not develop clinical signs of disease. Serological surveys demonstrated that several species of African wild ruminants possess antibodies to BEF. Unweaned mice, rats, and hamsters are the only laboratory rodents that can acquire the infection through intracerebral inoculation of white blood cell (WBC) suspensions. The virulence of BEF virus increases with serial passage through suckling mice, and there is a concurrent reduction in the animals' survival time. Experimental transmission through laboratory animals usually reduces the pathogenicity for cattle.

Literature

Blood was found to be infective from the latter part of the incubation period up to the fourth day after subsidence of fever. The virus is associated with the platelet–leukocyte fraction of the blood. The virus was not apparent in synovial fluid, nor did it occur in high concentrations in the spleen or lymph nodes. The disease could not be transmitted by contact or by inoculation into the cervix. During the viremic stage, the virus could only be transmitted efficiently by the intravenous route; subcutaneous and intradermal injections were unreliable (Burgess 1971, 1973; Mackerras *et al*. 1940). Blood retained its infectivity for 48 days when it was stored at −2 °C to 2 °C and for 5 years when frozen in dry ice (Henning 1956) and 12 years at −100 °C (T. D. St George, personal communication). It was also shown to be infective for 48 hours when held at room temperature or under refrigeration (MacFarlane and Haig 1955).

Very little is known about the growth and distribution of BEF virus in the host tissues between the time of infection and the advent of clinical signs. The intracerebral inoculation of calves with a strain of BEF virus resulted in fatal encephalitis. This virus was reisolated from the brains of calves by intracerebral innoculation of suckling mice. Homogenates made from the calf-brain material did not induce antibody formation in other susceptible calves when inoculated intravenously. The original isolate failed to produce viremia in calves after intravenous inoculation. The strain was shown to have a degree of tropism for brain tissue in laboratory animals (Tzipori 1975a). It is postulated that the vascular endothelium is the most likely site of the viral replication (Burgess 1971).

Bovine ephemeral fever virus caused clinical syndromes in cattle and could also infect other ruminants. Asian buffalo with natural infections developed neutralizing antibodies and clinical signs which were similar to those observed in cattle. The results of serological surveys indicate that BEF does not occur naturally in sheep. However, the virus could be transmitted experimentally to these animals, which developed viremia and neutralizing antibodies in response to the infection, and no antibodies to BEF virus were detected in the sera of feral pigs in Australia (St George 1981). Other domestic animals (e.g. horses, goats, rabbits, guinea pigs, and a camel) could not be infected (Burgess 1971). Experimental infection of buffalo between the ages of 8 and 10 months was accomplished by intravenous inoculation of blood from a calf. Clinical signs were not induced in the buffalo, although the virus could be isolated from some of the infected animals (Young 1979). Previously, it was thought that sheep were not susceptible to BEF virus, but further investigation showed that these animals could be temporarily infected.

Some sheep demonstrated a mild hematological response, and leukocytes collected from these animals on days 3 and 4 after inoculation caused BEF in susceptible cattle. However, it is questionable whether sheep became infected under field conditions (Hall *et al.* 1975).

Tzipori (1975c) stated that van der Westhuizen was the first to isolate BEF virus from cattle by intracerebral passage in suckling mice. Of the 82 isolates obtained from natural clinical cases, 21 caused paralysis in suckling mice which had been inoculated intracerebrally with a buffy-coat preparation; the remaining 61 paralyzed the mice after a single blind passage. The virus isolated from suspected clinical cases in suckling mice caused relatively low mortality on first passage. Further passages increased the mortality in mice and attenuated the virus for cattle; it was rendered nonimmunogenic for bovines after approximately six to nine passages. The isolation of the virus in mice from naturally infected vectors was less efficient, requiring several intracerebral passages in suckling mice to obtain an isolate. Suckling hamsters and rats were also successfully used to passage BEF virus which had been adapted to mice (St George 1981; Sasaki *et al.* 1968). Inaba *et al.* (1968a, b) further investigated the multiplication of the virus in suckling hamsters, mice, and rats, and hamster tissue cultures.

Adult rats inoculated intravenously or intracerebrally did not develop clinical signs but produced a neutralizing antibody (Matumoto *et al.* 1970). Although strains of BEF virus were readily adapted to grow in the brains of suckling rodents, pathogenicity for adult animals was not commonly observed. Strain 525 of BEF virus was lethal for adult mice and guinea pigs on intracerebral inoculation. Other strains of virus which were found to be pathogenic for adult mice on intracerebral inoculation were derived after seven to eight passages through suckling mice. These strains produced tremors, convulsions, paralysis, and death in adult mice in 4 to 6 days, and there was an associated bilateral conjunctivitis (Gaffar Elamin and Spradbrow 1978c). Bovine ephemeral fever virus propagated along myelinated nerve fibers in the brains of guinea pigs, and maturation took place predominantly in the cytoplasm or cytoplasmic vacuoles. The virus was also found in glial cells and neutrophils in the brains of unweaned mice (Tzipori 1975d). In studies on mouse brains, the virus was observed to bud from the marginal membranes of neurones, but intracytoplasmic development also occurred (Holmes and Doherty 1970).

Bovine ephemeral fever virus has been grown in other laboratory systems. The virus isolated from bovine blood by intravenous inoculation into chicken embryos killed most of the embryos, but some chicks hatched with abnormalities. The virus was detected by immunofluorescence in the lung, liver, heart, and brain of these infected chick embryos. Viremia was also demonstrated in the lung and liver of hatched chicks. It was proposed that the virus multiplied in the vascular endothelium before it infected the target cells in the brain. The authors also concluded that the distribution of BEF virus in experimentally infected chicken embryos was similar to that observed in experimentally infected cattle (Gaffar Elamin and Spradbrow 1978a).

The pathogenicity and antigenic relationship of various isolates of BEF virus obtained during the 1956 and 1967–68 epizootics in Australia were examined. There were no differences in the clinical signs and antibody response of cattle after infection with the 1956 stain and several isolates of the 1968 strain. Suckling mice and tissue cultures of BHK21 cells were of nearly equal sensitivity in detecting neutralizing antibodies in the sera of recovered cattle. There were also no antigenic differences between isolates from these two epizootics; after infection with an isolate of either strain, cattle were resistant to a heterologous challenge (Snowdon 1970). A strain of BEF virus rapidly lost its pathogenicity for calves after passage in unweaned hamsters, unweaned mice, and tissue cultures. In calves, the attenuated virus only stimulated antibody production and immunity to virulent virus after repeated inoculations (Inaba *et al.* 1969a). A strain of BEF virus which was pathogenic for both cattle and mice was developed by alternating passages through cattle and mice. When injected intracerebrally, this strain killed unweaned mice within 3 days of first passage. The third baby mouse brain passage of this virus was pathogenic for adult mice, day-old guinea pigs, unweaned rats, and 3-day-old kittens when inoculated intracerebrally, and for 10- to 11-day-old chick embryos when injected intravenously. The adult mice and day-old guinea pigs had bilateral conjunctivitis, and the infected chicks developed ataxia and incoordination. This strain was also more pathogenic for calves (Tzipori and Spradbrow 1974).

CLINICAL SIGNS

Cattle and Asian buffalo infected with BEF virus develop characteristic clinical signs which appear to be uniform in natural cases observed in Africa, Australia and Japan. The incubation period of BEF ranges from 2 to 10 days, with an average of 3 days. The most striking pathognomonic feature of the disease is the dramatic suddenness of onset and recovery. The main symptoms are high fever, inappetence, shivering, lameness, and nasal discharge. There is considerable individual variation in the severity of the clinical signs which are observed in an outbreak. All breeds are susceptible, with bulls and cows being affected more severely than young calves. The morbidity in individual herds may be from 75 to 100%. In regions where the incidence is seasonal, the disease is most commonly observed in young animals, the more mature animals presumably being immune. Although one attack of BEF generally confers lifelong immunity, it has been reported that particular animals may exhibit clinical signs of the disease two or three times during a single epidemic.

The infection causes either clinical or subclinical syndromes. The first sign observed is elevation of temperature 12 to 24 hours prior to the development of other symptoms. The pyrexia may last for 1 to 4 days, but most animals are febrile for only 1 to 2 days. One or two peaks of elevated temperature may occur during the course of the illness. In uncomplicated cases, the temperature returns to normal within 3 days. Lameness is another prominent sign of BEF. It develops on the second day and persists for about 2 days. The lameness may be constant or shifting, and one or more legs may be affected. Persistent lameness, which is indicative of permanent nervous damage, has been observed occasionally. Muscle fibrillation, shivering, and swelling of joints may occur. The animals appear to be depressed, stiff, in pain, and stand with drooping heads. The majority of the animals remain standing during the fever, but some of the more severe cases may become recumbent for 8 to 24 hours. A small proportion of these seriously affected animals develops permanent paresis. In the more severe cases, the fever is accompanied by increased heart and respiratory rates, râles, and ocular and nasal discharges. The initial nasal discharge is watery, but it rapidly becomes mucoid and then purulent. An ocular discharge may occur in conjunction with a mucopurulent nasal discharge, conjunctivitis, and periorbital swelling. Excessive salivation is also occasionally observed. The changes which may occur in the digestive system include cessation of rumination, ruminal stasis, diarrhea, and constipation.

Clinical recovery is rapid, usually taking 1 to 3 days. The mortality rate seldom exceeds 2 to 3%. Death is frequently due to the complications of secondary infections. Fatal pulmonary emphysema is a complication which may be evidenced by an accumulation of air under the skin over the backbone. The commonest sequela is prolonged lameness. Other possible complications include pneumonia, mastitis, infertility, and locomotory disturbances. The infertility is confined to the bull and is temporary unless there is residual locomotory dysfunction. Abortion may also occur. A reduction in milk production is associated with subclinical mastitis and lasts for about 2 weeks; occasionally, lactation may cease altogether in animals late in lactation. Meat production is not significantly affected because muscle wastage is temporary.

Literature

Detailed reviews of the clinical signs of BEF were presented by Mackerras *et al.* (1940), Henning (1956), Burgess (1971), and St George (1981). A number of other investigators discussed the prevalence of the more common clinical manifestations of the disease in either cattle or buffalo (Balachandran 1965; Combs 1978; Lawrence 1957; Malviya and Prasad 1977).

Bovine ephemeral fever virus caused clinical syndromes in cattle (*Bos taurus, B. indicus, B. javanicus*) and water buffalo (*Bubalus bubalis*) (St George 1981). All breeds of cattle are affected; indigenous and exotic animals are equally susceptible, although it has been reported that more severe clinical symptoms occur in the exotic animals and in those which are in good condition (Henning 1956).

During an outbreak, only a few animals in a herd were affected initially, and the symptoms were mild and indefinite. Additional cases appeared within 4 to 7 days, and a peak was reached during the third week. Thereafter, the incidence of new cases declined, and the course of the disease through the herd was complete within 6 to 8 weeks. The incidence and persistence of the disease in the herd varied and depended on whether there were favorable conditions for transmission. It was reported that some animals experienced a second attack of BEF 1 to 6 weeks after the first. Certain animals which acquired the disease during one outbreak also exhibited clinical signs during a subsequent outbreak. Although calves as young as 10 days old were affected, the incidence in young stock was lower than that in mature animals (Newton and Wheatley 1970). The incubation period in animals experimentally infected by the intravenous route ranged from 29 hours to 10 days; a 2- to 4-day incubation period was most commonly observed. The length of the incubation period was affected by the passage level and dose of the infective material. For example, the average incubation period was about 2.5 days during the first ten passages, but it gradually increased to an average of 4 days by the thirtieth passage (Burgess 1971).

Three stages of the disease were described. The first stage, at the onset, was characterized by a very rapid development of clinical signs. The animal stood with the back arched, the head lowered, and the muzzle extended, and saliva drooled from the mouth. The eyes were sunken and discharged, first serous, and then catarrhal exudate. The muscle tremors were marked and the fever was transient. The second stage consisted of stiffness, and fleeting and shifting or persistent lameness in one or more limbs. The recovery stage commenced 24 to 36 hours later when eating and drinking were resumed. Some animals recovered very rapidly, but a few remained lame for weeks and some became recumbent for long periods of time (Newton and Wheatley 1970). The incidence of each major clinical sign was as follows: fever, 100%; complete inappetence, 92%; nasal discharge, 67%; shivering, 53%; respirations over 50 per minute, 53%; lameness, 39%; and paresis, 4% (Mackerras *et al.* 1940). The lameness and incoordination are associated with acute pain, and muscle tremors were observed in the majority of cases (MacFarlane and Haig 1955). The clinical signs were usually temporary, passing from one limb to another with the animal assuming a characteristic attitude of standing with its back arched and its neck extended (Henning 1956). Cases which were either paralyzed or ataxic following acute infection had bilaterally symmetrical Wallerian degeneration in the spinal cords. In most of the animals, the area of primary damage was present in the first cervical segment of the cord. This pathology was not considered to be a primary result of the infection; experimental evidence indicated that trauma to the cord was the likely etiology (Hill and Schultz 1977).

Subcutaneous and pulmonary emphysema is a serious complication of BEF. The histopathological changes associated with this sequela included destruction of the bronchiolar epithelium and degeneration and necrosis of muscle fibers in the bronchi (Theodoridis and Coetzer 1979). The virus was detected in only one out of 118 semen samples collected from experimentally infected bulls, and a small proportion of these animals produced spermatozoa with morphological changes. The one positive sample was contaminated with blood. Intrauterine inoculation of heifers with semen and virus resulted in normal conception rates and pregnancies (Parsonson and Snowdon 1974a). T. D. St George (personal communication) noted that during outbreaks BEF virus neither interfered with estrus, fertilization, or subsequent fertility. Because in Australia Akabane virus is a complicating feature, there is some uncertainty as to the effect of BEF virus on pregnant cows. The evidence at present is that the virus does not cross the placenta.

The loss of milk production caused by BEF virus depended on the stage of lactation at the time of infection, but the average daily reduction in the yield was approximately 60%. The virus predisposed the udder to secondary infections with bacteria and affected the leukocyte barrier in the udder. It was also suggested that BEF had an effect on the estrus cycle and conception (Theodoridis *et al.* 1973b). The drop in milk production was associated with varying degrees of mastitis. The udders of affected animals exhibited additional changes that ranged from slight sensitivity while being milked to marked edema with watery milk which occasionally contained blood (MacFarlane and Haig 1955).

PATHOLOGY

Coincident with the temperature peak early in the disease is a rapidly developing leukocytosis due to neutrophilia with a shift to the left. However, leukopenia and a reduction in erythrocyte numbers during the early stages of infection is also reported and lasts only a few hours.

The gross lesions which have been observed are not really definitive. The main findings are accumulation of fluid in the pericardium, the peritoneal and pleural cavities, and in the joints. The lymph nodes are edematous, and there is generalized vascular engorgement which is occasionally associated with fibrinous exudate. Congestion of the abomasal mucosa, hydropericardium, and hydrothorax, and rhinitis, tracheitis, pulmonary emphysema with lobular consolidation, and subcutaneous emphysema have also been observed. On the serous surfaces there is evidence of inflammation with vascular lesions and exudation. In the respiratory system there are inflammatory and hemorrhagic lesions in the upper respiratory tract and fluid exudate in the lung parenchyma. The lesions observed in these various tissues and organs are characterized by dilatation and engorgement of small veins and capillaries. In addition, the capillary endothelium thickens and becomes more permeable, and this is accompanied by a loose infiltration of scattered neutrophils, lymphocytes, and occasional plasma cells in the surrounding connective tissue.

The changes observed in the joints and muscles are extremely variable, and this variability is equally great from case to case and from joint to joint in a given animal. Serofibrinous polysinovitis and periarthritis occur in the joints. Cellulitis affects the tendons and fascia, and localized necrosis of the skeletal muscles occurs in animals which become recumbent. The lesions observed on histological examination of the venules and capillaries in the synovial membranes, tendon sheaths, muscles, fascia, and skin include hyperplasia of the endothelium, perivascular neutrophilic infiltration, and edema, which is followed by hyperplasia of pericytes, infiltration of round cells, necrosis of vessel walls, thrombosis, and fibrosis. The synovial and articular surfaces are either normal or show varying degree of inflammation with fluid, fibrin, and inflammatory cell exudates. No degenerative or inflammatory changes occur which can be associated with the clinical signs of paresis.

In summary, BEF virus is essentially an intravascular parasite closely associated with the white cell fraction of the blood. In the bloodstream, the virus has probably two primary effects: it causes dilation of capillaries and small veins, and it stimulates the neutrophils. The virus effect, however, may not necessarily be by its direct action on tissues. The vascular dilation produces engorgement and stasis; the latter sequela results in increased permeability which leads to edema, and degeneration of the vessel wall which allows extravasation of red blood cells and fluids. The degree to which these vascular lesions develop depends on the tissue in which the vessel is located. In solid organs there is only mild vascular engorgement, while in the loose connective tissues there is obvious edema and extravasation of red blood cells. In the spleen and lymph nodes, erythrophagocytosis and hemosiderosis occur in association with these vascular lesions.

Literature

The most comprehensive description of the pathogenesis of BEF and of the gross and microscopic lesions associated with the disease was presented by Mackerras *et al*. (1940).

There were characteristic changes in the WBC population. The development of neutrophilia and lymphopenia was related to the temperature peak. In addition, there was a slight increase in the number of monocytes and a rise in plasma fibrinogen (Akhtar *et al* 1967; St George 1981), and leukocytosis was reported by Mackerras *et al* (1940).

The gross lesions were associated with dilatation and engorgement o[f] the blood vessels, swelling of the lymph nodes, and inflammation o[f] the serosal surfaces, the latter being most severe in the joints (Mackerras *et al.* 1940). The tissue reaction was characterized by a pronounced neutrophilia and an influx of neutrophils into the serosae and serosal fluids. The increased permeability and other histological changes associated with the development of pathological lesions and clinical signs were considered to be a result of the influx of large numbers of neutrophils. The tissue reaction was prevented by inducing neutropenia with an injection of antiserum to bovine neutrophils. However, the antiserum probably also contained antibodies to other tissue antigens and therefore the role of the neutrophil has not been definitively established. Infected calves depleted of neutrophils still exhibited a prolonged viremia, but there was no detectable tissue damage or development of clinical signs. These tissue reactions observed in BEF virus infection of cattle resembled those of bovine serum albumin-induced, acute Arthus reaction in rabbits (Young and Spradbrow 1980). Hemorrhages, edema, ischemia, and necrosis with accompanying inflammation resulted from various vascular changes which were regarded as the primary lesions in the pathogenesis of BEF. Histologically, these lesions consisted of hypertrophy and hyperplasia of the endothelium, hyperplasia of pericytes, fibrinoid necrosis of the muscular coat of small arteries, perivascular inflammatory cell reaction, perivascular fibrosis, and occasional thrombosis of blood vessels in the muscles (Basson *et al.* 1970).

Postmortem examination of animals killed at varying intervals after the onset of fever was conducted by Basson *et al.* (1970), who reported serofibrinous polysynovitis, polytendovaginitis, periarthritis, fasciitis, cellulitis, and focal necrosis of the skeletal muscles and skin. A mild lymphadenitis occurred in the regional lymph nodes of the affected limbs. These lesions varied in severity and distribution. In the more severely affected joints, the turbid, straw-colored synovial fluid contained small yellow-white flakes and plaques. The synovial membranes were edematous, contained petechial hemorrhages, and had fibrinous strands which adhered to the surface. In less severe lesions, there was diffuse reddening of the synovial membranes with a few petechiae and a slight increase in the synovial fluid. The lesions in the skeletal muscles were localized and occurred most commonly in the quadriceps group. Less frequently, the affected muscles were the longissimus dorsi, biceps femoris, triceps, semiteninosus, and semimembranous. The lesions were focal and located near muscle attachment. In the tissues examined 1 to 4 days after the onset of fever, the lesions appeared as focal, pale, well-circumscribed areas which often contained petechial or ecchymotic hemorrhages. Irregular areas of necrosis were apparent from day 6 onwards, and by day 15 the necrotic tissue was surrounded by a connective tissue capsule. Histologically, there was typical hyaline necrosis of muscle fibers associated with hemorrhages and an infiltration of neutrophils. During the latter part of the infection, there was an infiltration of round cells, predominantly macrophages, and a proliferation of fibrocytes (Basson *et al.* 1970). In fatal cases of BEF hemorrhages in the mucous membranes of the upper respiratory tract, emphysema and consolidation in the lungs were observed. The symptoms of pharyngo-laryngeal paralysis were associated with the hyaline degeneration of the surrounding striated muscles (Inaba 1973). However, this was later considered to be due to Ibaraki disease.

During the 1968 epizootic of BEF in Australia, numerous congenitally deformed calves were born. However, further investigation of the incidence of defective calves could not be correlated to the presence of neutralizing antibodies in the dams, suggesting that BEF virus was not responsible for the abnormalities. However, it was proposed that bovine fetal development could be adversely affected by the occurrence of fever in the dam during certain critical stages of gestation (Young 1969). Pregnant cattle at 4, 5, 6, and 7 months of gestation were experimentally infected with BEF virus. Although characteristic periods of hyperthermia resulted, there was no evidence of arthrogryposis or other congenital abnormalities in the calves produced by these animals. It was concluded that the virus probably does not cross the placental barrier and produce lesions in the fetus (Parsonson and Snowdon 1974b). The experimental infection of susceptible pregnant heifers and fetuses borne by heifers immune to BEF virus did not cause abnormalities in any of the calves (Tzipori and Spradbrow 1975). T. D. St George (personal communication) proposed that arthrogryposis in Australia and Japan were probably due to the Akabane and Aino viruses of the Simbu group which have comparable seasonal incidence to the BEF virus in the temporal areas of Australia. This has resulted in the inconsistencies in observations. Four members of the Simbu group of viruses have been isolated and antibodies surveyed in Australia (St George *et al.* 1978, 1979; Cybinski and St George 1978).

A consistent rise in the percentage of abnormal midpieces and a decrease in motility were seen in the spermatozoa of experimentally and naturally infected bulls. The number of abnormalities reached a maximum 35 days after the peak fever, and after 155 days the semen showed signs of returning to normal. It was not possible to determine whether these changes were due to viral multiplication in the testis or to the fever (Chenoweth and Burgess 1972; Burgess and Chenoweth 1975).

Although adult mice experimentally infected with BEF virus did not develop syndromes which resembled those observed in the natural hosts, they were used as models in studies undertaken to determine: (1) the pathogenesis of the disease resulting from neurotropic viral infection, and (2) the function of humoral and cell-mediated immune responses in the suppression or enhancement of the disease process. Infection of adult mice with neurotropic BEF virus resulted in a rapidly fatal encephalitis which could be prevented by the administration of antibody at the time of infection. The cellular immune response did not appear to play a role in the lesion formation or in the induction of resistance (Young and Spradbrow 1981). The necrotic encephalomyelitis which occurred in mice was found throughout the brain and spinal cord, and the neurons contained viral antigen. The lesion was due to a strict neurotropism which was not characteristic of the pathogenetic mechanisms observed in cattle (Murphy *et al.* 1972).

IMMUNOLOGY

Bovine ephemeral fever virus usually causes a prolonged immunity after a single infection. The neutralizing antibody is observed at about 2 weeks and persists for about 2 years after experimental infection; the time of its occurrence in natural disease has not been established. The antigenic composition of isolates from widely separated geographical areas is relatively homogeneous; one isolate is capable of inducing resistance to a heterologous challenge. However, antigenic differences between strains are observed in serological tests.

Literature

It has been generally accepted that single attacks of BEF confer solid and lasting immunity for at least 2 years, although occasionally some animals are affected in a subsequent outbreak (Mackerras *et al.* 1940). Neutralizing antibodies were demonstrated in the convalescent sera of both naturally and experimentally infected cattle (van der Westhuizen 1967). There were different levels of neutralizing antibody in natural and experimental cases; in the former, neutralizing antibody could be detected before the occurrence of the clinical disease, suggesting a prolonged incubation period in naturally transmitted infections or possibly the result of infection by heterologous strains (St George 1981). In serum samples collected from a cow inoculated experimentally with BEF virus, neutralizing activity was first observed 15 days after inoculation and was associated with the 19S globulin fraction. The neutralizing activity in the 7S globulin fraction was detected 22 days after inoculation and continued to rise until day 36. The neutralizing activity in serum samples collected in the interenzootic period was confined to the 7S fraction. Neutralizing antibodies were found in herds for up to 2 years after infection (Snowdon 1971). Serological examination of sentinel herds of cattle in Australia provided evidence of widespread infection with BEF virus as well as a number of other arboviruses. The neutralizing antibodies to BEF virus persisted in cattle for approximately 6 months (Doherty *et al.* 1973). A simple quantitative screening test for measuring the serum neutralizing antibody to BEF virus was developed using VERO cells and microtiter methods. The technique was of comparable sensitivity to the mouse neutralization test but was less sensitive than the tube culture neutralization test (Burgess 1974).

The adaptation of the BEF virus to laboratory animals and tissue cultures enabled the development of the serum neutralization and complement fixation tests. The serial passage of BEF virus in suckling mice caused a rapid loss of virulence and immunogenicity for cattle (van der Westhuizen 1967). This also occurred on serial passage of the virus through tissue culture systems. The development of a suitable vaccine may be difficult because the attenuated virus is not immunogenic. However, since there is no significant antigenic variation, one effective vaccine would be suitable in all areas where the disease occurs (Burgess 1971). When BEF virus strains from different geographical regions were compared by cross-neutralization tests, in tissue cultures, or in mice, they were found to be antigenically similar. However, there is evidence that strain variation does occur. Certain isolates fail to induce neutralizing antibody to heterologous strains but do so to the homologous strains. In addition, other strains show marked differences in mouse cross-protection tests even though they are serologically identical (St George 1981).

VACCINATION

Tissue culture vaccines are commercially produced in South Africa and Japan. The regime used in Japan involves inoculating cattle with an attenuated live vaccine prior to administering a formalin-inactivated adjuvant vaccine. The efficacy of this method is difficult to determine under field conditions. The use of live vaccines is limited by the possibility that there may be a reversion of virulence, and this cannot be tested since the vectors have not yet been clearly identified.

Literature

It was found that BEF virus passaged in cell cultures was attenuated and satisfactory for the immunization of cattle when multiple inoculations were given with adjuvant (Heuschele and Johnson 1969). The use and safety of live and killed vaccines against BEF was debated in Australian scientific literature (Della-Porta and Snowdon 1977). The safety of a live attenuated vaccine against BEF was discussed (Lascelles 1976), and it was found that inactivated viral vaccines were generally inferior immunologically to attenuated viral vaccines (Spradbrow 1977). It was concluded that, although attenuated vaccine against BEF has some shortcomings, it could be used when the advantages outweigh the possible disadvantages (Francis 1976, 1977).

The vaccines developed at the University of Queensland Veterinary School involved the use of two strains of BEF virus attenuated by passage in rodents or cell cultures and mixed with adjuvant immediately before inoculation. The response to the vaccine was determined by measuring the levels of neutralizing antibodies and by challenging calves with virulent virus through experimentally induced or naturally acquired infections (Spradbrow 1975). A vaccine was prepared from fluids harvested from the twelfth passage of BEF virus in VERO cell culture. A single subcutaneous administration of the virus mixed with Freund's complete adjuvant at least induced a neutralizing antibody response which persisted for at least 40 weeks. Two subcutaneous injections of virus mixed with aluminium hydroxide adjuvant induced higher titers of antibody than intravenous inoculation of the virus alone. These antibodies persisted for at least 12 months, and a third vaccination at 52 weeks slightly enhanced the existing levels of antibody. Aluminium hydroxide was considered a satisfactory adjuvant for vaccination purposes. Although vaccines containing Freund's complete adjuvant produced an adequate serological response, they were unacceptable because the inoculated animals developed clinical reactions to the adjuvant (Tzipori and Spradbrow 1973, 1978).

Additional work was undertaken in South Africa. Bovine ephemeral fever virus of the fifth and eighth tissue culture passage level was more antigenic in cattle than either the seventeenth to nineteenth passage level or mouse-brain-adapted virus. The neutralizing antibody response was transient and probably conferred inadequate protection. Comparable results were obtained after cattle were inoculated with either low or high passage level virus that had been adsorbed onto aluminium hydroxide. However, emulsions of virus of both high and low passage level in Freund's incomplete adjuvant stimulated the production of high neutralizing antibody titers which persisted for at least a year and protected the animals against subsequent challenge with the virus (Theodoridis *et al.* 1973a). Another strain of the virus produced from the third intracerebral passage in mice protected cattle against experimental challenge when it was mixed with aluminium hydroxide adjuvant; the results of field trials indicated that this vaccine conferred protection against natural infection. Increased antibody titers were detected in a number of the vaccinated animals exposed to natural challenge, suggesting that reinfection had occurred, but clinical disease developed in only a few cases (Tzipori and Spradbrow 1973; Tzipori *et al.* 1975).

In Japan, formalin-inactivated aluminium phosphate gel vaccine prepared in cell culture effectively stimulated the production of neutralizing antibody; vaccinated animals were resistant to challenge when inoculated twice at intervals of 1 to 4 weeks apart. This vaccine was made commercially available in Japan (Inaba 1973; Inaba *et al.* 1973). An effective method of vaccinating calves involved an initial injection of attenuated virus which had been serially passaged in tissue cultures. This avirulent virus did not induce significant neutralizing antibody, but it did prime the animal to produce high titers of neutralizing antibody following the inoculation of a second vaccine composed of formalin-inactivated aluminium phosphate gel-adsorbed virus. This method could be used in pregnant cows and had no adverse effect on milk production (Inaba *et al.* 1974). A lyophilized live vaccine produced by serial passage in chick embryo tissue culture cells was also tested, and neutralizing antibodies were demonstrated up to a year after vaccination (Yamada 1964d).

Experimental work was undertaken on vaccines that consisted of a neurotropic strain of BEF virus which was lethal for adult mice on intracerebral inoculation. This model was used to study different vaccines prepared from infected suckling mouse-brain or infected VERO cell cultures. After two doses of uninactivated mouse-brain vaccine, formalin-inactivated mouse-brain vaccine with adjuvant, or uninactivated VERO cell vaccine with adjuvant, the mice developed neutralizing antibodies and resisted intracerebral challenge administered 1 to 7 weeks later (Gaffar Elamin and Spradbrow 1979).

DIAGNOSIS

When a high incidence of classical clinical signs occurs during an epizootic, BEF can be diagnosed with reasonable certainty. However, in sporadic cases, a diagnosis of BEF has to be confirmed, and this is most readily accomplished using serological techniques during the early clinical phase and stage of the disease. A fluorescent antibody (FA) test can be used to demonstrate viral antigens in circulating leukocytes and in primary isolations in cultures as early as 24 hours after infection.

Literature

Currently, the most reliable method of diagnosis is the detection of a rise in the titers of neutralizing antibody in paired serum samples collected during early clinical disease and on recovery. The tissue culture neutralization test is superior to the mouse protection test for this purpose. The neutrophilia is a constant finding in BEF and may help make the diagnosis easier. The differential diagnosis of BEF in the first case in an outbreak may be a problem, but as the disease spreads through the herd, its rapid course and characteristic clinical signs facilitate diagnosis (St George 1981). The virus isolated in Japan was identified as BEF virus by cross-neutralization tests (Inaba *et al.* 1969b). Fluorescent antibody tests may be a method which can be utilized in the field. A highly specific FA test was used to identify BEF virus in the cytoplasm of tissue culture cells as well as in the leukocytes from infected cattle. In the tissue culture cells, the fluorescence was diffuse, but in the peripheral leukocytes it was granular and at times confined to the outer layers of the cytoplasm. The diffuse cytoplasmic fluorescence was observed in the tissue culture cells as early as 24 hours after infection and became granular by about 40 hours. The intensity of the fluorescence was sufficient to enable the detection of even small numbers of positively stained cells. The staining of peripheral leukocytes from infected cattle correlated well with the subsequent development of neutralizing antibody titers. The FA test was sensitive and accurate and could be readily conducted under field conditions (Theodoridis 1969). Many false positives have been obtained with the FA tests when used on leukocytes of cattle. The tests, however, were very specific when used on tissue cultures infected with BEF virus (St George, personal communication).

CONTROL AND TREATMENT

Since the vectors involved in the epizootiology of BEF are unknown, the disease cannot be controlled through an insect eradication program. Vaccination is the only reliable control method.

Supportive treatment is used to alleviate the pain, decrease the inflammation and prevent secondary infections.

Literature

Supportive therapy, elimination of stressful conditions such as movement, and protection from the elements are beneficial. Symptomatic treatment with anti-inflammatory drugs such as salicylates and butazolidine is beneficial, and antibiotics have been used to prevent the appearance of secondary bacterial infections (St George 1981). Tetracycline administered with salicylate mixture was found to be more effective than other forms of treatment (Phatak 1968). The prognosis for those animals which become paralyzed and remain recumbent for 1 to 2 days is uncertain (St George 1981).

BIBLIOGRAPHY

Akhtar, A. S., Ali, R. and Hussain, S., 1967. Clinical pathology and transmission of ephemeral fever in buffaloes, *Proc. 18th/19th Pakist. Sci. Conf. Jamshoro*, part III, p. G–25.

Balachandran, K., 1965. An outbreak of ephemeral fever of cattle in Jaffna, *Ceylon vet. J.*, **13**(2): 55–7.

Basson, P. A., Pienaar, J. G. and van der Westhuizen, B., 1970. The pathology of ephemeral fever: a study of the experimental disease in cattle, *J. S. Afr. vet. med. Ass.*, **40**(4): 385–97.

Burgess, G. W., 1971. Bovine ephemeral fever: a review, *Vet. Bull.*, **41**(11): 887–95.

Burgess, G. W., 1973. Attempts to infect cattle with bovine ephemeral fever by inoculation of virus into the cervix, *Aust. vet. J.*, **49**: 341–3.

Burgess, G. W., 1974. A microtitre serum neutralization test for bovine ephemeral fever virus, *AJEBAK* **52**(pt 5): 851–5.

Burgess, G. W. and Chenoweth, P. J., 1975. Mid-piece abnormalities in bovine semen following experimental and natural cases of bovine ephemeral fever, *Br. vet. J.*, **131**: 536–44.

Chenoweth, P. J. and Burgess, G. W., 1972. Mid-piece abnormalities in bovine semen following bovine ephemeral fever, *Aust. vet. J.*, **48**: 37–8.

Combs, G. P., 1978. Bovine ephemeral fever, *82nd Ann. Meet. US Anim. Hlth Ass.*, Buffalo, 1978. Carter Composition Corp. (Richmond, Va.), pp. 29–35.

Cybinski, D. H. and St George, T. D., 1978. A survey of antibody to Aino virus in cattle and other species in Australia, *Aust. vet. J.*, **54**: 371–3.

Cybinski, D. H. and Zakrzewski, H., 1983. The isolation and preliminary characterization of a rhabdovirus in Australia related to bovine ephemeral fever virus, *Vet. Microbiol.*, **8**: 221–35.

Davies, F. G., Shaw, T. and Ochieng, P., 1975. Observations on the epidemiology of ephemeral fever in Kenya, *J. Hyg., Camb.*, **75**: 231–5.

Davies, F. G. and Walker, A. R., 1974. The isolation of ephemeral fever virus from cattle and *Culicoides* midges in Kenya, *Vet. Rec.*, **95**: 63–4.

Della-Porta, A. J. and Brown, F., 1979. The physico-chemical characterization of bovine ephemeral fever virus as a member of the family Rhabdoviridae, *J. gen. Virol.*, **44**: 99–112.

Della-Porta, A. J. and Snowdon, W. A., 1977. Vaccines against bovine ephemeral fever, *Aust. vet. J.*, **53**: 50–1.

Della-Porta, A. J. and Snowdon, W. A., 1979. An experimental inactivated virus vaccine against bovine ephemeral fever. 1. Studies of the virus, *Vet. Microbiol.*, **4**: 183–95.

Doherty, R. L., 1978. Bovine ephemeral fever (BEF), *Am. J. trop. Med. Hyg.*, **27**(2): 380–2.

Doherty, R. L., Carley, J. G., Standfast, H. A., Dyce, A. L. and Snowdon, W. A., 1972. Virus strains isolated from arthropods during an epizootic of bovine ephemeral fever in Queensland, *Aust. vet. J.*, **48**: 81–6.

Doherty, R. L., St George, T. D. and Carley, J. G., 1973. Arbovirus infections of sentinel cattle in Australia and New Guinea, *Aust. vet. J.*, **49**: 574–9.

Francis, J., 1976. An attenuated vaccine against bovine ephemeral fever, *Aust. vet. J.*, **52**: 537–8.

Francis, J., 1977. Vaccines against bovine ephemeral fever, *Aust. vet. J.*, **53**: 198–9.

Gaffar Elamin, M. A. and Spradbrow, P. B., 1978a. Isolation and cultivation of bovine ephemeral fever virus in chickens and chicken embryos, *J. Hyg., Camb.*, **81**: 1–7.

Gaffar Elamin, M. A. and Spradbrow, P. B., 1978b. The growth of bovine ephemeral fever virus in primary cell cultures, *Acta virol.*, **22**: 341.

Gaffar Elamin, M. A. and Spradbrow, P. B., 1978c. Neurotropic strains of bovine ephemeral fever virus, *Zbl. vet. Med.*, **B25**: 425–30.

Gaffar Elamin, M. A. and Spradbrow, P. B., 1979. Bovine ephemeral fever virus vaccines in mice, *Zbl. Vet. Med.*, **B26**: 773–8.

Gard, G. P., Cybinski, D. H. and St George, T. D., 1983. The isolation in Australia of a new virus related to bovine ephemeral fever virus, *Aust. vet. J.*, **60**: 89.

Gee, R. W., Hall, W. T. K., Littlejohns, I. R. and Snowdon, W. A., 1969. The 1967–68 outbreak of ephemeral fever in cattle, *Aust. vet. J.*, **45**: 132.

Hall, W. T. K., Daddow, K. N., Dimmock, C. K., St George, T. D. and Standfast, H. A., 1975. The infection of merino sheep with bovine ephemeral fever virus, *Aust. vet. J.*, **51**: 344–6.

Henning, M. W., 1956. Ephemeral fever, three-day sickness, Drie-daesiekte (Lazy man's disease, stiff sickness, stywesiekte). In *Animal Diseases in South Africa. Being an Account of the Infectious Diseases of Domestic Animals.* Central News Agency (South Africa), pp. 1053–61.

Heuschele, W. P., 1970. Bovine ephemeral fever. I. Characteristics of the causative virus, *Arch. ges. Virusforsch.*, **30**: 195–202.

Heuschele, W. P. and Johnson, D. C., 1969. Bovine ephemeral fever. II. Responses of cattle to attenuated and virulent virus, *Proc. 73rd Ann. Meet. US Anim. Hlth Ass.*, Milwaukee, Wis., pp. 185–95.

Hill, M. W. M. and Schultz, K., 1977. Ataxia and paralysis associated with bovine ephemeral fever infection, *Aust. vet. J.*, **53**: 217–20.

Holmes, I. H. and Doherty, R. L., 1970. Morphology and development of bovine ephemeral fever virus, *J. Virol.*, **5**(1): 91–6.

Inaba, Y., 1973. Bovine ephemeral fever (three-day sickness). Stiff sickness, *Bull. Off. int. Epiz.*, **79**(5–6): 627–73.

Inaba, Y., Kurogi, H., Sako, K., Goto Y., Omori, T. and Matumoto, M., 1973. Formalin-inactivated, aluminum phosphate gel-adsorbed vaccine of bovine ephemeral fever virus, *Arch. ges. Virusforsch.*, **42**: 42–53.

Inaba, Y., Kurogi, H., Takahashi, A., Sata, K., Omori, T., Goto, Y., Hanaki, T., Yamamoto, M., Kishi, S., Kodama, K., Harada, K. and Matumoto, M., 1974. Vaccination of cattle against bovine ephemeral fever with live attenuated virus followed by killed virus, *Arch. ges. Virusforsch.*, **44**: 121–32.

Inaba, Y., Sata, K., Tanaka, Y., Ito, H., Omori, T. and Matumoto, M., 1969b. Serological identification of bovine epizootic fever virus as ephemeral fever virus, *Jap. J. Microbiol.*, **13**(4): 388–9.

Inaba, Y., Tanaka, Y. Sato, K., Ito, H., Omori, T. and Matumoto, M.,

1968a. Propagation in laboratory animals and cell cultures of a virus from cattle with bovine epizootic fever, *Jap. J. Microbiol.*, **12**(2): 253–5.

Inaba, Y., Tanaka, Y., Sato, K., Ito, H., Omori, T. and Matumoto, M., 1968b. Bovine epizootic fever. I. Propagation of the virus in suckling hamster, mouse and rat, and hamster kidney BHK21–W12 cell, *Jap. J. Microbiol.*, **12**(4): 457–69.

Inaba, Y., Tanaka, Y., Sato, K., Ito, H., Omori, T. and Matumoto, M., 1969a. Bovine epizootic fever. III. Loss of virus pathogenicity and immunogenicity for the calf during serial passage in various host systems, *Jap. J. Microbiol.*, **13**(2): 181–6.

Kemp, G. E., Mann, E. D., Tomori, O., Fabiyi, A. and O'Connor, E., 1973. Isolation of bovine ephemeral fever virus in Nigeria, *Vet. Rec.*, **93**: 107–8.

Lascelles, A. K., 1976. Ephemeral fever vaccination, *Aust. vet. J.*, **52**: 381.

Lawrence, D. A., 1957. Ephemeral fever or three-day sickness, *Bull. epiz. Dis. Afr.*, **5**: 469–73.

Lecatsas, G., 1969. The structure of bovine ephemeral fever virus, *J. S. Afr. vet. med. Ass.*, **40**: 230.

Lecatsas, G., 1970. Further observations on the ultrastructure of ephemeral fever virus, *Onderstepoort J. vet. Res.*, **37**(2): 145–6.

Lecatsas, G., Theodoridis, A. and Els, H. J., 1969a. Morphological variation in ephemeral fever virus strains, *Onderstepoort J. vet. Res.*, **36**(2): 325–6.

Lecatsas, G., Theodoridis, A. and Erasmus, B. J., 1969b. Electron microscopic studies on bovine ephemeral fever virus, *Arch. ges. Virusforsch.*, **28**: 390–8.

MacFarlane, I. S. and Haig, D. A., 1955. Some observations on three day stiffsickness in the Transvaal in 1954, *J. S. Afr. vet. med. Ass.*, **26**(1): 1–7.

Mackerras, I. M., Mackerras, M. J. and Burnet, F. M., 1940. *Experimental Studies of Ephemeral Fever in Australian Cattle.* Commonwealth of Australia Council for Scientific and Industrial Research Bull. 136 (Melbourne), pp. 1–116.

Malviya, H. K. and Prasad, J., 1977. Ephemeral fever – a clinical and epidemiological study in cross-bred cows and buffaloes, *Indian vet. J.*, **54**: 440–4.

Matumoto, M., Inaba, Y., Tanaka, Y., Ito, H. and Omori, T., 1970. Behavior of bovine ephemeral fever virus in laboratory animals and cell cultures, *Jap. J. Microbiol.*, **14**(5): 413–21.

Morgan, I. and Murray, M. D., 1969. The occurrence of ephemeral fever of cattle in Victoria in 1968, *Aust. vet. J.*, **45**: 271–4.

Murphy, F. A., Taylor, W. P., Mims, C. A. and Whitfield, S. S., 1972. Bovine ephemeral fever virus in cell culture and mice, *Arch. ges. Virusforsch.*, **38**: 234–49.

Murray, M. D., 1970. The spread of ephemeral fever of cattle during the 1967–68 epizootic in Australia, *Aust. vet. J.*, **46**: 77–82.

Newton, L. G. and Wheatley, C. H., 1970. The occurrence and spread of ephemeral fever of cattle in Queensland, *Aust. vet. J.*, **45**: 561–8.

Parsonson, I. M. and Snowdon, W. A., 1974a. Ephemeral fever virus: excretion in the semen of infected bulls and attempts to infect female cattle by the intrauterine inoculation of virus, *Aust. vet. J.*, **50**: 329–34.

Parsonson, I. M. and Snowdon, W. A., 1974b. Experimental infection of pregnant cattle with ephemeral fever virus, *Aust. vet. J.*, **50**: 335–7.

Phatak, A. P., 1968. The use of tetracycline against ephemeral fever in dairy cattle, *Indian vet. J.*, **45**: 881–2.

St George, T. D., 1980. A sentinel herd system for the study of arbovirus infections in Australia and Papua New Guinea, *Vet. Sci. Comm.*, **4**: 39–51.

St George, T. D., 1981. Ephemeral fever. In *Virus Diseases of Food Animals. A World Geography of Epidemiology and Control*, ed. E. P. J. Gibbs. Academic Press Disease Monographs, vol. 2, pp. 541–64.

St George, T. D., Cybinski, D. H., Filippich, C. and Carley, J. G., 1979. The isolation of three Simbu group viruses new to Australia, *Exp. Biol. Med. Sci.*, **57**(6): 581–2.

St George, T. D., Standfast, H. A., Armstrong, J. M., Christie, D. G., Irving, M. R., Knott, S. G. and Rideout, B. L., 1973. A report on the progress of the 1972/73 epizootic of ephemeral fever – 1 December 1972 to 30 April 1973, *Aust. vet. J.*, **49**: 441–2.

St George, T. D., Standfast, H. A., Christie, D. G., Knott, S. G. and Morgan, I. R., 1977. The epizootiology of bovine ephemeral fever in Australia and Papua New Guinea, *Aust. vet. J.*, **53**: 17–28.

St George, T. D., Standfast. H. A. and Cybinski, D. H., 1978. Isolations of Akabane virus from sentinel cattle and *Culicoides brevitarsis*, *Aust. vet. J.*, **54**: 558–61.

St George, T. D., Standfast, H. A. and Dyce, A. L., 1976. The isolation of ephemeral fever virus from mosquitoes in Australia, *Aust. vet. J.*, **52**: 242.

Sasaki, N., Kodama, K., Iwamoto, I., Izumida, A. and Matsubara, T., 1968. Serial transmission in suckling mice of a virus from cattle with bovine epizootic fever, *Jap. J. Microbiol.*, **12**(2): 251–2.

Snowdon, W. A., 1970. Bovine ephemeral fever: reaction of cattle to different strains of ephemeral fever virus and the antigenic

comparison of two strains of virus, *Aust. vet. J.*, **46**: 258–66.
Snowdon, W. A., 1971. Some aspects of the epizootiology of bovine ephemeral fever in Australia, *Aust. vet. J.*, **47**: 312–17.
Spradbrow, P. B., 1975. Attenuated vaccines against bovine ephemeral fever, *Aust. vet. J.*, **51**: 464–8.
Spradbrow, P. B., 1977. Vaccines against bovine ephemeral fever, *Aust. vet. J.*, **53**: 351–2.
Spradbrow, P. B. and Francis, J., 1969. Observations on bovine ephemeral fever and isolation of virus, *Aust. vet. J.*, **45**: 525–7.
Standfast, H. A. and Dyce, A. L., 1972. Potential vectors of arboviruses of cattle and buffalo in Australia, *Aust. vet. J.*, **48**: 224–7.
Standfast, H. A., Murray, M. D., Dyce, A. L. and St George, T. D., 1973. Report on ephemeral fever in Australia, *Bull. Off. int. Epiz.*, **79**(5–6): 615–25.

Tanaka, Y., Inaba, Y., Ito, Y., Sato, K., Omori, T. and Matumoto, M., 1972. Double strandedness of ribonucleic acid of bovine ephemeral fever virus, *Jap. J. Microbiol.*, **16**(2): 95–101.
Theodoridis, A., 1969. Fluorescent antibody studies on ephemeral fever virus, *Onderstepoort J. vet. Res.*, **36**(2): 187–90.
Theodoridis, A., Boshoff, S. E. T. and Botha, M. J., 1973a. Studies on the development of a vaccine against bovine ephemeral fever, *Onderstepoort J. vet. Res.*, **40**(3): 77–82.
Theodoridis, A. and Coetzer, J. A. W., 1979. Subcutaneous and pulmonary emphysema as complications of bovine ephemeral fever, *Onderstepoort J. vet. Res.*, **46**: 125–27.
Theodoridis, A., Giesecke, W. H. and Du Toit, I. J., 1973b. Effects of ephemeral fever on milk production and reproduction of diary cattle, *Onderstepoort J. vet. Res.*, **40**(3): 83–91.
Theodoridis, A. and Lecatsas, G., 1973. Variation in morphology of ephemeral fever virus, *Onderstepoort J. vet. Res.*, **40**(4): 139–44.
Theodoridis, A., Nevill, E. M., Els, H. J. and Boshoff, S. T., 1979. Viruses isolated from *Culicoides* midges in South Africa during unsuccessful attempts to isolate bovine ephemeral fever virus, *Onderstepoort J. vet. Res.*, **46**: 191–8.
Tzipori, S., 1975a. The susceptibility of young and newborn calves to bovine ephemeral fever virus, *Aust. vet. J.*, **51**: 251–3.
Tzipori, S., 1975b. The susceptibility of calves to infection with a strain of bovine ephemeral fever virus inoculated intracerebrally, *Aust. vet. J.*, **51**: 254–5.
Tzipori, S., 1975c. The isolation of bovine ephemeral fever virus in cell cultures and evidence for autointerference, *Aust. J. exp. Biol.*, **53** (pt 4): 273–9.
Tzipori, S., 1975d. Electron microscopic study of a strain of bovine ephemeral fever virus in mouse and guinea-pig brain, *Kajian Veterinar.*, **7**: 17–23.
Tzipori, S. and Spradbrow, P. B., 1973. Studies on vaccines against bovine ephemeral fever, *Aust. vet. J.*, **49**: 183–7.

Tzipori, S. and Spradbrow, P. B., 1974. Development and behaviour of a strain of bovine ephemeral fever virus with unusual host range, *J. Comp. Path.*, **84**: 1–8.

Tzipori, S. and Spradbrow, P. B., 1975. The effect of bovine ephemeral fever virus on the bovine foetus, *Aust. vet. J.*, **51**: 64–6.

Tzipori, S. and Spradbrow, P. B., 1978. A cell culture vaccine against bovine ephemeral fever, *Aust. vet. J.*, **54**: 323–8.

Tzipori, S., Spradbrow, P. B. and Doyle, T., 1975. Laboratory and field studies with a bovine ephemeral fever vaccine, *Aust. vet. J.*, **51**: 244–50.

Uren, M. F., St George, T. D. and Stranger, R. S., 1983. Epidemiology of ephemeral fever of cattle in Australia 1975–1981, *Aust. J. Biol. Sci.*, **36**: 91–100.

van der Westhuizen, B., 1967. Studies on bovine ephemeral fever. I. Isolation and preliminary characterization of a virus from natural and experimentally produced cases of bovine ephemeral fever, *Onderstepoort J. vet. Res.*, **34**(1): 29–40.

Yamada, S., 1964a. Epizootiological study on epizootic-fever-like disease of cattle by means of neutralization test. I. Neutralizing antibody distribution in the Kyushu and Chugoku districts in 1960, *Jap. J. vet. Sci.*, **26**: 83–90.

Yamada, S., 1964b. Epizootiological study on epizootic-fever-like disease of cattle by means of neutralization test. II. Neutralizing antibody in Jersey cattle, goats, and sheep, *Jap. J. vet. Sci.*, **26**: 147–50.

Yamada, S., 1964c. Epizootiological study on epizootic-fever-like disease of cattle by means of neutralization test. III. Neutralizing antibody response in the epizootic season in 1961, *Jap. J. vet. Sci.*, **26**: 267–71.

Yamada, S., 1964d. Epizootiological study on epizootic-fever-like disease of cattle by means of neutralization test. IV. Neutralizing antibody response to lyophilized live virus vaccine, *Jap. J. vet. Sci.*, **26**: 272–9.

Young, J. S., 1969. Ephemeral fever and congenital deformities in calves, *Aust. vet. J.*, **45**: 574–6.

Young, P. L., 1979. Infection of water buffalo (*Bubalus bubalis*) with bovine ephemeral fever virus, *Aust. vet. J.*, **55**: 349–50.

Young, P. L. and Spradbrow, P. B., 1980. The role of neutrophils in bovine ephemeral fever virus infection of cattle, *J. Infect. Dis.*, **142**(1): 50–5.

Young, P. L. and Spradbrow, P. B., 1981. The pathogenesis of bovine ephemeral fever virus infection of adult mice, *J. Comp. Path.*, **91**: 369–79.

Chapter

9

Equine arboviral encephalitides

CONTENTS

INTRODUCTION

The equine arboviral encephalitides presented include Venezuelan equine encephalomyelitis (VEE), eastern equine encephalomyelitis (EEE), western equine encephalomyelitis (WEE), Japanese encephalitis (JE), and Near East equine encephalitis (NEEE). The first four diseases are caused by togaviruses and are similar in many respects. These diseases affect horses and related species, man, wild animals, and birds and are principally transmitted by various species of mosquitoes. Clinical syndromes develop in horses, man, and a few species of birds. In horses, the disease syndromes vary in severity; there is usually central nervous system involvement in the most severe cases.

The arboviruses which cause equine encephalitides in North and South America have many features in common, including adaptability to numerous tissue culture systems and infectivity for laboratory animals. Equines and man are regarded as dead-end hosts of both EEE and WEE viruses because low or undetectable levels of virus are present in their blood. The WEE and EEE viruses have some immunological relationships but are different in cross-protection. The VEE virus complex consists of four antigenically different serotypes which vary markedly in their geographic distribution and pathogenicity for equine species. The disease caused by the JE virus is widespread throughout the Far East. In addition to inducing encephalitis in man and equidae, the JE virus is abortifacient in swine and causes diseases in neonatal pigs but not in adult pigs. Many of the characteristics of JE virus are comparable to those of the equine arboviruses found in the Americas. Relatively little is known about the NEEE virus; it has been isolated from animals in Egypt and Syria and appears to be related to the unclassified Borna virus.

Literature

The various equine arboviral encephalitides were described by Byrne (1972) and Walton (1981). The literature on VEE was reviewed by Kissling and Chamberlain (1967), and more recently, the zoonoses of EEE and WEE were discussed by Hayes (1979a, b). Extensive research on VEE virus was conducted in the USA during the 1971 outbreak of the disease in southwestern Texas. Johnson and Martin (1974) reviewed the etiology, clinical signs, pathology, epidemiology, prevention, and control of VEE. Information on the NEEE virus is limited to the publications of Daubney (1967) and Daubney and Mahlau (1957) who isolated a number of strains of a virus which caused encephalitis in horses, donkeys, sheep, and cattle in Egypt and Syria. It has been suggested that this virus is related to the Borna virus found in Germany. There was also a report on the occurrence of encephalomyelitis in donkeys in Egypt. The results of serological tests indicated that this condition was caused by a virus which was antigenically unrelated to either EEE, WEE, or VEE viruses (Sabban *et al.* 1961).

ETIOLOGY

The arthropod-borne equine encephalomyelitis viruses are classified in the family Togaviridae because of their physical and chemical characteristics and their biological behavior. The members of the family Togaviridae are divided into two taxonomic groups, the alphaviruses and the flaviviruses, according to their antigenic relationships. The alphaviruses are further grouped into six immunological complexes on the basis of serological tests and are unrelated serologically to the flaviviruses. The EEE, WEE and VEE viruses comprise three of these complexes; the JE virus is classified as a flavivirus. Based on limited laboratory investigations involving cross-immunity testing, the NEEE virus is thought to be similar to the Borna virus.

The EEE, WEE, and VEE viruses can be isolated in several laboratory host systems, including intracerebrally inoculated adult and suckling mice and hatched chicks. These viruses also proliferate in a variety of cell cultures where they induce cytopathic changes and form plaques. Plaques are useful in quantitating the virus, in cloning subpopulations, and in determining antigenic relationships and differences in pathogenicity.

Literature

The EEE, WEE, and VEE viruses have morphologically similar virions which consist of a ribonucleic acid (RNA) core, approximately 30 nm in diameter, surrounded by a lipid-containing envelope (Hanson 1973). The outer envelope of the virion has surface projections. Electron microscopy and ultracentrifugation demonstrated that EEE virions are 45–55 nm, WEE virions are 50–60 nm, and VEE virions are 60–75 nm in diameter (Walton 1981). Variation in virion size was also observed in different clones of VEE virus (Klimenko *et al*. 1965; Tsilinsky *et al*. 1971).

The ultrastructure and development of WEE virus were studied in tissue cultures (Morgan *et al*. 1961). The physical properties of EEE virus were examined (Fuscaldo *et al*. 1971). Comparative analysis of the structural polypeptides of various EEE virus strains representing North and South American types showed that there were seven distinct profiles among the strains studied, but patterns of these structural polypeptides could not be correlated with any known *in vivo* virulence or with *in vitro* biological characteristics (Walder *et al*. 1981). The ribonucleoproteins of VEE virus were investigated (Yershov *et al*. 1977). The virus-specific RNAs synthesized in VEE virus-infected cells were similar to those observed in cells infected with other arboviruses (Zhdanov *et al*. 1969).

The kinetics of thermal inactivation of VEE virus varied between strains of different virulence, but there was no correlation between virulence and thermostability at different temperatures (Walder and Liprandi 1976). In a study of the virucidal effects of light and SO_2 on aerosolized VEE virus, it was found that a combination of light and SO_2 was more toxic than either agent employed separately (Barendt *et al.* 1972). A 15-minute exposure to a concentration of 2 to 4 mg of beta-propiolactone per liter of air-inactivated VEE virus, suggesting that this compound could be used instead of formaldehyde for the decontamination of large areas (Dawson *et al.* 1959). The virus was also inactivated by gamma radiation (Reitman 1969).

The morphogenesis of VEE virus was studied in cell cultures by means of an immunofluorescent technique. Maximum binding of the virus to cells occurred only at specific salt concentrations and was dependent on pH but not on temperature. The penetration of the virus into the cell was complete in 30 minutes at 35 °C. The process was temperature-dependent but not affected by the ionic content of the medium. The VEE virus could be assayed by the fluorescent cell-counting technique as early as 12 hours after the infection of cell monolayers. This assay was comparable in sensitivity to, but more rapid than, the intracerebral inoculation of mice (Hahon and Cooke 1967). The temperature-sensitive steps in the biosynthesis of VEE virus were identified (Zebovitz and Brown 1967). Electron microscopic examination of VEE virus-infected cells revealed that virus-specific structures were present early in the infection. These structures were composed of fibrillar and cylindrical formations. Viral nucleoids, which emerged from such structures, aggregated in the cytoplasm and occasionally in the nucleus. The mature virions formed on the cell membrane and on the membranes of intracellular vacuoles (Bykovsky *et al.* 1969). After maturing on the membranes which surrounded the cytoplasmic vacuoles, the virus migrated to the membrane of the cell and was released (Mussgay and Weibel 1962).

Eight different cell culture systems from various mammalian host species were tested for their ability to support the multiplication of VEE virus. All of the cell lines studied were susceptible to the virus. The development of cytopathogenic effects was dependent on the size of the inoculum and on the particular cell line used (Hardy 1959; Hanson 1973). *Aedes albopictus* cell cultures supported the growth of EEE virus and were recommended for use in primary isolations (Ajello 1979).

Various laboratory animals and cell culture systems affected the biological properties of VEE virus (Hrusková *et al.* 1969). Passage through different laboratory host systems influenced the plaque size, virulence, and lipid content of the virus (Heydrick *et al.* 1966). Storage of an attenuated VEE virus population which contained small numbers of virulent particles resulted in an increase in the proportion of the latter because of the relatively poor stability of the attenuated virus (Hearn *et al.* 1969). The differences in virulence and other biological properties observed between wild-type and mutant strains of EEE virus were thought to be due to two or more mutations which resulted from nitrous acid treatment and/or selection during plaque purification (Brown and Officer 1975).

The EEE virus induced the formation of interferon both in cell cultures of chick embryo fibroblasts and in the brains of newborn mice

(Ognianov and Fernández 1972a). Interferon production could explain, in part, the interference observed between Newcastle disease virus and VEE virus in tissue cultures (Kono 1962). Nonviable hemagglutinin of VEE virus was also produced in cell cultures (Reitman 1969).

EPIZOOTIOLOGY

Geographic distribution

The geographical distribution of EEE virus includes the eastern half of North America, from Canada to the Caribbean, and Central and South America. Eastern equine encephalomyelitis virus activity, as detected by isolation and serological techniques, has also been reported in areas outside the eastern region of North America. The distribution of WEE virus appears to be wider than that of EEE virus, encompassing practically all of North and South America. Because the EEE and WEE viruses respectively are not restricted to the eastern and western regions of North America, the designations 'eastern' and 'western' do not accurately describe their distribution.

In addition, there have been reports documenting the presence of antibodies to EEE and WEE viruses in humans, birds, and mammals and the isolation of EEE viruses in Europe and Asia, but the validity of these findings has not been established. The EEE virus causes a serious disease problem in the equine and human populations of South America. In many regions of North America, particularly in the East, WEE virus is not associated with outbreaks of encephalitis in man and horses. During the interepizootic periods, the WEE and EEE viruses have been isolated and antibodies demonstrated in a variety of animals, indicating a persistent enzootic cycle.

The VEE virus is defined as a virus complex comprising four antigenic subtypes which have discrete geographical distributions and distinct serological and epidemiological properties. The strains are broadly grouped into enzootic and epizootic varieties; the latter variants have been responsible for recurrent epizootics of fatal disease in horses in South America, with devastating socioeconomic consequences.

Until 1969, the epizootic VEE virus extended only to the northern part of South America, after which it spread through Central America into North America but has not persisted in the latter continent. However, due to the fact that the enzootic variants are nonpathogenic for horses and restricted to sylvatic cycles, VEE virus is more widespread in the Western Hemisphere than is indicated by the number of equine epizootics.

The JE virus is present throughout the Far East, while the NEE virus occurs in Egypt and Syria.

Literature

The occurrences of WEE and EEE viruses have been documented since the early 1900s, and the epidemiology of the diseases was reviewed by Hanson (1973). In addition, there have been numerous reports on the position of the equine encephalomyelitis viruses in various regions. The epidemiology of EEE virus in Florida, USA, was analyzed between 1955 and 1974 (Bigler *et al.* 1976). Encephalitis caused by EEE virus occurred in Jamaica (Belle *et al.* 1964) and in Panama (Dietz *et al.* 1980). There have been numerous publications on the occurrence of virus and disease in the USA. The possible occurrence of EEE virus in Central Europe was discussed, and it was concluded that this virus has been isolated and that there is serological evidence of the infection in various animal species. However, additional work is required (Sprockhoff and Ising 1971). Outbreaks of WEE in horses and humans in the USA and Canada were investigated (Morgante *et al.* 1968; Potter *et al.* 1977; Reeves *et al.* 1964). The zoonosis of WEE was discussed by Artsob (1979a). In Canada, at least 17 major horse epizootics have occurred since 1935. The virus remains enzootic and, in spite of control measures involving vaccination and spraying, small outbreaks still occur in the country's western provinces; there is serological evidence that the infection was also present in some of the eastern provinces (Artsob 1979a). Additional information was published on the occurrence of epizootics in Alberta in 1965 (Morgante *et al.* 1968) and in Manitoba in 1975 (Waters 1976).

Table 9.1 The distribution of VEE virus and disease

VIRUS		DISEASE	
SYLVATIC	*EPIZOOTIC*	*HORSE/MAN*	*MAN*
Brazil	Argentina	Argentina	Panama
Guyana	Trinidad	Peru	Florida
Surinam	Venezuela	Ecuador	(sylvatic
Florida	Colombia	Colombia	virus)
Colorado	Peru	Venezuela	
Panama	Ecuador	Trinidad	
Trinidad	Costa Rica	Costa Rica	
Venezuela	Nicaragua	Nicaragua	
Colombia	Honduras	Honduras	
Peru	Belize	Belize	
Ecuador	El Salvador	El Salvador	
Panama	Guatemala	Guatemala	
Costa Rica	Mexico	Mexico	
Honduras	Texas	Texas	
Nicaragua			
Belize			
Mexico			
Guatemala			
El Salvador			

The epidemiology of the VEE virus complex has been reviewed (Eddy *et al.* 1973; Johnson and Martin 1974). The cycle of enzootic VEE viruses in rodents was not lethal for horses, while the epizootic strains produced high levels of equine mortality (Justines *et al.* 1980). Various serotypes of VEE virus caused outbreaks of disease throughout Central and South America (Spertzel and McKinney 1970). In the epidemiology of VEE the distribution of sylvatic and epizootic virus as well as the diseases in horses and man have to be considered. Information on the presence of viruses and/or diseases is presented in Table 9.1, and was provided by T. G. Walton (personal communication).

The VEE virus was 10 to 100 times more virulent than the EEE virus. The enzootic virus was isolated from mosquitoes and positive sera were obtained from rodents in Florida during the 1960s. There was also serological evidence that horses and humans in southern Florida had been exposed to the virus (McConnell and Spertzel 1979). Epizootiological studies of VEE outbreaks were also undertaken in Venezuela (Sellers *et al.* 1965). The epizootiology was also investigated in Brazil (Shope *et al.* 1964) and Panama (Grayson and Galindo 1969) where sylvatic virus only occurred. Epizootic VEE appeared in South America in 1967 and in Central America in 1969, extended into Mexico in 1970, and finally reached Texas, USA, in 1971 where approximately 1500 cases in horses were investigated and 142 deaths were documented. Subsequently, extensive epizootiological studies were undertaken in Peru (Scherer *et al.* 1975), Costa Rica (Martin *et al.* 1972) Haiti (McLean *et al.* 1979), and Texas (Sudia and Newhouse 1975). An investigation of the epidemiology of VEE in Central America provided evidence of possible methods of transmission of virulent VEE virus from one geographical area to another (Franck and Johnson 1971).

Japanese encephalitis virus has been reported in Japan, eastern Siberia, China, Korea, Taiwan, Malaysia, Singapore, and India. During the 1961 epizootic in Hokkaido (Japan) the morbidity and mortality rates were 62.3 and 25% respectively (Goto *et al.* 1969). Ecological and epizootiological studies of JE virus in Japan revealed the quantitative dynamics of mosquito–bird–swine infections and their epidemiological significance to human infections (Scherer and Buescher 1959; Buescher and Scherer 1959). The incidence of inapparent human infection by JE virus was also studied (Scherer *et al.* 1959c). The role of insect vectors and animal hosts in the epidemiology of JE was further investigated (Detels *et al.* 1970). The epidemiology and transmission of JE virus in Taiwan was also studied (Grayston *et al.* 1962; Hu and Grayston 1962; Wang *et al.* 1962a, b; Wang and Grayston 1962; Chu and Grayston 1962).

Transmission

Transmission of equine encephalomyelitis viruses depend on climatic conditions that favor the propagation of the vector. Climatic conditions that are adverse to the vector profoundly influence the epizootiology of all forms of equine encephalitis, restricting the outbreaks to clearly defined seasons. Under suitable climatic conditions the virus probably persists in reservoir hosts, but this has not been documented. Although mosquitoes are the primary vectors of EEE, WEE, and VEE viruses, there is evidence that other biting arthropods may also carry these agents.

The EEE, WEE and VEE viruses have both enzootic and epizootic cycles. The sylvatic cycle of EEE and WEE viruses is the basis of an enzootic situation and involves wild rodents and wild and domestic birds whose levels of viremia are sufficient to enable infection of the vectors. Mosquitoes transmit the virus from wild animals and birds to equines and man. The EEE and WEE enzootic viruses are pathogenic for horses and man and cause epizootics. The VEE enzootic virus does not cause clinical disease in horses but causes disease in man. The enzootic virus does not give rise to epizootics or the epizootic virus. The two viruses are different in their pathogenicity and epizootiology.

After the female mosquito ingests an infected blood meal, the virus multiplies in the cells of the midgut and then spreads to virtually all organs and tissues; its localization in the salivary glands results in transmission during feeding. The virus is not injurious to the vector, and the infection persists for the entire life span of the insect. The mosquito is infective 10 days after the ingestion of infective blood and can transmit the virus repeatedly through a series of bites. Infection of the mosquito is critically dependent on the level of viremia in the reservoir host. In some forms of equine encephalitis, the horse is usually a dead-end host and not a dominant factor in the spread of the infection.

The epizootiology of EEE virus involves swamp-dwelling birds along the Atlantic coast and the Gulf of Mexico. These swamp cycles produce epizootics when other birds acquire the infection and are subsequently attacked by various species of mosquitoes which spread the virus to man, the equidae, and other vertebrate hosts. Epizootics involving horses and humans usually occur in the vicinity of swamps during periods which favor increased infection rates in the enzootic cycle. Viremias of EEE in horses may be high and clinical cases act as amplifiers.

The epizootiology of VEE virus is more complex than that of EEE and WEE viruses. The sylvatic form of VEE virus is comparable to that of the other two viruses. The evolvement of VEE epizootics from the enzootic foci has not been shown to occur. The origin of the epizootic VEE virus has not been determined, but several mechanisms of persistence are possible, including mutation of sylvatic VEE virus, maintenance of epizootic virus in as yet unidentified mosquito–vertebrate cycles, and low-level transmission through horses. The horse is the most important amplifier of epizootic VEE virus activity because its level of viremia is sufficient to infect mosquitoes. Endemic VEE invariably results from the cycling of certain antigenic variants and subtypes between particular rodent and mosquito populations.

Literature

Efficient vectorial transmission of a virus depends on the vector's susceptibility to infection, relative abundance, and feeding habits. Because of the complex biological cycle of EEE, WEE, and VEE viruses, it is unlikely that they could readily become established in other parts of the world (Hanson 1973; McConnell and Spertzel 1979; Sudia *et al.* 1971). The isolation of EEE, VEE, and WEE viruses from mosquitoes was studied extensively (Karstad *et al.* 1957; Scherer *et al.* 1975; Galindo and Grayson 1971; Grayson and Galindo 1972).

The epizootiology of EEE virus is not completely defined, but it probably involves freshwater swamp mosquitoes such as *Culiseta melanura* (Byrne 1972). Although horses infected with EEE virus usually have low viremias, it was shown that *A. sollicitans* mosquitoes could be infected when allowed to feed on an inoculated horse. After a 2-week incubation period, the mosquitoes were able to transmit the infection, indicating that horses could occasionally play a role in transmission (Sudia *et al.* 1956).

The epizootiology of WEE has been investigated more extensively than that of the EEE. The mosquito *Culex tarsalis* appears to be the primary vector, with a wide range of wild birds, mammals, and reptiles being involved (Byrne 1972). It has also been shown that certain species of ectoparasites isolated from birds could support a WEE-related alphavirus and serve as an overwintering host for this agent (Hayes *et al.* 1977).

The NEEE virus was isolated from ticks, particularly *Hyalomma anatolicum anatolicum*, and transmitted transovarially (Daubney and Mahlau 1957).

Culex tritaeniorhynchus was the primary vector of JE virus. The host range of *C. tritaeniorhynchus* was determined, and it was found that infection of vertebrates was directly related to the time when the maximal density of infected mosquitoes occurred in a specific area (Buescher *et al.* 1959b; Hurlbut and Nibley 1964; Pennington and Phelps 1968; Scherer *et al.* 1959a, b, c). *Culex annulus* was identified as an important vector of JE virus in Taiwan (Cates and Detels 1969). It was shown that *C. gelidus* could transmit the virus after an incubation period of 6 days (Gould *et al.* 1962).

Enzootic strains of VEE virus have been recovered from 40 different species of mosquitoes representing 11 genera (Johnson and Martin 1974). A relatively low dose of an enzootic strain of VEE virus was necessary to infect *C.* (*Melanoconion*) *taeniopus* mosquitoes. Thus, the virus could be acquired from reservoir hosts with low levels of viremia (Scherer *et al.* 1981). The VEE virus differs from EEE and WEE viruses in that it does not multiply as well in birds as in mammals, indicating that birds play a lesser role in the epizootiology (Sidwell *et al.* 1967). To date, no epizootic strain of VEE virus has been shown to cycle enzootically in rodents (Justines *et al.* 1980). The search for epizootic VEE virus in enzootic areas of Guatemala was conducted by isolating strains from sentinel hamsters and mosquitoes, and one strain recovered from a sentinel hamster was considered to be an epizootic strain, but was isolated from a hamster held at the edge of an enzootic focus where the sylvatic virus was active at the time (Scherer *et al.* 1976). A serological survey was conducted to determine the presence and prevalence of VEE in about 30 wild and domestic species of animals in southern Texas. The presence of neutralizing antibodies to VEE virus suggested that the infection had been enzootic in this area prior to the epizootic which occurred in 1971 (Smart *et al.* 1975). The mechanism by which the equine-virulent strains of VEE virus are maintained between epizootic periods has not been determined, but it has been suggested that these strains may remain dormant or latent for long periods in mammalian hosts and then become activated later (Justines *et al.* 1980). However, the most likely mechanism of epizootic virus maintenance involves mosquito–vertebrate cycles which persist until conditions are favorable for the development of epizootics in horses (Johnson and Martin 1974). Cotton rats excreted sylvatic VEE virus in their urine and could be infected by intraoral exposure to feces. Thus, contact spread is a method by which the virus could be maintained in rodent populations without the involvement of a vector (Zarate and Scherer 1968). It has also been shown that aerosol exposure of ground squirrels to WEE virus caused fatal infections and resulted in viremia which attained levels sufficient to infect hematophagus arthropods. The recovery of the virus from the urine also indicated the possibility of transmission through contact or aerosol (Leung *et al.* 1978).

Because contact transmission of VEE was a potential hazard to people who work with infected material, the effects of relative humidity and temperature on airborne VEE virus were investigated (Ehrlich and Miller 1971). Airborne VEE virus was viable for up to 23 hours, with survival being dependent on both temperature and relative humidity (Harper 1961). It was shown that aerosolized VEE was highly infectious for man, and even small amounts of attenuated virus in aerosol form induced immunological responses in a variety of laboratory animals (Kuehne *et al.* 1962). Mice were readily infected with VEE virus by inhalation (Hrusková *et al.* 1969).

INFECTION

Infectivity and virulence

The infectivity and virulence of EEE, WEE, and VEE viruses for horses vary with the different serotypes. After infection, the virus multiplies in the regional drainage lymph nodes, then in the hematopoietic tissue, and in the brain. The virulence is associated, to a certain degree, with the level of viremia and the distribution of virus in the tissues. The strains of the VEE virus complex may be clearly divided on the basis of their antigenic composition into enzootic and epizootic serotypes which are associated with different levels of virulence. There is considerable evidence that a multiplicity of relatively avirulent variants exists. Surveys indicate that inapparent EEE, WEE, and VEE infections are common in horses. A few antigenically distinguishable strains of VEE virus are associated with epizootics, but the majority of the serological subtypes occur in rodents in enzootic situations. The level and duration of viremia in different forms of encephalitis vary and have an effect on the transmission of the disease.

The viremia of animals infected with NEEE virus is detectable for weeks.

A variety of domestic and wild animals are susceptible to infection by EEE, WEE, and VEE viruses, as determined by virus isolation, experimental infections, and serological examination. In the majority of cases, the infections are asymptomatic. Man is susceptible to infection and develops clinical disease but is considered a dead-end host. Many species of birds are also susceptible to infection, but clinical signs occur only in a few species, e.g. EEE virus-infected pheasants.

Natural or experimental VEE infections have been demonstrated in over 150 different animal species, primarily mammals and birds. Wild rodents are the reservior hosts in enzootic foci but usually do not show disease. During epizootics, the horse is the most significant amplifying host, while dogs and pigs, which also develop high levels of viremia, are of secondary importance. Other species of domestic animals are not thought to play a significant role. Although domestic ruminants can be infected with epizootic strains, they rarely show clinical disease and experience transient, low-level viremias.

The JE virus causes encephalitis in horses and man and may produce inapparent infection, abortion, or stillbirth in pigs, which have been incriminated as amplifiers of epizootic JE virus activity.

Literature

Following injection through the bite of a mosquito, the VEE virus multiplies in the regional lymph nodes and then spreads to the general circulation. Further proliferation in the visceral organs results in a second peak of viremia during which infection of the central nervous tissue occurs (Hanson 1973). Examination of VEE virus-infected cell cultures revealed that the first phase of cellular infection involved electrostatic absorption to the external membrane of the cell, with penetration occurring within 30 minutes. The virus develops in the cytoplasm of the cell. There is a latent period of 3 to 4 hours, and a sharp increase in virus titer from 8 to 14 hours followed by a period of constant virus production of up to 80 hours (Johnson and Martin 1974).

The enzootic strains of VEE virus did not cause high viremia, and such infections were not associated with clinical disease. Virulent VEE strains caused a viremia which occurred 24 to 48 hours after infection and persisted for 2 to 3 days in conjunction with fever, anorexia, and malaise. The disappearance of the viremia coincided with the appearance of circulating neutralizing antibodies. The period of peak viremia preceded the onset of clinical signs by 2 to 4 days. Symptoms indicative of central nervous system involvement were associated with high viremia and developed after the fifth day postinfection. Death usually occurred between days 6 and 8 (Kissling *et al.* 1956; Walton *et al.* 1973a). The VEE virus reached titers of more than $10^{5.5}$ and $10^{7.6}$ in horse and guinea pig blood respectively, and these levels could induce infection in mosquitoes. (Walton *et al.* 1973a). In comparison the concentrations of EEE virus usually attained in the blood of horses appeared to be below the threshold necessary to infect mosquitoes. The maximum titers of virus ranged from $10^{0.5}$ to $10^{4.5}$, and the period of the viremia varied from 24 to 66 hours (Kissling *et al.* 1954). The VEE virus was shed in the nasal, eye, and mouth secretions, urine and milk of an infected horse (Kissling *et al.* 1956). Thirteen strains of VEE virus were isolated from blood and nasal or throat swabs obtained from sick horses and humans in Guatemala in 1969. Titrations of virus in these specimens were performed by intracerebral inoculation of suckling mice (Scherer *et al.* 1972). Transplacental passage of an epizootic strain of VEE virus was demonstrated in mares with clinical disease. The virus was recovered in high titers from fetal blood and organs, but it was not demonstrated in the maternal blood (Justines *et al.* 1980).

In NEEE virus infections, the viremia was detected for weeks (Daubney 1967).

The infectivity and pathogenicity varied with the different viruses and with the different isolates or strains of each virus. When WEE virus was injected by a variety of peripheral routes, it did not cause clinical signs of central nervous system involvement. Intracerebral inoculation was necessary to induce this syndrome, in contrast to natural infections in which severe clinical signs and central nervous system involvement were reported (Walton 1981). Venezuelan equine encephalomyelitis could be transmitted to horses by intranasal instillation of the virus (Kissling *et al.* 1956). Following peripheral injection of horses with enzootic or epizootic VEE virus strains, low titers of virus were found in the cerebrospinal fluid; however, intrathecal inoculation produced higher titers. Enzootic strains injected by the intrathecal, but not the peripheral, route caused death. Horses with fatal infections had widespread histological changes and large amounts of virus in the brain tissue. The attenuated VEE virus vaccine strain TC-83 also multiplied in the brain after intrathecal injection but did not cause clinical disease or extensive histological changes (Dietz *et al.* 1978).

During the early stages of infection in horses, tissue tropisms other than the viremia have not been clearly demonstrated. In EEE, WEE, and VEE, the virus could be isolated from the brain during the latter stages of the disease, but success in isolating the virus from the central nervous system has varied and this tissue has been found to be a poor source of the virus. More EEE virus was recovered from the thalamus and basal ganglia than from other brain areas (Kissling *et al.* 1954).

The distribution of the viruses in the tissue has been investigated in laboratory rodents. Virulent VEE virus caused encephalitis and necrosis of the liver and lymphoid organs in hamsters. Infectious virus and viral antigens were detected in all tissues studied, with the greatest accumulation occurring in the brain. Although attenuated virus produced an inapparent infection in hamsters, lesions were observed in the brain, liver, and lymphoid tissues (Dremov *et al.* 1978). The multiplication of VEE virus in the myocardium of newborn mice and its passage through the endothelium were demonstrated (García-Tamayo 1973). The EEE virus could be demonstrated in the blood, brain, and internal organs of adult and newborn mice from 8 hours to 7 days after infection, with the maximum titers occurring between 48 and 72 hours (Ognianov and Fernández 1972b).

It has been established that the various strains of EEE, WEE, and VEE virus have different degrees of virulence. The virulence of a virus population was often determined by a subpopulation of infectious virions with greater virulence than the majority of the population. The proportion of virulent to avirulent subpopulations could be shifted by passages in various hosts and tissue culture systems. For example, the selective removal of small-plaque-forming WEE virus from a heterogeneous population enabled the demonstration of a small subpopulation of a virulent large-plaque-forming virus (Jahrling 1976). While plaque size and virulence were not irrevocably linked properties of VEE virus, deliberate selection and passage in specific laboratory systems could produce stable viral types whose plaque size and virulence characteristics were correlated (Hearn and Jameson 1971). After vaccination of mice with an attenuated strain of VEE, the virus isolated from 24-hour spleen, liver, and brain samples possessed the virulence and plaque characteristics of the attenuated vaccine virus strain, while the properties of the virus populations recovered from 72-hour spleen specimens resembled those of the virulent parent virus from which the attenuated strain was derived (Hearn 1961a).

In a comparative study of the pathogenesis of WEE and EEE viral infections in mice inoculated intracerebrally or subcutaneously, it was shown that the EEE virus was more virulent. The intracerebral inoculation of mice with EEE virus resulted in a rapidly fatal infection. The virus was present in all tissues, but the highest titers occurred in the brain. Subcutaneous injection also caused a generalized infection. The WEE virus caused fatal infections on intracerebral inoculation but did not produce a viremia. Subcutaneous injection of the WEE virus caused a transient low-grade viremia, and the virus persisted at the inoculation site for 3 to 4 days. In mice infected with WEE or EEE, viral antigens were detected by fluorescent antibody (FA) staining only in the central nervous system, primarily in the cytoplasm of neurons and glial cells (Liu *et al.* 1970). With the exception of the attenuated vaccine strain TC-83, all of the strains used in a study of the virulence of various VEE virus subtypes were highly pathogenic for suckling mice by the intracranial or intraperitoneal route of infection.

The pathogenicity for older mice and guinea pigs provided a means of distinguishing the virulence of strains as well as rapid method of separating epizootic subtypes from TC-83 VEE virus (Calisher and Maness 1974). Using the direct FA staining technique, attenuated and virulent strains of VEE virus were found to cause a pantropic infection in suckling mice regardless of the concentration of inoculum or the route of infection. Viral antigens were detected in many tissues, particularly in the pancreas and central nervous system (Kundin *et al.* 1966). Similar experiments in young adult mice indicated that tissue infectivity and viral lethality were comparable after intracerebral or subcutaneous inoculation of virulent VEE virus, but young adult mice were able to withstand massive doses of peripherally inoculated attenuated virus (Kundin 1966). The degree of homogeneity of the VEE virus with respect to virulence for hamsters varied with the strain, and that there was evidence that the avirulence property of some strains was not stable (Jahrling and Scherer 1973b). The virulence of VEE virus strains for humans appeared to correlate with the ability to cause mortality in hamsters. Virulent strains injected subcutaneously killed hamsters within 3 to 6 days and produced extensive necrosis of hematopoietic tissues and brain cells, focal hemorrhage in the cerebral cortex, and abundant viral antigens in hematopoietic tissues. Strains which caused a low level of mortality did not produce these lesions or detectable antigens in the tissues (Jahrling and Scherer 1973a). The virulence of VEE virus for guinea pigs also depended on the strain, and although exceptions occasionally occurred, there was a good correlation between virulence for equines and guinea pig lethality (Scherer and Chin 1977).

The propagation of virulent and attenuated strains of VEE virus and the development of lesions were investigated in hamsters. The virulent virus caused high mortality, whereas the attenuated virus rarely produced disease. In addition, the virulent strain began to multiply sooner and reached higher titers in the blood than the attenuated virus. Maximum titers of both viruses were similar in the brain, bone marrow, lymph nodes, and spleen, but the growth of the attenuated virus peaked almost a day later than that of the virulent virus. After intracranial inoculation, both viruses grew at the same rate. The virulent virus caused lesions in the hematopoietic system, brain, and intestine, while the attenuated virus did not produce distinct histopathologic lesions. The lesions induced in the hematopoietic tissues by the virulent virus were characterized by massive destruction of the cells. Virulence was not associated with selective growth in a particular tissue, since both viruses reached essentially equal maximum concentrations in target organs (Austin and Scherer 1971). A discrepancy was observed in that there were similar quantities of infectious virulent and benign viruses in the hematopoietic tissues, but there were dissimilar quantities of viral antigen and histopathological lesions. Further investigations of the behavior of virulent and avirulent VEE viruses revealed that the viral concentrations in the blood correlated directly and clearance rates inversely with the virulence for hamsters, whereas the rate and extent of growth of the viruses in hematopoietic and brain tissues did not correlate with the virulence (Jahrling and Scherer 1973a). More than 99% of the infectious benign VEE viruses was cleared from the circulation of hamsters within 30 minutes of inoculating, whereas only 0.8% of the virulent virus was removed. Only the benign virus was found in the phagocytic vacuoles of reticuloendothelial cells in the liver. Thus, the interaction between the virus and hepatic endothelial and Kupffer cells was critical in the determination of VEE viral virulence (Jahrling and Gorelkin 1975).

Infection in cattle, dogs, and pigs

Serological surveys using hemagglutination-inhibition and neutralization tests showed that cattle and pigs had antibodies to VEE virus, and it was proposed that these species could be involved in the enzootic cycle (Scherer *et al.* 1971a). Subcutaneous infection of cows with VEE virus did not cause clinical illness, but significant neutropenia developed and low levels of viremia were also observed. It was concluded that cattle did not play a significant role in the transmission of the virus during epizootics (Walton and Johnson 1972a). Young pigs and young cattle developed viremia between 0.5 and 3 days after experimental infection with VEE virus, but the different viral strains used varied in their ability to induce viremia. Hemagglutination-inhibiting and neutralizing antibodies developed in both species. Transient fever occurred in cattle with viremia or virus in the throat. It was concluded that these two species might be involved in the maintenance of VEE virus (Dickerman *et al.* 1973a). Eastern equine encephalomyelitis virus was isolated from a naturally infected 3-week-old pig which developed signs of central nervous system disturbance. The infection could be transmitted experimentally to pigs and resulted in brain lesions characterized by neutrophils in perivascular cuffs and in areas of necrosis. Western equine encephalomyelitis virus has also been isolated from pigs (Pursell *et al.* 1972). Near East equine encephalitis virus was isolated from encephalitic sheep and cattle in Syria (Daubney and Mahlau 1957).

During a serological survey in Guatemala, antibodies to VEE virus were detected in dogs, and it was proposed that this species played an important role in the endemic cycle of the VEE virus (Dickerman *et al.* 1973b). Dogs were shown to be susceptible to experimental infection by an intramuscular inoculation with VEE, which induced fever, viremia, hemagglutination-inhibition antibody formation, and some mortality (Davis *et al.* 1966). The latter infections, as well as those caused by the bite of infected mosquitoes, resulted in sufficient levels of viremia to enable mosquitoes to transmit the virus to other animals (Bivin *et al.* 1967). Attenuated VEE virus caused an inapparent infection in dogs, which had an immunological response (Taber *et al.* 1965). On the other hand, dogs were found to be relatively resistant to WEE virus (Furumoto 1969). In a study of the susceptibility of coyotes to VEE virus, most of the experimentally infected coyote pups developed clinical disease characterized by a viremia of 3 to 5 days' duration and antibody formation. The concentration of virus in the blood was sufficient for mosquito transmission. Approximately 25% of the 1- to 2-month-old animals died, but all of the 6- to 7-month-old pups survived, indicating that resistance to the virus developed with age (Lundgren and Smart 1969).

In Japan, serological surveys using the hemagglutination-inhibition test revealed a high incidence of inapparent JE virus infections in pigs (Konno *et al.* 1966). Pigs were identified as a major natural source of the virus for the vector mosquito, and during one period, nearly 100% of the pigs in an area were infected. The viremia persisted for up to 4 days after infection and occurred at levels sufficient to infect mosquitoes (Scherer *et al.* 1959d). Annual cycles of infection in Taiwan were correlated with the appearance of infection in pigs, and the transmission of infection to mosquitoes was related to the level and duration of viremia and to the antibody response in pigs of various ages (Hurlbut 1964).

Infection in wild mammals

A number of wild species of birds and mammals were found to be infected with WEE virus (Burton *et al.* 1966b). Western equine encephalomyelitis virus caused extensive lesions in suckling and adult Richardson's ground squirrels (*Spermophilus richardsonii*), and the viremia was of sufficient level to infect mosquitoes (Leung *et al.* 1976). The level and duration of the viremia induced in the snowshoe hare (*Lepus americanus*) by WEE virus infection increased when the animals were exposed to fluctuating temperatures and humidity. This species could be implicated in the maintenance of WEE virus in enzootic situations (Kiorpes and Yuill 1975). The Mongolian gerbil (*Meriones unguiculatus*) was also shown to be highly susceptible to WEE virus infection (Hayles 1972). Western equine encephalomyelitis virus was also found in frogs and snakes and could be transmitted to these animals experimentally (Burton *et al.* 1966a; Gebhardt *et al.* 1966).

Wild rodents, the reservoir hosts of sylvatic VEE virus, developed sufficient levels of viremia to infect mosquitoes for 2 to 4 days after inoculation. Other wild animals, such as marsupials, bats, rabbits, raccoons, and nonhuman primates, could be infected with the virus. However, because of their low viremia or low frequency of infection, these species did not appear to play major roles in the enzootic cycle of VEE (Johnson and Martin 1974). Eighty-three wild mammals of ten species collected in the USA were infected with VEE virus. Rodents were again shown to be highly susceptible to infection and developed high levels of viremia which could easily infect mosquitoes. High mortality was observed in several rodent species. In some species juvenile animals appeared to be more susceptible and had higher levels of viremia and mortality than adults. The lagomorphs were susceptible to infection, but the viremia was observed at thresholds infective for mosquitoes for only 1 day. Raccoons and opossums were relatively resistant (Bowen 1976). In Mexico, sylvatic VEE virus was isolated from four species of wild mammals, and six species were seropositive

(Scherer *et al.* 1971b). A vampire bat was also found to be infected during an equine epizootic of VEE in Mexico in 1970 (Correa-Girion *et al.* 1972). Rhesus monkey experimentally infected with some strains of VEE virus developed fever and other clinical signs. Both clinically ill and asymptomatic animals had high titers of circulating virus which appeared 1 day after infection and lasted for 4 to 6 days (Monath *et al.* 1974).

Infection in birds

Wild birds were a principal source of WEE and EEE virus infection for mosquitoes during the spring and summer months (Kissling *et al.* 1957b). Sixty-three birds from thirteen species collected in Georgia, USA, were experimentally infected with VEE virus; the viremia was moderately high and persisted for 2 to 6 days (Bowen and McLean 1977). Various species of wild birds were shown to be infected with VEE virus, and the infection was subsequently transferred by mosquitoes to other birds. In the majority of birds, these infections did not cause clinical signs (Chamberlain *et al.* 1956). The bobwhite quail was found to be susceptible to VEE virus and could be used as a sentinel animal (Watts and Williams 1972). Certain species of songbirds and northward-migrating birds captured on the Pacific coast of Guatemala were susceptible to infection with both epizootic and enzootic strains of VEE virus. They developed moderate levels of viremia which lasted for 2 to 4 days and were high enough to infect mosquitoes. However, because of the existence of antigenic subtypes with discrete geographical distributions, avian dissemination of these strains appeared to be of minimal importance (Dickerman *et al.* 1980).

An outbreak of EEE in 1977 killed more than 90 000 coturnix quail (*Coturnix coturnix*) on a farm in South Carolina, USA. Cannibalism was thought to be responsible for the rapid spread of the infection throughout the flock (Eleazer *et al.* 1978). Different isolates of EEE virus varied considerably in pathogenicity for pheasants 21 days old or older which had been inoculated subcutaneously, but 9-day-old chicks were highly susceptible to the virus (Weinack *et al.* 1978). Venezuelan equine encephalomyelitis infected pheasants and chukars but did not cause clinical disease (Proctor and Pearson 1975). In endemic areas of southern Alberta, indicator chickens were found to be serologically positive to WEE virus (Morgante *et al.* 1969). The effects of the behavior, bionomics, and population dynamics of birds on the ecology of JE virus were investigated (Scherer *et al.* 1959b), and the prevalence of the virus and antibodies in wild birds was studied (Buescher *et al.* 1959a). Clinically inapparent infection and viremia were induced experimentally in several species of birds (Buescher *et al.* 1959c).

CLINICAL SIGNS

The clinical signs and lesions in horses infected with EEE, WEE, or VEE virus are similar. Each of the three viruses can induce a variety of syndromes which range in severity from subclinical to generalized disease with central nervous system involvement. The severe syndromes are least common in cases of WEE and most often observed in VEE virus infections. In man, the disease syndrome is generally milder than that in horses, is usually systemic, and is rarely associated with a frank encephalitis. Severe syndromes occur in pheasants. Western equine encephalomyelitis resembles the eastern form with the exception that the mortality rate is lower; the course of the disease tends to be more chronic and subtle, and the infection is characterized by a febrile reaction and a systemic response.

The EEE, WEE, and VEE viruses cause three syndromes: (1) inapparent infection accompanied by fever with or without a transient, low-level viremia; (2) mild clinical disease marked by high fever and viremia without subsequent central venous system involvement; and (3) severe clinical disease characterized by high fever, viremia, and subsequent central nervous system involvement which can be fatal or cause sequelae in the survivors. Venezuelan equine encephalomyelitis virus differs significantly from EEE and WEE viruses in that it more often causes a fulminating systemic disease or an encephalitis, as well as a high level of infectivity in the blood. Clinical symptoms are usually associated with the development of an inflammatory response, and the neurological signs are observed subsequent to the appearance of a viremia and formation of neutralizing antibodies. Horses, pheasants, and man are the most severely affected species.

Literature

The clinical signs of the different syndromes caused by EEE, WEE, and VEE viruses have been presented in various reviews (Walton 1981; Byrne 1972; Johnson and Martin 1974; Gibbs 1976). Eastern equine encephalomyelitis virus caused a biphasic febrile reaction in horses with severe infections. The initial pyrexic response occurred about 1.5 to 2 days after infection and lasted for 1 day; the second febrile period began 4 to 6 days postinfection and persisted for 1 to 4 days. The first rise in temperature was accompanied by the development of viremia, while the second febrile phase occurred in conjunction with signs of central nervous system involvement. The severe syndrome was characterized by marked depression and high fever, had a short course of up to 3 days, and terminated in death. The type of neurological signs varied from one animal to another and changed with the course of infection. Depression, incoordination, hyperesthesia, and bizarre behavior developed. Frequently, there was evidence that the animals were blind and deaf and suffered from intense pruritus. Grinding of the teeth and aimless chewing were also observed (Walton 1981; Byrne

1972). Four distinct syndromes were recognized in horses experimentally infected with EEE virus either by inoculation or by the bite of infected mosquitoes. Animals that exhibited a biphasic febrile reaction either died or recovered with or without sequelae indicative of central nervous system damage. A second syndrome was characterized by a single temperature elevation and the presence of viremia, but there was no central nervous system involvement. The third syndrome was marked by low levels of viremia without a febrile reaction. In the fourth syndrome, no fever or viremia was detected, but a specific antibody was induced. A good correlation was observed between the dose of virus inoculated and the number of hours which elapsed until the first appearance of viremia (Kissling *et al.* 1954).

The WEE virus is less virulent than the EEE virus, although the case fatality rate may reach 50%, the average being 20 to 30% (Hayes 1979b). Experimental infection of horses with several strains of WEE virus by various routes produced syndromes which ranged from inapparent to severe disease characterized by central nervous system malfunction. The disease pattern was characterized by three phases: viremia, pyrexia, and signs of encephalitis, and there was considerable overlap of these phases. There was no evidence that the disease could be transmitted by contact (Sponseller *et al.* 1966).

The clinical disease caused by VEE was characterized by three forms: an asymptomatic infection accompanied by slight fever; a systemic disease characterized by fever, tachycardia, depression, anorexia, and in some cases diarrhea; and an encephalitic form, which may have symptoms in common with the systemic disease, but also has signs referable to central nervous system involvement, such as circling, ataxia, head pressing, continuous chewing movements, and hyperexcitability. There was evidence that equine neurovirulence was associated with certain antigenic types, which also induced high viremia. There was not much information regarding the sequelae of epizootic VEE, but there was evidence of permanent neurological damage (Johnson and Martin 1974).

The two severe forms of VEE were the acute febrile systemic disease of hematopoietic tissues and blood vessels, and the encephalitic form, in which the signs of nervous tissue involvement were dominant. Various clinical signs developed sequentially after the incubation period. Fever was usually the first sign of infection, followed by inappetance and mild excitability. Thereafter the disease progressed rapidly, and affected animals developed weakness, ataxia, and dramatic signs of encephalitis consisting of muscle spasms, incoordination, chewing movements, and convulsions. Encephalitic symptoms followed the peak of the viremia and occurred at the time when the circulating virus was disappearing and body temperature was returning to normal. Some animals were extremely depressed, somnolent, and unresponsive to stimuli, while others wandered aimlessly or pressed against solid objects. Late in the infection, a broad stance and circling were observed. At any point in the evolution of these clinical signs, an animal could recover or become prostrate and succumb. The course could be extremely rapid, with mortality occurring within hours after the first signs were observed. On the other hand, the development of clinical signs could be protracted and accompanied by severe loss of body weight before an encephalitic death or recovery finally occurred (McConnell and Spertzel 1979). In a number of experimental infections, approximately half of the animals developed clinical signs indicative of central nervous system involvement (Kissling and Chamberlain 1967). In the epizootic situation, it was estimated that 35% of the equines died of the infection, 5% were mildly infected, and 10% had inapparent infections (Scherer *et al.* 1972).

The disease caused by NEEE virus varied in its clinical severity. In the most severe syndrome, signs of central nervous system involvement developed, and there was evidence of paralysis of groups of muscles, hyperexcitability, frenzied action, muscle tremors, incoordination, and convulsions (Daubney and Mahlau 1957).

In other species of domestic and wild animals, the natural clinical diseases caused by EEE, WEE, and VEE viruses have not been well documented; mild clinical signs and low titers of circulating virus have been reported. Most of the investigations of wild mammals have been limited to rodents, which are susceptible to infection and develop clinical syndromes of varying severity (Johnson and Martin 1974). The outcome of an infection with VEE virus depends on the virus strain and the susceptibility of the host. Cattle, sheep, and goats presented a very mild form of the disease which was characterized by transient temperature elevation and leukopenia. The clinical signs were more obvious in experimentally infected dogs and pigs, which developed anorexia, depression, reluctance to move, and aggressive behavior terminating in death (McConnell and Spertzel 1979).

In transmission studies of VEE virus, six of the ten experimentally infected dogs died of an encephalitic syndrome characterized by neuronal degeneration, glial cell proliferation, and perivascular cuffing. In addition, two dogs in contact with the affected animals also became infected (Davis *et al.* 1966). In other experiments, virulent VEE virus caused fever, viremia, and leukopenia in three of the ten inoculated dogs. Two of the three affected animals died, but no evidence of encephalitis was observed upon microscopic examination (Taber *et al.* 1965).

A congenital disease of swine, characterized by stillbirth or death during the neonatal period, occurred concomitantly with an outbreak of JE in equidae and humans (Burns 1950).

Pheasants were also susceptible to infection with EEE virus and developed a clinical disease which was characterized by fever, ataxia, trembling, weakness, leg paralysis, and generalized paralysis terminating in death (Hayes 1979a).

PATHOLOGY

Relatively little information is available on the general pathology of the arboviral encephalitides in horses; most descriptions are concerned with the microscopic lesions in the central nervous tissue. The lesions caused by EEE, WEE, and VEE viruses are basically similar and depend on the virulence of the particular strain or serotype and the duration and severity of the clinical syndromes. The various signs of neurologic malfunction can occasionally be correlated with the distribution of lesions in the central nervous system. The lesions that occur in both the neutrophil and the meninges are comprised of vascular changes, cellular inflammatory infiltration, and degenerative and necrotic changes in the neurons. A diffuse necrotizing meningoencephalitis occurs, and the lesions involved range from a mild perivascular accumulation of cellular exudate to an extensive necrosis of blood vessels, hemorrhages, gliosis, and loss of neurons. These histopathological changes are most severe in the cortex. In acute cases, the inflammatory reaction is characterized by neutrophil infiltration, with accompanying vascular lesions consisting of endothelial proliferation, thrombi, hemorrhages, and perivascular accumulation of lymphocytes and neutrophils. In more chronic lesions, there is nodular formation by microglial cells as well as more extensive lymphocyte accumulation around blood vessels. While all three viruses cause severe vascular lesions, this type of damage predominates in VEE virus infections. Lesions are generalized in the brain and spinal cord, although the cerebral cortex, thalamus, hypothalamus, hippocampus, and dorsal nuclei of the medulla are most affected. The presence of intracytoplasmic and intranuclear inclusion bodies has not been definitely determined.

In other tissues, the development of lesions has not been clearly demonstrated. It would appear likely that the vascular changes, which are probably generalized, could be associated with lesions in various parenchymatous organs. Degenerative and necrotic changes have been observed in the liver, adrenals, heart, and pancreas and are associated with necrosis and vasculitis in small and medium blood vessels. Depletion of bone marrow cells and extensive necrosis of lymphocytes in major lymphoid organs have been reported. Lesions in the blood vessels and in the hematopoietic tissue are probably associated with the systemic syndromes observed. The attenuated cell culture vaccine virus causes slight reversible lesions in the brains of equidae. In laboratory animals, the development of lesions depends on the species of host and involves either necrosis of myeloid and lymphoid tissues, meningoencephalomyelitis, or a combination thereof.

Literature

Kissling *et al.* (1954, 1956) described the pathological lesions induced by EEE and VEE viruses. In the severe syndrome produced by VEE, encephalitis was not consistently expressed, while in EEE and WEE infections, the central nervous system involvement was usually the only manifestation of the disease which was clinically recognizable. The change caused by WEE and EEE in tissues other than those of the central nervous system have not been adequately described, and the lesions observed in causes of VEE were not discussed in great detail.

The brain lesions of EEE virus-infected animals surviving 1 day or less after the appearance of neurologic symptoms were characterized by diffuse neutrophil infiltration of the gray matter, endothelial degeneration, perivascular hemorrhage, and moderate perivascular fluid effusion. In animals surviving 2 days or longer, the infiltration of neutrophils diminished, and there were perivascular infiltrations of lymphocytes and cellular nodular formations which contained large mononuclear cells and stimulated microglia. The lesions were found almost exclusively in the gray matter, with the most extensive damage occurring in the cerebral cortex. The distribution of lesions varied in other areas and determined the nature of the clinical signs (Kissling and Rubin 1951).

In horses dying of VEE virus infection, congestion of mucous membranes and subserosal ecchymotic hemorrhages were observed. Early progressive leukopenia was associated with the presence of virus in the blood. In horses that recovered, the leukocyte count reverted to normal levels within 2 days of the termination of the viremia. In fatal cases, almost complete cellular depletion was observed in hematopoietic tissues, including the bone marrow, spleen, and lymph nodes. In the lymphoid organs, there was depletion of mature cells with only remnants of lymphoid follicles remaining. In the pancreas, multiple necrotic foci were found without an accompanying inflammatory response and involved acinar, but not islet, cells. The brain lesions induced in horses by VEE virus differed from those caused by WEE and EEE viruses in that they were primarily vascular and did not involve large numbers of inflammatory cells. In horses that died without central nervous system involvement, there were only minimal lesions in the brain, while horses with brain involvement had marked vascular lesions consisting of swollen endothelial cells, perivascular edema and hemorrhage, and a sparse lymphocytic infiltration into the perivascular spaces. Many of the cells in the perivascular exudate were undergoing lysis and fragmentation. Lesions in recovered cases consisted of atrophy of the acinar cells of the pancreas and lymphocytic perivascular infiltration in the cerebral cortex (Kissling *et al.* 1956). In another report, histopathological changes were described in the brains of 15 horses naturally infected with VEE virus. The inflammatory reactions were found to be similar to those produced by EEE virus. The characteristic lesion was a perivascular inflammatory reaction involving lymphocytes and neutrophils, and thrombosis and necrosis of small arteries often occurred. Glial nodules were also observed in some regions of the brain. Frequently, there was lysis of the infiltrating lymphocytes (Roberts *et al.* 1970). A pronounced necrotizing meningoencephalomyelitis was observed in burros with severe cases of

VEE. These diffuse lesions were characterized by extensive necrosis, hemorrhage, and intense neutrophil infiltration, with concomitant severe necrotizing vasculitis of small and medium-sized blood vessels. Necrotic foci were also observed in the kidneys, heart, adrenal glands, spleen, lymph nodes, and bone marrow (Gochenour *et al.* 1962).

After vaccination with the attenuated VEE vaccine virus, strain TC-83, slight perivascular cuffing with lymphocytes, swelling of vascular endothelial cells, and slight, acute hyperemia were found in some of the horses between the fifth and the ninth day after injection. These lesions were reversible and were not observed 10 days after infection. In the vaccinated animals there was slight evidence of a systemic effect and an increase in rectal temperature (Monlux *et al.* 1972a, b). During the first week after the vaccination of burros and ponies with strain TC-83 attenuated virus vaccine there was elevation of temperature, a 25% decrease in the leukocyte count, and an increase in serum glutamic oxaloacetic transaminase. All values returned to normal by 14 days postvaccination (Brown 1972).

In various species of laboratory animals, the VEE virus induced lesions in the major lymphoid organs and myelopoietic and central nervous tissues. The distribution of the lesions varied with the species of host. In guinea pigs and rabbits, lesions were observed only in the lymphoid and myelopoietic tissues, while in mice, there was also involvement of the central nervous system. The lesions in the lymphoid organs and myelopoietic tissues of these animals consisted of necrosis of all cellular elements. In the monkey, only the brain was affected by meningoencephalitis (Victor *et al.* 1956; Gleiser *et al.* 1962). In the brains of monkeys, this virus initially caused marked proliferation of glial cells and perivascular infiltration of lymphocytes with minimal damage to neurons. These responses were observed at the time when viremia was disappearing and antibody was first detected, suggesting that the inflammatory reaction was due to a combination of antibody and viral antigen in the brain and not neuronal damage inflicted directly by the virus. This conclusion was supported by experimental work on mice in which infection of the brain had already been established. Administration of VEE antiserum to these animals resulted in the early appearance of an inflammatory response in the brain. Therefore, the development of these lesions was dependent on the presence of a specific antibody (Berge *et al.* 1961). In hamsters, the VEE virus also caused extensive destruction of the lymphoreticular and hematopoietic cells (Walker *et al.* 1976). In rats infected with VEE virus, the placental and fetal damage varied with the stage of pregnancy. Inoculation before day 15 of pregnancy caused extensive necrosis and hemorrhages in the embryonic disks, with death of the embryo occurring 3 to 4 days after infection. Animals infected on the sixteenth day of pregnancy and sacrificed 2 days later had some viable fetuses and inflammatory reactions in the mesometrial and decidual vessels. Other rats sacrificed 3 to 4 days after inoculation developed large placental infarcts which were associated with fetal death (García-Tamayo *et al.* 1981).

There was no correlation between the clinical signs and the severity of histological induced in hamsters by WEE virus. Virulent and attenuated strains of WEE virus multiplied in the central nervous system and produced comparable encephalitic lesions, but the attenuated strain did not cause mortality. The administration of an immunosuppressant agent to hamsters that had been inoculated with the attenuated strain either delayed or partially eradicated the inflammatory action and enhanced the virulence (Zlotnik *et al.* 1972). The development of lesions in the central nervous system of mice infected by EEE virus was investigated. The initial changes consisted of interstitial and perivascular edema, which caused an increase in the extracellular space. The neuronal damage was characterized by disruption of the cytoplasmic organization and terminated in crenation, vacuolation, and membrane breakdown. Virus nucleoids formed in the cytoplasm of all brain cells except the endothelium (Murphy and Whitfield 1970).

In a human case of encephalitis caused by EEE virus, demyelinization and necrosis were observed throughout the white matter and brainstem (Bastian *et al.* 1975). In pheasants, the neuropathologic lesions caused by EEE virus consisted of vasculitis, patchy necrosis, microgliosis, focal meningitis, and neuronal degeneration. The lesions were myocardiotropic rather than neurotropic in chickens, a species less susceptible to EEE infection (Jungherr *et al.* 1957).

Near East equine encephalitis virus induced lesions in the cerebral cortex, hippocampus, nucleus caudatus, lateral ventricles, pons, basal nuclear area, and medulla. The disease is a lymphocytic meningoencephalomyelitis characterized by relatively mild perivascular infiltration, diffuse lymphocytic infiltration, marked microgliosis, satellitosis of neurons which show chromatolysis and neuronophagia, and formation of glial nodules (Daubney and Mahlau 1957).

IMMUNOLOGY

The EEE, WEE, and VEE virus complexes are related immunologically, and each complex comprises different antigenic variants. The EEE virus complex is composed of two main antigenic variants which have distinct geographical distributions and are characterized as North or South American types. At least three antigenic variants of WEE virus are recognized and appear to be associated with particular geographical locations. Serological techniques have shown that the VEE virus is a complex consisting of four antigenic subtypes (I to IV) and that VEE subtype I is composed of several antigenic variants (I-A to I-E). Variants I-A, I-B, and I-C are associated with epizootic VEE virus infections, whereas variants I-D and I-E and subtypes II, III, and IV have been identified in sylvatic cycles. Some of the enzootic subtypes and variants do not cause encephalitis. These features of VEE are of fundamental importance in the epizootiology of the disease.

The antigenic relationships which have been established among the EEE, WEE, and VEE viruses are dependent on the sensitivity of the serological tests used and on individual interpretation of the results. These viruses can be distinguished on the basis of neutralization tests undertaken either in laboratory animals, embryonated eggs, or tissue cultures. A commonly used method is the inhibition of plaque formation in cell cultures. Hemagglutination-inhibition, complement fixation (CF), immunodiffusion, and other tests have been used to differentiate the three viruses and demonstrate antigenic heterogeneity within each of the virus types.

Because the three viruses are serologically related, there is partial to complete cross-protection in natural and experimental infections and after vaccination. For example, in cross-challenge studies reciprocal protection is observed with different strains of VEE virus, even though serological tests demonstrated that antigens localized on the surface of the virions were not homologous.

Antibodies to the equine encephalomyelitis viruses develop rapidly and can be detected by the neutralization or hemagglutination-inhibition test within 2 weeks of infection and during the latter part of the clinical response. The level and persistence of antibodies vary with the virus, strain, and clinical response. There is evidence that antibodies may persist for 2 or 3 years.

Literature

The antigenic variation among different strains of WEE virus was determined by using the neutralization, hemagglutination-inhibition, and CF tests (Karabatsos *et al.* 1963). Using the plaque reduction neutralization test, it was demonstrated that strains of WEE virus were comprised of subpopulations of virions having antigenically distinct properties and that the quantitative distribution of common but distinct antigens determined in part the immunological properties of each strain. There seemed to be some localization in the geographic distribution of WEE variants (Henderson 1964). The molecular basis for the antigenic differences observed between strains of WEE virus was studied using the oligonucleotide fingerprint technique. The viruses isolated from western and central North America, Mexico, and South America were easily distinguished from the strains isolated from the eastern USA (Trent and Grant 1980).

By means of the hemagglutination-inhibition test, 19 strains of EEE virus were grouped into two main types, which were designated as North and South American (Casals 1964; Clarke and Casals 1958).

Antigenic differences between many field and laboratory strains of VEE virus have been demonstrated by serological tests. The hemagglutination-inhibition test was used to classify the antigenic variants in the VEE virus complex. All strains within a geographical region were identical and differed from those in other localities (Young and Johnson 1969; Shope 1972). The VEE virus complex comprises four subtypes, I to IV. Five antigenic variants have been classified within subtype I, but only three are thought to be of epizootiological importance (Walton *et al.* 1973a, b). Extensive serological investigation of 124 virus strains of the VEE complex was undertaken using a kinetic hemagglutination-inhibition technique which was more sensitive than the standard hemagglutination-inhibition technique. The antigenic specificity of each strain was shown to be stable upon passage through mice and cell culture and was not dependent on the host from which the virus was isolated. However, the locality from which a strain was obtained and, to some extent, the time of isolation were important in determining the antigenic variation. Based on these observations, it was postulated that some epizootics may not be due to the introduction of a new antigenic variant into an area but may result from the amplification of local enzootic cycles of virus activity (Young and Johnson 1969). Analyses of the antigenic and biological characteristics of strains of VEE virus recovered from the Amazon region of Peru showed that the majority of the isolates belonged in subtype I (Scherer and Anderson 1975). Serologically identical or closely related strains of VEE virus could be distinguished on the basis of a quantitative virulence gradient defined by different levels of host response. It was concluded that these populations were heterogeneous with respect to virulence, efficiency of infection, and immunogenicity (Walder and Bradish 1975).

Clinical reactions, levels and duration of viremia, and antibody responses varied in horses infected with different strains of VEE virus. These strains could be distinguished on the basis of the pattern of development and persistence of hemagglutination-inhibiting, complement-fixing, and neutralizing antibodies, although there was cross-neutralization between all three virus strains (Henderson *et al.* 1971). Horses inoculated with enzootic strains of VEE virus developed slight fever, mild leukopenia, and moderate levels of neutralizing, complement-fixing, and hemagglutination-inhibiting antibodies. The epizootic strains, however, caused high fever, severe leukopenia, depressed hematocrit, signs of encephalitis, and high levels of viremia, with survivors producing large amounts of neutralizing antibodies. The neutralizing antibodies were detected by the fifth or sixth day after infection when viremia ended and clinical encephalitis was observed (Walton *et al.* 1973a).

Varying degrees of cross-protection have been demonstrated in animals exposed to one or more of the equine encephalomyelitis viruses. Experimentally, neither the EEE or WEE virus provided protection against virulent VEE virus. The effect of prior exposure to EEE or WEE virus on subsequent immunization against VEE has not been fully determined, but the two viruses may significantly affect the efficacy of a TC-83 vaccination campaign (Johnson and Martin 1974). Burros which had been injected with VEE virus were resistant to challenge with EEE virus, but the reverse was not true. Prior infection with VEE or EEE virus modified the response to challenge with WEE virus (Byrne *et al.* 1964). The results of serological studies of sick, healthy, vaccinated, and unvaccinated horses during the 1971 epizootic of VEE indicated that the preexisting antibody to EEE and/or WEE virus modified or interfered with infection by VEE virus (Calisher *et al.* 1973). Cross-protection was demonstrated among viruses in the VEE complex (Scherer and Pancake 1970).

The duration of the humoral immunity induced in the host by the equine encephalomyelitis viruses has not been investigated extensively. Horses in Nicaragua had detectable neutralizing antibody to both the TC-83 vaccine strain and an epizootic strain of VEE virus 30 months after inoculation, whereas another group of horses in Panama produced neutralizing antibodies to these strains for 20 months postexposure (Walton and Johnson 1972b; Walton *et al.* 1973b).

The neutralizing ability of the fragment obtained from the isolated and purified IgG fraction of hyperimmune serum prepared against WEE virus was comparable to that of the 7S molecule (Cremer *et al.* 1975).

VACCINATION

Work on the development of vaccines against EEE and WEE was started in the 1930s. Inactivated vaccines against EEE, WEE, and VEE are now commercially available and are either monovalent, bivalent, or trivalent products. The antibody levels needed to maintain immunity to natural challenge are not known, so it is recommended that annual vaccinations be undertaken. Although the use of inactivated vaccines greatly simplifies control programs, their efficacy in certain epizootic situations is questionable. For example, the early use of formalin-inactivated VEE vaccine in epizootics in South America was not effective in bringing the outbreaks completely under control.

The live attenuated VEE vaccine, known as strain TC-83 vaccine, was originally developed to protect humans, but it was subsequently used to immunize horses. In equines, the vaccine produces very mild clinical signs, leukopenia, and transient lesions in the central nervous system. Strain TC-83 vaccine is produced by serial passage of equine-virulent, epizootic variant I-A in primary cultures of fetal guinea pig heart cells. The vaccine is extremely effective under field conditions. One dose induces solid immunity, causes 95% seroconversion, and provides significant protection within 3 days of vaccination, together with some heterologous protection against EEE and WEE. It appears that the circulating antibody to WEE or EEE virus antigens suppresses the development of antibodies to the VEE vaccine. Optimal antibody response is attained when strain TC-83 and inactivated EEE–WEE vaccine are administered simultaneously.

Inactivated vaccines

Literature

An inactivated cell culture-derived vaccine against EEE and WEE viruses was tested in both adults and foals and shown to produce hemagglutination-inhibiting antibodies at levels comparable to those observed in horses recovering from acute infection (Gutekunst *et al.* 1966). A bivalent cell culture vaccine was compared to a chick embryo vaccine, and it was found that the latter induced a fourfold rise in hemagglutination-inhibiting antibodies against EEE and WEE antigens in a significantly lower percentage of horses (Gutekunst 1969). A potency test for WEE virus vaccine involved immunizing mice with different dilutions of the vaccine and challenging them intracerebrally with virulent virus to establish the ED_{50} (i.e. the dose of vaccine capable of protecting 50% of the animals) (Robinson *et al.* 1972). While vaccination with inactivated VEE and EEE viruses did not engender cross-protection, the immunity induced by infection with live viruses was cross-protective (Hearn 1961b).

Because of the potential problems (e.g. reversion to equine virulence of the vaccine virus, teratogenicity and interference with vaccine virus replication by preexisting antibodies to group A arboviruses) associated with the use of attenuated live VEE vaccines, more work has recently been undertaken on inactivated vaccines. A VEE vaccine prepared by inactivation of the virus with formalin and Tween-80-tri(*n*-butyl) phosphate (TNBP) and addition of saponin was tested in donkeys. Vaccinated animals did not develop clinical signs or viremia on challenge 14 days after vaccination (Villasmil *et al.* 1975). Because inactivated virus vaccines tend to be weakly antigenic, the usefulness of employing antigen–antibody complexes for potentiating immunogenicity was investigated. It was found that complexes of formalinized VEE virus vaccine and specific IgG formed at antigen–antibody equivalence enhanced the immune responses of the rhesus monkey (*Macaca mulatta*) (Houston *et al.* 1977). In a series of experiments designed to determine the potencies of inactivated VEE vaccines, mice were inoculated with formalin-inactivated TC-83 or virulent virus that had been treated in various ways. Vaccines prepared by the treatment of inactivated virus with Tween 80-TNBP and saponin proved to be the most immunogenic (Mussgay *et al.* 1972). Gamma-irradiated VEE virus was highly effective in protecting guinea pigs against intraperitoneal or aerosol challenge with virulent VEE virus (Reitman and Tonik 1971).

Live, attenuated vaccines

A WEE variant of low pathogenicity was obtained by the clonal selection method and used experimentally as a live virus vaccine (Johnson 1963). Horses subcutaneously inoculated with this attenuated

WEE vaccine developed asymptomatic infections, low levels of viremia, and neutralizing antibodies. The vaccinated animals were resistant to challenge with a field strain of WEE virus. However, intracranial inoculation of the attenuated virus induced mild encephalitis, as determined by histological examination, but did not cause viremia or clinical signs of central nervous system involvement (Binn *et al.* 1966). The vaccine was tested in a field trial which included pregnant mares, and there was no abortion or disease in the foals. The passive transfer of antibody to the foals occurred through ingestion of the colostrum and persisted for up to 6 or 7 months (Hughes and Johnson 1967).

The development of the attenuated VEE vaccine and its use in the control of epizootics in Central America and the USA were reviewed by Spertzel (1973) and Johnson and Martin (1974). The strain TC-83 vaccine was obtained by passage of the virus through 83 serial cultures of fetal guinea pig heart cells (Berge *et al.* 1961a). The efficacy of the vaccine was shown in the field rather than through extensive laboratory trials in horses. It was found that the vaccine induced complete protection within 7 to 10 days. Following vaccination, the titers of circulating virus were low, and the duration of viremia was irregular. About 50% of the vaccinated animals developed a slight elevation of body temperature. Although there was generally no evidence of other clinical signs, listlessness and decreased appetite were occasionally observed. Seroconversion could be affected by previous immunization with EEE and WEE vaccines; only 71% of the EEE- or WEE-exposed animals were seropositive for VEE after inoculation with strain TC-83 vaccine, whereas 96% seroconversion was found in horses which lacked EEE and WEE neutralizing antibodies. It is not clear whether horses which fail to show an antibody response are protected (Spertzel 1973). However, the percentage of horses that developed VEE neutralizing antibodies exceeded the number considered adequate to suppress a VEE epizootic in a population (Ferguson *et al.* 1978).

After the initial work on the efficacy of the vaccine in burros was reported, studies were undertaken to determine the efficacy of strain TC-83 vaccine in horses which was found to be highly effective (Walton *et al.* 1972). Three different concentrations of strain TC-83 vaccine were used to immunize horses, and animals that had plaque-neutralizing serum antibody titers of 1 : 40 or more were found refractory to challenge. The recommended minimal dose of vaccine induced titers of 1 : 80 or greater (Jochim *et al.* 1973). Reconstituted vaccine held at 4 or 22 °C for 24 hours was still potent and effectively immunized horses (McManus and Robinson 1972). Horses were immune to virulent challenge 9 to 19 months after strain TC-83 vaccination, and a high concentration of neutralizing antibody to challenge virus developed in most animals (Walton *et al.* 1973b). The persistence of antibodies to VEE virus depended on the preexisting levels of antibody to EEE, WEE, and VEE. The immunological response also depended on the sequence of the vaccinations. Only 57% of the horses previously vaccinated against WEE and EEE had neutralizing antibodies to VEE 18 months after initial vaccination against VEE, whereas 100% of the VEE-immunized horses with no record of WEE–EEE vaccination developed VEE neutralizing antibodies, and their serum levels were much higher than those of the first group. There was also evidence that vaccination against WEE–VEE viruses had a depressant effect on VEE neutralizing antibodies which were already present. Horses immunized against all three viruses produced the best serological response to VEE vaccination when the VEE vaccine was given simultaneously with the bivalent WEE–EEE vaccine (Vanderwagen *et al.* 1975).

The simultaneous vaccination of horses with a combined EEE–WEE vaccine and TC-84 VEE vaccine resulted in the production of serum neutralizing VEE antibodies in concentrations equal to or greater than those observed in horses vaccinated with the VEE vaccine alone. Horses were refractory to challenge with virulent VEE virus 48 weeks after vaccination with the TC-84 vaccine whether or not neutralizing antibodies to VEE virus were present (Jochim and Barber 1974). Although antibodies to EEE and WEE could suppress homologous antibody stimulation by live virus of VEE vaccines, VEE antibodies did not affect hemagglutination-inhibition antibody stimulation by WEE or EEE–WEE vaccines. The results obtained from studies of the effect of VEE neutralizing antibody induction by the heterologous alphavirus vaccines were not conclusive (Ferguson *et al.* 1977). After the vaccination of horses with strain TC-83 of VEE virus, an anamnestic response of heterologous antibody to EEE and WEE viruses occurred and was presumed to be due to prior vaccination with these viruses (Grimes 1972). Maternal antibodies to EEE, WEE, and VEE viruses were transferred to foals through the colostrum. The passively acquired maternal antibodies had a half-life of 20 days and inhibited the development of antibodies to vaccines. Therefore, foals vaccinated when less than 6 months of age should be revaccinated when they are 1 year old (Ferguson *et al.* 1979).

Consideration has been given to the disadvantages of using an attenuated live vaccine against VEE. The attenuated TC-83 vaccine induced fever of variable duration during the first days after the injection, and mild leukopenia due to a reduction of lymphocytes and neutrophils (Walton *et al.* 1972). Irregular viremia was observed in most animals, with depression and anorexia developing in some (Spertzel and Kahn 1971). The vaccine induced mild, reversible perivascular cuffing, vascular endothelial swelling, and general hyperemia in the blood vessels of vaccinated horses (Monlux *et al.* 1972a). Some workers believe that liabilities of the attenuated TC-83 vaccine are sufficient to warrant the utilization of inactivated vaccines (Mussgay *et al.* 1972).

The results of field studies involving the vaccination of horses in south Texas confirmed earlier observations that the viremia produced by the TC-83 vaccine virus was below that necessary to infect vectors. The clinical reactions in animals were minimal and transient, with no observed abortions or death which could be attributed to the vaccine (Baker *et al.* 1978). Further studies showed that the attenuated VEE virus used in the TC-83 vaccine was not transmitted under natural conditions by three species of mosquitoes when vaccinated and unvaccinated ponies were pastured together (Taylor and Buff 1972). However, a virus isolated from a pool of *Psorophora confinnis* mosquitoes trapped in Louisiana during the vaccination campaign against the 1971 VEE epizootic was identified as the TC-83 vaccine strain on the basis of animal studies and serological techniques such as kinetic hemagglutination-inhibition, kinetic neutralization, and gel diffusion. This isolation was rare, suggesting that very few mosquitoes had been infected (Pedersen *et al.* 1972).

The question of reversion of attenuated strains of VEE virus to equine virulence has been explored. There has been no evidence to date that attenuated strains of VEE virus becomes more virulent on passage through horses (Monlux *et al.* 1972b). Virus populations recovered from different tissues in mice showed varying degrees of virulence. Virus isolated from the spleen, liver, and brain during the first 24 hours postinoculation resembled the attenuated vaccine virus, while virus in the spleen at 72 hours resembled the virulent parent virus in that it was lethal for normal mice and produced larger plaques in tissue culture (Hearn 1961a). Adult hamsters became more susceptible to the TC-83 vaccine strain of VEE virus after splenectomy or pretreatment with cyclophosphamide. These immunosuppressive procedures caused extensive necrosis of hematopoietic tissues and the development of hemorrhagic lesions in the central nervous system (Jahrling *et al.* 1974).

Additional work was undertaken in laboratory animals to determine the mechanism responsible for immunity following vaccination. The kinetics of the neutralizing antibody response was studied in donor mice immunized with inactivated VEE vaccine and in mice adoptively immunized by the transfer of spleen cells from donor animals. Although inactivated VEE vaccine protected donor mice against challenge with virulent virus, it did not provide them with the capacity to transfer adoptive immunity readily. It was shown that the ability of adoptively immunized recipients to produce neutralizing antibodies depended on the use of adjuvants in the vaccine administered to the donors (Rabinowitz 1976a, b; Rabinowitz *et al.* 1979). Spleen cells from immune donors were found to exert a potent, immunologically specific inhibitory effect on viral growth *in vitro* when cocultivated with VEE-virus-infected L-cells, but neither interferon nor neutralizing antibodies appeared to be involved in the antiviral activity. It was proposed that immunocompetent T-cells and activated macrophages were responsible for the inhibition of viral growth (Rabinowitz and Proctor 1974). However, the interference observed between virulent and vaccine strains of VEE virus in mixed infections in hamsters was correlated with the interferon concentrations in the spleen and bone marrow (Jahrling 1975). Mice passively immunized with heterogeneous gamma globulin from rabbits were effectively protected against fatal VEE infection (Danes and Hrusková 1969).

The efficacy of an inactivated vaccine against JE virus was evaluated in terms of its effect on the incidence of the disease in Hokkaido, Japan, from 1948 to 1966, and mass vaccination was associated with dramatic disease with morbidity and mortality (Goto 1976).

DIAGNOSIS

Presumptive diagnosis of the equine encephalomyelitides is made on the basis of clinical signs and the seasonal incidence of severe disease syndromes affecting the central nervous system. The less dramatic forms of these diseases require identification of the virus either directly by isolation or indirectly by the demonstration of a specific antibody response.

In EEE and VEE virus infections, the viremia usually terminates before clinical signs or central nervous system involvement can be recognized. Because isolation of these viruses from tissue is difficult, sera should be collected from animals during the febrile stage of the disease. Isolation from the central nervous system is not consistent. Isolation of the equine encephalomyelitis viruses is undertaken in various laboratory animals and tissue cultures. Differential plaque neutralization tests can be used to identify VEE virus subtypes and variants; the highest neutralizing antibody titer is produced to the infecting strain.

In cases where the virus cannot be isolated, a serological diagnosis can be made by comparing the titers of hemagglutination-inhibiting, complement-fixing, or neutralizing antibodies in paired acute and convalescent phase sera. The presence of characteristic histopathological lesions in the brains of affected animals is a useful criterion for making a diagnosis on postmortem examination.

Literature

The basic literature covering the isolation and propagation of the viruses in various laboratory animal and cell culture systems has been presented in the etiology and immunology sections. Some of the more recent methods used have involved refinements of basic techniques of virus propagation and identification. These methods are useful because they are rapid and eliminate the need to use susceptible laboratory animals. For the diagnosis of VEE infection by the intracerebral inoculation of suckling mice 3 to 7 days were required, and the use of the FA test enabled the identification of a virus isolated in cell culture within 48 hours. The goat VEE antiserum–fluorescein conjugate used in the test was specific and did not cross-react with EEE or WEE-virus-infected cells (Erickson and Maré 1975). The microprecipitation test is another method which has been developed for the rapid detection and identification of VEE, EEE, and WEE viruses. This technique involves precipitation of the virus after primary isolation in cell culture with specific fluorescein-conjugated gamma globulin, followed by cellulose acetate electrophoresis (Levitt *et al.* 1975).

CONTROL

Prevention and control are accomplished by the vaccination of horses and humans and by protecting susceptible individuals from the vector. Annual immunization of horses is conducted in enzootic areas. Because EEE and WEE viruses are not restricted geographically, inactivated bivalent vaccines are used. In an epizootic situation, susceptible animals should be protected from the vector. Both inactivated and attenuated vaccines are used widely in horses during VEE epizootics. The attenuated vaccine in particular is extensively used in regions where the virus is active and also in disease-free areas at high risk. Vaccination campaigns are supported by restriction of the movement of horses and by mosquito control. Quarantine is not required for EEE or WEE because the viremic titers which develop in susceptible hosts are usually below the threshold of infection for mosquitoes. However, this measure is important in the control of VEE since the relatively high levels of viremia enable large numbers of mosquitoes to become infected. Control of arboviral epizootics by the elimination of vectors is difficult with VEE because its spread depends on a variety of species of mosquitoes distributed over very wide geographical areas. Low-volume aerial spraying with insecticides has been used in heavily populated areas. However, vector control alone does little more than slow the transmission of these diseases; the essential component of control is large-scale vaccination of horses.

Literature

The prevention and control of the different forms of equine viral encephalomyelitis have been discussed in various review articles (Artsob 1979a, b; Hanson 1973; Hayes 1979a, b; McConnell and Spertzel 1979; Spertzel 1973). In addition the very large aerial spraying operation undertaken by the US government to control the VEE epizootic in Texas was described by Spears (1972). Byrne (1973) listed the cell-culture and chick-embryo-derived inactivated monovalent and bivalent vaccines which were available in the USA.

BIBLIOGRAPHY

Ajello, C. A., 1979. Evaluation of *Aedes albopictus* tissue culture for use in association with arbovirus isolation, *J. med. Virol.*, **3**: 301–6.

Artsob, H., 1979a. Arboviral zoonoses in Canada. Western equine encephalomyelitis (WEE). In *CRC Handbook Series in Zoonoses: Viral Zoonoses, Section B*, ed. G. W. Beran. CRC Press (Boca Raton, Fla.), vol. 1, pp. 143–6.

Artsob, H., 1979b. Arboviral zoonoses in Canada. Eastern equine encephalomyelitis (EEE). In *CRC Handbook Series in Zoonoses: Viral Zoonoses, Section B*, ed. G. W. Beran. CRC Press (Boca Raton, Fla.), vol. 1, pp. 146–7.
Austin, F. J. and Scherer, W. F., 1971. Studies of viral virulence. I. Growth and histopathology of virulent and attenuated strains of Venezuelan encephalitis virus in hamsters, *Am. J. Path.*, **62**: 195–210.

Baker, E. F. Jr, Sasso, D. R., Maness, K., Prichard, W. D. and Parker, R. L., 1978. Venezuelan equine encephalomyelitis vaccine (strain TC–83): a field study, *Am. J. vet. Res.*, **39**(10): 1627–31.
Bastian, F. O., Wende, R. D., Singer, D. B. and Zeller, R. S., 1975. Eastern equine encephalomyelitis. Histopathologic and ultrastructural changes with isolation of the virus in a human case, *Am. J. clin. Path.*, **64**: 10–13.
Belle, E. A., Grant, L. S. and Thorburn, M. J., 1964. An outbreak of eastern equine encephalomyelitis in Jamaica. II. Laboratory diagnosis and pathology of eastern equine encephalomyelitis in Jamaica, *Am. J. trop. Med. Hyg.*, **13**: 335–41.
Berendt, R. F., Dorsey, E. L. and Hearn, H. J., 1972. Virucidal properties of light and SO_2. I. Effect on aerosolized Venezuelan equine encephalomyelitis virus, *Proc. Soc. Exp. Biol. Med.*, **139**: 1–5.
Berge, T. O., Banks, I. S. and Tigertt, W. D., 1961. Attenuation of Venezuelan equine encephalomyelitis virus by *in vitro* cultivation in guinea-pig heart cells, *Am. J. Hyg.*, **73**: 209–18.
Bigler, W. J., Lassing, E. B., Buff, E. E., Prather, E. C., Beck, E. C. and Hoff, G. L., 1976. Endemic eastern equine encephalomyelitis in Florida: a twenty-year analysis, 1955–1974, *Am. J. trop. Med. Hyg.*, **25**: 884–90.
Binn, L. N., Sponseller, M. L., Wooding, W. L., McConnell, S. J., Spertzel, R. O. and Yager, R. H., 1966. Efficacy of an attenuated western encephalitis vaccine in equine animals, *Am. J. vet. Res.*, **27**(121): 1599–604.
Bivin, W. S., Barry, C., Hogge, A. L. Jr and Corristan, E. C., 1967. Mosquito-induced infection with equine encephalomyelitis virus in dogs, *Am. J. trop. Med. Hyg.*, **16**: 544–7.
Bowen, G. S., 1976. Experimental infection of North American mammals with epidemic Venezuelan encephalitis virus, *Am. J. trop. Med. Hyg.*, **25**(6): 891–9.
Bowen, G. S. and McLean, R. G., 1977. Experimental infection of birds with epidemic Venezuelan encephalitis virus, *Am. J. trop. Med. Hyg.*, **26**(4): 808–14.
Brown, A. and Officer, J. E., 1975. An attenuated variant of eastern encephalitis virus: biological properties and protection induced in mice, *Arch. Virol.*, **47**: 123–38.
Brown, D. G., 1972. Clinical changes in burros and Shetland ponies

after vaccination with Venezuelan equine encephalomyelitis vaccine, TC-83, *Vet. Med./Small Anim. Clin.*, **67**: 505–11.

Buescher, E. L. and Scherer, W. F., 1959. Ecologic studies of Japanese encephalitis virus in Japan. IX. Epidemiologic correlations and conclusions, *Am. J. trop. Med. Hyg.*, **8**: 719–22.

Buescher, E. L., Scherer, W. F., McClure, H. E., Moyer, J. T., Rosenberg, M. Z., Yoshii, M. and Okada, Y., 1959a. Ecologic studies of Japanese encephalitis virus in Japan. IV. Avian infection, *Am. J. trop. Med. Hyg.*, **8**: 678–88.

Buescher, E. L., Scherer, W. F., Rosenberg, M. Z., Gresser, I., Hardy, J. L. and Bullock, H. R., 1959b. Ecologic studies of Japanese encephalitis virus in Japan. II. Mosquito infection, *Am. J. trop. Med. Hyg.*, **8**: 651–64.

Buescher, E. L., Scherer W. F., Rosenberg, M. Z. and McClure, H. E., 1959c. Ecologic studies of Japanese encephalitis virus in Japan. III. Infection and antibody responses of birds, *J. Immunol.*, **83**: 605–13.

Burns, K. F., 1950. Congenital Japanese B encephalitis of swine, *Proc. Soc. Exp. Biol. Med.*, **75**: 621–5.

Burton, A. N., McLintock, J. R. and Rempel, J. G., 1966a. Western equine encephalitis virus in Saskatchewan garter snakes and leopard frogs, *Science*, **154**: 1029–31.

Burton, A. N., McLintock, J. R., Spalatin, J. and Rempel, J. G., 1966b. Western equine encephalitis in Saskatchewan birds and mammals 1962–1963, *Can. J. Microbiol.*, **12**: 133–41.

Bykovsky, A. F., Yershov. F. I. and Zhdanov, V. M., 1969. Morphogenesis of Venezuelan equine encephalomyelitis virus, *J. Virol.*, **4**(4): 496–504.

Byrne, R. J., 1972. Neurotropic viral diseases. In *Equine Medicine and Surgery*, eds E. J. Catcott, J. F. Smithcors. American Veterinary Publications (Ill.), pp. 46–57.

Byrne, R. J., 1973. The control of eastern and western arboviral encephalomyelitis of horses, *Proc. 3rd int. Conf. Equine infect. Dis.*, Paris 1972, eds J. T. Bryans, H. Gerber. Karger (Basle). pp. 115–23.

Byrne, R. J., French, G. R., Yancey, F. S., Gochenour, W. S., Russell, P. K., Ramsburg, H. H., Brand, O. A., Schneider, F. G. and Buescher, E. L., 1964. Clinical and immunological interrelationship among Venezuelan, eastern and western equine encephalomyelitis viruses in burros, *Am. J. vet. Res.*, **25**(104): 24–31.

Byrne, R. J., Hetrick, F. M., Scanlon, J. E., Hastings, J. W. Jr and Locke, L. N., 1961. Observations on eastern equine encephalitis in Maryland in 1959, *J. Am. vet. med. Ass.*, **139**(6): 661–4.

Calisher, C. H. and Maness, K. S. C., 1974. Virulence of Venezuelan equine encephalomyelitis virus subtypes for various laboratory hosts, *Appl. Microbiol.*, **28**(5): 881–4.

Calisher, C. H., Sasso, D. R. and Sather, G. E., 1973. Possible evidence for interference with Venezuelan equine encephalitis virus vaccination of equines by pre-existing antibody to eastern or western equine encephalitis virus, or both, *Appl. Microbiol.*, **26**(4): 485–8.

Casals, J., 1964. Antigenic variants of eastern equine encephalitis virus, *J. Exp. Med.*, **119**: 547–65.

Cates, M. D. and Detels, R., 1969. Japanese encephalities virus in Taiwan: preliminary evidence for *Culex annulus* Theob. as a vector, *J. med. Ent.*, **6**(3): 327–28.

Chamberlain, R. W., Kissling, R. E., Stamm, D. D., Nelson, D. B. and Sikes, R. K., 1956. Venezuelan equine encephalomyelitis in wild birds, *Am. J. Hyg.*, **63**: 261–73.

Chu, I-H. and Grayston, J. T., 1962. Encephalitis on Taiwan. VI. Infections in American servicemen on Taiwan and Okinawa, *Am. J. trop. Med. Hyg.*, **11**: 159–61.

Clarke, D. H. and Casals, J., 1958. Technique for hemagglutination-inhibition with arthropod-borne viruses, *Am. J. trop. Med. Hyg.*, **7**: 561–73.

Correa-Giron, P., Calisher, C. H. and Baer, G. M., 1972. Epidemic strain of Venezuelan equine encephalomyelitis virus from a vampire bat captured in Oaxaca, Mexico, 1970, *Science*, **175**: 546–7.

Cremer, N. E., Riggs, J. L. and Lennette, E. H. 1975. Neutralization kinetics of western equine encephalitis virus by antibody fragments, *Immunochemistry*, **12**: 597–601.

Danes, L. and Hrusková, J., 1969. Efficiency testing of passive immunization against Venezuelan equine encephalomyelitis in mice, *Acta virol.*, **13**: 554–6.

Daubney, R., 1967. Viral encephalitis of equines and domestic ruminants in the Near East – Part II, *Res. vet. Sci.*, **8**: 419–39.

Daubney R. and Mahlau, E. A., 1957. Near-Eastern equine encephalomyelitis, *Nature, Lond.*, **179**: 584–5.

Davis, M. H., Hogge, A. L. Jr, Corristan, E. C. and Ferrell, J. F., 1966. Mosquito transmission of Venezuelan equine encephalomyelitis virus from experimentally infected dogs, *Am. J. trop. Med. Hyg.*, **15**(2): 227–30.

Dawson, F. W., Hearn, H. J. and Hoffman, R. K., 1959. Virucidal activity of B-propiolactone vapor. I. Effect of B-propiolactone vapor on Venezuelan equine encephalomyelitis virus, *Appl. Microbiol.*, **7**: 199–201.

Detels, R., Cates, M. D., Cross, J. H., Irving, G. S. and Watten, R. H., 1970. Ecology of Japanese encephalitis virus on Taiwan in 1968, *Am. J. trop. Med. Hyg.*, **19**(4): 716–23.

Dickerman, R. W., Baker, G. J., Ordonez, J. V. and Scherer, W. F., 1973a. Venezuelan equine encephalomyelitis viremia and antibody responses of pigs and cattle, *Am. J. vet. Res.*, **34**(3): 357–61.

Dickerman, R. W., Martin, M. S. and Dipaola, E. A., 1980. Studies of Venezuelan encephalitis in migrating birds in relation to possible transport of virus from South to Central America, *Am. J. trop. Med. Hyg.*, **29**(2): 269–76.

Dickerman, R. W., Scherer, W. F., Navarro, E. M. and Ordonez, J. V., 1973b. The involvement of dogs in endemic cycles of Venezuelan encephalitis virus, *Am. J. Epidemiol.*, **98**(4): 311–14.

Dietz, W. H., Jr, Alvarez, O. Jr, Martin, D. H., Walton, T. E., Ackerman, L. J. and Johnson, K. M., 1978. Enzootic and epizootic Venezuelan equine encephalomyelitis virus in horses infected by peripheral and intrathecal routes, *J. Infect. Dis.*, **137**(3): 227–37.

Dietz, W. H. Jr, Galindo, P. and Johnson, K. M., 1980. Eastern equine encephalomyelitis in Panama: the epidemiology of the 1973 epizootic, *Am. J. trop. Med. Hyg.*, **29**(1): 133–40.

Dremov, D. P., Solyanick, R. G., Miryutova, T. L. and Laptakova, L. M., 1978. Attenuated variants of eastern equine encephalomyelitis virus: pathomorphological, immunofluorescence and virological studies of infection in Syrian hamsters, *Acta virol.*, **22**: 139–45.

Eddy, G. A., Martin, D. H. and Johnson, K. M., 1973. Epidemiology of the Venezuelan equine encephalomyelitis virus complex, *Proc. 3rd int. Conf. Equine infect. Dis.*, Paris 1972, eds J. T. Bryans, H. Gerber. Karger (Basle), pp. 126–45.

Ehrlich, R. and Miller, S., 1971. Effect of relative humidity and temperature on airborne Venezuelan equine encephalitis virus, *Appl. Microbiol.*, **22**(2): 194–9.

Eleazer, T. H., Blalock, H. G. and Warner, J. H. Jr, 1978. Eastern equine encephalomyelitis outbreak in coturnix quail, *Avian Dis.*, **22**(3): 522–5.

Erickson, G. A. and Maré, C. J., 1975. Rapid diagnosis of Venezuelan equine encephalomyelitis by fluorescence microscopy, *Am. J. vet. Res.*, **36**(2): 167–70.

Ferguson, J. A., Reeves, W. C. and Hardy, J. L., 1977. Antibody studies in ponies vaccinated with Venezuelan equine encephalomyelitis (strain TC-83) and other alphavirus vaccines, *Am. J. vet. Res.*, **38**(4): 425–30.

Ferguson, J. A., Reeves, W. C. and Hardy, J. L., 1979. Studies on immunity to alphaviruses in foals, *Am. J. vet. Res.*, **40**(1): 5–10.

Ferguson, J. A., Reeves, W. C., Milby, M. M. and Hardy, J. L., 1978. Study of homologous and heterologous antibody responses in California horses vaccinated with attenuated Venezuelan equine encephalomyelitis vaccine (strain TC-83), *Am. J. vet. Res.*, **39**(3): 371–6.

Franck, P. T. and Johnson, K. M., 1971. An outbreak of Venezuelan equine encephalomyelitis in Central America. Evidence for exogenous source of a virulent virus subtype, *Am. J. Epidemiol.*, **94**(5): 487–95.

Furumoto, H. H., 1969. Susceptibility of dogs to St. Louis encephalitis and other selected arthropod-borne viruses, *Am. J. vet. Res.*, **30**(8): 1371–80.

Fuscaldo, A. A., Aaslestad, H. G. and Hoffman, E. J., 1971. Biological, physical, and chemical properties of eastern equine encephalitis virus. I. Purification and physical properties, *J. Virol.*, **7**(2): 233–40.

Galindo, P. and Grayson, M. A., 1971. *Culex (Melanoconion) aikenii*: natural vector in Panama of endemic Venezuelan encephalitis, *Science*, **172**: 594–5.

García-Tamayo, J., 1973. Venezuelan equine encephalomyelitis virus in the heart of newborn mice, *Arch. Pathol.*, **96**: 294–7.

Garcıa-Tamayo, J., Esparza, J. and Martinez, A. J., 1981. Placental and fetal alterations due to Venezuelan equine encephalitis virus in rats, *Infect. Immun.*, **32**(2): 813–21.

Gebhardt, L. P., Stanton, G. J. and de St Jeor, S., 1966. Transmission of WEE virus to snakes by infected *Culex tarsalis* mosquitoes, *Proc. Soc. Exp. Biol. Med.*, **123**: 233–5.

Gibbs, E. P. J., 1976. Equine viral encephalitis, *Equine vet. J.*, **8**(2): 66–71.

Gleiser, C. A., Gochenour, W. S. Jr., Berge, T. O. and Tigertt, W. D., 1962. The comparative pathology of experimental Venezuelan equine encephalomyelitis infection in different animal hosts, *J. Infect. Dis.*, **110**: 80–97.

Gochenour, W. S. Jr., Berge, T. O., Gleiser, C. A. and Tigertt, W. D. 1962. Immunization of burros with living Venezuelan equine encephalomyelitis virus, *Am. J. Hyg.*, **75**: 351–62.

Goto, H., 1976. Efficacy of Japanese encephalitis vaccine in horses, *Equine vet. J.*, **8**(3): 126–7.

Goto, H., Shimizu, K. and Shirahata, T., 1969. Studies on Japanese encephalitis of animals in Hokkaido. I. Epidemiological observation on horses, *Res. Bull. Obihiro Univ.*, **6**: 1–8.

Gould, D. J., Barnett, H. C. and Suyemoto, W., 1962. Transmission of Japanese encephalitis virus by *Culex gelidus* Theobald, *Trans. Roy. Soc. trop. Med. Hyg.*, **56**(5): 429–35.

Grayson, M. A. and Galindo, P., 1969. Ecology of Venezuelan equine encephalitis virus in Panama, *J. Am. vet. med. Ass.*, **155**(12): 2141–5.

Grayson, M. A. and Galindo, P., 1972. Experimental transmission of Venezuelan equine encephalitis virus by *Deinocerites pseudes* Dyar and Knab, 1909, *J. Med. Ent.*, **9**(3): 196–200.

Grayston, J. T., Wang, S-P. and Yen, C-H., 1962. Encephalitis on Taiwan. I. Introduction and epidemiology, *Am. J. trop. Med. Hyg.*, **11**: 126–30.

Grimes, J. E., 1972. Serological response of horses vaccinated with the

TC-83 live attenuated Venezuelan equine encephalomyelitis virus, *SWest. Vet.*, **25**: 125–9.

Gutekunst, D. E., 1969. Immunity to bivalent tissue culture origin equine encephalomyelitis vaccine, *J. Am. vet. med. Ass.*, **155**(2): 368–74.

Gutekunst, D. E., Martin, M. J. and Langer, P. H., 1966. Immunization against equine encephalomyelitis with a new tissue culture origin vaccine, *Vet. Med./Small Anim. Clin.*, **61**: 348–51.

Hahon, N. and Cooke, K. O., 1967. Primary virus–cell interactions in the immunofluorescence assay of Venezuelan equine encephalomyelitis virus, *J. Virol.*, **1**(2): 317–26.

Hanson, R. P., 1973. Virology and epidemiology of eastern and western arboviral encephalomyelitis of horses, *Proc. 3rd int. Conf. Equine Infect. Dis.*, Paris 1972, eds J. T. Bryans, H. Gerber. Karger (Basle), pp. 100–14.

Hardy, F. M., 1959. The growth of Venezuelan equine encephalomyelitis virus in various tissue cultures, *Am. J. Hyg.*, **70**: 21–7.

Harper, G. J., 1961. Airborne micro-organisms: survival tests with four viruses, *J. Hyg., Camb.*, **59**: 479–86.

Hayes, R. O., 1979a. Eastern and western encephalitis. Eastern encephalitis. *The CRC Handbook Series in Zoonoses: Viral Zoonoses*, ed. G. W. Beran. CRC Press (Boca Raton, Fla.), pp. 29–37.

Hayes, R. O., 1979b. Eastern and western encephalitis. Western encephalitis. *The CRC Handbook Series in Zoonoses: Viral Zoonoses*, ed. G. W. Beran. CRC Press (Boca Raton, Fla.), pp. 37–57.

Hayes, R. O., Francy, D. B., Lazuick, J. S., Smith, G. C. and Gibbs, E. P. J., 1977. Role of the cliff swallow bug (*Oeciacus vicarius*) in the natural cycle of a western equine encephalitis-related alphavirus, *J. Med. Entomol.*, **14**(3): 257–62.

Hayles, L. B., 1972. Susceptibility of the Mongolian gerbil (*Meriones unguiculatus*) to western equine encephalitis, *Can. J. Microbiol.*, **18**: 941–4.

Hearn, H. J. Jr, 1961a. Differences among virus populations recovered from mice vaccinated with an attenuated strain of Venezuelan equine encephalomyelitis virus, *J. Immunol.*, **87**: 573–7.

Hearn, H. J. Jr, 1961b. Cross-protection between Venezuelan equine encephalomyelitis and eastern equine encephalomyelitis virus, *Soc. Exp. Biol. Med. Proc.*, **107**: 607–10.

Hearn, H. J. and Jameson, P., 1971. Plaque size and virulence of attenuated Venezuelan equine encephalomyelitis virus after passage in various hosts, *Am. J. Epidemiol.*, **94**(1): 56–61.

Hearn, H. J., Seliokas, Z. V. and Andersen, A. A., 1969. Factors influencing virulence and plaque properties of attenuated Venezuelan equine encephalomyelitis virus populations, *J. Virol.*, **4**(4): 545–6.

Henderson, B. E., Chappell, W. A., Johnston, J. G. Jr and Sudia,

W. D., 1971. Experimental infection of horses with three strains of Venezuelan equine encephalomyelitis virus. I. Clinical and virological studies, *Am. J. Epidemiol.*, **93**(3): 194–205.

Henderson, J. R., 1964. Immunologic characterization of western encephalomyelitis virus strains, *J. Immunol.*, **93**: 452–61.

Heydrick, F. P., Wachter, R. F. and Hearn, H. J. Jr, 1966. Host influence on the characteristics of Venezuelan equine encephalomyelitis virus, *J. Bact.*, **91**(6): 2343–8.

Houston, W. E., Kremer, R. J., Crabbs, C. L. and Spertzel, R. O., 1977. Inactivated Venezuelan equine encephalomyelitis virus vaccine complexed with specific antibody: enhanced primary immune response and altered pattern of antibody class elicited, *J. Infect. Dis.*, **135**(4): 600–10.

Hrusková, J., Danes, L., Jelinková, A., Kruml, J. and Rychterová, V., 1969. Experimental inhalation infection of mice with Venezuelan equine encephalomyelitis virus, *Acta virol.*, **13**: 560–3.

Hu, S. M. K. and Grayston, J. T., 1962. Encephalitis on Taiwan. II. Mosquito collection and bionomic studies, *Am. J. trop. Med. Hyg.*, **11**: 131–40.

Hughes, J. P. and Johnson, H. N., 1967. A field trial of a live-virus western encephalitis vaccine, *J. Am. vet. med. Ass.*, **150**(2): 167–71.

Hurlbut, H. S., 1964. The pig–mosquito cycle of Japanese encephalitis virus in Taiwan, *J. Med. Ent.*, **1**(3): 301–7.

Hurlbut, H. S. and Nibley, C. Jr, 1964. Virus isolations from mosquitoes in Okinawa, *J. Med. Ent.*, **1**(1): 78–83.

Jahrling, P. B., 1975. Interference between virulent and vaccine strains of Venezuelan encephalitis virus in mixed infections of hamsters, *J. gen. Virol.*, **28**: 1–8.

Jahrling, P. B., 1976. Virulence heterogeneity of a predominantly avirulent western equine encephalitis virus population, *J. gen. Virol.*, **32**: 121–8.

Jahrling, P. B., Dendy, E. and Eddy, G. A., 1974. Correlates to increased lethality of attenuated Venezuelan encephalitis virus vaccine for immunosuppressed hamsters, *Infect. Immun.*, **9**(5): 924–30.

Jahrling, P. B. and Gorelkin, L., 1975. Selective clearance of a benign clone of Venezuelan equine encephalitis virus from hamster plasma by hepatic reticuloendothelial cells, *J. Infect. Dis.*, **132**(6): 667–76.

Jahrling, P. B. and Scherer, W. F., 1973a. Growth curves and clearance rates of virulent and benign Venezuelan encephalitis viruses in hamsters, *Infect. Immun.*, **8**(3): 456–62.

Jahrling, P. B. and Scherer, W. F., 1973b. Homogeneity of Venezuelan encephalitis virion populations of hamster-virulent and benign strains, including the attenuated TC83 vaccine, *Infect. Immun.*, **7**(6): 905–10.

Jochim, M. M. and Barber, T. L., 1974. Immune response of horses after simultaneous or sequential vaccination against eastern, western and Venezuelan equine encephalomyelitis, *J. Am. vet. med. Ass.*, **165**(7): 621–5.

Jochim, M. M., Barber, T. L. and Luedke, A. J., 1973. Venezuelan equine encephalomyelitis: antibody response in vaccinated horses and resistance to infection with virulent virus, *J. Am. vet. med. Ass.*, **162**(4): 280–3.

Johnson, K. M., 1963. Selection of a variant of western encephalitis virus of low pathogenicity for study as a live virus vaccine, *Am. J. trop. Med. Hyg.*, **12**: 604–10.

Johnson, K. M. and Martin, D. H., 1974. Venezuelan equine encephalitis. In *Advances in Veterinary Science and Comparative Medicine*, eds C. A. Brandly, C. E. Cornelius. Academic Press (New York), vol. 18, pp. 79–116.

Jungherr, E. L., Helmboldt, C. F., Satriano, S. F. and Luginbuhl, R. E., 1957. Investigation of eastern equine encephalomyelitis. III. Pathology in pheasants and incidental observations in feral birds, *Am. J. Hyg.*, **67**: 10–20.

Justines, G., Sucre, H. and Alvares, O., 1980. Transplacental transmission of Venezuelan equine encephalitis virus in horses, *Am. J. trop. Med. Hyg.*, **29**(4): 653–6.

Karabatsos, N., Bourke, A. T. C. and Henderson, J. R., 1963. Antigenic variation among strains of western equine encephalomyelitis virus, *Am. J. trop. Med. Hyg.*, **12**: 408–12.

Karstad, L. H., Fletcher, O. K., Spalatin, J., Roberts, R. and Hanson, R. P., 1957. Eastern equine encephalomyelitis virus isolated from three species of Diptera from Georgia, *Science*, **125**: 395–6.

Kiorpes, A. L. and Yuill, T. M., 1975. Environmental modification of western equine encephalomyelitis infection in the snowshoe hare (*Lepus americanus*), *Infect. Immun.*, **11**(5): 986–90.

Kissling, R. E. and Chamberlain, R. W., 1967. Venezuelan equine encephalitis, *Adv. Vet. Sci.*, **11**: 65–84.

Kissling, R. E., Chamberlain, R.W., Eidson, M. E., Sikes, R. K. and Bucca, M. A., 1954. Studies on the North American arthropod-borne encephalitides. II. Eastern equine encephalitis in horses, *Am. J. Hyg.*, **60**: 237–50.

Kissling, R. E., Chamberlain, R. W., Nelson, D. B. and Stamm, D. D., 1956. Venezuelan equine encephalomyelitis in horses, *Am. J. Hyg.*, **63**: 274–87.

Kissling, R. E. and Rubin, H., 1951. Pathology of eastern equine encephalomyelitis, *Am. J. vet. Res.*, **12**: 100–5.

Kissling, R. E., Stamm, D. D., Chamberlain, R. W. and Sudia, W. D., 1957b. Birds as winter hosts for eastern and western equine encephalomyelitis viruses, *Am. J. Hyg.*, **66**: 42–7.

Klimenko, S. M., Yershov, F. I., Gofman, Y. P., Nabatnikov, A. P. and Zhdanov, V. M., 1965. Architecture of Venezuelan equine encephalomyelitis virus, *Virology*, **27**: 125–8.

Konno, J., Endo, K., Agatsuma, H. and Ishida, N., 1966. Cyclic outbreaks of Japanese encephalitis among pigs and humans, *Am. J. Epidemiol.*, **84**(2): 292–300.

Kono, Y., 1962. The interference between Newcastle disease virus and Venezuelan equine encephalomyelitis virus, *Nat. Inst. Anim. Hlth Quart.*, **2**(1): 1–9.

Kuehne, R. W., Sawyer, W. D. and Gochenour, W. S. Jr, 1962. Infection with aerosolized attenuated Venezuelan equine encephalomyelitis virus, *Am. J. Hyg.*, **75**: 347–50.

Kundin, W. D., 1966. Pathogenesis of Venezuelan equine encephalomyelitis virus. II. Infection in young adult mice, *J. Immunol.*, **96**(1): 49–58.

Kundin, W. D., Liu, C. and Rodina, P., 1966. Pathogenesis of Venezuelan equine encephalomyelitis virus. I. Infection in suckling mice, *J. Immunol.*, **96**(1): 39–48.

Leung, M. K., Iversen, J., McLintock, J. and Saunders, J. R., 1976. Subcutaneous exposure of the Richardson's ground squirrel (*Spermophilus richardsonii* Sabine) to western equine encephalomyelitis virus, *J. Wildl. Dis.*, **12**: 237–46.

Leung, M. K., McLintock, J. and Iversen, J., 1978. Intranasal exposure of the Richardson's ground squirrel to western equine encephalomyelitis virus, *Can. J. comp. Med.*, **42**: 184–91.

Levitt, N. H., Miller, H. V., Pedersen, C. E. Jr. and Eddy, G. A., 1975. A microprecipitation test for rapid detection and identification of Venezuelan, eastern, and western equine encephalomyelitis viruses, *Am. J. trop. Med. Hyg.*, **24**(1): 127–30.

Liu, C., Voth, D. W., Rodina, P., Shauf, L. R. and Gonzalez, G., 1970. A comparative study of the pathogenesis of western equine and eastern equine encephalomyelitis viral infections in mice by intracerebral and subcutaneous inoculations, *J. Infect. Dis.*, **122**: 53–63.

Lundgren, D. L. and Smart, K. L., 1969. Experimental infection of coyote pups with Venezuelan equine encephalomyelitis virus, *Am. J. trop. Med. Hyg.*, **18**(2): 268–72.

Martin, D. H., Eddy, G. A., Sudia, W. D., Reeves, W. V., Newhouse, V. F. and Johnson, K. M., 1972. An epidemiologic study of Venezuelan equine encephalomyelitis in Costa Rica, 1970, *Am. J. Epidemiol.*, **95**(6): 565–78.

McConnell, S. and Spertzel, R. O., 1979. Venezuelan equine encephalomyelitis (VEE). In *CRC Handbook Series in Zoonoses: Viral Zoonoses, Section B*, ed. G. W. Beran. CRC Press (Boca Raton, Fla.), pp. 59–69.

McLean, R. G., Trevino, H. A. and Sather, G. E., 1979. Prevalence of selected and zoonotic diseases in vertebrates from Haiti, 1972, *J. Wildl. Dis.*, **15**: 327–30.

McManus, A. T. and Robinson, D. M., 1972. Stability of live attenuated Venezuelan equine encephalitis vaccine, *Appl. Microbiol.*, **23**(3): 654–5.

Monath, T. P., Calisher, C. H., Davis, M., Bowen, G. S. and White, J., 1974. Experimental studies of rhesus monkeys infected with epizootic and enzootic subtypes of Venezuelan equine encephalitis virus, *J. Infect. Dis.*, **129**(2): 194–200.

Monlux, W. S., Luedke, A. J. and Bowne, J., 1972a. Central venous system response of horses to Venezuelan equine encephalomyelitis vaccine (TC-83), *J. Am. vet. med. Ass.*, **161**: 265–9.

Monlux, W. S., Luedke, A. J., Mercado, S., Rosales, J. C. and Rios, R., 1972b. Effect of back passage of Venezuelan equine encephalomyelitis vaccine on the central nervous system of horses, *J. Am. vet. med. Ass.*, **161**: 832–3.

Morgan, C., Howe, C. and Rose, H. M., 1961. Structure and development of viruses as observed in the electron microscope. V. Western equine encephalomyelitis virus, *J. exp. Med.*, 1., **113**: 219–34.

Morgante, O., Shemanchuk, J. A. and Windsor, R., 1969. Western encephalomyelitis virus infection in 'indicator' chickens in southern Alberta, *Can. J. comp. Med.*, **33**: 227–30.

Morgante, O., Vance, H. N., Shemanchuk, J. A. and Windsor, R., 1968. Epizootic of western encephalomyelitis virus infection in equines in Alberta in 1965, *Can. J. comp. Med.*, **33**: 403–8.

Murphy, F. A. and Whitfield, S. G., 1970. Eastern equine encephalitis virus infection: electron microscopic studies of mouse central nervous system, *Exper. Molec. Path.*, **13**: 131–46.

Mussgay, M., Bergold, G. H., Weiland, E. and Uberschar, S., 1972. Preparation and evaluation of inactivated Venezuelan equine encephalitis vaccines, *Zbl. Vet. Med.*, **B19**: 511–17.

Mussgay, M. and Weibel, J., 1962. Electron microscopic and biological studies on the growth of Venezuelan equine encephalitis virus in KB cells, *Virology*, **16**: 52–62.

Ognianov, D. and Fernández, A., 1972a. Isolation and characterization of interferon from chicken embryo fibroblasts and mouse brain infected with the virus of eastern equine encephalomyelitis (EEE), *Zbl. Vet. Med.*, **B19**: 94–8.

Ognianov, D. and Fernández, A., 1972b. Studies on the pathogenesis of eastern equine encephalomyelitis in mice, *Zbl. Vet. Med.*, **B19**: 89–93.

Pedersen, C. E. Jr., Robinson, D. M. and Cole, F. E., 1972. Isolation of the vaccine strain of Venezuelan equine encephalomyelitis virus from mosquitoes in Louisiana, *Am. J. Epidemiol.*, **95**(5): 490–6.

Pennington, N. E. and Phelps, C. A., 1968. Identification of the host range of *Culex tritaeniorhynchus* mosquitoes on Okinawa, Ryukyu

Islands, *J. Med. Ent.*, **5**(4): 483–7.

Potter, M. E., Currier, R. W. II., Pearson, J. E., Harris, J. C. and Parker, R. L., 1977. Western equine encephalomyelitis in horses in the northern Red River Valley, 1975, *J. Am. vet. med. Ass.*, **170**(12): 1396–9.

Proctor, S. J. and Pearson, J. E., 1975. Venezuelan equine encephalomyelitis in pheasants and chukars, *J. Wildl. Dis.*, **11**: 14–16.

Pursell, A. R., Peckham, J. C., Cole, J. R., Stewart, W. C. and Mitchell, F. E., 1972. Naturally occurring and artificially induced eastern encephalomyelitis in pigs, *J. Am vet. med. Ass.*, **161**(10): 1143–7.

Rabinowitz, S. G., 1976a. Host immune responses after administration of inactivated Venezuelan equine encephalomyelitis virus vaccines. I. Description and characterization of adoptive transfer by immune spleen cells, *J. Infect. Dis.*, **134**(1): 30–8.

Rabinowitz, S. G., 1976b. Host immune responses after administration of inactivated Venezuelan equine encephalomyelitis virus vaccines. II. Kinetics of neutralizing antibody responses in donors and adoptively immunized recipients, *J. Infect. Dis.*, **134**(1): 39–47.

Rabinowitz, S. G., Huprikar, J. and Whitacre, C., 1979. Host immune reponses after administration of inactivated Venezuelan equine encephalomyelitis virus vaccines. III. Kinetics for neutralizing antibody immunoglobulin class responses in donors and adoptively immunized recipients, *Comp. Immun. Microbiol. Infect. Dis.*, **1**: 295–303.

Rabinowitz, S. G. and Proctor, R. A., 1974. *In vitro* study of antiviral activity of immune spleen cells in experimental Venezuelan equine encephalomyelitis infection in mice, *J. Immunol.*, **112**(3): 1070–7.

Reeves, W. C., Bellamy, R. E., Geib, A. F. and Scrivant, R. P., 1964. Analysis of the circumstances leading to abortion of a western equine encephalitis epidemic, *Am. J. Hyg.*, **80**: 205–20.

Reitman, M., 1969. Nonviable Venezuelan equine encephalomyelitis hemagglutinin prepared from tissue cultures by gamma radiation, *Appl. Microbiol.*, **18**(2): 278–9.

Reitman, M. and Tonik, E. J., 1971. Immunity to aerosol challenge in guinea pigs immunized with gamma-irradiated Venezuelan equine encephalitis vaccines, *Appl. Microbiol.*, **21**(4): 688–92.

Roberts, E. D., Sanmartin, C., Payán, J. and Mackenzie, R. B., 1970. Neuropathologic changes in 15 horses with naturally occurring Venezuelan equine encephalomyelitis, *Am. J. vet. Res.*, **31**(7): 1223–9.

Robinson, D. M., Berman, S. and Lowenthal, J. P., 1972. Mouse potency assay for western equine encephalomyelitis vaccines, *Appl. Microbiol.*, **23**(1): 104–7.

Sabban, M. S., El Dahaby, H. and Hussein, N., 1961. An outbreak of encephalomyelitis in donkeys in Eygpt, *Bull. Off. int. Epiz.*, **55**: 1701–16.

Scherer, W. F. and Anderson, K., 1975. Antigenic and biologic characteristics of Venezuelan encephalitis virus strains including a possible new subtype, isolated from the Amazon region of Peru in 1971, *Am. J. Epidemiol.*, **101**(4): 356–61.

Scherer, W. F., Anderson, K., Pancake, B. A., Dickerman, R. W. and Ordonez, J. V., 1976. Search for epizootic-like Venezuelan encephalitis virus at enzootic habitats in Guatemala during 1969–1971, *Am. J. Epidemiol.*, **103**(6): 576–88.

Scherer, W. F. and Buescher, E. L., 1959. Ecologic studies of Japanese encephalitis virus in Japan. I. Introduction, *Am. J. trop. Med. Hyg.*, **8**: 644–50.

Scherer, W. F., Buescher, E. L., Flemings, M. B., Noguchi, A. and Scanlon, J., 1959a. Ecologic studies of Japanese encephalitis virus in Japan. III. Mosquito factors. Zootropism and vertical flight of *Culex tritaeniorhynchus* with observations on variations in collection from animal-baited traps in different habitats, *Am. J. trop. Med. Hyg.*, **8**: 665–77.

Scherer, W. F., Buescher, E. L. and McClure, H. E., 1959b. Ecologic studies of Japanese encephalitis virus in Japan. V. Avian factors, *Am. J. trop. Med. Hyg.*, **8**: 689–97.

Scherer, W. F. and Chin, J., 1977. Responses of guinea pigs to infections with strains of Venezuelan encephalitis virus, and correlations with equine virulence, *Am. J. trop. Med. Hyg.*, **26**(2): 307–12.

Scherer, W. F., Cupp, E. W., Lok, J. B., Brenner, R. J. and Ordonez, J. V., 1981. Intestinal threshold of an enzootic strain of Venezuelan encephalitis virus in *Culex* (*Melanoconion*) *taeniopus* mosquitoes and its implication to vector competency and vertebrate amplifying hosts, *Am. J. trop. Med. Hyg.*, **30**(4): 862–9.

Scherer, W. F., Dickerman, R. W., Campillo-Sainz, C., Zarate, M. L. and Gonzalez, E., 1971a. Ecologic studies of Venezuelan encephalitis virus in southeastern México. V. Infection of domestic animals other than equines, *Am. J. trop. Med. Hyg.*, **20**(6): 989–93.

Scherer, W. F., Dickerman, R. W., La Fiandra, R. P., Wong Chia, C. and Terrian, J., 1971b. Ecologic studies of Venezuelan encephalitis virus in southeastern México. IV. Infections of wild mammals, *Am. J. trop. Med. Hyg.*, **20**(6): 980–8.

Scherer, W. F., Kitaoka, M., Okuno, T. and Ogata, T., 1959c. Ecologic studies of Japanese encephalitis virus in Japan. VII. Human infection, *Am. J. trop. Med. Hyg.*, **8**: 707–15.

Scherer, W. F., Madalengoitia, J., Flores, W. and Acosta, M., 1975. Ecologic studies of Venezuelan encephalitis virus in Peru during 1970–1971, *Am. J. Epidemiol.*, **101**(4): 347–55.

Scherer, W. F., Moyer, T., Izumi, T., Gresser, I. and McCown, J., 1959d. Ecologic studies of Japanese encephalitis virus in Japan.

VI. Swine infection, *Am. J. trop. Med. Hyg.*, **8**: 698–706.

Scherer, W. F., Ordonez, J. V., Jahrling, P. B., Pancake, B. A. and Dickerman, R. W., 1972. Observations of equines, humans and domestic and wild vertebrates during the 1969 equine epizootic and epidemic of Venezuelan encephalitis in Guatemala, *Am. J. Epidemiol.*, **95**(3): 255–66.

Scherer, W. F. and Pancake, B. A., 1970. Cross-protection among viruses of the Venezuelan equine encephalitis complex in hamsters, *Am. J. Epidemiol.*, **91**(2): 225–9.

Sellers, R. F., Bergold, G. H., Suárez, O. M. and Morales, A., 1965. Investigations during Venezuelan equine encephalitis outbreaks in Venezuela, 1962–1964, *Am. J. trop. Med. Hyg.*, **14**(3): 460–9.

Shope, R. E., Causey, O. R., Homobono Paes de Andrade, A. and Theiler, M., 1964. The Venezuelan equine encephalomyelitis complex of group A arthropod-borne viruses, including Mucambo and Pizuna from the Amazon region of Brazil, *Am. J. trop. Med. Hyg.*, **13**: 723–7.

Shope, R. E. (discussant), 1972. In *Venezuelan Equine Encephalitis.* Pan-American Health Organization (Washington, DC), publ. No. 243, pp. 271–2.

Sidwell, R. W., Gebhardt, L. P. and Thorpe, B. D., 1967. Epidemiological aspects of Venezuelan equine encephalitis virus infections, *Bact. Rev.*, **31**(1): 65–81.

Smart, D. L., Trainer, D. O. and Yuill, T. M., 1975. Serologic evidence of Venezuelan equine encephalitis in some wild and domestic populations of southern Texas, *J. Wildl. Dis.*, **11**: 195–200.

Spears, J. F., 1972. Largest spray operation ever: the story of how government and industry combined forces to contain the VEE epidemic, *Ag. Chem. Comm. Fert.*, **26:** 12, 13, 14 and 30.

Spertzel, R. O., 1973. Venezuelan equine encephalomyelitis, vaccination and control, *Proc. 3rd int. Conf. Equine infect. Dis.*, Paris 1972, eds I. T. Bryans, H. Gerber. Karger (Basle), pp. 146–56.

Spertzel, R. O. and Kahn, D. E., 1971. Safety and efficacy of an attenuated Venezuelan equine encephalomyelitis vaccine for use in equidae, *J. Am. vet. Med. Ass.*, **159**(6): 731–8.

Spertzel, R. O. and McKinney, R. W., 1970. V. E. E., a disease on the move, *Proc. 74th Anim. Meet. US. Anim. Hlth Assoc.*, 1970, pp. 268–75.

Sponseller, M. L., Binn, L. N., Wooding, W. L. and Yager, R. H., 1966. Field strains of western encephalitis virus in ponies: virologic, clinical, and pathologic observations, *Am. J. vet. Res.*, **27**(121): 1591–8.

Sprockhoff, H. von and Ising, E., 1971. On the presence of viruses of the American equine encephalomyelitis in Central Europe, *Arch. ges. Virusforsch.*, **34:** 371–80.

Sudia, W. D. and Newhouse, V. F., 1975. Epidemic Venezuelan equine encephalitis in North America: a summary of virus–vector–host relationships, *Am. J. Epidemiol.* **101**(1): 1–13.

Sudia, W. D., Newhouse, V. F. and Henderson, B. E., 1971. Experimental infection of horses with three strains of Venezuelan equine encephalomyelitis virus. II. Experimental vector studies, *Am. J. Epidemiol.*, **93**(3): 206–11.
Sudia, W. D., Stamm, D. D., Chamberlain, R. W. and Kissling, R. E., 1956. Transmission of eastern equine encephalitis to horses by *Aedes sollicitans* mosquitoes, *Am. J. trop. Med. Hyg.*, **5**: 802–8.

Taber, L. E., Hogge, A. L. Jr and McKinney, R. W., 1965. Experimental infection of dogs with two strains of Venezuelan equine encephalomyelitis virus, *Am. J. trop. Med. Hyg.*, **14**(4): 647–51.
Taylor, W. M. and Buff, E., 1972. Transmissibility of an attenuated Venezuelan equine encephalomyelitis vaccine virus, *J. Am. vet. med. Ass.*, **161**(2): 159–63.
Trent, D. W. and Grant, J. A., 1980. A comparison of New World alphaviruses in the western equine encephalomyelitis complex by immunochemical and oligonucleotide fingerprint techniques, *J. gen. Virol.*, **47**: 261–82.
Tsilinsky, Y. Y., Gutshin, B. V., Klimenko, S. M. and Lvov, D. K., 1971. Variations of virion sized in different clones of Venezuelan equine encephalomyelitis virus, *Arch. ges. Virusforsch.*, **34**: 301–9.

Vanderwagen, L. C., Pearson, J. L., Franti, C. E., Tamm, E. L., Riemann, H. P. and Behymer, D. E., 1975. A field study of persistence of antibodies in California horses vaccinated against western, eastern and Venezuelan equine encephalomyelitis, *Am. J. vet. Res.*, **36**(1): 1567–71.
Victor, J., Smith, D. G. and Pollack, A. D., 1956. The comparative pathology of Venezuelan equine encephalomyelitis, *J. Infect. Dis.*, **98**: 55–66.
Villasmil, D. P., de Siger, J., Barrientos, M. P., Mussgay, M. and Mackenzie, R. B., 1975. Evaluation in donkeys of an inactivated Venezuelan equine encephalitis vaccine, *Zbl. Vet. Med.*, **B22**: 162–8.

Walder, R. and Bradish, C. J., 1975. Venezuelan equine encephalomyelitis virus (VEEV): strain differentiation and specification of virulence markers, *J. gen. Virol.*, **26**: 265–75.
Walder, R. and Liprandi, F., 1976. Kinetics of heat inactivation of Venezuelan equine encephalomyelitis virus, *Arch. Virol.*, **51**: 307–17.
Walder, R., Rosato, R. R. and Eddy, G. A., 1981. Virion polypeptide heterogeneity among virulent and avirulent strains of eastern equine encephalitis (EEE) virus, *Arch. Virol.*, **68**: 229–37.

Walker, D. H., Harrison, A., Murphy, K., Flemister, M. and Murphy, F. A., 1976. Lymphoreticular and myeloid pathogenesis of Venezuelan equine encephalitis in hamsters, *Am. J. Path.*, **84**(2): 351–69.

Walton, T. E., 1981. Venezuelan, eastern, and western encephalomyelitis. In *Virus Diseases of Food Animals. A World Geography of Epidemiology and Control*, vol. II. ed. E. P. J. Gibbs. Academic Press (London), Disease Monographs, pp. 557–625.

Walton, T. E., Alvarez, O. Jr, Buckwalter, R. M. and Johnson, K. M., 1972. Experimental infection of horses with an attenuated Venezuelan equine encephalomyelitis vaccine (strain TC-83), *Infect. Immun.*, **5**(5): 750–6.

Walton, T. E., Alvarez, O. Jr, Buckwalter, R. M. and Johnson, K. M., 1973a. Experimental infection of horses with enzootic and epizootic strains of Venezuelan equine encephalomyelitis virus, *J. Infect. Dis.*, **128**(3): 271–82.

Walton, T. E. and Johnson, K. M., 1972a. Experimental Venezuelan equine encephalomyelitis virus infection of the bovine, *Infect. Immun.*, **5**(2): 155–9.

Walton, T. E. and Johnson, K. M., 1972b. Persistence of neutralizing antibody in equidae vaccinated with Venezuelan equine encephalomyelitis vaccine strain TC-83, *J. Am. vet. med. Ass.*, **161**(8): 916–18.

Walton, T. E. and Johnson, K. M., 1972c. Epizootiology of Venezuelan equine encephalomyelitis in the Americas, *J. Am. vet. med. Ass.*, **161**(11): 1509–15.

Walton, T. E., Luedke, A. J., Jochim, M. M., Crenshaw, G. L. and Ferguson, J. A., 1973b. Duration of immunity of horses vaccinated with strain TC-83 Venezuelan equine encephalomyelitis virus vaccine, *Proc. 77th Ann. Meet. US Anim. Hlth Assoc.*, **77**: 196–202.

Wang, S-P. and Grayston, J. T., 1962. Encephalitis on Taiwan. IV. Human serology, *Am. J. trop. Med. Hyg.*, **11**: 149–54.

Wang, S-P., Grayston J. T. and Chu, I-H, 1962a. Encephalitis on Taiwan.V. Animal and bird serology, *Am. J. trop. Med. Hyg.*, **11**: 155–8.

Wang, S-P., Grayston, J. T. and Chu, I-H., 1962a. Encephalitis on Taiwan. III. Virus isolations from mosquitoes, *Am. J. trop. Med. Hyg.*, **11**: 141–8.

Waters, J. R., 1976. V. An epidemic of western encephalomyelitis in humans – Manitoba, 1975, *Can. J. Pub. Hlth*, Suppl. 1, **67**: 28–32.

Watts, D. M. and Williams, J. E., 1972. Experimental infection of bobwhite quail (*Colinus virginianus*) with western equine encephalitis (WEE) virus, *J. Wildl. Dis.*, **8**: 44–8.

Weinack, O. M., Snoeyenbos, G. H. and Rosenau, B. J., 1978. Pheasant susceptibility at different ages to eastern encephalitis virus from various sources in Massachusetts, *Avian Dis.*, **22**(3): 378–85.

Yershov, F. I., Sokolova, T. M. and Titenko, A. M., 1977. Properties of virions and ribonucleoproteins of Venezuelan equine encephalomyelitis virus, *Acta virol.*, **21**: 213–21.

Young, N. A. and Johnson, K. M., 1969. Antigenic variants of Venezuelan equine encephalitis virus: their geographic distribution and epidemiologic significance, *Am. J. Epidemiol.*, **89**(3): 286–307.

Zarate, M. L. and Scherer, W. F., 1968. Contact-spread of Venezuelan equine encephalomyelitis virus among cotton rats via urine or feces and the naso- or oropharynx. A possible transmission cycle in nature, *Am. J. trop. Med. Hyg.*, **17**(6): 894–9.

Zebovitz, E. and Brown, A., 1967. Temperature-sensitive steps in the biosynthesis of Venezuelan equine encephalitis virus, *J. Virol.*, **1**(1): 128–34.

Zhdanov, V. M., Yershov, F. I. and Uryvayev, L. V., 1969. Ribonucleic acids synthesized in Venezuelan equine encephalomyelitis virus-infected cells, *Virology*, **38**: 355–8.

Zlotnik, I., Peacock, S., Grant, D. P. and Batter-Hatton, D., 1972. The pathogenesis of western equine encephalitis virus (W. E. E.) in adult hamsters with special reference to the long and short term effects on the C. N. S. of the attenuated clone 15 variant, *Br. J. exp. Path.*, **53**: 59–77.

Chapter

10

Lumpy skin disease

CONTENTS

INTRODUCTION

Lumpy skin disease (LSD) is a viral disease of cattle confined to Africa, causing acute, subacute, or asymptomatic syndromes characterized by fever and development of firm, well-demarcated nodules affecting skin, subcutaneous connective tissue, mucosa of the respiratory and digestive systems, and, occasionally, skeletal muscles. The cutaneous lesions are associated with subcutaneous edema of the legs and ventral aspects of the body, and enlargement of local drainage lymph nodes.

Literature

A most comprehensive review on LSD was presented by Weiss (1968). The author included in his description a considerable amount of information both from his own unpublished work and from personal communication with other workers. This is referenced in this chapter under Weiss (1968). Lumpy skin disease has been reviewed earlier by Haig (1957), by Henning (1956) who presented the history of the first outbreaks of LSD and its spread throughout South Africa, and more recently by Davies (1981). The disease was first observed in 1929 in Northern Rhodesia; subsequently in 1943, it was identified in South Africa as being caused by an infectious agent (von Backstrom 1945). Since then it has been reported in many regions of Africa.

ETIOLOGY

On the basis of morphology, cytopathic effect in tissue culture cells, presence of inclusion bodies typical of pox viruses, and serology, LSD virus is considered to be a capripoxvirus. Two other viruses, a herpes virus referred to as 'Allerton' and an orphan herpes virus, are occasionally associated with LSD-like syndromes. The Allerton virus causes lesions which in the early stages are comparable to LSD lesions, and the syndrome is known as pseudo-LSD.

Lumpy skin disease virus can be propagated in a number of mammalian cell cultures, including tissues from lambs, calves, rabbits, monkeys, and hamsters, as well as in embryonated chicken eggs. In these cell cultures the virus causes a cytopathic effect (CPE) which results in plaque formation and the presence of intracytoplasmic inclusion bodies.

Literature

The morphology and biological properties of LSD virus have been undertaken primarily on the Neethling-type isolates, which have been associated with relatively severe syndromes of disease. The virions in tissue culture were structurally similar to the vaccinia virus and had two distinct forms, one with irregular threads on its surface, and the other with a capsule consisting of three components surrounding an inner body (Munz and Owen 1966). Other features which supported the classification of the virus in the pox group were presented by Weiss (1968) and included positive histochemical staining for deoxyribonucleic acid (DNA), development of macroscopic 'pocks' in chorioallantoic membranes of chick embryos, local skin reaction on intradermal inoculation in rabbits with subsequent generalized infection within 4 days, and antigenic relationship to sheeppox. A number of pox viruses, including sheeppox and LSD were highly ether sensitive, a characteristic of the majority of mammalian and avian pox viruses (Plowright and Ferris 1959). The LSD virus was also comparable in its resistance to environmental factors to other pox viruses. Lumpy skin disease virus in allantoic fluid was stable to a wide range of pH conditions, exposed for differing times and temperatures (Polson and Turner 1954).

Weiss (1968) summarized the growth and behavior of the LSD virus in tissue culture. With primary isolation, the cytopathic changes were evident on day 11, and the time of appearance decreased slowly with serial passage. The rate of appearance of cytopathic changes progressing to plaque formation depended on the composition of the medium, and with the adaptation of the virus to the culture system. The development of plaques first appeared as discrete foci or clumps of rounded or more refractile cells. Although some cells detached forming irregular holes, the majority adhered for a considerable period of time. Single or multiple intracytoplasmic inclusions, similar to those found in skin lesions, developed in association with the CPE. These inclusions first appeared as small round basophilic bodies when stained with hematoxylin and eosin, and later became eosinophilic with a central basophilic component remaining as they increased in size. The inclusions also stained positive for DNA by Feulgen reaction and acridine orange. Fluorescent antibody (FA) methods failed to demonstrate that the inclusion contained viral antigens. They were rounded or had an irregular outline with small protuberances. The host cell containing the inclusions became rounded and shrunken, and the cytoplasm became intensely eosinophilic. The nucleus underwent degenerative changes which terminated in cell necrosis.

For optimal conditions for propagation of the Neethling strain of LSD in embryonated eggs, the age of the embryo, route of inoculation, temperature, and period of incubation had to be taken into consideration. The growth characteristics of the virus were shown to differ considerably from those of other mammalian pox viruses, and the occurrence of the pock-like lesions in the chorioallantoic membrane was not a reliable indication of virus multiplication (van Rooyen *et al.* 1969).

Early work on the isolation of virus from LSD resulted in a description of three types which could be divided by the time of onset and severity of cytopathic effects in calf kidney cultures (Alexander *et al.* 1957). An increase in the growth and cytopathogenic effect of the virus was obtained by increasing the lactalbumin hydrolysate content of medium in kidney tissue culture (Weiss and Geyer 1959). One isolate grew well in testis tissue culture, and the growth was correlated with the progressive cytopathic changes with the formation of inclusion bodies (Plowright and Witcomb 1959). Cytopathic changes produced by Allerton and Neethling viruses in monolayers of calf and lamb kidney cells were compared. Allerton virus produced intranuclear acidophilic granules and inclusions, while Neethling-type virus caused acidophilic intracytoplasmic inclusions with a central basophilic inner body (de Lange 1959; Ramisse *et al.* 1969a, b).

Another of the three original viruses associated with LSD was the herpes virus BHV 2. The disease was shown to be relatively mild as compared to that caused by the pox virus but resembled LSD enough to be referred to as another pseudo-LSD. The disease syndromes it caused were found outside Africa and included mammilitis, stomatitis, and facial infections in bovine and buffalo calves (Gibbs and Rweyemamu 1977). Castrucci *et al.* (1975) summarized the characteristics of the common bovine herpes virus which included formation of multinucleated syncytiae, eosinophilic intranuclear inclusions in cell cultures, induction of skin lesions in cattle, and production of skin inflammation and necrosis in suckling mice. Another virus complicated the initial work on LSD in South Africa and caused unique and characteristic lesions in chick embryos. Subsequently, it was not shown to be the causative agent and was referred to as a cytopathogenic bovine orphan virus (Kipps *et al.* 1961).

EPIZOOTIOLOGY

Lumpy skin disease is found only in Africa and appears to have spread northward from South Africa after 1940. Although classified as a capripoxvirus, its geographical distributions are not identical to those of sheep- and goatpox. The disease is recognized in most countries of Africa south of 10 °N latitude and is associated with heavy rainfall.

Based on epizootical evidence of spread in South Africa, there is strong indication that LSD virus may be vector-borne. Within a herd it can also spread by direct contact. Experimental infection can be induced by injection of blood and material from extracts from skin nodules. Economic losses result from emaciation, decreased milk production, infertility, and damage to hides.

Literature

The incidence and severity of the syndrome has varied in different parts of Africa. Haig (1957) presented a detailed account of the epizootiology of outbreaks in South Africa, where up to 1949 it was estimated that approximately 8 million animals were affected with the disease. The morbidity in southern Africa was usually 50 to 100%, mortality was usually 1% but occasionally could reach 75% (Diesel 1952) Davies (1981) discussed the epizootiology of LSD in Kenya and addressed the possibility of a cattle to cattle cycle and the presence of infections in wild game populations. Lefevre *et al.* (1979) presented the dates when LSD was first detected in various countries of Africa and showed a sequential spread of the disease northward from South Africa. The occurrence of LSD and its clinical and histological manifestations were described in Mozambique by de Sousa Dias and Limpo-serra (1956). A localized outbreak of LSD was described in Madagascar in 1957 which was characterized by a relatively mild syndrome (Lalanne 1956). The first occurrence of LSD was reported in Nigeria in 1974 (Woods 1974). An epizootic of LSD in northern Nigeria and its regional spread has also been described (Nawathe *et al.* 1978). In the Kenya epizootics in 1957 a morbidity of 0.5% was reported and very few animals died (MacOwan 1959; Ayre-Smith 1960). Limited serological surveys undertaken in Kenya showed one-third of cattle with antibodies to Allerton type virus (Martin and Gwynne 1968). In the Ivory Coast the morbidity was 25% (Pierre 1978).

There has been circumstantial evidence that biting insects played a role in the spread of LSD virus. This was based on the observation that the disease was most prevalent during seasons when biting insects were numerous, i.e. during the wet summer months. Attempts to isolate the virus from mosquitoes, *Culicoides*, and various species of ticks, were unsuccessful. However, virus was isolated from *Stomoxys calcitrans* and *Biomyia fasciata* caught on infected animals. Recovery could also be made 3 days after the insects were artificially fed on infected material (Weiss 1968). Infections were also spread by direct and indirect contact between infected animals, which were either clinically sick or had inapparent infections, and susceptible cattle. In addition, experimental transmission by materials from nodules and blood was possible. It was proposed that, because the virus was found in the saliva of cattle, it could be a source of infective material and play a role as a method by which the virus was transmitted (Haig 1955, personal communication; cited by Henning 1956).

INFECTION

Cattle are the natural hosts of LSD virus. Zebu and exotic breeds are susceptible, but a large percentage of animals, irrespective of breed, have natural resistance and do not develop lesions. The imported breeds with thin skin, as opposed to the thick-skinned indigenous African breeds, are more susceptible. Lesions and systemic clinical signs are more severe in calves than in adults, and in very young calves mortality may be high. The virus is present in blood, spleen, saliva, semen, and skin lesions, where it is viable for days in the superficial exudates. Experimentally infected sheep and goats develop erythematous swelling which disappears quickly. It has been suggested that sheep may act as asymptomatic carriers of the virus. The disease has not been reported in game animals, although both giraffe and impala calves are highly susceptible to experimental infections.

Literature

Following the appearance of fever and generalized skin lesions, the virus was present in blood for 4 days, in saliva for 11 days, in the semen for 22 days, and in skin nodules for at least 33 days. It was also found in muscle and spleen, but could not be demonstrated in urine and feces. In the necrotic dried portion of the skin lesions, the virus remained viable for 18 days (Weiss 1968). Viremia was not detected following clinical recovery (Haig 1957). The virus was maintained for months at 4 °C and for years at −80 °C. In experimental infections, 40 to 50% of animals developed a localized painful swelling at the site of injection, or did not respond (Weiss 1968). Neither age, sex, color, nor breed could be associated with susceptibility, but animals with thinner skin were more predisposed to development of severe lesions (Pierre 1978). Giraffe and impala calves were susceptible with development of typical lesions, but neither wildebeest nor buffaloes could be infected (Young *et al.* 1970).

CLINICAL SIGNS

The clinical syndromes vary from a mild disease of a few days' duration to one which results in widespread dissemination of nodules and extensive tissue destruction. Asymptomatic infections also occur. Mortality is the highest in young calves and, occasionally, may also be high in mature animals. Severe acute disease is characterized by rapid eruption of cutaneous nodules at different sites with extensive edema of limbs, ventral thorax, and abdomen. The superficial lymph nodes are markedly enlarged. Nodules also develop in the mucosa of the upper respiratory system and the gastrointestinal tract and, more rarely, in the skeletal muscles, serous membranes, liver, and genital organs. When secondary bacterial infections complicate the skin lesions, extensive sloughing of skin and subcutaneous tissue takes place.

Literature

Various clinical syndromes, particularly the severe acute form, were described by Haig (1957), Henning (1956), Ayre-Smith (1960), and later by Weiss (1968) who also summarized the observations recorded in the earlier literature. The composite description included the following main clinical signs. After experimental infection clinical signs developed after an incubation period of 7 to 14 days, while after natural exposure the period was longer, varying from 2 to 5 weeks. A characteristic diphasic temperature response occurred, with skin nodules appearing during the second fever phase about a week to 10 days after the first febrile response. The swelling in both skin and underlying muscle was painful and developed early during the fever.

Fever was accompanied by inappetance, salivation, lachrymation, and nasal discharge. The nodules were more readily observed in short-haired animals. The skin lesions were either flat, rounded, or well circumscribed with an obvious intracutaneous localization, and varied in size from 0.5 to 5 cm in diameter. Generalized skin lesions were found over the entire body with some predilection for the skin on the neck, brisket, back, thighs, legs, perineum, udder, vulva, scrotum, and around the eyes and muzzle. The severity of the lesion ranged from the presence of a few nodules in mild cases to several hundred in severe cases. Nodules either regressed rapidly, underwent necrosis with skin ulceration, or persisted as hard lumps for months. Necrosis occurred after about 7 to 10 days, the tissue became dry and hard and was shed after 3 to 5 weeks. Granulation tissue and excessive inflammatory exudate due to secondary bacterial infection extended into the subcutaneous tissue. Subcutaneous edema of the limbs, dewlap, and external genitalia persisted for weeks, was usually associated with skin necrosis, and was often accompanied by lameness. The skin over the edema sloughed off, resulting in deep wounds.

A constant feature accompanying the cutaneous lesions was enlargement of the local drainage lymph nodes. Other complications observed were mastitis, anestrus, and abortion. Scrotal lesions were associated with infertility. Temporary infertility was also thought to result from fever and general debility rather than as a direct result of the virus on the genitalia. Soft, yellowish-gray, occasionally ulcerated nodules were observed in the mucous membranes of the mouth, nose, and external genitalia. In cases with extensive lesions in the respiratory tract pneumonia developed.

In large numbers of cases in Kenya there was no correlation observed between the severity of lesions and age, breed, color, and sex. Less than five skin lesions were detected in the mild forms syndrome without any systemic effect. Considerable difference in size of nodules occurred between animals, and within any one animal (Ayre-Smith 1960).

The Allerton virus caused a syndrome with an incubation period of 5 to 9 days, and the clinical signs were characterized by mild fever followed by the sudden appearance of skin nodules involving the superficial layers of the epidermis, which could not be distinguished from the early lesions caused by LSD virus. The swellings subsided in 7 to 8 days; occasionally the nodule underwent necrosis and the tissue sloughed off in 10 to 14 days (Alexander *et al.* 1957).

PATHOLOGY

The cutaneous lesions consist of firm masses of edematous whitish-gray tissue, affecting the skin and underlying connective tissue, occasionally extending into the muscle, and may also be more widely distributed throughout the skeletal muscles, lungs, rumen, and uterus. In the mucosa of the upper respiratory and gastrointestinal systems, soft, gray–yellow, ulcerated necrotic masses are formed.

Histologically, the nodule consists of an acute focal inflammatory reaction characterized by accumulation of histiocytes, plasma cells, neutrophils, and eosinophils, with proliferation of fibrocytes and infiltration of inflammatory exudate containing fibrin. Intracytoplasmic inclusions, varying greatly in size, are found in the histiocytes, smooth muscle, and epithelial cells.

There is some similarity in the early gross lesions of LSD and those caused by the Allerton virus, with nodule formation and superficial necrosis of the epidermis.

Literature

Subcutaneous and intradermal experimental LSD infection induced a firm, circumscribed, or diffuse swelling after 4 to 7 days which was 20 cm or more in diameter and occasionally involved the underlying muscle. The regional lymph nodes were enlarged. In early lesions, acute cellular and fluid inflammatory reaction affected the corium and the dermal papillae. Associated with the thrombosis of small blood vessels, there was perivascular infiltration of lymphocytes, histiocytes, plasma cells, and neutrophils, and proliferation of fibroblasts. The lesion progressed to coagulative necrosis of the superficial epidermis. Intracytoplasmic inclusions were found in epithelial and smooth muscle cells, as well as in the infiltrating macrophages, lymphocytes, and occasionally in the proliferating fibroblasts (Weiss 1968; Haig 1957). Inflammation and petechial hemorrhages with ulceration of circular flat-top nodules were observed in the abomasal mucosa and in the upper respiratory tract (Ayre-Smith 1960). Capstick (1959) compared experimental skin lesions in cattle caused by five strains of virus including the Allerton and Neethling types, and found that only the Allerton virus very frequently induced generalized lesions. The Neethling virus has been reported to produce generalized lesions in only a variable percentage of experimentally infected animals (Weiss 1968; Ali and Obeide 1977).

There has been little information on the susceptibility of laboratory animals to infection. It has been reported but not verified that rabbits injected intradermally with LSD virus from tissue cultures developed an erythematous swelling at the site of inoculation and lesions became generalized (Weiss 1968).

In experimental infections of giraffe and impala calves, the lesions resembled those in cattle with necrosis of blood vessels and lymphatics, accumulation of inflammatory fluid exudate, and skin necrosis. Intranuclear and intracytoplasmic inclusions were found in a variety of cells, including histiocytes and endothelial cells and particularly epidermal cells (Young *et al.* 1970). Allerton virus was proposed as causing severe lesions in the alimentary tract of buffalo (*Syncerus caffer*) (Schiemann *et al.* 1971).

IMMUNOLOGY

Isolates of LSD virus from various regions of Africa are antigenically similar and closely related to sheeppox viruses. Natural resistance to infection occurs in approximately 50% or more of all cattle exposed either to natural or experimental infection. The immunity engendered by infection is effective against a variety of isolates, lasts for several years, and is associated with the development of antibodies. Passive immunity can be transferred through colostrum and persists for 6 months. Early workers reported short-term immunity following infection, but this may have been due to subsequent infections by the antigenically unrelated Allerton virus.

Literature

Based on complete reciprocal cross-neutralization, as well as on cross-immunity tests, one basic immunological type of LSD virus has been identified. Antigenic relationship was demonstrated between LSD virus, sheeppox virus and cowpox virus (Davies and Otema 1981). Animals which recover from natural infection develop humoral antibodies capable of neutralizing the virus for up to 5 years, and antibody titers may be lifelong (Weiss 1968). Henning (1956) reported that immunity was of short duration, up to about 100 days. This was based on the observations made by early workers of the recurrent development of LSD lesions in animals. However, whether this could have resulted in reinfection with the antigenically unrelated Allerton virus was not clearly defined (Weiss 1968).

Three strains of bovine herpes virus (Allerton, bovine mammilitis, and the Italian isolate 69/1L0) were compared antigenically by cross-protection tests in calves. Following intradermal infection, homologous intravenous challenge did not induce either skin lesions or febrile response. Heterologous challenges did cause fever, but skin lesions did not develop (Castrucci *et al*. 1975).

Limited information has been published on the serology of LSD virus. Titration experiments using neutralizing antibodies have been undertaken in embryonated eggs (Van den Ende and Turner 1950).

VACCINATION

Kenya sheep- and goatpox virus and attenuated Neethling strain of LSD viruses are used as vaccines and induce effective immunity under experimental conditions. The usefulness of these vaccines in the face of an epizootic are not determined.

Literature

Two vaccines have been produced, a Kenyan vaccine of goat- and sheeppox viruses not attenuated for sheep and goats, and a South African vaccine using a strain of attenuated Neethling virus (Davies 1981). A sheeppox virus in lamb testes tissue culture was produced and used to vaccinate cattle against LSD and was protected from intradermal challenge by Neethling virus (Coackley and Capstick 1961; Capstick *et al.* 1959). The vaccine virus was not transmitted from cattle to sheep and was effective in field trials. However, there was no conclusive evidence as to the usefulness of this vaccine in the face of severe epizootics (Capstick and Coackley 1961). Serial passage of Neethling strain of LSD virus in embryonated eggs also resulted in attenuation. After the twentieth passage, the virus produced only a local skin swelling without evidence of necrosis, which disappeared within 4 to 6 weeks. Reversion of virulence was not evident. Immunized cattle developed circulating antibody by the tenth day with high titers on day 30 in those animals which showed a local skin reaction. Antibodies persisted for 3 years during which time animals were resistant to challenge. In those animals which did not develop skin reactions antibodies could not be demonstrated (Weiss 1968).

DIAGNOSIS

In epizootics, diagnosis of LSD is made on the basis of characteristic lesions in acute severe cases. Diagnosis of mild or atypical cases, especially under enzootic conditions, is difficult and requires laboratory confirmation demonstrating the virus. Cultures are examined for the characteristic inclusions, with final identification of LSD virus being made by the neutralization test. Histological examination of tissues from a number of affected animals is also helpful.

Literature

The diagnosis of LSD has been summarized by Haig (1957) and Weiss (1968). Differential diagnosis between LSD virus and lesions caused by the bovine herpes virus 2 were made by examination of tissues with the electron microscope and by FA techniques on 24-hour cultures (Davies *et al.* 1971). Because of nonspecific FA staining, cryostat sections of lesions did not give reliable results. Diagnosis of LSD could also be made by demonstrating intracytoplasmic inclusions in epithelial and mononuclear cells and characteristic inflammatory and vascular lesions (Burdin 1959).

After tanning, the appearance of hides from cattle affected with LSD virus could be differentiated from other skin diseases, particularly those associated with dermatophilosis (Green 1959).

BIBLIOGRAPHY

Alexander, R. A., Plowright, W. and Haig, D. A., 1957. Cytopathogenic agents associated with lumpy-skin disease of cattle, *Bull. epiz. Dis. Afr.*, **5**: 489–92.

Ali, B. H. and Obeidi, H. M., 1977. Investigation of the first outbreaks of lumpy skin disease in the Sudan, *Br. vet. J.*, **133**: 184–9.

Ayre-Smith, R. A., 1960. The symptoms and clinical diagnosis of lumpy skin disease, *Vet. Rec.*, **72**(24): 469–72.

Burdin, M. L., 1959. The use of histopathological examinations of skin material for the diagnosis of lumpy skin disease in Kenya, *Bull. epiz. Dis. Afr.*, **7**: 27–36.

Capstick, P. B., 1959. Lumpy skin disease, experimental infection, *Bull. epiz. Dis. Afr.*, **7**: 51–62.

Capstick, P. B. and Coackley, W., 1961. Protection of cattle against lumpy skin disease. I. Trials with a vaccine against Neethling type infection, *Res. vet. Sci.*, **2**: 362–8.

Capstick, P. B., Prydie, J., Coackley, W. and Burdin, M. L., 1959. Protection of cattle against the 'Neethling' type virus of lumpy skin disease, *Vet. Rec.*, **71**(20): 422–3.

Castrucci, G., Martin, W. B., Pedini, B., Cilli, V. and Ranucci, S., 1975. A comparison in calves of the antigenicity of three strains of bovid herpesvirus 2, *Res. vet. Sci.*, **18**: 208–15.

Coackley, W. and Capstick, P. B., 1961. Protection of cattle against lumpy skin disease. II. Factors affecting small scale production of a tissue culture propagated virus vaccine, *Res. vet. Sci.*, **2**: 369–74.

Davies. F. G., 1981. Lumpy skin disease. In *Virus Diseases of Food Animals*, disease monographs, vol. 2, ed. E. P. J. Gibbs. Academic Press (London), pp. 751–64.

Davies, F. G., Krauss, H., Lund, J. and Taylor M., 1971. The laboratory diagnosis of lumpy skin disease, *Res. vet. Sci.*, **12**: 123–7.

Davies, F. G. and Otema, C., 1981. Relationship of capripox viruses found in Kenya with two Middle Eastern strains of some orthopox viruses, *Res. vet. Sci.*, **31**: 253–5.

de Lange, M., 1959. The histology of the cytopathogenic changes produced in monolayer epithelial cultures by viruses associated with lumpy skin disease, *Onderstepoort J. vet. Res.*, **28**(2): 245–55.

de Sousa Dias, A. and Limpo-serra, J., 1956. Lumpy skin disease in Mozambique, *Bull. Off. int. Epiz.*, **46**: 612–25.

Diesel, A. M., 1952. The epizootiology of lumpy skin disease in South Africa, *Proc. XIVth Int. Vet. Congr.*, 1949. HMSO (London), vol. 1, pp. 492–500.

Gibbs, E. P. J. and Rweyemamu, M. M., 1977. Bovine herpesviruses. Part II. Bovine herpesviruses 2 and 3, *Vet. Bull.*, **47**(6): 411–25.
Green, H. F., 1959. Lumpy skin disease – its effect on hides and leather and a comparison in this respect with some other skin diseases, *Bull. epiz. Dis. Afr.*, **5**: 421–30.

Haig, D. A., 1957. Lumpy skin disease. *Bull. epiz. Dis. Afr.*, **5**: 421–30.
Henning, M. W., 1956. Knopvelsiekte, lumpy-skin disease. In *Animal Diseases in South Africa. Being an Account of the Infectious Diseases of Domestic Animals*. Central News Agency Ltd (South Africa), pp. 1023–37.

Kipps, A., Turner, G. S. and Polson, A., 1961. Some properties of a cytopathogenic bovine orphan virus (Van den Ende strain), *J. gen. Microbiol.*, **26**: 405–13.

Lalanne, A., 1956. Lumpy skin disease in Madagascar in relation to the leather industry, *Bull. Off. int. Epiz.*, **46**: 596–611.
Lefevre, P. C., Bonnet, J. B. and Vallat, B., 1979. Lumpy skin disease in cattle. I. Epizootiology in Africa, *Rev. Elev. Méd. vét. Pays trop.*, **32**(3): 227–31.

MacOwan, K. D. S., 1959. Observations on the epizootiology of lumpyskin disease during the first year of its occurrence in Kenya, *Bull. epiz. Dis. Afr.*, **7**: 7–70.
Martin, W. B. and Gwynne, M., 1968. Antibodies to the group II lumpy skin disease viruses in the sera of cattle in Kenya, *Bull. epiz. Dis. Afr.*, **16**: 217–22.
Munz, E. K. and Owen, N. C., 1966. Electron microscopic studies on lumpy skin disease virus type 'Neethling', *Onderstepoort J. vet. Res.*, **33**(1): 3–8.

Nawathe, D. R., Gibbs, E. P. J., Asagba, M. O. and Lawman, M. J.P., 1978. Lumpy skin disease in Nigeria, *Trop. Anim. Hlth Prod.*, **10**: 49–54.

Pierre, F., 1978. Bovine lumpy skin disease in the Ivory Coast, *Rev. Elev. Méd. vét. Pays trop.*, **31**(3): 281–6.
Plowright, W. and Ferris, R. D., 1959. Ether sensitivity of some mammalian poxviruses, *Virology*, **7**: 357–8.
Plowright, W. and Witcomb, M. A., 1959. The growth in tissue cultures of a virus derived from lumpy-skin disease of cattle, *J. Path. Bact.*, **78**: 397–407.

Polson, A. and Turner, G. S., 1954. pH stability and purification of lumpy skin disease virus, *J. gen. Microbiol.*, **11**: 228–35.

Ramisse, J., Serres, H. and Rakotondramary, E., 1969a. Isolation of viruses associated with bovine lumpy skin disease in Madagascar, *Rev. Elev. Méd. vét. Pays trop.*, **22**(3): 357–62.

Ramisse, J., Serres, H. and Rakotondramary, E., 1969b. Adaptation to the rabbit renal cells of viruses associated with bovine lumpy skin disease, *Rev. Elev. Méd. vét. Pays trop.*, **22**(3): 363–71.

Schiemann, B., Plowright, W. and Jessett, D. M., 1971. Allerton-type herpes virus as a cause of lesions of the alimentary tract in a severe disease of Tanzanian buffaloes (*Syncerus caffer*), *Vet. Rec.*, **89**: 17–22.

Van den Ende, M. and Turner, G. S., 1950. Further observations on a filtrable agent isolated from bovine lumpy skin disease, *J. gen. Microbiol.*, **4**: 225–34.

van Rooyen, P. J., Munz, E. K. and Weiss, K. E., 1969. The optimal conditions for the multiplication of Neethling-type lumpy skin disease virus in embryonated eggs, *Onderstepoort J. vet. Res.*, **36**(2): 165–74.

von Backstrom, U., 1945. Ngamiland cattle disease: preliminary report on a new disease, the etiological agent being probably of an infectious nature, *J. S. Afr. vet. med. Ass.*, **16**: 29–33.

Weiss, K. E., 1968. Lumpy skin disease virus. In *Virology Monographs*, eds S. Gard, C. Hallauer, K. F. Meyer. Springer-Verlag (New York), vol. 3, pp. 111–31.

Weiss, K. E. and Geyer, S. M., 1959. The effect of lactalbumin hydrolysate on the cytopathogenesis of lumpy skin disease virus in tissue culture, *Bull. epiz. Dis. Afr.*, **7**: 243–54.

Woods, J. A., 1974. A skin condition of cattle, *Vet. Rec.*, **95**: 326.

Young, E., Basson, P. A. and Weiss, K. E., 1970. Experimental infection of game animals with lumpy skin disease virus (Prototype strain Neethling), *Onderstepoort J. vet. Res.*, **37**(2): 79–88.

Chapter

11

Nairobi sheep disease

CONTENTS

INTRODUCTION

Nairobi sheep disease (NSD) is a tick-transmitted viral disease of sheep and goats in East Africa, characterized by high temperature, severe hemorrhagic gastroenteritis, and lymph node hyperplasia. Adult sheep and goats are gradually immune to NSD virus in enzootic areas, while those reared in areas free from the principal tick vector, or where the vector does not occur, are highly susceptible.

Literature

Relatively little information has been published on NSD. Montgomery (1917) published a comprehensive account of the epidemiology, clinical signs, and pathology of natural and experimental NSD which was then referred to as tick-borne gastroenteritis of sheep and goats. Exotic sheep were more resistant to NSD than the local breeds in which the mortality could be as high as 70%. Henning (1956) reviewed in detail the available information on NSD. In the review article by Davies *et al.* (1976), reference was made to a DVM thesis by C. Terpstra (1970), University of Utrecht, which probably also represents another major publication describing the disease.

ETIOLOGY

The NSD virus is considered to belong to the genus *Bunyavirus* and recently it is shown to have antigenic similarity to other arboviruses. The virus is relatively resistant to the adverse effects of environment and can be stored for long periods of time under refrigeration and in preservatives such as glycerin. It grows in tissue cultures and can be assayed in adult, and intracerebrally and intraperitoneally in suckling, mice.

Literature

Davies *et al.* (1978) referred to the work of Melnick (1973) who concluded that on the basis of physicochemical properties the virus belongs to the genus *Bunyavirus*, and on ultrastructural characteristics it has been shown to be a deoxyribonucleic acid virus (Terpstra 1970). Antigenically it was very closely related to the Ganjam virus isolated from ticks and mosquitoes in India, and it had some serological relationship to the Dugbe, Hazara, and Congo viruses as demonstrated by fluorescent antibody (FA) and indirect hemagglutination tests (Davies *et al.* 1978).

Isolation and identification of NSD virus could be undertaken by inoculation of tissue culture (baby hamster kidney, BHK21, c. 13) with infected organs and plasma with subsequent FA technique for identification of the virus. This system did not depend on the development of cytopathic effect (CPE). A slightly more sensitive method of isolation was intracerebral infection of infant mice. Impression smears and cryostat sections of mouse brains showed fine granular fluorescence in the cytoplasm of neurons (Davies *et al.* 1977). In tissue culture cells of goat testes, goat kidney, and hamster kidney, a consistent and uniform cytopathic effect occurred only in BHK cells and was found between 3 and 4 days postinoculation (Howarth and Terpstra 1965). The virus produced a cytopathic effect in lamb testes, lamb kidney, and BHK cells and pleomorphic eosinophilic cytoplasmic bodies were observed in hematoxylin and eosin stain (Coackley and Pini 1965). The virus was closely associated with the membrane of cytoplasmic vacuoles. The viral particles were spherical or slightly oval, with a diameter of 70 to 80 nm, but elongated forms also occurred (Terpstra 1970; Munz *et al.* 1981).

EPIZOOTIOLOGY

The presence of NSD, as determined either by evidence of clinical syndromes or serologically, is reported from Kenya, Uganda, Somalia, Tanzania, and Zaïre. The occurrence is related to the geographical distribution of certain *Rhipicephalus* ticks. Permanently infested areas are likely to be enzootic.

Literature

The economic importance of NSD has not been established in various parts of Africa. Davies (1978a) stated that NSD virus caused the most pathogenic virus infection in sheep and goats in Kenya with a mortality of up to 90%. Jessett *et al.* (1976) pointed out that survey work on the incidence of NSD in Kenya had been carried out using the indirect FA test. Serum samples collected from sheep and goats from various areas throughout Tanzania indicated that NSD was also enzootic in Tanzania (Jessett 1978). The disease was detected in a 1969–72 epizootic in sheep in Somalia where during this time 90% of the so-called 'tick-fever' cases were NSD; however, the virus was not isolated. The morbidity varied from 30 to 70% and mortality from 50 to 80%. Approximately 10% of the sheep had complicating bacterial pneumonia caused by *Pasteurella haemolytica*. The widespread distribution of disease in northern Somalia was associated with *R. pulchellus* (Edelstein 1975).

Although *Rhipicephalus* ticks other than *R. appendiculatus* could transmit the disease, this species was the most efficient vector in Kenya (Lewis 1949; Davies 1978b).

The infection was confined to the salivary glands (Henning 1956) and was transmitted both transstadially and transovarially (Montgomery 1917; Davies and Mwakima 1982). Infection was thought to be lost from ticks after feeding on susceptible, resistant, and immune animals, but these ticks could be subsequently reinfected (Neitz 1966). However, more recently it has been shown that the virus could be transmitted transstadially by the ticks after feeding on these three different types of hosts (Davies and Mwakima 1982). The virus survived for nearly 3 years in adult ticks, for at least a year in nymphs, and for up to 1 year in larvae. Pastures infected with infected ticks remained infective for sheep for at least 18 months (Lewis 1946, 1949). Experimentally, it was possible to transmit the disease by *A. variegatum*, but it was considered to be a far less efficient vector than *R. appendiculatus* (Daubney and Hudson 1934).

INFECTION

Sheep and goats are the species naturally susceptible to infection. Cattle can be infected experimentally, and in this species blood remains infective for only 24 hours. During the febrile period in sheep and goats, the virus is present in various organs as well as in urine, feces, and in fluid effusions in the abdominal cavity. It cannot usually be demonstrated in tissues 24 hours after temperature has returned to normal. Experimental infection can be induced by administering infective material by various routes, but transmission by contact does not occur.

Literature

During the first 8 days of infection the virus was isolated from plasma, spleen, liver, and mesenteric lymph nodes. Fine, granular fluorescent particles were seen in lymphoblasts, first in the regional lymph nodes adjacent to the site of the inoculation, and then in the spleen, mesenteric lymph nodes, and the mucosa, and submucosa of the ileum, jejunum, and abomasum. In the intestinal mucosa, fluorescence was also observed in the epithelial cells of the villi (Davies *et al.* 1977).

CLINICAL SIGNS

The disease is manifested by a syndrome varying in severity from acute bloody dysentery to a mild fever without evidence of diarrhea. After experimental infection, fever occurs within 48 hours. In the peracute cases, the fever drops off suddenly after 2 to 4 days, clinical signs develop, and mortality occurs quickly. In the less acute, it persists for a longer period of time and falls off gradually. Clinical signs consist of depression, inappetance, mucopurulent nasal discharge which may contain blood, and rapid respiration and pulse. A characteristic sign is the bright to dark green watery diarrhea accompanied by straining and grunting with evidence of considerable pain. The external genitalia of ewes may be swollen and abortions commonly occur. A second fever peak may occur from 3 to 7 days later and it may also terminate fatally, but is often followed by recovery without development of clinical signs.

In the less acute form, the clinical signs are milder and are limited to depression and diarrhea. If diarrhea develops, the prognosis is usually grave. Death occurs approximately 2 days after the fall of temperature, which is usually 4 to 8 days after infection. The mortality rate may be as high as 70%.

Literature

Henning (1956) presented the most complete description of the clinical signs. Neitz (1966) and Weinbren *et al.* (1958) also reported similar manifestations of disease which was characterized by the fever and diarrhea.

PATHOLOGY

The pathology of NSD is, as yet, not well defined and the pathogenesis is unknown. The main macroscopic lesions described are serosal and mucosal hemorrhages and evidence of enteritis. Histologically, glomerulonephritis is reported. Descriptions of microscopic lesions in either the gastrointestinal tract in association with the hemorrhages, ulcerations, and the diarrhea, or in the major lymphoid organs are not available.

Literature

The severity of macroscopic lesions varied with the syndromes and were characterized by mucosal and serosal hemorrhages, enlarged spleen with prominent Malpighian corpuscles, and characteristic changes in the gastrointestinal tract with hemorrhagic inflammation and ulceration of the mucosa of the abomasum, small intestine, with the most severe lesions occurring in the large intestine (Daubney and Hudson 1931). In the colon and rectum, the mucosa was edematous with characteristic striped appearance due to the linear hemorrhages (Weinbren *et al.* 1958). In ewes, there was inflammation of the uterus and vagina, and in pregnant animals the fetus had extensive hemorrhages (Henning 1956). In experimental infections, lesions in spleen and lymph nodes were enlarged 24 hours after infection. Congestion was obvious in the gastrointestinal tract at 72 hours, and at 96 hours the most constant lesion was congestion of the trachea and longitudinal hemorrhages in the colon. Epicardial hemorrhages were found during the latter stages of infection. By 96 hours most extensive hemorrhages were present in the lower gastrointestinal tract. Histologically, in addition to the hemorrhages in various tissues, hepatocytic necrosis occurred around central veins and acute glomerular nephritis was evident (Mugera and Chema 1967). The pathognomonic lesion was the glomerulonephritis which was detected

72 hours after the clinical syndrome commenced. The early acute lesions were glomerulonephritis, and later interstitial tissue was also affected (Neitz 1966; Weinbren *et al.* 1958). Intracerebral injection of adult mice resulted in coagulation necrosis of the brain with widespread loss of neurons but no perivascular inflammatory cell cuffing. In infant mice, brain lesions were much less severe and, in addition, there was a generalized myositis and myocarditis. The hematological picture was characterized by leukopenia and decreased total serum protein (Weinbren *et al.*, 1958; Mugera and Chema 1967).

IMMUNOLOGY

Recovery from infection results in solid immunity. Antibody response is detectable by complement fixation and precipitation, FA, and indirect hemagglutination tests, but not by the neutralization test.

Literature

Recovered animals were solidly immune and resistance was lifelong (Neitz 1966). Complement fixation, indirect fluorescent antibody (IFA), indirect hemagglutination, and serum neutralization tests were used to study the antibody responses in sheep for 15 months following infection with virulent NSD. Complement-fixing antibodies could be detected for 6 to 9 months, while the FA and indirect hemagglutination tests could be used for 15 months (Davies *et al.* 1976). Precipitating antibodies could be demonstrated 1 to 2 days after the disappearance of viremia (Terpstra 1970). The indirect hemagglutination test was developed, shown to be specific and highly sensitive, and was closely correlated with the IFA test (Jessett *et al.* 1976).

VACCINATION

The serial passage of virulent NSD virus through tissue culture or by intracerebral inoculation of mice results in attenuation. Vaccination with attenuated strains is as yet not available.

Literature

A number of techniques were used in the development of a vaccine against NSD. Formalinization of spleen and blood, irradiation of spleen and freezing and thawing of infected spleen material were the early methods tried and were generally ineffective. Intracerebral inoculation of adult mice resulted in development of a neurotropic strain which was partially attenuated between the fourteenth and twenty-second passage, and could be used to immunize sheep against the virulent virus although it was too virulent for field use (Ansell 1957). Virulent virus passaged through tissue culture also produced some attenuation but was not antigenic. Precipitated and killed virus, given in two doses with incomplete Freund's adjuvant, protected sheep. In vaccinated sheep, the virus could be isolated for several days after injection, and a few animals had a transient febrile response and leukopenia (Davies *et al.* 1974). This brain-adapted strain could not be transmitted by ticks, while the attenuated tissue culture strain was transmitted by the vector. The brain-adapted strain has not been tested in vaccines (Terpstra 1970).

CONTROL

The epizootiology of NSD is not defined for most of the enzootic regions of Africa. In enzootic situations, because of the expense of adequate tick control, no control measures can be undertaken. Vaccination has application only when introducing susceptible animals into enzootic areas or when there are extensions from enzootic areas following ecological changes which favor the tick vector.

BIBLIOGRAPHY

Ansell, R. H., 1957. Attenuation of Nairobi sheep disease virus in the mouse brain, *Vet. Rec.*, **69**: 410–12.

Coackley, W. and Pini, A., 1965. The effect of Nairobi sheep disease virus on tissue culture systems, *J. Path. Bact.*, **90**: 672–5.

Daubney, R. and Hudson, J. R., 1931. Nairobi sheep disease, *Parasitology*, **23**: 507–24.

Daubney, R. and Hudson, J. R., 1934. Nairobi sheep disease: natural and experimental transmission by ticks other than *Rhipicephalus appendiculatus*, *Parasitology*, **26**: 496–509.

Davies, F. G., 1978a. A survey of Nairobi sheep disease antibody in sheep and goats, wild ruminants and rodents within Kenya, *J. Hyg., Camb.*, **81**: 251–8.

Davies, F. G., 1978b. Nairobi sheep disease in Kenya. The isolation of virus from sheep and goats, ticks and possible maintenance hosts, *J. Hyg., Camb.*, **81**: 259–65.

Davies, F. G., Casals, J., Jessett, D. M. and Ochieng, P., 1978. The serological relationship of Nairobi sheep disease virus, *J. Comp. Path.*, **88**: 519–23.

Davies, F. G., Jessett, D. M. and Otieno, S., 1976. The antibody response of sheep following infection with Nairobi sheep disease virus, *J. Comp. Path.*, **86**: 497–502.

Davies, F. G., Mungai, J. and Shaw, T., 1974. A Nairobi sheep disease vaccine, *Vet. Rec.*, **94**: 128.

Davies, F. G., Mungai, J. N. and Taylor, M. 1977. The laboratory diagnosis of Nairobi sheep disease, *Trop. Anim. Hlth Prod.*, **9**: 75–80.

Davies, F. G. and Mwakima, F., 1982. Qualitative studies of the transmission of Nairobi sheep disease virus by *Rhipicephalus appendiculatus* (Ixodoidea, Ixodidae), *J. Comp. Path.*, **92**: 15–20.

Edelstein, R. M., 1975. The distribution and prevalence of Nairobi sheep disease and other tick-borne infections of sheep and goats in northern Somalia, *Trop. Anim. Hlth Prod.*, **7**: 29–34.

Henning, M. W., 1956. Nairobi sheep disease. In *Animal Diseases in South Africa. Being an Account of the Infectious Diseases of Domestic Animals*. Central News Agency (South Africa), pp. 1123–7.

Howarth, J. A. and Terpstra, C., 1965. The propagation of Nairobi sheep disease virus in tissue culture, *J. Comp. Path.*, **75**: 437–41.

Jessett, D. M., 1978. Serological evidence of Nairobi sheep disease in Tanzania, *Trop. Anim. Hlth Prod.*, **10**: 99–100.

Jessett, D. M., Davies, F. G. and Rweyemamu, M. M., 1976. An indirect hemagglutination test for the detection of antibody to Nairobi sheep disease virus, *Res. vet. Sci.*, **20**: 276–80.

Lewis, E. A., 1946. Nairobi sheep disease: the survival of the virus in the tick *Rhipicephalus appendiculatus*, *Parasitology*, **37**: 55–9.

Lewis, E. A., 1949. Nairobi sheep disease. In *Annual Report of the Department of Veterinary Services, Kenya*, p. 51.

Melnick, J. L., 1973. Classification and nomenclature of viruses. In *Ultrastructure of Animal Viruses and Bacteriophages. An Atlas*, eds A. J. Dalton, F. Haguenau. Academic Press (London and New York), pp. 1–20.

Montgomery, E., 1917. On a tick-borne gastroenteritis of sheep and goats occurring in British East Africa, *J. Comp. Path.*, **30**: 38–57.

Mugera, G. M. and Chema, S., 1967. Nairobi sheep disease: a study of the pathogenesis in sheep, goats and suckling mice, *Bull. epiz. Dis. Afr.*, **15**: 337–54.

Munz, E., Gobal, E., Krolopp, C., Reimann, M. and Davies, F. G., 1981. Electron microscopic studies on the morphology of Nairobi sheep disease virus, *Zbl. Vet. Med.*, **B28**: 553–63.

Neitz, W. O., 1966. Nairobi sheep disease, *Bull. Off. int. Epiz.*, **65**(9–10): 1743–8.

Terpstra, C., 1970. Nairobi sheep disease, studies on virus properties, epizootiology and vaccination in Uganda, *Tijdschr. Diergeneesk.*, **95**(13): 671–7.

Weinbren, M. P., Gourlay, R. N., Lumsden, W. H. R. and Weinbren, B. M., 1958. An epizootic of Nairobi sheep disease in Uganda, *J. Comp. Path.*, **68**: 174–87.

Chapter

12

Peste des petits ruminants

CONTENTS

INTRODUCTION

Peste des petits ruminants (PPR) is a contagious viral disease, resembling rinderpest, of goats and sheep in West Africa, and characterized by clinical signs and lesions of respiratory and alimentary systems involvement.

Literature

Scott (1981) presented a most comprehensive up-to-date review of PPR and its history, and compared the disease to rinderpest. Peste des petits ruminants was first observed in 1940 in sheep and goats in the Ivory Coast (Gargadennec and Lalanne 1942). The early work by Mornet *et al.* (1956a, b) showed that the virus was related to the rinderpest virus. They concluded that it actually was a rinderpest virus with adapted pathogenicity for goats and sheep.

In 1965 a syndrome was described in western Nigeria in dwarf goats, which closely resembled rinderpest and was known by the local name of *kata*, and characterized by high mortality with recovering animals developing prominent labial scabs on the mouth (Whitney *et al.* 1967). A comparative study of PPR and *kata* showed that on the basis of clinical signs, cross-protection, and lesions the syndrome produced by the PPR virus and the virus isolated from *kata* were indistinguishable. Similar intranuclear inclusions were also found in lymphoid and epithelial cells in *kata* as were seen in PPR (Rowland *et al.* 1971). Antibody responses in goats experimentally infected with either rinderpest virus or PPR virus were distinguishable by neutralizing antibody titration methods using PPR virus (Taylor 1979a). Further viral studies from animals dying from PPR resulted in isolation of two viruses: PPR virus and an adenovirus which was thought to be a commensal (Gibbs *et al.* 1977). It was concluded that PPR virus was enzootic in the small ruminant population of Nigeria (Durtnell 1972; Taylor 1979a).

Orf and pox viruses have to be considered in making a differential diagnosis of PPR. The incidence of orf in sheep and goats in Nigeria was reviewed, and it was considered to occur as either a complication of PPR or as a cause of mouth lesions which had to be distinguished from the lesions seen on lips in more chronic forms of PPR (Obi and Gibbs 1978).

ETIOLOGY

On the basis of morphology, growth in tissue culture, the nucleic acid composition antigens, and physicochemical properties, the PPR virus is classified as the fourth member of the genus *Morbillivirus* of Paramyxoviridae and grouped together with the canine distemper, human measles, and rinderpest viruses. Ovine and caprine kidney cell cultures are used for the isolation and assay of the virus. A cytopathic effect develops between 6 and 15 days after inoculation, resulting in large clock-faced syncytia which sometimes contain intranuclear inclusions.

Literature

The morphology, as observed by negative staining electron microscopy, was typical of paramyxoviruses, and staining with acridine orange and Feulgen reagents indicated that the genome was ribonucleic acid (Bourdin and Laurent-Vautier 1967; Gibbs *et al*. 1979). The structure of PPR virus is comparable to that of rinderpest and measles viruses in having an envelope with projections. The virions are enveloped in helical particles, usually exceeding 500 nm, which are pleomorphic, either spheres or filaments, and the envelopes bristle with minute projections (Bourdin and Laurent-Vautier 1967).

Multiplication of the PPR virus in tissue cultures was similar to that of rinderpest virus (Hamdy and Dardiri 1976). It grew in ovine embryo kidney cells and caused formation of multinucleated giant cells with eosinophilic inclusions. Single- or multiple-inclusion bodies were present in both the cytoplasm and in the nucleus (Johnson and Ritchie 1968; Hamdy and Dardiri 1976). In cultures maintained at 40 °C, but not at 37 °C the virus retained its pathogenicity. Virus grown at lower temperatures could be used to immunize animals (Gilbert and Monnier 1962).

EPIZOOTIOLOGY

In West Africa, PPR is a serious economic problem causing extensive losses in sheep and goats, especially when animals migrate or are transported from one region to another. The disease is most prevalent in animals less than 1 year of age.

Literature

Peste des petits ruminants is enzootic in West Africa. The epizootiology, clinical signs, and diagnostic methods were presented on an outbreak in the Sudan in 1974 by Bourdin and Doutre (1976). Serologically positive animals have been observed in Chad and the Sultanate of Oman (Hedger *et al*. 1980).

In Nigeria, up to 20% of sheep and goats had sera which neutralized rinderpest virus and these animals were determined as not having been in contact with rinderpest-infected cattle (Zwart and Rowe 1966). In another survey on samples collected from abattoirs, about 57% of sheep and 44% of goats had serological evidence of previous exposure to PPR virus. The proportion of positive animals increased with age. In the goat and sheep populations, approximately 25% of animals were positive and there was a large variation in the incidence from one region to another (Taylor 1979a).

INFECTION

The infection is transmitted by close contact, mainly by inhalation, and can be experimentally passaged by suspensions of splenic and lymph node tissues from infected animals. The virus is restricted in its host range, being confined in natural infections to sheep and goats, with the latter species being more often affected. Experimental infection has been shown to cause severe clinical disease in white-tailed deer (*Odocoileus virginianus*).

The virus is excreted by all routes once clinical signs appear after a short incubation period of up to 5 days and does not persist in the tissues of recovered animals. The existence of carriers is not known. On the basis of experimental work in white-tailed deer which, at times, develop infections without clinical signs, the possibility of a carrier state exists in the wild game populations of West Africa. The role of other domestic animals in the epizootiology is not defined.

Literature

The disease has been reported to be highly contagious and quickly spreads within a flock. With the onsert of fever and diarrhea, excretion of PPR virus has been reported to occur in the feces, and in the nasal, ocular, and buccal discharges (Abegunde and Adu 1977). In cattle, PPR virus was not pathogenic and, although neither replication nor excretion of the virus could be demonstrated, antibodies were produced (Gibbs *et al.* 1979). White-tailed deer (*O. virginianus*) have been infected experimentally with PPR virus, causing a variety of clinical syndromes ranging from asymptomatic infections to fatal disease. Clinical and pathological observations were comparable to those seen in goats, and antibodies were detected by the complement fixation (CF) and virus neutralization tests. Survivors were resistant to challenge with virulent rinderpest virus (Hamdy and Dardiri 1976).

CLINICAL SIGNS

Peste des petits ruminants has peracute, acute, and subacute syndromes. Morbidity is often as high as 100%, and mortality can be up to 90% in the most severe outbreaks. Severe PPR is characterized by fever, nasal catarrh, stomatitis, diarrhea, and death, with early development of lesions similar to those of rinderpest, while chronic lesions in the buccal mucosa resemble orf.

The acute syndrome has an incubation period of 5 days with a course of 5 to 6 days terminating in death. The first clinical sign is fever which lasts approximately 5 days in animals that die while in those which survive it lasts about 3 days. Fever is followed quickly by anorexia, with inflammation of the nasal and buccal mucosa which rapidly develops into ulcerative necrotic stomatitis. The exudates from eyes, nose, and mouth quickly become profuse and mucopurulent. During the latter stages of the disease, extensive encrustation by exudate occurs on nares and eyes. This characteristic encrustation on the lips, particularly at the commisures, consists of brown scab material covering patchy erosion, and ulcers of the buccal epithelium.

Literature

Comprehensive reviews of the clinical syndromes in sheep and goats caused by PPR virus were presented by Braide (1981) and Whitney *et al.* (1967). In an experimental infection on American goats, the virus caused 25% mortality. Cattle infected with direct contact with infected goats underwent a subclinical infection, with the development of antibodies which cross-reacted against rinderpest virus (Dardiri *et al.* 1976).

PATHOLOGY

Lesions which characterize PPR are confined to the upper alimentary and respiratory tracts. Degeneration and necrosis of the epithelium result in erosions, ulceration, and profuse initially serous and later mucopurulent exudate which forms the characteristic encrustation of the nares, lips, and around the eyes. Microscopically the lesions are characterized by the development of syncytia, with intranuclear and intracytoplasmic inclusion bodies. These lesions in the stratified squamous epithelium of the upper digestive tract and in the columnar epithelium of the respiratory tract are complicated by secondary bacterial infections, resulting in stomatitis, rhinitis, and bronchopneumonia with extensive inflammatory cell exudate. Necrotic lesions in the glandular mucosa of the lower alimentary tract also occur but are less pronounced than those in the stratified epithelium.

Literature

The lesions observed in the West African dwarf goat with *kata* and PPR were found to be indistinguishable (Rowland *et al.* 1969, 1971). The development of characteristic lesions in fatal acute syndromes was observed in the upper and lower alimentary and respiratory systems. In the upper alimentary tract, the first grossly observable lesions to develop were white foci 1 to 2 mm in diameter which became numerous, enlarged, and confluent, forming extensive areas of superficial erosion often involving the entire mucosa of the buccal cavities, and were covered by desquamated epithelium. Extension of the lesion to the lips resulted in a diffuse grayish deposit of necrotic epithelium forming a scab. The authors refer to the early work in which these lesions in the mouth were described as exudative labial dermatitis, characterized by hyperplasia of the epithelium, and formation of syncytia. The lesions extended to the pharynx and esophagus, where multiple linear erosions were present. Characteristic early microscopic changes involved degeneration, and necrosis occurred in the stratum granulosum of the stratified squamous epithelium. The lesion usually did not penetrate the stratum germinativum. Eosinophilic intracytoplasmic inclusions were constant but not numerous in the degenerating epithelium. Desquamation and accumulation of inflammatory debris occurred on the stratum spinosum. This lesion progressed to develop into small intraepidermal abscesses with extensive inflammatory cell reaction and acanthosis. Secondary bacterial invasion of the surface debris occurred.

In the buccal mucosa, the more chronic lesions were characterized by cytoplasmic vacuolation in the stratum granulosum and isolated syncytial formations. The mucosa of the gastrointestinal tract, from the abomasum to the rectum, often did not have macroscopic lesions. Occasionally, petechial hemorrhages and ulcers were found in the glandular mucosa of the stomach. In the small intestine there is a loss of villi with elongation of glands lined by degenerate cells with infrequent inclusions. The lamina propria was infiltrated by a mononuclear inflammatory cell reaction with macrophages containing intranuclear inclusions. In the large intestine, congestion and horizontal hemorrhage in the mucosa, referred to as 'zebra striping', were also observed. The microscopic lesion consisted of scattered, isolated, degenerated, and necrotic cells in the glandular epithelium and intracytoplasmic inclusions with accumulation of cell debris in the lumen of the glands. This was accompanied by focal increase of lymphocytes and eosinophils in the lamina propria.

In the upper respiratory tract there was rhinitis with profuse mucopurulent discharge. Secondary bacterial pneumonia associated with *Pasteurella* infection was a common feature affecting 25% of the animals. Degenerative, necrotic, and hyperplastic changes, which became metaplastic as the lesion progressed, were seen in the cells of the respiratory mucosa extending from the nasal turbinates to the terminal bronchiols. Eosinophilic intracytoplasmic inclusions were occasionally present in these cells. Associated with lesions in the terminal bronchiols was consolidation of the surrounding alveolar tissue, with formation of giant cells which contained intranuclear inclusion bodies. In the liver, there was focal fatty degeneration and necrosis.

Rowland *et al.* (1969) did not report specific lesions in the lymphoreticular system. In those lymph nodes draining the upper respiratory and digestive tracts, occasional necrosis of the medullary cords was observed and there were no changes in the lymphoid tissue in the mucosa of the digestive tract. However, Whitney *et al.* (1967) reported that throughout the entire gastrointestinal tract the Peyer's patches were necrotic. There was also enlargement, hemorrhage and edema of the lymph nodes throughout the body and, microscopically, lymphocytolysis and necrosis of lymphoid follicles were observed in the spleen and lymph nodes. In severe clinical cases Rowland *et al.* (1971) found intramuscular inclusions in reticuloendothelial cells of lymph node sinuses and germinal centers.

IMMUNOLOGY

The serological relationship between PPR and rinderpest viruses is close, but cross-neutralization tests can differentiate the two viruses. Peste des petits ruminants virus protects cattle against rinderpest, and conversely the rinderpest virus protects sheep and goats against PPR. The antigenic relationship as determined by cross-immunization tests established that the antigenic homology was not greater between the PPR virus and canine distemper, measles, and rinderpest viruses than the known homogeneity between these three viruses.

Literature

The virus has been regarded to be of one antigenic type and closely related to rinderpest. The antigen in infected cells was found around the virus particles at the budding stages (Hamdy *et al.* 1975). Complement fixation and particularly neutralization tests have shown that the viruses are not identical, based on titration methods (Taylor 1979b). The PPR virus was also related to measles and canine distemper by the CF test (Dardiri *et al.* 1976). Primary lamb kidney cell cultures were appropriate for the isolation of field strains of PPR virus. Further serology using cross-neutralization tests showed that four strains of virus were distinct but related to rinderpest virus (Taylor and Abegunde 1979). In the early work comparing the *kata* and PPR viruses, cross-challenge of goats infected with one virus challenged with another showed development of cross-immunity (Rowland *et al.* 1971; Rowland and Bourdin 1970).

VACCINATION

Because various isolates of PPR virus are of one antigenic type, use of the bovine tissue culture rinderpest vaccine is recommended. Although limited experimental work is encouraging, the efficacy of this method of vaccination in protecting sheep and goats against PPR has not been fully determined in the field. Only partial protection can be induced with either measles or canine distemper viruses.

Literature

Goats vaccinated with the Kabete 'O' strain of rinderpest virus, which had undergone serial passage in calf kidney cells, protected goats against virulent PPR virus challenge for at least 12 months. Neutralizing antibody against rinderpest was present prior to challenge and higher antibody titers developed to both viruses after challenge with PPR virus (Bourdin *et al.* 1970; Bourdin 1973; Taylor 1979b). Rinderpest vaccine was used to protect pregnant West African dwarf goats against PPR and there was no adverse reaction to the vaccine (Adu and Nawatha 1981). These workers quoted information presented by Nduaka and Ihemelandu (1978) who reported that the rinderpest vaccine precipitated the development of PPR in apparently healthy goats which were incubating the disease (Adu and Nawatha 1981). Cross-protection with other members of the genus *Morbillivirus* was also tested. The Schwarz strain vaccine of measles virus did not protect against PPR while canine distemper did have some cross-protection. The challenge PPR virus was found to multiply in those animals which had been immunized with either rinderpest, canine distemper, or measles viruses, but not in animals recovered from PPR (Gibbs *et al.* 1979).

BIBLIOGRAPHY

Abegunde, A. A. and Adu, F. D., 1977. Excretion of the virus of peste des petits ruminants by goats, *Bull. Anim. Hlth Prod.*, **25**: 307–11.

Adu, F. D. and Nawatha, D. R., 1981. Safety of tissue culture rinderpest vaccine in pregnant goats, *Trop. Anim. Hlth Prod.*, **13**: 166.

Bourdin, P. and Doutre, M. P., 1976. Pseudo-rinderpest of small ruminants in Senegal. New data, *Rev. Elev. Méd. vét. Pays trop.*, **26**(4): 71a–74a.

Bourdin, P. and Doutre, M. P., 1976. Pseudo-rinderpest of small ruminants in Senegal. New data, *Rev. Elev. Méd. vét. Pays trop.*, **29**(3): 199–204.

Bourdin, P. and Laurent-Vautier, A., 1967. Note on the structure of the small ruminants pest virus, *Rev. Elev. Méd. vét. Pays trop.*, **20**(3): 383–6.

Bourdin, P., Rioche, M. and Laurent, A., 1970. A tissue culture vaccine against pseudo-rinderpest of goats – field experiments in Dahomey, *Rev. Elev. Méd. vét. Pays trop.*, **23**(3): 295–300.

Braide, V. B., 1981. Peste des petits ruminants. A review. *Wld Anim. Rev.*, **39**: 25–28.

Dardiri, A. H., DeBoer, C. J. and Hamdy, F.M., 1976. Response of American goats and cattle to peste des petits ruminants virus, *Proc. 19th Ann. Meet. Am. Ass. Vet. Lab. Diagnost.*, 1976, pp. 337–44.

Durtnell, R. E., 1972. A disease of Sokoto goats resembling 'Peste des petits ruminants', *Trop. Anim. Hlth Prod.*, **4**: 162–4.

Gargadennec, L. and Lalanne, A., 1942. La peste des petits ruminants, *Bull. Serv. Zootech. Epiz.*, **5**(1): 16–21.

Gibbs, E. P. J., Taylor, W. P. and Lawman, M. J. P., 1977. The isolation of adenoviruses from goats affected with peste des petits ruminants in Nigeria, *Res. vet. Sci.*, **23**: 331–5.

Gibbs, E. P. J., Taylor, W. P., Lawman, M. J. P. and Bryant, J., 1979. Classification of peste des petits ruminants virus as the fourth member of the genus *Morbillivirus*, *Intervirology*, **11**: 268–74.

Gilbert, Y. and Monnier, J., 1962. Adaptation du virus de la peste des petits ruminants aux cultures cellulaires. Note préliminaire, *Rev. Elev. Méd. vét. Pays trop.*, **15**: 321–35.

Hamdy, F. M. and Dardiri, A. H., 1976. Response of white-tailed deer to infection with peste des petits ruminants virus, *J. Wildl. Dis.*, **12**: 516–22.

Hamdy, F. M., Dardiri, A. H., Breese, S. S. Jr and DeBoer, C. J., 1975. Immunologic relationship between rinderpest and peste des petits ruminants viruses, *Proc. Ann. Meet. US Anim. Hlth Assoc.*, 1975, **79**: 168–79.

Hedger, R. S., Barnett, I. T. R. and Gray, D. F., 1980. Some virus diseases of domestic animals in the Sultanate of Oman, *Trop. Anim. Hlth Prod.*, **12**: 107–14.

Johnson, R. H. and Ritchie, J. S. D., 1968. A virus associated with pseudo-rinderpest in Nigerian dwarf goats, *Bull. epiz. Dis. Afr.*, **16**: 411–17.

Mornet, P., Gilbert, Y., Orue, J., Thiery, G. and Mamadou, S., 1956a. 'La peste des petits ruminants' en Afrique Occidentale française. Ses rapports avec la peste bovine, *Rev. Elev. Méd. vét. Pays trop.*, **9**: 313–35.

Mornet, P., Orue, J. and Gilbert, Y., 1956b. Unicité et plasticité du virus bovipestique. A propos d'un virus naturel adapté sur petits ruminants, *Compte Rendus Hebdomadaires des Séances de l'Academie des Sciences*, **242**: 2886–9.

Nduaka, O. and Ihemelandu, E. C., 1978. *Ann. Conf. Nigerian vet. Med. Assoc.*

Obi, T. U. and Gibbs, E. P. J., 1978. Orf in sheep and goats in Nigeria, *Trop. Anim. Hlth Prod.*, **10**: 233–5.

Rowland, A. C. and Bourdin, P., 1970. The histological relationship between 'peste des petits ruminants' and kata in West Africa, *Rev. Elev. Méd vét. Pays trop.*, **23**: 301–7.

Rowland, A. C., Scott, G. R. and Hill, D. H., 1969. The pathology of an erosive stomatitis and enteritis in West-African dwarf goats, *J. Pathol.*, **98**: 83–7.

Rowland, A. C., Scott, G. R., Ramachandran, S. and Hill, D. H., 1971. A comparative study of peste des petits ruminants and Kata in West African dwarf goats, *Trop. Anim. Hlth Prod.*, **3**: 241–7.

Scott, G. R., 1981. Rinderpest and peste des petits ruminants. In *Virus Diseases of Food Animals. A World Geography of Epidemiology and Control*, ed. E. P. J. Gibbs. Academic Press (New York), Disease monographs, vol. II, pp. 401–32.

Taylor, W. P., 1979a. Serological studies with the virus of peste des petits ruminants in Nigeria, *Res. vet Sci.*, **26**: 236–42.

Taylor, W. P., 1979b. Protection of goats against peste des-petits-ruminants with attenuated rinderpest vaccine, *Res. vet. Sci.*, **23**: 321–4.

Taylor, W. P. and Abegunde, A., 1979. Isolation of peste des petits ruminants virus from Nigerian sheep and goats, *Res. vet. Sci.*, **26**: 94–6.

Whitney, J. C., Scott, G. R. and Hill, D. H., 1967. Preliminary observations on a stomatitis and enteritis of goats in southern Nigeria, *Bull. epiz. Dis. Afr.*, **15**: 31–41.

Zwart, D. and Rowe, L. W., 1966. The occurrence of rinderpest antibodies in the sera of sheep and goats in northern Nigeria, *Res. vet. Sci.*, **7**: 504–11.

Chapter

13

Pox viruses

CONTENTS

INTRODUCTION

Sheeppox, goatpox, buffalopox, and camelpox are contagious viral infections. The ovine and caprine syndromes are the most severe of the pox diseases which afflict domestic animals. In various tropical regions, sheeppox causes mortality in lambs and mastitis and abortion in ewes. Buffalopox virus causes a syndrome which clinically resembles that induced by cowpox virus. It is classified separately in the vaccinia–variola subgroup of pox viruses. Various characteristics of the camelpox virus are similar to those of the smallpox virus of man. It is believed that pox diseases originally came from one or more basic strains which, over the course of time, changed and became adapted to different hosts.

Literature

Sheeppox and goatpox infections were investigated most extensively in India and the Middle East (Davies 1981; Singh *et al.* 1979). Most of the work on buffalopox was undertaken in India, where it is considered to be a disease of economic importance (Lal and Singh 1973a).

ETIOLOGY

The viruses in the Poxviridae family have a characteristic morphology by which they are readily identified and assigned to pox virus groups. The classification of pox viruses depends on the following criteria: morphology, presence of double-stranded deoxyribonucleic acid (DNA) in the viral genome, antigenic relationship to other pox viruses, sensitivity to lipid solvents, acid lability, and induction of skin lesions. All the viruses are antigenically related, and the possession of common internal antigens is an important taxonomic criterion. Pox viruses survive for long periods of time in the environment, especially in the scab material from the skin lesions of recovered animals, which yield viable virus for at least 3 months.

Sheeppox and goatpox viruses grow in many ovine, caprine, and bovine cell tissue cultures and produce intracytoplasmic inclusion bodies and cytopathic effects (CPEs). The CPEs consist of increased cellular density, with the cell outline being clearly demarcated, followed by rounding and detachment from the monolayer. The intracytoplasmic eosinophilic inclusions stain positive for DNA. Only some isolates can be grown in embryonated chicken eggs, but buffalopox and camelpox viruses can be propagated in chicken embryos as well as in a number of different tissue cell lines.

Literature

In the *Manual of Standardized Methods for Veterinary Microbiology*, Cottral (1978) divided the members of the Poxviridae family into the genera and subgroups shown in Table 13.1.

The buffalopox and camelpox viruses have been added to the genus *Orthopoxvirus* (Baxby and Hill 1971; Tantawi *et al.* 1978).

Table 13.1

Genera and subgroups	Strain	Genera and subgroups	Strain
Orthopoxvirus (variola–vaccinia)	Vaccinia Cowpox Variola Alastrim Rabbitpox Monkeypox Ectromelia	*Avipoxvirus* (avianpox)	Fowlpox Turkeypox Canarypox Pigeonpox
		Leporipoxvirus (myxoma)	Myxoma (Brazil) Myxoma (Calif.) Rabbit fibroma Hare fibroma Squirrel fibroma
Parapoxvirus (orf)	Orf Bovine pseudopox Bovine papular stomatitis Sealpox	(Molluscum)	Molluscum contagiosum Yaba pox Yaba-like pox Tana pox
Capripoxvirus (sheeppox)	Sheeppox Goatpox Bovine lumpy skin disease	(Swinepox)	Swinepox

The structure of the pox viruses was reviewed in detail by Joklik (1966). The physicochemical properties of sheeppox and goatpox viruses were presented in tabular form (Singh *et al.* 1979). In electron micrographs, sheeppox virus morphologically resembled other animal pox viruses but was smaller and more elongated (Abdussalam 1957). The sensitivity of sheeppox and goatpox viruses to heat, chloroform, and ether was determined and it was found that the viruses were sensitive to both chloroform and ether (Pandey and Singh 1970a; Plowright and Ferris 1959).

The buffalopox virus was first isolated by Singh and Singh (1967) during an outbreak of disease in buffalo in India. The biological, physiochemical, and serological properties of the buffalopox virus justified its classification as a separate member of the variola–vaccinia group of pox viruses (Baxby and Hill 1969, 1971; Lal and Singh 1977). It appeared that the virus was less common in buffalo than the vaccinia virus (Baxby and Hill 1971). Electron-microscopic studies demonstrated that the ultrastructure of buffalopox virus in infected chorioallantoic membranes was comparable to that of the vaccinia virus (Bloch and Lal 1975). The results obtained from gel diffusion, immunoelectrophoretic and complement-fixation (CF) tests showed that the buffalopox virus was different from, but closely related to, the vaccinia and cowpox viruses (Lal and Singh 1973b).

Camelpox virus was classified as a pox virus on the basis of its morphological, biological, and physicochemical characteristics. It was found to be serologically and morphologically related to the vaccinia–variola subgroup (Mahnel and Bartenbach 1973). Despite the fact that the experimental host range and laboratory characteristics of camelpox and smallpox viruses were similar, *in vivo* studies confirmed epidemiological evidence that camels were unlikely to act as alternative hosts for smallpox virus (Baxby *et al.* 1975).

The growth characteristics of sheeppox and goatpox viruses in various tissues cultures were reported by Singh *et al.* (1979). The multiplication of sheeppox virus in lamb kidney and lamb testis cell cultures was described (Lang and Leftheriotis 1961; Kalra and Sharma 1981; Edlinger and Iftimovici 1973; Pandey *et al.* 1969). The cultivation of goatpox virus in sheep kidney, goat kidney, and goat testis cell cultures was also reported (Ramyar 1966). Although cell lines derived from testes and kidneys of very young lambs, kids, and calves were generally used for the propagation of sheeppox and goatpox viruses, thyroid cell tissue cultures obtained from mature animals had the advantage of being readily available and relatively easy to grow (Nitzschke *et al.* 1967). The optimum conditions for the replication of attenuated sheeppox virus in lamb kidney cell cultures were investigated. Primary cell cultures were best utilized 4 to 7 days after infection, and the optimum pH and incubation temperature were 8.2 and 36 to 37 °C respectively (Soman and Singh 1981).

In an in-depth review of the biochemical events which occur during the general pox virus infection cycle, Joklik (1966) described the uncoating of the viral genome, the synthesis and fate of viral messenger ribonucleic acid and virus-coded protein, the replication of viral DNA, and the maturation process. The growth curves of identical viruses were dependent on the cultural conditions, and pox viruses were generally not liberated readily from the cells in which they multiplied. Viruses of the variola subgroup caused two types of cytopathic effect: (1) cell rounding, which was thought to be a cellular response to the ingestion of virus particles; and (2) cell fusion, which led to the formation of giant syncytia and occurred when the viral DNA replicated (Joklik 1966). In some cell culture systems, camelpox and smallpox viruses could be differentiated by these cytopathic effects: the former virus produced multinucleated giant cells, whereas the latter caused rounding up of individual cells. However, in other cell lines, there was little or no difference between the cultural characteristics of these viruses (Baxby 1974; Bedson 1972). The CPEs induced by sheeppox and goatpox viruses in lamb and kid kidney and testicular cell monolayers were characterized by degenerative changes in the nucleus and cytoplasm and the formation of intracytoplasmic inclusions which stained positive for DNA (Cilli 1961; Pandey and Singh 1970b; Plowright and Ferris 1958; Soman and Singh 1980). Light and electron-microscopic examination of the staining properties of viral inclusions in infected cells confirmed that the inclusions are the site of DNA and protein synthesis (Joklik 1966).

Direct fluorescent antibody (FA) techniques were used to study the multiplication of sheeppox virus in sheep embryo cells, and viral proteins were demonstrated in the cytoplasm as early as 14 hours after infection. The number of infected cells and the amount of viral antigen increased with time (Vigário and Ferraz 1967). The infection cycle of sheeppox virus in embryo muscle cell cultures was investigated using autoradiographic and immunofluorescent methods. In these experiments, an inhibitor of DNA synthesis, 5-fluorodeoxyuridine, prevented the formation of infectious virus but did not suppress the virus-induced cytopathology or the synthesis of viral antigens (Vigário *et al.* 1968). The viral DNA contained in the intracytoplasmic inclusions resisted digestion by deoxyribonuclease (Vigário and Terrinha 1964). From comparative studies of the cytopathogenicity and immunogenicity of sheeppox virus in subcultures, it was concluded that the virus which was to be used for immunization should possess the property of intracytoplasmic replication (Soman and Singh 1980).

The pocks produced on the chorioallantoic membrane of chicken embryos by the variola–vaccinia group of pox viruses have been used in the identification of these viruses and in the study of their characteristics. Generally, these lesions have not been seen with sheeppox and goatpox viruses (Baxby 1969; Sen and Uppal 1972). It has been reported that a strain of sheeppox virus from Egypt was successfully cultivated on the chorioallantoic membrane of chicken embryos and could be passaged using the alternating method (Sabban 1957). Pock counting on the chorioallantoic membrane of chicken embryos was a more sensitive method of assaying buffalopox virus than plaque counting in chick embryo fibroblast monolayers (Bansal and Singh 1974). Various strains of camelpox virus from widely separated geographical areas produced white pock lesions on the chorioallantoic membranes of chicken embryos (Tantawi *et al.* 1978).

EPIZOOTIOLOGY

Sheeppox and goatpox are the two most important viral infections of domestic animals, causing significant economic losses because of the high morbidity and mortality, partial loss of reproductive potential, and effect on the wool and hair. The diseases are endemic and occur in the Near, Middle, and Far East and Africa. Buffalopox has been reported in India, Indonesia, Italy, Pakistan, the USSR and Egypt. In contrast, there have been only limited reports of camelpox epidemics. Pox diseases are relatively rare among domestic animals in Europe and North America. The transmission of pox viruses occurs through close contact and inhalation. Contaminated premises may be infective for up to 6 months.

Literature

There is little detailed information on the epizootiology and economic importance of the pox diseases affecting sheep, goats, buffalo and camels. Davies (1976) discussed to occurrence of sheeppox and goatpox in Kenya. These diseases were enzootic in some parts of the country since 82% of the animals sampled showed specific antibodies to the viruses. In enzootic areas, the morbidity was 5 to 10% with a very low mortality; young animals were predominantly involved. However, in regions where antibodies to sheeppox and goatpox viruses were not detected, there were massive epizootics affecting thousands of animals. In these susceptible flocks the morbidity was 60%; the rest of the animals developed inapparent infections. The mortality was usually below 2% in the indigenous hair sheep and goats, although it could be considerably higher in young lambs and kids during periods of drought. The course of the disease in the flocks was rapid, with infection involving most animals within 4 weeks (Davies 1976). An outbreak of sheeppox in Nigeria resulted in 100% morbidity and 30% mortality (Aasagba and Nawathe 1980). In recent years, the nodular form of sheeppox has caused serious problems in the Sudan, where a mortality rate of 6% has been observed. Some outbreaks of sheeppox coincided with outbreaks of bovine lumpy skin disease (LSD) (Muzichin and Ali 1979).

Because the nonvesicular forms of sheeppox and goatpox had been observed to spread rapidly in field epizootics, Davies (1981) proposed that an arthropod vector may be involved in the mechanical transmission of the viruses. In endemic areas, pox viruses are probably maintained through short-cycle transmission and their ability to resist desiccation and other hostile environmental factors. These viruses can survive in scab material for periods of 3 to 6 months (Singh *et al.* 1979). Thus, recovered animals are a source of infection to susceptible populations with which they come into contact during seasonal grazing and trade movements (Davies 1981).

The infection was readily transmitted experimentally by scarification and intradermal, subcutaneous, and intravenous injection (Katiyar 1961).

INFECTION

The sheeppox and goatpox viruses are generally host-specific, but in certain areas there may be cross-infection between sheep and goats. The viruses found in Kenya differ from those observed in India and the Middle East in that they are not host-specific and show some pathogenicity for both sheep and goats; in mixed flocks, both species are affected in natural outbreaks. Laboratory animals are refractory to these two pox viruses. All strains of camelpox virus are pathogenic for monkeys and for mice on intracerebral inoculation. The host specificity of the camelpox and buffalopox viruses is not known. The existence of nonhost-adapted pox virus strains has resulted in outbreaks of pox disease in a variety of species in zoological gardens.

In the World Health Organization scheme for the eradication of smallpox, attention is given to animal pox viruses which share properties with smallpox virus, (e.g. the ability to infect different species) and to the possible role of the animals as reservoirs.

Literature

Davies (1981) discussed the host specificity of sheeppox and goatpox viruses. The host specificity of these pox viruses has not been clearly established because of reports in the early literature of experimentally induced cross-infections. The viruses in Kenya were found to be host-specific for either sheep or goats; however, necrotic skin lesions could be produced experimentally in cattle. Many strains outside Africa were adapted to either sheep or goats, and although local skin reactions could be experimentally induced, there was no evidence of cross-infection under natural field conditions (Davies 1981). Inoculation of sheeppox virus into a variety of animals, including goats, indicated that it was host-specific (Khan 1960). Sheeppox and goatpox viruses were not infective for chick embryos, day-old mice, rabbits, guinea pigs, or hamsters. The sheeppox virus infected goats while the goatpox virus did not affect sheep (Sharma *et al.* 1966; Sharma and Dhanda 1972). During natural outbreaks of sheeppox and goatpox, Davies (1976) observed that skin lesions failed to develop in a large number of animals. The existence of silent infections was confirmed by serological studies using the indirect fluorescent antibody (IFA) technique (Davies 1976). The camelpox virus infects monkeys and infant mice (Baxby 1972; quoted by Baxby *et al.* 1975).

The information on cross-infections among captive wild animals was summarized by Baxby (1977). There have been reports of cowpox infection in okapies, cheetahs, and elephants in a zoological garden. Outbreaks of a pox disease in a Russian zoo primarily affected members of the family Felidae and caused high mortality. Rats acting as the reservoir hosts of a cowpox-like virus proved to be the source of these epidemics (Baxby 1977).

The campaign to eradicate smallpox in man depends on the assumption that this virus does not have an animal reservoir. A particular animal species is regarded as a reservoir of a given pox virus when (1) there is serological and clinical evidence of the involvement of the species, and (2) viral isolation indicates that the incidence of infection is sufficient to insure the survival and transmission of the virus under natural conditions (Baxby 1977).

After inoculation into the skin of African and Merino sheep, sheeppox virus exhibited a complete eclipse phase which was followed by a phase of logarithmic increase. Peak titers occurred in tissues sampled on the seventh or eighth day postinfection and were maintained until the fourteenth day, after which they slowly declined. A mild leukocytosis affecting predominantly the neutrophils was associated with the development of the local lesions. The viremia lasted for up to 7 days. The affinity of the virus for different tissues and organs has not been clearly defined; some workers have found that the virus is widely disseminated in the body (Plowright *et al.* 1959; Singh *et al.* 1979). The pox virus is associated with the white blood cells during viremia. Subsequently it is found in skin lesions, regional lymph nodes, the spleen, and lesions in various organs, particularly the kidney and the lungs. The virus is present in the secretions from the skin lesions and is also found in milk and saliva. The main source of virus for transmission is the scab material on healed lesions in which the virus may persist for 3 to 6 months (Davies 1981).

CLINICAL SIGNS

The pox diseases of sheep, goats, buffalo and camels are characterized by the formation of pustules on the skin; signs of systemic infection may also be present. The clinical syndromes exhibited by sheep and goats vary in different geographical regions according to the virus strain and host species involved. Although all age groups can be affected, pox infections are most severe in young animals. Secondary bacterial infections complicate the disease. In a severe epizootic, the morbidity may exceed 75% and 50% of the affected animals succumb. The mortality in animals under 4 months of age is approximately 100%.

In sheep, the incubation period varies from 4 to 7 days. The acute disease is characterized by a severe systemic response with widespread vesicular lesions affecting the head, nostrils, lips, and wool-free skin. The vesicular stage is followed by the development of pustules which eventually become covered by scabs. Skin lesions take up to 4 weeks to heal. Severe outbreaks of a variant form of sheeppox frequently occur and cause high morbidity and mortality. This disease differs from the classical form in that the affected sheep develop skin nodules which do not change into vesicles and pustules. The nodules become necrotic and are shed, leaving ulcers that heal very slowly. Approximately 35 to 40% of the affected animals develop secondary pneumonia and die.

Buffalopox is a comparatively benign contagious disease in which lesions localize mainly on the teats and udder. In the generalized form of the disease, other parts of the body are involved. Camelpox is characterized by the presence of typical pox vesicles and pustules which usually have a limited distribution.

Literature

The incubation period varied from 4 to 7 days in sheep (Singh *et al.* 1979) and from 4 to 7 days in goats (Kolayli *et al.* 1933; quoted by Rafyi and Ramyar 1959). The first signs of sheeppox and goatpox were rhinitis, conjunctivitis, fever, depression, and loss of appetite. Vesicular skin lesions erupted 1 to 2 days later and frequently affected the external nares, lips, and buccal surfaces. The extent of cutaneous involvement was variable, lesions being most prominent in areas where the wool or hair was shortest. In some cases, these skin lesions coalesced and affected large areas of the body. Mortality was high when the disease was systemic and lesions developed in the respiratory and alimentary canals (Davies 1981). Goats develop lesions that pass through the typical pock stages. Small grayish-red papules appeared a few days after the rise in temperature. These primary lesions were later transformed into lymph-filled vesicles which eventually become necrotic. A purulent fluid exuded from the vesicles formed scabs and crusts (Rafyi and Ramyar 1959).

There have been reports of outbreaks of a disease which differed from classical sheeppox in that vesicular and pustular lesions failed to develop. Clinically, the disease was characterized by elevated temperature, rough staring coat, loss of appetite, and extensive erythema. Within 24 hours, raised, circumscribed nodules formed in the erythematous areas. These lesions affected the entire body; in some cases even the skin between the hoof clefts and on the coronary bands was involved, resulting in lameness and stiffness of gait. The nodules were 5 to 18 mm in diameter and 1 to 3 mm in height. Within 8 to 12 days, the nodules became necrotic and sloughed off, leaving shallow, clearly demarcated ulcers. Complete healing took place in 5 to 7 weeks. In acute cases where large areas of the body were affected, death occurred in 3 to 5 days. However, in subacute cases, the disease had a course of 3 to 7 weeks and terminated in recovery or death (Katiyar 1961).

Both generalized and localized forms of buffalopox have been observed. In the pre-eruptive stage, there was fever, loss of appetite, conjunctivitis, and serous discharge from the eyes (Maqsood 1958). During the acute phase, localized lesions occurred predominantly on the teats, udder, medial aspect of the thighs, and, in a few cases, on the lips and nostrils. The lesions on the teats resulted in stenosis of the milk duct in 30 to 60% and mastitis in 15 to 20% of the affected buffalo. Occasionally, lesions were observed on the cornea and conjunctiva (Lal and Singh 1977). In uncomplicated cases, the animals recovered in 3 to 4 weeks (Maqsood 1958).

In 1973–74, an outbreak of cowpox occurred among carnivora of the family Felidae and anteaters housed in the same building in the Moscow Zoo. Pulmonary and dermal forms of the disease were observed. The pulmonary form was always fatal and was characterized by a serofibrinous bronchopneumonia with extensive exudate in the pleural cavity. In these cases there were no skin lesions, but the virus could be isolated from the pulmonary tissue and exudate. The dermal form seldom terminated in death (Marennikova *et al.* 1975).

PATHOLOGY

Sheep afflicted with a systemic pox infection develop lesions in parts of the body which are not well covered by hair, such as the ears, mouth, tail, perineum, axillae, and groin. The vesicular and pustular formations are characteristic of the disease, with necrotic nodules most commonly observed. Lesions are also regularly found in the respiratory and gastrointestinal tracts. Depressed gray areas up to 3 cm in diameter appear on the parietal surface of the lungs. Secondary bacterial bronchopneumonia is often a complication. Typical nodules are observed on the mucous membrane of the abomasum.

The histopathological changes include acanthosis, hyperkeratosis, and purulent exudate in the epithelium. The inflammatory reaction in the dermis consists of an accumulation of macrophage that contain spherical, homogeneous, pink, intracytoplasmic inclusions. The destruction of the dermis is due to severe necrotizing vasculitis and thrombosis.

There is little information on the pathogenesis and pathology of buffalopox and camelpox, but the lesions appear to be similar to those produced by the cowpox virus.

Literature

Plowright *et al.* (1959) stated that the sheeppox virus caused a severe systemic disease which had clinicopathological manifestations comparable to those observed in cases of variola, ectromelia, and myxomatosis. However, a number of workers (Vegad and Sharma 1973; Davies 1976; Katiyar 1961) described atypical sheeppox infections in which the vesicular and pustular stages of lesion development were absent. Instead of the characteristic pustule formation, there was an accumulation of purulent material between the necrosed crust of epidermis and the underlying granulation tissue (Vegad and Sharma 1973). The main histological changes occurred in the connective tissue under the epithelium and subcutis. Microvesicle formation in the epidermis was reported by Murray *et al.* (1973). In the dermis, there were the characteristic 'sheeppox cells' or *cellules claveleuses* of Borrel which have a vacuolated nucleus and large intracytoplasmic inclusions. The histological and ultrastructural features of these cells demonstrated that they included monocytes, macrophages, and fibrocytes. Both intracytoplasmic and intranuclear inclusions were observed in the macrophages. There was proliferation of the endothelial cells lining the small subcutaneous blood vessels. This change was followed by the development of a severe vasculitis which was characterized by necrosis of the vessel wall, aggregation of polymorphonuclear leukocytes in the lumen, wall, and surrounding adventitia, and thrombosis. This process resulted in extensive necrosis of the dermis. The increased thickness of the epidermis was due to acanthosis, hyperkeratosis, and hydropic degeneration of prickle cells in the Malpighian layer. Because the hydropic degeneration did not result in the rupture of the cells, there was no vesicle formation (Katiyar 1961; Krishnan 1968; Murray *et al.* 1973; Plowright *et al.* 1959; Vegad and Sharma 1973).

The nodules were present throughout the lungs and on the mucosa of the trachea, mouth, pharynx, and abomasum. These lesions occasionally appeared on the mucosa of the duodenum and large intestine. Desquamation of the nodules led to the formation of ulcers in the mucosa (Katiyar 1961). Ramachandran (1967) reported that pulmonary lesions developed in only 30 to 40% of the animals experimentally infected with sheeppox or goatpox virus, whereas pulmonary involvement was exhibited in 70 to 90% of the naturally infected sheep and goats. In a separate study in which one strain of goatpox virus and three strains of sheeppox virus were used, the incidence of pulmonary lesions in the experimental goats and sheep was approximately 36%. The nodules appeared in the latter stages of the disease and were between 0.5 and 3 cm in width, with a grayish or dull white opaque center and an erythematous margin. In the early lesions, there was hypertrophy and hyperplasia of the septal vascular endothelial cells and exudation of plasma and fibrin into the interalveolar stromal tissue and alveolar spaces, suggesting hematogenous invasion of the lung parenchyma by the infective agent. Subsequently, there was coagulation necrosis with neutrophil infiltration. The other salient histological features of pox pneumonitis in sheep and goats were focal hyperplasia of the bronchial epithelium, peribronchial cuffiing by mononuclear cells, fetalization of the alveolar lining, and a serofibrinous inflammation of the interstitial tissue in which macrophages predominated. Eosinophilic intracytoplasmic inclusions were occasionally observed in the mesenchymal cells of the interstitial tissue. The lesion healed by fibrosis, infiltration with mononuclear cells and fetalization (Ramachandran 1967).

IMMUNOLOGY

There is a close antigenic relationship between sheeppox and goatpox viruses, but the relationship of these viruses to other pox viruses has not been well defined because the serological methods used in such determinations vary in their specificity. Buffalopox and camelpox viruses are serologically related to viruses in the variola–vaccinia group. The immunity induced by infection with sheeppox or goatpox virus is lifelong and appears to depend on both humoral and cellular components.

Literature

The soluble antigens of sheeppox virus have been studied by immunodiffusion (Sambyal and Singh 1980a). The antigenic differences between the intracellular and extracellular forms of sheeppox virus grown in lamb tissue culture were demonstrated by cross-neutralization tests and by cross-protection tests in which immunoglobulins were passively transferred. Ninety-seven percent of the progeny virus was found to be intracellular (Srivastava and Singh 1980b).

The antigenic relationships among the various pox viruses were studied extensively. Davies (1981) reviewed the early literature concerning the determination of the antigenic composition of sheeppox and goatpox viruses by cross-protection tests. The antigenic relationship between sheeppox and goatpox viruses was determined using gel diffusion, CF and cross-protection tests, and it was found that the viruses shared one antigen (Sharma and Dhanda 1971b). Soluble antigens common to both sheeppox and goatpox viruses were detected by the double diffusion and immunoelectrophoretic techniques (Pandey and Singh 1972). The results of direct and indirect FA and serum neutralization tests demonstrated that sheeppox and goatpox strains isolated from Kenya and the Middle East were serologically identical with LSD virus. All of these viruses were shown to be distantly related to cowpox virus by the FA techniques but not by the neutralization test. There was no serological evidence that these viruses were related to the camelpox virus (Davies and Otema 1981). Cross-protection tests showed that sheeppox and goatpox viruses were not related to contagious pustular dermatitis virus. However, some cross-reactions were observed between these pox viruses and contagious pustular dermatitis virus in cross CF tests, but not in gel precipitation tests.

No relationship was established between sheeppox and goatpox viruses and vaccinia virus (Sharma and Dhanda 1971c). Sheeppox, goatpox, and contagious pustular dermatitis viruses could be differentiated by the cross-neutralization test, but goatpox hyperimmune serum neutralized the other two viruses (Rao and Malik 1979). Goatpox and contagious pustular dermatitis viruses were found to be serologically related by the cross agar-gel diffusion, immunoelectrophoretic, serum neutralization and capillary agglutination tests. In cross-precipitation reactions, six out of eight precipitable factors were common to both viruses (Dubey and Sawhney 1979). Cross-reactions between sheeppox and goatpox viruses were observed in neutralization, CF, and immunogel diffusion tests, but there was no indication that these viruses were antigenically related to either avianpox or vaccinia virus (Uppal and Nilakantan 1970). Buffalopox virus was distinguishable from vaccinia and cowpox viruses in cross agar-gel diffusion, immunoelectrophoretic, serum neutralization and CF tests. The patterns of cross-reaction obtained with double diffusion and immunoelectrophoresis suggested that buffalopox virus was more closely related to vaccinia virus than to cowpox virus (Kataria and Singh 1970; Sarkar *et al.* 1976).

The immunity acquired after infection with sheeppox virus is considered to be lifelong. In studies designed to determine the host mechanisms responsible for immunity to sheeppox, the following observations were made: (1) passive transfer of antiserum against sheeppox virus conferred partial protection on subsequent challenge by increasing the incubation period; and (2) lambs hyperimmunized with sheeppox virus developed delayed hypersensitivity reactions. It was therefore concluded that both humoral and cellular factors were involved in the development of immunity to sheeppox (Srivastava and Singh 1980a). There was no correlation between the titer of neutralizing antibody and the degree of immunity (Srivastava and Singh 1980b). Cell-mediated immunity was also demonstrated in buffalopox-infected guinea pigs (Kalra *et al*. 1977). An immediate type of cutaneous hypersensitivity was observed in sensitized sheep after intradermal challenge with sheeppox virus soluble antigens (Sambyal and Singh 1980b).

A number of serological tests have been used to study the antibody responses to different pox viruses. The agar-gel diffusion test was utilized to detect antibodies in experimentally infected sheep and goats (Uppal and Nilakantan 1967; Sharma and Dhanda 1971a). Neutralization (Davies and Otema 1978) and CF (Sharma and Dhanda 1971b) have also been employed. The use of antiglobulin in agglutination tests for sheeppox virus was investigated (Baharsefat and Yamini 1967). The conglutinating-complement-absorption test was found to be a useful serological technique (Sen *et al*. 1971). The IFA test was more reliable than the neutralization test (Davies 1976). Hyperimmune serum prepared from sheep was more effective in reducing the cytopathic effect of the virus in tissue culture than convalescent serum, which had poor neutralizing ability (Pandey and Singh 1970c).

VACCINATION

Vaccines against sheeppox and goatpox are produced from viruses propagated in animals or in tissue cultures. The old vaccines used small quantities of live virulent virus which had been grown in animals, but these are no longer administered exclusively. Two types of vaccines are currently used: attenuated live vaccine and formalin-inactivated vaccine adsorbed to aluminium hydroxide gel. Attenuation of the virus is accomplished by serial passage through lamb or calf kidney tissue cultures. The level of attenuation and the efficacy of these vaccines have been fully evaluated. There is no dependable, safe, and effective vaccine against sheeppox and goatpox which has been adequately standardized and is being used universally. The immunogenicity and pathogenicity of strains should be determined so that a more uniform approach to the control of these diseases through vaccination may be achieved.

Literature

The early methods of immunization against sheeppox involved chemically inactivated antigens, dilution of live virulent vaccine, or antigens combined with adjuvants. The widespread use of live vaccines had the disadvantage of causing a high incidence of generalized reactions (Khan 1961; Rafyi 1960). The Borrel-type vaccine consisted of aluminium hydroxide gel mixed with the fluid obtained after filtering homogenates of the subcutaneous tissue and fluid extracted from the lesions of experimentally infected sheep. The immunity produced by this vaccine varied considerably, but it was used extensively (Martin *et al.* 1973; Celiker and Arik 1962; Uppal *et al.* 1967). This method of immunization was discarded because it produced severe reactions in vaccinated animals. Moreover, vaccinated animals with localized skin lesions constituted a dangerous source of infection for unvaccinated animals (Rafyi and Mir Chamsy 1956). Another early vaccine consisted of a 1% suspension of sheeppox scab material in 50% normal saline glycerine. Kids and lambs inoculated by the sacrification method exhibited local skin redness, vesicle formation and a rise in the temperature by the seventh postvaccinal day. The efficacy of the vaccine varied, but young animals were protected against challenge with virulent virus 6 to 7 months after vaccination (Sharma and Malhotra 1959). The immunity induced by desiccated live virus vaccines commenced on the ninth day postinoculation and lasted for 14 months. The vaccinated sheep showed a local reaction and a mild febrile response (Sabban 1955, 1960). Sheeppox vaccine did not protect goats against goatpox, whereas a goatpox vaccine developed in embryonated chicken eggs induced protection against both sheeppox and goatpox (Rafyi and Ramyar 1959).

Some live attenuated tissue culture sheeppox virus vaccines were produced by consecutive passage of the virulent virus in lamb kidney cells. The inoculation of the virus at the forty-ninth and fiftieth lamb kidney cell passages resulted in the development of high fever and local reactions which varied in severity (Martin *et al.* 1973). Sheep inoculated with virus at the forty-sixth lamb kidney cell passage developed nodular lesions at the site of inoculation (Soman and Singh 1979). The live modified sheeppox virus vaccine strain RM/65 was shown to be completely innocuous after 30 consecutive passages in sheep kidney cells (Ramyar and Hessami 1965). The latter vaccine was safe, could be lyophilized, and protected sheep against challenge for up to 22 months. There was a poor correlation between the antibody titers detected by the serum neutralization and CF tests and the degree of immunity produced by the vaccine (Ramyar and Hessami 1970). An attenuated live virus vaccine propagated in lamb testicular cells conferred good protection against sheeppox for up to 1 year postvaccination. After the vaccine was injected into the abaxial surface of the tail, there was localized inflammation at the site of inoculation followed by the formation of a papule which became encrusted and sloughed off. Transient fever was also observed during this period. Four million doses of the vaccine were used without any reported side effects (Penkova *et al.* 1974). A vaccine produced from sheeppox virus attenuated by continuous passage in calf kidney cells caused local reactions and immunity but did not induce generalized infection. The local reaction involved the formation of firm nodules which underwent necrosis in a small number of sheep. There was a transient elevation of temperature seen in 10% of the sheep. These reactions varied between individual sheep and breeds (Martin *et al.* 1973). In sheep vaccinated against sheeppox virus, complement-fixing antibodies could be detected on the seventh day postvaccination in about 50% of the animals. The antibody titers became maximal on the twenty-first or twenty-eighth day and then gradually declined (Sharma and Dhanda 1970a). Two goatpox cell culture vaccines, one attenuated and one inactivated with phenol, protected against challenge with virulent goatpox virus. The capillary agglutination test was used to detect the antibody formation after immunization with either of these vaccines (Dubey and Sawhney 1978).

Because live attenuated tissue culture viruses may be contagious and have been known to cause severe reactions, the inactivation of vaccine strains by various chemical agents was deemed necessary. Beta-propiolactone-inactivated sheeppox virus combined with an adjuvant such as alumina gel, oil or sodium alginate gave good results in immunization trials. However, these vaccines did not protect goats against goatpox infection (Sharma and Dhanda 1970b). The formalized sheeppox vaccine produced from scab material was poorly antigenic: the administration of large doses resulted in short periods of immunity. Because of the possibility of strain variation in sheeppox virus, attempts were made to develop vaccines out of indigenous strains (Kalra and Sharma 1981). Further work showed that a formalized aluminium hydroxide gel-adsorbed goatpox vaccine induced solid protection (Prasad and Datt 1973). In other attempts to develop an inactivated sheeppox virus vaccine, it was found that formaldehyde, hydroxylamine, and *N*-acetyl ethyleneimine effectively destroyed viral infectivity without the loss of antigenicity (Goyal and Singh 1975). The cytopathic activity of sheeppox virus was reduced by rifampicin, a drug known to inhibit the multiplication of DNA-containing viruses (Bhatnagar *et al.* 1974). Soluble antigens of sheeppox virus injected with Freund's complete adjuvant have also been used as an experimental inactivated vaccine (Sambyal and Singh 1980b).

DIAGNOSIS

The clinical diagnosis of sheeppox and goatpox is not difficult when generalized infections occur during epizootics. In enzootic areas, however, these diseases clinically resemble orf, as they may be mild and produce lesions confined to the mouth and udder. The laboratory methods required for the definitive diagnosis of sheeppox and goatpox are isolation of the virus, detection of viral antigens in the skin lesions, demonstration of serum antibodies, and light- and electron-microscopic analysis of the histopathology. Isolation of the virus is accomplished by inoculating cultures with vesicular fluid or emulsified preparations of the cutaneous lesions. The virus can be identified within 24 hours by the direct FA technique. The typical CPEs and eosinophilic intracellular inclusions that develop after additional incubation also help to identify the infection. The classical elementary bodies, which are considered to be pathognomonic for the infection, can be demonstrated on microscopic examination of the lesions. Serological methods such as CF, indirect immunofluorescence, and serum neutralization can demonstrate antibodies 1 week after the development of skin lesions and are particularly useful for making a diagnosis on a herd basis.

Literature

The procedures used in diagnosing sheeppox and goatpox infections were reviewed by Davies (1981). A slide immunodiffusion test developed for the diagnosis of these diseases utilizes antigen prepared from the tissues of infected animals, but its reliability has not been established (Bhambani and Murty 1963).

CONTROL

Prophylactic immunization is an effective means of preventing disease in the face of an epizootic, especially when indigenous strains are used in the vaccines. In many of the endemic areas, control is difficult due to the practice of nomadic pastoralism.

BIBLIOGRAPHY

Aasagba, M. O. and Nawathe, D. R., 1980. Evidence of sheep pox in Nigeria, *Trop. Anim. Hlth Prod.*, **13**: 61.

Abdussalam, M., 1957. Elementary bodies of sheep pox, *Am. J. vet. Res.*, **18**: 614–17.

Baharsefat, M. and Yamini, B., 1967. Agglutination test for sheeppox virus using antiglobulin, *Cornell Vet.*, **57**: 558–63.

Bansal, R. P. and Singh, I. P., 1974. Plaque assay of buffalopox virus, *Indian J. Anim. Sci.*, **44**(1): 31–5.

Baxby, D., 1969. Variability in the characteristics of pocks produced on the chick chorioallantois by white pock mutants of cowpox and other pox viruses, *J. Hyg., Camb.*, **67**: 637–47.

Baxby, D., 1972. Smallpox-like viruses from camels in Iran, *Lancet*, **2**: 1063–5.

Baxby, D., 1974. Differentiation of smallpox and camelpox viruses in cultures of human and monkey cells, *J. Hyg., Camb.*, **72**: 251–5.

Baxby, D., 1977. Poxvirus hosts and reservoirs, *Arch. Virol.*, **55**: 169–79.

Baxby, D. and Hill, B. J., 1969. Buffalopox virus, *Vet. Rec.*, **85**: 315–16.

Baxby, D. and Hill, B. J., 1971. Characteristics of a new poxvirus isolated from Indian buffaloes, *Arch. ges. Virusforsch.*, **35**: 70–9.

Baxby, D., Ramyar, H., Hessami, M. and Ghaboosir, B., 1975. Response of camels to intradermal inoculation with smallpox and camelpox viruses, *Infect. Immun.*, **11**: 617–21.
Bedson, H. S., 1972. Camelpox and smallpox, *Lancet*, **2**: 1253.
Bhambani, B. D. and Murty, D. K., 1963. An immuno-diffusion test for laboratory diagnosis of sheep pox and goat pox, *J. Comp. Path.*, **73**: 349–60.
Bhatnagar, A., Husain, M. M. and Gupta, B. M., 1974. Comparative sensitivity of sheep pox and neurovaccinia viruses to rifampicin and marboran in tissue cultures, *Acta virol.*, **18**: 81–4.
Bloch, B. and Lal, S. M., 1975. A study of the ultrastructure of the buffalo pox virus. *Acta path. microbiol. scand. Sect. B*, **83**: 191–200.

Celiker, A. and Arik, F., 1962. Aluminium-gel-adsorbed sheep pox virus vaccine, *Br. vet. J.*, **118**: 159–61.
Cilli, V., 1961. Sur quelques aspects biologiques du virus de la clavelée, *Rec. Méd. Vét.*, **137**: 663–78.
Cottral, G. E., 1978. Poxviruses. In *Manual of Standardized Methods for Veterinary Microbiology*, ed. G. E. Cottral. Cornell University Press (Ithaca and London), pp. 273–91.

Davies, F. G., 1976. Characteristics of a virus causing a pox disease in sheep and goats in Kenya, with observations on the epidemiology and control, *J. Hyg., Camb.*, **76**: 163–71.
Davies, F. G., 1981. Sheep and goat pox. In *Virus Diseases of Food Animals. A World Geography of Epidemiology and Control*, ed. E. P. J. Gibbs. Academic Press (New York), disease monographs, vol. II, pp. 733–49.
Davies, F. G. and Otema, C., 1978. The antibody response in sheep infected with a Kenyan sheep and goat pox virus, *J. Comp. Path.*, **88**: 205–10.
Davies, F. G. and Otema, C., 1981. Relationship of capripox viruses found in Kenya with two Middle Eastern strains and some orthopox viruses, *Res. vet. Sci.*, **31**: 253–5.
Dubey, S. C. and Sawhney, A. N., 1978. Live and inactivated tissue culture vaccines against goat-pox, *Indian vet. J.*, **55**: 926–7.
Dubey, S. C. and Sawhney, A. N., 1979. Serological relationship between viruses of goat-pox and contagious pustular dermatitis, *Indian J. Anim. Sci.*, **49**(2): 135–9.

Edlinger, E. and Iftimovici, M., 1973. Etude de la multiplication du virus claveleux sur cultures cellulaires ovines, *Arch. Inst. Pasteur de Tunis.*, **50**: 373–86.

Goyal, S. M. and Singh, I. P., 1975. Inactivation of sheep-pox virus by formaldehyde, hydroxylamine and N-acetyl ethyleneimine, *Indian J. Anim. Sci.*, **45**(10): 748–53.

Joklik, W. K., 1966. The poxviruses, *Bacteriol. Rev.*, **30**: 33–66.

Kalra, S. K., Dogra, S. C., Singh, S. B. and Sharma, V. K., 1977. Demonstration of cell mediated immunity in (experimentally) buffalo pox infected guinea pigs by macrophage migration inhibition test, *Indian J. Microbiol.*, **16**: 185–8.

Kalra, S. K. and Sharma, V. K., 1981. Adaptation of Jaipur strain of sheeppox virus in primary lamb testicular cell culture, *Indian J. exp. Biol.*, **19**: 165–9.

Kataria, R. S. and Singh, I. P., 1970. Serological relationship of buffalopox virus to vaccinia and cowpox viruses, *Acta virol.*, **14**: 307–11.

Katiyar, R. D., 1961. An infectious disease of viral origin in sheep with anatomicopathological changes at slight variance with those of the classical sheep pox, *Indian J. vet. Sci.*, **31**: 132–40.

Khan, C. K. A., 1960. Cultivation of sheep-pox virus, *Indian vet. J.*, **37**: 296–302.

Khan, C. K. A., 1961. Sheep pox vaccination, *Indian vet. J.*, **38**: 233–40.

Kolayli, A. C., Marvidis, N. and Ilhami, 1933. Etude sur le virus de la variole des chevres. Vaccination du mouton et de la chevre. *Rec. Méd. vét.*, **109**: 920–32.

Krishnan, R., 1968. Pathogenesis of sheep pox, *Indian vet. J.*, **45**: 297–302.

Lal, S. M. and Singh, I. P., 1973a. Buffalopox virus, *Arch. ges. Virusforsch.*, **40**: 390–1.

Lal, S. M. and Singh, I. P., 1973b. Serological characterization of buffalopox virus, *Arch. ges. Virusforsch.*, **43**: 393–6.

Lal, S. M. and Singh, I. P., 1977. Buffalopox – a review, *Trop. Anim. Hlth Prod.*, **9**: 107–12.

Lang, R. and Leftheriotis, E., 1961. L'adaptation du virus de la clavelée sur les cellules rénales du mouton, *Bull. Acad. Vét.*, **34**: 337–43.

Mahnel, H. and Bartenbach, G., 1973. Classification of camelpox virus, *Zbl. Vet. Med.*, **B20**: 572–6.

Maqsood, M., 1958. Generalised buffalo-pox, *Vet. Rec.*, **70**: 321–2.

Marennikova, S. S., Maltseva, N. N., Korneeva, V. I. and Garanina, V. M., 1975. Pox infection in carnivora of the family Felidae, *Acta virol.*, **19**: 260.

Martin, W. B., Ergin, H. and Koylu, A., 1973. Tests in sheep of attenuated sheep pox vaccines, *Res. vet. Sci.*, **14**: 53–61.

Murray, M., Martin, W. B. and Koylu, A., 1973. Experimental sheep pox. A histological and ultrastructural study, *Res. vet. Sci.*, **15**: 201–8.

Muzichin, S. I. and Ali, B. H., 1979. A study of sheep pox in the Sudan, *Bull. Anim. Hlth Prod. Afr.*, **27**: 105–12.

Nitzschke, E., Buckley, L. S. and Ergin, H., 1967. Isolation and titration of sheep and goat pox viruses in sheep thyroid cell cultures, *Vet. Rec.*, **81**: 216–17.

Pandey, A. K., Malik, B. S. and Bansal, M. P., 1969. Studies on sheep pox virus. I. Adaptation and propagation of the virus in cell culture, *Indian vet. J.*, **46**: 925–9.

Pandey, R. and Singh, I. P., 1970a. A note on heat, chloroform and ether sensitivity of sheep pox and goat pox viruses, *Acta virol.*, **14**: 318–19.

Pandey, R. and Singh, I. P., 1970b. Cytopathogenicity and neutralization of goatpox virus in cell culture, *Res. vet. Sci.*, **11**: 195–7.

Pandey, R. and Singh, I. P., 1970c. Cytopathogenicity and neutralization of sheeppox virus in primary cell culture of ovine and caprine origin, *Indian J. Pathol. Bacteriol.*, **13**: 6–11.

Pandey, R. and Singh, I. P., 1972. Soluble antigens of sheep pox and goat pox viruses as determined by immunodiffusion in agar gel, *Acta virol.*, **16**: 41–6.

Penkova, V. M., Jassim, F. A., Thompson, J. R. and Al-Doori, T. M., 1974. The propagation of an attenuated sheep pox virus and its use as a vaccine, *Bull. Off. int. Epiz.*, **81**: 329–39.

Plowright, W. and Ferris, R. D., 1958. The growth and cytopathogenicity of sheep-pox virus in tissue cultures, *Br. J. Exp. Path.*, **39**: 424–35.

Plowright, W. and Ferris, R. D., 1959. Ether sensitivity of some mammalian pox viruses, *Virology*, **7**: 357–8.

Plowright, W., MacLeod, W. G. and Ferris, R. D., 1959. The pathogenesis of sheep pox in the skin of sheep, *J. Comp. Path.*, **69**: 411–13.

Prasad, I. J. and Datt, N. S., 1973. Observation on the use of live and inactivated vaccines against goat pox, *Indian vet. J.*, **50**: 1–10.

Rafyi, A., 1960. Progrès réalisés dans la lutte contre les varioles ovine et caprine par la vaccination, *Bull. Off. int. Epiz.*, **54**: 463–74.

Rafyi, A. and Mir Chamsy, H., 1956. Seven years' control of sheep pox in Iran with adsorbed tissue vaccine on aluminium gel, *Br. vet. J.*, **112**: 541–7.

Rafyi, A. and Ramyar, H., 1959. Goat pox in Iran. Serial passage in

goats and the developing egg, and relationship with sheep pox, *J. Comp. Path.*, **69**: 141–7.
Ramachandran, S., 1967. Observations on the histopathology of lung lesions in experimental pox infection of sheep and goats, *Ceylon vet. J.*, **15**: 78–81.
Ramyar, H., 1966. Propagation of goat pox virus on monolayer cell cultures, *Zbl. Vet. Med.* **B13**: 334–7.
Ramyar, H. and Hessami, M., 1965. Development of an attenuated live virus vaccine against sheep pox, *Zbl. Vet. Med.*, **B14**: 516–19.
Ramyar, H. and Hessami, M., 1970. Studies on the duration of immunity conferred by a live-modified sheep pox tissue culture virus vaccine, *Zbl. Vet. Med.*, **B17**: 869–74.
Rao, M. V. S. and Malik, B. S., 1979. Cross-neutralization tests on sheep pox, goat pox and contagious pustular dermatitis viruses, *Acta virol.*, **23**: 165–7.

Sabban, M. S., 1955. Sheep pox and its control in Egypt using a desiccated live virus vaccine, *Am. J. vet. Res.*, **16**: 209–13.
Sabban, M. S., 1957. The cultivation of sheep pox virus on the chorioallantoic membrane of the developing chicken embryo, *Am. J. vet. Res.*, **18**: 618–24.
Sabban, M. S., 1960. Sheep pox and its control in Egypt, *Bull. Off. int. Epiz.*, **53**: 1527–39.
Sambyal, D. S. and Singh, I. P., 1980a. A short note on sheep pox virus soluble antigens studied by immunodiffusion, *Zbl. Vet. Med.*, **B27**: 340–3.
Sambyal, D. S. and Singh, I. P., 1980b. Cutaneous hypersensitivity in sheep injected with sheep pox virus soluble antigens, *Zbl. Vet. Med.*, **B27**: 544–8.
Sarkar, P., Singh, S. P. and Pandey, A. K., 1976. A note on the studies of sheep pox virus by gel diffusion and immunoelectrophoresis, *Indian J. Anim. Hlth*, **15**: 19–21.
Sen, A. K. and Uppal, P. K., 1972. Adaptation of sheep-pox virus in embryonated eggs, *Indian J. Anim. Sci.*, **42**(6): 427.
Sen, A. K., Uppal, P. K. and Nilakantan, P. R., 1971. Complement-fixation and conglutinating-complement-absorption test in sheep-pox – a note, *Indian J. Anim. Sci.*, **41**(9): 862–3.
Sharma, R. M. and Malhotra, F. C., 1959. Protective value of sheep pox vaccines in Indian breeds of animals, *Indian J. Anim. Sci.*, **29**: 58–61.
Sharma, S. N. and Dhanda, M. R., 1970a. Serological studies of sheep- and goat-pox viruses, *Indian J. Anim. Sci.*, **40**: 522–8.
Sharma, S. N. and Dhanda, M. R., 1970b. Studies on sheep- and goat-pox viruses – immunization trials, *Indian J. Anim. Sci.*, **40**: 626–39.
Sharma, S. N. and Dhanda, M. R., 1971a. Immuno-diffusion studies on sheep- and goat-pox viruses, *Indian J. Anim. Sci.*, **41**(3): 166–71.
Sharma, S. N. and Dhanda, M. R., 1971b. Studies on the

inter-relationship between sheep- and goat-pox viruses, *Indian J. Anim. Sci.*, **41**(4): 267–72.

Sharma, S. N. and Dhanda, M. R., 1971c. Studies on sheep- and goat-pox viruses: relationship with contagious pustular dermatitis and vaccinia viruses, *Indian J. Anim. Sci.*, **41**(9): 864–7.

Sharma, S. N. and Dhanda, M. R., 1972. Studies on sheep and goat pox viruses: pathogenicity, *Indian J. Anim. Hlth*, **11**: 39–46.

Sharma, S. N., Nilakantan, P. R. and Dhanda, M. R., 1966. A preliminary note on pathogenicity and antigenicity of sheep and goat pox viruses, *Indian vet. J.*, **43**: 673–8.

Singh, I. P., Pandey, R. and Srivastava, R. N., 1979. Sheep pox: a review, *Vet. Bull.*, **49**: 145–54.

Singh, I. P. and Singh, S. B., 1967. Isolation and characterization of the aetiologic agent of buffalopox, *J. Res. (Ludhiana)*, **4**: 440–8.

Soman, J. P. and Singh, I. P., 1979. A note on immunogenicity of cell-culture-attenuated sheep-pox virus, *Indian J. Anim. Sci.*, **49**(8): 674–5.

Soman, J. P. and Singh, I. P., 1980. Cytopathic and immunogenic studies of sheep pox virus serially cultivated in cell culture, *J. Comp. Path.*, **90**: 99–106.

Soman, J. P. and Singh, I. P., 1981. Determination of optimum conditions for the growth of cell culture attenuated sheep pox virus, *Indian vet. J.*, **58**: 10–12.

Srivastava, R. N. and Singh, I. P., 1980a. A study on the role of cellular and humoral factors in immunity to sheep-pox, *Indian J. Anim. Sci.*, **50**(10): 861–6.

Srivastava, R. N. and Singh, I. P., 1980b. Antigenic difference between extracellular and intracellular sheep-pox virus, *Indian J. Anim. Sci.*, **50**(12): 1098–103.

Tantawi, H. H., El-Dahaby, H. and Fahmy, L. S., 1978. Comparative studies on poxvirus strains isolated from camels, *Acta. virol.*, **22**: 451–7.

Uppal, P. K. and Nilakantan, P. R., 1967. Serological reactions in sheep pox. II. Agar-gel diffusion test, *Indian vet. J.*, **44**: 374–82.

Uppal, P. K. and Nilakantan, P. R., 1970. Studies on the serological relationship between avian pox, sheep pox, goat pox and vaccinia viruses, *J. Hyg., Camb.*, **68**: 349–58.

Uppal, P. K., Nilakantan, P. R. and Sakkubai, P. R., 1967. Observations on the use of live and inactivated virus vacccines against sheep pox, *Indian vet. J.*, **44**: 815–27.

Vegad, J. L. and Sharma, G. L., 1973. Cutaneous and pulmonary lesions of sheep-pox, *Indian J. Anim. Sci.*, **43**(12): 1061–7.

Vigário, J. D. and Ferraz, F. P., 1967. Study of sheeppox virus synthesis by fluorescent antibody technique, *Am. J. vet. Res.*, **28**: 809–13.

Vigário, J. D. and Terrinha, A. M., 1964. Resistance of sheeppox viral deoxyribonucleic acid to deoxyribonuclease in intracytoplasmic inclusion bodies in sheep testicle cell cultures, *Am. J. vet. Res.*, **25**: 1690–4.

Vigário, J., Terrinha, A., Nunes, J., Bostos, A., Marques, D., Correia, D. and Silva, F., 1968. An autoradiographic and immunofluorescent study of the infection cycle of sheeppox virus in cell cultures exposed to 5-fluorodeoxyuridine, *Arch. ges. Virusforsch.*, **25**: 321–9.

Chapter
14

Rift Valley fever

CONTENTS

INTRODUCTION

Rift Valley fever (RVF) is an acute infectious, vector-transmitted, viral disease of sheep and cattle which is abortifacient and causes high mortality in young lambs and calves. It is characterized by a short incubation period, fever, leukopenia, focal or diffused necrotic changes in the liver, and acidophilic intranuclear inclusions in the hepatocytes. Rift Valley fever is a zoonosis which is assumed to have spread from the Rift Valley of Kenya to other regions of Africa where it causes serious disease in man and animals.

Literature

The most comprehensive review of RVF was published by Easterday (1965). The author presented the history of the discovery of the disease throughout Africa, and thoroughly reviewed the early literature. Murphy and Easterday (1962) summarized the review articles on RVF which had been published before 1961. Symposia and workshops on RVF were held more recently (Anon 1979; Rift Valley fever workshop 1981). The disease was described as a zoonosis by Peters and Meegan (1981) and McIntosh and Gear (1981).

Henning (1952, 1956) described another disease in South Africa which was very similar to RVF and caused by an agent called Wesselsbron virus. It was first reported in the Wesselsbron area of South Africa, and occurred in a flock of sheep where mortality was observed in newborn lambs, and abortions without any clinical signs in other sheep (Haig 1965). These two viruses were difficult to differentiate on the basis of epidemiology, clinical syndromes, and pathology, but they were antigenically distinct. Wesselsbron virus infections were observed in newborn lambs and pregnant ewes. In the ewes, the virus caused fatty changes in the liver and fever, whereas in the lambs there was focal necrosis of liver cells associated with neutrophil infiltration. The Wesselsbron virus was found to be infective for sheep, cattle, horses, pigs, mice, rabbits, guinea pigs, and human beings. The agent could be passaged intracerebrally in infant mice, and inoculation of pregnant rabbits and guinea pigs resulted in infection of the fetuses (Alexander 1951). A serological relationship has been demonstrated between RVF virus and Zinga virus, which possibly is a strain of RVF virus, and on this basis the two viruses could not be differentiated (Meegan *et al.* 1983).

ETIOLOGY

The virus has been placed in the family Bunyaviridae on the basis of its morphological and biochemical characteristics, and its serological cross-reaction with viruses in the phlebotomus fever group. The virus is spherical, 90 to 100 nm in diameter, and has surface projections which are similar to those found in the Bunyaviridae viruses. The virus grows in most commonly used cell cultures, except lymphoblastoid cell lines, and the growth can be demonstrated by fluorescent antibody (FA) techniques. Rift Valley fever virus can propagate in a variety of animals, embryonated eggs, and cell culture systems. The hepatotropic virus is grown most frequently in mice, sheep, and cell culture systems; the neurotropic virus can be grown in embryonated eggs as well.

Literature

The viruses in the Bunyaviridae family are characterized by the presence of a single-stranded ribonucleic acid (RNA) with three unique segments, a nucleocapsid protein associated with the RNA, and an envelope which contains at least one virus-specific glycopeptide. The biochemical properties of RVF virus polypeptides were similar to those of other members of the family Bunyaviridae. The molecular weights of major structural polypeptides of several diverse viral isolates were identical, and the proteins and RNA were closely related to those found in some members of the phlebotomus fever group. The size of the viscerotropic strains was investigated and was not found significantly different from that of the neurotropic form (Naudé *et al.* 1954).

The RVF virus had been grown in a variety of tissue culture systems and was cytolytic. The dose of the virus injected influenced the time and level of peak titer, and the time of complete cell destruction. The pH, type of medium, and temperature influenced the growth of the virus *in vitro* (Easterday and Murphy 1963a). A number of factors related to the growth of RVF in suspended cell cultures were studied in order to develop optimal conditions for the propagation of the virus (Walker *et al.* 1969). The growth of RVF virus in mouse fibroblast-like cells was characterized by a latent period of 6 hours, the occurrence peak viral titers of both cell-free and cell-associated virus between 16 and 20 hours, and a phase of viral release which lasted for 48 hours (Johnson and Orlando 1968). Two variants of RVF virus differed with respect to plaque size and other biological characteristics such as growth rate, thermal stability, and yield from monolayers of mouse fibroblast cells. In addition, the large-plaque variant was less virulent, requiring 100 times more plaque-forming units to kill mice by the intraperitoneal route than the small-plaque variant (Boyle 1967). Serial passage of a pantropic strain of RVF virus in tissue cultures of lamb testis cells resulted in neurotropic adaptation of the virus (Coackley 1965). Both the pantropic and neurotropic viruses could be propagated in 1-day-old embryonated eggs, and the viral multiplication declined with the age of the developing embryo (Matumoto *et al.* 1959).

An FA technique was used to detect RVF virus antigen in tissue cultures after 5 hours of incubation, as well as in tissues from experimentally infected lambs and mice. The fluorescent staining was always exclusively in the cytoplasm (Easterday and Jaeger 1963). However, the eosinophilic intranuclear filaments which appeared in RVF-virus-infected cells were stained specifically with fluorescein in an indirect technique, indicating that the filaments were associated with virus-specific antigen (Swanepoel and Blackburn 1977). Further support for the development of virus-associated intranuclear inclusions came from ultrastructural studies on the nucleus and the cytoplasm of cells obtained from humans infected with RVF virus. The viral particles were found in smooth endoplasmic reticular systems. Inclusion bodies occurred in the host cell nuclei as rods and fine granules and in the cytoplasm as aggregates of fine or coarse granules (Ellis *et al.* 1979).

EPIZOOTIOLOGY

Geographical distribution

The disease was first reported in the Rift Valley of Kenya and is confined to the African continent.

Literature

Sellers (1981) reviewed the occurrences of epizootics in domestic animals and epidemics in man in Africa up to 1979. Factors which affected the epizootics involved climate, vectors, movement of wild game reservoirs, and reservoirs among domestic animals. The 1977 outbreak of RVF in Egypt was considered to have possible origins through either importation of infected ruminants or camels from the Sudan, through infected insects carried in transportation vehicles or by wind (Sellers *et al.* 1982). It was considered that spread was most likely by wind-borne insects. Shope *et al.* (1982) reviewed the spread of RVF virus based on the 1977 epizootic in Egypt and considered control methods which could be implemented.

Epizootics of RVF occurred in Kenya in 1961–62 (Coackley *et al.* 1967a) and in 1978–79 (Davies and Highton 1980). During the earlier outbreak, the disease was primarily observed in cattle, but abortion in camels was also reported. Subsequent serological investigation revealed that approximately 50% of the young, adult, and aged camels had neutralizing antibodies for RVF virus. Because of the high rate of abortion observed during the outbreak, RVF was considered a possible cause (Scott *et al.* 1963). The epizootiology of RVF in Kenya between 1969 and 1974 was investigated by isolating the virus and conducting serological surveys of cattle and wild bovidae. The examination of sentinel herds indicated that the virus did not persist in cattle between epizootics. There was some evidence that the interepizootic maintenance cycle at certain forest and forest-edge situations appeared to involve cattle. Only a few wild animals close to the outbreaks of the disease in domestic animals were found to be positive. However, the basic maintenance cycle for the virus remained unknown (Davies 1975). Serological examination of birds in enzootic areas of Kenya showed a low percentage of animals with positive sera, but it was not determined whether the neutralizing antibody was specific for RVF (Davies and

Addy 1979). Davies and Onyango (1978) concluded that the vervet monkey (*Ceropithecus aethiops*) probably did not act as a reservoir host for RVF virus in Kenya. A survey of a number of wild rodent species in Zimbabwe showed that some of the murid species were capable of maintaining viral infections which could be infective for mosquitoes (Swanepoel *et al.* 1978). Ten percent of all the abortions investigated by a diagnostic laboratory in Zimbabwe within a period of 1 year were found to be due to RVF (Shone *et al.* 1958). In 1983 and 1976 outbreaks of RVF were reported in the Sudan (Eisa *et al.* 1980).

Until 1976–77, RVF as a zoonosis was reported only in sub-Saharan Africa, but in 1977 an outbreak occurred in Egypt in which extensive human involvement and numerous fatalities were observed for the first time, thus furnishing evidence that the virus had spread throughout Africa (Peters and Meegan 1981). The 1977 epizootic and the second outbreak in 1978 in Egypt were characterized by extensive human involvement; benign syndromes as well as acute ocular, encephalitic, and fatal hemorrhagic forms were reported. It was estimated that between 20 000 and 200 000 human cases occurred during the 1977 epizootic. Antibodies to RVF virus were detected in sheep, cattle, water buffalo, goats, camels, donkeys, and dogs (Meegan *et al.* 1979). During the 1977 outbreak, the virus was most commonly isolated from domestic animals, rats (*Rattus rattus frugivorus*), and man. A large number of isolates were obtained from sheep, and single isolates were recovered from cattle, camels, goats, horses, and rats (Imam *et al.* 1979).

Transmission

Rift Valley fever virus is transmitted to sheep and cattle by biting arthropods; mosquitoes are probably the most important vectors. Infections in man are caused by exposure to contaminated meat or laboratory materials.

Literature

Rift Valley fever virus might be transmitted both biologically and mechanically by hematophagous vectors. Although man has been infected by direct contact with infected animal tissues, most animals become infected through mosquito vectors (Meegan *et al.* 1980). The mosquito's involvement in the transmission of RVF was demonstrated when the virus was isolated from three *Aedes* and six *Eretmapocites* species collected in the Semliki forest of Uganda. Subsequently, the virus was isolated from several other mosquito species (Murphy and Easterday 1962).

During epizootics of RVF in Kenya in 1968 and 1978–79, virus was isolated from pools of *Culicoides* (Davies 1975; Davies and Highton 1980). Recently, transovarial transmission of RVF virus in *Aedes lineatopennis* was reported from the research work undertaken in Kenya

(R. F. Sellers, personal communication). The susceptibility of *Culicoides variipennis*, a North American species, to RVF virus infection was investigated and the virus did not multiply in this vector (Jennings *et al.* 1982). During the 1977–78 RVF epizootics in Egypt, two strains of virus were isolated from unengorged female *Culex pipiens*. This species became infected after feeding on viremic hamsters (Meegan *et al.* 1980). Rift Valley fever virus was isolated from *Culex theileri, Aedes lineatopennis, Anopheles coustani, Aedes dentatus*, and *Eretmapocites quinquevittatus* during epizootics in southern Africa. It was concluded that *C. theileri* was an important vector during epizootics in cattle and sheep. Multiple isolations of Wesselsbron virus and Middelburg virus were made from *A. lineatopennis* (McIntosh 1972). Seven species of mosquitoes were investigated for their ability to transmit RVF virus. Although the virus was experimentally transmitted by several species of mosquitoes, *C. theileri* was the most efficient vector (McIntosh *et al.* 1973a).

In the 1977–78 epidemic of RVF in man in Egypt, *C. pipiens* was incriminated as the chief vector. Humans also contracted the disease by handling infected meat and by inhaling virus aerosols. Various domestic animals were implicated as sources of the virus. For example, more than 30% of the camels tested were serologically positive for antibodies to RVF virus. It was postulated that camels from the south brought the infection into Egypt (Hoogstraal *et al.* 1979). The experimental transmission of RVF virus by *C. pipiens* confirmed that this species was an important vector in the 1977–78 RVF epizootic in Egypt (Meegan *et al.* 1980).

There has been ample evidence of transmission of RVF virus by nonentomological means. Although infection does not appear to be transmitted by ingestion, the disease has been transmitted by aerosols of RVF virus (Murphy and Easterday 1962). Rift Valley fever and yellow fever virus were found to be highly stable in aerosols at temperatures of 24 °C and at relative humidities of 50 or 85%. The loss of infectivity ranges between 1 and 5% per minute (Miller *et al.* 1963). Transmission through contact between infected lambs and susceptible lambs did not occur, and lambs did not become diseased when suckling infected dams (Murphy and Easterday 1962).

INFECTION

Rift Valley fever virus has a wide range of susceptible hosts, including domestic, wild, and laboratory animals, and man, but disease can be experimentally induced in mice, hamsters, rats, and very young dogs. Experimental infection can be induced by a variety of parenteral inoculations but not by ingestion. The infection can also be transmitted to laboratory animals by inhalation. In sheep and cattle, viremia develops with subsequent localization of virus in the liver. Most studies on infectivity, viral distribution in the tissues, and tropism have been undertaken in mice. Various isolates are antigenically identical but differ in pathogenicity and other behavioral characteristics. The virus develops neurotropic properties after intracerebral passage in mice.

Literature

Experimental infections in domestic and laboratory animals were induced by subcutaneous, intratesticular, intracerebral, intramuscular, intravenous, and intranasal inoculation, as well as by application of the virus to scarified skin and conjunctiva. The disease was transmitted to sheep by mosquitoes after an extrinsic incubation period of 3 to 4 weeks (Easterday 1965). The disease was transmitted to young lambs by various parenteral routes, but not by contact with infected lambs. Lambs showed an earlier onset of viremia and a greater maximum level of virus in the blood than adult sheep (Easterday *et al.* 1962b). Rift Valley fever virus was stored up to 30 days at 4 °C without loss of infectivity or antigenicity (Craig *et al.* 1967). The West African dwarf sheep was found to be highly susceptible to RVF virus (Tomori 1979a). When these animals were challenged with low-mouse-brain-passaged RVF virus, they developed viremia, mild fever, and neutralizing antibodies (Fagbami *et al.* 1975). In cattle inoculated with infected blood, viremia was detected between the first and fourth or seventh day, while in lambs it was observed during the first 3 days (McIntosh *et al.* 1973b). The susceptibility of cattle to RVF virus was assessed in terms of an animal's ability to develop pyrexia, viremia, and circulating neutralizing antibody. However, these response were variable and their severity did not appear to be dependent on the amount of virus inoculated. Thus, susceptibility could not be judged solely on the basis of the absence of neutralizing antibody in the pre-challenge sera (Coackley *et al.* 1967a). Although neutralizing antibodies were not found in 114 feral African buffalo (*Syncerus caffer*), experimental infection with a pantropic strain of virus grown in hamsters caused abortion in one of two pregnant animals, and viremia which persisted for at least 48 hours in four of the five animals infected. These results indicated that the species probably played a role in the epizootiology of RVF (Davies and Karstad 1981).

Dogs were shown to be susceptible to RVF virus. Death occurred in animals 1 to 7 days of age, and 50% of the adult dogs developed viremia. Transmission of virus between pups and dams was demonstrated, and antibodies were passed by colostrum to pups (Walker *et al.* 1970a). Eight- to ten-week-old puppies and kittens were susceptible to RVF virus administered by inhalation, but not by ingestion. Although none of these animals developed clinical signs, viremia was observed in some (Keefer *et al.* 1972). There was an 81% mortality in kittens (21 days old or younger) challenged with RVF virus, whereas the infection was subclinical in older cats (Walker *et al.* 1970b). Pigs were not susceptible to infection by RVF virus (Scott 1963). There is also evidence that even the attenuated virus is infective for man

(Henning 1952). The susceptibility of baboons (*Papio anubis*) seemed comparable to that of other monkeys. The viremia in baboons lasted for 3 to 4 days, and there were no overt clinical signs (Davies *et al.* 1972).

Mice were used extensively in investigations on the isolation, identification, multiplication, and pathogenesis of RVF virus. Detailed studies of the infectivity and pathogenesis of RVF virus in mice were published in a series of papers by Mims (1956a–f) and Mims and Mason (1956). The low infectivity of RVF virus in large inocula which were serially passaged was attributed to the presence of incomplete noninfective forms of the virus. These forms interfered with the growth of the infective virus in tissue by increasing the incubation period and by reducing the peak level of infectivity attained (Mims 1956d). Intravenous inoculations of a very large dose of RVF virus in mice produced a synchronous cycle of infection within 10 hours. The first changes occurred in the nucleus of the hepatic cells after 1 hour, and intranuclear inclusion bodies were present at the end of 3 hours (Mims 1957). The distribution of the virus in the blood and tissues of infected mice was investigated. High titers were observed in the blood, while the urine, bile, and milk were either devoid of virus or contained only small quantities of particles. Infected pregnant mice transmitted the disease to embryos, possibly as a result of the transfer of virus across the placental barrier at the site of small hemorrhages (Mims 1956a).

The respiratory infectivity of four strains of RVF virus was investigated in mice exposed to infectious aerosols. The four strains were found to be infective at comparable doses, and the virus underwent initial replication in the lungs without causing pneumonia. The virus multiplied in the lungs during the first 30 hours of infection; then virions established a primary viremia and localized in the liver over the next 24 hours. Massive viremia and concentrations of virus in all tissues developed after 54 hours (Brown *et al.* 1981). Mice and hamsters died after inhaling aerosols of RVF virus, but rats survived infection by the respiratory route (Easterday and Murphy 1963b).

Adult hamsters were more suitable than 6-day-old mice for use in transmission studies involving mosquitoes. Subcutaneously inoculated hamsters were more susceptible to infection than intracerebrally inoculated mice (McIntosh *et al.* 1973b). After intraperitoneal injection with a hepatotropic strain of RVF virus in mouse blood or liver, suckling rats up to 15 days of age were susceptible to the infection, while adult rats were resistant. However, animals in both age groups were susceptible to intracerebrally injected neurotropic virus (Findlay and Howard 1952). After reviewing the findings of studies on RVF in inbred strains of rats in which hepatic neurosis occurred with varying severity and susceptibility to encephalitis varied, Peters and Meegan (1981) concluded that there is a genetic basis for host resistance to the disease.

Most virus isolates are considered identical antigenically, but viral strains are known to differ with respect to pathogenicity in laboratory animals and other behavioral characteristics. When RVF virus was cloned and passed either in tissue cultures, by intracerebral inoculation in mice, or by other techniques, the viral populations developed different properties such as neurotropism and various degrees of attenuation (Easterday 1965). The strains of RVF virus isolated from animals and mosquitoes were hepatotropic (pantropic) and were occasionally capable of inducing encephalitis in mice. However, intracerebral passage of these strains through laboratory rodents simultaneously enhanced viral affinity for nervous tissue and decreased the hepatotropism. Neurotropic variants were produced gradually through successive intracerebral passages in young mice, and the hepatotropic character lasted until approximately the fifteenth passage. Between the fifteenth and twentieth transfers, both neuro- and hepatotropism were observed, but the hepatotropism disappeared with subsequent passages (Murphy and Easterday 1962). When inoculated into rhesus monkeys, the neuro-adapted RVF virus of early (twentieth to fiftieth) mouse-brain passages circulated and expressed hepatotropic as well as neurotropic attributes. However, the neurostability of the virus increased with the number of mouse-brain passages, so that by the eighty-first transfer the agent could not be detected in the bloodstream (Kitchen 1950).

The indirect fluorescent antibody (IFA) technique was used to detect pantropic and neurotropic RVF virus antigens in the organs of experimentally infected mice and sheep. Anti-sheep, anti-rabbit, and anti-human globulin conjugates were used; tissues from sheep were specifically stained only with the anti-rabbit conjugate. In infected sheep, the antigen was detected in the liver as early as 24 hours after infection, and it persisted there throughout the course of the disease. These FA techniques could be used to examine tissues which were stored for 13 days at 4 °C in glycerol buffered solution (Pini *et al.* 1970). Interference between hepatotropic and neurotropic viruses was demonstrated: inactivated virus of one tropism interfered with the infectivity of an active virus of the other tropism (Findlay and Howard 1948). Ultraviolet-irradiated pantropic RVF virus was thought to interfere with the active virus remaining in the inoculum, resulting in a prolongation of the incubation period (Naudé and Polson 1957). A virus-inactivating factor which affected the survival of the virus in the brain and its extracts was found in brain tissue (Polson and Madsen 1955).

Mice, embryonated eggs, and tissue cultures have been used in the assay of RVF virus. A method of titration of RVF virus by plaque count was developed for use in cultures of Chang's human liver cells (Iwasa 1959). A more sensitive method for quantifying the growth of RVF virus involved counting the cells containing fluorescent viral antigens after infection of L-cell monolayers. Centrifugation of the virus inoculum with the cell monolayers caused viral attachment to cells within 10 minutes and penetration within 30 minutes. The infected cells could be enumerated as early as 12 hours after inoculation, and a linear relationship was demonstrated between the number of infected cells and the viral concentration in the inoculum. This method was more precise, sensitive, and rapid than assays based on the intraperitoneal inoculation of mice or the determination of cytopathic effects in cell cultures (Hahon 1969).

CLINICAL SIGNS

The clinical syndromes are classified as peracute, acute, subacute, and mild. The severity of the signs depends on the species and age of the host. The most severe syndromes are observed in lambs, calves, and adult sheep. The main symptoms are not specific and consist of fever, nasal discharge, and abortion. The mortality rate may be 70% in lambs and calves. In both sheep and cattle, the only evidence of disease may be abortion.

In man, RVF may be manifested either as a benign disease marked by fever, headaches, and malaise, or as a severe syndrome characterized by hepatic, central nervous system, and ocular complications.

Literature

In adult sheep, irregularly appearing signs of the acute disease included vomiting, mucopurulent discharge from the nose, rapid pulse, unsteady gait, and abortion, and the mortality rate was 20 to 30%. The subacute form was also common in adult animals and was characterized by fever, anorexia, general weakness, and abortion. In the mild form, only a slight febrile reaction occurred. In lambs, the peracute form was most common. The syndrome had an incubation period of 12 hours and caused death within 36 hours, with a mortality rate of approximately 100%. The course of the disease was more variable in goats and appeared to be less severe (Easterday 1965). Three strains of RVF virus propagated in mice caused typical acute clinical signs in West African dwarf sheep. The severity of the response depended on the strain of virus used; Smithburn's neurotropic strain caused the mildest reaction. Sheep infected with virus in mouse-brain material had a mild febrile response and low viremia (Tomori 1979a).

The signs of RVF in cattle were indefinite; cessation of lactation, salivation, diarrhea, and fever were reported. In some cases abortion was the only sequela observed and the mortality was less than 10%. In calves, the mortality was as high as 70%, and the animals became recumbent at the height of the fever (Easterday 1965).

Infected serum from lambs was inoculated into calves, goats, and pigs. Viremia and leukopenia were observed in calves which received different doses of RVF virus by different routes of infection. The susceptibility of calves less than 1 week old was comparable to that of lambs of the same age, but the mortality rate was lower in calves (70%) than in lambs (90%). In goats of various ages, the course of the disease varied, while pigs were not infected (Easterday *et al.* 1962a).

Rift Valley fever in humans in an acute, febrile, self-limiting syndrome which on occasion may cause mortality due to hemorrhagic fever. The uncomplicated self-limiting illness has an incubation period of 2 to 6 days (Peters and Meegan 1981). In man, the disease is characterized by fever, headache, muscular pains, weakness, nausea, and malaise which lasts for 1 to 4 days. The sequelae associated with the more severe syndrome include hemorrhagic fever, hepatic necrosis, encephalitis, and ocular complications (Easterday 1965).

PATHOLOGY

Rift Valley fever virus causes similar pathological changes in most susceptible domestic and laboratory animals. The pathognomonic features of this syndrome include focal or confluent hepatic necrosis, intranuclear inclusions, and subcutaneous, serosal, and mucosal hemorrhages. The encephalitis which occurs in laboratory animals infected with the neurotropic strains is characterized by necrosis of neural tissue, development of acidophilic intranuclear inclusions, and gliosis. Ocular lesions with hemorrhage, vasculitis, and retinitis are observed in some human cases.

Literature

In a temporal study of the development of lesions in lambs experimentally infected with RVF virus, it was found that a gray to faintly yellow foci, 0.5 to 1.0 mm in diameter, formed in the parenchyma of the liver between 28 and 40 hours after inoculation. These foci enlarged during the next 12 hours to approximately 2 to 2.5 mm. The histological changes observed in the lesions included hepatocyte degeneration and necrosis, mural thrombi formation, development of acidophilic intranuclear inclusion bodies, and infiltration of leukocytes and histiocytes. The time at which the necrotic lesions appeared seemed to be related to the quantity of virus present in the inoculum. The necrotic foci became confluent in the most severe lesions (Easterday 1965). The levels of virus in the various tissues of lambs suggested that the liver was the primary site of virus replication; the presence of virus in other tissues could be associated with the virus circulating in the blood (Easterday *et al.* 1962c). Liver changes in newborn lambs progressed from focal, primary lesions involving a few sparsely affected degenerating and necrotic hepatocytes with acidophilic bodies at 6 to 12 hours to enlarged primary foci and degenerate parenchyma by 30 to 36 hours (Coetzer and Ishak 1982). Extensive destruction of the lymphocytes in the lymph nodes and spleen of the cells in the glomeruli and mucosa of the small intestine was observed in naturally infected lambs (Coetzer 1977). The spleen, lungs, and adrenals of infected sheep developed lesions which consisted of either hemorrhages, cellular degeneration, and necrosis, or accumulation of inflammatory infiltrate (Easterday 1965). In lambs and adult sheep the serosal surfaces, endocardium, and gastrointestinal mucosa developed ecchymotic and petechial hemorrhages in the disease. The spleen had subcapsular petechiae and the kidneys were congested. The gastrointestinal tract was inflamed, and cyanosis was evident in the visible mucous membranes and skin (Peters and Meegan 1981). Moribundity and death were associated with the hemorrhage and massive necrosis in the liver, and hemorrhages in the adrenals and gastrointestinal tract (Murphy and Easterday 1962). Hemorrhages were also observed in cutaneous, subcutaneous, and subperitoneal locations and throughout the muscles. These lesions were observed in sheep and cattle in the field as well as in experimentally infected mice and hamsters (Schulz 1951). There was a limited inflammatory reaction in the brains of lambs (Easterday 1965).

In other host species the hepatic lesions were similar but tended to remain focal (Easterday 1965). Upon histologic examination, the hepatic lesions in dogs and cats were identical to those observed in other species infected with RVF virus. However, there was lack of definite Councilman-like bodies, and the intranuclear inclusions were not as well defined. Myocarditis, necrosis of myocardial fibers, and encephalitis, which included gliosis and necrosis, occurred in addition to the lesions commonly observed in other species (Mitten *et al.* 1970). Ultrastructural studies of the development of hepatic lesions in mice showed that the virus multiplied in the cytoplasm. The acidophilic nuclear inclusions did not appear to be associated with the virus particles *per se* and possibly represented a degenerative phenomenon (McGavran and Easterday 1963).

Different strains of RVF virus caused identical histological changes in the liver and brain of mice. However, the inclusion bodies were not consistently seen with all strains, and there was no correlation between virus titers and the severity of the histological changes observed (Tomori and Kasali 1979). The histological changes in the livers of mice following the inoculation of a saturating dose of the virus were investigated. The saturating dose synchronized the cellular changes and enabled the temporal development of the histological lesions to be correlated to the adsorption, multiplication, and release of the virus. This single cell of viral growth was produced by the inoculation of large quantities of virus which infected all susceptible cells. Adsorption took place within 30 minutes, and within an hour the liver cell nuclei swelled, and the chromatin pattern became coarse and marginated in reaction to the infection. By 2 hours after inoculation, almost all of the nuclei showed these changes, and within 3 hours intranuclear inclusion bodies were visible. The latent or eclipse period, during which the virus was multiplying in a noninfective form, occurred between the first and third hours. The release of the virus betwen 3.5 and 5.5 hours postinfection was accompanied by extensive disintegration of hepatic cells involving rupture of the nucleus and breakdown of the cytoplasm. By the end of this period, the destruction of the cells was widespread. A coagulation defect was present at 5 hours and was associated with extensive hemorrhages (Mims 1957). The prothrombin deficiency detected in the plasma of mice infected with RVF virus was probably responsible for the prolongation of the clotting time. This coagulation malfunction was associated with the hemorrhagic syndromes (Mims 1956e). Mims and Mason (1956) described the properties of an RVF hemagglutinin that they isolated from the sera of infected mice. Rodents infected with the neurotropic strain of RVF virus developed lesions which were characteristic of a meningoencephalitis. Destruction of neurons and perivascular infiltration by inflammatory cells and intranuclear inclusion bodies were observed in the brains of these animals (Easterday 1965).

Fatal human cases which occurred during the 1977 RVF epidemic in Egypt had severe liver necrosis, interstitial pneumonia, and myocardial degeneration (Abdel-Wahab *et al.* 1978). Patients with ocular manifestations were also studied during this outbreak (Siam and Meegan 1980; Deutman and Klomp 1981). The ocular lesions were characterized by hemorrhage, edema, vasculitis, retinitis, and vascular occlusion. These lesions regressed, but permanent loss of visual acuity was observed (Siam *et al.* 1980).

IMMUNOLOGY

There is very limited information on the immune response of domestic and laboratory animals to RVF virus. The various strains isolated appear to be closely related antigenically. The antibodies which develop in both domestic and laboratory animals can be demonstrated by several standard serological tests. Antisera and colostrum have prophylactic and therapeutic value as they may be used to induce passive immunity in lambs and calves.

Literature

Weiss (1962) quoted earlier work in which resistance to RVF was transmitted to calves by ingestion of colostrum and lasted for 5 months after weaning. Immune serum was also prophylactic and therapeutic in mice and lambs infected with RVF virus. If serum therapy in mice was delayed until 11 to 25 hours after challenge, the pantropic nature of the virus was masked and the neurotropic features appeared. In lambs the serum was therapeutic when administered after the first appearance of viremia and clinical signs. The surviving lambs were immune to subsequent challenge (Bennett *et al.* 1965). The immunity produced in humans by an attack of RVF persisted for at least 20 years (Findlay and Howard 1948). The serum-virus neutralization test and the IFA technique were used to detect specific antibodies to RVF virus in sheep and cattle (Pini *et al.* 1973). Neutralization, complement-fixation (CF), hemagglutination/hemagglutination-inhibition, and agar-gel diffusion tests could be used to differentiate three strains of RVF virus (Tomori 1979b).

VACCINATION

The vaccine prepared from a neurotropic strain of virus propagated by serial intracerebral passage in mice is not sufficiently immunogenic and may cause abortions when administered to pregnant ewes. Humans are vaccinated with RVF virus which is grown in tissue cultures and then formalin-inactivated. In animals, single injections of similar vaccines induce low neutralizing antibody titers which do not always prevent abortion or the development of viremia. Therefore, multiple injections of vaccine consisting of virus and adjuvants are recommended. Developmental anomalies are associated with the use of a vaccine composed of attenuated RVF virus in combination with Wesselsbron virus; the latter virus is the causative agent.

Literature

The injection of an intracerebral mouse-passaged strain of virus at the 106th passage-level was one of the first methods used to vaccinate cattle and sheep. Vaccinated sheep which were challenged 30 days after inoculation with a pantropic strain developed neither pyrexia nor viremia. Control sheep developed high levels of neutralizing antibody, pyrexia, and viremia within 11 days of the challenge (Capstick and Gosden 1962). After 102 intracerebral passages in mice, neurotropic RVF virus could be safely administered to sheep and very young lambs, but it could not be used to immunize pregnant ewes because intrauterine infection of the fetus occurred (Weiss 1962). Vaccine produced passage through mouse brains or through embryonated eggs caused abortion in pregnant ewes and were weakly immunogenic (Easterday 1965). Cattle vaccinated with a neurotropic strain of RVF virus developed a low-level serum neutralizing antibody response, but still possessed some degree of immunity when challenged with the pantropic virus 28 months later. Some of the calves born to vaccinated mothers had demonstrable antibodies in their sera prior to ingesting colostrum, and antibody appeared in all the sera of calves after ingestion of colostrum. The sera of cattle and sheep infected with the pantropic virus contained high levels of antibody which persisted for 2.5 and 3 years respectively (Coackley *et al.* 1967a, b).

A safe, potent RVF vaccine was developed for use in humans. The vaccine was prepared from rhesus and African green monkey kidney stable (MS) cell cultures infected with the pantropic strain of the virus and inactivated by formalin. The addition of 2% human serum albumin increased the heat stability of the lyophilized vaccine. This vaccine was extremely stable with respect to immunogenic potency and proved effective in protecting high-risk laboratory workers (Randall *et al.* 1963, 1964). Formaldehyde-inactivated vaccine prepared from lamb kidney and hamster kidney primary cell cultures was comparable in efficacy to that derived from MS cell cultures (Binn *et al.* 1963).

A formalin-inactivated RVF virus vaccine prepared in tissue cultures for human use effectively protected sheep against challenge by inducing the formation of neutralizing antibodies (Harrington *et al.* 1980). Cattle, goats, and sheep were immunized with this vaccine, and the virus neutralization titers determined by plaque reduction tests were generally low in steers and sheep and high in goats. The sheep which were reinoculated with undiluted vaccine did not develop any clinical signs or viremia on challenge with virulent virus, indicating that solid immunity was produced in all of these animals (Yedloutschnig *et al.* 1979). A dose of 2 ml formalin-inactivated cell culture supernatant with alum adjuvant protected sheep against illness and viremia when the animals were challenged with RVF virus several months later. This effect was obtained even when the levels of serum neutralizing antibody were very low. It appeared that the titers of neutralizing antibody were not directly related to the level of immunity (Peters and Meegan 1981).

The effects of varying doses and combinations of live and inactivated vaccines were compared in cattle. The antibody response to the first injection of either vaccine was poor when measured by the serum-virus neutralization and hemagglutination-inhibition tests, but a booster dose of the inactivated vaccine evoked a good anamnestic response. Cattle vaccinated with the live vaccine but negative for RVF in serological tests were immune when challenged with virulent RVF virus (Barnard 1979). Sheep and cows which had been previously vaccinated with various doses of an RVF vaccine produced in cell cultures and inactivated with formalin were challenged with a virulent strain. A single dose did not protect sheep against challenge with virulent RVF virus; viremia developed in 86% of the ewes. There was no detectable difference between the vaccinated and unvaccinated animals. All of the ewes developed clinical signs and aborted between days 6 and 18. All of the ewes either aborted or had dead fetuses. Although all pregnant cows aborted on challenge after a single dose, two doses prevented abortion (Yedloutschnig *et al.* 1981). The vaccination of pregnant ewes with attenuated RVF virus alone or in combination with attenuated Wesselsbron virus vaccine resulted in the development of hydranencephaly, arthrogryposis, brachygnathy, inferior defects in the spinal cord, and neurogenic muscular atrophy in the fetuses, and accumulation of large volumes of amniotic fluid. The affected ewes usually had a prolonged gestation period and ultimately died. *Hydrops amnii* was observed in about 15% of the ewes in flocks in the field. It was proved experimentally that both the wild type and the attenuated Wesselsbron disease virus produced these uterine lesions and fetal malformations. Preliminary experimental work also showed that the attenuated RVF virus vaccine was responsible for several of these conditions (Coetzer and Barnard 1977).

DIAGNOSIS

A clinical diagnosis of RVF must be confirmed by serological tests and isolation of the virus. The features indicative of the disease are: (1) clinical illness, a high mortality in lambs and calves, and a much lower incidence of morbidity in adult animals; (2) high abortion rates; (3) hepatic lesions; and (4) infections in humans who had been in contact with infective material. In association with the epizootics in sheep and cattle, there may be high mortality rates among wild rodents. A variety of laboratory animals can be used for inoculation experiments and viral isolation, but mice, hamsters, ferrets, and lambs are preferred. The hepatic lesions and hemorrhages are important diagnostic signs. The serum neutralization, hemagglutination-inhibition, and CF tests are adequate for diagnostic purposes. Additional serological tests on paired sera from the acute and convalescent phases are useful. Fluorescent antibody techniques can detect the presence of RVF virus in infected tissue cultures within 6 hours of inoculation. This is the fastest method of diagnosis and is optimally undertaken 18 to 22 hours after the inoculation of cell cultures. Direct or indirect FA techniques can also be applied to frozen postmortem specimens. Another relatively sensitive laboratory system for virus isolation is the intracerebral injection of 1- to 2-day-old suckling mice. The adult mice should also be used to differentiate RVF virus from the many other viruses that cause similar diseases which are not lethal for adult mice.

Literature

The literature has been reviewed under other sections in this chapter, particularly those which deal with tissue culture methods, infection in laboratory animals, and serological techniques. The clinical features of RVF and the methods used for the diagnosis of this disease were described by Easterday (1965) and Peters and Meegan (1981).

CONTROL

Rift Valley fever can be controlled most effectively by vaccinating cattle and sheep. The screening of holding areas protects susceptible animals from the several species of mosquitoes which are capable of transmitting RVF virus. The vector can also be controlled by applying residual insecticides to the animals, pens, and barns.

BIBLIOGRAPHY

Abdel-Wahab, K. S. E., El Baz, L. M., El Tayeb, E. M., Omar, H., Ossman, M. A. M. and Yasin, W., 1978. Rift Valley fever virus infections in Egypt: pathological and virological findings in man, *Trans. R. Soc. trop. Med. Hyg.*, **72**(4): 392–6.

Alexander, R. A., 1951. Rift Valley fever in the Union, *J. S. Afr. vet. med. Ass.*, **22**: 105–12.

Anon., 1979. Symposium on Rift Valley fever held by the Veterinary Services in Tel Aviv on 26th April, 1979, *Refuah Vet.*, **36**: 119–25.

Barnard, B. J. H., 1979. Rift Valley fever vaccine – antibody and immune response in cattle to a live and an inactivated vaccine, *J. S. Afr. vet. med. Ass.*, **50**(3): 155–7.

Bennett, D. G., Glock, R. D. and Gerone, P. J., 1965. Protection of mice and lambs against pantropic Rift Valley fever virus, using immune serum, *Am. J. vet. Res.*, **26**(110): 57–62.

Binn, L. N., Randall, R., Harrison, V. R., Gibbs, C. J. Jr and Aulisio, C. G., 1963. Immunization against Rift Valley fever. The development of vaccines from nonprimate cell cultures and chick embryos, *Am. J. Hyg.*, **77**: 160–8.

Boyle, J. J., 1967. Biological characteristics of plaque variants of Rift Valley fever virus, *Am. J. vet. Res.*, **28**(125): 1027–31.

Brown, J. L., Dominik, J. W. and Morrissey, R. L., 1981. Respiratory infectivity of a recently isolated strain of Rift Valley fever virus, *Infect. Immun.*, **33**(3): 848–53.

Capstick, P. B. and Gosden, D., 1962. Neutralizing antibody response of sheep to pantropic and neurotropic Rift Valley fever virus, *Nature*, **195**: 583–4.

Coackley, W., 1965. Alteration in virulence of Rift Valley fever virus during serial passage in lamb testis cells, *J. Path. Bact.*, **89**: 123–31.

Coackley, W., Pini, A. and Gosden, D., 1967a. Experimental infection of cattle with pantropic Rift Valley fever virus, *Res. vet. Sci.*, **8**: 399–405.

Coackley, W., Pini, A. and Gosden, D., 1967b. The immunity induced in cattle and sheep by inoculation of neurotropic or pantropic Rift Valley fever viruses, *Res. vet. Sci.*, **8**: 406–14.

Coetzer, J. A. W., 1977. The pathology of Rift Valley fever. I. Lesions occurring in natural cases in new-born lambs, *Onderstepoort J. vet. Res.*, **44**(4): 205–12.

Coetzer, J. A. W. and Barnard, B. J. H., 1977. *Hydrops amnii* in sheep associated with hydranencephaly and arthrogryposis with Wesselsbron disease and Rift Valley fever viruses as aetiological agents, *Onderstepoort J. vet. Res.*, **44**(2): 119–26.

Coetzer, J. A. W. and Ishak, K. G., 1982. Sequential development of the liver lesions in new-born lambs infected with Rift Valley fever virus I. Macroscopic and microscopic pathology, *Onderstepoort J. vet. Res.*, **49**: 103–8.

Craig, D. E., Thomas, W. J. and DeSanctis, A. N., 1967. Stability of Rift Valley fever virus at 4 °C, *Appl. Microbiol.*, **15**(2): 446–7.

Davies, F. G., 1975. Observations on the epidemiology of Rift Valley fever in Kenya, *J. Hyg., Camb.*, **75**: 219–30.

Davies, F. G. and Addy, P. A. K., 1979. Rift Valley fever. A survey for antibody to the virus in bird species commonly found in situations considered to be enzootic, *Trans. R. Soc. trop. Med. Hyg.*, **73**(5): 584.

Davies, F. G., Clausen, B. and Lund, L. J., 1972. The pathogenicity of Rift Valley fever virus for the baboon, *Trans. R. Soc. trop. Med. Hyg.*, **66**: 363–5.

Davies, F. G. and Highton, R. B., 1980. Possible vectors of Rift Valley fever in Kenya, *Trans. R. Soc. trop. Med. Hyg.*, **74**(6): 815–16.

Davies, F. G. and Karstad, L., 1981. Experimental infection of the African buffalo with the virus of Rift Valley fever, *Trop. Anim. Hlth Prod.*, **13**: 185–8.

Davies, F. G. and Onyango, E., 1978. Rift Valley fever: the role of the vervet monkey as a reservoir or maintenance host for this virus, *Trans. R. Soc. trop. Med. Hyg.*, **72**: 213–14.

Deutman, A. F. and Klomp, H. J., 1981. Rift Valley fever retinitis, *Am. J. Ophthalmol.*, **92**: 38–42.

Easterday, B. C., 1961. Experimental Rift Valley fever, Diss., Wisconsin, Abstr. 22: 546,197 pp.

Easterday, B. C., 1965. Rift Valley fever. In *Advances in Veterinary Science*, eds C. A. Brandly, C. Cornelius. Academic Press (New York), vol. 10, pp. 65–127.

Easterday, B. C. and Jaeger, R. F., 1963. The detection of Rift Valley fever virus by a tissue culture fluorescein-labeled antibody method, *J. Infect. Dis.*, **112**(1): 1–6.

Easterday, B. C., McGavran, M. H., Rooney, J. R. and Murphy, L. C., 1962c. The pathogenesis of Rift Valley fever in lambs, *Am. J. vet. Res.*, **23**(94): 470–9.

Easterday, B. C. and Murphy, L. C., 1963a. The growth of Rift Valley fever virus in cultures of established lines of cells, *Cornell Vet.*, **53**: 3–11.

Easterday, B. C. and Murphy, L. C., 1963b. Studies on Rift Valley fever in laboratory animals, *Cornell Vet.*, **53**: 423–33.

Easterday, B. C., Murphy, L. C. and Bennett, D. G., 1962a. Experimental Rift Valley fever in calves, goats, and pigs, *Am. J. vet. Res.*, **23**(97): 1224–30.

Easterday, B. C., Murphy, L. C. and Bennett, D. G., 1962b.

Experimental Rift Valley fever in lambs and sheep, *Am. J. vet. Res.*, **23**: 1231–9.

Eisa, M., Kheir El Sid, E. D., Shomein, A. M. and Meegan, J. M., 1980. An outbreak of Rift Valley fever in the Sudan – 1976, *Trans. R. Soc. trop. Med. Hyg.*, **74**(3): 417–18.

Ellis, D. S., Simpson, D. I. H., Stamford, S. and Wahab, K. S. E. A., 1979. Rift Valley fever virus: some ultrastructural observations on material from the outbreak in Egypt 1977, *J. gen. Virol.*, **42**: 329–37.

Fagbami, A. H., Tomori, O., Fabiyi, A. and Isoun, T. T., 1975. Experimental Rift Valley fever in West African Dwarf sheep, *Res. vet. Sci.*, **18**: 334–5.

Findlay, G. M. and Howard, E. M., 1948. Notes on Rift Valley fever, *Archiv f. Virusforschung*, **4**: 411–23.

Findlay, G. M. and Howard, E. M., 1952. The susceptibility of rats to Rift Valley fever in relation to age, *Ann. trop. Med. Parasit.*, **46**: 33–7.

Hahon, N., 1969. Immunofluorescent cell-counting assay of Rift Valley fever virus, *Am. J. vet. Res.*, **30**: 1007–14.

Haig, D. A., 1965. Symposium: the smallest stowaways. II. The arboviruses, *Vet. Rec.*, **77**: 1428–31.

Harrington, D. G., Lupton, H. W., Crabbs, C. L., Peters, C. J., Reynolds, J. A. and Slone, T. W. Jr, 1980. Evaluation of a formalin-inactivated Rift Valley fever vaccine in sheep, *Am. J. vet. Res.*, **41**(10): 1559–64.

Henning, M. W., 1952. Rift Valley fever, *J. S. Afr. vet. med. Ass.*, **23**(2): 65–78.

Henning, M. W., 1956. Rift Valley fever. In *Animal Diseases in South Africa. Being an Account of the Infectious Diseases of Domestic Animals.* Central News Agency (South Africa), pp. 1115–21.

Hoogstraal, H., Meegan, J. M., Khalil, G. M. and Adham, F. K., 1979. The Rift Valley fever epizootic in Egypt 1977–78. 2. Ecological and entomological studies, *Trans. R. Soc. trop. Med. Hyg.*, **73**(6): 624–9.

Imam, I. Z. E., El-Karamany, R. and Darwish, M. A., 1979. An epidemic of Rift Valley fever in Egypt. 2. Isolation of the virus from animals, *Bull. Wld. Hlth Org.*, **57**: 441–3.

Iwasa, S., 1959. Multiplication of Rift Valley fever virus in human liver cell culture with special reference to production complement fixing antigen, *Jap. J. Exp. Med.*, **29**(4): 323–34.

Jennings, M., Platt, G. S. and Bowen, E. T., 1982. The susceptibility of *Culicoides variipennis* Coq. (Diptera: Ceratopogonidae) to laboratory infection with Rift Valley fever virus, *Trans. R. Soc. trop. Med. Hyg.*, **76**(5): 587–9.

Johnson, R. W. and Orlando, M. D., 1968. Growth of Rift Valley fever virus in tissue culture, *Am. J. vet. Res.*, **29**(2): 463–71.

Keefer, G. V., Zebarth, G. L. and Allen, W. P., 1972. Susceptibility of dogs and cats to Rift Valley fever by inhalation or ingestion of virus, *J. Infect. Dis.*, **125**(3): 307–9.

Kitchen, S. F., 1950. The development of neurotropism in Rift Valley fever virus, *Ann. trop. Med. Parasit.*, **44**: 132–45.

Matumoto, M., Saburi, Y. and Nishi, I., 1959. Rift Valley fever virus in the one-day-old chick embryo, *J. Immunol.*, **82**: 219–25.

McGavran, M. H. and Easterday, B. C., 1963. Rift Valley fever virus hepatitis. Light and electron microscopic studies in the mouse, *Am. J. Path.*, **42**: 587–607.

McIntosh, B. M., 1972. Rift Valley fever. 1. Vector studies in the field, *J. S. Afr. vet. med. Ass.*, **43**(4): 391–5.

McIntosh, B. M., Dickinson, D. B. and dos Santos, I., 1973b. Rift Valley fever. 3. Viraemia in cattle and sheep. 4. The susceptibility of mice and hamsters in relation to transmission of virus by mosquitoes, *J. S. Afr. vet. med. Ass.*, **44**(2): 167–9.

McIntosh, B. M. and Gear, J. H. S., 1981, Rift Valley fever. In *CRC Handbook Series in Zoonoses: Viral Zoonoses*. ed. G. W. Beran. CRC Press (Boca Raton, Fla.), vol. 1, pp. 230–3.

McIntosh, B. M., Jupp, P. G., Anderson, D. and Dickinson, D. B., 1973a. Rift Valley fever. 2. Attempts to transmit virus with seven species of mosquitoes, *J. S. Afr. vet. med. Ass.*, **44**(1): 57–60.

Meegan, J. M., Hoogstraal, H. and Moussa, M. I., 1979. An epizootic of Rift Valley fever in Egypt in 1977, *Vet. Rec.*, **105**: 124–5.

Meegan, J. M., Khalil, G. M., Hoogstraal, H. and Adham, F. K., 1980. Experimental transmission and field isolation studies explicating *Culex pipiens* as a vector of Rift Valley fever virus in Egypt, *Am. J. trop. Med. Hyg.*, **29**(6): 1405–10.

Meegan, J. M., Shope, R. E., Peters, C. J. and Digoutte, J. P., 1983. Zinga virus: a strain of Rift Valley fever virus, *Morbidity and Mortality Weekly Report, US Dept. Hlth Hum. Serv.*, **32**(7): 90–2.

Miller, W. S., Demchak, P., Rosenberger, C. R., Dominik, J. W. and Bradshaw, J. L., 1963. Stability and infectivity of airborne yellow fever and Rift Valley fever viruses, *Am. J. Hyg.*, **77**: 114–21.

Mims, C. A., 1956a, b, c. Rift Valley fever in mice. I. General features of the infection. II. Adsorption and multiplication of virus. III. Further quantitative features of the infective process, *Br. J. exp. Path.*, **37**(1): 99–109.

Mims, C. A., 1956d. Rift Valley fever in mice. IV. Incomplete virus; its production and properties, *Br. J. exp. Path.*, **37**: 129–43.

Mims, C. A., 1956e. The coagulation defect in Rift Valley fever and yellow fever virus infections, *Ann. trop. Med. Parasit.*, **50**: 147–9.

Mims, C. A., 1956f. Viruses as pathogenic agents, *Bull. epiz. Dis. Afr.*, **4**: 316–17.

Mims, C. A., 1957. Rift Valley fever in mice. VI. Histological changes in the liver in relation to virus multiplication, *Aust. J. exp. Biol.*, **35**: 595–604.

Mims, C. A. and Mason, P. J., 1956. Rift Valley fever in mice. V. The properties of haemagglutinin present in infective serum, *Br. J. exp. Path.*, **37**: 423–33.

Mitten, J. Q., Remmele, N. S., Walker, J. S., Carter, R. C., Stephen, E. L. and Klein, F., 1970. The clinical aspects of Rift Valley fever virus in household pets. III. Pathologic changes in the dog and cat, *J. Infect. Dis.*, **121**(1): 25–31.

Murphy, L. C. and Easterday, B. C., 1962. Rift Valley fever: A zoonosis. In *Proceedings Sixty-Fifth Annual Meeting of the United States Livestock Sanitary Association*. MacCrellish and Quigley (Trenton, NJ), pp. 397–412.

Naudé, W. du T., Madsen, T. and Polson, A., 1954. Different-sized infective particles of Rift Valley fever virus, *Nature*, **173**: 1051–2.

Naudé, W. du T. and Polson, A., 1957. Interference between active and ultraviolet-irradiated Rift Valley fever virus, *J. gen. Microbiol.*, **16**: 491–7.

Peters, C. J. and Meegan, J. M., 1981. Rift Valley fever. In *CRC Handbook Series in Zoonoses: Viral Zoonoses*. ed. G. W. Beran. CRC Press (Boca Raton, Fla.), vol. 1, pp. 403–20.

Pini, A., Lund, L. J. and Davies, F. G., 1970. Detection of Rift Valley fever virus by the fluorescent antibody technique in organs of experimentally infected animals, *Res. vet. Sci.*, **11**: 82–5.

Pini, A., Lund, L. J. and Davies, F. G., 1973. Fluorescent and neutralizing antibody response to infection by Rift Valley fever virus, *J. S. Afr. vet. med. Ass.*, **44**(2): 161–5.

Polson, A. and Madsen, T. I., 1955. A brain factor influencing the viability of neurotropic Rift Valley fever, *Nature*, **176**: 645–6.

Randall, R., Binn, L. N. and Harrison, V. R., 1963. Rift Valley fever virus vaccine, *Am. J. trop. Med. Hyg.*, **12**: 611–5.

Randall, R., Binn, L. N. and Harrison, V. R., 1964. Immunization. against Rift Valley fever virus. Studies on the immunogenicity of lyophilized formalin-inactivated vaccine, *J. Immunol.*, **93**: 293–9.

Rift Valley fever workshop, 1981. In *Contributions to Epidemiology and Biostatistics*, eds T. A. Swartz, M. A. Klingberg, N. Goldblum. Karger (Basle), vol. 3, 196 pp.

Schulz, K. C. A., 1951. The pathology of Rift Valley fever or enzootic hepatitis in South Africa, *J. S. Afr. vet. med. Ass.*, **22**(3): 113–20.

Scott, G. R., 1963. Pigs and Rift Valley fever, *Nature*, **200**: 919–20.

Scott, G. R., Coackley, W., Roach, R. W. and Cowdy, N. R., 1963. Rift Valley fever in camels, *J. Path. Bact.*, **86**: 229–31.

Sellers, R. F., 1981. Rift Valley fever. In *Virus Diseases of Food Animals, A World Geography of Epidemiology and Control*, ed. E. P. J. Gibbs, Academic Press (New York), Disease Monographs, vol. 2, pp. 674–80.

Sellers, R. F., Pedgley, D. E. and Tucker, M. R., 1982. Rift Valley fever, Egypt 1977: disease spread by windborne insect vectors?, *Vet. Rec.*, **110**: 73–7.

Shone, D. K., Philip, J. R., Roberts, R. M. and Christie, G. J., 1958. Some aetiological agents of bovine abortions in Southern Rhodesia, *J. S. Afr. vet. med. Ass.*, **29**(1): 55–62.

Shope, R. E., Peters, C. J. and Davies, F. G., 1982. The spread of Rift Valley fever and approaches to its control, *Bull. Wld Hlth Org.*, **60**(3): 299–304.

Siam, A. L. and Meegan, J. M., 1980. Ocular disease resulting from infection with Rift Valley fever virus, *Trans. R. Soc. trop. Med. Hyg.*, **74**(4): 539–41.

Siam, A. L., Meegan, J. M. and Gharbawi, K. F., 1980. Rift Valley fever ocular manifestations: observations during the 1977 epidemic in Egypt, *Br. J. Ophthalmol.*, **64**: 366–74.

Swanepoel, R. and Blackburn, N. K., 1977. Demonstration of nuclear immunofluorescence in Rift Valley fever infected cells, *J. gen. Virol.*, **34**: 557–61.

Swanepoel, R., Blackburn, N. K., Efstratiou, S. and Condy, J. B., 1978. Studies on Rift Valley fever in some African murids (Rodentia: Muridae), *J. Hyg., Camb.*, **80**: 183–96.

Tomori, O., 1979a. Clinical, virological and serological response of the West African dwarf sheep to experimental infection with different strains of Rift Valley fever virus, *Res. vet. Sci.*, **26**: 152–9.

Tomori, O., 1979b. Immunological reactions of Rift Valley fever virus strains from East and West Africa, *Res. vet. Sci.*, **26**: 160–4.

Tomori, O. and Kasali, O., 1979. Pathogenicity of different strains of Rift Valley fever virus in Swiss albino mice, *Br. J. exp. Path.*, **60**: 417–22.

Walker, J. S., Carter, R. C., Klein, F., Snowden, S. E. and Lincoln, R. E., 1969. Evaluation of factors related to growth of Rift Valley fever virus in suspended cell cultures, *Appl. Microbiol.*, **17**(5): 658–64.

Walker, J. S., Remmele, N. S., Carter. R. C., Mitten, J. Q., Schuh, L. G., Stephen, E. L. and Klein, F., 1970a. The clinical aspects of

Rift Valley fever virus in household pets. I. Susceptibility of the dog, *J. Infect. Dis.*, **121**(1): 9–18.
Walker, J. S., Stephen, E. L., Remmele, N. S., Carter, R. C., Mitten, J. Q., Schuh, L. G. and Klein, F., 1970b. The clinical aspects of Rift Valley fever virus in household pets. II. Susceptibility of the cat, *J. Infect. Dis.*, **121**(1): 19–24.
Weiss, K. E., 1962. Studies on Rift Valley fever – passive and active immunity in lambs, *Onderstepoort J. vet. Res.*, **29**(1): 3–9.

Yedloutschnig, R. J., Dardiri, A. H., Mebus, C. A. and Walker, J. S., 1981. Abortion in vaccinated sheep and cattle after challenge with Rift Valley fever virus, *Vet. Rec.*, **109**: 383–4.
Yedloutschnig, R. J., Dardiri, A. H., Walker, J. S., Peters, C. J. and Eddy, G. A., 1979. Immune response of steers, goats and sheep to inactivated Rift Valley fever vaccine, *Proc. US Anim. Hlth Assoc.* Carter Composition Corp. (Richmond, Va.), vol, 83, pp. 253–60.

Chapter

15

Rinderpest

CONTENTS

INTRODUCTION

Rinderpest is a contagious viral disease of cattle, buffalo, sheep, goats, pigs, camels, and wild game, characterized by a short period of fever, lymphocytolysis, erosive stomatitis, and gastroenteritis. It causes the most serious losses in cattle and buffalo.

Literature

Rinderpest is an ancient Asiatic plague of cattle and buffalo. Henning (1956) gave a full account of the history and described how it has been one of the most devastating diseases of cattle since ancient times. More recent comprehensive reviews on rinderpest were published by Plowright (1962a, 1968), by Scott (1964, 1981) and by Liess in German (1965).

An extensive recent review of the effects of rinderpest on wildlife in Africa and the influence on populations of game animals by rinderpest control undertaken in domestic stock was presented by Plowright (1982). The author pointed out that the presence of susceptible herds in East Africa required the development of specific plans to combat the occurrence of possible epizootics. The elimination of rinderpest from cattle in northeast Africa would be a major development to safeguard the wildlife populations of Africa. These concerns have been realistic because of the outbreaks of rinderpest which were reported to occur in the Serengeti, Tanzania, and other parts of Africa in 1982.

Attention should be drawn to the resurgence of rinderpest in various regions of Africa and the Near East in 1982 and 1983, probably as a result of insufficient veterinary services and of military strife.

ETIOLOGY

Rinderpest virus is classified with the canine distemper and human measles viruses in the *Morbillivirus* genus of the Paramyxoviridae. The virions of rinderpest are enveloped helical particles that are pleomorphic; the majority are spherical, but some particles are filamentous. The envelopes bristle with minute projections. Rinderpest virus is very fragile, and given its extreme sensitivity to ordinary environmental conditions such as sunlight, putrefaction, and thermal and chemical agents, it is unlikely to survive for many hours outside the host.

The ability of rinderpest virus to grow readily in various tissue culture systems enabled researchers to develop a most efficient vaccine and study the pathogenesis and transmission of the infection.

Literature

Infective tissues were readily inactivated by heat, and the rate of inactivation was dependent on the temperature. For example, the half-life of the virus in lymphoid tissues maintained at 56 °C was 5 minutes, but at 7 °C it was extended to 2 to 3 days. The reduction observed in the titers of virus in frozen infected tissues was ascribed to inactivation which occurred during the freezing and thawing process. Rinderpest virus was also destroyed by drying and exposure to ultraviolet irradiation. Putrefaction, pH, and salt concentration also affected the survival of the virus in tissues (Scott 1964). The heat sensitivity was influenced by the salt concentration, particularly that of sulfate ions. The virus is unstable below pH 3 and above pH 11 (De Boer and Barber 1964b; Liess and Plowright 1963). The resistance of the virus to light, heat, freezing, storage at low temperature, lyophilization, pH, and salt concentration was discussed (Plowright 1968). More recently, the inactivation of rinderpest virus by a temperature of 56 °C and by ultraviolet irradiation was shown to be influenced by the composition of the suspending medium (Hussain *et al.* 1980b).

The history of the cultivation of rinderpest virus in various tissue culture systems was reviewed, and the different types of host cells which support the propagation of bovine strains of the virus in primary monolayer cultures were listed in tabular form (Plowright 1968). Virulent rinderpest virus was adapted to growth in monolayers of bovine kidney cells. The cytopathogenic effects became prominent on the fifth passage, and peak titers of virus developed between 6 and 8 days after inoculation (Plowright and Ferris 1959a). Virulent strains could be isolated from the tissues of infected cattle and titrated in primary cultures of calf kidney cells. The time to appearance of the typical cytopathic changes varied from 3 to 12 days after seeding and depended on the amount of virus in the inoculant (Plowright and Ferris 1962a). Serially cultivated calf kidney cells were highly susceptible to rinderpest infection; a particular cell line proved capable of producing high-titer virus over many serial passages (Ferris and Plowright 1961). Monolayer cultures of calf thyroid could be used for culturing rinderpest virus as well as other viruses of sheep and cattle (Plowright and Ferris 1961). The growth characteristics of rinderpest virus in HeLa cells were investigated, and the titer of intracellular virus was consistently 10 to 100 times greater than that of free virus (Liess and Plowright 1963/64). The basic techniques developed by Plowright and his coworkers were generally adopted in other laboratories (De Boer 1962a; Gilbert and Monnier 1962; Johnson 1962a; Bansal and Joshi 1981). These culture systems were used to titrate the virus and demonstrate the virus-neutralizing antibody. Various modifications of the original techniques described were used to make the system more advantageous (Plowright and Ferris 1962a).

Virulent and attenuated strains of rinderpest virus were studied in calf kidney cells. The infection of calf kidney cells with a low multiplicity of rinderpest virus resulted in the development of large quantities of superficial virus which could readily be removed (Plowright 1964a). Caprinized and lapinized viruses did not induce the characteristic cytopathic effects (CPEs) in tissue cultures and could not be isolated in the system. Also, the re-isolation of the culture-attenuated virus from the blood of vaccinated cattle was rarely accomplished (Plowright 1962b). The direct immunoperoxidase test was used to detect rinderpest virus antigens in bovine kidney cell cultures. It was shown that viral multiplication, indicated by the increase in the number of affected cells, correlated well with the progressive virus-specific CPEs (Krishnaswamy *et al.* 1981).

The sequence of events involved in the process of viral multiplication was studied in cell cultures. In the initial phase the virus adsorbed to the cell within the first 8 hours, and the rate of adsorption depended on the conditions of the culture media. The adsorption stage was followed by the eclipse phase, which probably lasted for 14 to 20 hours and ended with the appearance of the progeny of the input virus. This was followed by the growth phase, during which the cell-associated virus reached peak levels after 48 to 72 hours. The time to maximum virus production depended on the conditions of the culture system and time of peak depended on the quantity of virus inoculated into the medium (Plowright 1968).

The propagation of the virus in tissue culture was associated with cytopathogenic effects. Two main cell changes occurred: (1) the formation of round, elongated, or stellate cells; and (2) the development of multinucleated syncytia. The first change was observed early in the infection, while the syncytia were found in the later stages. Both intranuclear and intracytoplasmic inclusions were observed in several cell lines. Attenuated vaccine strains did not proliferate or produce CPEs in the various cell cultures used (Plowright and Ferris 1957, 1959a). The first manifestation of infection in tissue culture cells were eosinophilic cytoplasmic inclusions and syncytia. These developments were followed 24 hours later by the formation of eosinophilic intranuclear inclusions. Both the cytoplasmic and intranuclear inclusions were composed of numerous tubular nuclear protein strands resembling the nucleocapsids within virions (Tajima and Ushijima 1971). The occurrence of these cytopathic changes depended on the cell type, the stage of infection, and the strain of the virus. The growth of the virus in monolayers produced round clearings of 1 mm in diameter when the dissemination of the virus through the fluid was prevented by incorporating immune serum into the medium. The number of plaques formed was proportional to the dilution of the virus used (Plowright 1962a). No differences were observed in the morphology of the plaques produced after 6 days of incubation by five strains of rinderpest virus known to differ in their virulence for cattle (Taylor and Perry 1970). Plaque formation by rinderpest and other viruses pathogenic for cattle was investigated (McKercher 1963, 1964). The CPEs of rinderpest virus as well as other bovine viruses which induce clinical syndromes comparable to those of rinderpest were described. It was concluded that these viruses could be tentatively identified on the basis of their CPEs in cell cultures. Tissue culture rinderpest vaccine virus interfered with the replication of bovine virus diarrhea, infectious bovine rhinotracheitis, bovine parainfluenza type 3, and foot-and-mouth disease Asia type 1 in bovine kidney cell cultures. These findings suggested that interferon-mediated auto-interference limited the development of rinderpest virus CPEs in tissue culture (Hussain *et al.* 1980a; Bansal *et al.* 1981).

EPIZOOTIOLOGY

Incidence and geographical distribution

Rinderpest is confined to Africa and parts of Asia where enzootic foci exist. The dissemination of the disease from enzootic areas results in devastating epizootics. In the past rinderpest was spread by military campaigns and, more recently, by the trade in livestock and the movement of wild game. A shipment of antelope from East Africa caused the last outbreak of the disease in Europe.

Literature

In enzootic areas, the incidence of rinderpest is age-related: calves have passive immunity and the adults are actively immune as a result of natural infection or vaccination. In addition, indigenous animals have a high innate resistance to the disease. Therefore, rinderpest spreads slowly and steadily through the immature and young animals at risk. Clinical disease is not intense, but the mortality rates may approach 30%. Epizootics in rinderpest-free areas are characterized by very high morbidity and high mortality in animals of all ages (Scott 1981). Rinderpest rapidly burns itself out in animals which have low innate resistance. These animals were important in the dissemination of rinderpest but were relatively insignificant in the maintenance of the disease (Branagan and Hammond 1965).

Scott (1981) defined the worldwide distribution of the disease in 1975. Enzootic infections persisted in northern equatorial Africa and India and the surrounding countries. In Africa, the disease persisted largely because of nomadism and the difficulties in conducting widespread vaccination campaigns. The last pandemic swept through the Middle East from Afghanistan to the Mediterranean in 1969–73. Minor epizootics continue in Yemen, the Gulf States, and Saudi Arabia following the importation of live ruminants from Somalia. Scott (1964) quoted the summation of data published by the Office International des Epizooties in which it was estimated that around 40 000 outbreaks and just over 1 million deaths had occurred in the decade before 1964. Using information known from little-known and unpublished documents, Mack (1970) recounted the history of the 1890 epizootic of rinderpest in Africa which resulted in a total loss of approximately 2.5 million head of cattle in South Africa alone. Branagan and Hammond (1965) reviewed the history of rinderpest in Tanzania and discussed the importance of wild ungulates in the epizootiology of the disease and the variations in virulence and invasiveness of different strains. The incidence and control of rinderpest in Africa between 1952 and 1962 was reviewed by Beaton (1963).

In the Sudan, a natural outbreak of rinderpest involving sheep, goats, and cattle was reported. In sheep and goat herds, the mortality rate was 60 to 70% among the young stock and 20 to 25% among the adult animals (Ali 1973). Recent examination of the virus isolated showed that it was the virus causing peste des petits ruminants (PPR) (G. R. Scott, personal communication). The occurrence of a rinderpest-like illness, which was probably a member of the complex of diseases known as mucosal diseases, was recorded in the Sudan and Ethiopia. The presence of this disease in Africa would have to be considered in making a differential diagnosis (Otte 1961). In a short review, Taylor and Ojeh (1981) discussed the incidence of rinderpest outbreaks and the vaccination campaigns conducted in Nigeria. Only 75% of Nigeria's 10 million cattle were immune to rinderpest, and contact among the 2.5 million susceptible cattle present in the general population could maintain the infection once it was introduced. In an outbreak of rinderpest involving sheep and cattle, the syndrome observed in artificial and natural infection in sheep was variable and the incidence of the natural disease was low (Johnson 1958). Hindsight now suggests that the outbreak in sheep was also caused by PPR virus (G. R. Scott, personal communication). Although a serological survey conducted in northern Nigeria revealed that 18.8% of the sheep and 15.2% of the goats had neutralizing antibodies to rinderpest, it was concluded that these antibodies resulted from infections with PPR virus and were not due to the spread of virulent or avirulent rinderpest virus from cattle to sheep and goats (Zwart and Rowe 1966).

The position of rinderpest and the diagnostic and control measures being applied in 1970 in the countries in the Near East were described in two reports issued by the FAO (Anon. 1970a, b). The epizootiology, diagnosis, and control of rinderpest and rinderpest-like diseases in India were reviewed (Rao 1969, 1973). The incidence of the disease in cattle and buffalo declined sharply with the introduction of a massive preventative vaccination program in India in 1956. However, outbreaks have occurred in sheep and goats since 1967, and there appeared to be an increase in the incidence of these outbreaks. The viruses isolated from different regions varied in their virulence (Rao *et al.* 1974). An outbreak of rinderpest was documented in Iran in 1969 (Rafyi and Afshar 1969). A contagious disease broke out among cattle and buffalo on the island of Bali in 1964. Thousands of animals were affected by this illness, which was considered a rinderpest-like disease. The epidemic was controlled by the use of a Japanese LA vaccine (Adiwinata 1968;

Anon. 1969). The disease locally known as *tembara* is now considered to be caused by a tick-borne pathogen, probably rickettsia.

In addition to the occurrence of rinderpest in cattle and buffalo, the disease or evidence of infection had been reported in sheep, goats, pigs, camels, and game animals. Scott (1955) presented a historical review of the incidence of rinderpest in sheep and goats and concluded that severe losses had occurred in the past. The isolation of rinderpest from sheep which had clinical signs of varying severity was reported more recently (Narayanaswamy and Ramani 1973; Rao *et al.* 1974). Scott *et al.* (1959) reviewed the literature on rinderpest in pigs and experimentally infected swine with the virus. Many of the resultant infections were clinically inapparent, and this probably explains the relative lack of information on the occurrence of rinderpest in pigs. The lack of apparent symptoms and the transmissibility of the virus through pig populations were considered important factors in the epizootiology of rinderpest (Scott *et al.* 1959). The occurrence of rinderpest in pigs in India was reported more recently and although natural infections were observed, they were not associated with high morbidity and mortality (Bansal *et al.* 1974; Ramani *et al.* 1974).

Antibodies to rinderpest virus were demonstrated in the sera of camels in Chad (Maurice *et al.* 1967), but none of the camels tested in Kenya during the 1962 epizootic of rinderpest in East Africa possessed antibodies to the disease (Scott and MacDonald 1962). The incidence of rinderpest in camels in one district in India was reviewed. The disease was diagnosed on the basis of clinical signs and the tendency to spread to other livestock. The course was acute and subacute, with a duration of 4 to 6 days; mild attacks leading to recovery were not infrequent (Dhillon 1959).

The spread of rinderpest through East, Central and southern Africa during the latter part of the nineteenth century was described by Simon (1962). Both domestic and wild ungulate populations were completely susceptible at the time and were thus severely affected. Among wild animals, buffalo (*Syncerus caffer* Sparrman), eland *Taurotragus oryx* Pallas) and warthog (*Phacochoerus aethiopicus* Pallas) were the first to be infected, followed by giraffe (*Giraffa camelopardalis* Linnaeus and *G. reticulata* De Winton), greater kudu (*Tragelaphus strepsiceros* Pallas), wildebeest (*Connochaetes taurinus* Burchell), and probably bongo (*Boocercus eurycerus* Ogilby) (Stewart 1964). The role game animals played in the epizootiology of rinderpest in East Africa over a period of 30 years was examined, and it was concluded that a mild type of rinderpest had been continuously enzootic in the cattle–game contact areas. Relatively stable strains of virus infected cattle, wildebeest, eland, and probably buffalo (Plowright 1963b). There was further evidence of the involvement of game animals in the transmission of rinderpest in Kenya (Stewart 1968). The species affected in various outbreaks recorded in Kenya during 1960–62 were listed (Stewart 1964). The epizootic which occurred during 1953–54 in game and cattle in the area centered on the junction between the Sudan, Uganda, and Zaïre was briefly described (Beaton 1954). Serological surveys of game animals were conducted in Kenya and Tanzania during 1960–63. The results of these investigations indicated that there was a high incidence of rinderpest infection in the wildebeest in some regions (Plowright and McCulloch 1967). Additional epizootiological studies on rinderpest in the blue wildebeest in Tanzania and Kenya during 1865–67 confirmed the importance of this species in the maintenance of the disease in the wild game population (Taylor and Watson 1967). The virus isolated from a natural case of the disease in eland caused a mild syndrome in cattle (Robson *et al.* 1959). The occurrence of rinderpest in impala was confirmed (Scott *et al.* 1960) In a study on the susceptibility of the hippopotamus (*Hippopotamus amphibius* Linnaeus) antibodies were observed only in the older animals, suggesting that these antibodies persisted for many years (Plowright *et al.* 1964). White-tailed deer (*Odocoileus virginianus*) experimentally infected with virulent rinderpest virus developed an acute, fatal disease which was comparable to that observed in cattle (Hamdy *et al.* 1975).

Transmission

The spread of the disease is most often due to the introduction of live infected animals into rinderpest-free areas. Transmission is usually effected by direct contact between infected and susceptible animals. There is no evidence that vectors such as biting insects are significant factors in the dissemination of rinderpest. Successful transmission by oral route in species other than wild and domestic pigs is erratic. Artificial transmission can be achieved by the parenteral or oral administration of infected materials such as blood, tissues, exudates, and discharges. The virus is readily transmitted experimentally by intranasal instillation and by inhalation. Infection also takes place following conjuctival instillation and vaginal deposition of the virus. The virus is excreted by the animal in all discharges, including conjunctival, nasal, and vaginal secretions, urine, and feces. Fields and contaminated stables are alleged to remain infective for up to 4 days. Feces are the source of the greatest amount of virus, which can be detected for up to 8 months after recovery. The virus has also been known to persist for up to 45 days in the milk of recovered animals.

The natural transmissibility of strains of rinderpest virus varies considerably under field conditions; no generalizations can be made with regard to the speed and consistency of spread, even when animals are at the height of infectivity. The ease of transmission of rinderpest varies with the host species and viral strain. Under laboratory conditions, strains which have been passaged by the subcutaneous route quickly lose their capacity to be transmitted by contact, but they revert to their original infectivity after a few passages in cell cultures. The artificially attenuated strains used in vaccines are not disseminated by contact because they do not proliferate in the alimentary and respiratory tracts which enable the excretion of the virus.

Experimental infections are not disseminated readily by contact from sheep to sheep or from sheep to cattle, but naturally occurring infections spread readily among sheep. It has also been demonstrated that pigs can acquire the disease by the ingestion of contaminated meat and that the infection can be spread by contact from pig to pig and pig to cattle or vice versa. Thus the importation of meat from enzootic areas may constitute a risk to rinderpest-free regions. However, this mode of dissemination is not considered a major factor in the epizootiology of the disease.

Literature

Under certain experimental conditions, the transmission of rinderpest virus by contact with donor animals in the initial stage of clinical disease was not consistent, and this was attributed to the considerable variation in the quantity of virus in nasal and other secretions produced during the early phase of infection (Taylor *et al.* 1965). Limited transmission to cattle was also effected using aerosols of virulent and attenuated viruses (Provost 1958). Rinderpest was transmitted to cattle housed in contact with experimentally infected goats which had a relatively mild form of the disease. The infection was conveyed from the reacting cattle to sheep (Macadam 1968). Contact transmission of rinderpest from experimentally infected indigenous African sheep to healthy sheep of the same variety occurred rarely, and the virus was not transmitted to cattle kept in close contact with reacting sheep (Plowright 1952). Contact transmission of rinderpest from cattle to sheep and goats was demonstrated (Zwart and Macadam 1967a). In further experiments, virus was isolated from the feces and nasal swabs of rinderpest-infected goats and sheep; only one bovine held in close contact with the goats developed the disease, while none of the susceptible cattle similarly exposed to infected sheep became ill (Zwart and Macadam 1967b).

Asiatic pigs were considered more susceptible to rinderpest than those of European origin. Contact transmission occurred in 25% of the pigs housed with infected pigs, and the virus was also transmitted by the ingestion of contaminated meat (Scott *et al.* 1959). Since the majority of infected pigs showed only mild fever, some depression, and anorexia, and many infections were clinically inapparent, pigs could be very dangerous disseminators of the disease to cattle (Scott *et al.* 1962). Rinderpest virus was detected in the tissues of pigs at 10 but not at 38 days after direct contact with experimentally infected cattle. However, cattle which had been exposed to rinderpest-convalescent pigs for 18 days did not contract the infection. Convalescent pigs developed neutralizing antibodies 31 days but not 10 days postinfection (DeLay and Barber 1963).

New rinderpest outbreaks were always associated with the importation of live animals; the transmission of the virus was rarely attributable to contact with infected materials. Thus, the risk incurred by rinderpest-free countries which imported meat from enzootic areas was considered relatively low (Scott 1957). However, it was pointed out that rinderpest could be transmitted by infected meat, and reference was made to earlier work which showed that freezing and other normal methods of preserving meat would allow the virus to persist. In the case of freezing, viable virus could be recovered for up to 57 days (Ademollo 1959; Scott 1959a). The risk of spread of rinderpest virus by fresh and frozen meat was examined further. It was concluded that the importation of meat from rinderpest-enzootic countries could be undertaken without risk, especially if a number of precautions were employed. However, further research into this potential mode of transmission was recommended.

INFECTION

All cloven-hoofed animals are susceptible to infection with rinderpest, but because host species show considerable variation in natural resistance and strains of rinderpest virus vary widely in their host affinities, there is marked variability in the incidence and severity of the disease among different host species in different regions. Cattle indigenous to the countries where the disease occurs enzootically are more resistant than those which are imported from rinderpest-free areas. Although goats, sheep, and pigs are susceptible to artificial infection, they seldom show severe clinical signs.

The virulence of a strain for a particular host can be altered by laboratory manipulations. After a variable number of passages in experimental hosts, strains reach a fixed level of virulence for cattle and other domesticated species, and because this characteristic is remarkably stable, these fixed attenuated strains are used in the production of live vaccines. Strains attenuated for cattle are highly virulent for experimental hosts such as rabbits and vary in the ease of their transmission between hosts. Some laboratory strains differ from field strains in that they have lost the ability to spread easily by contact, and this may be related to the lack of viral multiplication in the gastrointestinal tract and other sites from which the virus would normally be shed.

The multiplication of rinderpest virus in the host is described by a typical growth curve which delineates the eclipse, expansion, peak, and decline stages of the cycle; the expansion and decline phases are exponential. The duration of the eclipse phase is related to the size of the infecting dose, and the peak levels obtained depend on the extent to which the virus is adapted to the host. The level of infection attained is related to the virulence; high levels are associated with the development of clinical signs. Titration of the virus content of blood and various tissues collected throughout infection revealed that viral multiplication occurred primarily in the lymphoid tissue.

Cattle can be infected experimentally by any parenteral route of inoculation, but the virus appears to be incapable of passing through intact skin or other stratified squamous epithelia. This may be responsible for the frequent failure to infect cattle by drenching them with highly virulent material. Infection in cattle takes place readily via the respiratory tract. The virus passes through the epithelium of the upper and, less frequently, the lower portions of the respiratory tract to establish foci of proliferation in the draining lymph nodes from which it disseminates through the blood to other lymphoid tissues. The persistence of the virus in the blood and other tissues of cattle despite the presence of appreciable levels of circulating antibody is due to the association of the virus with leukocytes, particularly the mononuclear cells. The mechanism underlying the persistence of latency of rinderpest infection has not been determined. It is generally accepted that recovered animals do not become carriers, but there are instances where virus has been isolated from cases of so-called chronic rinderpest. It also appears that domestic pigs, which acquire the infection relatively easily by ingesting contaminated food, are an important factor in the maintenance of the virus.

Literature

The species of the order Artiodactyla in which natural rinderpest infections have been confirmed were listed in a table presented by Plowright (1968), who verified the statement by Scott (1964) that all and exclusively species of the order Artiodactyla are susceptible to rinderpest. The responses of local races and breeds of cattle to virulent infections and to attenuated virus in various forms of vaccines vary because of differences in their innate resistance (Henning 1956).

There have been numerous reports that field strains vary with respect to cattle pathogenicity. Certain strains produce severe syndromes and high mortality, while others cause relatively mild clinical signs and low mortality; strains of low virulence have been isolated frequently. Field isolates passaged one to three times in tissue culture were found to be of low virulence for cattle, which were viremic for 3 to 11 days. Mouth lesions developed in 68% of the cattle inoculated with culture isolates, and dysentery was observed in 18% of the animals. Febrile reactions were generally mild, and the rate (approximately 5%) was very low (Plowright 1963a). The separation of an avirulent strain of rinderpest virus from a heterogeneous population by the terminal dilution technique was described. Cattle inoculated with this avirulent strain developed immunity and did not transmit the virus to healthy cattle by contact (De Boer and Barber 1964a).

There was also considerable variability in the innate resistance of different host species. Water buffalo were found to have a higher resistance to rinderpest than cattle; experimental infections caused milder, more protracted clinical signs and lower mortality in water buffalo (Rao *et al.* 1975; Singh *et al.* 1967b). Joshi and Sinha (1961) reviewed the literature on the susceptibility of various types of water buffalo to rinderpest in different geographical regions. The susceptibility varied from one area to another. In India, the mortality among experimentally infected buffalo was between 25 and 30%, and an overall susceptibility of 90% was reported. Indigenous Red Masai sheep were susceptible to caprinized rinderpest virus and developed a mild disease, the only clinical sign being a transient fever (Scott 1962c). The reactions of susceptible purebred and crossbred Nigerian dwarf goats to caprinized rinderpest virus differed significantly, with the pure goats having shorter illnesses and a higher mortality rate. It was concluded that the variation in response was not associated with inherited innate resistance (Scott *et al.* 1970). Pigs of European origin were susceptible to virulent and attenuated strains of virus which were administered parenterally or by ingestion. The only overt manifestation of the disease in these animals was mild, transient fever; many infections were subclinical (Scott *et al.* 1962). A bovine-lethal strain of rinderpest virus was serially passaged through pigs, which developed pyrexia and leukopenia in response to the infection. After 15 passages, the virus did not increase in virulence for pigs but continued to be lethal for cattle (Barber and Heuschele 1964b). There was a very low incidence (10%) of disease among experimentally infected camels in Chad, and neutralizing antibodies were observed in the affected animals (Provost *et al.* 1968).

The literature on experimental rinderpest infection in goats, rabbits, dogs, ferrets, rodents, embryonated eggs, and chicks was reviewed by Scott (1964). The virus was maintained and attenuated by serial passage in rabbits. The virulence of the virus for rabbits increased and the reaction was characterized by the development of fever and grayish-white, granular, necrotic areas in the Peyer's patches of the intestine and in the mesenteric lymph nodes. The concentration of virus was highest in the intestinal lymph nodes, and less in the spleen and blood. The virus became attenuated for cattle after several hundred passages, and the safety depended on the strain used, the type of rabbit employed, and the breed of cattle tested (Henning 1956). The infectivity of rinderpest virus for rabbits depended on the route of exposure; higher doses were required to induce infection by the oral and rectal routes than by parenteral administration (Scott and Rampton 1962). A strain of caprinized rinderpest virus failed to infect rabbits (Scott 1959b).

Rinderpest virus proliferated in the pharyngeal and submaxillary lymph nodes and in the palatal tonsils of experimental cattle by the third day following contact exposure, but no infectivity was demonstrated in the mucosae associated with these lymphoid tissues (Taylor *et al.* 1965). The course of the infection was divided into four phases: incubation (days 1 to 4), prodromal (days 5 to 7), mucosal (days 8 to 12), and early convalescent (days 13 to 16). The prodromal period is defined as the phase between the onset of fever and the first appearance of mucosal lesions in the mouth. Low-level viremia began on the second and third days after infection, and generalization occurred by the end of the incubation period when the virus became established throughout the gastrointestinal tract. During the prodromal phase, high virus titers were detected in the lymphoid organs and in the gastrointestinal tract. Virus appeared in the turbinate mucosa on the fifth day postinfection, and high titers were evident in the lungs towards the end of this period. The mucosal phase was characterized by continued high titers of virus in all major sites of proliferation, but lower virus titers as well as neutralizing antibodies were observed from the ninth day onwards. During the early convalescent period, the virus disappeared from many animals (Plowright 1964b). The virus content of the nervous tissue and bone marrow of rinderpest-infected calves was studied, and both tissues had very low concentrations of virus (Bergeon 1952). Liess and Plowright (1964) investigated the relationships, clinical signs, viremia, and virus excretion by various routes in cattle experimentally infected with rinderpest virus.

Grade cattle, 'Zebu-crossbred cattle', inoculated with a highly attenuated strain of rinderpest virus did not develop clinical signs, but viral proliferation was investigated in 22 tissues harvested at daily intervals from the first to the tenth day of infection. The virus was generalized in the lymphoid tissues on the fourth day, and a low level of viremia was detected in some of the cattle killed between the fifth and eighth days. The virus was not recovered from the mucosa of the gastrointestinal tract. However, considerable growth of virus was observed in the prescapular, pharyngeal, and mesenteric lymph nodes, and in the palatal tonsils and Peyer's patches of the ileum. It was concluded that the lack of pathogenicity was primarily due to failure of the virus to proliferate in the mucosae of the gastrointestinal and respiratory tracts. The inability of the attenuated strain to spread by contact among susceptible cattle was probably the result of absence of the virus from mucosae and parenchymatous organs and hence from excretions (Taylor and Plowright 1965).

Tissue tropism was studied in cattle, rabbits, and goats infected with rinderpest. Different strains of the virus varied with respect to tissue tropism in cattle. The lapinized virus was lymphotropic, while the caprinized virus primarily localized in lymphoid tissues and affected epithelial tissues to a lesser degree. In contrast, field isolates of the virus in acute cases affected both types of tissues (Thiery 1956b). Further comparisons of the lesions in Zebu and non-humped cattle showed that in the latter the virus infected the lymphoid tissues more frequently. There were indications that the Zebus were more resistant to the development of the lesions. After many serial passages of the virus in Zebus, the epithelial tropism disappeared (Thiery 1956a). In infected rabbits, the titers of virus were highest in the major lymphoid organs (Scott 1954).

CLINICAL SIGNS

The clinical signs caused by rinderpest in cattle and other natural hosts differ with respect to intensity and frequency, and this variation is related to the virulence of the strain of virus involved and the resistance of the host. The syndromes may be peracute (death occurs within 1 to 2 days after the appearance of clinical signs), acute (the symptoms last 4 to 7 days), or mild (the animals may live up to 3 weeks or longer). Sometimes the disease is characterized by mild symptoms which may pass unnoticed. Isolates from some outbreaks have been shown to be of low virulence and fail to kill cattle; about 10% of the affected animals develop asymptomatic infection. Strains of low virulence for cattle have been recovered from game animals. In newly infected areas, the mortality may exceed 90% and the morbidity may be as high as 100%. The incubation period ranges from 3 to 9 days and is longer in those regions where the disease is enzootic. The first symptoms are fever (40 °C to 40.5 °C), restlessness, loss of appetite, cessation of rumination, dryness of muzzle, and constipation. This is followed within a day or two by nasal and ocular discharges, photophobia, thirst, anorexia, excessive salivation, rough coat, and leukopenia. The temperature peaks between the third and fifth days and then drops as diarrhea develops and the other clinical signs are accentuated. Although the oral lesions develop by the second or third day they are not usually observed until after the development of diarrhea. The increase in the severity of the diarrhea is accompanied by clinical signs of accelerated respiration, cough, dehydration, and emaciation. The animal arches its back, and there is grinding of the teeth and twitching of the superficial muscles. As the abdominal pain intensifies, restlessness becomes more pronounced and the diarrhea is fetid and bloodstained. Inflammation and exudate are also present in the female reproductive tract and are associated with abortion. There is cessation of milk production. The skin on certain parts of the body occasionally becomes red and moist, and protuberances and vesicles may develop which subsequently cause thickening of the skin and scab formation. The animals quickly lose condition and become extremely dehydrated, emaciated, and exhausted. In the terminal stages, there is prostration, subnormal temperature, and death within 6 to 12 days.

Literature

Comprehensive reports on the clinical signs and pathology of rinderpest were presented by Maurer *et al.* (1955, 1956), who observed at least 600 experimental bovine cases and examined more than 400 animals at postmortem. Aberrant clinical forms of rinderpest, which might be characterized by peracute encephalitis of as yet undetermined etiology, sudden death, or transient subacute diarrhea, were not uncommon. Infections which did not induce enteric or febrile responses were also observed.

Plowright (1968) divided the pathogenesis of the disease into four periods: incubation, prodromal, mucosal, and convalescent; Scott (1981) added a diarrheic phase between the mucosal and convalescent stages. These terms are used to relate the clinical events observed during the course of infection to the proliferation of virus in the tissues.

Liess and Plowright (1964) found that the development of clinical signs, viremia, and virus excretion by various routes were correlated. Plowright (1968) presented a very comprehensive description of the host–virus interaction and the sequence of events which resulted in the development of clinical signs and lesions. This information is presented here in detail. The incubation period, which extended from the time of infection to the development of the fever, lasted 3 to 9 days depending on the strain, dose, and route of administration. Short incubation periods were associated with virus strains adapted to laboratory conditions; in the field, the incubation period following natural contact transmission varied from 8 to 15 days. Strains which required this relatively long interval would not produce fulminating, rapidly spreading outbreaks like those caused by other viruses with shorter incubation periods. During the first incubation period the virus passed through the mucosa to the local drainage lymph nodes and then spread throughout the body. It multiplied rapidly in lymphoid tissues, including the major lymphoid organs and the peripheral components of the lymphoid system which are localized in various tissues and organs.

The prodromal phase persisted for approximately 3 days on the average and induced the time between the onset of pyrexia and the initial appearance of mouth lesions. Fever occurred after the virus had been disseminated throughout the body and was associated with the release of virus and tissue breakdown products into the circulation. Rinderpest could not be diagnosed on the basis of the clinical signs which developed during the prodromal period. Mucosal lesion formation commenced between the second and fifth days following the onset of fever, and the quantity of virus reached high levels in the tissues during this stage of the infection.

The mucosal phase started with high titers of virus and was characterized clinically by the appearance of lesions in the mucous membranes of the mouth, followed 1 to 2 days later by diarrhea and the development of the whole range of clinical signs which lasted 3 to 5 days. Vulvar and vaginal lesions occurred at the same time as those observed in the mouth. The mucosal period terminated either with the death of the animal or the beginning of the convalescent period. The first oral lesions consisted of small, raised, grayish foci of necrotic epithelium 1 to 2 mm in diameter, under which were small ulcers. As the disease progressed, these lesions enlarged and spread throughout the buccal cavity. The stomatitis and rhinitis became generalized after 6 to 7 days and were accompanied by a fetid odor resulting from secondary bacterial infections. During this time, the respiration was labored and painful, and coughing and grunting sometimes occurred. Diarrhea usually appeared on the fourth to the seventh day of fever, 1 to 2 days after the first appearance of the mouth lesions. The affected animal evacuated large watery feces which contained mucus and blood, and toward the end of this stage, the amounts of mucus, blood, and necrotic epithelium increased and had a characteristically fetid odor. The diarrhea resulted in dehydration and weakness and was directly related to the death of the animal. Skin lesions also developed during the mucosal phase, but they were not as common as the mucosal lesions (Mornet and Guerret 1950; Kataria *et al.* 1974; Joshi *et al.* 1977). The cutaneous lesions appeared predominantly on the udder and scrotum, inside the thighs, and in the perineal region and consisted of erythematous, thickened areas with serous exudation. The formation of pustules and scabs resulted in matting of the hair. The skin lesions were associated with milder forms of the disease in cattle (Mares 1956) and goats (Mohan and Bahl 1953). Thus, the appearance of skin lesions was associated with a favorable prognosis. In some cases the lesions were considered the result of a secondary infection, namely, cutaneous streptothricosis (Beaton 1966). The viral titers in the tissues fell rapidly on about the sixth day of fever, and by the time the various lesions began to heal, relatively little virus was detected.

The convalescent period was characterized by the rapid healing of epithelial lesions. The majority of the buccal mucosa cleared within a few days, but the buccal papillae remained red and eroded for longer periods of time. The virus disappeared from tissues and excretions from the ninth or tenth day following the first clinical reaction. Mortality was usually associated with the mucosal phase, and the incidence depended on the strain of the virus. Animals with mild syndromes exhibited one or more of the cardinal clinical signs (e.g. mouth lesions or transient diarrhea), but the clinical syndrome could be absent entirely. Central nervous system involvement in the disease had never been proved to be due to rinderpest virus because neither encephalitis nor meningitis had been demonstrated. Neurological clinical signs could have been associated with secondary infection by other pathogens. In a report on a rinderpest-like disease of cattle in Ethiopia, it was noted that nervous symptoms and abortion occurred in addition to the classical severe signs of rinderpest (Otte and Peck 1960).

In other species of animals such as camels, sheep, goats, and wild ungulates, the severity of the clinical response varied according to the level of innate resistance and the strain of virus. Experimental infection of sheep and goats resulted in a mild course of rinderpest characterized by a slight discharge and transient diarrhea (Zwart and Macadam 1967a). Clinical disease and diagnostic methods were investigated in experimentally infected sheep, and the disease which developed was mild and inapparent, thus confirming the findings of studies on artificial infection in sheep. These experimental syndromes were not comparable to the natural cases, which resembled those seen in cattle (Barber and Heuschele 1964a). Dhanda and Manjrekar (1951/52) reviewed the early work on experimental rinderpest among goats and sheep in India, where outbreaks characterized by high mortality had been recorded. Although large numbers of sheep and goats were affected in an outbreak, there was no evidence of disease in the cattle and buffalo which were in close contact. The importance of the disease in India in more recent times was pointed out (Narayanaswamy and Ramani 1973). Pigs experimentally infected with rinderpest virus also did not develop severe clinical signs, and only 2 of the 31 animals died. The virus was recovered from the tissues of pigs at 6 and 36, but not at 22 or

92 days postinfection. Cattle placed in contact with convalescent pigs at 41 days postinfection did not acquire the disease (DeLay *et al.*, 1962). Taylor (1968) reviewed some of the early work undertaken in India on the transmission of rinderpest to camels. These reports indicated that camels were susceptible to infection and generally developed a relatively mild form of the disease characterized by fever, diarrhea, and mouth lesions. There were also reports of outbreaks in which the mortality was high. Experimental infection of camels with virulent virus resulted in the development of neutralizing antibodies. Although camels proved susceptible to subclinical infection, Taylor (1968) concluded that they were unlikely to play a role in the transmission of rinderpest to other animals. In other studies, camels experimentally infected with virulent virus developed slight dermal reactions and neutralizing antibodies (Singh and Ata 1967). Rabbits inoculated with attenuated rinderpest virus developed fever, diarrhea, and lymphopenia (Yamanouchi *et al.* 1974a).

PATHOLOGY

The rinderpest virus has an affinity for lymphoid tissues and the epithelium of the upper respiratory and alimentary tracts. In these sites, there is extensive cellular necrosis as well as the development of characteristic multinucleated giant cells, or syncytia, which contain eosinophilic intranuclear and intracytoplasmic inclusions. The infection of lymphoid tissue causes necrosis of lymphocytes in the lymph nodes, spleen, and Peyer's patches. Although microscopic examination may reveal extensive destruction of lymphocytes, this may not be readily reflected in the gross appearance of the tissues.

The virus also selectively attacks the epithelium of the digestive tract, where it produces characteristic lesions. Small necrotic foci, which appear as pinpoints of grayish-white tissue surrounded by normal epithelium, first occur in the oral mucosa. These foci then develop into small erosions which may widen and coalesce to form large areas of desquamation throughout the buccal cavity, esophagus, and upper gastrointestinal tract. The pyloric region of the abomasum is one of the most common sites of lesion formation. The microscopic necrotic foci in the epithelium are accompanied by congestion and hemorrhage in the underlying lamina propria. These lesions appear grossly as irregularly outlined superficial streaks which range in color from bright red to dark brown. As the lesion enlarges, the epithelium sloughs off leaving sharply delineated, irregularly shaped ulcers which bleed. Severe lesions are less common in the small intestine than in other parts of the alimentary tract. The lesions vary from areas of discoloration and hemorrhage to obvious erosions and are usually found in the initial portion of the duodenum and terminal part of the ileum. The Peyer's patches are frequently black and friable. In the cecum and colon, streaks of congestion and hemorrhage along the crests of the folds of mucosa give it the characteristic 'zebra-striped' appearance. Erosions in the upper respiratory tract are uncommon, but there may be hemorrhages and discolorations.

Literature

A major contribution to the understanding of the pathogenesis of rinderpest was made by Maurer *et al.* (1955, 1956), who presented detailed descriptions of the lesions observed at postmortem examination of over 400 experimental cases of rinderpest produced in both African Zebu and European breeds of cattle by 16 distinct strains of the virus. Rinderpest virus had a specific tropism for lymphocytes, and the resulting destruction of the cells produced the lesions observed in the major lymphoid organs and in the peripheral lymphoid system, which included the lymph nodules and Peyer's patches in the gastrointestinal system. The necrosis of lymphocytes was first manifested by the fragmentation of the nuclei in the germinal centers and the disappearance of mature lymphocytes. The remaining tissue consisted of fibrillar, somewhat eosinophilic, acellular material. Edema of the lymph node was grossly visible at this stage. Since the capillary endothelium was not affected by the virus, there was no congestion or hemorrhage in the lymph nodes, which appeared to be grossly enlarged, soft, and edematous (Maurer *et al.* 1955, 1956). The sequential development of lesions in the lymph nodes of cattle was studied. The first change observed was a hyperplasia of reticuloendothelial elements such as macrophages, and in the lymph follicles this was soon followed by necrosis of the reticular cells, which gave the lymph nodule a 'washed-out' appearance. In the nonfollicular regions of the lymph nodes, histiocytes and macrophages accumulated, and multinucleated macrophages and giant cells appeared and contained eosinophilic inclusions. On about the eighth day postinfection, the macrophages, histiocytes, and lymphocytes underwent necrosis. Toward the terminal stages, there was evidence of fibrosis with focal lymphocytic regeneration (Khera 1958). The degenerative and necrotic lesions were accompanied by the development of inclusion bodies in the lymphocytes and were directly related to viral multiplication in the cells. The intranuclear and intracytoplasmic inclusions contained antigen of viral origin which stained specifically with fluorescent antibody (FA) (Tajima and Ushijima 1971). One type of cytoplasmic inclusion found in cultured calf kidney cells, lymphocytes, reticular cells, and mucosal epithelial cells infected with rinderpest virus was composed of numerous filaments with a tubular structure, while another type contained large quantities of fine granular and fibrillar material in addition to the filaments. The latter type of inclusion was observed primarily in the cells of infected cattle. There were no particles which resembled mature virus (Tajima *et al.* 1964).

In addition to the destruction of lymphoid tissues, the virus had an affinity for the epithelium of the gastrointestinal tract. Because the application of the virus to the oral mucosa did not induce infection, it appeared that the virus was carried to the mucosa by the bloodstream (Maurer *et al.* 1955, 1956). In the stratified squamous epithelium, syncytium formation began in the stratum spinosum as foci of ballooning cells with acidophilic cytoplasmic inclusions (Plowright 1968). The first changes were seen in the deep layers of the stratum malpighii just above the basal layer. The epithelial cells underwent necrosis but did not form vesicles. As the lesions increased in size and extended toward the surface, the cornified layer became raised and the necrotic areas were seen grossly as tiny, grayish-white, slightly elevated foci 1 mm in diameter. These lesions then coalesced, and the detachment of the overlying necrotic tissue from the underlying basal cell layer resulted in the formation of shallow erosions, but the basal layer was rarely penetrated. Once the erosions became more extensive, they were associated with congestion, hemorrhage, and cellular inflammatory exudate. The penetration of the basal cell layer and the subsequent development of true ulcers were considered to be due to secondary bacterial infections. The cheesy exudate observed in the mouth was due to the extensive destruction of the epithelium and to the accumulation of necrotic debris (Maurer *et al.* 1955, 1956).

The lesions in the oral mucosa were distributed in specific locations. They were first observed on the inside of the lower lip, on the adjacent gum, on the cheeks near the commissures, and on the ventral surface of the free portion of the tongue. As the disease progressed, other areas of the oral mucosa became affected. The severity of the oral lesions that developed depended on the virulence of the virus; only the more virulent field strains produced the lesions. Lesions could extend into the esophagus but were rarely found in the rumen, reticulum, and omasum (Maurer *et al.* 1955, 1956).

Lesions in the lower regions of the gastrointestinal system resulted from the necrosis of lymphoid as well as epithelial tissues. In the glandular mucosae of the abomasum and intestines, the necrosis of the columnar epithelium is accompanied by congestion and hemorrhage. The vascular response observed in the mucous membranes lined with a single layer of columnar cells was more severe than that found in tissues covered with stratified squamous epithelium because the highly vascular stroma was relatively closer to the necrosis of the overlying epithelium. The abomasum was one of the most common sites of lesion formation and the pyloric region was the most severely and consistently involved. The earliest lesions consisted of necrotic foci accompanied by capillary congestion and hemorrhage in the underlying lamina propria, and edema in the submucosa gave the tissue a thickened, gelatinous appearance. As the lesions increased in size, the epithelium sloughed off, leaving sharply outlined, irregularly shaped ulcers which bled and contained black-colored, clotted blood. Severe lesions were more frequent in the small intestine than in the mouth, abomasum, or large intestine (Maurer *et al.* 1955, 1956).

The respiratory epithelium, particularly in the trachea, responded to the virus in a manner which had features common to the reactions observed in the squamous and single columnar epithelia. Hemorrhagic areas could be distinguished grossly, but erosions were not particularly common. The lower respiratory system appeared to be involved only secondarily (Maurer *et al.* 1955, 1956). In some cases there was more severe inflammation of the upper respiratory system with extensive purulent discharge. In small ruminants, pneumonia was common and could be confused with pleuropneumonia (Henning 1956). Hemorrhages, interlobular and alveolar emphysema, congestion, and occasional small areas of consolidation were also observed in the lungs of animals with acute cases of rinderpest. Histologically, there was no evidence of cellular changes directly attributable to the effect of the virus (Maurer *et al.* 1955, 1956).

The changes in the heart and urinary system were nonspecific. In contrast to what has been reported in the early literature, more recent studies showed that skin lesions were rare. Of the several hundred field cases examined, cutaneous lesions were observed only in four cattle (Maurer *et al.* 1956).

Pigs with fatal cases of rinderpest developed fever, nasal and lacrymal discharges, congestion of the buccal mucosa, and acute gastroenteritis (Ramani *et al.* 1974). Characteristic lesions were also observed in the lymphatic tissues, particularly in the spleen and ileum. The occurrence of focal degeneration, necrosis, and phagocytosis resulted in the depletion of the mature lymphocytes with subsequent regeneration. The epithelium of the gastrointestinal tract was not affected in pigs with experimental syndromes.

The histological lesions of rinderpest and the mucosal disease complex were compared. There were no distinctive features which would differentiate the two diseases on gross postmortem examination. It was proposed that erosions in the interdigital cleft were diagnostic for mucosal disease. Histologically, the development of giant cells in rinderpest was thought to be less reliable (Ilchmann and Lehnert 1972).

In experimentally infected rabbits the main lesions were found in the Peyer's patches, sacculus rotundus, and appendix, wherein the lymphoid follicles were enlarged and chalk-white. The primary lesions consisted of necrosis of lymphoid follicles and formation of giant cells (Yamanouchi *et al.* 1974a; Maurer *et al.* 1956).

Changes in the blood of cattle infected with a highly virulent strain of rinderpest virus were characterized by an initial leukocytosis, followed by leukopenia and terminal hemoconcentration reflected in increased packed cell volume. This hematological picture persisted until death. Leukopenia occurred at the same time as the development of fever, and the terminal hemoconcentration and electrolyte imbalance were associated with the development of diarrhea (Heuschele and Barber 1966). Leukopenia was also observed in cattle infected with an avirulent strain which caused a slight transient decrease in the number of leukocytes (Robey and Hale 1946). Rinderpest-infected swine had a decrease in the total white blood cell counts without any other hematological changes (Heuschele and Barber 1963).

IMMUNOLOGY

Strains of rinderpest virus are immunologically homogeneous, which probably reflects the basic structural similarity of the surface antigens. It is not known how these serologically demonstrable antigens are associated with the production of immunity or how any of them are related to the structures in the virion or virus-specific products in infected cells. The antigens have not been characterized, but they are serologically related to canine distemper and measles viruses. The presence of one immunologic type enables protection against all known strains. Infection with virulent strains of rinderpest virus confers solid and lifelong immunity to either parenteral or natural challenge, and resistance is associated with the presence of humoral antibodies. Evidence for innate resistance being dependent on age and body condition is contradictory, as is the susceptibility to infection with different quantities of virus. Innate resistance, however, is one of the major factors which governs the pattern by which rinderpest spreads in any epizootiological situation. An important feature of infection with both virulent and certain attenuated experimental strains is the marked suppression of the humoral immune response and of cell-mediated immunity, which results in complications arising from secondary bacterial and protozoal infections.

Neutralization and complement-fixation (CF) tests are used to study antibody responses following infection with virulent and attenuated viruses. The first appearance of neutralizing antibody occurs from 6 to 21 days after infection, depending on the dose of the virus administered, and could persist for years. When the neutralizing levels of antibody are high, subsequent infections with virulent or attenuated viruses do not alter the titers, but an anamnestic boost occurs when the neutralizing antibody titers are low. Complement-fixing antibodies are detected in experimentally and naturally infected animals 1 week after infection, reach a peak within 2 to 3 weeks, and thereafter decline rapidly. However, there is wide individual variation with respect to the duration of these antibodies.

Literature

There appears to be little information on the biochemical composition of the virus. Recently it was shown that nine polypeptides specific for rinderpest virus were present in infected cells (Prakash *et al.* 1979).

A number of antigens were demonstrated by various workers using the agar-gel diffusion technique, and there were considerable differences in the reported properties of the complement-fixing antigens derived from rinderpest-infected tissues (Plowright 1968). The test showed heat-labile and heat-stable components (Stone 1960). Specific soluble precipitating antigens were present in the lymph nodes of animals infected with rinderpest and were detected by the

Ouchterlony gel diffusion precipitation technique, which is a valuable diagnostic procedure (White 1962).

The immunological relationships among measles, canine distemper, and rinderpest viruses were compared, and the nucleocapsid components could not be distinguished by the serological tests used. It was concluded that the three viruses shared envelope antigens which were more readily demonstrated by the hemolysis-inhibition technique than by the hemagglutination-inhibition test (Orvell and Norrby 1974). Each of the three viruses was grown in tissue culture and treated with ferritin-tagged antibodies to each virus. The resultant cross-reactions demonstrated that the viruses were morphologically indistinguishable and antigenically similar (Breese and De Boer 1973). The immunological relationships between distemper virus and normal or modified rinderpest virus were investigated in cattle and rabbits (Gilbert *et al.* 1960). The results of serological tests and experiments involving cross-immunization and challenge of dogs and cattle with distemper and rinderpest viruses showed that the two viruses were immunologically similar and capable of protecting the natural host against subsequent challenge with host-specific virulent virus (Mornet *et al.* 1960). There was no cross-protection between virus diarrhea and rinderpest as shown by the susceptibility of calves recovered from virus diarrhea to challenge with rinderpest virus (DeLay and Kniazeff 1966).

The results of a virus neutralizing test showed that the 19S and 7S antibodies developed sequentially during rinderpest infection. The time that antibody appeared depended on the challenge dose of the virus. The appearance of 19S antibody preceded that of 7S antibody by 3 to 4 days, irrespective of the route of inoculation and the strain of virus used. The duration of 19S antibody was 7 to 14 days and the 19S antibodies disappeared by 3 weeks after infection (Okuna and Rweyemamu 1974).

The innate resistance of various breeds of cattle in enzootic areas has not been conclusively established. Cattle populations which had been periodically exposed to the virus over time were less susceptible than those which had evolved in isolation. Thus, breed susceptibility would probably not be a significant factor in determining the severity of clinical features in an outbreak (Plowright 1968). The relationship between the resistance of calves to rinderpest and the immune status of the dam was discussed. Calves as young as 1 day old could produce antibodies to rinderpest antigen. The antibodies were transferred from the dam via the colostrum, and this maternally derived immunity in calves interfered with the production of active immunity. Calves 3 months of age or less did not respond to rinderpest vaccine, but calves about 8 months old developed antibodies (Brown 1958). A serious complication of natural infection, and particularly of vaccination with some attenuated virus vaccines, was the activation of latent protozoal infections such as babesiosis, theileriosis, and trypanosomiasis, as well as bacterial and rickettsial infections. The degree of attenuation of the virus vaccine influenced the incidence and the severity of these secondary complicating infections (Scott 1964). Rinderpest virus infection caused extensive suppression of both humoral and cell-mediated immunity in rabbits. In the primary antibody response, both the IgM and IgG antibodies were suppressed, but there was no effect on memory cells. Cell-mediated immunity was also decreased, but the phagocytic activity of the reticuloendothelial system was not affected (Yamanouchi *et al.* 1974b).

The neutralization test was useful in detecting active and passive immunity induced by rinderpest infections which were either naturally or artificially acquired. Virulent and attenuated strains of virus stimulated similar antibody titers (Scott and Brown 1958; Rowe 1966). The serum neutralization test was adapted for both qualitative and quantitative work using the strain of virus adapted from tissue culture and developed by Plowright and Ferris (1959a, b) (Johnson 1962b). This technique was used extensively for the screening of sera to detect animals which were resistant to rinderpest challenge (Brown and Scott 1959). Calves from rinderpest-immune dams had higher levels of neutralizing antibody than their dams, but the immune response to vaccination was adequate at 6 months of age (Bansal *et al.* 1978).

The CF test detected antibody in heat-inactivated bovine sera from 5 days after the fever peak for at least 50 days postinfection (Moulton and Stone 1961). The sensitivity of the CF test was greatly enhanced when the reaction was carried out overnight in the refrigerator rather than at 37 °C (MacLeod and Scott 1963). Rinderpest virus antigen could be demonstrated in the tissues of rabbits and cattle by the CF test (Boulanger 1957a, b). A procedure for obtaining high-potency rinderpest hyperimmune sera involved inoculating rabbits once with rinderpest hyperimmune serum and lapinized virus and then twice with a lapinized virus–oil adjuvant mixture; this was followed by one or two additional intravenous injections with the lapinized virus (Mohamed *et al.* 1977).

An indirect gel diffusion precipitation test was used to detect antibodies in rinderpest-convalescent cattle. These antibodies differed from neutralizing antibodies, and the development of antibody could be correlated with the severity of the clinical response (White and Scott 1960). Different concentrations of the virucidal agent beta-propiolactone did not significantly alter the complementing activity or the neutralizing capacity of anti-rinderpest rabbit serum. The use of this compound would limit the need for expensive animal safety tests (Stone and DeLay 1961). A comparison of rinderpest antibody levels assayed by the hemagglutination-inhibition test using measles antigen and by the neutralization test using rinderpest tissue culture virus showed that there was a 15% discrepancy between the tests with respect to the incidence of positive sera detected. The hemagglutination-inhibition test was used because it was easier to perform and gave a quantitative measurement of the level of antibodies (Rowe *et al.* 1967). The measles hemagglutination-inhibition test was only partially successful in detecting antibodies in cattle and sheep vaccinated against rinderpest. Animals which were serologically negative in this test had neutralizing antibodies and were resistant to challenge with virulent virus (Jayaraman *et al.* 1979). The discrepancy between the results obtained using the measles hemagglutination-inhibition test and the neutralization test were investigated, and it was shown that different groups of serum antibodies were involved in these tests (Provost *et al.* 1969a).

Recently, a microplate enzyme-linked immunosorbent assay (ELISA) was developed which detected antibodies to a soluble antigen prepared from sonicated rinderpest-infected cells. The antibodies were detected in cattle 3 weeks after immunization, indicating that the sensitivity of the ELISA was comparable to that of the neutralization test. The ELISA was a rapid and economical technique for screening large numbers of sera (Rossiter *et al.* 1981).

VACCINATION

Although cell-culture-adapted virus vaccines are superseding both the avianized and lapinized vaccines, different types of vaccines are still used in various regions of the world. In Africa and India, the cell-culture-adapted virus vaccine is employed. In southeast Asia, the attenuated lapinized virus is used to immunize cattle and buffalo, while lapinized–avianized vaccine is administered to pigs. In the USSR and Afghanistan, the LT strain of cell-culture-adapted lapinized virus is used. The duration of immunity following vaccination varies, but generally all of these vaccines are effective for several years. The virus has been shown to multiply in some challenged vaccinated animals. In Francophone Africa the cell-culture-adapted vaccine is mixed with the vaccine against contagious pleuropneumonia. The use of mixed vaccines facilitates the control of many infectious diseases in the tropics.

The cell-culture-adapted vaccine is produced in calf kidney cells after up to 100 passages of the virus. The stable characteristics of the cell-culture-adapted virus are its high level of attenuation for cattle and its failure to spread by contact. The reactions to the vaccine are limited to an occasional adverse effect in very susceptible animals. Serial back-passage of the culture vaccine in cattle does not alter the level of attenuation. Another very important feature of the vaccine is that it does not activate latent protozoal infections. However, the use of this vaccine has one disadvantage: the techniques require laboratory equipment and technical skills of a certain level of sophistication. It has been proposed that reliable and economical production of the vaccines would be in central, possibly international, laboratories rather than in small local facilities. The vaccine consists of infected culture fluids and equal volumes of protective and stabilizing additives containing 10% sucrose and 5% lactalbumin hydrolysate. This mixture is freeze-dried in vacuum ampules. In storage, cell culture vaccine has a half-life of 3 months at 20 to 22 °C and 3 weeks at 37 °C. After reconstitution, the stability depends on the use of saline, the temperature, and the amount of exposure to visible light. It confers solid resistance to experimental challenge with virulent virus for at least 10 years. In some animals, high titers of neutralizing antibody are present after 120 months, while in others the levels slowly decline and become low by 24 months.

Caprinized vaccine is produced from the spleens of goats infected with an adapted virus. This vaccine is not ideal, but it did revolutionize the control of rinderpest in enzootic areas. The degree of attenuation of the caprinized vaccine for cattle is constant, and the virus is not spread by contact between reacting cattle, buffalo, or goats. The host range of the caprinized vaccine virus is wide but less than that of virulent strains, and the goat-adapted virus cannot be grown in rabbits or tissue cultures. The response of cattle and buffalo vaccinated with goat-adapted virus may be severe and varies with the degree of innate resistance to rinderpest. Animals with low innate resistance or with latent protozoal infections have higher postvaccinal mortality. Therefore, the use of the vaccine should be restricted to cattle with high innate resistance such as East African Zebu and buffalo. In these animals the response consists of fever which begins 3 to 5 days after vaccination and persists for 4 to 5 days. Lacrimation and nasal discharges sometimes develop and diarrhea is also observed in about 1% of the animals. Cattle reacting to caprinized vaccine should not be used as virus donors since the resultant vaccine may be contaminated by anaplasms, bacteria, and other viruses which further increase the danger of adverse postvaccinal reactions.

The rabbit-adapted strain of rinderpest virus has been employed in Asia and Africa to immunize cattle possessing a moderate innate resistance to the disease. The lapinized vaccine was more extensively used than the caprinized vaccine, but its widespread use was limited by the difficulty of rearing rabbits in adequate numbers in these regions. It was prepared by harvesting spleen and mesenteric lymph nodes from infected rabbits and freeze-drying the tissues. The vaccine was characterized by its production of pathognomonic lesions in rabbits, its inability to spread by contact, its failure to grow in tissue culture, and its attenuation for moderately resistant cattle. Adverse reactions occasionally occurred, particularly when latent protozoal infections are activated. Lapinized vaccine prepared directly from rabbits is now no longer used. In the Far East, avianized versions of this type of vaccine are still used and in the USSR a tissue-culture-adapted version is used. Avianized vaccines are less virulent than caprinized vaccines, are simple and economical to produce, have good keeping properties, and provide cattle with a serviceable immunity. However, they are not used extensively.

Literature

Henning (1956) reviewed various methods of immunization such as passive immunization with serum, active immunization using the serum virus method, inactivated tissue vaccines, and goat- and rabbit-adapted viruses. The subject has been extensively discussed in more recent reviews by Scott (1964) and Plowright (1968).

Plowright and Ferris (1959a, b) produced an attenuated virus vaccine by serially passaging a strain of rinderpest virus in bovine kidney cell monolayers. This method was adopted in other regions of Africa (Johnson 1962c; Johnson and Smith 1962; De Boer 1962b). The passage of virulent rinderpest virus in calf-kidney monolayers resulted in a decline of virulence manifested by mild clinical signs, decreased mortality rate, and increased ease of contact transmission. A marked reduction in virulence occurred between the sixteenth and twenty-first passages, and no severe clinical signs were caused by vaccine at the sixteenth to forty-fifth passage level; however, the cattle were immunized against subsequent challenge by virulent virus. A proportion of these cattle developed mild temperature reactions, and the incidence of this response depended on the dose of the attenuated virus (Plowright and Ferris 1959b). After 70 to 90 passages the vaccine did not produce any clinical reaction. The neutralizing antibody response was dependent on the dose of the virus administered. Serial subinoculation of the attenuated ninetieth culture passage virus back through cattle did not enhance the pathogenicity of the virus. The cell-culture-adapted virus did not spread from inoculated cattle to susceptible contacts (Plowright and Ferris 1962b). Cattle that had been immunized with tissue culture rinderpest vaccine did not show any clinical reaction, viremia, nasal excretion of the virus, or anamnestic response after intranasal challenge with virulent virus 11 years later (Rweyemamu *et al.* 1974). Considerable effort was made to optimize and standardize the procedures used for the production of this type of vaccine. A number of factors, including temperature, handling of the medium, and the level of virus inoculated into the culture system, affected the optimal production of the virus in this system (Plowright *et al.* 1969a).

The reproducibility and accuracy of the vaccine potency test, which was based on infectivity titrations in cell cultures, were determined using different batches of cells, different dilution intervals, and varying numbers of replicate tubes. The major source of variation in the assay technique was the differing sensitivity of successive batches of cells (Plowright *et al.* 1969b). The stability of the lyophilized rinderpest culture vaccine was studied at different temperatures, and it was shown that the addition of certain ingredients to the culture media enhanced the keeping qualities. Batches of this vaccine which were stored at −20 °C for 4 to 4.5 years and at 4 °C for 3 years showed no detectable decline of titers, while storage at higher temperatures considerably reduced the half-life of the vaccine (Plowright *et al.* 1970).

The tissue culture vaccine was tested in various species of animals. The early work on the efficacy of tissue culture vaccine was confirmed, and this vaccine was shown to be an effective form of immunization in calves, sheep, and pigs (Barber and De Boer 1965). More recently, it was shown that the tissue culture vaccine did not cause any clinical reactions in buffalo, sheep, goats, and cattle, but there was a significant leukopenia in buffalo calves (Murty and Sharma 1974). It was effective in Egyptian cattle and water buffalo. The time to the immune response of cattle was related to the dose of the virus administered, and there was no transmission of the virus from vaccinated cattle and buffalo to in-contact animals (Singh *et al.* 1967a). The tissue culture vaccine was safe in European breeds of cattle imported into India (Singh and Osman 1970) and proved to be the vaccine of choice in Iran and Afghanistan (Ramyar 1968). Buffalo calves could be used for the standardization of this vaccine (Bansal and Joshi 1976). Vaccinated buffalo calves had a significant rise in the gamma globulin component between the thirteenth and twenty-fifth day after vaccination (Sharma and Murty 1974). The immunogenicity of tissue culture rinderpest vaccine was confirmed in cattle and buffalo, and the immunity appeared to be lifelong. It was thought that very low levels of circulating antibody in clinically immune cattle might permit temporary proliferation of virulent challenge virus locally in the upper respiratory tract and probably in the lymphoid tissues and blood as well, but this was not verified (Bansal and Joshi 1979). The vaccine adapted from tissue culture effectively immunized sheep over 6 months of age (Sankaran *et al.* 1976). The tissue culture rinderpest vaccine was titrated in goats to determine the dose which would adequately immunize goats against PPR (Taylor and Best 1977).

Virus-neutralizing antibody was investigated in various breeds of cattle which had been inoculated with rinderpest culture vaccine. The rate of decline of antibody and the resistance to challenge of animals with very low titers indicated that lifelong immunity occurred. Immune cattle with very low titers could contract inapparent infections which were transitory (Plowright 1957). The development of complement-fixing and virus-neutralizing antibodies occurred in the majority of vaccinated animals (Nakamura *et al.* 1955). The virus neutralization technique was also used to detect the immunological responses in cattle vaccinated with low and high doses. The tissue culture rinderpest vaccine could be successfully used in 9-month-old calves from immune dams. However, this was the average age at which the animals became susceptible, and there was considerable individual variation with respect to the persistence of the passive immunity (Smith 1966). Based on the assumption that maternally derived antibodies were not found in the nasal mucosa, an intranasal route of vaccination in calves was proposed (Provost *et al.* 1972a; Provost 1972). The effect of protozoal and rickettsial infections on the efficacy of tissue culture rinderpest vaccine has not been established. Cattle afflicted with severe cases of East Coast fever had a diminished response to rinderpest vaccination (Wagner *et al.* 1975).

Tissue culture rinderpest vaccine could be mixed with the broth culture of pleuropneumonia vaccine provided that the latter did not contain bovine serum from rinderpest-immune animals (Macadam *et al.* 1964). The rinderpest vaccine was quickly inactivated when it was reconstituted with other bacterial vaccines and failed to induce immunity (Macadam 1964). The use of a combined rinderpest–pleuropneumonia–anthrax vaccine in Central Africa was described (Provost *et al.* 1974). Some of the cattle which were simultaneously vaccinated against rinderpest and foot-and-mouth disease proved susceptible to subsequent challenge with either virulent virus (Kathuria *et al.* 1976).

The production of caprinized vaccine in West Africa was described (Mornet *et al.* 1957; Johnson *et al.* 1961). Edwards (1949) reviewed the use of caprinized virus to control rinderpest in the Near East. The keeping qualities of the caprinized and lapinized vaccine viruses were tested after storage in the deep-freeze for up to 1 year. No loss of titer occurred over this time (Purchase *et al.* 1953). Studies of various breeds of dairy cattle in India indicated that caprinized, lapinized, and lapinized–avianized vaccines conferred lifelong immunity (Bansal *et al.* 1971; Brown and Rashid 1965).

Certain breeds of indigenous African cattle (e.g. the Ankole of East Africa and the Maturu and N'Dama of West Africa) cannot be safely immunized with goat-adapted rinderpest vaccine. On occasion, this vaccine also caused severe reactions and death in the local Zebu cattle in West Africa. This necessitated the development of more highly attenuated vaccine strains like lapinized virus (Plowright 1957). Calves up to 4 months of age from immune dams did not respond to the caprinized vaccine, but the percentage of older calves which reacted steadily increased with time until all animals responded when 9 months old (Strickland 1962). The growth rate of calves 9 to 12 months of age was inhibited temporarily by the caprinized vaccine, but by the seventeenth week after inoculation, the vaccinated calves and the unvaccinated controls had comparable weight gains (Brown and Lampkin 1961). The mortality among vaccinated calves was 2%, and a high proportion of these deaths was associated with concurrent theilerial and trypanosomal infections (Branagan 1965). The vaccine enhanced the development of lesions in experimental contagious bovine pleuropneumonia (Brown 1963). Vaccinated bulls showed a loss of semen quality for up to 3 weeks (Radhakrishnan *et al.* 1975).

The postvaccinal reactions caused by the caprinized vaccine in sheep and goats included fever, loss of appetite, dullness, sluggish movement, and congested mucous membranes (Lall 1947). In goats and sheep, there was no significant difference in the severity of the response obtained by the scarification and subcutaneous methods of vaccination. The immunization of goats with caprinized virus resulted in a mortality of 25% whether the scarification or the subcutaneous procedure was employed (Sharma and Ram 1955). The major changes observed in goats used for the production of rinderpest vaccine were hematological. A progressive leukopenia developed; neutrophils were more abundant than lymphoid cells and eosinophils (Krishnan and Viswanathan 1965). There was also loss of body weight which was related to the rise in body temperature (Sapra *et al.* 1969).

Cambodian cattle, buffalo, and swine vaccinated with lapinized–avianized rinderpest virus developed adequate levels of neutralizing antibody without reacting to the vaccine (Sonoda 1971). The utilization of pigs in the production of lapinized rinderpest virus was proposed in order to avoid the use of rabbits which at the time were considered difficult to raise in quantity in the tropics (Hudson and Wongsongsarn 1950). The stability of lyophilized rinderpest cell culture vaccine reconstituted in saline was influenced by exposure to light (Plowright *et al.* 1971). A lyophilized rinderpest vaccine which was thought to have better keeping qualities was developed and could be used without refrigeration under field conditions (Provost *et al.* 1972b). Antibodies could be detected within 14 days in cattle and buffalo inoculated with various concentrations of caprinized, lapinized, or lapinized–avianized virus vaccine (Singh 1971). The adverse reactions to lapinized rinderpest virus included high mortality associated with the activation of latent protozoal infections, abortion, transient spermatolysis, and anaphylaxis (Scott 1963). Fetal involvement in rinderpest infection was observed after goats and rabbits had been inoculated with caprinized and lapinized rinderpest vaccines respectively (Chawla and Sinha 1961).

Rinderpest virus, whether virulent, caprinized, or lapinized, could not be recovered from cattle 1 month after vaccination, and massive doses of virulent virus inoculated into immune cattle disappeared immediately and permanently (Scott 1957). However, it was shown that vaccinates challenged by contact exposure could harbor virulent virus in the nasal mucosa and contaminate in-contact susceptible animals. The permanence of the immunity induced by the cell culture vaccine was questioned (Provost *et al.* 1969b). Cattle immunized with an inactivated vaccine excreted highly virulent challenge virus for 3 to 19 days after vaccination (Bourdin 1968).

Because rinderpest cannot be controlled in wild species by conventional methods of vaccination, the feasibility of an oral vaccine was investigated. Vaccine administered in salt licks was only partially successful (Scott 1976).

Although inactivated vaccines proved safe and efficacious, animals required multiple injections and the resultant immunity was short-lived. Cattle immunized with formalin-inactivated adjuvant rinderpest vaccine developed objectionable purulent lesions at or near the inoculation site (Scott and Ginsberg 1959). More modern formulations, however, have proven safe and efficacious (Mirchamsy *et al.* 1974).

DIAGNOSIS

The methods which are used for the diagnosis of rinderpest depend on the epizootiological situation; i.e. the disease is enzootic or suspected in a rinderpest-free area. Although a tentative diagnosis can be made on the basis of clinical and pathological findings, laboratory support is essential for confirmation. Partial confirmation of a provisional diagnosis can be made by examining impression smears or tissue sections for the presence of intracytoplasmic and intranuclear inclusions and syncytia. However, the interpretation of slides requires considerable experience. Laboratory diagnosis of rinderpest involves isolation of the virus, detection of virus-specific antigens in tissues, demonstration of antibodies, and identification of characteristic histological lesions. Fluorescent antibody methods effectively demonstrate virus antigens in cell cultures and infected animal tissues.

Serological diagnosis is made using immunodiffusion and CF tests, the latter technique being the more sensitive. Serological identification is achieved by incorporating immune serum in the cultures or by pinpointing viral antigens in cells by immunofluorescence. The detection of virus-specific antigens in tissues is the most rapid means of demonstrating the virus and can be accomplished in less than 24 hours. Rapid identification of rinderpest antigen in tissues is accomplished with the CF and agar-gel diffusion tests, the latter technique being the more sensitive. Both tests are ineffective early in the course of the disease and after the appearance of antibodies. A recently developed counter-immunoelectrophoresis technique is very sensitive and can detect antigens more quickly than the older methods.

Virus can be demonstrated by infecting tissue cultures or susceptible animals. The detection of antigen depends on adequate sampling, degree of postmortem change, and the stage of infection. In reacting animals, biopsy samples are taken from superficial lymph nodes. The optimal period for the collecting of samples is during the first days of fever before the onset of diarrhea. Animals in the latter stages of infection have low titers of virus, and samples from dead animals are often not satisfactory.

The demonstration of rinderpest-specific antibodies in enzootic areas necessitates the simultaneous examination of paired serum samples, one taken during the early acute stage of disease and the other 2 to 4 weeks later. The antibody test is the most reliable method.

Literature

A provisional diagnosis of rinderpest could be made on the basis of the clinical signs and lesions and should be verified by laboratory tests which involve virus recovery and identification, demonstration of viral antigens in lymphoid tissues, determination of the presence of syncytia and intranuclear and intracytoplasmic inclusions in the epithelial and lymphoid cells, and the demonstration of antibodies by serological tests (Plowright 1965).

Scott and Brown (1961) discussed the diagnosis of rinderpest with special reference to the agar-gel double diffusion test. They summarized the physical and biological properties of the virus as well as the clinical and pathological observations and provided details of the differential diagnoses. Provost and Joubert (1973) also reviewed the diagnostic methods. Liess and Bogel (1969) described the diagnostic procedure used to differentiate rinderpest from mucosal disease complex.

The agar-gel double diffusion test was of great practical value in the diagnosis of rinderpest under field conditions because of its ease, simplicity, and definite identification of rinderpest antigens in infected tissues. In addition, it was thought to be more readily applicable than the CF test (White and Cowan 1962). Biopsy samples of lymph nodes of infected cattle were examined using the agar-gel double diffusion technique, and rinderpest antigens were obtained from the first to the eighth day after the onset of fever (Brown and Scott 1960). Lymph nodes and salivary glands gave better results than other tissues collected at post-mortem (Kamel and El Ghaffar 1974). The distribution of rinderpest-diffusible precipitinogen in the tissues of susceptible cattle was specified; the lymph nodes and gastrointestinal tissues were the best sources (Scott and Brown 1961). The application of the agar-gel double diffusion test was investigated under field conditions. The technique proved to be an efficient method of demonstrating the virus in lymph nodes collected from dead animals between the third and twelfth day of fever (Joshi *et al.* 1972). The optimal time for reading the agar-gel double diffusion test was dependent on the ambient temperature (Scott 1962d). The use of bovine hyperimmune serum in this technique was described (Scott 1962a). The CF test was found to be a satisfactory method for diagnosing rinderpest on a herd basis, but it was not always effective in confirming infection in individual animals. The stage of infection and the freshness of the tissues were important considerations (Nakamura and Macleod 1959). More recently it was shown that counter-immunoelectrophoresis was 4 to 16 times more sensitive than immunodiffusion with respect to the detection of antigens in lymph node biopsies; positive reactions were observed within 40 minutes. This test could be used for rapid laboratory confirmation of rinderpest infections (Rossiter and Mushi 1980).

The usefulness of the measles hemagglutination inhibiting test in the diagnosis of rinderpest was considered (Maurice *et al.* 1969). Viral antigens could be detected in tissues and secretions by the passive hemagglutination test (Singh 1972). The blocking of measles hemagglutination-inhibition antibodies by antigens from lymph nodes infected with caprinized or lapinized rinderpest virus was found to be useful in the diagnosis of rinderpest (Gnanabaranam *et al.* 1980).

The FA test could be a useful diagnostic aid, but the technique was not as reliable as other methods (Provost 1970). In infected cell cultures, specific immunofluorescence was found as early as 18 hours postinfection, and the immunofluorescent areas became larger and brighter with time (Prabhudas and Sambamurti 1976). The direct immunoperoxidase test showed that the progressive virus-specific cytopathic changes could be directly correlated with the increase in the number of cells containing viral antigens. The test was sensitive and could detect the antigens 6 hours after infection. In addition, this technique was more advantageous than the immunofluorescent test because there was no nonspecific background fluorescence (Krishnaswamy *et al.* 1981).

The isolation and identification of the virus was achieved by inoculating susceptible cattle with infected tissues. Blood was used in acute cases, and the other preferred tissues were lymph nodes and spleen. Both rinderpest-immune cattle and susceptible cattle were used. The susceptible cattle reacted 1 to 11 days after infection. The nonreactors and surviving animals were challenged 2 to 3 weeks later by the inoculation of known virulent virus. The diagnosis was confirmed by the presence of rinderpest-neutralizing antibodies in the postinfection sera (Scott and Brown 1961). Subendocardial hemorrhages tended to be present in animals which died during or immediately after the acute febrile stage of rinderpest and could therefore be used to indicate those animals which might provide tissue samples for further diagnostic tests (Scott 1962b).

The histologic evidence of encephalitis found in cattle afflicted with malignant catarrhal fever distinguished the disease from rinderpest (Khater *et al.* 1964). The agar-gel diffusion test was used to differentiate rinderpest from bovine mucosal disease (Darbyshire *et al.* 1961).

CONTROL

Control measures include restricting the movement of domestic and wild animals between enzootic and high-risk areas. Domestic animals are vaccinated in the enzootic regions and the high-risk areas which usually border these regions. In spite of the widespread application of very effective vaccines, rinderpest is enzootic in Asia and Africa because the available financial and technical resources are insufficient for the implementation of appropriate control measures throughout these regions. The factors which impede the eradication of the disease include lack of understanding of the importance of continued immunization, the migratory nature of many of the husbandries, and, in Africa, large migratory herds of wild ungulates.

Literature

The control of rinderpest is relatively simple and the persistence of the disease in most countries was related inversely to the available technical and financial resources. However, recent attempts have been made to control the disease in some enzootic areas. For example, a nationwide rinderpest eradication program was launched in India in 1954, and by the end of 1978 775 million animals had been vaccinated. The morbidity rate plummeted from 2000 per million cattle to 7 per million. Another campaign, known as JP-15, took place in West Africa in 1962 and ended in 1969 after 81 million vaccinations had been carried out. The failure to eradicate the disease despite a dramatic decrease in the number of losses was probably related to the presence of wild game. The development of efficient measures for controlling the disease in game animals would be highly desirable. A lyophilized caprinized vaccine fed to cattle with salt was only partially effective (Scott 1976). The vaccination of wild game animals required immobilization, an impossible task even with relatively small numbers of animals (Harthoorn and Lock 1960). The vaccination techniques used in the massive eradication campaign in West Africa were described (Lepissier and MacFarlane 1967). The final report on phase 1 of the joint campaign against rinderpest in Africa was published by Lepissier and MacFarlane (1966). The extension of the JP-15 rinderpest control campaign to eastern Africa was discussed in relation to the epizootiology of the disease in the region (Atang and Plowright 1969). In northeast Africa, 8.5 million doses of caprinized vaccine were used in 1960 (Plowright 1968). The eradication campaign in India was described by Datta (1954). In India, 130 million head of cattle received the caprinized vaccine between 1964 and 1965.

BIBLIOGRAPHY

Ademollo, A., 1959. Introduction of rinderpest by imported meat, *Bull. epiz. Dis. Afr.*, **7**: 91–95.

Adiwinata, R. T., 1968. Some informative notes on a rinderpest-like disease on the island of Bali, *Bull. Off. int. Epiz.*, **69**(1–2): 7–14.

Ali, B. E. H., 1973. A natural outbreak of rinderpest involving sheep, goats and cattle in Sudan, *Bull. epiz. Dis. Afr.*, **21**(4): 421–8.

Anon., 1956. Cutaneous lesions in rinderpest, *Bull. epiz. Dis. Afr.*, **4**: 81–2.

Anon., 1969. Rinderpest-like disease on the Island of Bali (Indonesia), *Bull. Off. int. Epiz.*, **71**(11–12): 1305–6.

Anon., 1970a. Joint OIE–FAO consultative meeting on rinderpest in the Near East. Paris, 26 May 1970, *Bull. Off. int. Epiz.*, **73**: 817–32.

Anon., 1970b. Emergency meeting on rinderpest organized by the FAO Regional Animal Production and Health Commission for the Near East. Beirut (Lebanon), 12–13 October 1970, *Bull. Off. int. Epiz.*, **73**: 873–93.

Atang, P. G. and Plowright, W., 1969. Extension of the JP-15 rinderpest control campaign to eastern Africa: the epizootiological background, *Bull. epiz. Dis. Afr.*, **17**: 161–70.

Bansal, R. P., Chawla, S. K., Sharma, S. D. and Menon, M. S., 1971. Studies on the duration of immunity conferred by attenuated rinderpest vaccines, *Indian J. Anim. Sci.*, **41**(1): 18–26.

Bansal, R. P. and Joshi, R. C., 1976. Potency testing of tissue-culture rinderpest vaccine in buffalo calves. *Indian J. Anim. Sci.*, **46**(8): 413–16.

Bansal, R. P. and Joshi, R. C., 1979. Immunogenicity of tissue-culture rinderpest vaccine, *Indian J. Anim. Sci.*, **49**(4): 260–5.

Bansal, R. P. and Joshi, R. C., 1981. Production and standardization of tissue-culture rinderpest vaccine in lamb-kidney cell-cultures, *Indian J. Anim. Sci.*, **51**(8): 782–7.

Bansal, R. P., Joshi, R. C. and Kumar, S., 1974. Occurrence of rinderpest in pigs in India, *Bull. Off. int. Epiz.*, **81**(3–4): 305–12.

Bansal, R. P., Joshi, R. C. and Kumar, S., 1978. Active immunization of calves with tissue culture rinderpest vaccine, *Bull. Off. int. Epiz.*, **89**: 119–25.

Bansal, R. P., Joshi, R. C., Tandon, H. K. L. and Kumar, S., 1981. Production of interferon by rinderpest virus in calf kidney cell cultures, *Acta virol.*, **25**: 61.

Barber, T. L. and De Boer, C. J., 1965. Response of calves, sheep and pigs to a cell-culture-modified rinderpest virus, *Cornell Vet.*, **55**: 590–8.

Barber, T. L. and Heuschele, W. P., 1964a. Experimental rinderpest in sheep, *Proc. 67th Ann. Meet. US Livestock Sanit. Ass.*, Albuquerque, NM, pp. 155–62.

Barber, T. L. and Heuschele, W. P., 1964b. Experimental passage of rinderpest virus in North American pigs, *Bull. epiz. Dis. Afr.*, **12**: 277–85.

Beaton, W. G., 1954. Rinderpest. Summary of reports on the epizootic in game and cattle in the area centred on the junction between the Sudan, Uganda and Belgian Congo, *Bull. epiz. Dis. Afr.*, **2**: 413–15.

Beaton, W. G., 1963. Perspectives in incidence and control of rinderpest in Africa – 1952–62, *Bull. epiz. Dis. Afr.*, **11**: 339–45.

Beaton, W. G., 1966. Skin lesions in rinderpest, *Vet. Rec.*, **78**(11): 393–4.

Bergeon, P., 1952. Rinderpest virus content of nervous tissues and bone marrow, *Bull. Soc. Path. Exot.*, **45**: 148–52.

Boulanger, P., 1957a. The use of the complement-fixation test for the demonstration of rinderpest virus in rabbit tissue using rabbit antisera, *Can. J. comp. Med.*, **21**(11): 363–9.

Boulanger, P., 1957b. Application of the complement-fixation test to the demonstration of rinderpest in the tissue of infected cattle using rabbit antiserum. I. Results with the Kabete and Pendik strains of virus, *Can. J. comp. Med.*, **21**(11): 379–88.

Bourdin, P., 1968. Duration of rinderpest virus excretion in cattle immunized with an inactivated vaccine, *Rev. Elev. Méd. vét. Pays trop.*, **21**(2): 141–4.

Branagan, D., 1965. Observations on post-vaccinal sequelae to rinderpest vaccination using caprinised vaccine on cattle in Tanganyika Masailand, *Bull. epiz. Dis. Afr.*, **13**: 5–10.

Branagan, D. and Hammond, J. A., 1965. Rinderpest in Tanganyika: a review, *Bull. epiz. Dis. Afr.*, **13**: 225–46.

Breese, S. S. Jr and De Boer, C. J., 1973. Ferritin-tagged antibody cross-reactions among rinderpest, canine distemper, and measles viruses, *J. gen. Virol.*, **20**: 121–5.

Brown, R. D., 1958. Rinderpest immunity in calves – a review, *Bull. epiz. Dis. Afr.*, **6**: 127–33.

Brown, R. D., 1963. The effect of caprinised rinderpest virus on the experimental production of contagious bovine pleuropneumonia, *Vet. Rec.*, **75**(48): 1306–7.

Brown, R. D. and Lampkin, G. H., 1961. Effect of caprinized rinderpest vaccine on the growth of weaner calves, *East Afr. Agric. and For. J.*, **26**: 156–57.

Brown, R. D. and Rashid, A., 1965. Duration of rinderpest immunity in cattle following vaccination with caprinised rinderpest virus, *Bull. epiz. Dis. Afr.*, **13**: 311–15.

Brown, R. D. and Scott, G. R., 1959. A screening procedure for the detection of rinderpest-immune cattle, *Bull. epiz. Dis. Afr.*, **7**: 169–71.

Brown, R. D. and Scott, G. R., 1960. Diagnosis of rinderpest by lymph node biopsy, *Vet. Rec.*, **72**(47): 1055–6.

Chawla, S. K. and Sinha, K. C., 1961. Detection of the virus of rinderpest in goat and rabbit foetuses after inoculation during pregnancy, *Indian vet. J.*, **38**: 273–80.

Darbyshire, J. H., Brown, R. D., Scott, G. R. and Huck, R. A., 1961. A serological differentiation of rinderpest and bovine mucosal disease by agar gel diffusion, *Vet. Rec.*, **73**(10): 255–6.

Datta, S., 1954. The national rinderpest eradication plan, *Indian J. vet. Sci.*, **24**: 1–9.

De Boer, C. J., 1962a. Adaptation of two strains of rinderpest virus to tissue culture, *Arch. ges. Virusforsch.*, **11**: 534–43.

De Boer, C. J., 1962b. Studies with tissue culture-modified rinderpest virus as an immunizing agent, *J. Immunol.*, **89**: 170–6.

De Boer, C. J. and Barber, T. L., 1964a. Segregation of an avirulent variant of rinderpest virus by the terminal dilution technique in tissue culture, *J. Immunol.*, **92**: 902.

De Boer, C. J. and Barber, T. L., 1964b. pH and thermal stability of rinderpest virus, *Arch. ges. Virusforsch.*, **15**: 98–108.

DeLay, P. D. and Barber, T. L., 1963. Transmission of rinderpest virus from experimentally infected cattle to pigs, *Proc. 66th Ann. Meet. US Livestock Sanit. Assoc.*, Washington, pp. 132–6.

DeLay, P. D. and Kniazeff, A. J., 1966. Response of virus diarrhea-mucosal disease-convalescent calves and rinderpest-vaccinated calves to inoculation with heterologous virus, *Am. J. vet. Res.*, **27**(117): 512–18.

DeLay, P. D., Moulton, W. M. and Stone, S. S., 1962. Survival of rinderpest virus in experimentally infected swine, *Proc. 65th Ann. Meet. US Livestock Sanit. Assoc.*, Minneapolis, pp. 376–83.

Dhanda, M. R. and Manjrekar, S. L., 1951/52. Observations on rinderpest amongst sheep and goats in the state of Bombay, *Indian vet. J.*, **28**: 306–19.

Dhillon, S. S., 1959. Incidence of rinderpest in camels in Hissar district, *Indian vet. J.*, **36**: 603–7.

Edwards, J. T., 1949. The uses and limitations of the caprinized virus in the control of rinderpest (cattle plague) among British and Near-eastern cattle, *Br. vet. J.*, **105**(7): 209–53.

Ferris, R. D. and Plowright, W., 1961. The serial cultivation of calf kidney cells for use in virus research, *Res. vet. Sci.*, **2**: 387–95.

Gilbert, Y., Mornet, P. and Goueffon, Y., 1960. Comportement humoral du bœuf et du lapin evers l'inoculation de virus de Carré: ses rapports avec l'immunisation contre le virus bovipestique normal ou modifié, *Bull. Acad. Vet. France*, **33**: 305–15.

Gilbert, Y. and Monnier, J., 1962. Adaptation d'une souche de virus bovipestique à la culture cellulaire. Premiers résultats, *Rev. Elev. Méd. vét. Pays trop.*, **15**(4): 311–20.

Gnanabaranam, J. F., Padmanaban, V. D., Jayaraman, M. S., Nachimuthu, K. and Balaprakasam, R. A., 1980. Diagnosis of rinderpest by blocking measles haemagglutination inhibition antibody with infected lymph nodes, *Indian vet. J.*, **57**: 792–5.

Hamdy, F. M., Dardiri, A. H., Ferris, D. H. and Breese, S. S. Jr, 1975. Experimental infection of white-tailed deer with rinderpest virus, *J. Wildl. Dis.*, **11**: 508–15.

Harthoorn, A. M. and Lock, J. A., 1960. A note on the prophylactic vaccination of wild animals, *Br. vet. J.*, **116**: 252–4.

Henning, M. W., 1956. Rinderpest, cattle plague, runderpest (Pestis bovina). In *Animal Diseases in South Africa*, 3rd edn. Central News Agency (South Africa), pp. 828–67.

Heuschele, W. P. and Barber, T. L., 1963. Hematological studies of rinderpest-infected swine, *Can. J. comp. Med.*, **27**: 56–60.

Heuschele, W. P. and Barber, T. L., 1966. Changes in certain blood components of rinderpest-infected cattle, *Am. J. vet. Res.*, **27**(119): 1001–6.

Hudson, J. R. and Wongsongsarn, C., 1950. The utilisation of pigs for the production of lapinised rinderpest virus. *Br. vet. J.*, **106**: 454–72.

Hussain, S. F., Rweyemamu, M. M., Kaminjolo, J. S., Akhtar, A. S. and Mugera, G. M., 1980a. Studies on viral interference induced by rinderpest virus: interference and interferon induction by tissue culture rinderpest vaccine (TCRV) virus *in vitro, Zbl. Vet. Med.*, **B27**: 181–9.

Hussain, S. F., Rweyemamu, M. M., Kaminjolo, J. S., Akhtar, A. S. and Mugera, G. M., 1980b. Studies on viral interference induced by rinderpest virus: inactivation of tissue culture rinderpest vaccine virus by heat treatment at 56 °C and by ultraviolet irradiation, *Zbl. Vet. Med.*, **B27**: 233–42.

Ilchmann, G. and Lehnert, T., 1972. Pathological and histological differentiation of rinderpest and mucosal disease, *Archiv. fur Experimentelle Veterinarmedizin*, **26**: 559–68.

Jayaraman, M. S., Masillamony, P. R., Nachimuthu, K. and Padmanaban, V. D., 1979. The usefulness of measles haemagglutination inhibition test in detecting rinderpest antibodies in cattle and sheep after inoculation of tissue culture rinderpest vaccine, *Indian vet. J.*, **56**: 816–20.

Johnson, R. H., 1958. An outbreak of rinderpest involving cattle and sheep, *Vet. Rec.*, **70**(22): 457–61.

Johnson, R. H., 1962a. Rinderpest in tissue culture. I. Methods for virus production, *Br. vet. J.*, **118**: 107–16.

Johnson, R. H., 1962b. Rinderpest in tissue culture. II. Serum neutralization tests, *Br. vet. J.*, **118**: 133–40.

Johnson, R. H., 1962c. Rinderpest in tissue culture. III. Use of the attenuated strain as a vaccine for cattle, *Br. vet. J.*, **118**: 141–50.

Johnson, R. H. and Smith, V. W., 1962. The production and use of tissue culture rinderpest vaccine in Nigeria, *Bull. epiz. Dis. Afr.*, **10**: 417–22.

Johnson, R. H., Thorne, A. L. C. and Chifney, S. T. E., 1961. The production of caprinised rinderpest vaccine in Nigeria, *Bull. epiz. Dis. Afr.*, **9**: 233–40.

Joshi, R. C., Chaudhary, P. G. and Bansal, R. P., 1977. Occurrence of cutaneous eruptions in rinderpest outbreak among bovine, *Indian vet. J.*, **54**: 871–3.

Joshi, R. C., Shukla, D. C. and Bansal, R. P., 1972. Rinderpest diagnosis by agar gel double diffusion test, *Indian vet. J.*, **49**: 449–56.

Joshi, T. P. and Sinha, K. C., 1961. Observations on the susceptibility of adult buffaloes to rinderpest, *Indian vet. J.*, **38**: 527–35.

Kamel, J. and El Ghaffar, S. A., 1974. Immunodiffusion technique for diagnosis of rinderpest, *Egyptian vet. Med. Assoc. J.*, **34**(3/4): 367–76.

Kataria, R. S., Majumdar, S. S. and Shrivastava, S. N., 1974. Demonstration of specific precipitinogen in skin lesions in a case of rinderpest, *Indian vet. J.*, **51**: 736–7.

Kathuria, B. K., Uppal, P. K. and Kumar, S., 1976. Studies on simultaneous vaccination of cattle against rinderpest and foot and mouth disease, *Indian vet. J.*, **53**: 571–6.

Khater, A. R., Messow, C. and Stober, M., 1964. The histopathological lesions of the brain as a means for differential diagnosis of mucosal disease, malignant catarrh and rinderpest, *Dt. Tierarztl. Wschr.*, **71**(5): 127–31.

Khera, K. S., 1958. Histological study of rinderpest. I. Pathogenesis of rinderpest virus in lymph nodes, *Rev. Elev.*, **11**: 399–405.

Krishnan, R. and Viswanathan, S., 1965. Tissue changes in goats used for rinderpest vaccine production, *Indian vet. J.*, **42**: 480–3.

Krishnaswamy, S., Keshavamurthy, B. S. and Sundararajan, S., 1981. The use of the direct immunoperoxidase test to detect the multiplication of rinderpest virus in bovine kidney cell culture, *Vet. Microbiol.*, **6**: 23–9.

Lall, H. K., 1947. Some observations on the immunization of sheep and goats against rinderpest, *Indian J. vet. Sci.*, **17**: 11–22.

Lepissier, H. E. and MacFarlane, I. M., 1966. OAU/STRC joint campaign against rinderpest. Final report of the coordinators on Phase I, *Bull. epiz. Dis. Afr.*, **14**: 194–224.

Lepissier, H. E. and MacFarlane, I. M., 1967. Techniques of mass vaccination in the control of rinderpest in Africa. (Joint campaign against rinderpest), *Bull. Off. int. Epiz.*, **68**: 665–89.

Liess, B., 1965. The rinderpest problem in East Africa, *Berl. Munch. Tierarztl. Wschr.*, **78**: 266–9.

Liess, B. and Bogel, K., 1969. Differential diagnosis of rinderpest virus diarrhoea-mucosal disease and malignant catarrh, *Dt. Tierarztl. Wschr.*, **76**(6): 138–41.

Liess, B. and Plowright, W., 1963. Studies in tissue culture on the pH-stability of rinderpest virus, *J. Hyg., Camb.*, **61**: 205–11.

Liess, B. and Plowright, W., 1963/64. The propagation and growth characteristics of rinderpest virus in HeLa cells, *Arch. ges. Virusforsch.*, **14**: 27–38.

Liess, B. and Plowright, W., 1964. Studies on the pathogenesis of rinderpest in experimental cattle. I. Correlation of clinical signs, viraemia and virus excretion by various routes, *J. Hyg., Camb.*, **62**: 81–100.

Macadam, I., 1964. The response of zebu cattle to tissue culture rinderpest vaccine mixed in (1) blackquarter vaccine and (2) anthrax spore vaccine, *Bull. epiz. Dis. Afr.*, **12**: 401–3.

Macadam, I., 1968. Transmission of rinderpest from goats to cattle in Tanzania, *Bull. epiz. Dis. Afr.*, **16**: 53–60.

Macadam, I., Ezebuiro, E. O. and Oreffo, V. O. C., 1964. The response of zebu cattle to mixed contagious pleuropneumonia and tissue culture rinderpest vaccines, *Bull. epiz. Dis. Afr.*, **12**: 237–40.

Mack, R., 1970. The great African cattle plague epidemic of the 1890s, *Trop. Anim. Hlth Prod.*, **2**: 210–19.

MacLeod, A. K. and Scott, G. R., 1963. Time and temperature of complement-fixation in the diagnosis of rinderpest, *J. Comp. Path.*, **73**: 88–92.

Mares, R. G., 1956. Cutaneous lesions in rinderpest, *Bull. epiz. Dis. Afr.*, **4**: 81–2.

Maurer, F. D., Jones, T. C., Easterday, B. and DeTray, D., 1955. Pathology of rinderpest – an abstract, *J. Am. vet. med. Ass.*, **127**: 512–14.

Maurer, F. D., Jones, T. C., Easterday, B. and DeTray, D., 1956. The pathology of rinderpest, *Proc. 92nd Ann. Meet. Am. Vet. Med. Ass.*, Minneapolis, 1955, pp. 201–11.

Maurice, Y., Provost, A. and Borredon, C., 1967. Presence of antibodies against rinderpest virus in dromedary in Chad, *Rev. Elev. Méd. vét. Pays trop.*, **20**(4): 537–42.

Maurice, Y., Provost, A. and Borredon, C., 1969. Possibilities and limits of the measles haemagglutination inhibition test in the serology of rinderpest. I. Interpretation and usefulness of this test (M.H.I. test), *Rev. Elev. Méd. vét. Pays trop.*, **22**(1): 1–8.

McKercher, P. D., 1963. Plaque production by rinderpest virus in bovine kidney cultures: a preliminary report, *Can. J. comp. Med.*, **27**: 71–2.

McKercher, P. D., 1964. A comparison of the viruses of infectious bovine rhinotracheitis (IBR), infectious pustular vulvo-vaginitis (IPV) and rinderpest. Part II. Plaque assay, *Can. J. comp. Med.*, **28**: 113–20.

Mirchamsy, H., Shafyi, A., Bahrami, S., Nazari, P. and Akburzadeh, J., 1974. Active immunization of cattle with killed vaccines prepared from cell-cultured rinderpest virus, *Res. vet. Sci.*, **17**: 242–7.

Mohamed, Z. E., Hafez, S. M. and Ozawa, Y., 1977. Studies on the methods of preparation of rinderpest hyperimmune sera in rabbits, *Trop. Anim. Hlth Prod.*, **9**: 25–8.

Mohan, R. and Bahl, M. R., 1953. Cutaneous eruptions of rinderpest in goats, *Indian J. vet. Sci.*, **23**(1): 39–42.

Mornet, P., Gilbert, Y. and Mahou, R., 1957. Prophylaxie de la peste bovine. Nouvelle methode économique de préparation du virus-vaccine bovipestique caprinise sur bœuf réagissant, *Rev. Elev. Méd. vét. Pays trop.*, **10**: 333–9.

Mornet, P., Goret, P., Gilbert, Y. and Goueffon, Y., 1960. Sur les relations croisées des caractères antigènes et immunigènes des virus de la maladie de Carré et de la peste bovine. Etat actuel des recherches, *Rev. Elev. Méd. vét. Pays trop.*, **13**(1): 5–25.

Mornet, P. and Guerret, M., 1950. Skin lesions in rinderpest, *Bul. Acad. Vét.*, **23**: 283–5.

Moulton, W. M. and Stone, S. S., 1961. A procedure for detecting complement-fixing antibody to rinderpest virus in heat-inactivated bovine serum, *Res. vet. Sci.*, **2**: 161–6.

Murty, D. K. and Sharma, S. K., 1974. Studies on reactogenicity and immunogenicity of cell-culture rinderpest vaccine in different species of ruminants, *Indian J. Anim. Sci.*, **44**(6): 359–65.

Nakamura, J., Kishi, S., Kiuchi, J. and Reisinger, R., 1955. An investigation of antibody response in cattle vaccinated with rabbit-passaged LA rinderpest virus in Korea, *Am. J. vet. Res.*, **16**: 71–5.

Nakamura, J. and Macleod, A. J., 1959. The complement fixation test and its application to the diagnosis of rinderpest, *J. Comp. Path.*, **69**: 11–19.

Narayanaswamy, M. and Ramani, K., 1973. Preliminary studies on rinderpest virus isolated from outbreaks in sheep in Mysore State, *Indian vet. J.*, **50**(8): 829–32.

Okuna, N. and Rweyemamu, M. M., 1974. Observations on the development of serum neutralizing antibody in rinderpest infection, *Bull. epiz. Dis. Afr.*, **22**(3): 185–94.

Orvell, C. and Norrby, E., 1974. Further studies on the immunologic relationships among measles, distemper, and rinderpest viruses, *J. Immunol.*, **113**(6): 1850–8.

Otte, E., 1961. A note on a 'rinderpest-like disease' in the Sudan and in Ethiopia, *Bull. epiz. Dis. Afr.*, **9**: 215–26.

Otte, E. and Peck, E. F., 1960. A note on a rinderpest-like disease of cattle in Ethiopia, *Bull. epiz. Dis. Afr.*, **8**: 203–16.

Plowright, W., 1952. Observations on the behaviour of rinderpest virus in indigenous African sheep, *Br. vet. J.*, **108**: 450–7.

Plowright, W., 1957. Recent observations on rinderpest immunisation and vaccines in northern Nigeria, *Br. vet. J.*, **113**: 385–99.

Plowright, W., 1962a. Rinderpest virus, *Ann. N.Y. Acad. Sci.*, **101**: 548–73.

Plowright, W., 1962b. The application of monolayer tissue culture techniques in rinderpest research. I. Introduction. Use in serological investigations and diagnosis, *Bull. Off. int. Epiz.*, **57**: 1–23.

Plowright, W., 1963a. Some properties of strains of rinderpest virus recently isolated in E. Africa, *Res. vet. Sci.*, **4**: 96–108.

Plowright, W., 1963b. The role of game animals in the epizootiology of rinderpest and malignant catarrhal fever in East Africa, *Bull. epiz. Dis. Afr.*, **11**: 149–62.

Plowright, W., 1964a. The growth of virulent and attenuated strains of rinderpest virus in primary calf kidney cells, *Arch. ges. Virusforsch.*, **14**: 431–48.

Plowright, W., 1964b. Studies on the pathogenesis of rinderpest in experimental cattle. II. Proliferation of the virus in different tissues following intranasal infection, *J. Hyg., Camb.*, **62**: 257–81.

Plowright, W., 1965. III – Rinderpest, *Vet. Rec.*, **77**(48): 1431–7.

Plowright, W., 1968. Rinderpest virus. In *Monographs in Virology*, eds J. Parker, R. F. Stape. Springer-Verlag (Vienna and New York), vol. 3, pp. 25–110.

Plowright, W., 1982. The effects of rinderpest and rinderpest control on wildlife in Africa, *Symp. zool. Soc. Lond.*, No. 50: 1–28.

Plowright, W. and Ferris, R. D., 1957. Cytopathogenicity of rinderpest virus in tissue culture, *Nature*, **179**: 316.

Plowright, W. and Ferris, R. D., 1959a. Studies with rinderpest virus in tissue culture. I. Growth and cytopathogenicity, *J. Comp. Path.*, **69**: 152–72.

Plowright, W. and Ferris, R. D., 1959b. Studies with rinderpest virus in tissue culture. II. Pathogenicity for cattle of culture-passaged virus, *J. Comp. Path.*, **69**: 173–84.

Plowright, W. and Ferris, R. D., 1961. The preparation of bovine thyroid monolayers for use in virological investigations, *Res. vet. Sci.*, **2**: 149–52.

Plowright, W. and Ferris, R. D., 1962a. Studies with rinderpest virus in tissue culture. A technique for the detection and titration of virulent virus in cattle tissues, *Res. vet. Sci.*, **3**: 94–103.

Plowright, W. and Ferris, R. D., 1962b. Studies with rinderpest virus in tissue culture. The use of attenuated culture virus as a vaccine for cattle, *Res. vet. Sci.*, **3**: 172–82.

Plowright, W., Herniman, K. A. J. and Rampton, C. S., 1969a. Studies on rinderpest culture vaccine. I. Some factors affecting virus production, *Res. vet. Sci.*, **10**: 373–81.

Plowright, W., Herniman, K. A. J. and Rampton, C. S., 1969b. Studies on rinderpest culture vaccine. II. Factors influencing the accuracy of vaccine potency tests, *Res. vet. Sci.*, **10**: 502–8.

Plowright, W., Herniman, K. A. J. and Rampton, C. S., 1971. Studies on rinderpest culture vaccine. IV. The stability of the reconstituted product, *Res. vet. Sci.*, **12**: 40–6.

Plowright, W., Laws, R. M. and Rampton, C. S., 1964. Serological evidence for the susceptibility of the hippopotamus (*Hippopotamus amphibius* Linnaeus) to natural infection with rinderpest virus, *J. Hyg., Camb.*, **62**: 329–36.

Plowright, W. and McCulloch, B., 1967. Investigations on the incidence of rinderpest virus infection in game animals of N. Tanganyika and S. Kenya 1960/63, *J. Hyg., Camb.*, **65**: 343–58.

Plowright, W., Rampton, C. S., Taylor, W. P. and Herniman, K. A. J., 1970. Studies on rinderpest culture vaccine. III. Stability of the lyophilised product, *Res. vet. Sci.*, **11**: 71–81.

Prabhudas, K. and Sambamurti, B., 1976. A note on fluorescent antibody technique for rapid diagnosis of rinderpest, *Indian J. Anim. Sci.*, **46**(8): 454–7.

Prakash, K., Antony, A. and Ramakrishnan, T., 1979. Polypeptides of rinderpest virus and virus-specific polypeptide synthesis in infected cells, *Indian J. exp. Biol.*, **17**: 1287–9.

Provost, A., 1958. Attempts to transmit rinderpest by means of infective aerosols, *Bull. epiz. Dis. Afr.*, **6**: 79–85.

Provost, A., 1970. Rinderpest and immunofluorescence. Application in the differential diagnosis of rinderpest infection, *Bull. Off. int. Epiz.*, **73**: 915–922.

Provost, A., 1972. Rinderpest transmission by calves with maternal residual colostral immunity, *Rev. Elev. Méd. vét. Pays trop.* **25**(2): 155–9.

Provost, A., Borredon, C. and Bocquet, P., 1974. Trivalent vaccine against rinderpest, contagious pleuropneumonia and anthrax, *Rev. Elev. Méd. vét. Pays trop.*, **27**(4): 385–95.

Provost, A., Borredon, C., Dufau, G. and N'Galdam, M. Z., 1972a. Trials of rinderpest nasal vaccination of calves with or without colostral immunity, *Rev. Elev. Méd. vét. Pays trop.*, **25**(2): 141–53.

Provost, A., Borredon, C., Dufau, G. and N'Galdam, M. Z., 1972b. A combined lyophilised rinderpest–CBPP vaccine to be used in the field without refrigeration. I. Selection of rinderpest virions with delayed thermal inactivation properties, *Rev. Elev. Méd. vét. Pays trop.*, **25**(4): 507–20.

Provost, A. and Joubert, L., 1973. Modern methods of laboratory diagnosis of rinderpest, *Rev. Elev. Méd. vét. Pays trop.*, **26**(4): 383–96.

Provost, A., Maurice, Y. and Borredon, C., 1968. A note on experimental rinderpest in the dromedary, *Rev. Elev. Méd. vét. Pays trop.*, **21**(3): 293–6.

Provost, A., Maurice, Y. and Borredon, C., 1969a. Possibilities and limits of the measles haemagglutination inhibition test in the serology of rinderpest. II. Dissimilarity between the results obtained with this test and the rinderpest virus seroneutralization, *Rev. Elev. Méd. vét. Pays trop.*, **22**(1): 9–15.

Provost, A., Maurice, Y. and Borredon, C., 1969b. Clinical and immunological reactions to exposure to rinderpest in cattle vaccinated several years previously against rinderpest with cell culture vaccines, *Rev. Elev. Méd. vét. Pays trop.*, **22**(4): 453–64.

Purchase, H. S., Burdin, M. L., Scott, G. R. and Brotherton, J. G., 1953. Keeping qualities of live rinderpest vaccines, *Vet. Rec.*, **65**: 590–2.

Radhakrishnan, R., Venkataswami, V. and Pattabiraman, S. R., 1975. Further report on the effect of protective vaccination on the semen quality of breeding bulls, *Indian vet. J.*, **52**: 620–5.

Rafyi, A. and Afshar, A., 1969. Recent outbreak of rinderpest in Iran, *Bull. Off. int. Epiz.*, **71**(11–12): 1289–91.

Ramani, K., Charles, Y. S., Srinivas, R. P., Narayanaswamy, M. and Ramachandran, S., 1974. Isolation of rinderpest virus from an outbreak in domestic pigs in Karnataka, *Indian vet. J.*, **51**: 36–41.

Ramyar, H., 1968. The use of live-modified tissue culture vaccine in immunisation of Iranian cattle against rinderpest, *Vet. Rec.*, **82**: 779–80.

Rao, C. K., 1969. Rinderpest and rinderpest-like diseases in India, *Bull. Off. int. Epiz.*, **71**: 1297–1301.

Rao, C. K., 1973. Rinderpest and rinderpest-like disease in India. Epizootiology, diagnosis and control, *Bull. Off. int. Epiz.*, **79**(5–6): 513–18.

Rao, D. V. R., Sundaram, S., Ramani, K., Ramachandran, S. and Scott, G. R., 1975. Observations on the resistance of the domestic buffalo and graded zebu to rinderpest, *Indian vet. J.*, **52**: 201–8.

Rao, M., Devi, T. I., Ramachandran, S. and Scott, G. R., 1974. Rinderpest in sheep in Andhra Pradesh and its control by vaccination, *Indian vet. J.*, **51**: 439–50.

Receveur, R., 1957. Risques de dispersion de la peste bovine par les viandes fraîches ou congelées provenant des pays contaminés?, *Bull. Off. int. Epiz.*, **48**: 148–58.

Robey, T. O. and Hale, M. W., 1946. Rinderpest. XV. Morphological changes in the blood of young cattle during rinderpest and after vaccination with attenuated virus vaccine, *Am. J. vet. Res.*, **7**: 222–7.

Robson, J., Arnold, R. M., Plowright, W. and Scott, G. R., 1959. The isolation from an eland of a strain of rinderpest virus attenuated for cattle, *Bull. epiz. Dis. Afr.*, **7**: 97–102.

Rossiter, P. B., Jessett, D. M. and Holmes, P., 1981. MicroELISA test for detecting antibodies to rinderpest virus antigens, *Trop. Anim. Hlth Prod.*, **13**: 113–16.

Rossiter, P. B. and Mushi, E. Z., 1980. Rapid detection of rinderpest virus antigens by counter-immunoelectrophoresis, *Trop. Anim. Hlth Prod.*, **12**: 209–16.

Rowe, L. W., 1966. A screening survey for rinderpest neutralising antibodies in cattle in northern Nigeria. *Bull. epiz. Dis. Afr.*, **14**: 49–52.

Rowe, L. W., Zwart, D. and Kouwenhoven, B., 1967. A comparison of the haemagglutination-inhibition and neutralization test in the assay of rinderpest antibodies in cattle, *Bull. epiz. Dis. Afr.*, **15**: 301–6.

Rweyemamu, M. M., Reid, H. W. and Okuna, N., 1974. Observations on the behaviour of rinderpest virus in immune animals challenged intranasally, *Bull. epiz. Dis. Afr.*, **22**: 1–9.

Sankaran, N., Masillamony, P. R., Thilagarajan, N. and Balaprakasam, R. A., 1976. A study on the efficacy of tissue culture rinderpest virus (Kabete 'O' strain) vaccine in sheep, *Cheiron, Tamil Nadu J. vet. Sci. Anim. Husb.*, **5**(2): 82–7.

Sapra, K. L., Bhatnagar, V. K. and Kalia, M. L., 1969. Loss of body weight in relation to rise in body temperature in goats, *Indian vet. J.*, **46**: 668–74.

Scott, G. R., 1954. The virus content of the tissues of rabbits infected with rinderpest, *Br. vet. J.*, **110**: 152–7.

Scott, G. R., 1955. The incidence of rinderpest in sheep and goats, *Bull. epiz. Dis. Afr.*, **3**(2): 117–19.

Scott, G. R., 1957. The risk associated with the importation of meat from countries where rinderpest control measures are still required, *Bull. epiz. Dis. Afr.*, **5**: 11–13.

Scott, G. R., 1959a. Heat inactivation of rinderpest-infected bovine tissues, *Nature*, **184**: 1948–9.

Scott, G. R., 1959b. Effect of caprinized rinderpest virus in rabbits, *J. Comp. Path.*, **69**: 423–6.
Scott, G. R., 1962a. Bovine hyperimmune serum in the diagnosis of rinderpest, *Vet. Rec.*, **74**(13): 409.
Scott, G. R., 1962b. Subendocardial haemorrhage in rinderpest infected cattle, *Vet. Rec.*, **74**: 567–8.
Scott, G. R., 1962c. Experimental rinderpest in Red Masai sheep, *Bull. epiz. Dis. Afr.*, **10**: 423–6.
Scott, G. R., 1962d. Optimal incubation temperature for the rinderpest agar gel double diffusion test, *Bull. epiz. Dis. Afr.*, **10**: 457–60.
Scott, G. R., 1963. Adverse reactions in cattle after vaccination with lapinized rinderpest virus, *J. Hyg., Camb.*, **61**: 193–203.
Scott, G. R., 1964. Rinderpest, *Adv. vet. Sci.*, **9**: 113–224.
Scott, G. R., 1976. Oral vaccination against rinderpest, *Trans. Roy. Soc. trop. Med. Hyg.*, **70**: 287.
Scott, G. R., 1981. Rinderpest and peste des petits ruminants. In *Virus Diseases of Food Animals: A World Geography of Epidemiology and Control*, ed. E. P. J. Gibbs. Academic Press (New York), Disease Monographs, vol. II, pp. 401–32.
Scott, G. R. and Brown, R. D., 1958. A neutralization test for the detection of rinderpest antibodies, *J. Comp. Path.*, **68**: 308–14.
Scott, G. R. and Brown, R. D., 1961. Rinderpest diagnosis with special reference to the agar gel double diffusion test, *Bull. epiz. Dis. Afr.*, **9**: 83–125.
Scott, G. R., Cowan, K. M. and Elliott, R. T., 1960. Rinderpest in impala, *Vet. Rec.*, **72**(38): 787–8.
Scott, G. R., Currie, D. E., Ramachandran, S. and Hill, D. H., 1970. Resistance of purebred and crossbred Nigerian Dwarf goats to rinderpest, *Trop. Anim. Hlth Prod.*, **2**: 13–17.
Scott, G. R., DeTray, D. E. and White, G., 1959. A preliminary note on the susceptibility of pigs of European origin to rinderpest, *Bull. Off. int. Epiz.*, **51**: 694–8.
Scott, G. R., DeTray, D. E. and White, G., 1962. Rinderpest in pigs of European origin, *Am. J. vet. Res.*, **23**: 452–6.
Scott, G. R. and Ginsberg, A., 1959. Adjuvant rinderpest vaccine: adverse sequelae, *Vet. Rec.*, **71**(8): 151–2.
Scott, G. R. and MacDonald, J., 1962. Kenya camels and rinderpest, *Bull. epiz. Dis. Afr.*, **10**: 495–7.
Scott, G. R. and Rampton, C. S., 1962. Influence of the route of exposure on the titre of rinderpest virus in rabbits, *J. Comp. Path.*, **72**: 299–302.
Sharma, R. M. and Ram, T., 1955. Scarification *versus* subcutaneous method of vaccination against rinderpest in goats and sheep, *Indian J. vet. Sci.*, **25**: 129–42.
Sharma, S. K. and Murty, D. K., 1974. Serum electrophoretic pattern of buffalo calves vaccinated with cell culture rinderpest vaccine, *Indian J. exp. Biol.*, **12**: 535–6.
Simon, N., 1962. *Between the Sunlight and the Thunder: The Wild Life of Kenya*. (London).

Singh, G., 1971. Antibody response in animals inoculated with three different types of live rinderpest vaccine, *Indian J. Anim. Hlth*, **10**: 133–44.

Singh, K. V., 1970. Cytopathic effect in cell cultures in rinderpest virus and some other viruses causing rinderpest-like diseases, *Bull. epiz. Dis. Afr.*, **18**: 111–15.

Singh, K. V. and Ata, F., 1967. Experimental rinderpest in camels. A preliminary report, *Bull. epiz. Dis. Afr.*, **15**: 19–23.

Singh, K. V. and Osman, O. A., 1970. Response of pregnant Danish Friesian cows to tissue culture rinderpest vaccine, *Nord. Vet.-Med.*, **22**: 410–13.

Singh, K. V., Osman, O. A., Baz, T. I. and El Cicy, I. F., 1967a. The use of tissue culture rinderpest vaccine for Egyptian cattle and water buffaloes, *Cornell Vet.*, **57**: 465–79.

Singh, K. V., Osman, O. A., El Cicy, I. F., Ata, F. A. and Baz, T. I., 1967b. Response of water buffaloes to experimental infection with rinderpest virus, *Cornell Vet.*, **57**: 638–48.

Singh, S. N., 1972. Application of passive haemagglutination test in diagnosis of rinderpest, *Indian vet. J.*, **49**: 759–60.

Smith, V. W., 1966. Active immunisation of calves with tissue-cultured rinderpest vaccine, *J. Comp. Path.*, **76**: 217–24.

Sonoda, A., 1971. Susceptibility of cattle buffaloes and swine in Cambodia to lapinized–avianized rinderpest virus, *Nat. Inst. Anim. Hlth Quart.*, **11**: 134–44.

Stewart, D. R. M., 1964. Rinderpest among wild animals in Kenya, 1960–62, *Bull. epiz. Dis. Afr.*, **12**: 39–42.

Stewart, D. R. M., 1968. Rinderpest among wild animals in Kenya, 1963–1966, *Bull. epiz. Dis. Afr.*, **16**: 139–40.

Stone, S. S., 1960. Multiple components of rinderpest virus as determined by the precipitin reaction in agar gel, *Virology*, **11**: 638–40.

Stone, S. S. and DeLay, P. D., 1961. The inactivation of rinderpest virus by Beta-propiolactone and its effect on homologous complement-fixing and neutralizing antibodies, *J. Immunol.*, **87**: 464–7.

Strickland, K. L., 1962. Vaccination of calves against rinderpest, *Vet. Rec.*, **4**(22): 630–1.

Tajima, M. and Ushijima, T., 1971. The pathogenesis of rinderpest in the lymph nodes of cattle. Light and electron microscopic studies, *Am. J. Pathol.*, **62**: 221–36.

Tajima, M., Ushijima, T., Kishi, S. and Nakamura, J., 1964. Electron microscopy of cytoplasmic inclusion bodies in cells infected with rinderpest virus, *Virology*, **31**: 92–100.

Taylor, W. P., 1968. The susceptibility of the one-humped camel (*Camelus dromedarius*) to infection with rinderpest virus, *Bull. epiz. Dis. Afr.*, **16**: 405–10.

Taylor, W. P. and Best, J. R., 1977. Simultaneous titrations of tissue culture rinderpest vaccine in goats and cell cultures, *Trop. Anim. Hlth Prod.*, **9**: 189–90.

Taylor, W. P. and Ojeh, C. K., 1981. Rinderpest in Nigeria, *Vet. Rec.*, **108**: 127.

Taylor, W. P. and Perry, C. T., 1970. A plaque assay system for rinderpest virus and its use in characterizing virus adsorption, *Arch. ges. Virusforsch.*, **32**: 269–82.

Taylor, W. P. and Plowright, W., 1965. Studies on the pathogenesis of rinderpest in experimental cattle. III. Proliferation of an attenuated strain in various tissues following subcutaneous inoculation, *J. Hyg., Camb.*, **63**: 263–75.

Taylor, W. P., Plowright, W., Pillinger, R., Rampton, C. S. and Staple, R. F., 1965. Studies on the pathogenesis of rinderpest in experimental cattle. IV. Proliferation of the virus following contact infection, *J. Hyg., Camb.*, **63**: 497–506.

Taylor, W. P. and Watson, R. M., 1967. Studies on the epizootiology of rinderpest in blue wildebeest and other game species of northern Tanzania and southern Kenya, 1965–7, *J. Hyg., Camb.*, **65**: 537–45.

Thiery, G., 1956a. Influence of virus strains and of species affected on the lesions of rinderpest, *Rev. Elev. Méd. vét. Pays trop.*, **9**: 109–15.

Thiery, G., 1956b. Studies on haematology and histopathology and histochemistry of rinderpest with special reference to cellular inclusion bodies, *Rev. Elev. Méd. vét. Pays trop.*, **9**: 117–40.

Wagner, G. G., Jessett, D. M., Brown, C. G. D. and Radley, D. E., 1975. Diminished antibody response to rinderpest vaccination in cattle undergoing experimental East Coast fever, *Res. vet. Sci.*, **19**: 209–11.

White, G., 1962. Gel diffusion test in the diagnosis of rinderpest, *Vet. Rec.*, **74**(50): 1477–8.

White, G. and Cowan, K. M., 1962. Separation of the soluble antigens and infectious particles of rinderpest and canine distemper, *Virology*, **16**: 209–11.

White, G. and Scott, G. R., 1960. An indirect gel diffusion precipitation test for the detection of rinderpest antibody in convalescent cattle, *Res. vet. Sci.*, **1**: 226–9.

Yamanouchi, K., Chino, F., Kobune, F., Fukada, A. and Yoshikawa, Y., 1974a. Pathogenesis of rinderpest virus infection in rabbits. I. Clinical signs, immune response, histological changes, and virus growth patterns, *Infect. Immun.*, **9**(2): 199–205.

Yamanouchi, K., Fukuda, A., Kobune, F., Yoshikawa, Y. and Chino, F., 1974b. Pathogenesis of rinderpest virus infection in rabbits. II. Effect of rinderpest virus on the immune functions of rabbits, *Infect. Immun.*, **9**(2): 206–11.

Zwart, D. and Macadam, I., 1967a. Transmission of rinderpest by contact from cattle to sheep and goats, *Res. vet. Sci.*, **8**: 37–47.
Zwart, D. and Macadam, I., 1967b. Observations on rinderpest in sheep and goats and transmission to cattle, *Res. vet. Sci.*, **8**: 53–7.
Zwart, D. and Rowe, L. W., 1966. The occurrence of rinderpest antibodies in the sera of sheep and goats in northern Nigeria, *Res. vet. Sci.*, **7**: 504–11.

PART

III

BACTERIAL DISEASES

Chapter

16

Contagious bovine and caprine pleuropneumonia

CONTENTS

INTRODUCTION

Contagious bovine pleuropneumonia (CBPP) is a mycoplasmal disease of cattle and water buffalo caused by the organism *Mycoplasma mycoides* var. *mycoides* and characterized by extensive fibrinous pneumonia and pleuritis. The acute clinical syndrome consists of fever, dyspnea, coughing, and nasal discharge. Contagious caprine pleuropneumonia (CCPP) is one of the most common pneumonias in goats in the tropics. However, there is a great deal of confusion with regard to differentiation between CCPP, pasteurellosis, and pulmonary syndromes caused by other microorganisms. The causative significance of the mycoplasma is established with difficulty and involves several species of mycoplasma.

Literature

In 1971, Hudson presented a comprehensive account of the state of knowledge on CBPP and included appendices which gave detailed information of various laboratory techniques and experimental procedures. In earlier literature Adler (1965) reviewed all forms of mycoplasmosis of animals, while Lobry summarized some of the publications on CBPP up to 1964. The CBPP investigations in Australia were reported by Gregory (1957).

The diseases caused by mycoplasmas in goats were reviewed by Hudson *et al.* (1967a). The etiology of caprine pneumonias was discussed by Ojo (1977). Recently, information on CCPP was reviewed by McMartin *et al.* (1980) and by Cottew (1982).

ETIOLOGY

Classification

Mycoplasmas are the smallest and simplest of the self-replicating procaryotes and are placed in the class Mollicutes; only some are pathogenic, causing disease in animals, plants, and insects. Cattle are infected by 19, and goats and sheep by 17, species or subspecies; of these, only 3 are common to large and small ruminants. These animal microorganisms are associated with lesions in the mammary glands, joints, eyes, and respiratory and urogenital tracts. The diseases of major economic importance are CBPP, CCPP, and contagious agalactia.

Mycoplasma m. mycoides is the causative agent of CBPP in cattle, and in addition to the pleuropneumonia is associated with arthritis and synovitis. The organism was thought until recently to be responsible for natural disease only in cattle and buffalo. However, isolation of *M. mycoides*-types of organisms, indistinguishable in many characteristics from those of cattle, have been made from goats with clinical disease associated with either pleuropneumonia or septicemia with lesions in various tissues.

There is considerable controversy and confusion about the identity and classification of the various mycoplasmas involved in CCPP. To date, five species are to some extent characterized but other isolates are still inadequately identified. The etiology of CCPP is further complicated by pasteurella which has been commonly associated with caprine pneumonias. *Mycoplasma m. capri* was shown to be the first causative agent of CCPP of goats. Two others are *M.m. mycoides* and an organism isolated in Kenya known by the number F38. More recently, it is now known that *M.m. mycoides* is also responsible for severe outbreaks of septicemia and polyarthritis in goats. Caprine and bovine strains of *M. mycoides* cannot be easily differentiated with current taxonomical procedures. Differences are described in the size of colonies in culture and various other tests. Isolates which grow as large colonies are infectious for goats while those with small colonies produce lesions in both goats and cattle. Several of the agents originally isolated in different areas of the world and identified as *M.m. capri* are now reclassified as *M.m. mycoides*.

Literature

The most comprehensive information on human and animal mycoplasmas was published in a monograph edited by Tully and Whitcomb (1979) and was one of three volumes edited by Barile and co-editors entitled *The Mycoplasmas*. This volume included chapters on mycoplasmas of cattle by Gourlay and Howard (1979) and of sheep and goats by Cottew (1979).

Although biochemical tests have been useful in characterization, speciation of mycoplasma depended primarily on immunological methods. Growth-inhibition and immunofluorescence tests have been considered to be specific (Freundt 1981).

Early classification and nomenclature of organisms in the pleuropneumonia group were presented by Edward and Freundt (1956) and established the order, family, and genus of mycoplasma.

In the classification of mycoplasmas isolated from cattle and goats, reliance was placed on serological methods, notably the metabolism-inhibition and growth-inhibition tests, but these have often failed to distinguish between the isolates from goats and those from cattle (Davies and Read 1968; Hooker *et al.* 1979). Other methods have also been used including the identification of *M.m. mycoides* and *M.m. capri* species by fluorescent antibody (FA) techniques (Tessler and Yedloutschnig 1972). Defining the species of *M. mycoides* and related organisms by these tests did not agree with the hybridization studies, creating a problem in the classification of this group of mycoplasmas (Askaa *et al.* 1978). Cross-protection tests showed that the seven goat strains of *M.m. mycoides* could be differentiated from *M.m. capri* (Hooker *et al.* 1979). Double-diffusion together with metabolic-inhibition techniques were considered to provide the basis for definition of species and subspecies of bovine mycoplasmas (Erno and Jurmanova 1973; Erno and Stipkovits 1973). Two-dimensional polyacrylamide gel electrophoresis also showed that the degree of relationship differed between various strains of *M.m. mycoides* and the subspecies *capri* (Rodwell and Rodwell 1978). Protein fingerprinting of these species was an effective method of characterization. Many proteins were found to be strongly conserved within all strains of a given species or subspecies, while considerable variation occurred in other protein patterns and was related to strain variation (Rodwell 1982).

Separation of *M. mycoides* into subspecies *mycoides* and *capri* on the nature of the carbohydrate antigenic determinants, growth rate, clinical signs, and other characteristics has been only partially successful. The main difference has been shown to be the formation of small and large colony types. Large colony strains were closely related to the subspecies *capri* while small colony types of *M. mycoides* caused CBPP (Rodwell and Rodwell 1978). These small and large colony strains of *M. mycoides* could not be readily distinguished by the serological test. Antigenic differences, however, were demonstrated by the cross-protection test in mice. Large colony strains partially protected against challenge with subspecies *capri* and small colony strains, both from CBPP and from goats, induced weak partial cross-protection against subspecies *capri* (Smith and Oliphant 1981a, b).

There has been considerable confusion and controversy concerning the causative agents of CCPP even in the most current literature and this was discussed in detail by Cottew (1979). Classification and identification of ovine and caprine mycoplasmas on the basis of biochemical and serological tests was reviewed by Erno *et al.* (1978). McMartin *et al.* (1980) made the point that various clinical descriptions of CCPP in the more recent literature did not conform to the syndrome described by Duncan and Hutcheon in the original publications on CCPP in 1881 and 1889, and proposed that *M.m. capri* and *M.m. mycoides* and other recent isolates were not the causative agents of classical CCPP. The main characteristic of the classical disease was that it was highly contagious for goats, causing an acute disease with the incidence of morbidity and mortality being 100% and 80% respectively. In addition the agent did not affect sheep or cattle and did not cause local reactions when administered subcutaneously. In the pathology, CCPP differed from CBPP in that the sequestra did not develop in the lungs. A new mycoplasma, identified as F38 and isolated from CCPP in Kenya, produced typical classical CCPP lesions by endobronchial intubation and was found to be highly contagious to animals in contact (MacOwan and Minette 1976; MacOwan 1976). This agent was isolated from 57 acute cases in 46 outbreaks of CCPP in Kenya (MacOwan and Minette 1977). Although *M.m. capri* and *M.m. mycoides* have been incriminated as agents causing CCPP, they have not been associated with the acute contagious outbreaks seen with F38. The original classical description of CCPP was probably due to the unclassified mycoplasma F38 (Cottew 1982).

In goats, both *M.m. capri* and *M.m. mycoides* have been isolated from a variety of disease syndromes from various parts of the world. *Mycoplasma m. capri* has been identified as one of the agents responsible for CCPP and the so-called edema disease of goats characterized by acute fatal cellulitis (Smith 1967). *Mycoplasma m. mycoides* was first isolated from goats by Laws (1956) and has been reported from various countries with increasing frequency to be associated not only with CCPP but with other diseases, including mastitis, arthritis, abortion, and peritonitis (Bar-Moshe and Rappaport 1981). An agent identified as *M.m. capri* was isolated in North America in 1966 from a case of conjunctivitis. Subsequently, *M.m. mycoides* was isolated from goats with septicemia, polyarthritis, conjunctivitis, keratitis, pneumonia, and abscesses. Goats and sheep infected intravenously with *M.m. mycoides* developed septicemia terminating in death (Rosendal 1981). Goats harbored two groups of mycoplasma, both classified serologically as *M.m. mycoides*, one inducing large colonies which were not pathogenic for cattle and one causing small colonies which were pathogenic for cattle (Cottew and Yeats 1978). Highly pathogenic strains of *M.m. capri* have been isolated in the USA (Yedloutschnig *et al.* 1971) and some induced lung lesions comparable to CCPP (Jonas and Barber 1969).

Ojo (1977) concluded from his work in Nigeria that on the basis of etiological, clinical, pathological, and epidemiological grounds it was difficult to classify the various forms of pneumonia in goats. In his work, the majority of mycoplasma isolates from caprine pneumonia were *M.m. mycoides* (Ojo 1973). The species *M.m. capri* was also pathogenic, and experimentally both organisms caused typical CCPP lesions (Ojo 1982). Both agents have also been isolated in Australia (Littlejohns and Cottew 1977). *Mycoplasma m. capri* has been identified from outbreaks in Mexico and was associated with pleuritis and pneumonia; experimental subcutaneous injection caused cellulitis at the site of injection as well as lung lesions (Solana and Rivera 1967). An unidentified mycoplasma caused keratoconjunctivitis, arthritis, and pneumonia in Iraq (Al-Shammari and Al-Aubaidi 1977). In India a number of different species of mycoplasma were isolated from lung lesions from naturally infected sheep and goats, but were not identified as species which have been associated with CCPP-type lesions from other countries (Banerjee *et al.* 1979). The isolation of *M.m. mycoides* from maned sheep (*Ammotragus lervia*) in a zoo in Germany was reported by Erno *et al.* (1972).

Serological identification of mycoplasma isolates from CCPP has required the use of proper basic reference strains of *M.m. mycoides* and *M.m. capri* for comparison (Tully *et al.* 1974). Confusion has occurred in identification of strains based on improperly characterized reference strains (Lemcke 1974). New species of mycoplasmas isolated from goats have to be based on antigenic relationship, biochemical, and biological properties (Tully *et al.* 1974).

Culture and morphology

Mycoplasmas grow well *in vitro* and their various properties are readily studied in various culture systems. Colony morphology is variable, depending on the composition of the medium which usually has specialized nutritional additives, particularly serum. The organisms grow readily both aerobically and anaerobically on solid and liquid media. Because of the relatively slow growth, antibiotics are used to suppress contaminating bacteria. The organism also grows on a chorio-allantois of embryonated hen eggs, and this method of cultivation is used in the production of some vaccines.

Because mycoplasma are pleomorphic organisms without a rigid wall, they appear as either round, ovoid, coccoid, ring, or filamentous forms. The basic reproductive unit is the elementary body which gives rise in broth culture to the homogeneous filament which subsequently develops spherical bodies, leading to formation of coccoid forms of between 125 and 250 nm. In solid media the organisms develop into typical colonies with a central denser core.

Literature

Razin (1981) presented a comprehensive summary of the cell biology of mycoplasmas. The structure and function of mycoplasma membranes was reviewed by Archer (1981).

Relatively little definitive information, specifically on the structure and biochemistry, is available on the various agents associated with CBPP and CCPP. The growth characteristic of *M.m. mycoides* included a growth phase of both filamentous and single bodies and the replication of cells involved budding, forming multinucleated cells (Furness and De Maggio 1972, 1973). A solid medium used for measuring growth inhibition and neutralization of *M. mycoides* by immune bovine serum was described by Domermuth and Gourlay (1967). The active transport of K^+ in the *M.m. capri* was investigated (Leblanc and Grimellec 1979). Isolation and analysis of deoxyribonucleic acid from *M.m. capri* was reported by Jones and Walker (1963).

EPIZOOTIOLOGY

Geographic distribution

Contagious bovine pleuropneumonia persists in the Iberian Peninsula, Africa, Asia and China. This chronic insidious disease of cattle is considered of major economic importance in various parts of Africa. There is little information on the economic impact of CBPP from other parts of the world.

Contagious caprine pleuropneumonia is widely distributed in

tropical regions where goats are reared in any significant numbers and is one of the two most important mycoplasmal diseases of goats. It is reported in about 35 countries, mostly in Africa, the Middle East, Asia, and to a lesser extent in Europe, North and Central America.

Literature

Henning (1956) reviewed the history of the distribution of CBPP in the USA, Africa, and Australia. Before 1890 the disease had worldwide distribution, originating in Europe and being disseminated with the export of animals to South Africa, Australia, and the Far East in the middle of the nineteenth century (Hudson 1971). The history of the introduction of CBPP from England in 1858 and its spread was presented by McIntosh (1969). In Australia, CBPP was restricted by 1969 to the quarantine areas of Queensland, the Northern Territory, and Western Australia (Lloyd 1969).

There have been reports at various times from different countries on the history, incidence, and economic importance of CBPP. In Africa, the history of CBPP in the Sudan was presented by Abdulla (1969). A summary on the research work undertaken in Chad from 1964 to 1966 was reported by Provost (1967). In Nigeria, the incidence of CBPP from 1924 to 1964 was discussed by Griffin and Laing (1966) and between 1960 and 1963 by Ezebuiro *et al.* (1964), and methods of control were evaluated. In eastern Africa, the history of CBPP in Kenya was summarized by Kariuki (1971). In Tanganyika, the situation up to 1965 was described by Hammond and Branagan (1965) with additional information up to 1969 presented by Lwebandiza (1969). Santiago Duarte (1969) reviewed the situation in Angola.

Outside Africa reports were made from India (Rao 1969) and from Egypt and Syria (Zaki Abdel Hai 1969).

Information on the incidence of CCPP has been complicated by the complexity of multiple etiological agents being associated with the disease in goats and the difficulty of diagnosing the disease. An outbreak occurred in 1964 in Mexico (Solana and Rivera 1967). Serological surveys of slaughtered goats in Nigeria showed CCPP not to be prevalent (Goni and Onoviran 1973). The occurrence of CCPP in Arizona was recorded by Pearson *et al.* (1972). Harbi *et al.* (1981) reported from the Sudan the occurrence of the F38 strain in association with CCPP lesions.

Transmission

The mycoplasmas causing CBPP are transmitted by aerosol from clinical and carrier cases. Infection results through the inhalation of droplets which are expelled from the respiratory tract of infected animals by coughing. Organisms are present in the nasal cavity during the incubation and clinical periods. Various types of sequestra in the lungs are the source of organisms in the expired air. The ease of transmission depends on the closeness of contact between animals and on the level of infection. Transmission can occur over a distance of 20 m. Outbreaks of CBPP usually have a slow course and clinical signs are detected within 4 to 6 weeks after the introduction of an infected animal into a herd. The infection spreads very slowly and several months elapse before many animals are affected.

The susceptibility varies considerably between individuals and 10 to 60% of cattle may be resistant to infection with only up to 8% developing acute clinical signs. A number of factors play a role in natural dissemination and include individual and breed susceptibility and husbandry conditions. Resistance is probably partly dependent on the fact that healthy, normally functioning respiratory systems are usually resistant to mycoplasma infection.

Literature

The possible role of contaminated environment was investigated in an experimental system which involved applying cultures to placenta and urine. The organism was recovered from the placenta for up to 72 hours and from urine for up to 96 hours. In urine, survival was affected by exposure to direct sunlight and the organisms could be killed within 24 hours. In contaminated hay the organism was viable for 216 hours in the shade and for 144 hours in direct sunlight (Windsor and Masiga 1977).

Ticks have also been considered as a possible indirect method of transmission. Although *M.m. mycoides* was isolated from *Rhipicephalus pulchellus* removed from infected cattle, infected nymphs placed as adults failed to infect susceptible cattle (Shifrine *et al.* 1972).

INFECTION

Innate resistance of individuals and breeds of cattle to CBPP is observed. Stress and virulence of strains are important factors in the development of acute disease. Although the organism is basically of one antigenic type, various isolates differ considerably in virulence.

Water buffalo, yak, and bison are also susceptible to infection by *M. myocoides*. On occasion, goats and sheep can be infected experimentally by parenteral injection with organisms isolated from CBPP. In these species the susceptibility varies and, as in cattle, there is great difference in individual susceptibilities with the prominent lesion being fibrinous serositis. Opinion varies as to the susceptibility of camels to infections and to development of lesions.

It has been difficult to induce typical pulmonary lesions in cattle experimentally. Lung lesions can be produced experimentally by intravenously inoculating cultures mixed with melted agar to produce emboli in the small pulmonary vessels. Lesions typical of acute CBPP can also be induced, but not consistently, by intratracheal intubation of virulent cultures. A reasonably reliable method is by inhalation of air in which the culture is in a fine aerosol. Endobronchial intubation to produce donor animals is used as a method of challenge to test the development of immunity following vaccination. Of major importance in all experimental procedure is the variable susceptibility of individual animals. Other routes of infection (subcutaneous, intradermal, intramuscular, intracerebral or intravenous) do not result in pulmonary lesions. In these experimental infections, the organism often becomes mycoplasmemic but it does not induce systemic lesions except in calves where occasionally arthritis develops. Subcutaneous injection may induce local inflammatory reaction known as Willem's reaction and the development of this lesion is used to study both the infectivity and pathogenicity of various isolates and the resistance of the host. The severity of this characteristic local inflammatory reaction depends on the virulence of a particular strain and the susceptibility of the host. It varies from a small necrotic nodule to diffuse serofibrinous cellulitis, which may be severe enough to result in death.

The transmission of natural CCPP is by contact, and infectivity by artificial means depends on the differences in virulence between different species and strains of mycoplasma. Both *M.m. capri* and *M.m. mycoides* induce, by intratracheal intubation, lesions characteristic of CCPP but do not produce the contagious pneumonia seen in natural field syndromes. Subcutaneous infections cause cellulitis and arthritis. Strains of *M.m. mycoides* isolated from polyarthritis in goats when injected intravenously can cause fatal septicemia.

A major obstacle in the study of the etiology, kinetics of infection, and pathogenesis of CBPP and CCPP is the relative difficulty of uniformly and repeatedly causing infections and clinical syndromes which are similar to those observed in the field. Contagious bovine pleuropneumonia can be produced experimentally at varying degrees of consistency by endobronchial intubation, aerosol spray, or by contact with infected cattle. Endobronchial inoculation of cattle with various strains results in small acute necrotic lesions in the lungs. More diffuse tissue involvement can be produced by stresses such as by simultaneous infection with caprinized rinderpest vaccine. Goats are less susceptible to infection by inhalation of aerosol cultures than by parenteral routes. Mortality can be readily caused by experimental intramuscular and subcutaneous infections.

Literature

Bos indicus cattle were found to be more susceptible to CBPP than *B. taurus* which supported the concept that the disease originated in Europe and spread to those continents where *B. indicus* cattle were indigenous. The contact between the organism and these tropical breeds of cattle was more recent resulting in increased susceptibility (Francis 1973). However, other work has failed to support this conclusion and there were no observable differences in susceptibilities of *B. indicus* and *B. taurus* cattle together in contact exposure to the infection or in the efficacy of responses to T_1 vaccine (Masiga and Read 1972). Some evidence has been presented that cattle over 3 years of age were more resistant than younger animals (Masiga and Windsor 1978).

The incidence of infection in wild ruminants, as indicated by serology, has been studied to a limited degree. The antibodies to *M. mycoides* were found in the buffalo, impala, and in the camel, but not in other species of wild antelope in Kenya (Paling *et al.* 1978). Sera from 645 animals representing 8 species of wildlife were tested using the complement-fixation (CF) test. Seven percent of the sera from wildebeest and hippopotami were positive. Because these sera did not inhibit the growth of organisms it was concluded that the antibodies were not specific and that CBPP probably was not present in the wildlife population tested (Shifrine and Domermuth 1967). White-tailed deer (*Odocoileus virginianus*) experimentally infected with *M. mycoides* did not develop the typical lesions observed in cattle (Yedloutschnig and Dardiri 1976).

Adhesion of the organism to the cell, enabling colonization of the surfaces of mucous membranes, has been considered to be central to the pathogenicity of mycoplasmas. The adherence mechanisms differed depending on the species of mycoplasma and host involved (Bredt *et al.* 1981). Attachment of mycoplasmas to erythrocytes was proposed as a model to study attachment of these organisms to epithelium cells (Kahane *et al.* 1981). Because the cell membrane of the organism has been involved in the adhesion, its antigenic composition was analyzed. Quantitative but not qualitative differences were observed in the membrane proteins of virulent and avirulent strains of *M.m. mycoides* using immunoelectrophoretic analysis (Stone and Razin 1973).

The virulence of *M. mycoides* has not been shown to be a stable feature. A strain grown through the first few passages in culture evoked acute inflammatory reaction on subcutaneous injection (Das 1968). On subsequent subculture, virulence was diminished and by the twenty-fifth passage remained constant; the organism produced a much less severe inflammatory reaction (Hudson 1971). It has been suggested that there could be a correlation between the virulence of the strain of *M. mycoides* as detected by subcutaneous reaction and its ability to cause lesions by endobronchial intubation (Brown 1964). Three attenuated vaccine strains of *M.m. mycoides,* when passaged through cattle for three to five times, induced subcutaneous lesions which were comparable to those caused by virulent strains. These originally attenuated strains also could not be differentiated by their growth characteristics from virulent strains (Davies *et al.* 1969). Cultures of virulent and attenuated strains of *M.m. mycoides* and *M.m. capri* were shown to be mixtures of both virulent and avirulent organisms based on differences in the colony types produced on culture (Nasri 1966).

Dissemination during the course of infections and the tissue tropism of pathogenic and attenuated strains of various stages of infection have been studied. Mycoplasmemia in CBPP has been well documented and its occurrence appeared to be related to the severity and the stage of infection. Serum, plasma, lysed blood cells, urine pleural fluid, and inflammatory exudates were examined for organisms by culture techniques, for antigens by the agar-gel precipitation test, and for antibodies by CF and slide agglutination tests. Viable organisms were found in the serum and lymph and antigens were demonstrated in all fluids (Gourlay 1964b; Gourlay 1965a, b; Gourlay and Palmer 1965a). Organisms were detected in the urine of 14 of 19 naturally infected cases and their secretion was related to the severity of the disease, being observed only in acute clinical cases (Scudamore 1976). Following infection by endobronchial intubation 2 to 4 weeks before calving, mycoplasmas were isolated from tissues of cows and those from calves which developed extensive lung lesions. This indicated that transplacental transmission of *M. mycoides* could occur (Stone *et al.* 1969).

The attenuated T_1 strain organism has been recovered only intermittently from the blood within 24 hours after vaccination. Supporting *in vitro* experiments suggested phagocytosis of organisms by circulating leukocytes (Masiga and Boarer 1973). Organisms persisted for up to 14 days after vaccination in regional lymph nodes draining the site of vaccination. In animals which were previously vaccinated with caprinized rinderpest virus, the mycoplasmas persisted in the lymph nodes for a longer period of time. Persistence of the organism was associated with the CF and agglutination titers (Davies 1969b). In other investigations, cattle vaccinated with T_1 strain harbored the organisms for up to 71 days in the local drainage lymph nodes. Antigens, but not viable organisms, were also widespread in the tissues by day 11 and were still detectable up to day 204 (Masiga and Mugera 1973).

In reviewing the experimental reproduction of CBPP, endobronchial inoculation using cultures or infected material has been the most consistent method, producing lesions comparable to those observed in natural cases. The success of this method has varied with the particular group of research workers (Gourlay 1964a). Fulminating CBPP has been induced by nasal inoculation of lung material infected with a highly virulent strain (Karst 1970b; Shifrine and Moulton 1968). Early attempts to use spray systems which aerosolized virulent cultures were inconsistent, resulting in the development of clinical signs in about 45% and subclinical infection in approximately 90% of cattle (Hyslop 1963). The subcutaneous inoculation of caprinized rinderpest virus vaccine, given at the time of endobronchial inoculation, enhanced the production of lesions (Brown 1963). A caprine strain of *M.m. mycoides* given by endobronchial inoculation also caused infection in calves, and typical CBPP lesions developed when there was a concurrent infection with *Trypanosoma vivax* (Ojo *et al.* 1980).

The occurrence of CBPP in species other than domestic cattle was reviewed by Leach (1957) and reference was made to the disease occurring in water buffalo and yaks. Shifrine *et al.* (1970) summarized the information on water buffalo. This species has been shown to be susceptible to experimental induction of CBPP by endobronchial intubation and aerosol methods, but was more resistant than cattle. Lesions were resolved more rapidly and cattle in contact with these buffalo did not become infected. Of the important animal mycoplasmas, only *M.m. mycoides* has been shown to be infective for both cattle and sheep and goats (Gourlay 1981).

Experimental CCPP infections have been produced by aerosols. Subcutaneous injections caused acute and often fatal cellulitis spreading from the injection site (Smith 1967). Both *M.m. mycoides* and *M.m. capri* were infective to goats by endobronchial intubation and the gross lesions were characteristic of CCPP (Ojo 1976). In goats, polyarthritis was the predominant feature of spontaneous disease caused by large colony type of *M.m. mycoides*, and in calves this strain produced slight fever and arthritis (Rosendal 1981).

Laboratory animals were not susceptible unless the *M.m. mycoides* was incorporated in an agar base (Gourlay 1964a). Successful infections, resulting in bacteremia and occasionally in death, were induced intraperitoneally into mice by incorporating mucin in the inoculum (Smith 1967). Repeated passage through mice did not affect the virulence for mice. Intraperitoneal infection of mice resulted in mycoplasmemia, the duration of which depended on the virulence of the strain and the number of organisms injected. This was used to monitor the attenuation of the organisms as a result of passaging through cultures (Dyson and Smith 1976). Induction of lesions in rabbits by using *M.m. capri* in mucin had only limited success (Smith 1965).

CLINICAL SIGNS

Contagious bovine pleuropneumonia is characterized by acute, subacute, chronic, and asymptomatic syndromes. The incubation period varies greatly under different husbandry conditions, the shortest period being 3 to 6 weeks. In the acute form, the first signs observed are dullness, listlessness, anorexia, and accelerated respiration with grunts and a soft cough. As the disease becomes more severe, coughing becomes frequent, painful, and exaggerated when the animals are exercised. Animals are reluctant to move, standing with their heads down and front legs spread apart. In the final stages, there is pronounced abdominal respiration, extension of the neck, extrusion of the tongue with excess mucus secretion and frothy saliva. At this stage pleural exudate can be detected by auscultation and percussion, but the degree of pleuritis varies. The nasal discharge becomes mucopurulent and subcutaneous edema develops over the chest and abdomen. The sequela to the acute syndrome is either death with accompanying severe terminal symptoms or slow clinical recovery which takes months, and relapses do occur. The organism persists in the sequestra lungs, resulting in chronic carriers. Subacute and chronic syndromes are associated with less severe clinical signs and lesions.

Subclinical syndromes dominate the incidence of clinical disease because large volumes of lung tissue may be affected by focal lesions without obvious evidence of clinical signs such as temperature elevation and respiratory malfunction. Small and localized lesions cannot be located by percussion and auscultation, the only symptom may be an occasional cough.

In calves less than 6 months of age, infection causes arthritis, often without involvement of the respiratory system. A proportion of calves also develop vegetative endocarditis and myocarditis.

Experimental subcutaneous injection of organisms causes a local inflammatory reaction which may be extensive and results in necrosis and sloughing of skin. Severe reactions are accompanied by fever and anorexia.

The disease syndromes in CCPP vary considerably in the severity of clinical signs. Some are comparable to those observed with CBPP. Outbreaks of the disease may be more contagious than CBPP and acute syndromes predominate. The major differences probably reflect the complex etiology and virulence of the species of mycoplasma incriminated in CCPP.

Literature

The most detailed descriptions of the clinical syndromes seen in CBPP were presented by Henning (1956) and Hudson (1971). Reports on outbreaks of CBPP have been available from various countries. The most extensive report has been from East Africa and included a summary on clinical signs and lesions observed in 2541 animals (Bygrave *et al.* 1968). Clinical manifestations of CBPP in a dairy herd of Zebu cattle in Nigeria were described by Hill (1956). Outbreaks of CBPP in herds of humpless cattle in the Ivory Coast were described by Lindley (1973). Clinical and pathological observations in an outbreak of CCPP in Ethiopia were presented by Otte and Peck (1960).

PATHOLOGY

The pathogenicity of infections caused by various animal mycoplasmas depends on the primary tissues affected, and these include mucous membranes of the respiratory and urogenital tracts, eyes, alimentary canal, mammary glands, and joints. The ability of mycoplasma to adhere to epithelial lining is of major importance in its ability to cause tissue injury, enabling the establishment of infection. This adherence is firm enough to prevent elimination of the organism by mucous secretions. A microenvironment develops with local concentration of mildly toxic excreted byproducts of mycoplasma. The direct effect of the mycoplasma and its metabolites and immunologically induced injury probably play a role in the pathogenesis. Pathogenicity and virulence is not stable and can be altered by both serial passage in culture and in animals.

The most pronounced lesions are found in animals dying from the acute form of CBPP. The carcass is emaciated and there is subcutaneous edema of the lower abdomen and chest. The thoracic cavity contains clear or yellowish-gray turbid fluid and fibrin associated with fibrinous pleuritis. Parietal and visceral pleura is covered by a thick layer of yellow or yellowish-gray fibrinous exudate. Fibrinous pneumonia is usually characterized by unilateral focal or diffuse necrotic consolidation with large amounts of gray, pale red, or brownish fluid in the interlobular tissue, resulting in the often described 'marbling' effect. Accompanying the lesions in the thorax and lungs are inflammatory changes in the pericardium, peritoneum, and in the joints. Resolution of the fibrinous pleuritis results in fibrinous and fibrous adhesions between visceral and parietal pleura. The local drainage lymph nodes, in either experimental subcutaneous infection or in natural respiratory infection, are hyperplastic and undergo necrosis. In the acute syndrome in calves the carpus and tarsus are the joints which are most frequently affected, and may be accompanied by vegetative endocarditis and myocarditis.

Lesions become less severe in the chronic and carrier animals and consist of small localized areas of consolidation and necrosis surrounded by thick fibrous capsule. These sequestra vary in size from 1 to 30 cm in diameter.

Microscopic lesions depend on the severity and stage of infection. Acute cases are characterized by fibrinous pneumonia with early necrosis and extensive accumulation of serofibrinous exudate. The lesion starts as a terminal bronchiolitis with involvement of surrounding alveolar tissue. This progresses to extensive accumulation of fibrinous and polymorphonuclear cell inflammatory exudate in the parenchyma and interlobular connective tissue with dilated lymphatics containing fibrinous and inflammatory cell thrombosis. An alternate sequence of events in the pathogenesis is the organism passing through the bronchial epithelium without causing damage to infect the lymphatics, producing primary necrotic lymphadenitis, lymphangitis, and secondary parenchymal involvement of the lungs. A predisposition for the lymph vessels is evident following intradermal injections of the virulent organism which passes quickly into lymph channels without causing any localized lesions at the site of injection into connective tissue. Galactan increases the invasiveness of *M. mycoides* but does not enhance its virulence. Extensive necrosis occurs during the later stages and is accompanied by surrounding fibrosis. In longstanding chronic cases, the sequestra consist of a connective tissue enclosing necrotic material which may be calcified. In the calves, the acute, nonpurulent, serofibrinous polyarthritis and tendosinovitis is characterized by lymphatic and vascular thrombosis. This is accompanied by perivascular edema and eventually by fibrosis. Necrotic myocardial and valvular lesions are accompanied by extensive inflammatory reactions.

The gross and microscopic lesions in CCPP resemble those reported in CBPP. Septicemic disease in goats is characterized by leukopenia, coagulopathy, and widely disseminated lesions which include pneumonia, myocarditis, renal infarcts, adrenal cortical necrosis, enteritis, focal splenic necrosis, polyarthritis, and lymphadenitis.

Factors other than the mere presence of mycoplasmas in lung tissue appear necessary for the development of lesions. Mechanical trauma assists in the induction of the lesion in experimental infections caused by aerosols or by large volumes of material intubated into the bronchus. The host inflammatory and immunological responses also play an important role in the pathogenesis. There is some evidence that transfer of antigens between the mycoplasma and the host cell wall takes place, which enables the organisms to escape the immunological responses and induces autoimmune and hypersensitivity reactions to the host cells.

Literature

Hudson (1971) presented a comprehensive description of the pathology of CBPP. Bygrave *et al.* (1968) reported on the clinical, serological, and pathological findings of CBPP in East Africa, involving examination of 2541 animals. The cases were divided into early, acute, subacute, chronic, and those which were infected but had no visible lesions. Acute lesions affecting one entire lung with extensive fibrinous exudate and pleuritis were observed to make up 50% of all lesions encountered. Subacute lesions made up about 9% and affected less than 50% of one lung. In these, there was some sequestra formation and less exudate. Chronic lesions were those which were completely sequestered and persisted for up to 18 months after clinical signs (Stone and Bygrave 1969).

Subcutaneous and intravenous injection of calves up to 50 days of age with *M.m. mycoides* resulted in arthritis in 28% of the animals 3 to 4 weeks after infection. Vegetative endocarditis and myocarditis were also observed in 20% of these cases (Trethewie and Turner 1961). In an experimental CBPP, fibrinogen levels, platelet counts, clotting times, and fibrinolytic activity were related to thrombosis, which was an early event in the pathogenesis and considered to be responsible for the subsequent parenchymal lesions developing in the lungs (Lloyd *et al.* 1975).

The pathology of CCPP has not been clearly established because it varied with the pathogenicity of the species of mycoplasma involved. A number of microorganisms besides mycoplasmas have also been isolated from various types of pneumonia of sheep and goats in the tropics (Abu Bakr *et al.* 1980, 1981). Both *M.m. mycoides* and *M.m. capri* produced lung lesions comparable to the fibrinous pleuropneumonia seen in natural CCPP. Isolates of *M.m. mycoides* also produced septicemic disease in goats (Rosendal 1981). The characteristic lesions in goats and sheep experimentally infected were cellulitis at the site of inoculation, pleural hemorrhages, pneumonia, myocarditis, renal infarcts, glomerulitis, adrenal cortical necrosis, enteritis and focal splenic necrosis, polyarthritis, and lymphadenitis (Bar-Moshe and Rappaport 1981; Rosendal 1981).

Evidence for immunologically mediated injury involved in pathogenesis has been supported by experimental work. Anaphylactic response was observed in young calves exposed to two inoculations of inactivated suspension of *M. mycoides* (Piercy 1970a). Immunoconglutinin detected in cattle with CBPP was taken as indicating that autoimmunity played a role in the pathogenesis of CBPP (Kakoma *et al.* 1973). Galactan, a haptenic polysaccharide isolated from washed organisms, affected the development of mycoplasmemia in experimental infection of *M. mycoides* as well as immunological responses. Galactan was thought to have a direct effect on the host, rather than in some way modulating the behavior of the mycoplasma (Hudson *et al.* 1967b). Soluble factors from the organisms in diffusion chambers implanted intramuscularly in immune cattle produced extensive inflammatory exudates, increased swelling, vascularity, and greater connective tissue response than in nonimmune cattle. Galactan could also have been associated with this response (Buttery *et al.* 1980). Mycoplasmal lipopolysaccharide induced an immediate allergic reaction in cattle previously infected, but the material was not specific and had antigens in common with other bacteria isolated from cattle (Shifrine and Gourlay 1965). Cattle injected with inactivated cultures, together with adjuvant, were sensitive and were immune to subsequent subcutaneous challenge with virulent organisms (Shifrine and Beech 1968).

Some evidence has been available for a toxic effect caused by the mycoplasma. Elevated plasma fibrinogen and focal necrosis of tissues were present in the fibrinous synovitis caused by killing *M. mycoides* in joints. It was postulated that a factor analogous to bacterial endotoxin was released (Piercy 1970b; Piercy and Bingley 1972). Further evidence of involvement of a diffusible toxin was obtained from the observation that necrosis was produced by *M. mycoides* in intraperitoneal diffusion chambers in rabbits (Lloyd 1966).

IMMUNOLOGY

Cattle naturally or experimentally infected with virulent strains of *M. mycoides* develop detectable agglutinating, precipitating and complement-fixing antibodies. After recovery from clinical disease, antibody levels fall within a few months and subsequent challenge leads to a transient appearance of antibodies. Recovered animals develop immunity against reinfection.

Immunity to *M. mycoides* in cattle can also be induced by infection with living organisms of low virulence and their immunizing power is directly related to virulence. The role of humoral and cell-mediated responses in resistance is not established. Some resistance can be transferred on occasion by convalescent sera. The organisms responsible for CBPP are an antigenically homogeneous species. Various strains isolated cannot be differentiated serologically by the commonly used serological tests which include the tube and slide agglutination, gel diffusion, indirect hemagglutination, precipitation and CF tests.

There is relatively little information on the serological and cellular responses in CCPP. The immunology probably varies with the species and subspecies involved, and the severity of the clinical syndromes induced.

Literature

Significant passive immunity was transferred by sera from CBPP-recovered cattle (Masiga *et al.* 1975; Masiga and Windsor 1975). However, increased resistance by passive immunity was not demonstrated by other workers (Lloyd 1967). Blood from cattle with CBPP was highly bacteriocidal for *M.m. mycoides* and hyperimmune rabbit serum inhibited growth (Domermuth and Gourlay 1967; Priestley 1952). However, there was no relationship between growth inhibition and the immunity (Davies and Hudson 1968). Cell-mediated immune response occurred in immunized cattle but its role in resistance was not established (Roberts *et al.* 1973). Immunosuppression also occurred in CBPP and the limited information on the mycoplasma-induced suppression was reviewed (Adegboye 1978).

Different immunoglobulins were induced in cattle during the hyperacute, acute, chronic, and recovered stages of CBPP. Complement-fixing and agglutinating antibodies were detected in the IgM fraction. Complement-fixing antibodies were also found in IgG at later stages of the disease (Pearson and Lloyd 1972). Complement fixation antibodies were detected from 7 to 154 days after infection. Initial antibodies were of the 19S variety and 7S antibodies were found toward the end. Agglutination antibodies were found both in the IgG and IgM fractions (Barber *et al.* 1970). Vaccination with *M.m. mycoides* also induced development of Forssman antibody, primarily a macroglobulin, which was detected before complement-fixing antibodies (Kakoma and Stone 1974).

Little work has been undertaken on the type of antibodies induced in CCPP. The electrophoretic pattern of serum protein fractions in clinical cases showed a significant increase in gamma and decrease in beta globulins (Sharma and Vyas 1975).

Serological tests have been commonly used in field and laboratory work, but were of limited diagnostic value following the cessation of clinical CBPP (Stone and Bygrave 1969). Positive CF reaction was well correlated with lesions in lungs and, on a herd basis, had acceptable specificity (Ladds 1965). The test was useful, even under difficult field conditions, in the detection of carriers in herds where CBPP had been brought under control (Gambles 1956; Golding 1958). A field test had a sensitivity of 40% and the microtiter test one of 89%, both methods having a specificity of approximately 98% (Scudamore 1975). Although the CF test has been routinely used, it was found to be relatively cumbersome under field conditions, requiring many reagents and many pieces of equipment (Rurangirwa 1976). Various methods have been used to improve and standardize the CF test (Campbell and Turner 1953; Provost 1972). A main problem has been the preparation of the antigens (Griffin 1969) and methods have been developed improving the specificity and yield (Etheridge and Buttery 1976). Increased sensitivity was achieved by preserving sera with phenol (Etheridge and Lloyd 1968).

The slide agglutination test was not as sensitive as the CF test and was of only limited use as a screening procedure of herds (Adler and Etheridge 1964). Cattle with severe disease were negative, as were animals in which the lung lesions were sequestered, which occurred approximately 6 weeks after infection. Postvaccination titers were detected for long periods of time by this test, further limiting its diagnostic value (Turner and Etheridge 1963).

Precipitating antibodies have been more rarely detected in sera of cattle with acute CBPP. Circulating antigens have been detected more often which has led to the development of the agar-gel diffusion precipitant test (Gourlay 1965a). Using one of the newer serological tests, the enzyme-linked immunosorbent assay (ELISA), antibodies were detected 20 months after recovery from infection and 23 months after vaccination. During these periods, antibodies were rarely detectable by the other serological tests (Onoviran and Taylor-Robinson 1979). Although the ELISA was sensitive, interpretation of the results was difficult in the absence of disease syndromes in enzootic areas where cattle are vaccinated (Gee 1979). Complement fixation, agglutination, lymphocyte transformation, leukocyte migration, and intradermal allergic tests failed to differentiate immune cattle, vaccinated 15 months earlier with T_1 strain of *M.m. mycoides*, from susceptible cattle (Roberts and Windsor 1974). The reverse radial immunodiffusion test detected 30% more reactors than the CF test and 75% more when the test was used on cattle 1 year after vaccination (Rurangirwa 1976). Fluorescent antibody techniques have also been used to detect both antigens and antibodies (Masiga and Stone 1968a).

Neither the antigenic composition nor antigenic similarities of mycoplasmas from CBPP and CCPP have been clearly established. Attempts have been made to determine the antigenic relationship between *M.m. mycoides* and *M.m. capri* and other species of mycoplasma by using the various serological tests, and some antigenic relationships were demonstrated. The antigenic relationship of *M.m. mycoides* and *M.m. capri* has required standardized serological techniques for adequate identification (Al-Aubaidi *et al.* 1972). The CF test showed a cross-reaction of about 25% identity between *M.m. mycoides* and *M.m. capri* (Griffin 1969). Common precipitant antigens were present in both infected lungs and bronchial lymph nodes in cases of CCPP caused by *M.m. capri* and in CBPP (Lindley and Abdulla 1969). *Mycoplasma mycoides* isolated from cattle and goats had an antigenic relationship by immunoelectrophoretic techniques (Stone and Yedloutschnig 1973).

An antigenic relationship has been shown between *M. pneumoniae* and *M.m. mycoides* by the CF test and to a lesser extent by immunofluorescent and growth-inhibition tests (Buttery and Etheridge 1971; Lemcke *et al.* 1965). A serological relationship was also found between two unidentified mycoplasmas isolated from horses and *M.m. mycoides* (Lemcke *et al.* 1981). Because, on occasion, cattle free of CBPP had CF antibodies, antigens of *M. mycoides* were compared with those from *Escherichia coli* and some cross-reactions were demonstrated, suggesting a possible cause of these false positive results (Stone and Shifrine 1968).

VACCINATION

Attenuated egg- and broth-grown strains of *M.m. mycoides* are used in vaccination procedures and are protective in 80 to 90% of cattle of different breeds. Inactivated vaccines are not effective. Immunization can also be undertaken under certain conditions by using virulent organisms. Currently, the most common vaccine against CBPP is a live attenuated broth culture of *M.m. mycoides* which is administered subcutaneously. The efficacy of the vaccine depends on adequate methods of production, storage, distribution, and veterinary supervision in the field. Adverse side effects can occur and include extensive local inflammation at the site of vaccination, development of arthritis and heart lesions in young animals, and anaphylactic reactions, particularly with vaccines containing egg proteins.

Literature

The first vaccines which were developed were inactivated and these were not adequately protective (Brown 1966; Mendes 1957; Shifrine and Beech 1968). Adjuvants were of some use in vaccination procedures (Provost *et al.* 1963). Recently, further investigations on the development of inactivated vaccines were undertaken in mice, rabbits, and cattle. Subcutaneous inoculation of heat-killed *M.m. mycoides* emulsified in Freund's incomplete adjuvant gave encouraging results (Hooker *et al.* 1980).

The early developmental work of vaccines also involved use of virulent cultures. Dried organisms reconstituted in agar, but not in other fluids, were an efficient method (Priestley 1955). Dry vaccines in adjuvants were also recommended and required smaller doses of the organisms (Priestley and Dafaalla 1957).

Egg-propagated CBPP vaccines have been used extensively in the past, but have now been replaced by broth culture type of vaccines. The preparation, titration, and testing of these avianized vaccines was well established (Piercy and Knight 1957, 1958; Sheriff and Piercy 1952). This type of vaccine has been used in some regions of Africa since 1957 and was shown to be effective with immunity persisting for up to 8 months, vaccination being recommended to be undertaken annually (Provost *et al.* 1959). Avianized and broth culture vaccines were compared and both vaccines induced 80 to 90% protection and, in an outbreak, decreased considerably the death rate and severity of clinical signs and increased the incidence of complete recovery (Hudson and Turner 1963). A major adverse effect following the use of avianized vaccine was the development of lung lesions in a low percentage of animals (Hudson and Leaver 1965). This response was associated with the severe local postvaccination reaction at site of vaccination and not with any component *per se* of the embryonated eggs (Hudson 1965a).

Because of the adverse responses to avianized vaccines, a broth culture technique was developed using as seed culture the forty-sixth egg passage of a strain known as T_1 which was isolated from a clinical case in Tanzania and its growth was characterized (Davies *et al.* 1968). Vaccination against CBPP in East Africa using the T_1 strain was reviewed by Davies and Gilbert (1969). The vaccine consisted of a 3-day culture in tryptose broth (Davies 1969a). A concentration of 10^7 organism was required as the immunizing dose (Gilbert and Windsor 1971). The methods and equipment required for the efficient production of T_1 vaccine were developed in Kenya (Brown *et al.* 1965). Vaccines were produced from broth cultures with a high viable count and routine lyophilization was recommended.

The viability and immunizing potency of vaccines after storage and freeze-drying has been investigated. The shelf life of wet T_1 broth vaccine stored at 4 °C was reported to be 4 months by Garba (1980) and 4 weeks by Windsor (1978). Freeze-drying reduced the original number of viable organisms to 1% but the vaccine could still be used successfully (Gray and Turner 1954). The effect of lyophilization on vaccines in different reconstitution fluids was determined by Palmer and Gourlay (1964). Diluted with sterile water, the vaccine had to be used within half an hour because of the rapid drop of titer. Chlorinated water had an immediate effect on the viability of organisms. The drop of titer was negligible within 3 hours using phosphate buffered saline as diluent (Karst 1972).

Vaccinated cattle challenged by contact 1 month after vaccination with T_1 vaccine had good immunity (Davies *et al.* 1968). At 6 months a high level of immunity persisted and by 12 months it decreased (Gilbert *et al.* 1970). Challenge at 6 months after vaccination with virulent organisms in an aerosol resulted in the development of CF antibody titers postulated to be due to a temporary infection of tissues which was quickly eliminated (Turner 1964). Two years after vaccination significant immunity was still persistent, with only some of the animals developing after challenge CF antibody titers and small sequestra in the lungs (Windsor and Masiga 1972). Following challenge of recovered animals by either endobronchial or intravenous routes, mycoplasmemia did not result, but both methods caused elevation of CF antibody titers (Rurangirwa *et al.* 1976). Revaccination with T_1 culture vaccines induced an anamnestic response after 3 months, but not after 1 month (Shifrine *et al.* 1968).

Treatment with antibiotics and other chemotherapeutic drugs in association with the vaccination against CBPP reduced the efficacy of the vaccines and must be avoided. Treatment with tylosin, following vaccination with T_1 vaccine, significantly interfered with the development of immunity as determined by increased susceptibility to challenge (Windsor and Masiga 1976). Calves born to vaccinated cows received antibodies in the colostrum which also suppressed the response to T_1 vaccine for up to 60 days (Stone 1969, 1970; Gilbert and Stone 1970).

Vaccination into the tail tip with 0.5 ml of strain T_1 lyophilized CBPP vaccine has occasionally resulted in adverse reactions. Loss of the tail tip from necrotic reaction with swellings in the perineal region occurred in 17% of the adult cattle. Revaccination 6 to 8 months later resulted in a further tail loss in 0.3% of the animals but no reaction occurred after the third vaccination. The most optimal time to observe the postvaccination responses was 4 weeks after the injection (Revell 1973). The tail lesions have not been considered as a major problem by the owners (Minor 1967). Large vaccination schemes in the Sudan (Daleel 1972) and in Nigeria (Karst 1971) did not reveal any significant adverse postvaccinal reactions. Postvaccinal lesions were more severe in the humpless cattle common in West Africa than in the Zebu cattle (Lindley 1971).

Another CBPP vaccine was developed in Australia using the strain known as KH_3J which was selected because of the absence of local reaction. The original strain was isolated from the Sudan and attenuated through passages in broth culture (Lindley 1965; Hudson 1965b, 1968a). This strain produced small lesions in 2 of 20 cattle when inoculated endobronchially (Brown 1964). As with the T_1 strain the immunogenicity of KH_3J vaccine also depended on the presence of live organisms, and loss of viability from both frozen and nonfrozen vaccines was associated with the composition of the media (Pearson and Lloyd 1971). A vaccine containing 20% of bovine brain suspension was found to be efficient and could be maintained in a freeze-dried state (Hudson 1968c). A dried egg adjuvant KH_3J vaccine was as good as the wet tissue culture vaccine (Lindley 1967b). The efficacy of KH_3J and T_1 vaccines administered into different sites, the KH_3J behind the shoulder and the T_1 into the tail, was compared and the T_1 vaccine was superior in development of protection to in-contact challenge (Karst 1971).

Other vaccine strains have also been investigated and shown to have limited application. A vaccine using V5 strain was developed during the early vaccination campaigns in Australia (Hudson 1968b). In calves up to 50 days of age lesions developed, and were most severe in 7-day-old calves which developed myocarditis, endocarditis, and polyarthritis. The severity and incidence of lesions decreased rapidly with age (Turner 1961). Postvaccination reactions in the tail were more prevalent in adult cattle than in calves (Turner 1961; Turner and Trethewie 1961). In another vaccine tried in Australia, the Gladysdale strain was used. On endobronchial inoculation of cattle this strain produced clinical cases of CBPP in 80% of animals. Intranasal vaccination with the Gladysdale strain attenuated in bovine kidney cell culture had an efficacy rate of 70 to 80% on challenge up to 6 months after vaccination (Karst and Mitchell 1972).

In large vaccination campaigns, which are often undertaken in the tropics, applying more than one vaccine at the same time has been important economically and logistically. Mixing rinderpest and CBPP vaccines was discussed and shown to be advantageous (Provost 1969; Provost *et al*. 1969). Simultaneous inoculation with caprinized rinderpest vaccine, either mixed directly with CBPP vaccine or injected into different sites, gave comparable results to using the two vaccines at different times (Brown and Taylor 1966; Lindley 1967a; Macadam *et al*. 1964).

There has been relatively little information on the vaccination of goats against organisms causing CCPP. Goats which had survived infection with virulent *M.m. capri* were immune to subsequent homologous intranasal and subcutaneous challenge (Onoviran 1972). *Mycoplasma m. capri* could be adapted to embryonated chicken eggs but was not attenuated even after 154 passages (Sharma *et al*. 1965). Inactivated antigens from the F38 strain of mycoplasma with Freund's adjuvant protected against homologous challenge by contact with animals clinically affected with CCPP (Rurangirwa *et al*. 1981).

DIAGNOSIS

Diagnosis of CBPP in acute outbreaks is not difficult by serological methods and postmortem examination. In clinically acute cases the typical acute lung lesions and serological responses provide definitive diagnosis. When only the first few cases are detected clinically in a herd early diagnosis may be more difficult. History of the introduction or contact with new animals is an important consideration. Diagnosis of acute CBPP and CCPP on clinical grounds alone is not possible because they cannot be differentiated from other forms of acute pneumonia. The majority of the cases of CBPP cannot be detected clinically and require postmortem and serological examinations. Confirmation of diagnosis requires isolation and identification of the organism. Isolations are made from blood and nasal exudate. The CF test is the most common serological test used. Other tests which can be used are agglutination, precipitation, and allergic skin tests but give variable results. Serological tests are relatively efficient in detecting the active clinical disease, but are inadequate during incubation periods and in chronic infections. The main field problem is the recognition of carrier animals with low titers and the CF test is the test of choice. The agglutination test, which is easier for the field diagnosis, is limited by its lack of specificity and sensitivity.

Postmortem examination of representative animals exhibiting clinical signs is advisable in enzootic areas. The diagnosis is made on the basis of the characteristic lesions and isolation of the organisms in culture. Pasteurellosis, causing fibrinous pneumonia, is the disease which most closely resembles both CBPP and CCPP. In the more chronic forms of CBPP and CCPP the lesions have to be differentiated from abscesses caused by other organisms.

Literature

The general principles of diagnosis of animal mycoplasmal infections were presented by Freundt (1981), including methods of direct microscopic examination of tissues for organisms and antigens, isolation and culture, and techniques for identification and classification by biochemical and serological methods. Various combinations of laboratory techniques have been used, depending on the types of mycoplasmas and diseases they cause. Laboratory diagnosis of infections presented problems not common to other bacterial infections. Direct examination of excretions for the presence of mycoplasmas is usually not practical (Razin 1981). Mycoplasmas could be demonstrated in tissues by immunofluorescence and immunoperoxidase techniques. Isolation and cultivation of mycoplasmas has to take into consideration the source, method of collection, transportation of the material, inhibition of contaminants, elimination of growth-inhibiting factors in tissues, and providing media with special nutrients (Freundt 1981). Colonies are first identified by the growth characteristic and further classified with homologous fluorescein-conjugated antibody or by inhibiting growth by a specific antiserum. Further identification of isolates has been done routinely by more exact chemical and serological techniques and by using electrophoresis and ELISA (Razin 1981).

Routine diagnosis of CBPP has been undertaken by the culture-precipitation test to detect specific antigen in lesions, histological examination, and the CF test (Lloyd 1969). Various bacteriocidal mixtures of antibiotics have been used to suppress contamination in cultures (Davies and Read 1969). A direct FA has been applied to organisms grown in semi-solid media and the method was species specific, without cross-reaction and with minimal background fluorescence (Karst 1969). Fluorescent antibody and the agar-gel diffusion techniques have also been applied to formalin fixed and fresh lung specimens to detect antigens; the principal antigen was considered to be galactan (Masiga and Stone 1968b).

The CF has been the most widely used serological technique and was shown to detect most cases of disease (Griffin 1969). Adaptation of the CF test to the field diagnosis of CBPP was described by Provost (1972).

A plate test was developed for field use and was highly specific and able to detect acute, subacute, and chronic carriers (Chima and Onoviran 1975). There was a close relationship between the presence of the organism and the CF antibody, with the exception being in chronic well-encapsulated sequestra where antibodies would not necessarily be stimulated. Six weeks after the commencement of the clinical reaction, antibodies always indicated the presence of lesions in the lungs. At 4 to 6 months after infection the presence of antibody was not consistent in some animals with small sequestra (Hudson 1971). Absolute correlation has not been shown to occur between either the CF or the agglutination tests and the presence of lesions (Shifrine and Moulton 1968).

Simple diagnostic tests, dependent on the skin hypersensitivity reaction, have been attempted but false negatives occur in various disease syndromes (Gourlay 1964c; Gourlay and Palmer 1965b). Using an antigen which did not contain galactan, the intradermal allergic test was positive in infected and negative in control animals (Windsor and Boarer 1973).

CHEMOTHERAPY

Chemotherapy is generally not used in the control of CBPP. Because chronic carriers develop following therapy, antibiotics should be used only in very limited circumstances. There is justification in using chemotherapy in the control of CCPP because of the lack of any other efficient method of control. In CCPP, unlike in CBPP, there appears to be no sequestration following chemotherapy. The efficacy of treatments is not uniform in CCPP because of the different causative agents involved and secondary bacteriological complications.

Literature

The main principles in the chemotherapy of mycoplasmal diseases were presented by Razin (1981). Mycoplasmas are sensitive to most of the broad spectrum of antibiotics, such as tetracycline and chloramphenicol, but are resistant to antibiotics that specifically inhibit bacterial cell wall synthesis. Treatment often does not result in eradication of the organism and can result in development of antibiotic-resistant strains.

In treatment trials on CCPP tylocin tartrate, oxytetracycline, chloramphenicol, and a combination of streptomycin and penicillin were used. Tylocin tartrate at a dose of 11 mg/kg body weight was very effective and oxytetracycline at 15.4 mg/kg body weight was of some value (Onoviran 1974). Lung lesions associated with *M.m. mycoides* in goats treated with tylosin at 4 mg/kg daily for 4 days resulted in slow recovery (Thigpen *et al.* 1981). Tylosin was also found to be bacteriostatic against the organism *in vitro*. Experimental subcutaneous inflammatory reactions in cattle were controlled, but the organisms were not eliminated by seven 12-hourly intramuscular injections at doses of 7.5 or 15 mg/kg (Hudson and Etheridge 1965).

Antibiotics have been used in CBPP to control adverse local postvaccinal reactions, the severity of which depended on the dose of the organisms injected and on the immunological status of the animal (Lindley 1979).

CONTROL

Control CBPP depends on the epizootiological situation, livestock husbandry procedures, and the availability of veterinary services. Testing to detect infected cattle in the various stages of disease, vaccination, and slaughter policies are the principal methods. Use of quarantine varies with different countries. In enzootic regions control is primarily by vaccination and restriction of cattle movement. In disease-free zones, quarantine, testing, slaughter, and vaccination are used.

Literature

The geographical distribution and control of CBPP in Africa was reviewed by Atang (1968, 1969). An FAO/OIE/OAU panel of experts of CBPP was set up to coordinate research and field investigations in Africa (Lobry 1973). A major control program was the OAU/STRC CP 16 project which involved national and international funding organizations with objectives to the control and eradication of CBPP in Africa, and its achievements were summarized by Masiga (1972). The basic laboratory work and logistics of vaccination necessary in eradicating campaigns in Africa were summarized by Hudson (1964). One of the main problems has been the maintenance of viable vaccines under field conditions. In these campaigns the use of stable T_1 vaccine and slaughter policies were often difficult to administer and enforce (Lindley 1967c, 1979). Eradication of CBPP from Nigeria was reviewed by Osiyemi (1981) and the problems were discussed. Based on the experience gained in the successful control of CBPP in Nigeria from 1973 to 1974, it was emphasized that prevention of reinfection was most important and required strict control of movement of trade cattle. Success of the campaigns has been greatly influenced by economics and politics. To increase the success rate of eradication and control campaigns, plans had to be made on a regional basis rather than for an entire country (Karst 1970a).

In Australia, the progress in the campaigns to eradicate CBPP from various regions have been presented (Pierce 1969; Lloyd 1969). The eradication of CBPP from the focus in Spain which occurred in 1966 was reviewed by Diaz Montilla *et al.* (1969). The regulatory aspects of caprine mycoplasmosis in the USA were discussed by Yedloutschnig (1982).

BIBLIOGRAPHY

Abdulla, A. E. D., 1969. A note on contagious bovine pleuropneumonia in the Sudan, *Bull. Off. int. Epiz.*, **72**: 95–101.

Abu Bakr, M. I., Abdalla, S. A., El Faki, M. E. and Kamal, S. M., 1980. Pathological studies on sheep and goat pneumonia in the Sudan – Part I. Natural infection, *Bull. Anim. Hlth Prod. Afr.*, **28**: 288–93.

Abu Bakr, M. I., El Faki, M. E., Abdalla, S. A. and Kamal, S. M., 1981. Pathological studies on sheep and goat pneumonia in the Sudan – Part II. Experimental infection, *Bull. Anim. Hlth Prod. Afr.*, **29**: 85–94.

Adegboye, D. S., 1978. A review of mycoplasma-induced immunosuppression, *Br. vet. J.*, **134**: 556–60.

Adler, H. E., 1965. Mycoplasmosis in animals, *Adv. vet. Sci.*, **10**: 205–44.

Adler, H. E. and Etheridge, J. R., 1964. Contagious bovine pleuropneumonia: a comparison of two slide agglutination blood tests with the complement fixation test, *Aust. vet. J.*, **40**: 38–43.

Al-Aubaidi, J. M., Dardiri, A. H. and Fabricant, J., 1972. Biochemical characterization and antigenic relationship of *Mycoplasma mycoides* subsp. *mycoides* Freundt and *Mycoplasma mycoides* subsp. *capri* (Edward) Freundt, *Int. J. Syst. Bact.*, **22**(3): 155–64.

Al-Shammari, A. J. N. and Al-Aubaidi, J. M., 1977. Occurrence of caprine and ovine mycoplasma in Iraq, *Iraqi Med. J.*, **25**(3–4): 36–44.

Archer, D. B., 1981. The structure and function of the mycoplasma membrane, *Int. Rev. Cyt.*, **69**: 1–44.

Askaa, G., Erno, H. and Ojo, M. O., 1978. Bovine mycoplasmas: classification of groups related to *Mycoplasma mycoides*. *Acta vet. scand.*, **19**: 166–78.

Atang, P. G., 1968. The geographical distribution and control of contagious bovine pleuropneumonia in Africa today, *Bull. epiz. Dis. Afr.*, **16**: 173–81.

Atang, P. G., 1969. Review and progress on joint project (J.P.) 16. Research on contagious bovine pleuropneumonia (C.B.P.P.), *Bull. epiz. Dis. Afr.*, **17**: 301–3.

Banerjee, M., Singh, N. and Gupta, P. P., 1979. Isolation of mycoplasmas and acholeplasmas from pneumonia lesions in sheep and goats in India, *Zbl. Vet. Med.*, **B26**: 689–95.

Barber, T. L., Stone, S. S. and DeLay, P. D., 1970. Antibody in cattle experimentally infected with contagious bovine pleuropneumonia, *Infect. Immun.*, **2**(5): 617–22.

Bar-Moshe, B. and Rappaport, E., 1981. Observations on *Mycoplasma mycoides* subsp. *mycoides* infection in Saanen goats, *Isr. J. Med. Sci.*, **17**: 537–9.

Bredt, W., Feldner, J. and Kahane, I., 1981. Adherence of mycoplasmas to cells and inert surfaces: phenomena, experimental models and possible mechanisms, *Isr. J. Med. Sci.*, **17**: 586–8.

Brown, R. D., 1963. The effect of caprinised rinderpest virus on the experimental production of contagious bovine pleuropneumonia, *Vet. Rec.*, **75**(48): 1306–7.

Brown, R. D., 1964. Endobronchial inoculation of cattle with various strains of *Mycoplasma mycoides* and the effects of stress, *Res. vet. Sci.*, **5**: 393–404.

Brown, R. D., 1966. A note on inactivated contagious bovine pleuropneumonia vaccines, *Bull. epiz. Dis. Afr.*, **14**: 281–3.

Brown, R. D., Gourlay, R. N. and MacLeod, A. K., 1965. The production of T_1 broth culture contagious bovine pleuropneumonia vaccine, *Bull. epiz. Dis. Afr.*, **13**: 149–55.

Brown, R. D. and Taylor, W. P., 1966. Simultaneous vaccination of cattle against rinderpest and contagious bovine pleuropneumonia, *Bull. epiz. Dis. Afr.*, **14**: 141–6.

Buttery, S. H., Cottew, G. S. and Lloyd, L. C., 1980. Effect of soluble factors from *Mycoplasma mycoides* subsp. *mycoides* on the collagen content of bovine connective tissue, *J. Comp. Path.*, **90**: 303–14.

Buttery, S. H. and Etheridge, J. R., 1971. Observations on the cross reaction between *Mycoplasma pneumoniae* antigen and bovine antisera to *Mycoplasma mycoides* var. *mycoides*, *Aust. J. exp. Biol. med. Sci.*, **49**: 233–6.

Bygrave, A. C., Moulton, J. E. and Shifrine, M., 1968. Clinical, serological and pathological findings in an outbreak of contagious bovine pleuropneumonia. *Bull. epiz. Dis. Afr.*, **16**: 21–46.

Campbell, A. D. and Turner, A. W., 1953. Studies on contagious pleuropneumonia of cattle. IV. An improved complement fixation test, *Aust. vet. J.*, **29**: 154–63.

Chima, J. C. and Onoviran, O., 1975. Complement fixation test in the diagnosis and control of contagious bovine pleuropneumonia (J.P. 28) in Nigeria. *Bull. Off. int. Epiz.*, **83**(11–12): 1107–12.

Cottew, G. S., 1979. Caprine–ovine mycoplasmas. In *The Mycoplasmas*, eds J. G. Tully, R. F. Whitcomb. Academic Press (London and New York), vol. 2, pp. 103–32.

Cottew, G. S., 1982. Significance of mycoplasmoses in goats, *Proc. Int. Conf. on Goat Reproduction and Diseases*, pp. 221–5.

Cottew, G. S. and Yeats, F. R., 1978. Subdivision of *Mycoplasma mycoides* subsp. *mycoides* from cattle and goats into two types, *Aust. vet. J.*, **54**: 293–6.

Daleel, E. E., 1972. Report: contagious bovine pleuropneumonia (CBPP) T_1 broth vaccine safety trials in Sudanese cattle, *Bull. epiz. Dis. Afr.*, **20**: 197–202.

Das, C., 1968. Study on the virulence of contagious bovine pleuropneumonia organism (Assam strain) on subcutaneous pathogenicity test, *Indian vet. J.*, **45**: 816–18.

Davies, G., 1969a. Growth characteristics of the T_1 strain of *Mycoplasma mycoides*, *Trop. Anim. Hlth Prod.*, **1**: 7–12.

Davies, G., 1969b. The persistence of *Mycoplasma mycoides* in the host after vaccination with T_1 broth vaccine, *Res. vet. Sci.*, **10**: 225–31.

Davies, G. and Gilbert, F. R., 1969. Contagious bovine pleuropneumonia vaccination in East Africa, *Bull. epiz. Dis. Afr.*, **17**: 21–6.

Davies, G. and Hudson, J. R., 1968. The relationship between growth-inhibition and immunity in contagious bovine pleuropneumonia, *Vet. Rec.*, **83**: 256–8.

Davies, G., Masiga, W. N., Shifrine, M. and Read, W. C. S., 1968. The efficacy of T_1 strain broth vaccine against contagious bovine pleuropneumonia: preliminary in-contact trials, *Vet. Rec.*, **83**: 239–44.

Davies, G. and Read, W. C. S., 1968. A modification of the growth-inhibition test and its use in detecting *Mycoplasma mycoides* var. *mycoides*, *J. Hyg., Camb.*, **66**: 319–24.

Davies, G. and Read, W. C. S., 1969. The use of bacteriocidal agents in the primary isolation of *Mycoplasma mycoides*, *J. Comp. Path.*, **79**: 121–5.

Davies, G., Stone, S. S. and Read, W. C. S., 1969. Comparative characteristics of various strains of *Mycoplasma mycoides*, *Trop. Anim. Hlth Prod.*, **1**: 13–18.

Diaz Montilla, R., Garcia Ferrero, J. L. and Panos Marti, P., 1969. Un foco de perineumonia en Llivia: su erradicación, *Bull. Off. int. Epiz.*, **72**: 17–23.

Domermuth, C. H. and Gourlay, R. N., 1967. A solid medium test for measuring growth inhibition and neutralization of *Mycoplasma mycoides* by immune bovine serum. *J. gen. Microbiol.*, **47**: 289–294.

Dyson, D. A. and Smith, G. R., 1976. Virulence of established vaccine strains and artificially passaged field strains of *Mycoplasma mycoides* subsp. *mycoides*, *Res. vet. Sci.*, **20**: 185–90.

Edward, D. G. ff. and Freundt, E. A., 1956. The classification and nomenclature of organisms of the pleuropneumonia group, *J. gen. Microbiol.*, **14**: 197–207.

Erno, H., Al-Aubaidi, J. M., Ojo, M. O., Minga, U. M. and Sikdar, A., 1978. Classification and identification of ovine and caprine mycoplasmas, *Acta vet. scand.*, **19**: 392–406.

Erno, H., Freundt, E. A., Krogsgaard-Jensen, A. and Rosendal, S., 1972. The identification of an organism isolated from maned sheep as *Mycoplasma mycoides* subsp. *mycoides*, *Acta vet. scand.*, **13**: 263–5.

Erno, H. and Jurmanova, K., 1973. Bovine mycoplasmas: serological studies by double immunodiffusion, growth precipitation and growth inhibition. *Acta vet. scand.*, **14**: 524–37.

Erno, H. and Stipkovits, L., 1973. Bovine mycoplasmas: cultural and biochemical studies II, *Acta vet. scand.*, **14**: 450–63.

Etheridge, J. R. and Buttery, S. H., 1976. Improving the specificity and yield of the contagious bovine pleuropneumonia complement fixation test antigen, *Res. vet. Sci.*, **20**: 201–6.

Etheridge, J. R. and Lloyd, L. C., 1968. Increased sensitivity of the complement fixation test for contagious bovine pleuropneumonia on sera preserved with phenol, *Bull. epiz. Dis. Afr.*, **16**: 295–301.

Ezebuiro, E. O., Griffin, R. M. and Peers, F. G., 1964. Studies on contagious bovine pleuropneumonia in Nigeria, *Bull. epiz. Dis. Afr.*, **12**: 171–80.

Francis, J., 1973. Susceptibility of *Bos indicus* and *Bos taurus* cattle to pleuropneumonia, *Vet. Rec.*, **12**: 401.

Freundt, E. A., 1981. General principles of laboratory diagnosis of mycoplasma infections, *Isr. J. Med. Sci.*, **17**: 641–3.

Furness, G. and De Maggio, M., 1972. Binucleate classical mycoplasmas pathogenic for goats, *Infect. Immun.*, **5**(4): 433–41.

Furness, G. and De Maggio, M., 1973. The growth cycle of *Mycoplasma mycoides* var. *mycoides*, *J. Infect. Dis.*, **127**(5): 563–6.

Gambles, R. M., 1956. Studies on contagious bovine pleuropneumonia with special reference to the complement fixation test, *Br. vet. J.*, **112**: 34–40.

Garba, S. A., 1980. Shelf life of wet T_1 broth vaccine for contagious bovine pleuropneumonia, *Trop. Anim. Hlth Prod.*, **12**: 189–91.

Gee, R. W., 1979. ELISA detection of antibody against mycoplasma, *Vet. Rec.*, **94**: 360.

Gilbert, F. R., Davies, G., Read, W. C. S. and Turner, G. R. J., 1970. The efficacy of T_1 strain broth vaccine against contagious bovine pleuropneumonia: in-contact trials carried out six and twelve months after primary vaccination, *Vet. Rec.*, **86**: 29–32.

Gilbert, F. R. and Stone, S. S., 1970. Serological response to T_1 strain *Mycoplasma mycoides* in calves born of previously vaccinated dams, *Trop. Anim. Hlth Prod.*, **2**: 204–9.

Gilbert, F. R. and Windsor, R. S., 1971. The immunizing dose of T_1 strain *Mycoplasma mycoides* against contagious bovine pleuropneumonia, *Trop. Anim. Hlth Prod.*, **3**: 71–6.

Golding, N. K., 1958. The application of the complement fixation test to the control of contagious pleuropneumonia of bovines, *Aust. vet. J.*, **34**: 361–6.

Goni, M. and Onoviran, O., 1973. Contagious caprine

pleuropneumonia: a reassessment of the disease situation in Nigeria, *Trop. Anim. Hlth Prod.*, **5**: 114–18.
Gourlay, R. N., 1964a. Artificial reproduction of contagious bovine pleuropneumonia, *Bull. epiz. Dis. Afr.*, **12**: 229–35.
Gourlay, R. N., 1964b. Antigenicity of *Mycoplasma mycoides* I. Examination of body fluids from cases of contagious bovine pleuropneumonia, *Res. vet. Sci.*, **5**: 473–82.
Gourlay, R. N., 1964c. The allergic reaction in contagious bovine pleuropneumonia, *J. Comp. Path.*, **74**: 286–99.
Gourlay, R. N., 1965a. Antigenicity of *Mycoplasma mycoides* II. Further studies on the precipitating antigens in the body fluids from cases of contagious bovine pleuropneumonia, *Res. vet. Sci.*, **6**: 1–8.
Gourlay, R. N., 1965b. The antigenicity of *Mycoplasma mycoides* IV. Properties of the precipitating antigens isolated from urine, *Res. vet. Sci.*, **6**: 263–73.
Gourlay, R. N., 1965c. Comparison between diagnostic tests for contagious bovine pleuropneumonia, *J. Comp. Path.*, **75**: 97–109.
Gourlay, R. N., 1981. Mycoplasmosis in cattle, sheep and goats, *Isr. J. Med. Sci.*, **17**: 531–6.
Gourlay, R. N. and Howard, C. J., 1979. Bovine mycoplasmas. In *The Mycoplasmas*, eds J. G. Tully, R. F. Whitcomb. Academic Press (London and New York), vol. 2, pp. 49–102.
Gourlay, R. N. and Palmer, R. F., 1965a. The antigenicity of *Mycoplasma mycoides* III. Isolation of precipitating antigens for urine, *Res. vet. Sci.*, **6**: 255–62.
Gourlay, R. N. and Palmer, R. F., 1965b. Further studies on the allergic reaction in contagious bovine pleuropneumonia, *J. Comp. Path.*, **75**: 89–95.
Gray, D. F. and Turner, A. W., 1954. Viability and immunizing potency of freeze-dried bovine contagious pleuropneumonia culture-vaccine, *J. Comp. Path.*, **64**: 116–26.
Gregory, T. S., 1957. Contagious bovine pleuropneumonia report of investigations in Australia, *Bull. epiz. Dis. Afr.*, **5**: 187–98.
Griffin, R. M., 1969. Antigenic relationship among strains of *Mycoplasma mycoides* var. *mycoides*, *M. capri* and *M. laidlawii* revealed by complement-fixation tests, *J. gen. Microbiol.*, **57**: 131–42.
Griffin, R. M. and Laing, D. F., 1966. Contagious bovine pleuropneumonia in northern Nigeria, 1924–64, *Bull. epiz. Dis. Afr.*, **14**: 255–79.

Hammond, J. A. and Branagan, D., 1965. Contagious bovine pleuropneumonia in Tanganyika, *Bull. epiz. Dis. Afr.*, **13**: 121–47.
Harbi, M. S. M. A., El Tahir, M. S., Macowan, K. J. and Nayil, A. A., 1981. Mycoplasma strain F38 and contagious caprine pleuropneumonia in the Sudan, *Vet. Rec.*, **21**: 261.
Henning, M. W., 1956. Pleuro-pneumonia contagious bovium, lung-sickness of cattle, longsiekte. In *Animal Diseases in South*

Africa. Central News Agency (South Africa), pp. 204–29.
Hill, D. H., 1956. Some clinical and serological observations on an outbreak of contagious pleuropneumonia in a dairy herd of zebu cattle in Nigeria, *Br. vet. J.*, **112**: 63–70.
Hooker, J. M., Smith, G. R. and Milligan, R. A., 1979. Differentiation of *Mycoplasma mycoides* subsp. *mycoides* from certain closely related caprine mycoplasmas by mycoplasmaemia and cross-protection tests in mice, *J. Hyg., Camb.*, **82**: 407–18.
Hooker, J. M., Smith, G. R. and Milligan, R. A., 1980. Immune response of mice, rabbits and cattle to inactivated *Mycoplasma mycoides* subspecies *mycoides* vaccines containing adjuvants, *J. Comp. Path.*, **90**: 363–72.
Hudson, J. R., 1964. Contagious bovine pleuropneumonia: laboratory work in relation to the eradication campaign, *Aust. vet. J.*, **40**: 95–8.
Hudson, J. R., 1965a. Contagious bovine pleuropneumonia: studies in the pathogenesis of lung lesions following vaccination with egg vaccines, *Aust. vet. J.*, **41**: 36–42.
Hudson, J. R., 1965b. Contagious bovine pleuropneumonia: the immunizing value of the attenuated strain KH_3J, *Aust. vet. J.*, **41**: 43–9.
Hudson, J. R., 1968a. Contagious bovine pleuropneumonia: experiments on the susceptibility and protection by vaccination of different types of cattle, *Aust. vet. J.*, **44**: 83–9.
Hudson, J. R., 1968b. Contagious bovine pleuropneumonia: development of a satisfactory safe vaccine, *Bull. epiz. Dis. Afr.*, **16**: 165–72.
Hudson, J. R., 1968c. Contagious bovine pleuropneumonia: the keeping properties of the V5 vaccine used in Australia, *Aust. vet. J.*, **44**: 123–9.
Hudson, J. R., 1971. Contagious bovine pleuropneumonia. In *FAO Agricultural Studies No. 86*. FAO/UN (Rome), pp. 1–120.
Hudson, J. R., Buttery, S. and Cottew, G. S., 1967b. Investigations into the influence of the galactan of *Mycoplasma mycoides* on experimental infection with that organism, *J. Path. Bact.*, **94**: 257–73.
Hudson, J. R., Cottew, G. S. and Adler, H. E., 1967a. Diseases of goats caused by mycoplasma: a review of the subject with some new findings, *Ann. N.Y. Acad. Sci.*, **143**: 287–97.
Hudson, J. R. and Etheridge, J. R., 1965. Contagious bovine pleuropneumonia: experiments with the antibiotic tylosin, *Aust. vet. J.*, **41**: 130–5.
Hudson, J. R. and Leaver, D. D., 1965. Contagious bovine pleuropneumonia: the occurrence of lesions following vaccination with egg vaccine, *Aust. vet. J.*, **41**: 29–36.
Hudson, J. R. and Turner, A. W., 1963. Contagious bovine pleuropneumonia: a comparison of the efficacy of two types of vaccine, *Aust. vet. J.*, **39**: 373–85.
Hyslop, N. St G., 1963. Experimental infection with *Mycoplasma mycoides*, *J. Comp. Path.*, **73**: 265–76.

Jonas, A. M. and Barber, T. L., 1969. *Mycoplasma mycoides* var. *capri* isolated from a goat in Connecticut, *J. Infect. Dis.*, **119**: 126–31.

Jones, A. S. and Walker, R. T., 1963. Isolation and analysis of the deoxyribonucleic acid of *Mycoplasma mycoides* var. *capri*, *Nature*, **198**(4880): 588–9.

Kahane, I., Pnini, S., Banai, M., Baseman, J. B., Cassell, G. H. and Bredt, W., 1981. Attachment of mycoplasmas to erythrocytes: a model to study mycoplasma attachment to the epithelium of the host respiratory tract, *Isr. J. Med. Sci.*, **17**: 589–92.

Kakoma, I., Masiga, W. N. and Windsor, R. S., 1973. Detection of immunoconglutinin in cattle with contagious bovine pleuropneumonia: evidence of autoimmunity, *Res. vet. Sci.*, **15**: 101–5.

Kakoma, I. and Stone, S. S., 1974. The development of Forssman antibody in the sera of cattle following vaccination and infection with contagious bovine pleuropneumonia, *Res. vet. Sci.*, **16**: 143–6.

Kariuki, D. P., 1971. History of contagious bovine pleuropneumonia in Kenya, *Bull. epiz. Dis. Afr.*, **19**: 111–16.

Karst, O., 1969. Identification of *Mycoplasma mycoides varias mycoides* colonies by immunofluorescence, *Bull. epiz. Dis. Afr.*, **17**: 287–93.

Karst, O., 1970a. Contagious bovine pleuropneumonia: considerations in connection with a future interAfrican eradication campaign, *Bull. epiz. Dis. Afr.*, **18**: 105–10.

Karst, O., 1970b. Contagious bovine pleuropneumonia: artificial reproduction, *Vet. Rec.*, **86**: 506–7.

Karst, O., 1971. A comparison of 2 vaccines against contagious bovine pleuropneumonia, *Res. vet. Sci.*, **12**: 18–22.

Karst, O., 1972. Contagious bovine pleuropneumonia: lyophilized (T_1) vaccine, *Bull. epiz. Dis. Afr.*, **20**: 69–76.

Karst, O. and Mitchell, S., 1972. Intranasal vaccination of cattle with an attenuated Gladysdale strain of *Mycoplasma mycoides* var. *mycoides*, *J. Comp. Path.*, **82**: 171–8.

Ladds, P. W., 1965. The value of complement fixation testing of slaughter cattle in surveying the incidence of bovine contagious pleuropneumonia, *Aust. vet. J.*, **41**: 387–90.

Laws, L., 1956. A pleuropneumonia-like organism causing peritonitis in goats, *Aust. vet. J.*, **32**: 326–9.

Leach, T. M., 1957. The occurrence of contagious bovine pleuropneumonia in species other than domesticated cattle, *Bull. epiz. Dis. Afr.*, **5**: 325–8.

Leblanc, G. and Grimellec, C., 1979. Active K^+ transport in *Mycoplasma mycoides* var. *capri*. Relationships between K^+ distribution, electrical potential and ATPase activity, *Biochim. Biophys. Acta*, **554**: 168–79.

Lemcke, R. M., 1974. The relationship of a caprine mycoplasma to PG3, the type strain of *Mycoplasma mycoides* subsp. *capri*, *Res. vet. Sci.*, **16**: 119–21.

Lemcke, R. M., Erno, H. and Gupta, U., 1981. The relationship of two equine mycoplasmas to *Mycoplasma mycoides*, *J. Hyg., Camb.*, **87**: 93–100.

Lemcke, R. M., Shaw, E. J. and Marmion, B. P., 1965. Related antigens in *Mycoplasma pneumoniae* and *Mycoplasma mycoides* var. *mycoides*, *Aust. J. exp. Biol. med. Sci.*, **43**: 761–70.

Lindley, E. P., 1965. Experiments with an attenuated culture vaccine against contagious bovine pleuropneumonia, *Br. vet. J.*, **121**: 471–8.

Lindley, E. P., 1967a. Simultaneous vaccination of cattle with contagious bovine pleuropneumonia and goat-adapted rinderpest vaccine, *Bull. epiz. Dis. Afr.*, **15**: 221–6.

Lindley, E. P., 1967b. An immunity test in cattle to compare two contagious bovine pleuropneumonia vaccines, *Bull. epiz. Dis. Afr.*, **15**: 307–11.

Lindley, E. P., 1967c. Contagious bovine pleuropneumonia and the problems associated with its control, *J. Am. vet. med. Ass.*, **151**(12): 1810–15.

Lindley, E. P., 1971. Experience with a lyophilised contagious bovine pleuropneumonia vaccine in the Ivory Coast, *Trop. Anim. Hlth Prod.*, **3**: 32–42.

Lindley, E. P., 1973. Representation of the course of an outbreak of contagious bovine pleuro-pneumonia in a sedentary herd of humpless cattle, *Bull. epiz. Dis. Afr.*, **21**: 389–92.

Lindley, E. P., 1979. Control of contagious bovine pleuropneumonia with special reference to the Central African Empire, *Wld Anim. Rev.*, **30**: 18–22.

Lindley, E. P. and Abdulla, A. E. D., 1969. Some notes on the host specificity of the etiological agents of contagious caprine pleuropneumonia and contagious bovine pleuropneumonia, *Bull. epiz. Dis. Afr.*, **17**: 153–8.

Littlejohns, I. R. and Cottew, G. S., 1977. The isolation and identification of *Mycoplasma mycoides* subsp. *capri* from goats in Australia, *Aust. vet. J.*, **53**: 297–8.

Lloyd, L. C., 1966. Tissue necrosis produced by *Mycoplasma mycoides* in intraperitoneal diffusion chambers, *J. Path. Bact.*, **92**: 225–9.

Lloyd, L. C., 1967. An attempt to transfer immunity to *Mycoplasma mycoides* infection with serum, *Bull. epiz. Dis. Afr.*, **15**: 11–17.

Lloyd, L. C., 1969. Contagious bovine pleuropneumonia aspects of eradication in Australia, *Bull. Off. int. Epiz.*, **71**(11–12): 1329–34.

Lloyd, L. C., Piercy, D. W. T. and Bingley, J. B., 1975. Changes in fibrinogen levels, platelet counts, clotting times and fibrinolytic activity in relation to thrombosis in contagious bovine pleuropneumonia, *J. Comp. Path.*, **85**: 583–95.

Lobry, M. A., 1964. A review of recent publications on contagious bovine pleuropneumonia, *Bull. epiz. Dis. Afr.*, **12**: 209–17.

Lobry, M. A., 1973. The expert panel on contagious bovine pleuropneumonia and its role in the control of the disease, *Trop. Anim. Hlth Prod.*, **5**: 46–51.

Lwebandiza, T. S., 1969. Contagious bovine pleuropneumonia in Tanzania, *Bull. Off. int. Epiz.*, **72**: 71–8.

Macadam, I., Ezebuiro, E. O. and Oreffo, V. O. C., 1964. The response of zebu cattle to mixed contagious bovine pleuro-pneumonia and tissue culture rinderpest vaccines, *Bull. epiz. Dis. Afr.*, **12**: 237–40.

MacOwan, K. J., 1976. A mycoplasma from chronic caprine pleuropneumonia in Kenya, *Trop. Anim. Hlth Prod.*, **8**: 28–36.

MacOwan, K. J. and Minette, J. E., 1976. A mycoplasma from acute contagious caprine pleuropneumonia in Kenya, *Trop. Anim. Hlth Prod.*, **8**: 91–5.

MacOwan, K. J. and Minette, J. E., 1977. The role of mycoplasma strain F38 in contagious caprine pleuropneumonia (CCPP) in Kenya, *Vet. Rec.*, **101**(19): 380–1.

Masiga, W. N., 1972. Achievements of OAU/STRC CP 16 project, *Bull. epiz. Dis. Afr.*, **20**: 5–11.

Masiga, W. N. and Boarer, C. D. H., 1973. *In vivo* and *in vitro* studies with T_1 strain of *Mycoplasma mycoides* in cattle, *Res. vet. Sci.*, **14**: 180–6.

Masiga, W. N. and Mugera, G. M., 1973. Fate of the T_1 strain of *Mycoplasma mycoides* in cattle following vaccination, *J. Comp. Path.*, **83**: 473–9.

Masiga, W. N. and Read, W. C. S., 1972. Comparative susceptibility of *Bos indicus* and *Bos taurus* to contagious bovine pleuropneumonia, and the efficacy of the T_1 broth culture vaccine, *Vet. Rec.*, **90**: 499–502.

Masiga, W. N., Roberts, D. H., Kakoma, I. and Rurangirwa, F. R., 1975. Passive immunity to contagious bovine pleuropneumonia, *Res. vet. Sci.*, **19**: 330–2.

Masiga, W. N. and Stone, S. S., 1968a. Application of a fluorescent-antibody technique for the detection of *Mycoplasma mycoides* antigen and antibody, *J. Bact.*, **96**(5): 1867–9.

Masiga, W. N. and Stone, S. S., 1968b. Fluorescent antibody and agar gel diffusion techniques to detect *Mycoplasma mycoides* in fresh and formalin-fixed lung lesions of cattle, *Bull. epiz. Dis. Afr.*, **16**: 399–424.

Masiga, W. N. and Windsor, R. S., 1975. Immunity to contagious bovine pleuropneumonia, *Vet. Rec.*, **97**: 350–1.

Masiga, W. N. and Windsor, R. S., 1978. Some evidence of an age susceptibility to contagious bovine pleuropneumonia, *Res. vet. Sci.*, **24**: 328–33.

McIntosh, K. S., 1969. Progress towards eradication of contagious bovine pleuropneumonia from Australia, *Bull. Off. int. Epiz.*, **72**: 25–34.

McMartin, D. A., MacOwan, K. J. and Swift, L. L., 1980. A century of classical contagious caprine pleuropneumonia: from original description to aetiology, *Br. vet. J.*, **136**: 507–15.

Mendes, A. M., 1957. A dead vaccine against bovine pleuropneumonia, *Bull. epiz. Dis. Afr.*, **5**: 175–6.

Minor, R., 1967. Observations on the use of T_1 broth culture vaccine in the control of contagious bovine pleuropneumonia, *Bull. epiz. Dis. Afr.*, **15**: 115–19.

Nasri, M. E., 1966. The virulence and protective properties of cultures from single colonies of *Mycoplasma mycoides* and *Mycoplasma capri*, *Vet. Rec.*, **78**(7): 232–6.

Ojo, M. O., 1973. Isolation of 2 strains of *Mycoplasma* serologically closely related to *Mycoplasma mycoides* var. *mycoides* from pneumonic lungs of goats, *Bull. epiz. Dis. Afr.*, **21**: 319–23.

Ojo, M. O., 1976. Caprine pneumonia IV: pathogenicity of *Mycoplasma mycoides* subsp. *capri* and caprine strains of *Mycoplasma mycoides* subsp. *mycoides* for goats, *J. Comp. Path.*, **86**: 519.

Ojo, M. O., 1977. Caprine pneumonia, *Vet. Bull.*, **47**(8): 573–8.

Ojo, M. O., 1982. Contagious caprine pleuropneumonia in Africa, *Proc. Int. Conf. on Goat Reproduction and Disease*, pp. 209–11.

Ojo, M. O., Kasali, O. B. and Ozoya., S. E., 1980. Pathogenicity of a caprine strain of *Mycoplasma mycoides* subsp. *mycoides* for cattle, *J. Comp. Path.*, **90**: 209–15.

Onoviran, O., 1972. Immunity in contagious caprine pleuropneumonia, *Res. vet. Sci.*, **13**: 599–600.

Onoviran, O., 1974. The comparative efficacy of some antibiotics used to treat experimentally induced mycoplasma infection in goats, *Vet. Rec.*, **94**: 418–20.

Onoviran, O. and Taylor-Robinson, D., 1979. Detection of antibody against *Mycoplasma mycoides* subsp. *mycoides* in cattle by an enzyme-linked immunosorbent assay, *Vet. Rec.*, **105**: 165–7.

Osiyemi, T. I. O., 1981. The eradication of contagious bovine pleuropneumonia in Nigeria: prospects and problems, *Bull. Anim. Hlth Prod. Afr.*, **29**: 95–8.

Otte, E. and Peck, E. F., 1960. Observations on an outbreak of a contagious pleuropneumonia in goats in Ethiopia, *Bull. epiz. Dis. Afr.*, **8**: 131–40.

Paling, R. W., MacOwan, K. J. and Karstad, L., 1978. The prevalence of antibody to contagious caprine pleuropneumonia (mycoplasma strain F38) in some wild herbivores and camels in Kenya, *J. Wildl. Dis.*, **14**: 305–8.

Palmer, R. F. and Gourlay, R. N., 1964. Lyophilisation of *Mycoplasma mycoides* culture vaccine, *Bull. epiz. Dis. Africa.*, **12**: 397–400.

Pearson, C. W. and Lloyd, L. C., 1971. Freeze-drying of the KH_3J vaccine strain of *Mycoplasma mycoides*, *Bull. epiz. Dis. Afr.*, **19**: 117–22.

Pearson, C. W. and Lloyd, L. C., 1972. Immunoglobulins of cattle affected by contagious bovine pleuropneumonia, *Res. vet. Sci.*, **13**(3): 230–5.

Pearson, J. E., Rokey, N. W., Harrington, R., Proctor, S. J. and Cassidy, D. R., 1972. Contagious caprine pleuropneumonia in Arizona, *J. Am. vet. med. Ass.*, **161**(11): 1536–8.

Pierce, A. E., 1969. Progress in the campaign to eradicate contagious bovine pleuropneumonia from Australia, *Bull. Off. int. Epiz.*, **71**(11–12): 1313–28.

Piercy, D. W., 1970a. Anaphylaxis in young calves inoculated with heat-inactivated *Mycoplasma mycoides*, *Res. vet. Sci.*, **11**: 481–3.

Piercy, D. W., 1970b. Synovitis induced by intra-articular inoculation of inactivated *Mycoplasma mycoides* in calves, *J. Comp. Path.*, **80**: 549–60.

Piercy, D. W. and Bingley, J. B., 1972. Fibrinous synovitis in calves inoculated with killed *Mycoplasma mycoides*, *J. Comp. Path.*, **82**: 279–90.

Piercy, S. E. and Knight, G. J., 1957. Studies with avianised strains of the organisms of contagious bovine pleuropneumonia. IV. The preparation, titration and challenge of avianised bovine pleuropneumonia vaccines, *Bull. epiz. Dis. Afr.*, **5**: 161–73.

Piercy, S. E. and Knight, G. J., 1958. Studies with avianised strains of the organism of contagious bovine pleuropneumonia. V. Experiments with avianised vaccines at various levels of attenuation, *Br. vet. J.*, **114**: 245–53.

Priestley, F. W., 1952. Observations on immunity to contagious bovine pleuropneumonia, with special reference to the bactericidal action of blood, *Br. vet. J.*, **108**: 153–61.

Priestley, F. W., 1955. Immunisation against contagious bovine pleuropneumonia with special reference to the use of a dried vaccine, *J. Comp. Path.*, **65**: 168–82.

Priestley, F. W. and Dafaalla, E. N., 1957. Immunisation against contagious bovine pleuropneumonia using dried organisms and adjuvant, *Bull. epiz. Dis Afr.*, **5**: 177–86.

Provost, A., 1967. Recherches enterprises sur la péripneumonie contagieuse des bovidés au Laboratoire de Recherches Vétérinaires de Farcha, Fort-Lamy, Tchad, de 1964 à 1966, *Bull. Off. int. Epiz.*, **67**(1–2): 199–246.

Provost, A., 1969. Principes de production d'un vaccin mixte associe antibovipestique–antipéripneumonique inoculé en seul temps, *Bull. epiz. Dis. Afr.*, **17**: 7–10.

Provost, A., 1972. Adaption sur plaques de la réaction de fixation du complément pour la péripneumonie. Application à la decentralisation du diagnostic, *Bull. epiz. Dis. Afr.*, **20**: 13–22.

Provost, A., Borredon, C. and Queval, R., 1969. Recherches immunoliques sur la péripneumonie. XI. Un vaccin vivant mixte antibovipestique antipéripneumonique inoculé en un seul temps. Conception – production – contrôles, *Bull. Off. int. Epiz.*, **72**: 165–203.

Provost, A., Perreau, P. and Queval, R., 1963. Essais de vaccination antipéripneumonique a l'aide de corps microbiens lyses-echec, *Bull. epiz. Dis. Afr.*, **11**: 375–80.

Provost, A., Villemot, J. M. and Queval, R., 1959. Immunological research on pleuropneumonia. VII. Immunisation with a live avianised vaccine inoculated into the muzzle, *Rev. Elev. Méd. vét. Pays trop.*, **12**: 381–404.

Rao, C. K., 1969. Contagious bovine pleuropneumonia in India, *Bull. Off. int. Epiz.*, **71**(11–12): 1309–12.

Razin, S., 1981. Mycoplasmas: the smallest pathogenic procaryotes, *Isr. J. Med. Sci.*, **17**: 510–15.

Revell, S. G., 1973. Local reactions following CBPP vaccination in Zambia, *Trop. Anim. Hlth Prod.*, **5**: 246–52.

Roberts, D. H. and Windsor, R. S., 1974. Attempts to differentiate *Mycoplasma mycoides* var. *mycoides* immune cattle from susceptible cattle, *Res. vet. Sci.*, **17**: 403–5.

Roberts, D. H., Windsor, R. S., Masiga, W. N. and Kariavu, C. G., 1973. Cell-mediated immune response in cattle to *Mycoplasma mycoides* var. *mycoides*, *Infect. Immun.*, **8**(3): 349–54.

Rodwell, A. W., 1982. The protein fingerprints of mycoplasmas, *Rev. Infect. Dis.*, **4**, suppl.: S8–S17.

Rodwell, A. W. and Rodwell, E. S., 1978. Relationship between strains of *Mycoplasma mycoides* subsp. *mycoides* and *capri* studied by two-dimensional gel electrophoresis of cell proteins, *J. gen. Microbiol.*, **109**: 259–63.

Rosendal, C., 1981. Experimental infection of goats, sheep and calves with the large colony type of *Mycoplasma mycoides* subsp. *mycoides*, *Vet. Pathol.*, **18**: 71–81.

Rurangirwa, F. R., 1976. Single reverse radial immunodiffusion of sera from cattle after exposure to *Mycoplasma mycoides* var. *mycoides*, *J. Comp. Path.*, **86**: 45–50.

Rurangirwa, F. R., Masiga, W. N. and Mtui, B., 1976. An anamnestic response to challenge with virulent *Mycoplasma mycoides* subsp. *mycoides* of cattle immune to contagious bovine pleuropneumonia, *J. Comp. Path.*, **36**: 381–6.

Rurangirwa, F. R., Masiga, W. N. and Muthomi, E., 1981. Immunity to contagious caprine pleuropneumonia caused by F-38 strain of mycoplasma, *Vet. Rec.*, **109**: 310.

Santiago Duarte, V. M., 1969. La péripneumonie contagieuse des bovins en Angola, *Bull. Off. int. Epiz.*, **72**: 89–94.

Scudamore, J. M., 1975. Evaluation of the field complement fixation test in the diagnosis and control of contagious bovine

pleuropneumonia, *Trop. Anim, Hlth Prod.*, **7**: 73–9.
Scudamore, J. M., 1976. Observations on the epidemiology of contagious bovine pleuropneumonia: *Mycoplasma mycoides* in urine, *Res. vet. Sci.*, **20**: 330–3.
Sharma, G. L., Bhalla, N. P. and Negi, M. S., 1965. Studies on the development of avianised contagious caprine pleuropneumonia vaccine. I. Adaptation of virulent contagious caprine pleuropneumonia organism (*Mycoplasma caprae*) to grow in developing chick embryo and its influence on the virulence of the organism, *Indian J. vet. Sci.*, **35**: 355–7.
Sharma, S. N. and Vyas, C. B., 1975. A note on electrophoretic pattern of serum protein fraction in contagious caprine pleuro-pneumonia, *Indian vet. J.*, **52**: 158.
Sheriff, D. and Piercy, S. E., 1952. Experiments with an avianised strain of the organism of contagious bovine pleuropneumonia, *Vet. Rec.*, **64**(42): 615–21.
Shifrine, M., Bailey, K. P. and Stone, S. S., 1972. Contagious bovine pleuropneumonia: isolation of *Mycoplasma mycoides* var. *mycoides* from ticks collected from infected cattle and infection attempts using these ticks, *Bull. epiz. Dis. Afr.*, special issue: pp. 43–5.
Shifrine, M. and Beech, J., 1968. Preliminary studies on living culture and inactivated vaccines against contagious bovine pleuropneumonia, *Bull. epiz. Dis. Afr.*, **16**: 47–52.
Shifrine, M. and Domermuth, C. H., 1967. A contagious bovine pleuropneumonia in wildlife, *Bull. epiz. Dis. Afr.*, **15**: 319–22.
Shifrine, M. and Gourlay, R. N., 1965. The immediate type allergic skin reaction in contagious bovine pleuropneumonia, *J. Comp. Path.*, **75**: 381–5.
Shifrine, M. and Gourlay, R. N., 1967. Evaluation of diagnostic tests for contagious bovine pleuropneumonia, *Bull. epiz. Dis. Afr.*, **15**: 7–10.
Shifrine, M. and Moulton, J. E., 1968. Infection of cattle with *Mycoplasma mycoides* by nasal instillation, *J. Comp. Path.*, **78**: 383–6.
Shifrine, M., Stone, S. S. and Davis, G., 1968. Contagious bovine pleuropneumonia: serologic response of cattle after single and double vaccination with T_1 culture vaccine, *Rev. Elev. Méd. vét. Pays trop.*, **21**(1): 49–58.
Shifrine, M., Stone, S. S. and Staak, C., 1970. Contagious bovine pleuropneumonia in African buffalo (*Syncerus caffer*), *Bull. epiz. Dis. Afr.*, **18**: 201–5.
Smith, G. R., 1965. Infection of small laboratory animals with *Mycoplasma mycoides* var. *capri* and *Mycoplasma mycoides* var. *mycoides*, *Vet. Rec.*, **77**(50): 1527–8.
Smith, G. R., 1967. Experimental infection of mice with *Mycoplasma mycoides* var. *capri*, *J. Comp. Path.*, **77**: 21–7.
Smith, G. R. and Oliphant, J. C., 1981a. The ability of *Mycoplasma mycoides* subspecies *mycoides* and closely related strains from goats and sheep to immunize mice against subspecies *capri*, *J. Hyg., Camb.*, **87**: 321–9.

Smith, G. R. and Oliphant, J. C., 1981b. Observations on the antigenic differences between the so-called SC and LC strains of *Mycoplasma mycoides* subsp. *mycoides*, *J. Hyg., Camb.*, **87**: 437–42.

Solana, P. and Rivera, E., 1967. Infection of goats in Mexico by *Mycoplasma mycoides* var. *capri*, *Ann. N.Y. Acad. Sci.*, **143**(1): 357–63.

Stone, S. S., 1969. Comparison of bovine serum and colostral antibody: effect of colostral antibody on vaccination of calves for contagious bovine pleuropneumonia, *Bull. Off. int. Epiz.*, **72**: 131–46.

Stone, S. S., 1970. Comparison of bovine serum and colostral antibody: effect of colostral antibody on vaccination of calves for contagious bovine pleuropneumonia, *Immunology*, **18**: 369–77.

Stone, S. S. and Bygrave, A. C., 1969. Contagious bovine pleuropneumonia: comparison of serological tests and post-mortem observations in cattle with resolving lung lesions, *Bull. epiz. Dis. Afr.*, **17**: 11–19.

Stone, S. S., Masiga, W. N. and Read, W. C. S., 1969. *Mycoplasma mycoides* transplacental transfer in cattle, *Res. vet. Sci.*, 368–72.

Stone, S. S. and Razin, S., 1973. Immunoelectrophoretic analysis of *Mycoplasma mycoides* var. *mycoides*, *Infect. Immun.*, **7**(6): 922–30.

Stone, S. S. and Shifrine, M., 1968. Comparative studies of antigens from *Mycoplasma mycoides* and *Escherichia coli*, *J. Bacteriol.*, **95**(4): 1254–9.

Stone, S. S. and Yedloutschnig, R. J., 1973. Immunoelectrophoretic comparison of *Mycoplasma mycoides* isolated from cattle and goats with four mycoplasmas isolated from goats in the United States, *Ann. N.Y. Acad. Sci.*, **225**: 382–94.

Tessler, J. and Yedloutschnig, R. J., 1972. Immunofluorescence for identifying *Mycoplasma mycoides* var. *mycoides* and *M. mycoides* var. *capri* strains, *Can. J. comp. Med.*, **36**: 403–5.

Thigpen, J. E., Kornegay, R. W., Chang, J., McGhee, C. E. and Thierry, V. L., 1981. Pneumonia in goats caused by *Mycoplasma mycoides* subspecies *mycoides*, *J. Am. vet. med. Ass.*, **178**(7): 711–12.

Trethewie, E. R. and Turner, A. W., 1961. Preventative tail-tip inoculation of calves against bovine contagious pleuropneumonia. II. Vegetative endocarditis (valvulitis) and myocarditis sequelae to post-inoculation arthritis, *Aust. vet. J.*, **37**: 27–36.

Tully, J. G., Barile, M. F., Edward, D. G. ff., Theodore, T. S. and Erno., H., 1974. Characterization of some caprine mycoplasmas, with proposals for new species, *Mycoplasma capricolum* and *Mycoplasma putrefaciens*, *J. gen. Microbiol.*, **85**: 102–20.

Tully, J. G. and Whitcomb, R. F. (eds), 1979. *The Mycoplasmas.* Academic Press (London and New York).

Turner, A. W., 1961. Preventative tail-tip inoculation of calves against bovine contagious pleuropneumonia. III. Immunity in relationship to age at inoculation, *Aust. vet. J.*, **37**: 259–64.

Turner, A. W., 1964. The significance of positive complement fixation reactions in immune cattle after exposure to pleuropneumonia, *Aust. vet. J.*, **40**: 345–8.

Turner, A. W. and Etheridge, J. R., 1963. Slide agglutination tests in the diagnosis of contagious bovine pleuropneumonia, *Aust. vet. J.*, **39**: 445–51.

Turner, A. W. and Trethewie, E. R., 1961. Preventative tail-tip inoculation of calves against bovine contagious pleuropneumonia. I. Influence of age at inoculation upon tail reactions, serological responses, and the incidence of swollen joints, *Aust. vet. J.*, **37**: 1–8.

Windsor, R. S., 1978. An investigation into the viability of broth cultures of the T_1 strain of *Mycoplasma mycoides* subspecies *mycoides*, *Res. vet. Sci.*, **24**: 109–12.

Windsor, R. S. and Boarer, C. D. H., 1973. A new intradermal test antigen for the diagnosis of contagious bovine pleuropneumonia, *Res. vet. Sci.*, **15**: 125–8.

Windsor, R. S. and Masiga, W. N., 1972. The efficacy of T_1 strain broth vaccine against contagious bovine pleuropneumonia, *Vet. Rec.*, **90**: 2–5.

Windsor, R. S. and Masiga, W. N., 1976. The effect of postvaccinal treatment with the antibiotic tylosin on the immunity produced by the T_1 strain of *Mycoplasma mycoides* subspecies *mycoides*, *J. Comp. Path.*, **86**: 173–81.

Windsor, R. S. and Masiga, W. N., 1977. Investigations into the epidemiology of contagious bovine pleuropneumonia: the persistence of *Mycoplasma mycoides* sub-species *mycoides* in placenta, urine and hay, *Bull. Anim. Hlth Prod.*, **25**: 357–70.

Yedloutschnig, R. J., 1982. Regulatory aspects of caprine mycoplasmosis, *Proc. Int. Conf. on Goat Production and Disease*, pp. 217–18.

Yedloutschnig, R. J. and Dardiri, A. H., 1976. Experimental infection of white-tailed deer with *Mycoplasma mycoides* var. *mycoides*, *Proc. 80th Ann. Meet. US Anim. Hlth Assoc.*, **80**: 262–7.

Yedloutschnig, R. J., Taylor, W. D. and Dardiri, A. H., 1971. Isolation of *Mycoplasma mycoides* var. *capri* from goats in the United States, *Proc. 75th Ann. Meet. US Anim. Hlth. Assoc.*, pp. 166–75.

Zaki Abdel Hai, H., 1969. Contagious bovine pleuropneumonia in U.A.R, *Bull. Off. int. Epiz.*, **72**: 55–9.

Chapter

17

Dermatophilosis

CONTENTS

INTRODUCTION

Dermatophilosis is either an acute or chronic bacterial disease caused by *Dermatophilus congolensis* and is characterized by infections of the epidermis resulting in an exudative dermatitis. In the tropics, syndromes are most prevalent in cattle and sheep and, to a lesser extent, in horses, donkeys, goats, pigs, wild animals, and man. Dermatophilosis is known by a variety of names, the most common of which are lumpy wool disease, mycotic dermatitis, and cutaneous streptothricosis. The latter term is used in cattle and is applied to the severe syndrome observed in Africa and other tropical regions. Syndromes in cattle and sheep in the tropics will be discussed in this chapter.

Literature

An early account of the occurrence of dermatophilosis in cattle, known locally as Senkobo skin disease, in South Africa was presented by Schulz (1955). Comprehensive reviews of dermatophilosis as a skin condition of animals throughout the world was published by Stewart (1972a, b). More recently, a monograph edited by Lloyd and Sellers was published in 1976 on the dermatophilus infections of animals and man.

ETIOLOGY

Dermatophilus congolensis is Gram-positive, pleomorphic, and appears in culture as filamentous hyphae and spore-like cocci, the zoospores. The branching hyphae septate both transversely and longitudinally to form the flagellated cocci from 0.5 to 1.1 μm in diameter. These motile cocci are infective and develop rapidly in the skin to form hyphae. The organism grows best on blood agar plates at 37 °C in an atmosphere of 10 to 20% CO_2. Because colony formation is slow, isolation of colonies may be difficult because of overgrowth by other contaminating organisms. The colony morphology and color vary considerably, depending on the pigment in the zoospores. Colonies are either orange yellow or whitish, depending on the composition of the culture media and to some degree on the strain.

Classification of *D. congolensis* has been difficult and initially it was considered to be a fungus.

Literature

Classification and nomenclature of *D. congolensis* isolated from the various clinical syndromes was reviewed by Austwick (1958). More than one species were considered to be involved in the different clinical syndromes in various species of domestic animals. *Dermatophilus congolensis* was thought to be responsible for the cutaneous dermatophilus of cattle, while *D. dermatonomus* and *D. pedis* were considered to be species responsible for mycotic dermatitis and strawberry foot rot of sheep and goats. The three species were grouped in the family Dermatophilaceae of the order Actinomycetales. Evidence that these isolates responsible for the various syndromes should be regarded as a single species in the genus was presented by Abu-Samra (1978b, 1980). *Dermatophilus congolensis* had many characteristics of the *Actinomycetales* and morphologically was similar to *Geodermatophilus*, a soil-dwelling microorganism (Gordon 1976).

The culture, biochemical characteristics, antigenicity, and pathogenic properties of the organism have been compared (Mémery 1961; Plowright 1958; Vigier and Balis 1967; Meyer 1971). Growth characteristics, hemolytic activity and other features of isolates from bovine, equine, ovine, and caprine dermatophilosis from temperate and tropical regions were also studied (Abu-Samra 1978a; Macadam and Haalstra 1971). Various behavioral properties of strains from different hosts were closely related but not identical, and the minor differences observed were not related to a host species (El-Nageh 1971) nor were they sufficiently constant to be considered in speciation or in identifying an isolate as being of a particular strain type (Abu-Samra 1978a).

In addition to organisms found on the skin and soil which often overgrew *D. congolensis* in culture, *Bacillus pumilus* also actively inhibited the growth of *D. congolensis* (Ojo 1975).

Factors which influenced the cycle in cultures were similar to those which played a role in determining invasiveness, infectivity, and pathogenicity (Roberts 1961). Carbon dioxide affected the growth and sporulation in culture, and similarly the different rate of CO_2 diffusion at various depths in sheepskin stimulated the germination of the zoospores and invasion by the hyphae of the epidermis. Sporulation was also under the influence of CO_2 content of the infected tissues (Roberts 1963a). Oxygen requirements of various strains have been investigated (da Cruz 1975a, b).

EPIZOOTIOLOGY

Geographic distribution and incidence

Dermatophilosis is worldwide, but the most severe clinical syndromes occur in the tropics with the heaviest economic losses in sheep and cattle. The incidence and severity of disease is related to periods of heavy rainfall. Intercurrent diseases also predispose animals to development of dermatophilosis. Severe forms of disease in cattle occur in Africa where dermatophilosis is of major economic importance, particularly in those programs where exotic breeds are introduced to improve indigenous stock. In other tropical regions, for example Australia, it is of primary importance in sheep. The incidence and severity of clinical syndromes and the resulting economic losses depend on geographical distribution, being particularly devastating under certain husbandry practices. Losses occur in production of hides, beef, and milk, as well as through the high mortality in introduced exotic breeds.

Literature

The economic aspects of bovine dermatophilosis in livestock in East Africa was summarized by Bwangamoi (1976b). The incidence in cattle, goats, and sheep was presented and ranged from below 1 to 16% with the highest frequency being observed in cattle, then in goats, and lowest in sheep (Bwangamoi 1976a). A report on incidences in Ruanda and Burundi was presented by Braibant (1962). A short review of the various factors which play significant roles in the epizootiology and pathogenesis of *D. congolense* infections was presented by Abu-Samra (1980). The various aspects of dermatophilosis in Africa, including epizootiology and treatment, were summarized by Vandemaele (1961).

The economic importance of dermatophilosis of cattle and sheep in the hide and wool trade in Australia and Africa has been considered (Roberts and Vallely 1962). In a review of the economic importance of dermatophilosis in cattle, loss in meat and milk production was observed in moderate and severe forms of the disease and resulted from emaciation, debility, and mortality. The most devasting effects were observed in imported breeds and in the crosses with indigenous cattle, where in many instances the severity of the disease prevented the raising of these types of cattle (Lloyd 1976).

In Nigeria, the incidence of bovine dermatophilosis was seasonal, varying from 5 to 10% (Bida and Dennis 1976; Kurtze 1964; Lloyd 1976). An incidence of 5 to 6% occurred during the rainy season and 2 to 4% during the dry season (Oduye 1975). In the northern states the incidence was from 3 to 15%, with an average of about 11% which varied considerably from one district to another and between herds (Oduye and Lloyd 1971). In another study in northern Nigeria, disease was observed during the wet season in about 78% of the herds and affected approximately 12% of the animals (Kelley and Bida 1970). Severity of clinical signs and incidence of disease were related to climate, type of husbandry, and external parasitic infections (Oduye 1976a).

From other parts of Africa there has been less information on the incidence and economic importance of dermatophilosis. In some districts of the Sudan the incidence in cattle was 0.25 to 0.84% (Obeid 1976). In Ghana, an incidence of approximately 5% was reported during the dry season and this varied from 5 to 35% during the rainy season (Oppong 1973). In another report the incidence was 4.8% in the dry season and 12.8% in the wet season (Oppong 1976). In The Gambia the prevalence and chemotherapy of dematophilosis in sheep confined to the haired parts of the body was reported by Macadam (1976). In the Congo, dermatophilosis occurred in both cattle and horses (Balabanov and Boussafou 1977; Bugyaki 1959).

Moreira *et al.* (1974) reviewed the information available from various countries in South America and concluded that the disease in cattle, horses, sheep and goats was of economic importance and that the incidence was affected by husbandry and age. The disease was first reported in 1959 from Uruguay (Moreira and Barbosa 1976). The limited number of reports on dermatophilosis in horses, cattle, and sheep available from South America did not give a true picture of the distribution, severity, and importance of the various syndromes (Londero 1976). The condition in Brazil was first diagnosed by Barbosa *et al.* (1967). In cattle in Argentina the incidence was 20% with a mortality of 3% (Gallo *et al.* 1973).

In other tropical parts of the world, bovine dermatophilosis is generally of considerably less importance. In the Mediterranean countries, dermatophilosis in cattle was considered to be a relatively benign disease and outbreaks could be associated with a 20% drop in milk production (Nobel *et al.* 1976). However, severe clinical syndromes have been occasionally reported. Dermatophilosis was first diagnosed in the USA in 1961 (Kelley 1976). Isolation of *D. congolensis* was reported from about 11% of the skin samples presented for diagnosis (Jarnagin and Thoen 1977). The occurence of mild forms probably meant that the incidence was higher than that reported in the literature.

Transmission

Infection occurs in carrier animals either without any clinical manifestations or with lesions that are so mild that they are not readily detected. Based on field observations, clinically demonstrable lesions are usually associated with wet climatic conditions. The abundance of flies and ticks during this season are also important in transmission of infection and development of severe lesions. The disease in cattle is not contagious by contact. The role of humidity in transmission is not defined, but conditions resulting in wet skin appear to be significant in establishing infections. Infective zoospores are resistant to desiccation and remain viable in the scabs. Once the scab is wet, motile zoospores are released in large numbers.

Literature

Fifty percent of Tourine of Zebu cattle in Chad were reported to be healthy carriers of *D. congolensis* (Graber 1969). Organisms were not found in soil, but samples contaminated by scab material were infective for 4 months (Roberts 1963b). The nutrient requirements and environmental factors necessary for transmission of zoospores were determined. Infective motile zoospores in wet scabs did not survive well in the environment and the viability was highest during the first few hours after release from the hyphae (Roberts 1963b, c).

Although flies and humidity have been suspected to play a role in development of natural lesions of dermatophilosis in cattle, experimental investigations have on occasion not been conclusive (Macadam 1964a). Humidity did not appear to be a factor in the spread of the lesions but the biting insects were considered important in initiating the skin lesions (Macadam 1964b). A relationship between rainfall and dermatophilosis of sheep has also been proposed, and under favorable conditions infections were highly contagious (Austwick 1976). An association between tick infestation and development of clinical bovine dermatophilosis was made (Plowright 1956). Infection could be transmitted from cattle to rabbits by *A. variegatum* and the lesions were similar to those produced by other experimental methods. On ears of cattle a localized lesion could be produced by tick bite and application of cultures of *D. congolensis* (Macadam 1962). *Musca* and *Stomoxys* species of flies did not efficiently transmit infection even after the sebaceous barrier was removed from the skin by washing and swabbing with methyl alcohol. It was suggested that a challenge by larger numbers of organisms was required (Philpott and Ezeh 1978; Richard and Pier 1966).

INFECTION

Dermatophilus congolensis causes infections in many species of animals and man. Susceptibility to infection is governed by the environmental conditions. In cattle, breed differences, length of hair coat, age, skin thickness, plane of nutrition , and intercurrent diseases are considered to have a role in enabling infections to establish and to develop into syndromes of various severities. The N'Dama and Muturu breeds indigenous to West Africa are resistant, but exotic cattle and crosses with local breeds are very susceptible and all age groups are affected.

The organism invades the skin and induces infection only when this tissue is either injured or compromised in some way. It is difficult to reproduce experimentally the typical naturally occurring clinical syndrome characterized by extensive exudative lesions spreading over large areas of the body. Experimental infections result in localized nonspreading, self-limiting lesions. The pathogenesis of the natural fulminating infections is not determined but probably involves factors, both local and systemic, which compromise the resistance of the epidermis to infection. In the skin the stratum corneum is important in defense against invading organisms. The natural protective barriers of the epidermis also include hair or wool and a film of sebaceous wax which have to be overcome by the organisms to cause infection. Prolonged wetting and trauma disrupts these barriers and enables the organism to multiply and invade tissues. Growth of the organism occurs between the cells of the epidermis and does not invade the dermis.

Literature

Dermatophilus congolensis has been recognized to have a remarkably wide and diverse host range which included lower primates, man, and lizards (Kaplan 1976; Roberts 1965b). Disruption of the protective mechanisms of the skin predisposed the various animal species to infection (Lloyd *et al.* 1979).

Comprehensive investigation on infectivity was undertaken in sheep and laboratory animals by Roberts (1963d). This subject has been comprehensively reviewed by Lloyd (1984). Removal of the natural barriers consisting of greasy fleece and a film of sebaceous wax resulted in severe local infections following application of the organism. The organisms colonized the epidermis but did not attack either the keratin of the stratum corneum, hair, or wool, and did not penetrate into the dermis. Deeper invasion under the epidermis was inhibited by the inflammatory reaction which consisted of granulocytic accumulations beneath the infected epidermis. Beneath this protective inflammatory layer, the epidermis regenerated and was again reinfected by the hyphae extending from residual infections in hair follicles. This cycle of epidermal replacement and reinfection ended once infections in the follicles were eliminated. Chronic infections have been associated with persistence of organisms in the follicles (Roberts 1965b).

Variation in susceptibility has been associated with environmental and pasture conditions. Differences in resistance were expressed by incidences of infections in a herd, severity of the clinical syndrome, and occurrence of spontaneous recoveries. Considerable individual variability was observed between animals and was dependent on breed, degree of cross-breeding, particular blood lines, age, and sex (Blancou, 1976a, b). Crossbred cattle from Brahman bulls were considerably more susceptible than the indigenous stock found in Cameroon and Madagascar (Dumas *et al.* 1971).

Pathogenicity determinations and biochemical tests were undertaken on strains of *D. congolensis* isolated in the Sudan (Adlan and Obeid 1977). Growth of the hyphae and their penetration depended on CO_2 and nutrients in media. Hyphae invaded the epidermis by exerting a chemical force but production of toxins was not demonstrated. The inflammatory reaction was attributed to the mechanical tissue damage caused by the hyphae (Roberts 1965a). Resistance to infection depended on phagocytosis of zoospores by inflammatory cells (Roberts 1966b). Organisms were found in the hair follicle sheaths, hair papillae, and sebaceous glands, but were not found deeper than the basement membrane. If the basement membrane was not intact, infection of the dermis occurred. This structure was considered to be an important protective barrier preventing tissue invasion (Amakiri 1976).

The size and persistence of experimentally induced lesions in skin of cattle was dependent on the susceptibility of individual animals and the infectivity and virulence of a particular strain (Macadam 1961). Application of culture to scarified skin resulted in transient scab formation and resembled early stages of natural lesions. Local humidity, increased by application of local moist chambers or by frequent showers, enhanced the development of lesions and there was some evidence of spread (Chodnik 1956). Under other experimental conditions, high humidity was associated with healing of experimental lesions (Macadam 1961, 1970). These localized experimental infections in cattle and laboratory animals were characterized by spontaneous healing (Makinde and Ezeh 1981). Pathogenicity and virulence of strains was tested and isolates from equine dermatophilosis in Nigeria were identical bacteriologically and pathogenically to bovine strains. In horses, the typical 'paint brush' lesions were not very extensive (Macadam 1964c).

Infectivity and virulence of *D. congolensis* was discussed by Lloyd (1981) in the light of more recent information. Based on experimental work, environmental temperature and humidity were not thought to have a significant effect on the susceptibility of cattle. However, this did not exclude the possibility that under natural circumstances heavy rains could alter the microenvironment of the skin enabling both invasion and spread of organisms. Trauma of varying degrees of severity to the epidermis enabled extensive infection to occur. Severity of the experimental lesions used to demonstrate pathogenicity was dependent on methods by which the skin was prepared, which included removal of hair, application of solvents, and scarification. Resistance to infection was not related to the degree of trauma to the skin but appeared to be associated with an impermeable surface barrier, postulated to be hardening of the sebum in the follicles and between the superficial squames of the interfollicular regions. Microflora of the skin also influenced the ability of *D. congolensis* to become established and induce infections (Lloyd and McEwan Jenkinson 1980). In mice experimental lesions can be prevented by simultaneous application of staphylococci which produce antibiotics (Noble *et al.* 1980). Local experimental lesions in small numbers of cattle, goats, horses, sheep, rabbits, and pigs did not induce immunity, and infections could be reestablished at the same site (Macadam and Haalstra 1971). Inflammatory reaction to infection was not influenced by previous immunological response to antigen of *D. congolensis*.

Infections have been readily transmitted to both natural hosts and to many laboratory animals (Gordon 1976). Parenteral injection into rabbits and guinea pigs did not produce lesions. Subcutaneous infections caused localized abscesses which healed spontaneously (Chodnik 1956). Topical experimental induction of lesions in rabbits was comparable to the sequence of events observed in natural cases (Mémery and Mémery 1962). Lesions in rabbits were produced by clipping, washing, and scraping of the skin, and applying broth cultures. An acute ulcerative pustular dermatitis developed principally in the hair follicles and healing started within a week and spontaneous cure was completed by the second week (Gordon and Perrin 1971).

Following treatment with prednisolone trimethylacetate, mice could be infected intravenously, intraperitoneally, and by exposure of both intact and scarified skin to cultures. Subcutaneous and internal lesions were observed after parenteral administration. Application of culture to scarified skin resulted in scab formation over the entire traumatized area, while on unscarified skin only a localized lesion developed (Abu-Samra 1978c). In white mice, subcutaneous nodules 5 to 10 mm in diameter were caused by injection of organisms containing coccoid forms (Vanbreuseghem *et al.* 1976). Based on experimental procedure in rabbits in which nitrogen mustard was used to deplete granulocytes, it was concluded that control of local infection was dependent on the presence of circulating polymorphonuclear cells which were responsible for infiltrating into the local lesion. Resistance was due to phagocytosis of the zoospores during the first 3 hours after infection and to the layer of granulocytes which formed beneath the scarified skin which the hyphae could not penetrate. Granulocytes were responsible for restricting the lesion to the epidermis and limiting the growth of organisms within the epidermis. Other components of the inflammatory process did not inhibit multiplication and spread of organisms (Roberts 1965c). Delayed hypersensitivity to the organism accelerated the neutrophil response but did not appear directly to affect hyphal invasion (Roberts 1966a).

CLINICAL SIGNS

Clinical signs in cattle vary in severity according to the site and extent of skin lesions. In some outbreaks, sites of predilection occur and involve either the neck, dewlap, body and lower extremities, or are found around muzzle, face, udder, and tail. Unless large areas of the skin are affected or the lesions affect the feet, udder, or eyes, the systemic clinical signs are minimal. Lameness, emaciation, and debility result from extensive lesions particularly of the feet, mouth, and eyes. Syndromes last from 15 days to many months. Severe chronic forms in cattle are often complicated by other local and systemic infections and their role in pathogenesis has not been defined. When lesions are mild they recede spontaneously. The incubation period varies from a few days to weeks and often cannot be determined under field conditions. The 'paint brush' lesions, consisting of focal matting of hair by exudate, appear early and the tufts at first firmly adhere to the underlying skin, but later can be readily removed leaving a pinkish raw moist surface covered by grayish exudate and hemorrhage. During the early stages of the disease there is no systemic effect accompanying the skin lesions. Well-established clinical disease is characterized by chronic exudative dermatitis with accumulation of crusts. Lesions range from a small, nodule-like formations to large patches, and in advanced cases whole regions of the body are covered by hard crusts. In cases which terminate in death, the entire body may be covered. Lesions around the mouth, ears, and the perineal region may resemble papillomas.

In sheep, lesions are variable in severity and depend largely on climate, pathogenicity of the strain of organism, and to some degree on the geographic locality. Three clinical syndromes are identified and include mycotic dermatitis, also known as lumpy wool disease, affecting the wool-covered regions of the body; a dermatitis affecting primarily ears, commisures of lips and the nose; and a condition affecting the legs and known as strawberry foot rot.

Literature

Descriptions of severe forms of dermatophilosis in cattle occurring in Africa have been summarized by various authors (Chodnik 1956; Mornet and Thiery 1955; Macadam 1970; Schulz 1955; Stewart 1972a; Soltys 1965). There have been numerous additional reports on either single cases or outbreaks from many other regions of the world. Clinical cases of bovine dermatophilosis were described in South America from Chile (Kruze *et al.* 1975), Colombia (Adams *et al.* 1970; Navarrete and Trheebilcock 1979), and from Guatemala (Kubes and Ruiz 1972). Clinical signs in outbreaks of dermatophilosis in cattle in England were presented by Roberts and Vallely (1962). A particularly severe disease for a temperate zone was observed in cattle in Kansas, with mortality occurring in 50% of the animals. In addition to severe skin lesions, oral lesions were observed in calves. Predominantly shorthorn cattle were affected and the syndrome resembled the disease observed in Africa (Kelley *et al.* 1964a, b). In India, oral lesions in buffalo and cattle calves were also observed in cases of general skin involvement (Kharole *et al.* 1975). Dermatophilosis in cattle has also been reported from Israel (Nobel *et al.* 1971).

In Australia, the clinical disease in sheep affected the skin generally and occurred commonly in the Merino breed 3 to 12 months of age after shearing or at parturition. Lesions localized on the face and ears served as reservoirs of infections (Roberts 1963d). In the UK infections were also regarded to be widespread and lesions were aggravated by shearing, long wool, and housing (Hart 1976). Simultaneous outbreak of orf and dermatophilosis was reported from Kenya in goats and sheep which were splenectomized for 20 days. The lesions were localized primarily around the head affecting eyes, mouth, and ears (Munz 1969, 1976). In goats, lesions were characterized by being localized on the head, scrotum, and lower parts of the legs (Mémery 1960; Munro 1978; Nicolet *et al.* 1967).

PATHOLOGY

In cattle lesions start as small papules involving a few hair follicles and surrounding dermis with matted tufts of hair standing up above the surface. These localized lesions coalesce into an extensive exudative dermatitis. Detection of early lesions requires careful palpation. First predilection sites of lesions are often areas of the body where ticks localize, from where lesions spread to other parts of the body. Fully developed lesions are characterized by thick dry crusts covering the epidermis. Lesions are formed by separation of the layers of epidermis by inflammatory cell and fluid exudate with desquamation occurring in layers to form a thick, porous, cornified mass which contains masses of organisms. The organisms invade the epidermis which is shed with the underlying protective cellular inflammatory exudate. Continuous regeneration of the epidermis and its reinvasion by the organisms results in the typical lamellar microscopic structure of the scab. Deeper underlying layers of the epidermis are vacuolated, undergo proliferation, and are infiltrated by neutrophils. During recovery from the disease, the encrustation falls off and the underlying raw hemorrhagic lesions heal spontaneously.

Literature

The pathogenesis has been based on the hyphae of *D. congolensis* invading the uncornified epidermis by the mechanical penetrative ability observed both in skin and in culture systems (Roberts 1966a). Hyphae were found in the upper epidermis, especially in the stratum corneum, the hair follicles and in the sebaceous glands. When the basement membrane was injured organisms were also found in the papillary layers of the dermis (Amakiri 1974). The earliest lesions occurred 4 hours after infection and consisted of edema of the subepidermal tissue and accumulation of few neutrophils. By 24 hours after infection a layer of neutrophils separated the epidermis from the underlying dermis. The epidermis regenerated from adjacent hair follicles, forming a new layer of epidermis under the neutrophils. The desquamated epidermis and the underlying inflammatory cellular debris formed layers. Hyphae were observed in clusters 12 hours after infection in the epidermis. Although there was rarely a break in stratum germinativum of the epidermis, the dermis contained marked cellular and fluid inflammatory reactions (Oduye 1976b). The earliest histological lesions reported by Schulz (1955) consisted of proliferation of prickle cells which became swollen and eventually vesicles and spongiosis was formed accompanied by infiltration of mononuclear and polymorphonuclear cells. These developed into pustules (Schulz 1955). Based on the distribution of alkaline phosphatase in healthy skin and infected skin it was concluded that the infection induced proliferative rather than degenerative lesions (Amakiri 1972). Invasion of the keratinized layers of hair follicles occurred by the fourth day and in this location infection persisted and resulted in the development of a carrier state (Bida and Dennis 1977).

Mechanisms of tissue injury have not been determined. A necrotizing agent has been found in crude fractions of *D. congolensis* which caused necrosis of normal rabbit skin (Makinde 1979). In other studies using diffusion chambers implanted into the peritoneal cavity of rabbits toxic products were not found (Perreau 1968). Hypersensitivity has been associated both with the spontaneous recovery and with pathogenesis of lesions (Abu-Samra 1980).

Clinical biochemistry was studied in cattle to define the systemic effects of infection. Serum magnesium, copper, calcium, zinc, sodium, and potassium levels were not affected (Gbodi 1980). An increase in fibrinogen, a fall in cholesterol and in calcium potassium ratio, and changes in the protein component were also shown (Gaulier *et al.* 1972). Serum zinc, copper, magnesium, calcium, and potassium were low, but in general serum zinc, calcium, and magnesium levels in Nigerian Zebu cattle were significantly lower than normal (Kapu 1975). Protein, albumin, and globulin levels in healthy and diseased White Fulani and N'Dama cattle were studied and it was proposed that these serum components were not associated with the higher resistance observed in N'Dama cattle (Amakiri 1977).

IMMUNOLOGY

Dermatophilosis congolensis infection does not give rise to protective immunity in cattle, sheep, horses, goats, and rabbits. Both humoral antibodies and cellular responses develop early, but in spite of these potentially protective responses chronic lesions develop and animals can be reinfected experimentally and natural clinical diseases can reoccur in the same animal. Delayed hypersensitivity is indirectly involved in the prevention of epidermal invasion and initiation of healing.

Literature

The immunology of dermatophilosis including local, humoral responses and prospects for vaccination were reviewed by Lloyd (1984).

On recovery from dermatophilosis, cattle were not resistant to reinfection, and animals with lesions in one year could develop clinical disease in the following rainy season (Bida and Dennis 1976; Macadam 1970). The presence of antibodies did not prevent the development of lesions (Makinde and Ezeh 1981). In guinea pigs, somatic and flagellar antigens induced agglutination, precipitation, and hemagglutination antibodies, but the response did not influence resistance to infection by the scarification methods (Bida and Kelley 1976). Circulating antibodies also did not protect either rabbits or deer against reinfection (Richard *et al.* 1976). It has been postulated that in sheep primary infection was overcome as soon as the delayed hypersensitivity was fully developed. However, in chronically infected sheep, lesions persisted in spite of the delayed hypersensitivity reaction (Roberts 1966a).

A single injection of *D. congolensis* induced delayed hypersensitivity in rabbits without producing circulating antibody. Two injections 14 days apart caused somatic and flagellar agglutinins, precipitins, and an immediate cutaneous anaphylactic hypersensitivity. Vaccination, like the double infection, also induced hypersensitivity and circulating antibodies. Antibodies affected the course of infection, but the delayed hypersensitivity increased the inflammatory response which controlled hyphal invasion of tissue (Roberts 1966a). Merkal *et al.* (1972) reported that treatment of experimental infections in rabbits with methotrexate, an inhibitor of immediate and delayed hypersensitivity reactions, did not affect the development of lesions. It was concluded that a nonspecific as compared to an immunologically induced inflammatory reaction was involved.

Agglutination, agar-gel precipitation, and indirect hemagglutination tests were used to detect antibodies in naturally and experimentally infected cattle and in experimentally infected rabbits (Pulliam *et al.* 1967). Serological tests were considered to be useful in the detection of the mild forms of infection which could not be detected clinically (Bida and Kelley 1976). Different antigenic extracts used in the reverse single radial immunodiffusion technique gave variable results (Makinde 1980). Experimental lesions in cattle caused an antibody response detectable by the passive hemagglutination test. Second infections induced an anamnestic response which was associated with more rapid healing (Makinde and Ezeh 1981). Enzyme-linked immunosorbent assay could detect low levels of antibody which enabled detection of asymptomatic infections (Lloyd 1981).

A serological relationship was observed between different strains of *D. congolensis* (Richard *et al.* 1976). Various antigens isolated from the organisms induced cell-mediated immune response in rabbits but only exo-antigens caused antibody responses (Makinde and Wilkie 1979). Various methods for the preparation of antigens were compared by Aghomo and Lloyd (1983). The fluorescent antibody (FA) test was specific and useful in the demonstration and identification of the organism in lesions (Richard *et al.* 1976).

VACCINATION

Vaccination with whole cell antigen is used to a limited degree, but the usefulness of this method in control of natural diseases is not established. Some workers advocate immunization, while others have shown that neither natural infection nor vaccination protects against reinfection.

Literature

Vaccination against dermatophilosis was reviewed by Lloyd (1984) in a paper on immunology. The development of humoral and surface antibodies following intradermal vaccination of cattle has been described (Lloyd and McEwan Jenkinson 1981). Live adjuvant vaccine using mineral oil was effective against natural dermatophilosis in cattle while cultures, injected intradermally, protected only against experimental infection (Chamoiseu *et al.* 1973). In another study, intradermal inoculation of young lyophilized and nonlyophilized cultures into Zebu cattle protected against natural challenge with the vaccinated having lower and less severe lesions (Provost *et al.* 1974, 1976). Vaccines induced antibodies but not protection against the disease (Perreau *et al.* 1966). After vaccination of sheep and guinea pigs, increased resistance to infection developed by the zoospores of scarified skin. Resistance was demonstrated only when the infecting zoospores came in contact with phagocytes and antibodies increased the destructive capability of the phagocytes (Roberts 1966b). Rabbits vaccinated by intradermal inoculation of young cultures were protected against subsequent experimental challenge (Chamoiseau and Lefevre 1973).

CHEMOTHERAPY

There is relatively little information on the variability in susceptibility of various strains to chemotherapeutic agents. The organism is susceptible to many antibiotics including penicillin and chloromycetin. Treatment is effective with topical application of ointments, sprays, and dips in the early stages. Antibiotics must penetrate the exudate and come in contact with the organisms to be effective. Mild clinical cases usually undergo spontaneous healing and do not require treatment. Systemic medication involving antibiotics and supportive therapy is used in severe forms of disease. Extensive use of expensive antibiotics on a herd basis is not economically possible.

Literature

Bacteriostatic and bactericidal actions of dipping compounds on *D. congolensis* were tested *in vitro* (Presler 1973). The organism was also susceptible *in vitro* to large numbers of antibiotics (Abu-Samra *et al.* 1976), but drugs active *in vitro* were not necessary effective *in vivo*. The ability of a chemotherapeutic agent to come in contact with the causative agent located within the inflammatory exudates, particularly in severe clinical cases with massive lesions, has been related to its efficacy. Removal of inflammatory exudates has been difficult, resulting in additional trauma and pain to the animal and should not be undertaken indiscriminately (Coleman 1967).

Treatment of bovine dermatophilosis was reviewed by Coleman (1967) and Blancou (1976a). Topical and systemic treatments in chronic severe cases were generally shown not to be effective (Coleman 1967).

Prophylactic measures were the only adequate method of combating the disease in the field (Thiéry and Mémery 1961). Some treatments did not eliminate either the lesion or infection but did reduce the severity of clinical manifestations of disease (Mammerick 1961). The successful use of aureomycin chlorohydrate and cleaning of skin alternately with hydrogen peroxide and with a solution of novarsenobenzol was described by Mémery (1960). Intramuscular injections of penicillin and streptomycin were also reported to be effective in treatment of dermatophilosis in cattle (Blancou 1969). More recently, Ilemobade (1984) presented a summary of experience in Nigeria and found that most successful treatments usually involve parenteral administration of antibiotics using a variety of regimes and combinations. A single administration of a long-acting oxytetracycline was found to be highly effective. Acaricides were bactericidal in culture and in exudates (Vanbreuseghem *et al.* 1976).

DIAGNOSIS

In the tropics, dermatophilosis is usually diagnosed clinically, particularly when a number of animals in a herd are affected, and is confirmed by demonstrating the organism in stained smears. Differentiation of mild atypical lesions from local mycotic and other bacterial infection is necessary. Fluorescent antibody techniques are used to identify organisms in exudates. Growth and morphological characteristics of colonies in culture also identify the organisms.

Literature

A method of collecting and handling field samples for diagnosis was described by Haalstra (1965). A simple diagnostic procedure was the microscopic examination of smears from lesions using Seller's stain which contained basic fuchsine and methylene blue (Nobel and Klopfer 1978). Organisms could also be demonstrated in smears stained with either methylene blue or Giemsa's stain with the latter being the best routine method. Isolations were made on blood agar incubated in 10% CO_2 (Weber *et al.* 1982). The FA technique has been used to confirm infection by *D. congolensis* (Pier *et al.* 1964). Organisms were readily demonstrated in stained smears from acute exudates, but in chronic lesions they were difficult to detect (Richard *et al.* 1976).

CONTROL

Dermatophilosis is controlled by measures being taken against ectoparasites and limiting other mechanical trauma to the skin during rainy seasons. Good husbandry and control of intercurrent diseases are also important.

Literature

Prophylactic injections of antibiotics and dipping as well as vaccination of Brahman cattle had some beneficial effect in controlling the disease (Blancou 1976b). Development of satisfactory controls was postulated to depend on preventing optimum condition in the skin for growth, development, and invasion by the organisms. The microenvironment of the skin surface, which played a role in susceptibility to infection, included structure, microclimate, chemical composition, and resident bacterial flora (McEwan Jenkinson 1976).

BIBLIOGRAPHY

Abu-Samra, M. T., 1978a. Morphological, cultural and biochemical characteristics of *Dermatophilus congolensis*, *Zbl. Vet. Med.*, **B25**: 668–88.

Abu-Samra, M. T., 1978b. *Dermatophilus* infection: the clinical disease and diagnosis, *Zbl. Vet. Med.*, **B25**: 641–51.

Abu-Samra, M. T., 1978c. The effect of prednisolone trimethylacetate on the pathogenicity of *Dermatophilus congolensis* to white mice, *Mycopathologia*, **66**(1–2): 1–9.

Abu-Samra, M. T., 1980. The epizootiology of *Dermatophilus congolensis* infection (a discussion article), *Rev. Elev. Méd. vét. Pays trop.*, **33**(1): 23–32.

Abu-Samra, M. T., Imbabi, S. E. and Mahgoub, E. S., 1976 *Dermatophilus congolensis*. A bacteriological, *in vitro* antibiotic sensitivity and histopathological study of natural infection in Sudanese cattle, *Br. vet. J.*, **132**: 627–34.

Adams, L. G., Hipolito, O., Morales, H., Gongora, S. and Jones, L. P., 1970. Dermatofilosis bovina (Estreptotricosis cutánea) en Colombia, *ICA Revta.*, **5**: 3–16.

Adlan, A. M. and Obeid, H. M., 1977. Bacteriological study of Sudanese strains of *Dermatophilus congolensis*, *Bull. Anim. Hlth Prod. Afr.*, **25**(4): 381–3.

Aghomo, H. O. and Lloyd, D. H., 1983. Comparison of *Dermatophilus congolensis* precipitating antigens prepared by three methods, *Br. vet. J.*, **139**: 325–9.

Amakiri, S. F., 1972. Alkaline phosphatase activity in normal and *Dermatophilus congolensis* infected bovine skin, *Nigerian Vet. J.*, **1**(2): 46–9.

Amakiri, S. F., 1974. Extent of skin penetration by *Dermatophilus congolensis* in bovine streptothricosis, *Trop. Anim. Hlth Prod.*, **6**: 99–105.

Amakiri, S. F., 1976. Anatomical location of *Dermatophilus congolensis* in bovine cutaneous streptothricosis. In *Dermatophilus Infection in Animals and Man*, eds D. H. Lloyd, K. C. Sellers. Academic Press (London, New York, San Francisco), pp. 163–72.

Amakiri, S. F., 1977. Electrophoretic studies of serum proteins in healthy and streptothricosis infected cattle *Br. vet. J.*, **133**: 106–7.

Austwick, P. K. C., 1958. Cutaneous streptothricosis, mycotic dermatitis and strawberry foot rot and the genus *Dermatophilus* van Saceghem, *Vet. Rev. Annot.*, **4**: 33–48.

Austwick, P. K. C., 1976. The probable relationship of rainfall to *Dermatophilus congolensis* infection in sheep. In *Dermatophilus Infection in Animals and Man*, eds D. H. Lloyd, K. C. Sellers. Academic Press (London, New York, San Francisco), pp. 87–97.

Balabanov, V. A. and Boussafou, D., 1977. Cattle dermatophilosis in the People's Republic of the Congo, *Rev. Elev. Méd. vét. Pays trop.*, **30**(4): 363–8.

Barbosa, M., de Carvalho, C. M. F. and Neves da Rocha, F., 1967. Cutaneous streptothricosis in cattle in Brazil, *Arq. Esc. Vet. minas Gerais*, **19**: 15–17.

Bida, S. A. and Dennis, S. M., 1976. Dermatophilosis in northern Nigeria, *Vet. Bull.*, **46**(7): 471–8.

Bida, S. A. and Dennis, S. M., 1977. Sequential pathological changes in natural and experimental dermatophilosis in Bunaji cattle, *Res. vet. Sci.*, **22**: 18–22.

Bida, S. A. and Kelley, D. C., 1976. Immunological studies of antigenic components of *Dermatophilus congolensis*. In *Dermatophilus Infection in Animals and Man*, eds D. H. Lloyd, K. C. Sellers. Academic Press (London, New York, San Francisco), pp. 229–43.

Blancou, J. M., 1969. Treatment of bovine streptothricosis by only a high dose antibiotic injection, *Rev. Elev. Méd. vét. Pays trop.*, **22**(1): 33–40.

Blancou, J. M., 1976a. The treatment of infection by *Dermatophilus congolensis* with particular reference to the disease in cattle. In *Dermatophilus Infection in Animals and Man*, eds D. H. Lloyd, K. C. Sellers. Academic Press (London, New York, San Francisco), pp. 246–60.

Blancou, J. M., 1976b. Control of *Dermatophilus congolensis* infection in Brahman cattle. Results after seven years, *Rev. Elev. Méd. vét. Pays trop.*, **29**(3): 211–15.

Braibant, E., 1962. La streptothricose cutanée au Rwanda et au Burundi, *Bull. epiz. Dis. Afr.*, **10**: 517–21.

Bugyaki, L., 1959. Dermatose contagieuse des ruminants et du cheval (streptotrichose, actinomycose cutanée), *Bull. Off. int. Epiz.*, **51**: 237–49.

Bwangamoi, O., 1976a. Dermatophilus infection in cattle, goats and sheep in East Africa. In *Dermatophilus Infection in Animals and Man*, eds D. H. Lloyd, K. C. Sellers. Academic Press (London, New York, San Francisco), pp. 49–57.

Bwangamoi, O., 1976b. Economic aspects of streptothricosis in livestock in East Africa. In *Dermatophilus Infections in Animals and Man*, eds D. H. Lloyd, K. C. Sellers. Academic Press (London, New York, San Francisco), pp. 292–7.

Chamoiseau, G. and Lefevre, E., 1973. Immunological research on bovine cutaneous dermatophilosis. I. Immunization trials of rabbits against experimental dermatophilosis, *Rev. Elev. Méd. vét. Pays trop.*, **26**(1): 1–5.

Chamoiseau, G., Provost, A. and Touade, M., 1973. Immunological research on bovine cutaneous dermatophilosis. II. Immunization trial of cattle against natural dermatophilosis, *Rev. Elev. Méd. vét. Pays trop.*, **26**(1): 7–11.

Chodnik, K. S., 1956. Mycotic dermatitis of cattle in British West Africa, *J. Comp. Path.*, **66**: 179–85.

Coleman, C. H., 1967. Cutaneous streptothricosis of cattle in West Africa, *Vet. Rec.*, **81**: 251–4.

da Cruz, L. C. H., 1975a. *Dermatophilus congolensis* III. Comportamento em relaçao oxigênio, *Pesq. agropec. bras., Sér. Vet.*, **10**: 21–4.

da Cruz, L. C. H., 1975b. *Dermatophilus congolensis* IV. Manutençao de amostras em laboritório, *Pesq. agropec. bras., Sér. Vet.*, **10**: 25–6.

Dumas, R., Lhoste, P., Chabeuf, N. and Blancou, J., 1971. Note on hereditary predisposition of cattle to streptothricosis, *Rev. Elev. Méd. vét. Pays trop.*, **24**(3): 349–53.

El-Nageh, M. M., 1971. Comparison of strains of *Dermatophilus congolensis* van Saceghem 1915 isolated from different species of animals, *Ann. Soc. belge Méd. trop.*, **51**(2): 239–46.

Gallo, G. G., Audisio, S. N., Bouissou, R. G. and Elichiri, N., 1973. *Dermatophilus congolensis* in cattle. Detection in Buenos Aires and La Pamapa provinces, Argentina, *Revta Med. Vet.*, **54**(3): 197–203.

Gaulier, R., Blancou, J. M., Bourdin, P., Ribot, J. J., Ramisse, J., Serres, H. and Alexandre, F., 1972. Contribution to the serological and physio-pathological study of bovine streptothricosis, *Rev. Elev. Méd. vét. Pays trop.*, **25**(2): 171–85.

Gbodi, T. A., 1980. Serum mineral status of normal and *Dermatophilus congolensis* infected Friesian calves, *Bull. Anim. Hlth Prod. Afr.*, **28**: 348–50.

Gordon, M. A., 1976. Characterization of *Dermatophilus congolensis*: its affinities with the *Actinomycetales* and differentiation from *Geodermatophilus*. In *Dermatophilus Infections in Animals and Man*, eds D. H. Lloyd, K. C. Sellers. Academic Press (London, New York, San Francisco), pp. 187–202.

Gordon, M. A. and Perrin, U., 1971. Pathogenicity of *Dermatophilus* and *Geodermatophilus*, *Infect. Immun.*, **4**(1): 29–33.

Graber, M., 1969. Tourine and zebu cattle healthy carriers of *Dermatophilus congolensis* in Chad, *Rev. Elev, Méd, vét. Pays trop.*, **22**(1): 41–5.

Haalstra, R. T., 1965. Isolation of *Dermatophilus congolensis* from skin lesions in the diagnosis of streptothricosis, *Vet. Rec.*, **77**(28): 824–5.

Hart, C. B., 1976. Dermatophilus infection in the United Kingdom. In *Dermatophilus Infection in Animals and Man*, eds D. H. Lloyd, K. C. Sellers. Academic Press (London, New York, San Francisco), pp. 77–87.

Ilemobade, A. A., 1984. Clinical experiences in the use of chemotherapy for bovine dermatophilosis in Nigeria. In *Impact of Diseases on Livestock Production in the Tropics*, eds H. P. Riemann, M. J. Burridge. Elsevier (Amsterdam, Oxford, New York, Tokyo), pp. 83–92.

Jarnagin, J. L. and Thoen, C. O., 1977. Isolation of *Dermatophilus congolensis* and certain mycotic agents from animal tissues: a laboratory summary, *Am. J. vet. Res.*, **38**(11): 1909–11.

Kaplan, W., 1976. Dermatophilosis in primates. In *Dermatophilus Infection in Animals and Man*, eds D. H. Lloyd, K. C. Sellers. Academic Press (London, New York, San Francisco), pp. 128–39.

Kapu, M. M., 1975. Mineral compositions of serum from *Dermatophilus* infected zebu cattle under grazing conditions in Nigeria, *Nigerian J. Anim. Prod.*, **2**(2): 247–51.

Kelley, D. C., 1976. *Dermatophilus* infections in the United States. In *Dermatophilus Infection in Animals and Man*, eds D. H. Lloyd, K. C. Sellers. Academic Press (London, New York, San Francisco), pp. 116–24.

Kelley, D. C. and Bida, S. A., 1970. Epidemiological survey of streptothricosis (Kirchi) in northern Nigeria, *Bull. epiz. Dis. Afr.*, **18**: 325–8.

Kelley, D. C., Huston, K., Imes, G. D. and Weide, K. D., 1964a. Part I: Cutaneous streptothricosis in Kansas cattle. *Vet. Med./Small Anim. Clin.*, **59**: 73–8.

Kelley, D. C., Huston, K., Imes, G. D. and Weide, K. D., 1964b. Part II: Cutaneous streptothricosis in Kansas cattle, *Vet. Med./Small Anim. Clin.*, **59**: 175–8.

Kharole, M. U., Chauhan, H. V. S., Dixit, S. N. and Kaul, P. L., 1975. Oral streptothricosis in cow calves and a buffalo calf, *Indian J. Anim. Sci.*, **45**(3): 119–22.

Kruze, J., Zamora, J. and Norambuena, L., 1975. Bovine dermatophilosis in Chile. Clinical, bacteriological and histopathological aspects, *Zbl. Vet. Med.*, **B22**: 230–8.

Kubes, V. and Ruiz, J. A., 1972. Bovine dermatophilosis in Guatemala, *Rev. Fac. Med. Vet. y Zoot.*, **4**(1): 49–52.

Kurtze, H., 1964. Contribution to streptothricosis of cattle, *Deut. Tierarztl. Eschr.*, **7**(13): 358–9.

Lloyd, D. H., 1976. The economic effects of bovine streptothricosis. In *Dermatophilus Infection in Animals and Man*, eds D. H. Lloyd, K. C. Sellers. Academic Press (London, New York, San Francisco), pp. 274–92.

Lloyd, D. H., 1981. Measurement of antibody to *Dermatophilus congolensis* in sera from cattle in the west of Scotland by enzyme-linked immunosorbent assay, *Vet. Rec.*, **109**: 426–7.

Lloyd, D. H., 1984. Immunology of dermatophilosis: recent developments and prospects for control, *Preventive Vet. Med.*, **2**: 93–102.

Lloyd, D. H., Dick, W. D. B. and McEwan Jenkinson, D., 1979. The effects of some surface sampling procedures on the stratum corneum of bovine skin, *Res. vet. Sci.*, **26**: 250–2.

Lloyd, D. H. and McEwan Jenkinson, D., 1980. The effect of climate on experimental infection of bovine skin with *Dermatophilus congolensis*, *Br. vet. J.*, **136**: 122–34.

Lloyd, D. H. and McEwan Jenkinson, D., 1981. Serum and skin surface antibody responses to intradermal vaccination of cattle with *Dermatophilus congolensis*, *Br. Vet. J.*, **137**: 601–7.

Lloyd, D. H. and Sellers, K. C. (eds), 1976. *Dermatophilus Infection in Animals and Man*. Academic Press (London, New York, San Francisco).

Londero, A. T., 1976. *Dermatophilus* infection in the subtropical zone of South America. In *Dermatophilus Infection in Animals and Man*, eds D. H. Lloyd, K. C. Sellers. Academic Press (London, New York, San Francisco), pp. 110–16.

Macadam, I., 1961. The effect of humidity on the lesions of streptothricosis, *Vet. Rec.*, **73**(42): 1039–40.

Macadam, I., 1962. Bovine streptothricosis: production of lesions by the bite of the tick *Amblyomma variegatum*, *Vet. Rec.*, **74**(23): 643–6.

Macadam, I., 1964a. Observations on the effects of flies and humidity on natural lesions of streptothricosis, *Vet. Rec.*, **76**(7): 194–8.

Macadam, I., 1964b. The effects of ectoparasites and humidity on natural lesions of streptothricosis, *Vet. Rec.*, **76**(12): 354.

Macadam, I., 1964c. Streptothricosis in Nigerian horses, *Vet. Rec.*,

76(15): 420–2.
Macadam, I., 1970. Some observations on bovine cutaneous streptothricosis in northern Nigeria, *Trop. Anim. Hlth Prod.*, **2**: 131–8.
Macadam, I., 1976. Some observations on *Dermatophilus* infection in The Gambia with particular reference to the disease in sheep. In *Dermatophilus Infection in Animals and Man*, eds D. H. Lloyd, K. C. Sellers. Academic Press (London, New York, San Francisco), pp. 33–41.
Macadam, I. and Haalstra, R. T., 1971. Bacteriology of Nigerian strains of *Dermatophilus congolensis, Trop. Anim. Hlth Prod.*, **3**: 225–31.
Makinde, A. A., 1979. Necrotizing properties of some crude fractions of *Dermatophilus congolensis*. A preliminary report, *Bull. Anim. Hlth Prod. Afr.*, **27**: 159–61.
Makinde, A. A., 1980. The reverse single radial immunodiffusion technique for detecting antibodies to *Dermatophilus congolensis, Vet. Rec.*, **106**: 383–5.
Makinde, A. A. and Ezeh, A. O., 1981. Primary and secondary humoral immune responses in cattle experimentally infected with *Dermatophilus congolensis, Bull. Anim. Hlth Prod. Afr.*, **29**: 19–23.
Makinde, A. A. and Wilkie, B. N., 1979. Humoral and cell-mediated immune response to crude antigens of *Dermatophilus congolensis* during experimental infection of rabbits, *Can. J. comp. Med.*, **43**: 67–77.
Mammerick, M., 1961. Observations sur la Dermatose contagieuse des ruminants au Congo, *Ann. Soc. belge Med. trop.*, **41**: 133–44.
McEwan Jenkinson, D., 1976. The skin surface: an environment of *Dermatophilus congolensis*. In *Dermatophilus Disease in Animals and Man*, eds D. H. Lloyd, K. C. Sellers. Academic Press (London, New York, San Francisco), pp. 146–59.
Mémery, G., 1960. Cutaneous streptothricosis. II. Note on several cases of spontaneous infection in goats in the region of Dakar, *Rev. Elev. Méd. vét. Pays trop.*, **13**(2–3): 143–53.
Mémery, G., 1961. Cutaneous streptothricosis. III. Bacteriology, *Rev. Elev. Méd. vét. Pays trop.*, **14**(2): 141–63.
Mémery, G. and Mémery L., 1962. Cutaneous streptothricosis. Pathogenicity of the causal microorganism of bovine streptothricosis. *Rev. Elev. Méd. vét. Pays trop.*, **15**(1): 5–9.
Merkal, R. S., Richard, J. L., Thurston, J. R. and Ness, R. D., 1972. Effect of methotrexate on rabbits infected with *Mycobacterium paratuberculosis* or *Dermatophilus congolensis, Am. J. vet. Res.*, **33**: 401–7.
Meyer, E., 1971. Bacteriological investigations of nine strains of the virus of the skin streptothricosis in Tanzania, *Beit. Trop. Subtrop. Landwirtschaft. Trop. Veterinarmed.*, **4**: 311–18.
Moreira, E. C. and Barbosa, M., 1976. Dermatophilosis in tropical South America. In *Dermatophilus Infection in Animals and Man*, eds D. H. Lloyd, K. C. Sellers. Academic Press (London, New York, San Francisco), pp. 102–10.

Moreira, E. C., Barbosa, M. and Moreira, Y. K., 1974. Dermatophilosis in South America, *Arq. Esc. Vet. UFMG*, **26**(1): 77–84.
Mornet, P. and Thiery, G., 1955. Cutaneous bovine streptothricosis, *Bull. epiz. Dis Afr.*, **3**: 302–24.
Munro, R., 1978. Caprine dermatophilosis in Fiji, *Trop. Anim. Hlth Prod.*, **10**: 221–2.
Munz, E., 1969. Simultaneous occurrence of orf and streptothricosis in goats and sheep in Kenya, *Berl. Münch. Tierarztl. Wschr.*, **82**(12): 221–40.
Munz, E., 1976. Double infection of sheep and goats in Kenya with orf virus and *Dermatophilus*. In *Dermatophilus Infection in Animals and Man*, eds D. H. Lloyd, K. C. Sellers. Academic Press (London, New York, San Francisco), pp. 57–67.

Navarrete, S. M. and Trheebilcock, E., 1979. Bovine dermatophilosis in the department of Córdoba, *ICA Revta.*, **14**(2): 123–7.
Nicolet, J., Klingler, K. and Fey, H., 1967. *Dermatophilus congolensis*, agent de la streptothricose du chamois, *Path. Microbiol.*, **30**: 831–7.
Nobel, T. A. and Klopfer, U., 1978. Laboratory procedures for the diagnosis of dermatophilosis (cutaneous streptothricosis), *Refuah Vet.*, **35**(4): 171–2.
Nobel, T. A., Klopfer, U. and Neumann, F., 1976. Cutaneous streptothricosis (dermatophilosis) of cattle in Israel. In *Dermatophilus Infection in Animals and Man*, eds D. H. Lloyd, K. C. Sellers. Academic Press (London, New York, San Francisco), pp. 70–6.
Nobel, T. A, Klopfer, U. and Shavel, M., 1971. Streptothricosis in Israeli cattle, *Refuah Vet.*, **28**(3): 102–5.
Noble, W. C., Lloyd, D. H. and Appiah, S. N., 1980. Inhibition of *Dermatophilus congolensis* infection in a mouse model by antibiotic-producing staphylococci, *Br. J. exp. Path.*, **61**: 644–7.

Obeid, H. M. A, 1976. Cutaneous streptothricosis in Sudanese cattle. In *Dermatophilus Infection in Animals and Man*, eds D. H. Lloyd, K. C. Sellers. Academic Press (London, New York, San Francisco), pp. 44–9.
Oduye, O. O., 1975. Bovine cutaneous streptothricosis in Nigeria, *Wld Anim. Rev.*, **16**: 13–17.
Oduye, O. O., 1976a. Bovine streptothricosis in Nigeria. In *Dermatophilus Infection in Animals and Man*, eds D. H. Lloyd, K. C. Sellers. Academic Press (London, New York, San Francisco), pp. 2–17.
Oduye, O. O., 1976b. Histopathological changes in natural and experimental *Dermatophilus congolensis* infection of the bovine skin. In *Dermatophilus Infection in Animals and Man*, eds D. H. Lloyd, K. C. Sellers. Academic Press (London, New York, San Francisco), pp. 172–82.

Oduye, O. O. and Lloyd, D. H., 1971. Incidence of bovine cutaneous streptothricosis in Nigeria, *Br. vet. J.*, **127**(11): 505–10.
Ojo, M. O., 1975. *Bacillus pumilus*, an inhibitor of *Dermatophilus congolensis* and other micro-organisms: a preliminary report, *Bull. Anim. Hlth Prod. Afr.*, **23**: 43–4.
Oppong, E. N. W., 1973. Bovine streptothricosis in the Accra plains, *Ghana J. Sci.*, **13**(1): 44–62.
Oppong, E. N. W., 1976. Epizootiology of dermatophilus infection in cattle in the Accra plains of Ghana. In *Dermatophilus Infection in Animals and Man*, eds D. H. Lloyd and K. C. Sellers. Academic Press (London, New York, San Francisco), pp. 17–33.

Perreau, P., 1968. Is the pathogenicity of *Dermatophilus congolensis* related with a toxin production?, *Rev. Elev. Méd. vét. Pays trop.*, **21**(1): 59–69.
Perreau, P., Chambron, J. and Gayt, P., 1966. Immunology of bovine cutaneous streptothricosis of cattle. Vaccination trials, *Rev. Elev. Méd. vét. Pays trop.*, **21**(1): 59–69.
Philpott, M. and Ezeh, A. O., 1978. The experimental transmission by *Musca* and *Stomoxys* species of *D. congolensis* infection between cattle, *Br. vet. J.*, **134**: 515–20.
Pier, A. C., Richard, J. L. and Farrell, E. F., 1964. Fluorescent antibody and cultural techniques in cutaneous streptothricosis, *Am. J. vet. Res.*, **25**(107): 1014–20.
Plowright, W. 1956. Cutaneous streptothricosis of cattle: I. Introduction and epizootiological features in Nigeria, *Vet. Rec.*, **68**: 350–5.
Plowright, W., 1958. Cutaneous streptothricosis of cattle in Nigeria. II. The aerobic actinomycete (*Nocardia* sp.) associated with the lesions, *J. Comp. Path.*, **68**: 133–47.
Presler, D., 1973. Contribution to the study of bovine streptothricosis, *Ann. Soc belge Méd. trop.*, **53**(3): 187–94.
Provost, A., Touade, M. M., Guillaume, M., Peleton, H. and Damsou, F., 1974. Vaccination tests against bovine dermatophilosis in the southern region of Chad, *Bull. epiz. Dis. Afr.*, **22**(3): 223–9.
Provost, A., Touade, M. P., Guillaume, M., Peleton, H. and Damsou, F., 1976. Vaccination trials against bovine dermatophilosis in southern Chad. In *Dermatophilus Infection in Animals and Man*, eds D. H. Lloyd, K. C. Sellers. Academic Press (London, New York, San Francisco). pp. 260–9.
Pulliam, J. D., Kelley, D. C. and Coles, E. H., 1967. Immunologic studies of natural and experimental cutaneous streptothricosis infections in cattle, *Am. J. vet. Res.*, **28**(123): 447–55.

Richard, J. L. and Pier, A. C., 1966. Transmission of *Dermatophilus congolensis* by *Stomoxys calcitrans* and *Musca domestica*, *Am. J. vet. Res.*, **27**: 419–23.
Richard, J. L., Thurston, J. R. and Pier, A. C., 1976. Comparison of

antigens of *Dermatophilus congolensis* isolates and their use in serological tests in experimental and natural infections. In *Dermatophilus Infection in Animals and Man*, eds D. H. Lloyd, K. C. Sellers. Academic Press (London, New York, San Francisco), pp. 216–29.

Roberts, D. S., 1961. The life cycle of *Dermatophilus dermatonomus*, the causal agent of ovine mycotic dermatitis, *Aust. J. exp. Biol.*, **39**: 463–76.

Roberts, D. S., 1963a. The influence of carbon dioxide on the growth and sporulation of *Dermatophilus dermatonomus, Aust. J. Agric. Res.*, **14**(3): 412–23.

Roberts, D. S., 1963b. The release and survival of *Dermatophilus dermatonomus* zoospores, *Aust. J. Agric. Res.*, **14**(3): 386–99.

Roberts, D. S., 1963c. Properties of *Dermatophilus dermatonomus* zoospores in relation to the transmission of mycotic dermatitis, *Aust. J. Agric. Res.*, **14**(3): 373–85.

Roberts, D. S., 1963d. Barriers to *Dermatophilus dermatonomus* infection on the skin of sheep, *Aust. J. Agric. Res.*, **14**: 492–508.

Roberts, D. S., 1965a. Penetration and irritation of the skin by *Dermatophilus congolensis, Br. J. Exp. Path.*, **46**: 635–42.

Roberts, D. S., 1965b. The histopathology of epidermal infection with the actinomycete *Dermatophilus congolensis, J. Path. Bact.*, **90**: 213–16.

Roberts, D. S., 1965c. The role of granulocytes in resistance to *Dermatophilus congolensis, Br. J. Exp. Path.*, **46**: 643–8.

Roberts, D. S., 1966a. The influence of delayed hypersensitivity on the course of infection with *Dermatophilus congolensis, Br. J. Exp. Path.*, **47**: 9–16.

Roberts, D. S., 1966b. The phagocytic basis of acquired resistance to infection with *Dermatophilus congolensis, Br. J. Exp. Path.*, **47**: 372–82.

Roberts, D. S. and Vallely, T. F., 1962. Streptothricosis in cattle, *Vet. Rec.*, **74**(25): 693–6.

Schulz, K. C. A., 1955. Mycotic dermatitis (Senkobe skin-disease) of cattle in the Union of South Africa, *Bull. epiz. Dis. Afr.*, **3**: 244–61.

Soltys, M. A., 1965. Cutaneous streptothricosis in cattle in the Sudan, *Sudan J. Vet. Sci. Anim. Husb.*, **5**(1): 20–3.

Stewart, G. H., 1972a. Dermatophilosis: a skin disease of animals and man. Part I, *Vet. Rec.*, **91**: 537–44.

Stewart, G. H., 1972b. Dermatophilosis: a skin disease of animals and man, Part II, *Vet. Rec.*, **91**(23): 555–61.

Thiéry, G. and Mémery, G., 1961. Cutaneous streptothricosis. Etiology – treatment – prophylaxis, *Rev. Elev. Méd. vét. Pays trop.*, **14**: 413–27.

Vanbreuseghem, R., Takashio, M., El Nageh, M. M., Presler, D., Selly, M. and van Wettere, P., 1976. Some experimental research on *Dermatophilus congolensis*. In *Dermatophilus Infection in Animals and Man*, eds D. H. Lloyd, K. C. Sellers. Academic Press (London, New York, San Francisco), pp. 202–13.

Vandemaele, F. P., 1961. Enquete sur la streptothricose cutanée en Afrique, *Bull. epiz. Dis. Afr.*, **9**: 251–8.

Vigier, M. and Balis, J., 1967. Variability and antigenicity of *Dermatophilus congolensis*, *Rev. Elev. Méd. vét. Pays trop.*, **20**(1): 67–76.

Weber, A., Hofmann, W. and Frese, K., 1982. Zur Dermatophilose des Rindes – Diagnose und Differential – diagnose unter besonderer Berucksichtigung der Rinder trichophytie, *Mykosen*, **20**(2): 75–82.

Chapter

18

Hemorrhagic septicemia

CONTENTS

INTRODUCTION

Hemorrhagic septicemia is a form of pasteurellosis caused by *Pasteurella multocida* and characterized by acute septicemia and high mortality in cattle, buffalo, and pigs. In the tropics it occurs mainly during the rainy season and subclinical infections are often found in carriers.

Literature

Bain (1959) summarized the important information which had been published on hemorrhagic septicemia in cattle. In 1963 he published a comprehensive review on the disease, particularly as it occurred in Asia (Bain 1963). Ochi (1957) reviewed the reports on the occurrence of hemorrhagic septicemia in Japan. Dhanda and Sen (1972) published a monograph on hemorrhagic septicemia and comparable clinical syndromes in sheep, goats, pigs, and poultry in India.

ETIOLOGY

Strains causing hemorrhagic septicemia have the general morphology of the *Pasteurella* species, being small encapsulated bacilli with some coccobacillary forms and bipolar staining affinity with either methylene blue or Romaowsky's stains. These morphological characteristics are evident *in vivo* but are quickly lost in subcultures.

Cultural characteristics are also those of other members of the *Pasteurella* group. Blood agar is the most commonly used medium. Growth *in vitro* for a relatively short time preserves the viability and virulence of the organisms, but culture characteristics change quickly on subculture. After initial isolation and subculturing the capsule may be lost, altering the pathogenicity of the organism.

On the basis of capsular antigens, *P. multocida* isolates can be serologically typed and are classified as types A, B, D, and E. This classification is reliable and is widely used internationally. Causative organisms of hemorrhagic septicemia are types B and E, and based on these serological and other biological characteristics are readily distinguishable from other types of *Pasteurella*. Organisms isolated in Asia are type B, while those from Africa are type E. Type B strains are occasionally isolated from southern Europe and rarely from North America and Africa. Serological tests used for the classification are the mouse cross-protection, indirect hemagglutination, tube agglutination, and gel diffusion tests. Biochemical reactions are shared with other species of *Pasteurella*, and types B and E isolates cannot be differentiated on the basis of biochemical tests done. Some reactions differ between strains isolated from various regions. Occasionally cattle, sheep, and goats die from a septicemic condition caused by serotypes other than B and E. However, pneumonic pasteurellosis is most often associated with these serotypes. These syndromes are sporadic and not common, and are not included in the classical disease known as hemorrhagic septicemia.

Literature

Carter and Bain (1960) and Carter (1981) reviewed the classification of organisms in the *Pasteurella* group isolated from various animal hosts. Roberts (1947) using the mouse protection tests was the first to demonstrate four distinct types of *P. multocida* isolated from cases of pasteurellosis which he classified as types I, II, III, and IV. Carter (1955) using the hemagglutination tests also identified four distinct serological types which he designated as A, B, C, and D, with type E being added and type C being subsequently dropped. These classifications were based on the antigenic composition of the capsular material present in freshly isolated organisms. More recently counterimmunoelectrophoresis has been used for the identification of types B and E (Carter and Changappa 1981). A standard system for serotyping of organisms has been recommended using uncomplicated and available procedures identifying the capsular and somatic antigens (Carter and Changappa 1981). Namioka (1970) reviewed the antigenic analysis of *P. multocida* and, based on Carter's method, classified the organisms found in Japan. The somatic antigens were also examined and were combined with Carter's capsular type in the classification (Namioka 1967). Serological and biochemical properties of 155 isolates of *P. multocida* from hemorrhagic septicemia throughout Malaysia were tested using both the passive mouse protection and the hemagglutination tests. The majority were classified as belonging to Carter's type B, a few were type D, and a number were untypable by either method. Biochemical properties of these strains were relatively uniform (Chandrasekaran *et al.* 1981). Biochemical and serological comparisons were also undertaken in the Sudan on 42 strains of *P. multocida* isolated from healthy cattle and from outbreaks of hemorrhagic septicemia. Thirty-eight strains belonged to either types B or E (Shigidi and Mustafa 1979). Although there has been no evidence of hemorrhagic septicemia occurring in Australia, type B, but with a different somatic antigen, was isolated from wound infection (Bain 1959; Bain and Jones 1958). Pasteurellae isolated from healthy cattle and those with shipping fever were serotyped according to the Carter classification of A, B, and D. No differences were observed in the morphology, biochemistry and pathogenicity in mice of the isolates from normal cattle and cattle with shipping fever (Huq 1976).

EPIZOOTIOLOGY

Geographic distribution and incidence

Hemorrhagic septicemia occurs in southern Europe, the USSR, Africa, the Near East, and Asia. The disease is particularly important in cattle and buffalo in southeast Asia. It is found to a lesser extent in the Near and Middle East and Africa. The disease is most prevalent during the rainy season, and other factors such as increased work, nutrition, changes in management, temperature, and seasonal variations predispose to development of clinical disease. Outbreaks are often associated with the rainy season. The incidence and mortality vary greatly from one region to another, depending on environmental factors and control measures. In southern Asia, the mortality is highest among buffalo and at levels varying from 1 to 10%. Animals of all ages are affected and there is no difference in susceptibility between various breeds. Currently the incidence is reduced substantially through the wide use of vaccines.

Literature

In a report from the Regional Commission for Asia, the Far East, and Oceania, the incidences of hemorrhagic septicemia were presented for 1975 to 1977 in cattle, buffalo, and swine which died. Mortality in cattle and buffalo in these 3 years varied from 46 to 2172, while numbers of animals vaccinated were from about 0.5 to 1.5 million per annum (Subharngkasen 1977). Husbandry and climatic conditions which decreased resistance and predisposed to infection were important (Vittoz 1952).

The epizootiology of pasteurellosis in India was described by Bhattacharya (1968) and Dhanda and Sen (1972), where hemorrhagic septicemia caused considerable losses in buffalo and cattle. It was estimated that 40 000 cattle and buffalo were lost each year (Dhanda 1960). Dhanda and Sen (1972) cited Lall (1963) who stated that the economic loss in cattle and buffalo in India was 10 million rupees per year. The authors summarized the number of outbreaks and incidences of deaths which occurred in various regions of the country during 1964. The disease was a serious problem with 6307 outbreaks affecting about 29 000 animals with mortality occurring in 19 000. In the State of Madras between 1957 and 1964 temperature and rainfall influenced the incidence of the disease (Gajapathi and D'Souza 1968). More recently, sporadic outbreaks of the disease were reported from Assam (Sarma and Boro 1980).

Perreau (1960) reported on the occurrence and control of hemorrhagic septicemia through vaccination in Central Africa. Wang *et al.* (1969) cited a report that 10% of cattle on the government farms in Ethiopia were killed by hemorrhagic septicemia. Shirlaw (1957a, b) pointed out the relative absence of epizootics in Kenya. Isolation of serotype E from Tanzania was reported by Hummel (1970). A case report on the occurrence of hemorrhagic septicemia in the African buffalo (*S. caffer*) was reported in Nigeria in an animal kept in a zoological garden (Kasali 1972). A serological survey of camels, a species occasionally considered to develop hemorrhagic septicemia, in northern areas of Chad showed that type *A P. multocida* infections were prevalent (Perreau *et al.* 1968).

In the USA, three epizootics in buffalo and one in young dairy cattle have been reported since 1911. Buffalo had significant levels of antibody and although the infection was endemic few outbreaks occurred (Heddleston and Gallagher 1969). Hemorrhagic septicemia caused by serotype B in young dairy cattle was reported from the USA by Kradel *et al.* (1969). The outbreak was characterized by sudden onset, rapid clinical course, and high mortality. The occurrence of hemorrhagic septicemia in Mexico was discussed by López-Mayagoitia (1977) and, although it was considered to be relatively common, actual incidence and economic importance has not been established.

Ochi (1957) reported on the epizootiology of hemorrhagic septicemia in Japan and it has been regarded to be responsible for considerable economic losses (Ogata 1968).

Transmission

Outbreaks of disease occur when there is a decrease in resistance in animals harboring the *Pasteurella* as occurs in cattle in poor condition at end of season. Transmission of organisms which result in clinical disease does not occur to normal in-contact animals and animals develop a clinical syndrome only when stressed. Normal carrier animals maintain the organisms, and inapparent infections are probably readily transmitted either by inhalation or ingestion of the organisms. Species other than cattle, buffalo, and swine are not known to play a role in the epizootiology. The organism does not survive long in the soil and stable environments.

Literature

The main features of transmission of *P. multocida* responsible for hemorrhagic septicemia were discussed by Bain (1963) and were the same as those which applied in general to the transmission of *Pasteurella* serotypes and species which made up part of the upper respiratory tract flora of animals. An apparatus to produce an aerosol of *P. multocida* was used in experimental infections of buffalo calves (Prince 1969b).

INFECTION

In clinical cases the infection is a fulminating septicemia which probably starts with infection of the tonsils. The organisms are excreted in the feces, urine, and milk. Pathogenicity is associated with the presence of the capsule, and the virulence of isolates is quickly decreased by subculture in an artificial media which results in loss of capsular substance.

In addition to buffalo, cattle, and pigs, natural disease syndromes are occasionally observed in the elephant, deer, bison, and camel. Susceptibility of goats and sheep is variable and these species generally are not susceptible to either natural or experimental infection. Experimentally, infections are induced by either feeding or by inhalation.

Literature

Bain (1963) summarized the information available on infectivity, virulence, and host susceptibilities. The carrier animal was the most likely source of organisms. Over 10% of cattle and buffalo in India and southeast Asia had naturally acquired immunity to hemorrhagic septicemia which was probably related to the carrier state. Virulent type B organisms were cultured from the nares and pharynx of buffalo slaughtered in abattoirs in India, Thailand, and Malaysia (Bain 1963). In another study 3% of apparently healthy cattle harbored various types of *P. multocida* (Huq 1976). Pathogenic strains of *Pasteurella* have been commonly isolated from the tonsils of healthy cattle (Chandrasekaran *et al.* 1981).

Various strains of *P. multocida* isolated from different lesions were studied and the growth of smooth, mucoid, and round colonies in cultures was correlated with virulence. Isolates from chronic lesions and diseases had characteristics which indicated lower virulence (Carter and Bigland 1953). Carter and Bain (1960) produced experimental infection in swine with organisms recovered from hemorrhagic septicemia in cattle, but this required 10^4 more organisms than required to kill cattle. The pathogenicity of three strains of *P. multocida* from isolates from Asia, Africa, and North America were compared in calves exposed by aerosol and intramuscular injections (Heddleston *et al.* 1967).

CLINICAL SIGNS

The frequency and duration of outbreaks in enzootic areas are dependent on the prevalence of infections, stress factors, and the immune status of the population. Fever, salivation, dullness, and bacteremia are detectable within 12 hours after experimental infection. As the disease progresses the animals lie down, are reluctant to move, and develop respiratory stress, with edema of the throat and brisket and occasionally of the forelegs. Once clinical signs appear mortality in natural or experimental disease is close to 100%. There is little information on less acute syndromes. Localized tissue infection damage probably occurs, as for example in the lungs with development of pneumonia. These syndromes are then classified as different forms of pasteurellosis.

Literature

Clinically affected animals invariably died, with buffalo usually dying within 24 hours and cattle surviving longer (Bain 1966). In buffalo the syndromes were septicemic, whereas in cattle localization in the respiratory system could occur. The subcutaneous edematous swellings were more prevalent in buffalo than in cattle; in some outbreaks up to 90% of cattle did not develop the characteristic swelling of the throat (Huilgol 1962). Occasionally the syndrome in buffalo calves was so severe that animals died suddenly without development of the edema. Animals were found dead with protrusion of the rectum and tongue and bleeding from the nostrils and rectum (Khare 1956).

Predisposing factors have been related to climate, livestock-rearing procedures, and other concurrent stresses. In Sri Lanka, an outbreak was associated with physical strain, nutritional deficiencies, and water deprivation (Dassanayake 1957). In Nigeria, an outbreak in Holstein cattle was related to heavy rainfall and a marked drop in atmospheric temperature (Anosa and Isoun 1975). Following vaccination with freeze-dried goat rinderpest tissue vaccine, outbreaks were observed in both buffalo and cattle in India with animals dying within 3 days after vaccination (Dillon *et al.* 1974). Secondary infections due to chronic debilitating diseases such as dermatophilosis, trypanosomiasis, anaplasmosis, and theileriosis were also considered to have a predisposing effect (Anosa and Isoun 1975).

PATHOLOGY

There is very little published information on the pathology of hemorrhagic septicemia. Lesions are those of general toxic changes associated with septicemic conditions without development of pathognomonic lesions. The main grossly observable lesions are edema of the larynx and petechiation of the mucosa of the upper respiratory system. Hemorrhages are also found on the heart and there may be excess bloodstained fluid in the pericardium and thoracic cavity. Lungs are congested and have variable evidence of pneumonia. Lymph nodes are also congested. Development of other lesions, which indicate localization of the circulating organism in either the respiratory or gastrointestinal systems, depends on the duration of infection.

Endotoxin is an important factor in pathogenesis. Release of endotoxin occurs during the terminal phase in the acute syndrome and is precipitated by chemotherapy.

Literature

In an outbreak of hemorrhagic septicemia in a dairy herd, affecting primarily calves and buffalo, the lesions were consistently found in the gastrointestinal tract of cattle and in the respiratory tract of buffalo (Siew *et al.* 1970). In a report on hemorrhagic septicemia in southwest Africa the pathological features were described and, in addition to the generalized congestion and subcutaneous edema of the submandibular area, fibrinous arthritis, tendovaginitis, and myositis with accompanying lymphadenitis were found (Bastianello and Jonker 1981). Gross and histologic lesions observed in acute infections in calves and pigs were comparable to those resulting from endotoxin administration. The lesions consisted of widely distributed hemorrhages, edema, and general hyperemia, particularly in the lungs, and indicated widespread changes in the vascular system (Rhoades *et al.* 1967).

IMMUNOLOGY

A variety of serological methods are used to detect the serotypes involved in pasteurellosis and include the mouse protection, slide agglutination, hemagglutination, and precipitation tests. The agar-gel diffusion test, used for somatic or O antigens, is used most extensively to demonstrate the antigenic type found in infected cattle. Antigens of serotypes B and E are found in capsulated strains.

Naturally occurring immunity occurs in 10% of cattle and buffalo in enzootic countries, and this immunity is probably closely correlated with the carrier state. Capsular antigens are the main protective substances, but somatic antigens also appear to have an influence on immunity. Although the mechanism of immunity is not fully defined, resistance in cattle and buffalo is related to the presence of circulating antibody.

Literature

Antigens in the capsule were either protein or polysaccharide. Using immunoelectrophoresis 18 soluble antigens were identified, some of which were capsular. Some of the antigens observed were similar to those found in other Gram-negative species of bacteria (Prince and Smith 1966a, b). Type B in phase 1 of growth contained protein which was immunogenic and nontoxic to mice, and carbohydrates which were toxic (Mukkur and Nilakantan 1972). The antigenic relationship among strains of *P. multocida* was investigated by immunodiffusion techniques. Sixteen soluble somatic antigens were shared between bovine and avian strains. Some capsular antigens in the lipopolysaccharide fraction were type-specific for serotypes B and E (Prince and Smith 1966c).

In cattle, both capsular and somatic antigens were important in stimulating efficient protection (Bain 1955a; Prince and Smith 1966c). Antibodies to both antigens were present in sera from naturally occurring immune cattle and buffalo and in experimentally infected rabbits (Prince 1969a). There was a correlation between the mouse protection and the serum bactericidal opsonizing tests and the resistance of cattle and buffalo to subcutaneous injection of *Pasteurella*. Phagocytosis had a role in bactericidal activity of immune sera but bactericidal antibodies were not clearly demonstrated (Bain 1960a). The occurrence of natural immunity in water buffalo was related to the high incidence of corners of *P. multocida* type B (Bain 1954).

The mouse passive immunization test and the indirect hemagglutination test have been used in the serological identification of isolates from hemorrhagic septicemia, but have not been used routinely in the diagnostic laboratory. A coagulation test using antibody-coated staphylococci was simple, rapid, inexpensive, and applicable for diagnostic work. The sero-groups B and E were readily differentiated by this test (Rimler 1978). A simple, improved, indirect hemagglutination test has been developed for the recognition of type A strains of *P. multocida* (Carter 1972).

VACCINATION

A number of vaccines are used against hemorrhagic septicemia and include antigens, bacterins, and attenuated live organisms, and are used with a variety of adjuvants. Immunization with intact bacteria is better than with various isolated antigens. Immunity is improved by various adjuvants such as oil, lanolin, alum, and alumina gel. Recently isolated encapsulated strains are superior in vaccine production and are related to the antigenic composition of organisms in the early growth phase.

Plain bacterins and alum adjuvant bacterins are now replaced by oil adjuvant bacterins which provide the most effective immunization method. These vaccines are used extensively and confer immunity for 9 to 12 months. To some degree the choice of type of vaccine depends on the requirements of a particular geographical region and on the technical facilities available. Animals are challenged following vaccination to detect development of resistance by subcutaneous injection of virulent organisms in the middle of the neck. In immune animals, a sharply circumscribed local reaction occurs within 24 hours, while in nonimmune animals a soft, diffuse, hot swelling develops which spreads steadily to the lower neck and brisket. Vaccines can also be evaluated by indirect means using the mouse protection and serum bactericidal test. Systemic postvaccination reactions occur with an incidence of up to 0.001%. Local reactions at site of vaccination are, however, more common.

Antisera is occasionally used prophylactically and therapeutically.

Literature

The early experimental work on vaccination was concerned with vaccines against pasteurellosis in general as well as against septicemia. Vaccination against hemorrhagic septicemia was found to be effective, while against pneumonic syndromes it was not successful (Ochi 1952). First vaccinations against pasteurellosis of fowl, swine, and sheep consisted of an initial injection of killed cultures and subsequent inoculation of live organisms (Vaysse and Zottner 1952). Bacterins and soluble antigens were effective and protection was usually persistent for up to 6 months (Delpy 1952; Danielson and Bolton 1950; Rau and Govil 1950).

Methods of producing vaccines against hemorrhagic septicemia were described in detail by Bain (1963) and there have been short accounts from various countries on the use of various forms of vaccine. Vaccination of cattle and buffalo against hemorrhagic septicemia was also discussed by Jacotot (1958). While various vaccines incorporating different adjuvants and using purified antigens have been used experimentally, they have not been applied extensively in the field (de Alwas and Carter, 1980). Adjuvants enhanced protection in cattle against a higher challenge dose of virulent organisms than bacterins alone (Iyer *et al.* 1955). One basic method consisted of a special medium to which formalin and alum was added (Iyigoren and Batu 1962). These vaccines were effective for a minimal period of up to 6 months after a single injection and up to 16 months after double vaccination (Israil *et al.* 1965). Aluminium hydroxide adjuvant vaccines containing endotoxin-free capsular antigens of serotypes B and E were effective, and passive mouse protection and indirect hemagglutination tests were related to the degree of protection (Nagy and Penn 1976).

In the early work on oil adjuvant vaccine against hemorrhagic septicemia, extensive laboratory and field trials indicated that capsular antigens were responsible for the protective antibodies (Dhanda 1959). Various oil emulsions in vaccines have been tried (Tacu 1969). Sodium alginate and oil adjuvant vaccines gave comparable protection, but the former was simpler to prepare and easier to administer (Bhatty 1973). Alum precipitated, oil adjuvant, and aluminum gel vaccines were also gamma-globulin responses, aluminum gel induced the highest gamma-globulin responses, aluminium gel induced the highest response (Paul *et al.* 1974). Immunizations using multiple emulsion and oil adjuvant vaccines were carried out in mice, rabbits, and calves.

Multiple emulsion vaccines were effective and were easily administered in the field as compared to the oil adjuvant vaccines which, because of their thick consistency, were difficult to inject (Mittal *et al.* 1979). Comparisons of the complete and incomplete Freund's adjuvants with oil adjuvants showed that a higher titer was obtained with Freund's adjuvant (Rao and Sambamurti 1972).

Production of oil adjuvant vaccine has been described in various laboratory facilities (Bain and Jones 1955; Jones 1967; Geneidy *et al.* 1967). An efficient method by the continuous culture system produced 100 000 doses per day (Sterne and Hutchinson 1958). Testing of various systems was undertaken to increase efficiency and decrease the cost (Shivdekar and Beri 1969). Methods using multiple strains were not ideal and a single strain possessing wide immunizing properties was practical (Thomas 1968). Oil adjuvant vaccine stored at 45 °C for about 800 days or at 37 to 42 °C for 20 days still conferred immunity following vaccination of cattle (Nangia *et al.* 1966).

Effective immunity lasted for 18 months in cattle protected with oil adjuvant vaccine (Quader and Hyder 1974; Geneidy *et al.* 1967). Water buffalo were also successfully vaccinated (Cerruti and Quesada 1966). Immunity was conferred for at least 35 days following vaccination (Thomas *et al.* 1969). American buffalo were successfully vaccinated against serotype 2 of *P. multocida* following an outbreak of hemorrhagic septicemia (Heddleston and Wessman 1973). Sheep and goats could also be protected against certain strains of *P. multocida* (Dua *et al.* 1977).

In the vaccination program against hemorrhagic septicemia, 0.001% of calves developed anaphylactic reaction to a vaccine and this appeared to be related to pepton content (Batu 1965). Persistent subcutaneous swelling at the site of vaccination was another complication (Thomas *et al.* 1969). Vaccination with both broth bacterin and oil adjuvant vaccines also affected antibody levels to *Brucella* organisms. In certain circumstances this had to be taken into consideration in the diagnosis of brucellosis on a serological basis (Panda *et al.* 1963).

Serological tests such as agglutination, mouse protection, and complement fixation were used to detect immunity in vaccinated cattle. The mouse protection test was the best indicator of immunity and the agar-gel agglutination test was also useful (Bain 1955b). Contrary to other opinions the slide agglutination test had certain advantages over the agar agglutination and mouse protection tests in demonstrating immunity (Dhanda *et al.* 1959). Although agglutinins and protective antibodies were indicative of resistance, their absence did not necessarily indicate susceptibility. Following vaccination, 30 to 50% of the animals had antibodies 1 week after vaccination, and these were still detectable 11 months after vaccination (Thomas 1970). Following immunization by a potassium thiocyanate extract of the antigen in oil adjuvant, the antibodies measured by the indirect hemagglutination technique played only a limited role in protecting against challenge (Mukkur and Nilakantan 1969).

Assessment of vaccines has always been complicated by the

occurrence of natural immunity in cattle and buffalo which has been reported to be as high as 10% of animals in enzootic areas. The oil adjuvant vaccines were effective, with good correlation between levels of protection developing in buffalo calves and that induced in the mouse protection test (Gupta and Sareen 1976). Rabbits have been used to test the potency of vaccines and responded comparably to buffalo calves and cattle (Mittal and Jaiswal 1976; Thomas and Saroja 1972).

Live vaccines have been found to have greater efficacy due to the preservation of the entire intact organism and its critical antigens which were lost during laboratory manipulation. Multiplication of the organism in a host has also induced a greater immune response than by its antigens alone. Live streptomycin-dependent *P. multocida* mutant vaccine was developed and was shown to be effective in protecting both mice and rabbits (Wei and Carter 1978). In cattle and buffalo calves a single dose of the vaccine conferred immunity from 60 to approximately 80% of cattle and 100% of buffalo. A booster dose given 3 weeks later enhanced immunity in cattle. There were no adverse reactions in cattle to this form of vaccination (de Alwis and Carter 1980).

Vaccination against pasteurellosis in cattle and sheep has been undertaken in combination with other bacterial vaccines in order to increase cost efficiency (Tropa 1952). Simultaneous vaccination at different sites against hemorrhagic septicemia and rinderpest was effective (El-Ghaffar *et al.* 1968). Also, a combination of hemorrhagic septicemia and black-quarter vaccines conferred dependable levels of immunity in cattle as well as in mice, the level of protection depending on the composition of the vaccines (Sinha and Prasad 1973; Srivastava *et al.* 1976).

CHEMOTHERAPY

Very early treatment with antibiotics is successful. During well-developed clinical stages of the acute disease chemotherapy is ineffective although the organisms are eliminated. Tissue damage has already occurred and massive release of dead organism greatly aggravates the pathophysiology.

Literature

Treatment of hemorrhagic septicemia has generally been considered to be ineffectual because of the sudden onset and short duration of the disease and the lack of response to treatment undertaken at any point other than during the very initial stages of infection (Prince and Smith 1966a). Sulfadimidine sodium and oxytetracycline hydrochloride have been the two drugs most commonly used in Malaysia (Thomas 1972). In comparing treatment of natural cases with either penicillin G, terramycin, or streptopenicillin, the latter was found to be most effective with about 73% of the animals recovering (Ansari 1968). Administration of antisera to animals exhibiting clinical signs as well as in-contact animals has been of questionable efficacy and currently is not used (Thomas 1972). Following intranasal experimental infection of buffalo, immune serum had no prophylactic or curative value, but daily sulfamezathine administration was effective (Kheng and Phay 1963). Although evidence has been presented that sulfamezathine and terramycin are useful in some instances, the wide use of chemotherapeutic agents, both prophylactically and in the face of an outbreak, have often failed (Thomas 1972).

DIAGNOSIS

Clinically, diagnosis is dependent on the presence of edema of the throat, but the irregularity and infrequency of this sign, particularly in cattle, together with the very short course of the acute syndrome make clinical diagnosis difficult. Microorganisms are often found in smears of blood or in fluid exudates. The best source of infected tissue uncontaminated by other bacteria is the bone marrow. Diagnosis is confirmed by culture and serotyping of the organisms. Serological tests are of limited value and useful only in confirming in part previous exposure to the antigens.

Literature

Bain (1963) summarized the diagnostic procedures to be followed which basically rely on identification of septicemia and the *Pasteurella* organism both in body fluids and through culture techniques. Other techniques include inoculation of rabbits and identification of specific antigens in tissues of infected animals.

CONTROL

Hemorrhagic septicemia is controlled by vaccines directed against the two specific *Pasteurella* serotypes and it is an effective method of prophylaxis. Failure to control the disease is due to the inadequate timing of vaccination programs and the poor quality of the vaccine. Oil adjuvant vaccines are effective, while broth vaccines should be limited to providing immediate protection during an outbreak and have to be followed by revaccination with oil adjuvant vaccines to induce long-lasting immunity.

Literature

The use of vaccines in the control of hemorrhagic septicemia was discussed by Bain (1960b). More recently, effective control of clinical disease by vaccination of buffalo, cattle, pigs, sheep, goats, and horses was undertaken in Indonesia (Anon. 1977). The epidemiological situation in Malaysia was reviewed and the effectiveness of chemotherapy and vaccination programs was established (Joseph 1979; Thomas 1972). In Thailand, where hemorrhagic septicemia has been considered to be an important disease of cattle and buffalo, it has been effectively controlled (Wongsongsarn *et al.* 1968). The control methods used in Iran were presented by Baharsefat and Firouzi (1977).

BIBLIOGRAPHY

Anon., 1977. Haemorrhagic septicaemia and eradication programme in Indonesia, *Bull. Off. int. Epiz.*, **87**(7–8): 609–12.

Anosa, V. O. and Isoun, T. T., 1975. An outbreak of haemorrhagic septicaemia in Holstein cattle in Nigeria: possible role of associated factors, *Bull. Anim. Hlth Prod. Afr.*, **23**: 337–40.

Ansari, M. Y., 1968. Chemotherapeutic trials of some antibiotics in clinical cases of bovine pasteurellosis (haemorrhagic septicaemia): I, *Sci. Indy.*, **6**(4): 420–4.

Baharsefat, M. and Firouzi, Sh., 1977. Progress in control of haemorrhagic septicaemia (pasteurellosis) in cattle in Iran, *Bull. Off. int. Epiz.*, **87**(7–8): 621–5.

Bain, R. V. S., 1954. Studies on haemorrhagic septicaemia of cattle I. Naturally acquired immunity in Siamese buffaloes, *Br. vet. J.*, **110**: 481–4.

Bain, R. V. S., 1955a. Studies on haemorrhagic septicaemia in cattle IV. A preliminary examination of the antigens of *Pasteurella multocida* Type I, *Br. vet. J.*, **111**: 492–8.

Bain, R. V. S., 1955b. Studies on haemorrhagic septicaemia of cattle V. Tests for immunity in vaccinated cattle, *Br. vet. J.*, **111**: 511–18.

Bain, R. V. S., 1959. Haemorrhagic septicaemia of cattle. Observations on some recent work, *Br. vet. J.*, **115**: 365–9.

Bain, R. V. S., 1960a. Mechanism of immunity in haemorrhagic septicaemia, *Nature*, **186**: 734–5.

Bain, R. V. S., 1960b. Recherches sur le vaccin contre la septicémie hémorragique, *Bull. Off. int. Epiz.*, **53**: 192–5.

Bain, R. V. S., 1963. Hemorrhagic septicemia. In *FAO Agricultural Studies No. 62*. FAO/UN (Rome) pp. 1–78.

Bain, R. V. S., 1966. Haemorrhagic septicaemia, *Proc. Aust. Vet. Assoc. NSW Div.*, 1965, pp. 38–9.

Bain, R. V. S. and Jones, R. F., 1955. Studies on haemorrhagic septicaemia of cattle III. Production of adjuvant vaccine, *Br. vet. J.*, **111**: 30–4.

Bain, R. V. S. and Jones, R. F., 1958. The production of dense cultures of *Pasteurella multocida*, *Br. vet. J.*, **114**: 215–20.

Bastianello, S. and Jonker, M. R., 1981. A report on the occurrence of septicaemia caused by *Pasteurella multocida* type E in cattle from southern Africa, *J. S. Afr. vet. med. Ass.*, **52**: 99–104.

Batu, A., 1965. Anaphylactic reactions in cattle septicaemia in 1964, *Turk. Veteriner Hekimieri Dernegi Dergisis*, **35**: 459–63.

Bhattacharya, P., 1968. Regional epizootiology and prophylaxis of pasteurellosis (India), *Bull. Off. int. Epiz.*, **69**(1–2): 95–7.

Bhatty, M. A., 1973. A preliminary comparison of sodium alginate and oil adjuvants haemorrhagic septicaemia vaccines in cattle, *Bull. Epiz. Dis. Afr.*, **21**: 171–4.

Carter, G. R., 1955. Studies on *Pasteurella multocida*. I. A hemagglutination test for the identification of serological types, *Am. J. vet. Res.*, **16**: 481–4.

Carter, G. R., 1972. Improved hemagglutination tests for identifying type A strains of *Pasteurella multocida*, *Appl. Microbiol.*, **24**(1): 162–3.

Carter, G. R., 1981. The genus *Pasteurella*. In *The Prokaryotes. A Handbook of Habits, Isolation, and Identification of Bacteria*, eds M. P. Starr, H. Stolo, H. G. Truedfr, A. Balows, H. G. Schlegel. Springer-Verlag (Berlin, Heidelberg, New York)., pp. 1383–91.

Carter, G. R. and Bain, R. V. S., 1960. Pasteurellosis (*Pasteurella multocida*); a review stressing recent developments, *Vet Res. Annot.*, **6**: 105–8.

Carter, G. R. and Bigland, C. H., 1953. Dissociation and virulence in strains of *Pasteurella multocida* isolated from a variety of lesions, *Can. J. comp. Med.*, **17**: 473–9.

Carter, G. R. and Changappa, M. M., 1981. Recommendations for a standard system of designating serotypes of *Pasteurella multocida*, *Proc. 24th Ann. Meet. Am. Ass. Vet. Lab. Diag.*, pp. 37–42.

Cerruti, C. and Quesada, A., 1966. Richerche sulla vaccinazione dei bufali contro il barrone bufalino, *La Clinical Veterinaria*, **89**(8): 233–9.

Chandrasekaran, S., Yeap, P. C. and Chuink, B. H., 1981. Biochemical and serological studies of *Pasteurella multocida* isolated from cattle and buffaloes in Malaysia, *Br. vet. J.*, **137**: 361–7.

Danielson, I. S. and Bolton, R., 1950. Laboratory studies on the immunizing value of hemorrhagic septicemia bacterin and blackleg bacterin, *Proc. 54th Ann. Meet. US Livestock Sanit. Ass.*, pp. 259–71.

Dassanayake, L., 1957. The haemorrhagic septicaemia outbreak of 1955–56, *Ceylon vet. J.*, **5**: 56–8.

de Alwais, M. C. L. and Carter, G. R., 1980. Preliminary field trials with a streptomycin-dependent vaccine against haemorrhagic

septicaemia, *Vet. Rec.*, **106**: 435–7.
Delpy, L. P., 1952. Méthodes d'immunisation active contre les pasteurelloses septicémiques, *Bull. Off. int. Epiz.*, **38**: 209–18.
Dhanda, M. R., 1959. Immunization of cattle against haemorrhagic septicaemia with purified capsular antigens (a preliminary communication), *Indian vet. J.*, **36**: 6–8.
Dhanda, M. R., 1960. Haemorrhagic septicaemia in India, *Bull. Off. int. Epiz.*, **53**: 128–32.
Dhanda, M. R., Lall, J. M., Seth, R. N. and Chandrasekariah, P., 1959. Immunological studies on *Pasteurella septica* III. Indirect tests as indicators of immunity in haemorrhagic septicaemia, *Indian vet. J.*, **29**: 30–46.
Dhanda, M. R. and Sen, G. P., 1972. *Haemorrhagic Septicaemia and Allied Conditions in Sheep, Goats, Pigs, and Poultry*, eds P. L. Jaiswal, R. R. Lokeshwar. Indian Council of Agricultural Research (New Delhi), pp. 1–40.
Dillon *et al.*, 1974. Incidence of haemorrhagic septicaemia in cattle and buffaloes in course of rinderpest vaccination, *JNKVV Res. J.*, **8**(3–4): 283–9.
Dua, S. K., Pandurangareo, C. C. and Khera, S. S., 1977. Studies on the use of bovine haemorrhagic septicaemia vaccine in sheep and goats, *Indian vet. J.*, **54**: 421–4.

El-Ghaffar, M. M. A., El-Ghaffar, S. A., Lotfy, O., Geneidy, A. A., El-Affandy, A. M., Maker, W. and Aly, A. M., 1968. The simultaneous immunization against haemorrhagic septicaemia and rinderpest, *Egypt. Vet. Med. Assoc. J.*, **28**: 139–43.

Gajapathi, V. S. and D'Souza, B. A., 1968. Epidemiological studies on haemorrhagic septicaemia, black-quarter and foot and mouth disease in Madras state for the period 1957–1964, *Indian vet. J.*, **45**: 175–86.
Geneidy, A. A., Lotfy, O. and El-Affandy, A. M., 1967. Control of haemorrhagic septicaemia with special reference to the new oil adjuvant vaccine, *Egypt. Vet. Med. Assoc. J.*, **27**: 121–6.
Gupta, M. L. and Sareen, R. L., 1976. Evaluation of haemorrhagic septicaemia oil adjuvant vaccine by mouse protection test, *Indian vet. J.*, **53**: 489–92.

Heddleston, K. L. and Gallagher, J. E., 1969. Septicemic pasteurellosis (hemorrhagic septicemia) in the American bison: a serologic survey, *Proc. Ann. Conf. Bull. Wildl. Dis. Assoc.*, **5**: 205–7.
Heddleston, K. L., Rhoades, K. R. and Rebers, P. A., 1967. Experimental pasteurellosis: comparative studies on *Pasteurella multocida* from Asia, Africa and North America, *Am. J. vet. Res.*, **28**(125): 1003–12.

Heddleston, K. L. and Wessman, G., 1973. Vaccination of American bison against *Pasteurella multocida* serotype 2 infection (hemorrhagic septicemia), *J. Wildl. Dis.*, **9**: 306–10.
Huilgol, N.S., 1962. Observations on haemorrhagic septicaemia in bovines, *Indian vet. J.*, **39**: 450–4.
Hummel, P. H., 1970. Isolation of *Pasteurella multocida* Carter type E in Tanzania, *Vet. Rec.*, **86**: 42–3.
Huq, A. Y. Md. A., 1976. A comparison of *Pasteurella multocida* isolated from healthy cattle and cattle with shipping fever. III. The comparison with reference to Carter's type A, B, C, and D, *Indian vet. J.*, **53**: 319–22.

Israil, M., Quader, M. A. and Hyder, G., 1965. Haemorrhagic septicaemia alum precipitated vaccines, *Bull. Off. int. Epiz.*, **64**: 791–800.
Iyer, S. V., Gopalakrishnan, K. S. and Ramani, K., 1955. Studies on haemorrhagic septicaemia vaccines. The effect of adjuvants upon the immunizing value of formalin-killed *Pasteurella boviseptica* organisms, *Indian vet. J.*, **31**: 379–91.
Iyigoren, B. and Batu, A., 1962. A vaccine against haemorrhagic septicaemia in cattle. *Turk. Veteriner Hekimeiri Dernegi Dergisis*, **32**: 144–51.

Jacotot, H., 1958. Vaccination against pasteurellosis of cattle and buffaloes, *Rev. Elev. Méd. vét. Pays trop.*, **11**: 143–6.
Jones, R. F., 1967. *The Production of Vaccine for the Control of Haemorrhagic Septicaemia. Report to the Government of Ceylon*. United Nations Development Program, TA 2329, pp. 1–18.
Joseph, P. G., 1979. Haemorrhagic septicaemia in peninsular Malaysia, *Kajian Veterinar*, **11**: 65–79.

Kasali, O. B., 1972. A case of haemorrhagic septicaemia in an African buffalo (*Syncerus nanus*) in Nigeria. *Bull. epiz. Dis. Afr.*, **20**: 203–4.
Khare, V. G., 1956. Haemorrhagic septicaemia – some unusual aspects of the disease, *Indian vet. J.*, **32**: 287–9.
Kheng, C. S. and Phay, C. P., 1963. Haemorrhagic septicaemia. Sulphamezathine and immune serum therapy in buffaloes infected by the intranasal spray method, *Vet. Rec.*, **75**(7): 155–8.
Kradel, D. C., Heddleston, K. L., Risser, J. V. and Manspeaker, J. E., 1969. Septicemic pasteurellosis (hemorrhagic septicemia) in young dairy cattle, *Vet. Med. Small Anim. Clin.*, **64**: 145–7.

Lall, J. M., 1963. Haemorrhagic septicaemia – a serious scourge of cattle, *Indian Livestock*, **1**(4): 37.
López-Mayagoitia, A., 1977. Septicemia hemorrágica, *Veterinaria Méx.*, **8**: 111–18.

Mittal, K. R. and Jaiswal, T. N., 1976. Potency testing of haemorrhagic septicaemia oil adjuvant vaccine in rabbits, *Indian vet. J.*, **53**: 393–5.

Mittal, K. R., Jaiswal, T. N. and Gupta, B. K., 1979. Studies on haemorrhagic septicaemia oil adjuvant and multiple emulsion adjuvant vaccines II. Immunity trials in mice, rabbits and calves, *Indian vet. J.*, **56**: 449–54.

Mukkur, T. K. S. and Nilakantan, P. R., 1969. The relationship of hemagglutinating antibody with protection in cattle immunized against hemorrhagic septicemia, *Cornell Vet.*, **59**: 643–7.

Mukkur, T. K. S. and Nilakantan, P. R., 1972. Preliminary characterization of the crude capsular extracts of *Pasteurella multocida* var. bovine, type I in phase I, *Cornell Vet.*, **62**: 289–96.

Nagy, L. K. and Penn, C. W., 1976. Protection of cattle against experimental haemorrhagic septicaemia by the capsular antigens of *Pasteurella multocida*, types B and E, *Res. vet. Sci.*, **20**: 249–53.

Namioka, S., 1967. Pathogenicity and aetiology of *Pasteurella multocida* – with special reference to hemorrhagic septicemia and fowl cholera, *Jap. Agr. Res. Quart.*, **1**(4): 26–34.

Namioka, S., 1970. Antigenic analysis of *Pasteurella multocida, Nat. Inst. Anim. Hlth Quart.*, **10**: 97–108.

Nangia, S. S., Baxi, K. K., Gulrajani, T. S. and Seetharaman, C., 1966. Haemorrhagic septicaemia oil adjuvant vaccine-study of potency test in rabbits – duration of immunity and keeping quality, *Indian vet. J.*, **43**: 279–87.

Ochi, Y., 1952. La septicémie hémorragique et sa prophylaxie, *Bull. Off. int. Epiz.*, **38**: 226–32.

Ochi, Y., 1957. Septicémie hémorrhagique au Japon, *Bull. Off. int. Epiz.*, **47**(9–10): 703–8.

Ogata, M., 1968. Pasteurellosis in Japan: recent progress in the research of *Pasteurella multocida* in this country, *Bull. Off. int. Epiz.*, **69**(1–2): 99–115.

Panda, S. N., Misra, B. and Acharya, B. N., 1963. The effect of haemorrhagic septicaemia vaccination on *Brucella* agglutination test in cattle, *Indian vet. J.*, **40**: 45–9.

Paul, W. M., Moses, J. S. and Balaprakasam, R. A., 1974. An electrophoretic analysis of the efficiency of alum precipitated, oil adjuvant and alumina gel adsorbed vaccine against haemorrhagic septicaemia, *Cheiron*, **3**(2): 100–6.

Perreau, P., 1960. La septicémie hémorrhagique des bovidés dans le Centre-Afrique français, *Bull. Off. int. Epiz.*, **53**: 116–27.

Perreau, P., Maurice, Y., Botto, M. T. and Gayt, P., 1968. Epizootologie de la pasteurellose des chameaux au Tchad enquête sérologique, *Rev. Elev. Méd. vét. Pays trop.*, **21**(4): 451–4.

Prince, G. H., 1969a. Production of antigens of *Pasteurella multocida* and detection of antibodies against them in bovine sera, *J. Comp. Path.*, **79**: 173–86.

Prince, G. H., 1969b. Use of apparatus for controlled infection of buffalo calves with an aerosol of *Pasteurella multocida*, *J. Comp. Path.*, **79**: 187–96.

Prince, G. H. and Smith, J. E., 1966a. Antigenic studies on *Pasteurella multocida* using immunodiffusion techniques I. Identification and nomenclature of the soluble antigens of a bovine haemorrhagic septicaemia strain, *J. Comp. Path.*, **76**: 303–14.

Prince, G. H. and Smith, J. E., 1966b. Antigenic studies on *Pasteurella multocida* using immunodiffusion techniques II. Relationships with other Gram-negative species, *J. Comp. Path.*, **76**: 313–21.

Prince, G. H. and Smith, J. E., 1966c. Antigenic studies on *Pasteurella multocida* using immunodiffusion techniques III. Relationships between strains of *Pasteurella multocida*, *J. Comp. Path.*, **76**: 321–32.

Quader, M. and Hyder, G., 1974. Haemorrhagic septicaemia oil adjuvant vaccine-1, *Bang. Vet. J.*, **8**(1–4): 21–4.

Rao, N. M. and Sambamurti, B., 1972. Immunological studies on Freund's type vaccines against haemorrhagic septicaemia in calves, *Indian vet. J.*, **49**: 25–32.

Rau, K. G. and Govil, J. L., 1950. An improved haemorrhagic septicaemia vaccine, *Indian vet. J.*, **27**: 105–13.

Rhoades, K. R., Heddleston, K. L. and Rebers, P. A., 1967. Experimental hemorrhagic septicemia: gross and microscopic lesions resulting from acute infections and from endotoxin administration, *Can. J. comp. Med. Vet. Sci.*, **31**: 226–7.

Rimler, R. B., 1978. Coagglutination test for identification of *Pasteurella multocida* associated with hemorrhagic septicemia, *J. Clin. Microbiol.*, **8**(2): 214–18.

Roberts, R. S., 1947. An immunological study of *Pasteurella septica*, *J. Comp. Path.*, **57**: 261–78.

Sarma, G. and Boro, B. R., 1980. Isolation of *Pasteurella multocida* from sporadic outbreaks of bovine pasteurellosis in Assam, *Vet. Rec.*, **106**: 57–8.

Shigidi, M. T. A. and Mustafa, A. A., 1979. Biochemical and serological studies on *Pasteurella multocida* isolated from cattle in the Sudan, *Cornell Vet.*, **69**: 77–84.

Shirlaw, J. F., 1957a. Some observations on bovine pasteurellosis in Kenya, *Br. vet. J.*, **113**: 35–46.

Shirlaw, J. F., 1957b. Some observations on bovine pasteurellosis in

Kenya Part II, *Br. vet. J.*, **113**: 71–89.

Shivdekar, D. S. and Beri, S. P., 1969. Possibilities of preparation of an oil adjuvant vaccine against haemorrhagic septicaemia of cattle using a medium containing papain digest of beef, *Indian vet. J.*, **46**: 367–70.

Siew, T. W., Hadi, N. A. and Thomas, J., 1970. Outbreak of haemorrhagic septicaemia in a dairy herd, *Kajian Vet. Malaysia–Singapore*, **2**(3): 139–44.

Sinha, A. K. and Prasad, L. B. M., 1973. An experimental study with combined vaccines against haemorrhagic septicaemia and black quarter, *Br. vet. J.*, **129**: 175–83.

Srivastava, N. C., Harbola, P. C. and Khera, S. S., 1976. Preliminary observations on combined vaccination against haemorrhagic septicaemia and black quarter, *Indian vet. J.*, **53**: 168–74.

Sterne, M. and Hutchinson, I., 1958. The production of bovine haemorrhagic septicaemia vaccine by continuous culture, *Br. vet. J.*, **114**: 176–9.

Subharngkasen, S., 1977. Haemorrhagic septicaemia, *Bull. Off. int. Epiz.*, **87**(7–8): 607–8.

Tacu, D., 1969. Oil emulsion vaccine against bovine pasteurellosis, *Lucrarile Institului de Cerciltare Veterinair si Bio-preparate Pasteur*, **6**: 481–7.

Thomas, J., 1968. Studies on haemorrhagic septicaemia oil-adjuvant vaccine I. Methods of production of vaccine, *Kajian Vet. Malaysia–Singapore*, **1**(3): 152–8.

Thomas, J., 1970. Studies on haemorrhagic septicaemia oil-adjuvant vaccine III. Serological studies. *Kajian Vet. Malaysia–Singapore*, **2**(3): 103–12.

Thomas, J., 1972. The control of haemorrhagic septicaemia in west Malaysia, *Trop. Anim. Hlth Prod.*, **4**: 95–101.

Thomas, J., Omar, A. R., Fadzil, M., Mustaffa-babjee, A. and Vendargon, X. A., 1969. Studies on haemorrhagic septicaemia oil-adjuvant vaccine II. Field and laboratory trials, *Kajian Vet. Malaysia–Singapore*, **2**(1): 4–12.

Thomas, J. and Saroja, S., 1972. The evaluation of haemorrhagic septicaemia vaccines in rabbits, *Kajian Vet. Malaysia–Singapore*, **4**(2): 49–59.

Tropa, E., 1952. Les pasteurelloses et les méthodes d'immunisation les concernant, *Bull. Off. int. Epiz.*, **38**: 196–208.

Vaysse, J. and Zottner, G., 1952. Les pasteurelloses au Maroc méthodes d'immunisation, *Bull. Off. int. Epiz.*, **38**: 219–25.

Vittoz, R., 1952. Importance en Asie des facteurs géographiques et climatiques dans l'épizootologie et la prophylaxie des pasteurelloses, *Bull. Off. int. Epiz.*, **38**: 240–86.

Wang, C. T., Wu, M. H., Mahari, Y., Abate, F. and Tesema, A., 1969. An outbreak of hemorrhagic septicemia of cattle in Gorgora and Guramba Begemder Province, Ethiopia, *J. Taiw. Ass. Anim. Husb. Vet. Med.*, **14**: 44–51.

Wei, B. D. and Carter, G. R., 1978. Live streptomycin-dependent *Pasteurella multocida* vaccine for the prevention of hemorrhagic septicemia, *Am. J. vet. Res.*, **39**(9): 1534–7.

Wongsongsarn, C., Bhuchongsmutta, C. and Dissamarn, R., 1968. The eradication of haemorrhagic septicaemia in Thailand, *Bull. Off. int. Epiz.*, **69**(1–2): 119–21.

PART
IV
RICKETTSIAL DISEASES

Chapter

19

Anaplasmosis

CONTENTS

INTRODUCTION

Rickettsial diseases

The rickettsiae are a group of organisms classified in the order Rickettsiales with 17 genera distributed in the 3 families – Rickettsiaceae, Bartonellaceae, and Anaplasmataceae. Nineteen species parasitize domestic animals and have a worldwide distribution in both temperate and tropical zones. The following rickettsial diseases are considered of veterinary importance in tropical and subtropical regions and are reviewed: (1) anaplasmosis, (2) heartwater, (3) ehrlichiosis, (4) Q fever.

Rickettsial diseases of domestic animals of tropical veterinary importance comprise a heterogeneous group whose members share only a few common characteristics and differ significantly in their pathogenesis. A common characteristic is that the organisms are obligate intracellular parasites and multiply in membrane-lined vacuoles in the cytoplasm of infected cells. Infections differ in the cell tropism – *Cowdria ruminantium* causing heartwater localizes in the cytoplasm of reticuloendothelial cells, the *Anaplasma* species invade erythrocytes, and *Ehrlichia* species infect leukocytes.

The distribution of the rickettsiae is governed by vector activity. *Anaplasma* species have a wide range of arthropod vectors and cause the most widely distributed rickettsial disease in ruminants. *Coxiella burnetti*, the causative agent of Q fever, although not an important cause of clinical syndromes in domestic animals, has the widest range of animal species being infected. The most important are the domestic ruminants which serve as reservoir hosts.

Literature

A list of rickettsial diseases of specific tropical interest, excluding anaplasmosis, was presented by Bruner and Gillespie (1973) who briefly reviewed their distribution, tissue tropism and species of animal affected (see Table 19.1).

Scott (1978) presented a comprehensive review of tick-borne rickettsial diseases of domestic animals. In earlier literature there have been brief summaries of rickettsial diseases of domestic animals with 12 species considered of veterinary importance. The syndromes were divided according to whether they were local lesions or systemic

Table 19.1

Disease	Geographical distribution	Causative organism	Cell or tissues affected: natural hosts
Heartwater	East and South Africa	*Cowdria ruminantium*	Sheep, cattle, goats, and some wild ungulates; vascular endothelium
Benign bovine rickettsiosis	North and South Africa	*Ehrlichia bovis*	Cattle; lymphocytes and monocytes
Benign ovine rickettsiosis	North and South Africa	*Ehrlichia ovina*	Sheep; lymphocytes and monocytes
Canine ehrlichiosis	North and East Africa, India, Sri Lanka, Aruba, USA	*Ehrlichia canis*	Dogs and jackals; lymphocytes and monocytes
Equine ehrlichiosis	California	*Ehrlichia* sp.	Horses and burrows; granulocytes

diseases (Khera 1962; Manjrekar 1954). Ristic (1977) discussed the immunology of the diseases caused by *C. ruminantium* and the *Anaplasma* and *Ehrlichia* species.

Compared to the large amount of information which has been available on the rickettsial diseases of man, there is relatively little published information on most rickettsial diseases of domestic animals, on either the biology of the organisms or the mechanisms of pathogenesis involved in diseases. The morphology, growth, and physiology of rickettsiae causing diseases in man have been reviewed (Ormsbee 1969; Weiss 1973). Epidemiology, control, and public health significance of rickettsiosis in man have also been extensively discussed (Brezina *et al.* 1973; Weyer 1978).

Anaplasmosis

Anaplasmosis is a tick-borne disease of cattle, sheep, goats, buffalo, and some wild ruminants, caused by the hemotropic rickettsiae *A. marginale*, *A. centrale*, and *A. ovis* and characterized by progressive anemia. In tropical and subtropical regions of the world, anaplasmosis is an important economic disease of cattle, causing losses through mortality, reduction of weight gains and of milk production. Prevention of disease through chemotherapy, vaccination, and vector control is expensive and has an effect on the economics of livestock production.

Literature

Ristic (1960a, 1968, 1977, 1980) has reviewed the history of anaplasmosis and described in detail the causative organism, its epidemiology and transmission, and the pathogenesis, immunology, diagnosis, chemotherapy, and prophylaxis of the disease it caused. In another publication, Ristic (1976) discussed the diseases caused by species of *Theileria, Babesia*, and rickettsia. Kuttler (1979) summarized information on the diagnosis, treatment, immunization, and vector control of anaplasmosis in the USA. A review of ovine and caprine anaplasmosis included information on etiology, transmission, epidemiology, clinical signs, and pathology (Neitz 1968).

ETIOLOGY

Anaplasma organisms belong to the genus *Anaplasma* of the family Anaplasmataceae, order Rickettsiales. The organisms are obligate intraerythrocytic parasites and are referred to as marginal, inclusion, or anaplasma bodies in the cells. Transmission is by arthropod vectors, predominantly the tick, in which they undergo cyclic development. Three *Anaplasma* species are important in veterinary medicine. *Anaplasma marginale* is most pathogenic for cattle, *A. centrale* causes a relatively mild form of bovine anaplasmosis, and *A. ovis* causes infections and limited disease in sheep and goats. *Paranaplasma* is another genus found in cattle and deer in North America. The species in this genus differ from *Anaplasma* species in that the inclusion bodies have appendages and infections are usually asymptomatic.

In blood smears, *A. marginale* is spherical, 0.2 to 1.0 μm in diameter and stains bluish purple with Giemsa stain. Other shapes occur and include comma, rod, and ring forms. The organism is composed of up to eight subunits or initial bodies which are the basic infectious particles and are surrounded by a membrane. The morphology of *A. centrale* is comparable but the organism is found towards the centre of the erythrocytes. Morphologically, anaplasmas sometimes resemble other hemotropic rickettsiae in the genera *Haemobartonella* and *Eperythrozoon*.

Literature

On the basis of morphology and antigenicity, two distinct genera in the family Anaplasmataceae, represented by *A. marginale* and *P. caudatum*, were identified (Kreier and Ristic 1963b, c, 1972). The latter organism was first found in erythrocytes of cattle in the USA in a mixed infection with *A. marginale*. Inclusion bodies of *P. caudatum* differed in that the organism had appendages, usually in the form of a tapering tail, loop, or ring which appeared only in bovine erythrocytes (Carson *et al.* 1974).

The morphological characteristics of the *Anaplasma* and *Paranaplasma* species in the erythrocytes of different hosts were compared by Ristic (1980). The variable morphology of *Anaplasma* sometimes makes identification and classification difficult (Kreier and Ristic 1972).

There have been numerous studies of the morphology of *Anaplasma* as observed by light microscopy but relatively few on *Paranaplasma* (Brock 1962; Carson *et al.* 1974; Scott *et al.* 1961, Espana *et al.* 1959). In addition to being stained by Giemsa's stain it was Gram negative and stained with acridine orange (Amerault *et al.* 1973). The limiting membrane of inclusions was observed by immunoferritin labeling to be derived from the erythrocyte membrane (Francis *et al.* 1979).

The ultrastructure of *A. marginale* in erythrocytes has been studied extensively with the observation of the subunits making up the inclusion bodies (De Robertis and Epstein 1957; Foote *et al.* 1958; Ristic 1960a, b, 1967; Kocan *et al.* 1978a; Amerault *et al.* 1975). The inclusion body consisted of one to eight initial bodies embedded in a homogeneous matrix demarcated from the erythrocytes by a well-defined irregular lining membrane with several extensions into the erythrocyte (Gates *et al.* 1967). Intracytoplasmic vesicles contained subunits and fibrillar strands and bodies appeared to be food vacuoles (Simpson *et al.* 1967). The initial bodies were round or oval, 0.3 to 0.4 μm in diameter, and enclosed in a double membrane (Ristic and Watrach 1961; Ristic 1967; Francis *et al.* 1979). The ultrastructure of *A. marginale* in cytoplasm of *Aedes albopictus*-cultured cells was comparable to that observed in the erythrocytes (Mazzola *et al.* 1979).

Paranaplasma species in erythrocytes of cattle appeared as dumbbell, comet, ring, and bipolar discoid forms with the tail of the organisms appearing as distinct cylindrical structures (Keeton and Jain 1973).

Biochemistry

The organism contains both deoxyribonucleic acid (DNA), ribonucleic acid (RNA), and proteins. The metabolism of the organism has been studied to a limited degree by the measuring of enzymatic activity and amino acid incorporation of the erythrocytes of cattle infected with *Anaplasma marginale.*

Literature

The histochemical properties of *A. marginale* indicated the presence of DNA, RNA, protein, and organic iron (Moulton and Christensen 1955). Studies with ^{14}C-labeled amino acids showed that protein synthesis occurred when organisms were outside the erythrocyte (Johns and Dimopoullos 1974). Increased incorporation of various nucleic and amino acids also occurred in red blood cells infected with *A. marginale* (Billups *et al.* 1973). Increased incorporation of glycine by bovine erythrocytes infected with *A. marginale* was also reported (Mason and Ristic 1967).

Tissue culture

Various techniques have been used in attempts to cultivate *A. marginale* in tissue culture systems of mammalian and arthropod origins. Currently a culture system using red blood cells is available, in which the organisms multiply and can be maintained for up to 60 days although they are not always infective for cattle. This system is important for various *in vitro* research applications, especially in immunology and chemotherapy.

Literature

Short *in vitro* cultivation of *A. marginale* for 1 to 5 days in bovine erythrocytes and in peripheral blood lymphocytes has been used for metabolic and antigen studies (Davis *et al.* 1978, 1981). Attenuated *A. marginale* could be cultured in suspensions of ovine erythrocytes and bovine erythrocytes for 42 days. The organism had a period of rapid growth followed by gradual decrease in the percentage of parasitized erythrocytes. A threefold increase occurred in the primary culture during the first 8 days and further slight increases were observed in the second and third subcultures. During the process of invasion, growth, and multiplication the organism was studied and infection was transferred from ovine to bovine erythrocytes (Kessler and Ristic 1979; Kessler *et al.* 1979). In cultures of bovine erythrocytes infected with *A. marginale* a 4.5-fold increase occurred by day 3 and a 3.3-fold increase by day 11, and these cultures were pathogenic for calves up to day 12 (Mazzola and Kuttler 1980). Work on continuous *in vitro* cultures showed that the marginal bodies leave red blood cells without the lysis of host cells (Erp and Hahrney 1975).

Other cell culture systems have also been tried. In cells from bovine lymph nodes the organism multiplied within 6 hours, reaching the highest levels at 12 to 24 hours; after 24 hours numbers decreased rapidly but a few were still detected for at least 7 days (Hidalgo 1975). In this sytem the organism has been cultured through three serial passages, but continuous *in vitro* cultivation has not yet been achieved (Kuttler and Hidalgo 1980). A rabbit bone marrow tissue culture system was found to be infective for up to 140 days (Marble and Hanks 1972).

EPIZOOTIOLOGY

Geographic distribution and economic importance

Anaplasma marginale is widespread through tropical and subtropical regions and infects cattle, water buffalo, sheep, goats, and a variety of wild ruminants. *Anasplasma centrale* occurs naturally only on the African continent and causes a benign form of anaplasmosis. The organism has been introduced into Australia and Latin America in vaccination procedures. *Anaplasma ovis* has a comparable distribution to *A. marginale*. *Paranaplasma* is reported only in North America. A carrier state exists in domestic and many species of wild ruminants.

The incidence of anaplasmosis is determined by serological survey and hematologic examination. Although infection rates can be high, anaplasmosis in many tropical countries does not always cause significant economic losses. The prevalence of clinical syndromes depends on the maintenance of enzootic stability. The incidence and economic importance varies from one region and country to another depending on climatic conditions and movement of livestock. Unless new susceptible cattle are introduced into an enzootic region, the problem of anaplasmosis, as with some other tick-borne diseases, is usually relatively minor. Introduction of highly susceptible cattle, particularly those imported from temperate climates to improve local industry, results in the outbreak of severe clinical disease.

Literature

The epidemiology and control of anaplasmosis in Australia was reviewed by Rogers and Shiels (1979). *Anaplasma marginale* was studied in two endemic areas of Queensland, and the incidence of infection in calves was 46 to 90%. Infections were diagnosed by the complement fixation (CF) test and occurred most frequently after a wet summer. Infected calves were asymptomatic and their growth rates were comparable to those of vaccinated animals (Paull *et al.* 1980).

On the African continent there has been considerable variation in the prevalence of infection in different regions. In East Africa, 52% of the cattle surveyed were either identified as infected by hematological examination or had antibody activity as determined by the CF test. Of the 117 samples tested from wild ruminants, 15 were either positive or suspicious (Kuttler 1965). A survey of Nigerian Zebu trade cattle, using the card agglutination test, revealed a reaction rate of 34% (Obi 1978).

A survey undertaken in India showed that, on the basis of the capillary tube agglutination test, approximately 60% of cattle, 30% of buffalo, 60% of sheep and 70% of goats were infected with *A. marginale* (Gautam and Singh 1971).

The epizootiology of bovine anaplasmosis in Latin America is influenced by the variations in tropical, subtropical, and cool climates and prevalence rates of up to 90% have been reported. Extensive losses occurred when either susceptible cattle were imported (Knowles *et al.* 1982) or when indigenous cattle were moved from the cold mountainous areas to subtropical regions. Relapsing cases also occurred in indigenous cattle in enzootic areas precipitated by nutritional and environmental stress (Corrier *et al.* 1978). In Colombia, serologic surveys have shown 90% prevalence of infection in cattle (Kuttler *et al.* 1970; Patarroyo *et al.* 1978). In Bolivia, a prevalence rate of 80 to 90% was also demonstrated by the indirect fluorescent antibody (IFA) test (Nicholls *et al.* 1980). A group of calves was followed serologically from birth to 87 days of age; the titers did not reflect a recognized trend of infections (Berry *et al.* 1981). Similar serologic surveys of cattle in other countries have shown a 78.5% prevalence of *A. marginale* infection in El Salvador (Payne and Scott 1982), 25% in St Lucia (Knowles *et al.* 1982), and 80 to 90% in Jamaica (Bundy *et al.* 1983).

A list of the known country distribution of ovine and caprine anaplasmosis in Africa, America, Asia, and Europe was presented by Neitz (1968). There have not been any recent reports on large surveys of anaplasmosis in these species. Goksu (1965) reviewed anaplasmosis in sheep and goats in Turkey. The prevalence was low, under 5% in both sheep and goats on hematological examination, but latent infections were probably higher. The detection of *A. ovis* in sheep in the USA was presented by Splitter *et al.* (1955).

Extensive surveys of the prevalence of *Anaplasma* infections in game animals have been undertaken in North America. The occurrence of anaplasmosis in some of the larger game animals of North America was reported by Howe *et al.* (1964). Approximately 15% of mule deer (*Odocoileus hemionus hemionus*) and cattle in Idaho were positive, as determined by the card agglutination test (Renshaw *et al.* 1977). Mule deer were found to be carriers of a strain which caused acute anaplasmosis in recipient calves (Magonigle *et al.* 1975a). On the basis of a large serological survey undertaken in white-tailed deer (*O. virginianus*) in Missouri, approximately 1% of the animals were positive (Maas and Buening 1981a). American bison were not infected, suggesting natural resistance (Peterson and Roby 1975). Numerous species of African wild ruminants were found to carry *A. marginale* (Lohr and Meyer 1973; Augustyn and Bigalke 1972).

Information on the economic losses has been available from North America. Anaplasmosis was regarded by the American National Cattlemen's Association to be the second most important disease of cattle (McCallon 1973). The importance of anaplasmosis in the USA in 1963 was stressed by pointing out the wide distribution of infections and the involvement of 19 species of ticks under natural and experimental conditions (Anon. 1963). Annual losses which have been often quoted amount to $100 million with a mortality of 50 000 to 100 000 animals (Amerault *et al.* 1978; McCallon 1973; Ristic 1980). The disease has continued to spread to new areas, increasing the size of the enzootic regions of the USA.

Anaplasmosis has been of primary importance in beef cattle raised on range land (Christensen *et al.* 1962). The economic losses due to anaplasmosis in Californian beef cattle have been also analyzed and were approximately $5.2 million in 1976, which was part of an estimated $300 million loss due to livestock diseases in general (Goodger 1978; Goodger *et al.* 1979; Henderson 1969). A more recent, similar, study of beef cattle in Texas estimated losses of $9 million in 1980 (Alderink and Dietrich 1982).

Transmission

Ticks and biting flies are incriminated in the transmission of *A. marginale*. Some 29 species of ticks in various parts of the world are found experimentally to be capable of transmitting the rickettsia, although not all of them may be vectors in nature. Ticks are true vectors enabling the organism to undergo cyclic development. Except in *Dermacentor andersoni*, the development of the various tick species is not defined. In tropical regions, the one-host ticks, *Boophilus annulatus* and *B. microplus*, are primary vectors and transmission is mainly transstadial, but there is also some evidence for transovarial transmission. In North America, transstadial transmission occurs with *D. andersoni* and *D. occidentalis*.

Biting flies transmit the organisms within a few minutes after feeding by the direct transfer of infected blood to susceptible animals. Experimental transmission occurs with stable, deer, and horseflies.

A common and highly sensitive experimental procedure to induce infection or test for infectivity of blood from a donor is the subinoculation of blood into susceptible hosts. *Anaplasma marginale* can be transmitted to susceptible splenectomized calves by blood which is microscopically negative and has only traces of antibody activity as detected by a CF test. Man is also a major vector, through the use of veterinary instruments contaminated with blood from an infected animal that are not cleaned and disinfected before use on a susceptible animal.

Literature

Numerous articles appeared in the early literature on the experimental attempts to transmit *A. marginale* by a variety of ticks and biting flies and the available information was reviewed by Dikmans (1950). More recent literature has been reviewed by Yeruham and Braverman (1981).

In North America *D. andersoni*, not biting flies, was identified as the principal vector of *Anaplasma* (Peterson *et al*. 1977). Males of *D. variabilis* and *D. andersoni* maintained the infection for 42 days and 108 days respectively, and the latter remained infective for more than 6 months in a hibernating state (Anthony and Roby 1966). *Dermacentor occidentalis* and *lxodis pacificus* also could transmit the agent from deer to splenectomized calves (Osebold *et al*. 1962). Experimental transmission by the brown dog tick (*Rhipicephalus sanguineus*) was demonstrated (Parker and Wilson 1979), but not by *Amblyomma* species *americanus* and *cajennense* (Miller *et al*. 1976).

In Australia, the significant vector for *Anaplasma marginale* was *B. microplus* which favors a warm, moist environment (Callow 1974; Connell 1974). *Anaplasma* could not be transmitted by the three-host tick *Haemaphysalis longicornis* (Connell 1978).

In a review of the epizootiology and control of anaplasmosis in South Africa, five species of tick were identified as playing an important role in transmitting *A. marginale* intrastadially (Potgieter 1979).

The role of transstadial and transovarial transmissions has been investigated. The reports in the early literature of transovarial transmission occurring in *B. microplus* have not been verified more recently by a number of workers (Leatch 1973; Connell and Hall 1972; Thompson and Roa 1978). Transovarial transmission has also not been observed in *D. andersoni* and *D. variabilis* (Kocan *et al.* 1981). Transstadial transmission has been readily demonstrated in larval to nymph and nymph to adult transfers by feeding the first stage on an infected host and transferring the infection to a susceptible splenectomized recipient by the following stage (Connell 1974). Experimental intrahost transmission of *A. marginale* by males of *D. albipictus* and *D. occidentalis* has also been achieved (Stiller *et al.* 1983).

Relatively little has been published on the development of infections in ticks. Recent work on infections in *D. andersoni*, using fluorescent antibody (FA) techniques, has shown organisms only in the gut contents up to 24 hours after feeding, contrary to the early reports that organisms were present in Malpighian tubules 5 days after detachment (Bram and Romanowski 1970). In gut homogenates, organisms were demonstrated by the ferritin-conjugated antibody technique on day 6 after detachment (Kocan *et al.* 1980b). *Anaplasma marginale* was also demonstrated in salivary gland homogenates by fluorescent antibodies and by inoculation into animals (Kocan *et al.* 1980c). The organisms in the midgut epithelium could be labeled with peroxidase-antiperoxidase techniques (Staats *et al.* 1982) and were usually found near the basement membrane (Oberst *et al.* 1981). The organisms in the midgut epithelial cells of *D. andersoni* and *D. variabilis* were pleomorphic (Kocan *et al.* 1980a). The colonies were characterized by variable morphology involving five structural types of organisms which appeared to represent various developmental stages (Kocan *et al.* 1982b). Development of *A. marginale* in the tick depended on temperature and duration of the incubation period (Kocan *et al.* 1982a). Homogenate from gut tissues from fed and unfed incubated adults caused different prepatent periods in *A. marginale* infections induced in animals, being shortest with ticks which were either fed or incubated at 37 °C for 3 days (Kocan *et al.* 1981).

A variety of hematophagous arthropods have been incriminated in the mechanical transmission of *Anaplasma*, including flies of the genus *Chrysops, Tabanus, Hematobius,* and *Stomoxys,* and mosquitoes of the genera *Phorophora* (Yeruham and Braverman 1981). Organisms could be transmitted from acutely infected cattle by the stablefly, *S. calcitrans,* but not by the cattle louse fly, *Hippobosca rufipes* (Potgieter *et al.* 1981). Mechanical transmission by insects has played a significant role in the epizootiology of anaplasmosis in Zimbabwe (Lawrence 1977). Also based on the correlation of seasonal fluctuations of tabanids, it was concluded that *T. taeniola* was the principal mechanical vector for *A. marginale* on a dairy farm in Tanzania (Wiesenhutter 1975). Biting flies, notably tabanids, have been thought to be infective for up to 6 hours (Malherbe 1963). Recently it was found that *A. marginale* was viable for 3 days after ingestion by the eye gnat, *Hippalates pusio*, and 2 days after ingestion by tabanids (Roberts and Love 1977).

Transplacental transmission of *A. marginale* in cattle has been observed in the third trimester of gestation (Swift and Paumer 1976). A case of congenital transmission of *A. centrale* in cattle has also been reported (Uilenberg 1968; Paine and Miller 1977).

Intact cattle were not found to be susceptible to *A. ovis* but sheep could be infected with *A. marginale*. Transmission through sheep did not result in loss of virulence of *A. marginale* for cattle (Ryff *et al.* 1964). Infection of splenectomized calves with *A. ovis* resulted in parasitemia which was detected only after 177 days and could be demonstrated only by subinoculation into sheep (Kuttler 1981). *Anaplasma ovis* was infective for goats and had greater virulence for goats than for sheep (Splitter *et al.* 1956). Infection of splenectomized goats with *A. marginale* resulted in latent carriers for 75 days (Maas and Buening 1981b). White-tailed deer (*O. virginianus*) could be infected with *A. ovis* (Kreier and Ristic 1963a). Bob-tailed deer infected by blood from bovine carriers resulted in a patent infection and rise in complement-fixing antibodies (Christensen *et al.* 1958).

INFECTION

Anaplasma are strict, intracellular, obligate parasites infecting mature erythrocytes. Organisms are rarely observed extracellularly. Entry into cells is by an endocytotic process which consists of invagination of the cell membrane and formation of a vacuole around the organism. The organism interacts with the erythrocytic membrane, but is able to enter and leave the cell without incurring destruction. In the vacuoles, the initial body multiplies by binary fission to form the inclusion body.

Infection is divided into an incubation or prepatent period of 3 to 5 weeks, the duration of which is dependent on the quantity of infecting organisms, and is followed by the patent period when organisms multiply to a peak population. Maximum anemia occurs 1 to 6 days after the peak of parasitemia and persists for 4 to 15 days, during which time 75% of the circulating erythrocytes may be lost. Inclusion bodies are numerous during the acute phase of the infection and can be at very low levels in chronic and carrier states. Parasitemia and associated anemia are milder in calves than in adult animals. Infected red blood cells are rapidly removed from circulation by phagocytosis in the reticuloendothelial system, particularly in the spleen. Removal by phagocytosis of anaplasma-free erythrocytes suggests the involvement of an autoimmune process. The convalescent period lasts for 1 to 2 months, is accompanied by increased hematopoiesis and may be complicated by recurrence of parasitemia. The hematogical parameters then return to normal, but organisms continue to be present in the peripheral circulations.

There is little information on the virulence of various isolates of anaplasma. Infectivity and pathogenicity are often related to the age of the host. In splenectomized animals the organism is more virulent. Infection occurs in a variety of animal species; however, the development of clinical disease is restricted to some species.

Viable organisms can be preserved in blood and tick material for years in a frozen state (stabilates) with the addition of perservatives such as glycerin and dimethylsulfoxide.

Literature

Multiplication of the *Anaplasma* followed entry of the initial body into the erythrocyte. A vacuole formed by a membrane derived from erythrocytic plasmalemma surrounded the organism and entry and departure did not disrupt the cells (Francis *et al.* 1979). Multiplication occurred by binary fission, and four developmental stages were described on the basis of numbers of organisms and their position in the red blood cells. A marginal body comprising two or three initial bodies was observed by the tenth day with subsequent increase in their number (Ristic and Watrach 1963). It was proposed that the transit between erythrocytes by the organism takes place through intracellular tissue bridges (Ristic 1968). Immature red blood cells were more resistant to infection than mature erythrocytes (Williams and Jones 1968).

The spleen plays a central role in the control of the levels of infection. Splenectomized calves had high parasitemia and more severe clinical signs (Jones *et al.* 1968b; Ristic *et al.* 1958). Following an acute infection, parasitemia levels decreased markedly, but recrudescent infections could be induced by immunosuppression by either corticosteroid or cyclophosphamide and were characterized by increased parasitemia, decreased packed cell volume (PCV), and mortality (Kuttler and Adams 1977; Corrier *et al.* 1981).

Infectivity of blood during the acute and carrier stages of infection was investigated and correlated to the complement-fixing titers. High antibody levels were related to increased infectivity (Gates *et al.* 1957). The virulence of *A. marginale* and *A. centrale* was compared in splenectomized and intact cattle of different ages. Major differences between the two species were observed in intact animals but only minor differences were seen in splenectomized animals (Kuttler 1966).

Anaplasma have been observed in mixed infections with other rickettsia and with intracellular and extracellular protozoa. Mixed infections of *Anaplasma* and *Paranaplasma* have been reported (Kreier and Ristic 1963b). In splenectomized calves, interference between anaplasmosis and eperythrozoonosis was observed (Foote *et al.* 1957). In other mixed infections the virulence of the *Anaplasma* could be affected and be either increased or depressed.

Experimental infections have been routinely induced by infected whole blood from donor animals. Infectivity of blood was sensitive to temperatures and was reduced as time and temperature of incubation were increased (Bedell and Dimopoullos 1962). Sonic energy at temperatures of 33 to 35 °C, but not all lower temperatures, also affected the infectivity (Bedell and Dimopoullos 1963). The duration of infectivity of blood stored at 25 and 37 °C was enhanced by addition of tissue culture medium. Addition of glycerin to infected blood and storage at –70 °C was a most reliable method for preservation of the viable organism for long periods of time (Summers 1967). Infected red blood cells have been concentrated by centrifugation (Davis and Bowman 1952). Homogenates of *R. sinus* infected with *A. marginale* have also been used to induce infections in cattle (Potgieter and van Rensburg 1980).

CLINICAL SIGNS

Clinical syndromes are divided into mild, chronic, acute, and peracute forms. In acute disease the most significant clinical signs are fever, pallor, weakness, constipation, normal urine, watery blood, and occasionally icterus. The development of the syndromes occurs in four stages: incubation, clinical signs, convalescence, and the carrier state. Severity of clinical signs during anaplasmosis is dependent on the susceptibility of the animal. Although all ages are susceptible to infection, syndromes are most severe in mature animals. Disease is generally mild in calves up to 1 year of age and becomes progressively more severe as the animal gets older, being frequently peracute and fatal in cattle more than 3 years of age. Severity depends on the level and duration of parasitemia which is related to the rate of multiplication of the organism and the ability of the animal to suppress the levels of infection by immune responses.

Literature

Anaplasmosis is primarily a disease of mature cattle. The nature of resistance in calves has not been established but it could be overcome by splenectomy, and probably at least in part is due to immunological responses. Anti-inflammatory and immunosuppressive dexamethasone administered in large amounts to splenectomized carrier calves for prolonged periods of time caused relapsing infections (Kuttler and Adams 1977, 1978). The intensity of anemia and the levels and duration of the parasitemia are directly related to the age of the host (Jones *et al.* 1968a). In animals less than 1 year of age, infections were usually subclinical, in yearlings and 2-year-olds signs were of moderate intensity, and in older cattle the disease was severe and often fatal (Jones and Brock 1966). Natural exposure of calves to both *Anaplasma* and *Babesia* infections in an enzootic environment resulted in the appearance of parasitemias on the average at 11 weeks of age. There was an associated anemia which returned to normal within 4 weeks

(Corrier and Guzman 1977). Splenectomy caused a recrudescence of *Anaplasma* infection and development of severe clinical signs in indigenous and crossbred calves (Singh and Gautam 1971). In a dairy herd the disease was severe with mortality of 28%. Recovered cows had an average loss in milk yield of 26% (McDowell *et al.* 1964). In pregnant cows, abortion and occasionally transplacental transmission of organism have been reported (Fowler and Swift 1975).

Susceptibility of various breeds has been shown to vary. Based on clinical signs, hematology, and mortality, indigenous Boran, a Zebu type, were found more resistant than Ayrshire cattle (Lohr *et al.* 1975). Susceptibility of *Bos indicus* and *B. taurus* cattle was comparable in other climates based on body weights, parasitemia, hematology, and antibody and serum transaminase levels (Otim *et al.* 1980; Wilson *et al.* 1980a). The age resistance in these two breed types of cattle was also similar (Wilson *et al.* 1979). Poor nutrition was associated with less severe disease syndromes (Wilson 1979). Brahman-cross steers maintained on two planes of nutrition responded differently to intravenous challenge with *A. marginale*. Animals on higher levels of nutrition were more severely affected (Ajayi *et al.* 1978).

Jones and Norman (1962) provided a comprehensive description of the clinical signs. Characteristic features were anemia, weakness, fever, normal urine, and constipation. Other clinical signs observed were gastrointestinal atony, lowered production, and recumbency. In the most severe cases there was also depression, dehydration, labored respiration, muscle tremor, and irrational behavior due to cerebral anoxia. Animals in advanced pregnancy often aborted. Fever was the first clinical evidence of disease and anemia followed. However, the clinical recognition of anemia required the loss to be about 40 to 50%. The prognosis was grave in mature animals in which the red blood cell count fell to levels less than 2 million per cubic millimeter (Jones and Norman 1962). Some of the clinical signs were related to the acute anemia which, in turn, caused physiological adjustments of the respiratory and circulatory systems. Icterus usually developed late in the course of the disease and could frequently be observed during convalescence. Myocardial anoxia resulted in cardiac failure and death (Jones and Brock 1966). The convalescent period was of 1 to 2 months' duration or longer. Relapses occurred and the recovered animals became carriers for life and were resistant to new reinfections (Anon. 1963). Clinical and hematological responses of water buffalo (*Bubalus bubalis*) calves were similar to those observed in cattle (Sharma *et al.* 1978).

Ovine and caprine anaplasmosis caused by *A. ovis* was usually a mild disease characterized by mild fever, variable degrees of anemia, icterus, and only sometimes accompanied by digestive disturbances. Recovered animals developed premunity for life (Neitz, 1939). As with cattle, splenectomized sheep and goats were more susceptible to infection (Goksu 1965). A highly susceptible breed of goats to *A. ovis* was reported in India, and sheep on the same premises served as carriers (Sinha and Pathak 1966). Clinical anaplasmosis in goats was also reported by Mallick *et al.* (1979). A strain of *A. ovis* isolated from Nigerian goats was shown to be more pathogenic for goats than for sheep, based on height of parasitemia, anemia, and mortality in splenectomized animals (Zwart and Buys 1968). In splenectomized sheep anemia occurred between 15 and 20 days after infection, and in goats between 25 and 30 days and followed 2 or 3 days of maximum parasitemia. In addition to other commonly observed signs there was constipation followed by diarrhea, but most of the animals survived without treatment (Singh and Gautam 1972). After splenectomy of naturally infected animals, the onset of infection, levels of parasitemia, and immunological and clinical responses varied considerably between individuals (Kuil and Folkers 1968).

PATHOLOGY

Anaplasma causes a progressive anemia which is initially normocytic and later becomes macrocytic, with compensatory hyperplasia of bone marrow, granulocytosis, reticulocytosis, increased mean corpuscular cell volume, and increased osmotic fragility of erythrocytes. Red blood cells are removed by phagocytosis by the reticuloendothelial system, primarily in the spleen. Removal of the red blood cells rather than intravascular hemolysis accounts for the absence of hemoglobinemia and hemoglobinuria. Rapid destruction of red blood cells and low hematocrit levels are accompanied by degeneration of parenchymatous organs.

In some syndromes, there is no direct correlation between the level of infection and rate of destruction of erythrocytes. An autoimmune response is thought of as the mechanism which plays an important role in the pathogenesis.

Lesions are typical of acute anemia with pallor, icterus, and hepato- and splenomegaly. Histologically, the lesions are characterized by hepatic, renal, and myocardial degeneration, widespread hemosiderosis, and erythrophagocytosis. The bone marrow is usually hyperplastic, but in chronic cases there may be evidence of cellular depletion.

Literature

The principal pathological manifestation in acute cases was severe anemia with PCVs below 10% occurring rapidly within 4 to 5 days after the onset of parasitemia (Allen and Kuttler 1981). Maximum anemia has been associated with parasitemia occurring 1 to 3 days after the peak which was usually observed 2 to 3 weeks after infection. Reticulocytosis, macrocytopenia, and granulopoiesis indicated increased hematopoiesis (Jones and Brock 1966; Ristic 1961). During the period of increasing numbers of *Anaplasma*-infected erythrocytes, progressive normocytic normochromic anemia developed. During the convalescent period and decreasing parasitemia, a macrocytic anemia was observed (Brock *et al.* 1959). Convalescence usually took 1 to 2 months, and in calves and young adults replacement of the 75% of the preinfection blood values after maximal anemia required 2 to 3 weeks (Jones and Brock 1966). A significant increase in the ratio of total plasma to red blood cell iron was accompanied by increased turnover rate and decreased utilization. Iron was utilized during recovery and the short-lived red blood cells were produced (Hansard and Foote 1959). The selective removal of HbA-containing erythrocytes, rather than those with HbF, suggested that inherited erythrocyte factors could be associated with resistance to anemia (Anderson *et al.* 1972). The anemia was considered to be hemolytic with increases in conjugated bilirubin and serum aspartate aminotransferase during the acute phase (Ajayi *et al.* 1978). Following splenectomy of infected calves, the globulin levels and bilirubin and icterus indices were increased during the anemic phase (Galhotra *et al.* 1979).

Changes in the erythrocytes of cattle infected with *A. marginale* have been investigated (Medina 1959–60). The survival of erythrocytes in splenectomized calves during the hemolytic crisis with *A. marginale* was reduced by eight to tenfold (Baker *et al.* 1961). Chemical and physical changes occurred in infected erythrocytes with a decrease in the total phospholipids, the concentration being inversely proportional to the osmotic fragility of the cells (Dimopoullos and Bedell 1962). Enzyme activity also underwent significant changes which were related to the appearance of immature cells (Smith *et al.* 1972). Acetylcholinesterase activity was lost in infected erythrocytes and occurred before there was a decrease in PCV and an increase in osmotic fragility (Wallace 1967).

With peak parasitemia and accompanying anemia, serum protein concentration increased with increases in the alpha and beta globulins and total globulins. As the parasitemia decreased, the total serum protein and the albumin–globulin ratio decreased, alpha- and beta-globulin levels returned to normal, and gamma globulins increased (Dimopoullos and Bedell, 1960). Parasitemia induced hypolipoidemia and hypergammaglobulinemia, with the decreases in the lipoproteins occurring in the alpha fraction (Buening 1974). The degree of these changes was related to the severity of the disease.

Further studies on the clinical chemistry in mature cattle infected with either virulent or attenuated strains showed that severe anemia caused by virulent strains was associated with increases in the serum total bilirubin, direct bilirubin, urea nitrogen, alkaline phosphatase, and serum aspartate aminotransferase, while attenuated strains caused only mild anemia and an increase in the alkaline phosphatase (Allen *et al.* 1981a). Differences were also observed in the immunoglobulin concentrations and white blood cell (WBC) counts. Virulent strains caused a decrease in albumin and an increase in WBC counts and gamma globulins. The latter increased after peak parasitemia and during recovery. With the attenuated strains, increase in gamma globulin occurred only during the recovery period (Allen *et al.* 1981b).

In the bone marrow, a shift to erythroid production, resulting in erythroid hyperplasia started with the appearance of severe anemia. Plasma erythropoietin titers were elevated early during infections of calves and sheep, and peak titers occurred during maximum anemia and recovery periods (Jatkar and Kreier 1967a, b; Kreier *et al.* 1964). In fatal forms of the disease, increase in bone-marrow activity did not occur (Jones and Brock 1966). Absorption and physiological movement of iron, erythropoietin levels and hematopoiesis have been investigated in cattle throughout the course of infections (Hansard and Foote 1961; Hansard *et al.* 1972).

The pathogenesis of anemia could not be directly correlated to the cell injury due to invasion of erythrocytes by the *Anaplasma*, but loss of red blood cells was closely correlated to the level of infection in severely anemic animals (Jones *et al.* 1968a, b). Removal of erythrocytes was due in part to autoimmune antibodies bound to erythrocytes (Schroeder and Ristic 1965a; Ristic 1961). *Anaplasma* antigen–antibody complexes were detected in erythrocytes of infected cattle (Ristic and White 1960). Some initial investigations using hemolytic and direct antiglobulin tests did not reveal evidence of autoimmune mechanism in anemia (Brock *et al.* 1965b). Other work, however, conclusively showed involvement of autoimmune mechanisms. Autohemagglutinin was demonstrated in the serum of experimentally infected calves and in erythrocytes during the acute stages of infection and was associated with agglutination of erythrocytes (Mann and Ristic 1963a). The presence of autoantibody was associated with PCV in both acute and convalescent stages (Schroeder and Ristic 1965a, 1968). Autohemagglutinins and opsonins were directed against membrane antigens and were associated with erythrophagocytosis of both infected and noninfected erythrocytes by the reticuloendothelial system without evidence of intravascular hemolysis (Ristic *et al.* 1972). The pigment released from this destruction was excreted as urobilinogen. Autoantibodies were shown to react with erythrocyte membranes forming antigen–antibody complexes (Cox and Dimopoullos 1972). Maximum concentration of autoantibodies attached to erythrocytes was correlated with maximum anemia (Ristic 1961). Opsonins were associated with IgM and IgG fractions. Opsonin titers coincided with the highest levels occurring at the time of anemic crisis (Morris *et al.* 1971). The autohemaglobulins were demonstrated to be due to the beta$_2$ M-globulin in the euglobulin fraction and reacted with autologous, homologous, and heterologous erythrocytes, but not with *Anaplasma* antigens. Autoantibodies to soluble antigens obtained from normal and infected erythrocytes were also observed (Schroeder and Ristic 1965b; Mann and Ristic 1963b). Both antiparasitic and antierythrocytic antibodies appeared in infections, with the latter occurring earlier and persisting only during anemia (Jatkar and Kreier 1969). Based on infection of platelets, it was proposed that their destruction was associated with disruptions in the blood-clotting mechanisms (Ristic and Watrach 1962).

A nonspecific phagocytosis-stimulating serum factor was also elevated five- to tenfold at the time of the anemic crisis (Erp and Hahrney 1976). Changes in flocculating properties were due to alterations in the isoelectric point brought about by total phospholipid content (Dimopoullos and Bedell 1960).

Severity of anemia was not always related to the severity of the disease (Schroeder and Ristic 1965a). Mortality in acute cases has often been directly related to the severity of anemia, but prognosis based on the level of anemia was difficult. Lowered plasma potassium, lack of reticulocytosis, and uncompensated metabolic acidosis were regarded to be associated with mortality (Allen and Kuttler 1981). Liver degeneration was related to the circulatory failure due to anemia (Allbritton and Seger 1962; Schmidt 1973).

Animals dying of anaplasmosis were emaciated, dehydrated, the blood was watery and accompanied accumulation of fluid in the pleural and pericardial cavities. Lymph nodes were wet, lungs edematous and yellow, and the liver was enlarged and brownish yellow with the gall bladder distended. The spleen was enlarged, dark red, almost black, with soft pulpy consistency of tissue (Schmidt 1973; Galhotra *et al.* 1977b). Petechial hemorrhages were found on the serosal surfaces, especially on the pericardium. The heart was pale and flabby (Jones and Brock 1966). Brown discoloration was observed in the hepatic and mediastinal lymph nodes (Ristic and Sippel 1958). In pregnant animals fetal anoxia accompanied maternal anemia and resulted in fetal death (Swift and Paumer 1978). There has been a case report of a calf infected *in utero* showing icterus, anemia, opisthotonus, and nervous symptoms 2 days after birth (Bird 1973).

There have been relatively few reports on the histopathology of the disease syndromes of varying severity in cattle caused by *A. marginale*. A common feature in severe forms was hepatic necrosis, varying from loss of a few cells to extensive necrosis around central veins. This was usually accompanied by infiltration of mononuclear cells and large deposits of hemosiderin in Kupffer cells. Hemosiderosis was also found in the lungs, lymph nodes, and, to a lesser degree, in the kidney. The spleen was congested and contained large numbers of plasma cells. Erythrophagocytosis was observed in the spleens and medullary sinuses of lymph nodes (Trueman and Wilson 1979). Degeneration and necrosis of the liver and kidney parenchyma occurred only when hematocrit values dropped to 25% of normal (Seger and White 1962).

IMMUNOLOGY

Antigens

Antigens of *A. marginale* are found in the erythrocytes and soluble antigens are found in the serum. *Anaplasma* organisms have species-specific and common antigens and antigenic variation does not occur.

Strain-antigenic differences are not detected. Humoral responses and cross-protection studies with *A. marginale, A. centrale, A. ovis,* and *P. caudatum* show both antigenic differences and similarities.

Particulate antigens from infected erythrocytes are used in serological tests and contain erythrocyte membrane bound antigens. Soluble *Anaplasma* antigens are also found in serum and red blood cells.

Literature

The chemical composition of the antigens of *Anaplasma* species has not been extensively investigated, but appeared to be associated with glycoproteins and a soluble protein (Ristic and Carson 1977). Antigens were localized using ferritin-conjugated antibody on the chromatin of the initial body, inclusion appendage, and on the outer surface of the pellicle (Kocan *et al.* 1978b). Soluble antigens from infected erythrocytes were similar chemically but not antigenically to those observed from normal erythrocytes (Ristic *et al.* 1963; Ristic and Mann 1963). These soluble antigens from three *A. marginale* strains were similar when compared by agar-gel diffusion and immunoelectrophoretic techniques (Carson *et al.* 1970). Two-dimensional gel electrophoresis revealed apparent differences in protein structure between two geographically different *A. marginale* isolates (Barbet *et al.* 1983). Soluble antigen induced precipitating antibodies but not immunity to challenge infection (Amerault and Roby 1964, 1967). In cross-protection trials with two strains of *A. marginale* there was some evidence of antigenic differences, although cross-protection was observed (Taylor 1969).

Various methods have been used for the preparation of antigens from blood for serological tests. The stability and specificity of the antigen for the capillary and tube agglutination test was determined (Welter and Zuschek 1962; Welter 1964). Antigens were preserved by lyophilization (Malhotra *et al.* 1982). The stroma of infected erythrocytes was present in most antigen preparations and preferentially reacted with antibody in the capillary agglutination test (Budden and Dimopoullos 1977; Dimopoullos and Budden 1978). Antigens have also been prepared from the spleen of infected animals and used in the tube agglutination test (Banerjee *et al.* 1978b). Large-scale production of antigens from blood for the CF test using improved methods was developed (Franklin *et al.* 1962; Price *et al.* 1952).

Purified *A. marginale*, prepared free of bovine erythrocyte stroma, was shown to be nonreactive as an antigen in the capillary agglutination test (Budden and Dimopoullos 1977; Dimopoullos and Budden 1978) although the antigen could react in a precipitin test (Hart *et al.* 1981).

Immunity

Protective immunity is associated with the presence of infective organisms and has been termed 'premunity' or 'coinfectious immunity'. A degree of immunity also occurs after elimination of the organisms by chemotherapy. Resistance to infection is associated with the presence of antibody and particularly with development of cell-mediated immunity. Passive immunization with sera does not always confer resistance. Antibodies are thought to act as cytophilic agents, increasing the capacity of macrophages to ingest the organisms. Transfer of antibodies through the colostrum occurs, but its role in protection of calves from infection is not established.

Cell-mediated responses to *Anaplasma* antigens develop prior to or after the onset of parasitemia. The level of cell response is possibly related to the degree of resistance to the development of clinical disease on challenge by virulent organisms.

Literature

The ability of *Anaplasma* to escape the host's cellular and humoral immunological responses depends on the intracellular localization, a feature which is common to other rickettsial and protozoal parasites which infect leukocytes and erythrocytes (Ristic 1976). Although it has been established that protective immunity was mainly dependent on the maintenance of the carrier state, recent information indicated that considerable protection existed, even 8 months after sterilization through chemotherapy (Magonigle and Newby 1984). Protective immunity involved interaction between antibody and cell-mediated response with the latter having a principal role (Ristic and Sippel 1958; Ristic and Carson 1977). Antibody detected by the CF and other serologic tests were not directly related to resistance (Jones *et al.* 1968a). Injections of anti-erythrocyte serum into infected calves reduced and delayed the severity of infection (McHardy 1974). Based on cytotoxicity test results, both leukocytes and antibodies were active in clearance of infected erythrocytes from the blood (Carson *et al.* 1980). Both cell- and antibody-mediated protection appeared to be involved in immunity to anaplasmosis caused by virulent and avirulent strains (Carson *et al.* 1978; Francis *et al.* 1980a, b). Cell-mediated responses, as determined by leukocyte migration inhibition, were positively correlated with protection in one study (Carson *et al.* 1977b) but not in another (Eckblad and Magonigle 1983). Cutaneous hypersensitivity and development of isoantibodies were demonstrated in cattle infected with live or inactivated *A. marginale* in bovine and ovine erythrocytes (Carson *et al.* 1976). Both *in vivo* and *in vitro* tests demonstrated cell response in vaccinated and carrier animals (Banerjee *et al.* 1981). Cell-mediated responses to virulent and attenuated *A. marginale* were demonstrated by leukocyte migration and lymphocyte transformation tests (Carson *et al.* 1977a). Leukocyte migration inhibition was observed after antibodies were detected by the CF test but was not related to the titer (Buening 1973). There was no correlation between cell-mediated cytotoxicity and leukocyte migration inhibition tests (Buening 1976).

Serology

The contribution of the various classes of immune globulins and the kinetics of the humoral responses are not well defined in the disease syndromes caused by *Anaplasma* infections in cattle. Both specific and nonspecific antibodies are induced. The nonspecific immunoglobulins include autohemagglutinins and opsonins which react with nonparasitic antigens on the erythrocytes and other heterogeneous antigens. Demonstration of specific antibodies in a particular class of globulins depends on the serologic tests used. Infections stimulate IgM early, and later induce increases in IgG. Commonly used tests include CF and card agglutination. Other tests used include IFA, precipitation and capillary agglutination. There are advantages with each. The card agglutination test is most useful in monitoring anaplasmosis on a large scale and is used in control programs. The card agglutination, CF and IFA tests are reliable indicators of carrier animals.

Literature

Immunoglobulin responses during acute syndromes in intact and splenectomized calves have been investigated. In intact calves the IgM levels increased 7 days after infection and persisted for a long period of time. The IgG levels became elevated 11 days after the initial increase of IgM, but the levels were neither pronounced nor prolonged. In splenectomized calves which died during the acute phase of infection only the IgM increased and its onset was significantly delayed (Klaus and Jones 1968). After the acute anemic phase, the antibodies were made up of one-fourth IgG and three-fourths IgM which persisted for many months. Complement-fixing and agglutinating antibodies were heterogeneous, in that early complement-fixing antibodies consisted exclusively of IgM which after 45 days was augmented by IgG. Transfer of maternal antibody via colostrum involved IgG rather than IgM (Murphy *et al.* 1966a, b). In peracute and acute cases, conglutinin levels decreased following infection and disappeared at peak parasitemia. In those animals which survived, the levels returned to normal after 7 weeks. Complement levels in both acute and peracute syndromes did not change (Rose *et al.* 1978).

Immunoglobulin responses during recrudescent parasitemias of chronic carrier *A. marginale* infections have also been studied (Wagner 1981). Both splenectomized and intact calves were examined at weekly intervals over a 12-month period. Generally, splenectomized calves had diminished responses compared to intacts. After recovery from the primary infection, recrudescent parasitemias were accompanied by an anamnestic response in both IgM and IgG classes. Complement-fixing and indirect hemagglutinating antibody activities tended to rise and fall according to recrudescent episodes, especially in splenectomized calves. The IFA and card agglutination test activities, on the other hand, remained high throughout the observation period.

Various tests have been used in the serology and diagnosis of bovine anaplasmosis, but only some have been adapted to practical field use. Various CF methods have been used and generally gave acceptable uniformity (Boulanger *et al.* 1966). Complement-fixing microprocedures were established as reliable techniques (Hidalgo and Dimopoullos 1967), as were other rapid CF screening tests (Franklin and Huff 1964). Complement-fixing antibody activity was demonstrated before the onset of parasitemia, and the level and time of occurrence was similar in calves and young adult cattle but was delayed in aged cows (Jones *et al.* 1968b). Seventy percent of newborn calves from carrier cows were positive with maximum titers occurring at 6 to 10 days and then gradually declining (Kuttler *et al.* 1962).

The card agglutination procedure was recommended as the test of choice in field surveys and diagnosis, and has been used extensively in various species of animals (Amerault and Roby 1968; Franklin *et al.* 1966). The advantages of this test were that it was rapid, the antigen was stable, and untreated plasma could be used (Ristic 1980). The test was accurate and practical (Amerault *et al.* 1969, 1972). Some problems occurred with the test in detecting acute stages of the infection and when sera were stored. Addition of normal bovine serum brought out the activity in stored samples and in those from acute infections. This factor supplementing the reactivity had the properties of conglutinin (Rose *et al.* 1974; Madden and Kuttler 1980). Addition of phenol to sera partially inhibited the detection of antibody activity by the card agglutination and CF tests (Amerault *et al.* 1980). Modified tests were also used in species other than cattle, including Colombian black-tailed deer (*O. hemionus colombianus*) (Howarth *et al.* 1976; Renshaw *et al.* 1979).

Other serologic tests have developed, although they have not been extensively used. Precipitating antibodies, as detected by the agar double diffusion technique were demonstrated in acutely infected and carrier cattle. These antibodies appeared later than those demonstrated by the CF test (Amerault and Roby 1964). The specificity of the capillary agglutination test has been investigated and found to involve antigen–antibody reactions other than those specific for the organism (Dimopoullos and Bedell 1974; Pipano *et al.* 1972). Fluorescent antibody techniques were used to study the structure of *A. marginale* (Madden 1962), and in detecting carrier infections (Gonzalez *et al.* 1978). Enzyme immunoassays have also been developed (Thoen *et al.* 1980; Long and Wagner 1981).

The efficiency of many of the tests has been compared. The agglutination technique was considered to be at least as accurate as the CF test, but was simpler to perform and was less expensive (Ristic 1963). Antibody activity detectable by the card agglutination test developed several days after CF activity and persisted at relatively high titers (Todorovic *et al.* 1977). Following the elimination of the *Anaplasma* in the carrier state, the agglutination test was negative by day 95 and the CF by day 181 (Jatkar *et al.* 1966). An improved card agglutination test detected antibody levels at comparable sensitivity to the CF test (Amerault *et al.* 1981). Both CF and capillary agglutination tests had an accuracy around 98 to 99% with a correlation between the tests of 60% (Rogers 1971). A 90% agreement between these tests was also reported by Hibbs *et al.* (1966). In a comparison of the capillary agglutination, CF, plate agglutination, and IFA tests there was an 86.6% correlation, CF was the most sensitive and the plate agglutination the least. Antibody activity was first detected 7 days after infection with *A. marginale,* rose to a peak by day 29, and was still present on day 200. Antibodies to *A. centrale* were also first detected by day 29, rose to a peak by day 50, and disappeared by day 100 (Wilson *et al.* 1978). In another study, the accuracy of the CF test was 84%, the IFA test 97%, and the card agglutination test 79%, but the most efficient test identifying noninfected animals was the CF test (Gonzalez *et al.* 1978).

Serologic tests have been used to differentiate responses induced by the *Anaplasma* species. Antibody activity to *A. marginale* and *A. centrale* could be differentiated by CF (Kuttler 1967a) and IFA tests (Schindler *et al.* 1966; Lohr *et al.* 1975). Indirect fluorescent antibody and capillary agglutination tests were both used to study the homologous and heterologous responses in both infections (Lohr *et al.* 1975). Although cross-reaction occurred, there were quantitative differences in the immunofluorescent antibody activity (Schindler *et al.* 1966). Significantly higher titers with homologous antigens were obtained with the CF and capillary agglutination tests (Kuttler 1967a). Antigenic relationships between *A. marginale* and *A. centrale* were established by cross-protection tests (Kuttler 1967b). Anaplasma was distinct from *Paranaplasma* based on IFA tests and cross-immunity studies (Kreier and Ristic 1963d). The appendage-related antigen in *P. caudatum* in deer erythrocytes could be specifically stained by a FA technique (Carson *et al.* 1974). A serologic cross-reaction was observed in the CF test between *A. ovis* and *A. marginale* (Splitter *et al.* 1956; Welter 1964). Using the passive agglutination test, cross-reactivity between *A. marginale* and two *Plasmodium* species was demonstrated, which either indicated that there was antigenic similarity between these organisms or that antigens of the erythrocytes were involved in the reactions (Dimopoullos and Finerty 1976).

VACCINATION

A major obstacle to the development of standardized vaccination procedures against *Anaplasma* is the lack of an adequate *in vitro* culture technique. Various live vaccines are currently used and include small doses of virulent, avirulent, or attenuated *A. marginale* organisms, and *A. centrale*. Protection is dependent on establishing a chronic asymptomatic infection (premunization). This carrier status is a disadvantage in certain epidemiological situations. The use of virulent field isolates for premunization has certain risks and may require control of the initial infection by chemotherapy. Attenuated and avirulent strains have varying degrees of efficacy. Mildly pathogenic isolates cause a moderate parasitemia and slightly reduced PCV and in some instances may require treatment. Immunized calves become seropositive and develop cell-mediated responses. Live vaccines generally induce strong cell-mediated responses of long duration. Killed vaccines are less effective, possibly because of the relatively low level of cell-mediated immunity induced.

One form of vaccination involves laboratory attenuation of *A. marginale* by irradiation, and further selection of avirulent organisms by serial passage of irradiated organisms in splenectomized sheep. Immunogenicity, the growth pattern of the organism, and the safety of these attenuated organisms has been established in experimental animals. The prepatent period following vaccination is from 4 to 6 weeks with a level of parasitemia of 0.5 to 0.8%, and a slight decrease not exceeding 15% in the hematocrit values which lasts from 1 to 2 weeks. Specificity and immunogenicity of these vaccines in highly susceptible animals was tested in South America and the USA and a commercial vaccine is now available in many Latin American countries and in California. Infection with *A. centrale* does not prevent infection with *A. marginale,* but reduces the severity of the disease caused by the superimposed virulent infection.

Inactivated vaccines provide a lesser degree of protection and produce undesirable isoantibody, and have been used to some extent in Africa and the USA. Two doses given 6 weeks apart induce immunity 2 weeks after the second vaccine. Following field challenge animals are infected and become carriers. An annual booster vaccine may be required. The level of protection engendered by inactivated vaccines is reflected mainly in reduced parasitemia and a milder anemia following challenge. The antibody response as measured by CF is of 2 to 8 months' duration. A disadvantage is the isohemolytic anemia which develops in calves of vaccinated dams.

Literature

Three commonly used methods of immunization, including the use of diluted virulent stabilate, diluted, *Anaplasma*-infected bovine blood, and attenuated strains of ovine origin have been tested (Corrier *et al.* 1980). These three methods have been used successfully, and under field challenge neither clinical anaplasmosis nor mortality were observed in immunized cattle (Vizcaino *et al.* 1980; Vilas Novas and Viana 1980). Minimum doses without treatment resulted in 12½% mortality (Franklin and Huff 1967). Controlling virulent infections by treatment was still considered a dangerous form of immunoprophylaxis (Gonzalez *et al.* 1976; Ristic and Carson 1977). Postpremunition reactions were controlled by oxytetracycline alone. Premunization of adult cattle by virulent *A. marginale* with oxytetracycline in combination with dithiosemicarbazone was not effective (Todorovic and Tellez 1975).

Vaccination methods have been tried with a combination of *Anaplasma* and *Babesia*. *Anaplasma marginale, B. argentina,* and *B. bigemina* cryopreserved together in blood were administered by various regimes using different routes of injection, multiple injections, and chemotherapy. The safety and protection engendered by these methods has not been established (Todorovic *et al.* 1975, 1978). In earlier studies it was concluded that premunization against the piroplasms first and against *Anaplasma* 3 weeks later was advisable to avoid heavy losses (Dumag *et al.* 1962).

Because of the complications in using virulent organisms, an attenuated strain was developed by irradiation and by adapting an isolate of *A. marginale* to grow in sheep erythrocytes. This attenuated organism produced sufficient immunogenic response and was a safe vaccine for cattle (Ristic and Carson 1977; Henry *et al.* 1983). The adaptation of the organism to sheep resulted in a loss of virulence which was not dependent on a decrease in the rate of multiplication. The attenuation appeared stable after passage in cattle, although one report showed reversion to virulence following 12 cattle passages (Kuttler 1969). The organism could not be experimentally transmitted by ticks. After challenge, vaccinated animals had a mild response characterized by low parasitemia and slight, temporary hematocrit drop at approximately 4 to 5 weeks after infection with no other obvious clinical signs. The vaccine provided protection against the development of high parasitemia and severe anemia after exposure (Garcia 1978; Vizcaino *et al.* 1978). Serological responses were detected between 3 and 4 weeks and persisted for 2 to 3 years. Cell-mediated immunity was also demonstrated after 2 to 4 weeks (Ristic and Carson 1977). Different doses of vaccine in calves did not affect the degree of protection against challenge, (Vizcaino *et al.* 1978). Attenuated organisms were more easily destroyed by tetracycline than the virulent strains, and a dose of 18.7 mg/kg body weight for 4 days completely eliminated the infection, as opposed to 22 mg/kg which was required for 7 days to destroy the virulent organisms (Ristic and Carson 1977).

The trials using this vaccine were undertaken under laboratory and field conditions in the USA, Peru, Venezuela, Colombia, and Mexico (Ristic *et al.* 1968; Ristic and Carson 1977, 1978). Ribeiro *et al.* (1980) also reported the use of attenuated vaccine in South America. The efficacy of the vaccine under natural challenge in enzootic area of Mexico was tested and this method was useful in adapting high-quality young cattle to the tropics (Osorno *et al.* 1975). In another study, vaccinated cattle appeared to be immune to virulent challenge using a Texas isolate of *A. marginale*, but susceptible to challenge with a Colombian isolate (Kuttler and Zaraza 1969).

Anaplasma centrale infection as a vaccine did not prevent reinfection with *A. marginale* but the severity of the subsequent disease was decreased (Ristic 1980). Charolais cattle were successfully vaccinated and only rarely was treatment required to control challenge infections (Lohr 1969). *Bos indicus*-cross calves vaccinated with *A. marginale* were refractory to challenge but only a portion vaccinated with *A. centrale* were immune. After challenge a weak secondary antibody response occurred in the resistant animals and organisms were not detected in the blood (Wilson *et al.* 1980b). Similarly, when cross-bred *B. taurus* calves were vaccinated with *A. centrale* only partial protection was observed with virulent *A. marginale* challenge (Potgieter and van Rensburg 1983).

Various degrees of transient protection have been induced by inactivated *Anaplasma* derived from blood and used with adjuvants. Increased resistance to onset of clinical anaplasmosis required two injections and annual revaccination. The first vaccine induced transient CF antibodies, and a second vaccine given 6 weeks later resulted in an antibody titer for 1 to 10 months (Brock *et al.* 1965a, 1966).

A commercial vaccine, the Anaplaz vaccine (Fort Dodge), was first marketed in 1965 and consisted of a freeze-dried preparation of erythrocytes from infected cattle. It caused isohemolytic anemia in calves after ingestion of colostrum from immunized dams (Dimopoullos and Budden 1978). Because of this problem it was recommended that vaccine should be given while the breeding females were not pregnant and injections should be limited to an initial dose and one booster only (Searl 1980). However, the antibodies to erythrocytes did not develop using preparations similar to that of Anaplaz but incorporating ovine erythrocytic stroma. The ovine *Anaplasma* did not induce positive skin sensitivity when tested with bovine erythrocytes (Ristic and Carson 1977). Because of the incompatibility reactions between vaccinated cows and their calves, the use of the vaccine has been discontinued in some areas (Carson and Buening 1979; Loyacano *et al.* 1981).

Other attempts have been made to protect cattle with inactivated vaccines. Antigens prepared from washed infected bovine erythrocytes and used with saponin as the adjuvant resulted, following challenge, in a delay of infection and reduction in some cases of the severity of the clinical signs (McHardy and Simpson 1973). Chemically modified *Anaplasma* antigens induced cell-mediated but not antibody responses. On challenge, these vaccinated animals developed lower parasitemia (Buening 1978). The hypersensitivity reaction elicited by killed vaccines indicated that cell-mediated immunity was correlated with protection (Banerjee *et al.* 1978a).

The efficacy of the various vaccines has been compared. Attenuated *A. marginale* and *A. centrale* vaccines were used in cattle of different age groups. The former produced significantly more severe reactions in adult cattle and splenectomized calves, and slightly greater response in intact cattle (Kuttler 1972a). The Anaplaz vaccine and the attenuated vaccine of ovine origin induced a CF antibody response which persisted at least 6 weeks after the second dose of vaccine. Cell-mediated responses were also activated by the two procedures (Ristic and Carson 1977). The attenuated vaccine of ovine origin offered protection which approached the absolute immunity afforded by premunization with virulent *Anaplasma* strains of US origin (Carson and Buening 1979). In another report attenuated organisms, the killed adjuvant vaccine, and premunition using virulent *A. marginale* were compared. All methods induced CF antibodies. After field challenge in Colombia, the calves premunized with live organisms were protected, while those vaccinated with the inactivated antigens and the attenuated organisms developed severe clinical signs (Zaraza and Kuttler 1971). Partial resistance has been observed for 6 months after the latent infection was eliminated (Richey *et al.*, 1977).

CHEMOTHERAPY

Anaplasmosis in cattle is successfully treated with tetracyclines, imidocarb, and dithiosemicarbazone. Treatment is most effective during the early stages of infection, and a single dose of any of these drugs does not cause sterilization. Recrudescence of infections following single treatment usually occurs. Tetracyclines are most commonly used prophylactically, in treatment of disease, and in elimination of carriers. Supportive therapy is used in severe clinical cases. In latent infection, several treatments are required to eliminate the organism completely. Effective regimes for eliminating the carrier state are either by a daily dose of 10 mg/kg of short-acting tetracycline given intramuscularly or intravenously for 10 consecutive days, or 20 mg/kg of long-acting oxytetracycline given four times 3 to 7 days apart.

Literature

The chemotherapy of anaplasmosis, babesiosis, and theileriosis was reviewed by Joyner and Brocklesby (1973) and included the use of tetracyclines, dithiosemicarbazones (alpha-ethoxyethylglyoxaldithiosemicarbazone), and imidocarb ((3,3′-bis(2-imidazolin-2-yl) carbanilide dihydrochloride). Treatment with commercially available drugs was effective during the early stages of infection (Galhotra *et al.* 1977a). The drugs of choice for prophylaxis, therapy, and for elimination of the carrier state were oxytetracycline, chlortetracycline, and tetracycline (Roby 1972). However, the expense involved has restricted their wide use in many tropical countries. In the USA tetracyclines are the only drugs currently approved (Brock *et al.* 1959). Oxytetracycline caused suppression of the multiplication and degeneration of the organism which became enlarged and vacuolated, then became small and dense (Simpson 1975).

Prophylactically, long-acting tetracyclines given singly or in multiple injections after exposure significantly increased the prepatent periods and inhibited development of clinical signs in some of the animals (Eckblad *et al.* 1979). Feeding of 1.1 mg/kg of chlortetracyclines, usually as a medicated salt mineral block, was also sufficient to prevent anaplasmosis (Richey and Kliewer, 1981). A common practice in the field, once diagnosis has been made, has been to treat the entire herd with parenteral tetracyclines and to repeat the treatment 4 to 6 weeks later (Kuttler 1979). Sustained-release oxytetracycline boluses at a dose of 2.5 mg/kg prevented infection (Byford *et al.* 1981). It was found that feeding of 0.5 mg/kg of chlortetracycline for 120 days decreased the incidence of cattle with CF reactions from 60 to 8% (Franklin *et al.* 1966).

Treatment of clinical cases has been practical and effective when given early in the course of infection, before the onset of severe anemia (Ristic 1980). Both long- and short-acting tetracyclines were effective (Stewart *et al.* 1979). Oxytetracycline and chlortetracycline have been commonly used. Oxytetracycline at the rate of 6.6 to 11 mg/kg of body weight given one to three times, either intramuscularly or intravenously, effectively moderated the course of infection. Chlortetracycline administered orally in dosages as small as 1.1 mg/kg prevented infection, and in dosages ranging from 2.2 to 11 mg/kg for 30 to 90 days eliminated the carrier state (Kuttler 1980). Following therapy in calves and sheep, the hematocrit improved and the parasitemia was reduced (Singh *et al.* 1978). The high doses of chlortetracycline were found to be only partially effective (Brock *et al.* 1953). The effect of low multiple doses of oxytetracycline at 1, 2, or 3 mg/kg body weight caused marked reduction in clinical signs and parasitemia (Arline and Mamelli 1958). A single intramuscular dose of 2.0 to 2.5 mg/kg inhibited the development of parasitemia. The recrudescing and persistent post-treatment parasitemias also occurred after higher doses (Adams and Todorovic 1974a).

Long-acting oxytetracycline was compared to short-acting tetracycline in therapy. One treatment with 20 mg/kg of long-acting oxytetracycline was as effective as two injections of 10 mg/kg of short-acting formulation in moderating the course of infection and preventing severe clinical signs (Kuttler *et al.* 1978; Magonigle *et al.* 1978; Todorovic *et al.* 1979). In another report 20 mg/kg of long-acting oxytetracycline was equivalent to two daily injections of 50 mg/kg of standard oxytetracycline (Kutter *et al.* 1978; Magonigle *et al.* 1978). The efficacy of two oxytetracycline formulations and doxycycline in single and multiple injections were evaluated in treatment of the early stages of anaplasmosis in splenectomized calves (Kuttler and Simpson 1978).

Dithiosemicarbazone and imidocarb have been used only in development trials. They have been used successfully either singly or in combination with oxytetracycline in prophylactic, therapeutic, and carrier sterilization procedures (Kuttler 1971a, b). Dithiosemicarbazone caused degenerative changes with swelling and vacuolation of initial bodies and ballooning of the vesicular membrane (Simpson and Neal 1982). Imidocarb at 3 mg/kg was found to be a more effective therapeutic agent than oxytetracycline or chlortetracycline (Mishra and Sharma 1979). Development of an acute infection in splenectomized calves was inhibited by subcutaneous injection of imidocarb in a single dose of 2.5, 5.0, or 10.0 mg/kg (Roby 1972). Two intramuscular administrations 14 days apart at a level of 5 mg/kg was therapeutically effective but did not eliminate the infection (Kuttler 1971a, b). Repeated dosing with imidocarb – with the second injection given at the time of onset of the relapse – delayed and reduced the severity of the infection (McHardy and Simpson 1975). Imidocarb at 2.5 or 3.0 mg/kg given subcutaneously was effective, but dithiosemicarbazone was toxic in lactating cows (McHardy *et al.* 1980). Subcutaneous administration of two doses of amicarbalide (another derivative of carbanilide) at 20 mg/kg controlled acute infections of *A. marginale* and *A. centrale* in intact and splenectomized animals, but carriers were not sterilized. At doses of 40 mg/kg the compound was toxic causing lesions in the liver and in the kidneys (De Vos *et al.* 1978). Dithiosemicarbazone inhibited multiplication of *A. marginale* at levels of 50 and 10 mg/kg given intravenously, but only doses of 5 to 10 mg/kg were required to control clinical anaplasmosis (Brown *et al.* 1968).

Supportive therapy in acute anemia included blood transfusion. Transfusion was contraindicated when the restraint was difficult or the animals were restless. The presence of icterus indicated hepatic and myocardial damage, making transfusion hazardous (Jones and Brock 1966).

A variety of regimens have been used to sterilize the carrier animals. In the early investigations, 11 mg/kg of tetracycline daily for 10 consecutive days was recommended (Pearson *et al.* 1957). Chlortetracycline given intravenously at 33 mg/kg for 16 days was also successful (Splitter and Miller 1953). Long-acting oxytetracycline at 20 mg/kg body weight, given either four times at 3- to 4-day intervals or three times at 7-day intervals, eliminated the infections under experimental conditions. However, similar treatment regimens under field conditions in Texas generally failed to eliminate the infections (Kuttler *et al.* 1980). In another study, treatment with 20 mg/kg of long-acting oxytetracycline given two, three, or four times at 7 days apart eliminated an experimental carrier state (Roby *et al.* 1978). Also, in a field study in Indiana, four injections administered at 3-day intervals eliminated naturally acquired chronic infection (Magonigle and Newby 1982). These cattle retained immunity to *A. marginale* challenge for up to 8 months (Magonigle and Newby 1984). Intravenous administration of oxytetracycline hydrochloride at the rate of 22 mg/kg per day for 5 days also eliminated the infection. Four months after chemotherapy, challenge with a virulent strain caused transient hematological changes and a carrier state (Magonigle *et al.* 1975b; Renshaw *et al.* 1976). An effective treatment was daily feeding of chlortetracycline at 11 mg/kg for 30 to 60 days (Franklin *et al.* 1965), and at 11 mg/kg for 45 days (Sweet and Stauber 1978). Low levels (1.1 mg/kg) of fed chlortetracycline for 120 days also eliminated carriers and the animals were resistant to reinfection (Richey *et al.* 1976a, b). It may be important to keep animals in an *Anaplasma*-free environment during treatment to prevent reinfection (Kuttler 1983; Lincoln *et al.* 1983).

Imidocarb at 5 mg/kg administered either subcutaneously or intramuscularly in two injections 14 days apart eliminated the parasite from carrier cattle (Roby and Mazzola 1972), and the immunity persisted after the organisms were eliminated (Roby *et al.* 1974). Carrier calves treated intramuscularly five to ten times with 2.5 mg/kg of imidocarb in a period of 48 hours did not eliminate the organisms and toxicity and mortality were observed (Adams and Todorovic 1974b). Toxic effects of imidocarb were also studied in calves injected intramuscularly with 5, 10, or 20 mg/kg doses. The dosage-dependent clinical signs were transient and included excessive salivation, serous nasal discharge, diarrhea and dyspnea. There was an elevation in blood urea nitrogen and serum glutamic oxalacetic transaminase. Mortality occurred at 20 mg/kg dosage, and at postmortem examination there was hyperemia, hepatomegaly, pulmonary congestion and edema, hydrothorax, hydropericardium, and hydroperitoneum. Microscopic lesions consisted of acute necrosis of renal tubules and liver cells. At the site of injection there was necrotizing myositis (Adams *et al.* 1980). Combined treatments with 5 to 10 mg/kg of dithiosemicarbazone and 11 mg/kg oxytetracycline given three times at 24- to 48-hour intervals were successful in eliminating infection. Lower levels of the drugs, fewer injections, and greater time intervals between treatments and drugs given individually failed to eliminate infection (Kuttler 1971a, 1972b).

DIAGNOSIS

Diagnosis during the acute stage of the infection is made on the basis of clinical signs, hematological changes, and demonstration of the organism in erythrocytes. In well-defined epizootics, a tentative diagnosis can be made on the basis of fever and anemia without hemoglobinuria. However, demonstration of the organism and serologic confirmation are necessary for definitive diagnosis. In contrast to the relative ease of making a diagnosis during the acute phase, the detection of a chronic infection is difficult, requiring serologic tests because the organisms cannot be readily demonstrated. Giemsa stain is most commonly used and the organisms appear as homogeneous dense bodies 0.5 to 1 μm in size. Microscopic diagnosis is usually presumptive because only a very few *Anaplasma*-like inclusion bodies may be present and differentiation from other stained particulate material is difficult. Indirect fluorescent antibody, CF, capillary agglutination, and card agglutination tests are commonly used. In enzootic areas of *A. centrale* infection, cross-reactions in serologic tests between *A. centrale* and *A. marginale* must be taken into consideration.

Literature

Amerault *et al.* (1978) summarized the latest developments in the serologic diagnostic tests which were being used in the USA. Diagnosis of the carrier state by the CF test proved to be sufficiently accurate and enabled elimination of the disease problem in a number of regions of the USA (Brock 1963). The card agglutination test developed later had advantages in its relative simplicity with the need for minimum equipment (Amerault and Roby 1977).

Comparisons between the incidence of serologically positive animals and those with patent parasitemias were made. Eighteen percent of cattle and clinically normal water buffalo were found to be positive serologically by the tube agglutination test, the detection rate of organisms being 42% in the blood (Michael and El Refaii 1977). In earlier studies, the correlation between the CF test and parasitemia varied from 26 to 62% (Gainer 1961). Complement-fixing antibody activity demonstrated in latent *A. ovis* infections were not considered to be diagnostic of the carrier status (Magonigle *et al.* 1981).

A variety of stains were used to detect *Anaplasma* in smears (Galhotra *et al.* 1977a). The fluorescent dye acridine orange was a simple method to demonstrate *A. marginale* in formalin-fixed erythrocytes, but all particulate nucleic acid material, including Howell–Jolly bodies, stained with this dye (Gainer 1961). A direct FA technique was a specific method for demonstrating the inclusion bodies even in low numbers (Ristic *et al.* 1957). Direct FA technique was more sensitive than Giemsa stain. The blood smears prepared from subcutaneous tissues in the legs provided better diagnostic material than those made from kidneys, heart, or lungs (Johnston *et al.* 1980).

Only under special circumstances did diagnosis of the carrier stage require injection of blood into splenectomized calves (Simpson and Sanders 1953).

CONTROL

Control of anaplasmosis is undertaken either by eliminating the *Anaplasma* or by establishing widespread immunity in populations of animals by inducing low levels of infection. The efficacy of these two approaches depends on epidemiologic and economic considerations. Endemic situations are usually complex involving multiple arthropod vectors and frequent domestic and wild ruminant carriers, thus making control difficult and expensive. The time and money required to eliminate infections *per se* by treatment with available drugs has discouraged the use of the test and treatment techniques on a large scale in most tropical regions. Control of the clinical disease is more realistic and economically viable, but is dependent on the availability of adequate trained manpower and close veterinary supervision.

Literature

A number of reviews have been published on the different control measures implemented in various parts of the world. The diagnosis and control of *Anaplasma* were discussed by Anthony (1970). Malherbe (1963) reviewed the approaches to control which were undertaken in the USA and in South Africa. The control of tick-borne diseases in Australia, particularly anaplasmosis and babesiosis, was directed toward the tick and prevention of its spread throughout the continent (Gee 1976). A report of the control of the first outbreak in Canada by serologic identification and slaughter was made by Boulanger *et al.* (1971).

Cost–benefit analysis is of central importance in making a decision on the methods to be used in the control. Estimation of the losses must be defined and evaluated against the cost of various control measures and their effectiveness in a prolonged control program (Goodger 1978; Alderink and Dietrich 1982). One approach has been the elimination of the bovine carriers, vectors, and reservoirs in wild ruminant populations. The opposite approach has been the deliberate widespread production of carriers to ensure early and continuous exposure in all animals and thus prevent incidences of severe clinical disease (Malherbe 1963). Control has to begin with an accurate serologic diagnosis to determine the prevalence of infection and define the population at risk (Amerault *et al.* 1978). The elimination of carriers by chemotherapy depends on identifying infected cattle (Kuttler 1975). The reservoirs of infection, the mode of transmission, innate and acquired resistance, and the place of therapy have also to be considered (Jones and Brock 1966).

The current techniques used in the control of anaplasmosis in the USA were discussed by Kuttler (1979). Central to the efficient control measures was diagnosis by serologic tests to detect chronically infected animals. The use of live attenuated vaccine has not been approved in the USA because of the induction of latent infection and persistence of serologic reactions in vaccinated animals. The recent development of new long-acting tetracyclines which has enabled sterilization presented the possibility for combining vaccination followed by sterilizing treatment (Ristic 1980).

BIBLIOGRAPHY

Adams, L. G., Corrier, D. E. and Williams, J. D., 1980. A study of toxicity of imidocarb dipropionate in cattle, *Res. vet. Sci.*, **28**: 172–7.

Adams, L. G. and Todorovic, R. A., 1974a. The chemotherapeutic efficacy of imidocarb dihydrochloride on concurrent bovine anaplasmosis and babesiosis. I. The effects of a single treatment, *Trop. Anim. Hlth Prod.*, **6**: 71–8.

Adams, L. G. and Todorovic, R. A., 1974b. The chemotherapeutic efficacy of imidocarb dihyrochloride on concurrent bovine anaplasmosis and babesiosis. II. The effects of multiple treatments, *Trop. Anim. Hlth Prod.*, **6**: 79–84.

Ajayi, S. A., Wilson, A. J. and Campbell, R. S. F., 1978. Experimental bovine anaplasmosis: clinico-pathological and nutritional studies. *Res. vet. Sci.*, **25**: 76–81.

Alderink, F. J. and Dietrich, R. A., 1982. Economic and epidemiological implications of anaplasmosis in Texas cattle herds, *Proc. 86th Ann. Meet. US Anim. Hlth Assoc.*, pp. 65–75.

Allbritton, A. R. and Seger, C. L., 1962. The transport and excretion of bile pigments in anaplasmosis, *Am. J. vet. Res.*, **23**(96): 1011–18.

Allen, P. C. and Kuttler, K. L., 1981. Effect of *Anaplasma marginale* infection upon blood gases and electrolytes in splenectomized calves, *J. Parasitol.*, **67**(6): 954–6.

Allen, P. C., Kuttler, K. L. and Amerault, T. E., 1981a. Clinical chemistry of anaplasmosis: blood chemical changes in infected mature cows, *Am. J. vet. Res.*, **42**(2): 322–5.

Allen, P. C., Kuttler, K. L. and Amerault, T. E., 1981b. Clinical chemistry of anaplasmosis: comparative serum protein changes elicited by attenuated and virulent *Anaplasma marginale* isolates, *Am. J. vet. Res.*, **42**(2): 326–8.

Amerault, T. E., Mazzola, V. and Roby, T. O., 1973. Gram-staining characteristics of *Anaplasma marginale*, *Am. J. vet. Res.*, **34**(4): 552–5.

Amerault, T. E. and Roby, T. O., 1964. An exo-antigen of *Anaplasma marginale* in serum and erythrocytes of cattle with acute anaplasmosis, *Am. J. vet. Res.*, **25**(109): 1642–7.

Amerault, T. E. and Roby, T. O., 1967. Preparation and characterization of a soluble *Anaplasma marginale* antigen, *Am. J. vet. Res.*, **28**(125): 1067–72.

Amerault, T. E. and Roby, T. O., 1968. A rapid card agglutination test for bovine anaplasmosis, *J. Am. vet. med. Ass.*, **153**(12): 1828–31.

Amerault, T. E. and Roby, T. O., 1977. Card test. An accurate and simple procedure for detecting anaplasmosis, *Wld Anim. Rev.*, **22**: 34–8.

Amerault, T. E., Roby, T. O., McCallon, B. R. and Schilf, E. A., 1969. Current field and laboratory studies of the anaplasmosis card test, *Proc. 73rd Ann. Meet. US Anim. Hlth Ass.*, pp. 115–21.

Amerault, T. E., Roby, T. O., Rose, J. E. and Frerichs, W. M., 1978. Recent advances in the serologic diagnosis of anaplasmosis and babesiosis. In *Tick-borne Diseases and their Vectors*, ed. J. K. H. Wilde. Lewis Reprints (Tonbridge), pp. 122–9.

Amerault, T. E., Roby, T. O. and Sealock, R. L., 1975. Ultrastructure of *Anaplasma marginale* after freeze-fracture, *Am. J. vet. Res.*, **36**(10): 1515–19.

Amerault, T. E., Rose, J. E. and Kuttler, K. L., 1981. Comparative titration of *Anaplasma marginale* antibodies by card agglutination and complement-fixation tests, *Am. J. vet. Res.*, **42**(6): 1055–6.

Amerault, T. E., Rose, J. E., Martin, W. E. and Roby, T. O., 1980, Effects of phenol on card-agglutination and complement-fixation tests for bovine anaplasmosis, *Am. J. vet. Res.*, **41**(3): 435–8.

Amerault, T. E., Rose, J. E. and Roby, T. O., 1972. Modified card agglutination test for bovine anaplasmosis: evaluation with serum and plasma from experimental and natural cases of anaplasmosis, *Proc. 76th Ann. Meet. US Anim. Hlth Ass.*, pp. 736–44.

Anderson, I. L., Jones, E. W., Morrison, R. D., Holbert, D. and Lee, C. K., 1972. *Anaplasma marginale*: hemoglobin patterns in experimentally infected young calves, *Exp. Parasitol.*, **32**: 265–71.

Anon., 1963. Anaplasmosis. A costly disease of cattle, *US Agric. Res. Serv.*, **ARS 22–86**: 1–9.

Anthony, H. D., 1970. The diagnosis and control of anaplasmosis, *Proc. 74th Ann. Meet. US Anim. Hlth Ass.*, pp. 633–6.

Anthony, D. W. and Roby, T. O., 1966. The experimental transmission of bovine anaplasmosis by 3 species of North American ticks, *Am. J. vet. Res.*, **27**(116): 191–8.

Arline, R. E. and Mamelli, J. A., 1958. Laboratory studies of anaplasmosis in cattle treated with oxytetracycline, *J. Am. vet. med. Ass.*, **133**: 517–19.

Augustyn, N. J. and Bigalke, R. D., 1972. Anaplasma infection in a giraffe, *Onderstepoort J. vet. Res.*, **32**: 229.

Baker, N. F., Osebold, J. W. and Christensen, J. F., 1961. Erythrocyte survival in experimental anaplasmosis, *Am. J. vet. Res.*, **22**: 590–6.

Banerjee, D. P., Sarup, S., Gautam, O. P. and Singh, B., 1978a. Demonstration of cell mediated immune response in anaplasmosis in cattle. In *Tick-borne Diseases and their Vectors*, ed. J. K. H. Wilde. Lewis Reprints (Tonbridge), pp. 564–7.

Banerjee, D. P., Sarup, S., Gautam, O. P. and Singh, B., 1981. Cell-mediated immune response in anaplasmosis of cattle, *Z. Tropenmed. Parasit.*, **32**: 105–8.

Banerjee, D. P., Sharma, S. K., Gautam, O. P. and Sarup, S., 1978b. The use of spleen antigen in the tube agglutination test for diagnosis of anaplasmosis in cattle, *Trop. Anim. Hlth Prod.*, **10**: 83–6.

Barbet, A. F., Anderson, L. W., Palmer, G. H. and McGuire, T. C., 1983. Comparison of proteins synthesized by two different isolates of *Anaplasma marginale, Infect. Immun.*, **40**(3): 1068–74.

Bedell, D. M. and Dimopoullos, G. T., 1962. Biologic properties and characteristics of *Anaplasma marginale*. I. Effects of temperature on infectivity of whole blood preparations, *Am. J. vet. Res.*, **23**: 618–25.

Bedell, D. M. and Dimopoullos, G. T., 1963. Biologic properties and characteristics of *Anaplasma marginale*. II. The effects of sonic energy on the infectivity of whole blood preparations, *Am. J. vet. Res.*, **24**(99): 278–82.

Berry, S., Ibata, G. and Edwards, S., 1981. Antibody formation to *Babesia bovis* and *Anaplasma marginale* in calves in Bolivia, *Trop. Anim. Hlth Prod.*, **13**: 240–1.

Billups, M. E., Johns, R. W. and Dimopoullos, G. T., 1973. Amino acid and nucleic acid metabolic studies of RBC in bovine anaplasmosis, *Am. Soc. Microbiol.*, **73**: 180.

Bird, J. E., 1973. Neonatal anaplasmosis in a calf, *J. S. Afr. vet. med. Ass.*, **44**(1): 69–70.

Boulanger, P., Bannister, G. L., Avery, R. J., Gray, D. P., Barrett, B. B. and Ruckerbauer, G. M., 1966. Anaplasmosis: comparison of complement fixation methods and study of the cattle population of southern Alberta, *Can. J. comp.* Med., **30**: 102–6.

Boulanger, P., Ruckerbauer, G. M., Bannister, G. L., MacKay, R. R. and Peter, N. H., 1971. Anaplasmosis: control of the first outbreak in Canada by serological identification and slaughter, *Can. J. comp. Med.*, **35**: 249–57.

Bram, R. A. and Romanowski, R. D., 1970. Recognition of *Anaplasma marginale* Theiler in *Dermacentor andersoni* Stiles (= *D. venustus* Marx) by the fluorescent antibody method. I. Smears of nymphal organs, *J. Parasitol.*, **56**(1): 32–8.

Brezina, R., Murray, E. S., Tarizzo, M. L. and Bogel, K., 1973. Rickettsiae and rickettsial diseases, *Bull. Wld Hlth Org.*, **49**: 433–42.

Brock, W. E., 1962. Recent research on the characteristics of the etiologic agent of anaplasmosis, *Proc. 4th Nat. Anaplasmosis Conf.*, pp. 11–13.

Brock, W. E., 1963. Anaplasmosis – an up-to-date look at transmission, diagnosis, and immunization, *Sci. Proc. 100th Ann. Meet. Am. Vet. Med. Ass.*, pp. 258–61.

Brock, W. E., Kliewer, I. O., Jones, E. W. and Pearson, C. C., 1966. Vaccine studies in bovine anaplasmosis, *Pan. Am. Congr. Vet. Med. Zootech.*, **1**: 260–3.

Brock, W. E., Kliewer, I. O. and Pearson, C. C., 1965a. A vaccine for anaplasmosis, *J. Am. vet. med. Ass.*, **147**(9): 948–51.

Brock, W. E., Norman, B. B., Kliewer, I. O. and Jones, E. W., 1965b. Autoantibody studies in bovine anaplasmosis, *Am. J. vet. Res.*, **26**(111): 250–3.

Brock, W. E., Pearson, C. C. and Kliewer, I. O., 1953. High-level aureomycin dosage in anaplasmosis, *Am. J. vet. Res.*, **14**: 510–13.

Brock, W. E., Pearson, C. C., Kliewer, I. O. and Jones, E. W., 1959. The relation of treatment to hematological changes in anaplasmosis, *Proc. US Livestock Sanit. Ass.*, pp. 61–7.

Brown, C. G. D., Wilde, J. K. H. and Berger, J., 1968. Chemotherapy of experimental *Anaplasma marginale* infections, *Br. vet. J.*, **124**: 325–34.

Bruner, D. W. and Gillespie, J. H., 1973. The Rickettsiae. In *Hagan's Infectious Diseases of Domestic Animals*. Comstock Publishing Associates (Ithaca, N.Y. and London), pp. 747–73.

Budden, J. R. and Dimopoullos, G. T., 1977. Finite purification of *Anaplasma marginale*: serologic inactivity of the anaplasma body, *Am. J. vet. Res.*, **38**(5): 633–6.

Buening, G. M., 1973. Cell-mediated immune responses in calves with anaplasmosis, *Am. J. vet. Res.*, **34**(6): 757–63.

Buening, G. M., 1974. Hypolipoidemia and hypergammaglobulinemia associated with experimentally induced anaplasmosis in calves, *Am. J. vet. Res.*, **35**(3): 371–4.
Buening, G. M., 1976. Cell-mediated immune response in anaplasmosis as measured by a micro cell-mediated cytotoxicity assay and leukocyte migration-inhibition test, *Am. J. vet. Res.*, **37**(10): 1215–18.
Buening, G. M., 1978. Immune responses of cows to a chemically modified anaplasma antigen, *Am. J. vet. Res.*, **39**(6): 925–30.
Bundy, D. A. P., Hylton, G. A. and Wagner, G. G., 1983. Bovine haemoparasitic diseases in Jamaica, *Trop. Anim. Hlth Prod.*, **15**: 47–8.
Byford, R. L., Riner, J. L., Kocan, K. M., Stratton, L. G. and Hair, J. A., 1981. Chemoprophylaxis of vector-borne anaplasmosis with sustained release boluses, *Am. J. vet. Res.*, **42**(12): 2088–9.

Callow, L. L., 1974. Epizootiology, diagnosis and control of babesiosis and anaplasmosis. Relevance of Australian findings in developing countries, *Bull. Off. int. Epiz.*, **81**(9–10): 825–35.
Carson, C. A., Adams, L. G. and Todorovic, R. A., 1970. An antigenic and serologic comparison of two virulent strains and an attenuated strain of *Anaplasma marginale*, *Am. J. vet. Res.*, **31**(6): 1071–8.
Carson, C. A. and Buening, G. M., 1979. The immune response of cattle to live and inactivated *Anaplasma* vaccines and response to challenge, *J. S. Afr. vet. med. Ass.*, **50**: 330–1.
Carson, C. A., Kakoma, I. and Ristic, M., 1980. Use of peripheral blood leukocytes in the study of cell-mediated immunity in bovine anaplasmosis – a review, *Comp. Immun. Microbiol. infect. Dis.*, **3**: 277–81.
Carson, C. A., Ristic, M. and Lee, A. J., 1978. Immunologic responses in anaplasmosis. In *Tick-borne Diseases and their Vectors*, ed. J. K. H. Wilde, Lewis Reprints (Tonbridge), pp. 549–50.
Carson, C. A., Sells, D. M. and Ristic, M., 1976. Cutaneous hypersensitivity and isoantibody production in cattle injected with live or inactivated *Anaplasma marginale* in bovine and ovine erythrocytes, *Am. J. vet. Res.*, **37**(9): 1059–63.
Carson, C. A., Sells, D. M. and Ristic, M., 1977a. Cell-mediated immune response to virulent and attenuated *Anaplasma marginale* administered to cattle in live and inactivated forms, *Am. J. vet. Res.*, **38**(2): 173–9.
Carson, C. A., Sells, D. M. and Ristic, M., 1977b. Cell-mediated immunity related to challenge exposure of cattle inoculated with virulent and attenuated strains of *Anaplasma marginale*, *Am. J. vet. Res.*, **38**(8): 1167–71.
Carson, C. A., Weisiger, R. M., Ristic, M., Thurmon, J. C. and Nelson, D. R., 1974. Appendage-related antigen production by *Paranaplasma caudatum* in deer erythrocytes, *Am. J. vet. Res.*, **35**(12): 1529–31.

Christensen, J. F., Osebold, J. W. and Douglas, J. R., 1962. Bovine anaplasmosis in the Coast Range area of California, *J. Am. vet. med. Ass.*, **141**(8): 952–7.

Christensen, J. F., Osebold, J. W. and Rosen, M. N., 1958. Infection and antibody response in deer experimentally infected with *Anaplasma marginale* from bovine carriers, *J. Am. vet. med. Ass.*, **132**: 289–92.

Connell, M. L., 1974. Transmission of *Anaplasma marginale* by the cattle tick *Boophilus microplus*, *Queensland J. Agric. Anim. Sci.*, **31**(3): 185–93.

Connell, M. L., 1978. Attempted transmission of *Anaplasma marginale* by *Haemaphysalis longicornis*, *Aust. vet. J.*, **54**: 92–3.

Connell, M. and Hall, W. T. K., 1972. Transmission of *Anaplasma marginale* by the cattle tick *Boophilus microplus*, *Aust. vet. J.*, **48**: 477.

Corrier, D. E., Gonzalez, E. F. and Betancourt, A., 1978. Current information on the epidemiology of bovine anaplasmosis and babesiosis in Colombia. In *Tick-borne Diseases and their Vectors*, ed. J. K. H. Wilde. Lewis Reprints (Tonbridge), pp. 114–20.

Corrier, D. E. and Guzman, S., 1977. The effect of natural exposure to *Anaplasma* and *Babesia* infections on native calves in an endemic area of Colombia, *Trop. Anim. Hlth Prod.*, **9**: 47–51.

Corrier, D. E., Vizcaino, O., Carson, C. A., Ristic, M., Kuttler, K. L., Trevino, G. S. and Lee, A. J., 1980. Comparison of three methods of immunization against bovine anaplasmosis: an examination of postvaccinal effects, *Am. J. vet. Res.*, **41**(7): 1062–5.

Corrier, D. E., Wagner, G. G. and Adams, L. G., 1981. Recrudescence of *Anaplasma marginale* induced by immunosuppression with cyclophosphamide, *Am. J. vet. Res.*, **42**(1): 19–21.

Cox, F. R. and Dimopoullos, G. T., 1972. Demonstration of an autoantibody associated with anaplasmosis, *Am. J. vet. Res.*, **33**(1): 73–6.

Davis, L. R. and Bowman, G. W., 1952. Preliminary report on a concentration method for detecting *Anaplasma marginale*, *J. Parasitol.*, **38**: 26–7.

Davis, W. C., McGuire, T. C., Anderson, L. W., Banks, K. L., Seifert, S. D. and Johnson, M. I., 1981. Development of monoclonal antibodies to *Anaplasma marginale* and preliminary studies on their application, *Proc. 7th Nat. Anaplasmosis Conf.*, 1981, pp. 285–305.

Davis, W. C., Talmadge, J. E., Parish, S. M., Johnson, M. I. and Vibber, S. D., 1978. Synthesis of DNA and protein by *Anaplasma marginale* in bovine erythrocytes during short-term culture, *Infect. Immun.*, **22**(2): 597–602.

De Robertis, E. and Epstein, B., 1957. Electron microscope study of anaplasmosis in bovine red blood cells, *Proc. Soc. Exp. Biol. Med.*, **77**: 254–8.

De Vos, A. J., Barrowman, P. R., Coetzer, J. A. W. and Kellerman, T. S., 1978. Amicarbalide: a therapeutic agent for anaplasmosis, *Onderstepoort J. vet. Res.*, **45**: 203–8.

Dikmans, G., 1950. The transmission of anaplasmosis, *Am. J. vet. Res.*, **11**(38): 5–16.

Dimopoullos, G. T. and Bedell, D. M., 1960. Studies of bovine erythrocytes in anaplasmosis. I. Flocculating properties of stromata in water (26142) *Proc. Soc. Exp. Biol. Med.*, **105**: 463–6.

Dimopoullos, G. T. and Bedell, D. M., 1962. Studies of bovine erythrocytes in anaplasmosis. II. Role of chemical and physical changes in erythrocytes in the mechanism of anemia in splenectomized calves, *Am. J. vet. Res.*, **23**: 813–20.

Dimopoullos, G. T. and Bedell, D. M., 1974. Mechanism and specificity of the capillary tube-agglutination test for diagnosis of anaplasmosis, *Am. J. vet. Res.*, **35**(12): 1567–70.

Dimopoullos, G. T. and Budden, J. R., 1978. Finite purification of *Anaplasma marginale* by affinity chromatography. In *Tick-borne Diseases and their Vectors*, ed. J. K. H. Wilde. Lewis Reprints (Tonbridge), pp. 551–6.

Dimopoullos, G. T. and Finerty, J. F., 1976. Cross reactivity between *Anaplasma marginale* and two *Plasmodium* species as demonstrated by passive hemagglutination, *Am. J. vet. Res.*, **37**(6): 693–5.

Dumag, P. U., Reyes, P. V. and Castillo, A. M., 1962. Observations on the premunition of Santa Gertrudis cattle against *Piroplasma* spp. and *Anaplasma marginale*, *Philippine J. Anim. Ind.*, **23**(1–4): 1–20.

Eckblad, W. P., Lincoln, S. D. and Magonigle, R. A., 1979. Efficacy of terramycin/LA-200 administered during the prepatent period of anaplasmosis, *Proc. 83rd Ann. Meet. US Anim. Hlth Assoc.*, pp. 44–52.

Eckblad, W. P. and Magonigle, R. A., 1983. Acquired cellular responsiveness in cattle cleared of *Anaplasma marginale* 28 months earlier, *Vet. Immunol. Immunopath.*, **4**: 659–63.

Erp, E. E. and Hahrney, D., 1975. Exit of *Anaplasma marginale* from bovine red blood cells, *Am. J. vet. Res.*, **36**(5): 707–9.

Erp. E. E. and Hahrney, D., 1976. Changes in serum concentration of phagocytosis-stimulating factor in experimentally induced bovine anaplasmosis: preliminary findings, *Am. J. vet. Res.*, **37**(5): 607–9.

Espana, C., Espana, E. M. and Gonzalez, D., 1959. *Anaplasma marginale*. I. Studies with phase contrast and electron microscopy, *Am. J. vet. Res.*, **20**: 795–805.

Folsch, D. W. and Liau, M-Y., 1971. Experimental infection, clinical hematological course, and isolation of *Anaplasma marginale* and *Paranaplasma* of Taiwan origin, *Acta trop.*, **28**(1): 1–16.

Foote, L. E., Geer, J. C. and Stich, Y. E., 1958. Electron microscopy of the *Anaplasma* body: ultrathin sections of bovine erythrocytes, *Science*, **128**: 147–8.

Foote, L. E., Levy, H. E., Torbert, B. J. and Oglesby, W. T., 1957.

Interference between anaplasmosis and eperythrozoonosis in splenectomized cattle, *Am. J. vet. Res.*, **18**: 556–9.

Fowler, D. and Swift, B. L., 1975. Abortion in cows inoculated with *Anaplasma marginale, Theriogenology*, **4**(2–3): 59–67.

Francis, D. H., Buening, G. M. and Amerault, T. E., 1980a. Characterization of immune responses of cattle to erythrocyte stroma, *Anaplasma* antigen, and dodecanoic acid-conjugated *Anaplasma* antigen: humoral immunity, *Am. J. vet. Res.*, **41**(3): 362–7.

Francis, D. H., Buening, G. M. and Amerault, T. E., 1980b. Characterization of immune responses of cattle to erythrocyte stroma, anaplasma antigen, and dodecanoic acid-conjugated *Anaplasma* antigen: cell-mediated immunity, *Am. J. vet. Res.*, **41**(3): 368–71.

Francis, D. H., Kinden, D. A. and Buening, G. M., 1979. Characterization of the inclusion limiting membrane of *Anaplasma marginale* by immunoferritin labeling, *Am. J. vet. Res.*, **40**(6): 777–82.

Franklin, T. E., Cook, R. W. and Anderson, D. J., 1966. Feeding chlortetracycline to range cattle to eliminate the carrier state of anaplasmosis. *Proc. 70th Ann. Meet. US Livestock Sanit. Ass.*, pp. 85–90.

Franklin, T. E. and Huff, J. W., 1964. A rapid complement fixation screening procedure for anaplasmosis testing, *Am. J. vet. Res.*, **25**(107): 1321–2.

Franklin, T. E. and Huff, J. W., 1967. A proposed method of premunizing cattle with minimum inocula of *Anaplasma marginale, Res. vet. Sci.*, **8**: 415–18.

Franklin, T. E., Huff, J. W. and Grumbles, L. C., 1965. Chlortetracycline for elimination of anaplasmosis in carrier cattle, *J. Am. vet. med. Ass.*, **147**(4): 353–6.

Franklin, T. E., Huff, J. W. and Heck, F. C., 1962. Large scale production of anaplasmosis antigen, *SWest. Vet.*, **15**: 131–9.

Gainer, J. H., 1961. Demonstration of *Anaplasma marginale* with the fluorescent dye, acridine orange; comparisons with the complement-fixation test and Wright's stain. *Am. J. vet. Res.*, **22**: 882–6.

Galhotra, A. P., Gautam, O. P. and Banerjee, D. P., 1977a. Trial of some chemotherapeutic agents in bovine anaplasmosis, *Indian vet. J.*, **54**: 522–7.

Galhotra, A. P., Gautam, O. P., Banerjee, D. P., Chauban, H. V. S., Singh, R. P. and Kalra, D. S., 1977b. Pathological changes in bovine anaplasmosis, *Indian vet. J.*, **54**: 599–601.

Galhotra, A. P., Singh, R. P., Banerjee, D. P. and Gautam, O. P., 1979. Effect of splenectomy on the course of parasitaemia and consequent biochemical and bone marrow changes in *Anaplasma marginale* infection in calves, *Indian vet. J.*, **56**: 466–9.

Garcia, A. O., 1978. Immunizacion contra babesiosis y anaplasmosis bovina en el Valle del Cauca. Evaluacion de sistemas de vacunacion mono y bivalentes contra babesiosis en condiciones naturales, *Rev. Inst. Colombiano Agro.*, **13**(4): 739–40.

Gates, D. W., Madden, P. A., Martin, W. H. and Roby, T. O., 1957. The infectivity of blood from anaplasma-infected cattle as shown by calf inoculation, *Am. J. vet. Res.*, **18**: 257–60.

Gates, D. W., Roby, T. O., Amerault, T. E. and Anthony, D. W., 1967. Ultrastructure of *Anaplasma marginale* fixed with gluteraldehyde and osmium tetroxide, *Am. J. vet. Res.*, **28**: 1577–80.

Gautam, O. P. and Singh, B., 1971. Anaplasmosis – I: Incidence in cattle, sheep, and goats in Punjab and Haryana, *Haryana Agri. Univ. J. Res.*, **1**(1): 86–91.

Gee, R. W., 1976. Control of tick-borne diseases (anaplasmosis and babesiosis) of cattle in Australia, *Bull. Off. int. Epiz.*, **86**: 61–6.

Goksu, K., 1965. A review of anaplasmosis and observations of infections in sheep and goats, *Turk Veteriner Heklimeri Dernigi Dergisis*, **35**: 399–417.

Gonzalez, E. F., Long, R. F. and Todorovic, R. A., 1978. Comparisons of the complement-fixation, indirect fluorescent antibody, and card agglutination tests for the diagnosis of bovine anaplasmosis, *Am. J. vet. Res.*, **39**(9): 1538–41.

Gonzalez, E. F., Todorovic, R. A. and Thompson, K. C., 1976. Immunization against anaplasmosis and babesiosis: Part I. Evaluation of immunization using minimum infective doses under laboratory conditions, *Z. Tropenmed. Parasit.*, **27**(4): 427–37.

Goodger, W. J., 1978. Economic losses associated with anaplasmosis in California beef cattle utilizing three methods of economic analysis, *Calif. Vet.*, **32**(1): 12–14.

Goodger, W. J., Carpenter, T. and Riemann, H., 1979. Estimation of economic loss associated with anaplasmosis in California beef cattle, *J. Am. vet. med. Ass.*, **174**(12): 1333–6.

Hansard, S. L. and Foote, L. E., 1959. Anemia of induced anaplasmosis in the calf, *Am. J. Physiol.*, **197**: 711–16.

Hansard, S. L. and Foote, L. E., 1961. Absorption and physiological movement of iron in calves induced with anaplasmosis, *J. Anim. Sci.*, **20**: 395.

Hansard, S. L., McDonald, T. P. and Foote, L. E., 1972. Erythropoietin levels and hemopoiesis in bovine anaplasmosis, *Federation Proc.*, **31**: 630.

Hart, L. T., Larson, A. D., Decker, J. L., Weeks, J. P. and Clancy, P. L., 1981. Preparation of intact *Anaplasma marginale* devoid of host cell antigens, *Current Microbiol.*, **5**: 95–100.

Henderson, F. E., 1969. Anaplasmosis, *Proc. 73rd Ann. Meet. US Anim. Hlth Ass.*, pp. 113–14.

Henry, E. T., Norman, B. B., Fly, D. E., Wichmann, R. W. and York,

S. M., 1983. Effects and use of a modified live *Anaplasma marginale* vaccine in beef heifers in California, *J. Am. vet. med. Ass.*, **183**(1): 66–9.

Hibbs, C. M., Weide, K. D. and Marshall, M., 1966. Comparison of anaplasmosis tests, *J. A. vet. med. Ass.*, **148**(1): 545–6.

Hidalgo, R. J., 1975. Propagation of *Anaplasma marginale* in bovine lymph node cell culture, *Am. J. vet. Res.*, **36**(5): 635–40.

Hidalgo, R. J. and Dimopoullos, G. T., 1967. Complement-fixation micro-procedures for anaplasmosis, *Am. J. vet. Res.*, **28**(122): 245–51.

Howarth, J. A., Hokama, Y. and Amerault, T. E., 1976. The modified card agglutination test: an accurate tool for detecting anaplasmosis in Colombian black-tailed deer, *J. Wildl. Dis.*, **12**: 427–34.

Howe, D. L., Hepworth, W. G., Blunt, F. M. and Thomas, G. M., 1964. Anaplasmosis in big game animals: experimental infection and evaluation of serologic tests, *Am. J. vet. Res.*, **25**: 1271–6.

Jatkar, P. R. and Kreier, J. P., 1967a. Relationship between severity of anemia and plasma erythropoietin titer in anaplasma-infected calves and sheep, *Am. J. vet. Res.*, **28**: 107–13.

Jatkar, P. R. and Kreier, J. P., 1967b. Pathogenesis of anaemia in *Anaplasma* infection, *Indian vet. J.*, **44**: 393–9.

Jatkar, P. R. and Kreier, J. P., 1969. Pathogenesis of anaemia in anaplasma infection. Part II – auto-antibody and anaemia, *Indian vet. J.*, **46**: 560–6.

Jatkar, P. R., Kreier, J. P., Akin, E. L. and Tharp, V., 1966. Comparative persistence of capillary tube-agglutination and complement fixation test reactions in cattle treated to destroy the carrier state of anaplasmosis, *Am. J. vet. Res.*, **27**(116): 372–4.

Johns, R. W. and Dimopoullos, G. T., 1974. *In vitro* uptake of ^{14}C-labeled amino acids by preparations of partially purified *Anaplasma marginale* bodies, *Infect. Immun.*, **9**(4): 645–7.

Johnston, L. A. Y., Trueman, K. F., Leatch, G. and Wilson, A. J., 1980. A comparison of direct fluorescent antibody and Giemsa staining for the post-mortem diagnosis of anaplasmosis, *Aust. vet. J.*, **56**(3): 116–18.

Jones, E. W. and Brock, W. E., 1966. Bovine anaplasmosis: its diagnosis treatment, and control, *J. Am. vet. med. Ass.*, **149**(12): 1624–33.

Jones, E. W., Kliewer, I. O., Norman, B. B. and Brock, W. E., 1968a. *Anaplasma marginale* infection in young and aged cattle, *Am. J. vet. Res.*, **29**(3): 535–44.

Jones, E. W. and Norman, B. B., 1962. Bovine anaplasmosis. The disease, its clinical diagnosis and prognosis, *Proc. 4th Nat. Anaplasmosis Conf.*, pp. 3–6.

Jones, E. W., Norman, B. B., Kliewer, I. O. and Brock, W. E., 1968b. *Anaplasma marginale* infection in splenectomized calves, *Am. J. vet. Res.*, **29**(3): 523–33.

Joyner, L. P. and Brocklesby, D. W., 1973. Chemotherapy of anaplasmosis, babesiasis, and theileriasis, *Adv. Pharmacol. Chemother.*, **11**: 321–55.

Keeton, K. S. and Jain, N. C., 1973. Scanning electron microscopic studies of *Paranaplasma* sp. in erythrocytes of a cow, *J. Parasit.*, **59**(2): 331–6.

Kessler, R. H. and Ristic, M., 1979. *In vitro* cultivation of *Anaplasma marginale*: invasion of and development in noninfected erythrocytes, *Am. J. vet. Res.*, **40**(12): 1774–6.

Kessler, R. H., Ristic, M., Sells, D. M. and Carson, C. A., 1979. *In vitro* cultivation of *Anaplasma marginale*: growth pattern and morphologic appearance, *Am. J. vet. Res.*, **40**(12): 1767–73.

Khera, S. S., 1962. Rickettsial infections in animals: a review, *Indian J. vet. Sci.*, **32**: 283–301.

Klaus, G. G. B and Jones, E. W., 1968. The immunoglobulin response in intact and splenectomized calves infected with *Anaplasma marginale, J. Immunol.*, **100**(5): 991–9.

Knowles, R. T., Montrose, M., Craig. T. M., Wagner, G. G. and Long, R. F., 1982. Clinical and serolocal evidence of bovine babesiosis and anaplasmosis in St Lucia, *Vet. Parasitol.*, **10**: 307–11.

Kocan, K. M., Barron, S. J., Holbert, D., Ewing, S. A. and Hair, J. A., 1982a. Influence of increased temperature on *Anaplasma marginale* Theiler in the gut of *Dermacentor andersoni* Stiles, *Am. J. vet. Res.*, **43**(1): 32–4.

Kocan, K. M., Ewing, S. A., Holbert, D. and Hair, J. A., 1982b. Morphologic characteristics of colonies of *Anaplasma marginale* Theiler in midgut epithelial cells of *Dermacentor andersoni* Stiles, *Am. J. vet. Res.*, **43**(4): 586–93.

Kocan, K. M., Hair, J. A. and Ewing, S. A., 1980a. Ultrastructure of *Anaplasma marginale* Theiler in *Dermacentor andersoni* Stiles and *Dermacentor variabilis* (Say), *Am. J. vet. Res.*, **41**(12): 1966–76.

Kocan, K. M., Hair, J. A., Ewing, S. A. and Stratton, L. G., 1981. Transmission of *Anaplasma marginale* Theiler by *Dermacentor andersoni* Stiles and *Dermacentor variabilis, Am. J. vet. Res.*, **42**(1): 15–18.

Kocan, K. M., Hsu, K. C., Hair, J. A. and Ewing, S. A., 1980b. Demonstration of *Anaplasma marginale* Theiler in *Dermacentor variabilis* (Say) by ferritin-conjugated antibody technique, *Am. J. vet. Res.*, **41**(12): 1977–81.

Kocan, K. M., Teel, K. D. and Hair, J. A., 1980c. Demonstration of *Anaplasma marginale* Theiler in ticks by tick transmission, animal inoculation, and fluorescent antibody studies, *Am. J. vet. Res.*, **41**(2): 183–6.

Kocan, K. M., Venable, J. H. and Brock, W. E., 1978a. Ultrastructure of anaplasmal inclusions (Pawhuska isolate) and their appendages in intact and hemolyzed erythrocytes and in complement-fixation antigen, *Am. J. vet. Res.*, **39**(7): 1123–9.

Kocan, K. M., Venable, J. H., Hsu, K. C. and Brock, W. E., 1978b. Ultrastructural localization of anaplasmal antigens (Pawhuska isolate) with ferritin-conjugated antibody, *Am. J. vet. Res.*, **39**(7): 1131–5.

Kreier, J. P. and Ristic, M., 1963a. Anaplasmosis. VII. Experimental *Anaplasma ovis* infection in white-tailed deer (*Dama virginiana*), *Am. J. vet. Res.*, **24**: 567–72.

Kreier, J. P. and Ristic, M., 1963b. Anaplasmosis. X. Morphologic characteristics of the parasites present in the blood of calves infected with the Oregon strain of *Anaplasma marginale*, *Am. J. vet. Res.*, **24**: 676–87.

Kreier, J. P. and Ristic, M., 1963c. Anaplasmosis. XI. Immunoserologic characteristics of the parasites present in the blood of calves infected with the Oregon strain of *Anāplasma marginale*, *Am. J. vet. Res.*, **24**(101): 688–96.

Kreier, J. P. and Ristic, M., 1963d. Anaplasmosis. XII. The growth and survival in deer and sheep of the parasites present in the blood of calves infected with the Oregon strain of *Anaplasma marginale*, *Am. J. vet. Res.*, **24**: 697–702.

Kreier, J. P. and Ristic, M., 1972. Definition of taxonomy of *Anaplasma* species with emphasis on morphologic and immunologic features, *Z. Tropenmed. Parasit.*, **23**: 88–98.

Kreier, J. P., Ristic, M. and Schroeder, W., 1964. Anaplasmosis. XVI. The pathogenesis of anemia produced by infection with *Anaplasma*, *Am. J. vet. Res.*, **25**: 363–52.

Kuil, H. and Folkers, C., 1968. Studies on *Anaplasma ovis* infection. I. Course of spontaneous infections in splenectomised Nigerian sheep and goats, *Bull. epiz. Dis. Afr.*, **16**: 65–70.

Kuttler, K. L., 1965. Serological survey of anaplasmosis incidence in East Africa, using the complement-fixation test, *Bull. epiz. Dis. Afr.*, **13**: 257–62.

Kuttler, K. L., 1966. Clinical and hematologic comparison of *Anaplasma marginale* and *Anaplasma centrale* infections in cattle, *Am. J. vet. Res.*, **27**: 941–7.

Kuttler, K. L., 1967a. Serological relationship of *Anaplasma marginale* and *Anaplasma centrale* as measured by the complement-fixation and capillary tube agglutination tests, *Res. vet. Sci.*, **8**: 207–11.

Kuttler, K. L., 1967b. A study of the immunological relationship of *Anaplasma marginale* and *Anaplasma centrale*, *Res. vet. Sci.*, **8**: 467–71.

Kuttler, K. L., 1969. Serial passage of an attenuated *Anaplasma marginale* in splenectomized calves, *Proc. 73rd Ann. Meet. US Anim. Hth Assoc.*, 1969, pp. 131–5.

Kuttler, K. L., 1971a. Efficacy of oxytetracycline and a dithiosemicarbazone in the treatment of bovine anaplasmosis, *Am. J. vet. Res.*, **32**(9): 1349–52.

Kuttler, K. L., 1971b. Promising therapeutic agents for the elimination of *Anaplasma marginale* in the carrier animal, *Proc. 75th Ann. Meet. US Anim. Hlth Ass.*, pp. 92–8.

Kuttler, K. L., 1972a. Comparative response to premunization using attenuated *Anaplasma marginale*, virulent *A. marginale* and *A. centrale* in different age groups, *Trop. Anim. Hlth Prod.*, **4**: 197–203.
Kuttler, K. L., 1972b. Combined treatment with a dithiosemicarbazone and oxytetracycline to eliminate *Anaplasma marginale* infections in splenectomized calves, *Res. vet. Sci.*, **13**: 536–439.
Kuttler, K. L., 1975. Use of imidocarb to control anaplasmosis, *SWest. Vet.*, **28**(1): 47–52.
Kuttler, K. L., 1979. Current anaplasmosis control techniques in the United States, *J. S. Afr. vet. med. Ass.*, **50**: 314–20.
Kuttler, K. L., 1980. Pharmacotherapeutics of drugs used in treatment of anaplasmosis and babesiosis. *J. Am. vet. med. Ass.*, **176**(10(2)): 1103–8.
Kuttler, K. L., 1981. Infection of splenectomized calves with *Anaplasma ovis*, *Am. J. vet. Res.*, **42**(12): 2094–6.
Kuttler, K. L., 1983. Influence of a second *Anaplasma* exposure on the success of treatment to eliminate *Anaplasma* carrier infections in cattle, *Am. J. vet. Res.*, **44**(5): 882–3.
Kuttler, K. L. and Adams, L. G., 1977. Influence of dexamethasone on the recrudescence of *Anaplasma marginale* in splenectomized calves, *Am. J. vet. Res.*, **38**(9): 1327–30.
Kuttler, K. L. and Adams, L. G., 1978. Influence of dexamethasone therapy on *Anaplasma* carrier, splenectomized calves. In *Tick-borne Diseases and their Vectors*, ed. J. K. H. Wilde. Lewis Reprints (Tonbridge), pp. 557–63.
Kuttler, K. L., Adams, L. G. and Zaraza, H., 1970. Study of the epizootiology of *Anaplasma marginale* and *Trypanosoma theileri* in Colombia, *Inst. Colombiano Agro. Rvta.*, **5**: 127–48.
Kuttler, K. L. and Hidalgo, R. J., 1980. Recent progress in the control of anaplasmosis, *Texas Agric. Exp. Station/Coll. Station Progr. Rep., No. 3594–/3644*, pp. 97–101.
Kuttler, K. L., Johnson, L. W. and Simpson, J. E., 1980. Chemotherapy to eliminate *Anaplasma marginale* under field and laboratory conditions, *Proc. 84th Ann. Meet. US Anim. Hlth Ass.*, pp. 73–82.
Kuttler, K. L., Marble, D. W. and Matthews, N. J, 1962. Anaplasmosis complement-fixation response in calves from anaplasmosis-infected dams, *Am. J. vet. Res.*, **23**: 1007–10.
Kuttler, K. L. and Simpson, J. E., 1978. Relative efficacy of two oxytetracycline formulations and doxycycline in the treatment of acute anaplasmosis in splenectomized calves, *Am. J. vet. Res.*, **39**(2): 347–9.
Kuttler, K. L., Young, M. F. and Simpson, J. E., 1978. Use of an experimental long-acting oxytetracycline (Terramycin/LA) in the treatment of acute anaplasmosis, *Vet. Med./Small Anim. Clin.*, **73**: 187–92.
Kuttler, K. L. and Zaraza, H., 1969. Premunization with an attenuated *Anaplasma marginale*, *Proc. 73rd Ann. Meet. US Anim. Hlth Ass.*, pp. 104–12.

Lawrence, J. A., 1977. The mechanical transmission of *Anaplasma* under Rhodesian conditions, *Rhod. Vet. J.*, **8**: 74–6.
Leatch, G., 1973. Preliminary studies on the transmission of *Anaplasma marginale* by *Boophilus microplus*, *Aust. vet. J.*, **49**: 16–19.
Lincoln, S. D., Eckblad, W. P. and Magonigle, R. A., 1983. Bovine anaplasmosis: clinical, hematologic, and serologic manifestations in cows given a long-acting oxytetracycline formulation in the prepatent period, *Am. J. vet. Res.*, **43**(8): 1360–2.
Lohr, K.-F., 1969. Immunisierung gegen Babesiose und Anaplasmose von 40 nach Kenya importierten Charollais-Rindern und Bericht uber Erscheinungen der Photosensibilitat bei diesen Tieren, *Z. Veterinarmed.*, **B16**: 40–6.
Lohr, K.-F. and Meyer, H., 1973. Game anaplasmosis: the isolation of *Anaplasma* organisms from antelope, *Z. Tropenmed. Parasit.*, **24**: 192–7.
Lohr, K.-F., Otieno, P. S. and Gacanga, W., 1975. Susceptibility of Boran cattle to experimental infections with *Anaplasma marginale* and *Babesia bigemina*, *Zbl. Vet. Med.*, **B22**: 842–9.
Long, R. F. and Wagner, G. G., 1981. Antigen binding buffers in the enzyme-linked immunospecific assay (ELISA) for *Anaplasma marginale* antibody activity in bovine serum, *Proc. 7th Nat. Anaplasmosis Conf.*, 1981, pp. 321–32.
Love, J. N., 1972. Cryogenic preservation of *Anaplasma marginale* with dimethyl sulfoxide, *Am. J. vet. Res.*, **132**: 2257–60.
Loyacano, A. F., Nipper, W. A. and Blakewood, B. W., 1981. Effects of vaccination of beef cattle for anaplasma. Livestock producer's day – Louisiana, Agricultural Station. Animal Science Department, **21**: 185–6.
Luther, D. G., Cox, H. U. and Nelson, W. O., 1980. Comparisons of serotests with calf inoculations for detection of carriers in anaplasmosis-vaccinated cattle, *Am. J. vet. Res.*, **41**(12): 2085–6.

Maas, J. and Buening, G. M., 1981a. Serologic evidence of *Anaplasma marginale* infection in white-tailed deer (*Odocoileus virginianus*) in Missouri, *J. Wildl. Dis.*, **17**(1): 45–7.
Maas, J. and Buening, G. M., 1981b. Characterization of *Anaplasma marginale* infection in splenectomized domestic goats, *Am. J. vet. Res.*, **42**(1): 142–5.
Madden, P. A., 1962. Structure of *Anaplasma marginale* observed by using fluorescent antibody technique, *Am. J. vet. Res.*, **23**(95): 921–4.
Madden, P. A. and Kuttler, K. L., 1980. Factors affecting the rapid card agglutination test for anaplasmosis, *Proc. 84th Ann. Meet. US Anim. Hlth Ass.*, pp. 83–93.
Magonigle, R. A., Eckblad, W. P., Lincoln, S. D. and Frank, F. W., 1981. *Anaplasma ovis* in Idaho sheep, *Am. J. vet. Res.*, **42**(2): 199–201.
Magonigle, R. A. and Newby, T. J., 1982. Elimination of naturally

acquired chronic *Anaplasma marginale* infections with a long-acting oxytetracycline injectable, *Am. J. vet. Res.*, **43**(12): 2170–2.

Magonigle, R. A. and Newby, T. J., 1984. Response of cattle upon reexposure to *Anaplasma marginale* after elimination of chronic carrier infections, *Am. J. vet. Res.*, **45**: 695–7.

Magonigle, R. A., Renshaw, H. W., Stauber, E., Vaughn, H. W. and Frank, F. W., 1975a. Latent anaplasmosis infection in Idaho mule deer demonstrated by calf inoculation, *Proc. 79th Ann. Meet. US Anim. Hlth Ass.*, pp. 64–9.

Magonigle, R. A., Renshaw, H. W., Vaughn, H.W., Stauber, E. and Frank, F. W., 1975b. Effect of five daily intravenous treatments with oxytetracycline hydrochloride on the carrier status of bovine anaplasmosis, *J. Am. vet. med. Ass.*, **167**(12): 1080–3.

Magonigle, R. A., Simpson, J. E. and Frank, F. W., 1978. Efficacy of a new oxytetracycline formulation against clinical anaplasmosis, *Am. J. vet. Res.*, **39**(9): 1407–10.

Malherbe, W. D., 1963. Some observations on anaplasmosis, *Cornell Vet.*, **53**: 71–7.

Malhotra, M. N., Ristic, M. and Levy, M. G., 1982. Preservation by lyophilization of anaplasmosis capillary tube-agglutination test antigen, *Am. J. vet. Res.*, **43**(2): 368–9.

Mallick, K. P., Dwivedi, S. K. and Malhotra, M. N., 1979. Anaplasmosis in goats: report on clinical cases, *Indian vet. J.*, **56**: 693–4.

Manjrekar, S. L., 1954. *Rickettsia* of domesticated animals (a short review), *Indian J. vet. Sci.* **24**(4): 217–22.

Mann, D. K. and Ristic, M., 1963a. Anaplasmosis. XIII. Studies concerning the nature of autoimmunity, *Am. J. vet. Res.*, **24**(101): 703–7.

Mann, D. K. and Ristic, M., 1963b. Anaplasmosis. XIV. The isolation and characterization of an autohemagglutinin, *Am. J. vet. Res.*, **24**(101): 709–12.

Marble, D. W. and Hanks, M. A., 1972. A tissue culture method for *Anaplasma marginale*, *Cornell Vet.*, **62**: 196–205.

Mason, R. A. and Ristic, M., 1967. *In vitro* incorporation of glycine by bovine erythrocytes infected with *Anaplasma marginale*, *J. Infect. Dis.*, **116**: 335–42.

Mazzola, V., Amerault, T. E. and Roby, T. O., 1979. Electron microscope studies of *Anaplasma marginale* in an *Aedes albopictus* culture system, *Am. J. vet. Res.*, **40**(12): 1812–15.

Mazzola, V. and Kuttler, K. L., 1980. *Anaplasma marginale* in bovine erythrocyte cultures, *Am. J. vet. Res.*, **41**(12): 2087–8.

McCallon, B. R., 1973. Prevalence and economic aspects of anaplasmosis, *Proc. 6th Nat. Anaplasmosis Conf.*, pp. 1–3.

McDowell, R. E., Roby, T. O., Fletcher, J. L., Foote, L. F., Brandon, C. and High, J. W., 1964. Impact of anaplasmosis in a diary herd, *J. Anim. Sci.*, **23**: 168–71.

McHardy, N., 1974. The effects of injecting anti-erythrocyte serum into calves infected with *Anaplasma marginale*, *Ann. Trop. Med.*

Parasitol., **68**(1): 51–7.

McHardy, N., Berger, J., Taylor, R. J., Farebrother, D. and James, J. A., 1980. Comparison of gloxazone, an effective but toxic anaplasmacide, with imidocarb hydrochloride, *Res. vet. Sci.*, **29**: 198–202.

McHardy, N. and Simpson, R. M., 1973. Attempts at immunizing cattle against anaplasmosis using a killed vaccine, *Trop. Anim. Hlth Prod.*, **5**: 166–73.

McHardy, N. and Simpson, R. M., 1975. Repeated dosing in the treatment of Kenyan anaplasmosis, using imidocarb dyhydrochloride, *Trop. Anim. Hlth Prod.*, **7**: 139–48.

Medina, L. J. L., 1959–60. Changes in erythrocytes of cattle with anaplasmosis, *Rev. Med. Vet. y Paras. Maracay.*, **18**(1–8): 95–109.

Michael, S. A. and El Refaii, A. H., 1977. Serological diagnosis of anaplasmosis in Egyptian buffaloes, *El Assiut Vet. Med. J.*, **4**(7): 85–9.

Miller, R. M., Price, M. A. and Kuttler, K. L., 1976. Investigations on transstadial transmission of bovine anaplasmosis and benign bovine theileriosis in cattle by two species of *Amblyomma* (Acarina: Ixodidae), *Southwestern Entomol.*, **1**(3): 107–9.

Mishra, A. K. and Sharma, N. N., 1979. Comparative efficacy of drugs in bovine anaplasmosis, *Trop. Anim. Hlth Prod.*, **11**: 222–6.

Morris, H., Ristic, M. and Lykins, J., 1971. Characterization of opsonins eluted from erythrocytes of cattle infected with *Anaplasma marginale*, *Am. J. vet. Res.*, **32**(8): 1221–8.

Moulton, J. E. and Christensen, J. F., 1955. The histochemical nature of *Anaplasma marginale*, *Am. J. vet. Res.*, **16**: 377–80.

Murphy, F. A., Osebold, J. W. and Aalund, O., 1966a. Kinetics of the antibody response to *Anaplasma marginale* infection, *J. Infect. Dis.*, **116**: 99–111.

Murphy, F. A., Osebold, J. W. and Aalund, O., 1966b. Hyper-γM-globulinemia in experimental anaplasmosis, *Am. J. vet. Res.*, **27**(119): 971–4.

Neitz, W. O., 1939. Ovine anaplasmosis: the transmission of *Anaplasma ovis* and *Eperythrozoon ovis* to the Blesbuck (*Damaliscus albifrons*). *Onderstepoort J. Vet. Sci. Anim. Ind.*, **13**(1): 9–16.

Neitz, W. O., 1968. *Anaplasma ovis* infection, *Bull. Off. int. Epiz.*, **70**: 359–65.

Nicholls, M. J., Ibata, G. and Vallejas Rodas, F., 1980. Prevalence of antibodies to *Babesia bovis* and *Anaplasma marginale* in dairy cattle in Bolivia, *Trop. Anim. Hlth Prod.*, **12**: 48–9.

Oberst, R. D., Kocan, K. M., Hair, J. A. and Ewing, S. A., 1981. Staining characteristics of colonies of *Anaplasma marginale* Theiler in *Dermacentor andersoni* Stiles, *Am. J. vet. Res.*, **42**(11): 2006–9.

Obi, T. U., 1978. Survey of the incidence of anaplasmosis among Nigerian zebu trade cattle, *Trop. Anim. Hlth Prod.*, **10**: 87–90.

Ormsbee, R. A., 1969. Rickettsiae (as organisms), *Ann. Rev. Microb.*, **2B**: 275–92.
Osebold, J. W., Douglas, J. R. and Christensen, J. F., 1962. Transmission of anaplasmosis to cattle by ticks obtained from deer, *Am. J. vet. Res.*, **23**: 21–3.
Osorno, M. B., Solana, P. M., Perez. J. M. and Lopez, T. R., 1975. Study of an attenuated *Anaplasma marginale* vaccine in Mexico – natural challenge of immunity in enzootic area, *Am. J. vet. Res.*, **36**(5): 631–3.
Otim, C., Wilson, A. J. and Campbell, R. S. F., 1980. A comparative study of experimental anaplasmosis in *Bos indicus* and *Bos taurus* cattle, *Aust. vet. J.*, **56**: 262–6.

Paine, G. D. and Miller, A. S., 1977. Anaplasmosis in a newborn calf, *Vet. Rec.*, **100**: 58.
Parker, R. J. and Wilson, A. J., 1979. The experimental transmission of *Anaplasma marginale* by the brown dog tick *Rhipicephalus sanguineus* in Australia, *Aust. vet. J.*, **55**: 606.
Patarroyo, J. H., Villa, O. and Diazgranados, H., 1978. Epidemiology of cattle anaplasmosis in Colombia: I. Prevalence and distribution of agglutinating antibodies, *Trop. Anim. Hlth Prod.*, **10**: 171–4.
Paull, N. I., Parker, R. J., Wilson, A. J. and Campbell, R. S. F., 1980. Epidemiology of bovine and anaplasmosis in beef calves in northern Queensland, *Aust. vet. J.*, **56**: 267–71.
Payne, R. C. and Scott, J. M., 1982. Anaplasmosis and babesiosis in El Salvador, *Trop. Anim. Hlth Prod.*, **14**: 75–80.
Pearson, C. C., Brock, W. E. and Kliewer, I. O., 1957. A study of tetracycline dosage in cattle which are anaplasmosis carriers, *J. Am vet. med. Ass.*, **130**: 290–2.
Peterson, K. J., Raleigh, R. J., Stroud, R. K. and Goulding, R. L., 1977. Bovine anaplasmosis transmission studies conducted under controlled natural exposure in a *Dermacentor andersoni* = (*venustus*) indigenous area of eastern Oregon, *Am. J. vet. Res.*, **38**(3): 351–4.
Peterson, K. J. and Roby, T. O., 1975. Absence of *Anaplasma marginale* infection in American bison raised in an anaplasmosis endemic area, *J. Wildl. Dis.*, **11**: 395–7.
Pipano, E., Klinger, I. and Weisman, Y., 1972. Application of the capillary agglutination test for anaplasmosis in cattle vaccinated with *Anaplasma centrale*, *Refuah Vet.*, **29**(4): 166–9.
Potgieter, F. T., 1979. Epizootiology and control of anaplasmosis in South Africa, *J. S. Afr. vet. med. Ass.*, **50**: 367–72.
Potgieter, F. T., Sutherland, B. and Biggs, H. C., 1981. Attempts to transmit *Anaplasma marginale* with *Hippobosca rufipes* and *Stomoxys calcitrans*, *Onderstepoort J. Vet. Res.*, **48**: 119–22.
Potgieter, F. T. and van Rensburg, L., 1980. Isolation of *Anaplasma marginale* from *Rhipicephalus simus* males, *Onderstepoort J. vet. Res.*, **47**: 285–6.
Potgieter, F. T. and van Rensburg, L., 1983. Infectivity virulence and

immunogenicity of *Anaplasma centrale* live blood vaccine, *Onderstepoort J. vet. Res.*, **50**: 29–31.
Price, K. E., Poelma, L. J. and Faber, J. E., 1952. Preparation of an improved antigen for anaplasmosis complement-fixation tests, *Am. J. vet. Res.*, **13**: 149–51.

Renshaw, H. W., Magonigle, R. A., Eckblad, W. P. and Frank, F. W., 1976. Immunity to bovine anaplasmosis after elimination of the carrier status with oxytetracycline hydrochloride, *Proc. 80th Ann. Meet. US Anim. Hlth. Ass.*, pp. 79–88.
Renshaw, H. W., Magonigle, R. A. and Vaughn, H. W., 1979. Evaluation of the anaplasmosis rapid card agglutination test for detecting experimentally infected elk, *J. Wildl. Dis.*, **15**(3): 379–86.
Renshaw, H. W., Vaughn, H. W., Magonigle, R. A., Davis, W. C., Stauber, E. H. and Frank, F. W., 1977. Evaluation of free-roaming mule deer as carriers of anaplasmosis in an area of Idaho where bovine anaplasmosis is enzootic. *J. Am. vet. med. Ass.*, **170**(3): 334–9.
Ribeiro, M. F. B., Reis, R. and Salcedo, J. H. P., 1980. Evaluation of attenuated *Anaplasma marginale* vaccine in calves maintained in small pasture. *Arq. Esc. Vet. UFMG, Belo Horizonte*, **32**(2): 251–8.
Richey, E. J., Brock, W. E., Kliewer, I. O. and Jones, E. W., 1976a. The effect of feeding low levels of chlortetracycline for extended periods on the carrier state of anaplasmosis. *Bovine Practitioner*, **11**: 73–5.
Richey, E. J., Brock, W. E., Kliewer, I. O., Jones, E. W. and White, R. G., 1976b. Low levels of chlortetracycline for anaplasmosis. *J. Anim. Sci.*, **43**: 232.
Richey, E. J., Brock, W. E., Kliewer, I. O. and Jones, E. W., 1977. Resistance to anaplasmosis after elimination of latent *Anaplasma marginale* infections. *Am. J. vet. Res.*, **38**(2): 169–70.
Richey, E. J. and Kliewer, I. O., 1981. Efficacy of chlortetracycline against bovine anaplasmosis when administered free choice to cattle in a medicated feed block and salt-mineral mix. *Proc. 7th Nat. Anaplasmosis Conf.*, pp. 635–47.
Ristic, M., 1960a. Anaplasmosis. *Adv. Vet. Sci.*, **6**: 111–92.
Ristic, M., 1960b. Structural characterization of *Anaplasma marginale* in acute and carrier infections, *J. Am. vet. med. Ass.*, **136**(9): 417–25.
Ristic, M., 1960c. Studies of anaplasmosis. I. Filtration of the causative agent, *Am. J. vet. Res.*, **21**: 890–4.
Ristic, M., 1961. Studies in anaplasmosis. III. An autoantibody and symptomatic macrocytic anemia, *Am. J. vet. Res.*, **22**: 871–6.
Ristic, M., 1963. Economics of the CA anaplasmosis test, *Vet. Econ.*, **4**(4): 36–41.
Ristic, M., 1967. Anaplasmosis. XX. Electron microscopy of the causative agent stained by the negative contrast technique, *Am. J. vet. Res.*, **28**: 63–70.
Ristic, M., 1968. Anaplasmosis. In *Infectious Blood Diseases of Man and*

Animals, eds D. Weinman, M. Ristic. Academic Press (New York), pp. 478–542.

Ristic, M., 1976. Immunologic systems and protection in infections caused by intracellular blood protista, *Vet. Parasitol.*, **2**: 31–47.

Ristic, M., 1977. Bovine anaplasmosis. In *Parasitic Protozoa*, ed. J. P. Kreier. Academic Press (New York, San Francisco, London), vol. IV, pp. 235–50.

Ristic, M., 1980. Anaplasmosis. In *Bovine Medicine and Surgery*, ed. H. E. Amstutz. American Veterinary Publications (Santa Barbara, Calif.), vol. 1, pp. 324–48.

Ristic, M. and Carson, C. A., 1977. Methods of immunoprophylaxis against bovine anaplasmosis with emphasis on the use of the attenuated *Anaplasma marginale* vaccine. In *Immunity to Blood Parasites of Animals and Man*, eds L. H. Miller, J. A. Pino, J. J. McKelvey, Jr. Plenum Press (New York and London), pp. 151–88.

Ristic, M. and Carson, C. A., 1978. An attenuated *Anaplasma marginale* vaccine with emphasis on the mechanism of protective immunity. In *Tick-borne Diseases and their Vectors*, ed. J. K. H. Wilde. Lewis Reprints (Tonbridge), pp. 541–8.

Ristic, M., Lykins, J. D. and Morris, H. R., 1972. Anaplasmosis: opsonins and hemagglutinins in etiology of anemia, *Exp. Parasitol.*, **31**: 2–12.

Ristic, M. and Mann, D. K., 1963. Anaplasmosis. IX. Immunoserologic properties of soluble *Anaplasma* antigens, *Am. J. vet. Res.*, **24**(100): 478–82.

Ristic, M., Mann, D. K. and Kodras, R., 1963. Anaplasmosis. VIII. Biochemical and biophysical characterization of soluble *Anaplasma* antigens, *Am. J. vet. Res.*, **24**: 472–7.

Ristic, M., Sibinovic, S. and Welter, C. J., 1968. An attenuated *Anaplasma marginale* vaccine, *Proc. 72nd Ann. Meet. US Livestock Sanitary Ass.*, pp. 56–69.

Ristic, M. and Sippel, W. L., 1958. Effect of cortisone on the mechanism of *Anaplasma* immunity in experimentally infected calves. II. Studies of pathological changes, *Am. J. vet. Res.*, **19**: 44–50.

Ristic, M. and Watrach, A. M., 1961. Studies in anaplasmosis. II. Electron microscopy of *Anaplasma marginale* in dear, *Am. J. vet. Res.*, **22**: 109–16.

Ristic, M. and Watrach, A. M., 1962. Studies in anaplasmosis. V. Occurrence of *Anaplasma marginale* in bovine blood platelets, *Am. J. vet. Res.*, **23**(94): 626–31.

Ristic, M. and Watrach, A. M., 1963. Anaplasmosis. VI. Studies and a hypothesis concerning the cycle of development of the causative agent, *Am. J. vet. Res.*, **24**: 267–77.

Ristic, M. and White, F. H., 1960. Detection of an *Anaplasma marginale* antibody complex formed *in vivo*, *Science*, **131**: 987–8.

Ristic, M., White, F. H., Green, J. H. and Sanders, D. A., 1958. Effect of cortisone on the mechanism of *Anaplasma* immunity in experimentally infected calves. I. Hematological and immunoserological studies, *Am. J. vet. Res.*, **19**: 37–43.

Ristic, M., White, F. H. and Sanders, D. A., 1957. Detection of *Anaplasma marginale* by means of fluorescein-labeled antibody, *Am. J. vet. Res.*, **18**: 924–8.

Roberts, R. H. and Love, J. N., 1977. Infectivity of *Anaplasma marginale* after ingestion by potential insect vectors, *Am. J. vet. Res.*, **38**(10): 1629–30.

Roby, T. O., 1960. A review of studies on the biological nature of *Anaplasma marginale, Proc. US Livestock Sanit. Ass.*, pp. 88–94.

Roby, T. O., 1972. The inhibitory effect of imidocarb on experimental anaplasmosis in splenectomized calves. *Res. vet. Sci.*, **13**: 519–22.

Roby, T. O., Amerault, T. E., Mazzola, V., Rose, J. E. and Ilemobade, A., 1974. Immunity in bovine anaplasmosis after elimination of *Anaplasma marginale* infections with imidocarb, *Am. J. vet. Res.*, **35**(7): 993–5.

Roby, T. O., Gates, D. W. and Mott, L. O., 1961. The comparative susceptibility of calves and adult cattle to bovine anaplasmosis, *Am. J. vet. Res.*, **22**: 982–5.

Roby, T. O. and Mazzola, V., 1972. Elimination of the carrier state of bovine anaplasmosis with imidocarb, *Am. J. vet. Res.*, **33**(10): 1931–3.

Roby, T. O., Simpson, J. E. and Amerault, T. E., 1978. Elimination of the carrier state of bovine anaplasmosis with a long-acting oxytetracycline, *Am. J. vet. Res.*, **39**: 1115–6.

Rogers, R. J., 1971. Bovine anaplasmosis: an evaluation of the complement-fixation and capillary tube-agglutination tests and the incidence of antibodies in northern Queensland cattle herds, *Aust. vet. J.*, **47**: 364–9.

Rogers, R. J. and Shiels, I. A., 1979. Epidemiology and control of anaplasmosis of Australia *J. S. Afr. vet. med. Ass.*, **50**: 363–6.

Rose, J. E., Amerault, T. E. and Roby, T. O., 1974. Roles of conglutinin, complement, and antibody size in the card agglutination test for bovine anaplasmosis, *Am. J. vet. Res.*, **36**(9): 1147–51.

Rose, J. E., Amerault, T. E., Roby, T. O. and Martin, W. H., 1978. Serum levels of conglutinin, complement, and immunoconglutinin in cattle infected with *Anaplasma marginale*, *Am. J. vet. Res.*, **39**(5): 791–3.

Ryff, J. F., Weibel, J. L. and Thomas, G. M., 1964. Relationship of ovine to bovine anaplasmosis, *Cornell Vet.*, **54**: 407–14.

Schindler, R., Ristic, M. and Wokatsch, R., 1966. Vergleichende untersuchungen mit *Anaplasma marginale* und *A. centrale*, *Z. Tropenmed. Parasit.*, **17**: 337–60.

Schmidt, H., 1973. Anaplasmosis in cattle, *J. Am. vet. med. Ass.*, **90**: 723–36.

Schroeder, W. F. and Ristic, M., 1965a. Anaplasmosis. XVII. The relation of autoimmune processes to anemia, *Am. J. vet. Res.*, **26**(111): 239–43.

Schroeder, W. F. and Ristic, M., 1965b. Anaplasmosis. XVIII. An analysis of autoantigens in infected and normal bovine erythrocytes, *Am. J. vet. Res.*, **26**(112): 679–82.

Schroeder, W. F. and Ristic, M., 1968. Blood serum factors associated with erythrophagocytosis in calves with anaplasmosis, *Am. J. vet. Res.*, **29**(10): 1991–5.

Scott, G. R., 1978. Tick-borne rickettsial diseases of domestic livestock. In *Tick-borne Diseases and their Vectors*, ed. J. K. H. Wilde. Lewis Reprints (Tonbridge), pp. 451–74.

Scott, W. L., Geer, J. C. and Foote, L. E., 1961. Electron microscopy of *Anaplasma marginale* in the bovine erythrocyte, *Am. J. vet. Res.*, **22**: 877–81.

Searl, R. C., 1980. Use of an anaplasma vaccine as related to neonatal isoerythrolysis, *Vet. Med./Small Anim. Clin.*, **75**: 101–4.

Seger, C. L. and White, D., 1962. The histopathology of anaplasmosis, *Proc. 4th Nat. Anaplasmosis Conf.*, pp. 26–8.

Sharma, S. K., Banerjee, D. P. and Gautam, O. P., 1978. *Anaplasma marginale* infection in Indian water buffalo (*Bubalus bubalis*), *Indian J. Anim. Hlth*, **17**: 105–10.

Shmulevich, A. I., 1958. Chemotherapy and chemical prevention of hematozoic diseases in farm stock in the USSR, *Bull. Off. int. Epiz.*, **49**: 255–64.

Simpson, C. F., 1975. Morphologic alterations of *Anaplasma marginale* in calves after treatment with oxytetracycline, *Am. J. vet. Res.*, **36**(10): 1443–6.

Simpson, C. F. and Neal, F. C., 1982. Morphologic alteration of *Anaplasma marginale* in calves treated with a dithiosemicarbazone, *Am. J. vet. Res.*, **43**(11): 1903–6.

Simpson, C. F., Kling, J. M. and Love, J. N., 1967. Morphologic and histochemical nature of *Anaplasma marginale*, *Am. J. vet. Res.*, **28**(125): 1055–65.

Simpson, C. F. and Sanders, D. A., 1953. Diagnosis of the carrier stage of anaplasmosis under experimental conditions, *Vet. Med.*, **48**: 182–4.

Singh, B. and Gautam, O. P., 1971. Anaplasmosis – III. Experimental anaplasmosis induced by splenectomisation in indigenous and crossbred calves, *Indian vet. J.*, **48**: 1215–22.

Singh, B. and Gautam, O. P., 1972. Anaplasmosis – IV. Experimental anaplasmosis induced by splenectomization in sheep and goats, *Haryana Vet.*, **11**: 4–10.

Singh, B., Gautam, O. P. and Banerjee, D. P., 1978. Oxytetracycline therapy and blood changes in anaplasmosis in calves and sheep, *Haryana agric. Univ. J. Res.*, **8**(1): 35–9.

Sinha, G. K. and Pathak, R. C., 1966. Anaplasmosis in goats and sheep, *Indian vet. J.*, **43**: 490–3.

Smith, J. E., McCants, M. and Jones, E. W., 1972. Erythrocyte enzyme

activity during experimental anaplasmosis, *Int. J. Biochem.*, **3**: 345–50.
Splitter, E. J., Anthony, H. D. and Twiehaus, M. J., 1956. *Anaplasma ovis* in the United States. Experimental studies with sheep and goats, *Am. J. vet. Res.*, **17**: 487–91.
Splitter, E. J. and Miller, J. G., 1953. The apparent eradication of the anaplasmosis carrier state with antibiotics, *Vet. Med.*, **48**: 486–8.
Splitter, E. J., Twiehaus, M. J. and Castro, E. R., 1955. Anaplasmosis in sheep in the United States, *J. Am. vet. med. Ass.*, **127**: 244–5.
Staats, J. J., Kocan, K. M., Hair, J. A. and Ewing, S. A., 1982. Immunocytochemical labeling of *Anaplasma marginale* Theiler in *Dermacentor andersoni* Stiles with peroxidase-antiperoxidase technique, *Am. J. vet. Res.*, **43**(6): 983–7.
Stewart, C. G., Immelman, A., Grimbeek, P. and Grib, D., 1979. The use of a short and long acting oxytetracycline for the treatment of *Anaplasma marginale* in splenectomized calves, *J. S. Afr. vet. med. Ass.*, **50**: 83–5.
Stiller, D., Johnson, L. W. and Kuttler, K. L., 1983. Experimental transmission of *Anaplasma marginale* Theiler by males of *Dermacentor albipictus* (Packard) and *Dermacentor occidentalis* Marx (Acare: Ixodidae), *Proc. 87th Ann. Meet. US Anim. Hlth Ass.*, pp. 59–64.
Summers, W. A., 1967. Infectivity of *Anaplasma marginale* in bovine blood after prolonged freezing, *Am. J. vet. Res.*, **28**(124): 880–2.
Sweet, V. H. and Stauber, E. H., 1978. Anaplasmosis: a regional serological survey and oral antibiotic therapy in infected herds, *J. Am. vet. med. Ass.*, **172**(11): 1310–12.
Swift, B. L. and Paumer, R. J., 1976. Vertical transmission of *Anaplasma marginale* in cattle, *Theriogenology*, **6**(5): 515–21.
Swift, B. L. and Paumer, R. J., 1978. Bovine fetal anoxia observed in pregnant beef heifers experimentally inoculated with *Anaplasma marginale*, *Theriogenology*, **10**(5): 395–403.

Taylor, R. L., 1969. Immunogenic differences between two *Anaplasma marginale* isolates, *Am. J. vet. Res.*, **30**(11): 1999–2002.
Thoen, C. O., Blackburn, B., Mills, K., Lomme, J. and Hopkins, M. P., 1980. Enzyme-linked immunosorbent assay for detecting antibodies in cattle in a herd in which anaplasmosis was diagnosed, *J. Clin. Microbiol.*, **11**(5): 499–502.
Thompson, K. C. and Roa, J. C., 1978. Transmission (mechanical/biological) of *Anaplasma marginale* by the tropical cattle tick *Boophilus microplus*. In *Tick-borne Diseases and their Vectors*, ed. J. K. H. Wilde. Lewis Reprints (Tonbridge), pp. 536–9.
Todorovic, R. A., Gonzalez, E. F. and Adams, L. G., 1975. *Babesia bigemina, Babesia argentina*, and *Anaplasma marginale*: coinfectious immunity in bovines, *Exp. Parasitol.*, **37**: 179–92.
Todorovic, R. A., Gonzalez, E. F. and Garcia, O., 1979. Evaluation of

a new long-acting oxytetracycline formulation against anaplasmosis in Colombian cattle, *Z. Tropenmed. Parasit.*, **30**: 236–8.

Todorovic, R., Gonzalez, E. and Lopez, G., 1978. Immunization against anaplasmosis and babesiosis. Part II. Evaluation of cryo-preserved vaccines using different doses and routes of inoculation, *Z. Tropenmed. Parasit.*, **29**: 210–14.

Todorovic, R. A., Long, R. F. and McCallon, B. R., 1977. Comparison of rapid card agglutination test with the complement fixation test for diagnosis of *Anaplasma marginale* infection in cattle in Colombia, *Vet. Microbiol.*, **2**: 167–77.

Todorovic, R. A., Lopez, L. A., Lopez, A. G. and Gonzalez, E. F., 1975. Bovine babesiosis and anaplasmosis: control by premunition and chemoprophylaxis, *Exp. Parasitol.*, **37**: 92–104.

Todorovic, R. A. and Tellez, C. H., 1975. The premunition of adult cattle against babesiosis and anaplasmosis in Colombia, South America, *Trop. Anim. Hlth Prod.*, **7**: 125–31.

Trueman, K. F. and Wilson, A. J., 1979. Observation on the pathology of *Anaplasma marginale* infections in cattle, *Aust. Adv. Vet. Sci.*, **5**: 75.

Uilenberg, G., 1968. Notes on bovine babesioses and anaplasmosis in Madagascar. I. Introduction. Transmission, *Rev. Elev. Méd. vét. Pays trop.*, **21**(4): 467–74.

Vilas Novas, J. C. and Viana, F. C., 1980. Field evaluation of attenuated *Anaplasma marginale* vaccine in calves, *Arq. Esc. Vet. UFMG, Belo Horizonte*, **32**(1): 57–62.

Vizcaino, O., Carson, C. A., Lee, A. J. and Ristic, M., 1978. Efficacy of attenuated *Anaplasma marginale* vaccine under laboratory and field conditions in Colombia, *Am. J. vet. Res.*, **39**(2): 229–33.

Vizcaino, O., Corrier, D. E., Terry, M. K., Carson, C. A., Lee, A. J., Kuttler, K. L., Ristic, M. and Trevino, G. S., 1980. Comparison of three methods of immunization against bovine anaplasmosis: evaluation of protection afforded against field challenge exposure, *Am. J. vet. Res.*, **41**(7): 1066–8.

Wagner, G., 1981. Immunoglobulin responses of cattle associated with recrudescent *Anaplasma marginale* infections, *Proc. 7th Nat. Anaplasmosis Conf.*, pp. 307–20.

Wallace, W. R., 1967. Loss of erythrocytic acetlycholinesterase activity and its relationship to osmotic fragility of erythrocytes in bovine anaplasmosis, *Am. J. vet. Res.*, **28**(122): 55–61.

Weiss, E., 1973. Growth and physiology of rickettsiae, *Bact. Rev.*, **37**(3): 259–83.

Welter, C. J., 1964. Serologic stability and specificity of agglutinating

Anaplasma marginale antigen, *Am. J. vet. Res.*, **25**(107): 1058–61.
Welter, C. J. and Zuschek, F., 1962. Properties of *Anaplasma marginale* antigen used in a capillary tube-agglutination test, *J. Am. vet. med. Ass.*, **141**(5): 595–9.
Weyer, F., 1978. Progresses in ecology and epidemiology of rickettsioses. A review, *Acta trop.*, **35**: 5–21.
Weisenhutter, E., 1975. Research into the relative importance of Tabanidae (Diptera) in mechanical disease transmission. III. The epidemiology of anaplasmosis in a Dar-es-Salaam dairy farm. *Trop. Anim. Hlth Prod.*, **7**: 15–22.
Williams, E. I. and Jones, E. W., 1968. Blood transfusions during patent bovine anaplasmosis, *Am. J. vet. Res.*, **29**(3): 703–10.
Wilson, A. J., 1979. Observations on the pathogenesis of anaplasmosis in cattle with particular reference to nutrition, breed and age, *J. S. Afr. vet. med. Ass.*, **50**: 293–4.
Wilson, A. J., Parker, R. J. and Trueman, K. F., 1979. Anaplasmosis in *Bos indicus* cattle, *Aust. Adv. Vet. Sci.*, **5**: 76.
Wilson, A. J., Parker, R. and Trueman, K. F., 1980a. Susceptibility of *Bos indicus* crossbred and *Bos taurus* cattle to *Anaplasma marginale* infection, *Trop. Anim. Hlth Prod.*, **12**: 90–4.
Wilson, A. J., Parker, R. and Trueman, K. F., 1980b. Experimental immunization of calves against *Anaplasma marginale* infection: observations on the use of living *A. centrale* and *A. marginale*, *Vet. Parasitol.*, **7**: 305–11.
Wilson, A. J., Trueman, K. F., Spinks, G. and McSorley, A. F., 1978. A comparison of 4 serological tests in the detection of humoral antibodies to anaplasmosis in cattle, *Aust. vet. J.*, **54**: 383–6.
Wilson, B. H. and Meyer, R. B., 1966. Transmission studies of bovine anaplasmosis with the horseflies, *Tabanus fuscicostatus* and *Tabanus nigrovittatus*, *Am. J. vet. Res.*, **27**(116): 367–9.

Yeruham, I. and Braverman, Y., 1981. The transmission of *Anaplasma marginale* to cattle by blood-sucking arthropods, *Refuah vet.*, **38**(1–2): 37–44.

Zaraza, H. and Kuttler, K. L., 1971. Comparative efficacy of different immunization systems against anaplasmosis, *Trop. Anim. Hlth Prod.*, **3**: 77–82.
Zwart, D. and Buys, J., 1968. Studies on *Anaplasma ovis* infection. II. Pathogenicity of a Nigerian goat strain for Dutch sheep and goats, *Bull. epiz. Dis. Afr.*, **16**: 73–80.

Chapter

20

Ehrlichiosis

CONTENTS

INTRODUCTION

Ehrlichiosis is a group of diseases in dogs, horses, cattle, and sheep caused by species of rickettsia in the genus *Ehrlichia*. Various forms occur in different climatic regions, and those syndromes occurring in tropical climates are of primary importance and are discussed in this chapter. The type of disease produced differs with the species of organism and species of host. Canine ehrlichiosis is caused by *E. canis* and is manifested by progressive pancytopenia, particularly thrombocytopenia, epistaxis, anorexia, emaciation, dehydration, and fever. It was first observed in 1935 in Algeria and reported in 1957 in North America. A fatal hemorrhagic syndrome reported later from southeast Asia was particularly severe and given the name tropical canine pancytopenia. *Ehrlichia equi* causes a disease in horses and was first recognized in California in 1969; it is characterized by edema of the legs, ataxia, depression, anorexia, and fever. In cattle, bovine petechial fever (BPF), also called Ondiri disease, is caused by *Cytoecetes ondiri,* was first reported in Kenya in the 1930s, and is characterized by pyrexia and hemorrhages. Another form of bovine ehrlichiosis is caused by *E. bovis* and was first identified in Iran and Algeria in the 1930s and resembles heartwater. *Ehrlichia ovine* causes a mild form of ehrlichiosis in sheep. These two infections in cattle and sheep cause what are known as benign forms of ehrlichiosis.

Literature

Smith and Ristic (1977) reviewed in detail the various forms of ehrlichiosis including the species which occur in temperate regions. Henning (1956) described rickettsiosis of dogs found in Africa and included information on *Rickettsia conori* which caused primarily a disease affecting man (Boutonneuse fever) in the Mediterranean basin. In dogs it produced a mild, often inapparent, infection. The organism differed from *E. canis* in that it invaded the endothelial cells, while *E. canis* infected primarily monocytes. Boole (1959) reported on some of the early studies of *E. canis*. The most comprehensive review on canine ehrlichiosis was presented by Ewing (1969). In a short, concise review the various features of canine ehrlichiosis were discussed and a distinction was made of the clinical syndrome characteristic of canine ehrlichiosis and tropical canine pancytopenia (Wilkinson 1976). These two syndromes have to be regarded as a single disease entity differing in severity and possibly related to breed susceptibility (Seamer and Snape 1970). The two diseases in dogs caused by *E. canis* and *Neorickettsia helminthoeca* were compared by Philip (1959). In equine ehrlichiosis clinical manifestations, pathology, and transmission to sheep, goats, and dogs were reviewed by Gribble (1969). Danskin and Burdin (1963) reviewed the etiology, distribution, and pathogenesis of BPF.

ETIOLOGY

Genus *Ehrlichia* includes species of rickettsiae of similar morphology found in leukocytes of a variety of wild and domestic animals. Organisms are classified in the genus *Ehrlichia,* order Rickettsiales, family Rickettsiacae, and tribe Ehrlichiae. The classification of organisms found in different species of host is not completely determined because there is relatively little information available. The speciation is at best tenuous pending addition of more information. It is proposed that *Ehrlichia*-like parasites found in granulocytes should be included in a separate genus, *Cytoecetes*.

Most of the Ehrlichiae of veterinary importance in the tropics are host-specific, the exception being *E. equi* which has a wide host range. *Ehrlichia canis* is found primarily in circling monocytes but may also be observed in granulocytes. It produces well-defined clinical syndromes in dogs.

Differentiation of species parasitizing ruminants is based on tropism for either mononuclear or polymorphonuclear leukocytes, and to some degree by the geographical distribution and the severity of the disease. *Ehrlichia* (*Cytoecetes*) *phagocytophilia* causes tick-borne fever in Europe and is found primarily in circulating neutrophils and eosinophils. *Cytoecetes ondiri*, the cause of BPF in the tropics, resembles *E. phagocytophilia* in its tropism for circulating granulocytes, but based on the pathogenesis and immunological properties it is distinguished from *E. phagocytophilia*. *Ehrlichia ovina* occurs in circulating monocytes of sheep and is only slightly pathogenic. There is little information on this species.

Organisms in all species are observed in three different forms which are considered to represent the developmental stage in a life cycle. Initial bodies occur in the cytoplasm of the cells during the febrile response. This form subsequently undergoes reproduction and passes through the morula stage which fragments to form elementary bodies which leave the cell and invade other cells. The elementary bodies range from 0.2 to 0.6 μm, the initial bodies from 0.4 to 2 μm, and the morulae from 3 to 6 μm. More than one morula may be found in one cell and may be pleomorphic, but its morula shape is a characteristic form in all ehrlichiae species. This structure is contained in a membrane-lined vacuole which separates the organism from the host cytoplasm by a surrounding outer wall and plasma membrane. There is no metabolic and biochemical information on these organisms.

Laboratory animals are uniformly resistant to infection as are most tissue culture systems.

Literature

Ehrlichia canis in the morula form in monocytes was surrounded by single membrane which contained many elementary forms (Simpson 1972). Comparable morphology was observed with *E. equi* in neutrophils and eosinophils and contained 1 to 33 elementary bodies (Sells *et al.* 1976). *Cytoecetes ondiri* was highly pleomorphic and was found in the granulocytes, large lymphocytes, and monocytes. Colonies varied from small single elementary bodies of 0.3 μm to large structures 2 μm in diameter. Staining properties were lost rapidly after the death of the animal, making recognition difficult (Haig and Danskin

1962). *Cytoecetes ondiri* has been identified only in Kenya (Snodgrass 1978). It was proposed that it should be placed in a separate genus within the tribe Ehrlichiae because of the morphological and cell tropism observations (Krauss *et al.* 1972).

Limited information is available on propagation of the organisms *in vitro*. *Ehrlichia canis* multiplied in monocyte cell cultures derived from the blood and remained infective for dogs (Nyindo *et al.* 1971) and could be serially passaged (Hemelt *et al.* 1980). Somatic cell hybrids of canine peritoneal macrophages and transformed human fibroblasts could also be infected (Stephenson and Osterman 1980).

EPIZOOTIOLOGY

Geographic distribution

The distribution of canine ehrlichiosis is dependent on the host tick *Rhipicephalus sanguineus* and occurs in both the tropics and in temperate regions. It is reported from North and South America, the Caribbean, Africa, the Middle East, and throughout the Orient. Distribution of equine ehrlichiosis is restricted, occurring only in a few areas of the USA. Bovine petechial fever has to date been reported only in Kenya where it has a sporadic occurrence, and it is assumed to be vector-borne. *Ehrlichia bovis* occurs in North and Central Africa and is also reported to be found in Sri Lanka. The benign ehrlichiosis of sheep caused by *E. ovine* is found in North and South Africa.

Literature

There have been numerous case reports of canine ehrlichiosis from various regions and countries. The epizootiology of tropical canine pancytopenia in southeast Asia was presented by Nims *et al.* (1971). A brief summary of the various outbreaks of a hemorrhagic disease in dogs in southeast Asia, Puerto Rico, and the Virgin Islands was presented, with the conclusion being drawn that these syndromes were similar throughout the world and are caused by *E. canis* (Huxsoll *et al.* 1969). Reports on the occurrence of canine ehrlichiosis were made from Singapore (Wilkins *et al.* 1967), Thailand (Davidson *et al.* 1975), Israel, (Klopfer and Nobel 1972) and India (Raghavachari and Reddy 1958; Smith *et al.* 1975a, b).

In the Western Hemisphere the disease was reported first from Aruba (Netherlands Antilles) near Venezuela (Boole 1959). In the USA, more attention has been given recently to the distribution of canine ehrlichiosis (Pyle 1980). Reports have come from various states on cases of ehrlichiosis: Florida (Harper 1975), Texas (Pierce 1971), and Oklahoma (Ewing and Philip 1966). The first case of *E. canis* infection in South America was reported from Brazil (Costa *et al.* 1973).

Following the initial detection of the clinical cases of equine ehrlichiosis in California in 1968 the disease was found in 46 clinical cases between 1968 and 1980 (Madigan and Gribble 1982). A case report of equine ehrlichiosis in Mississippi was presented by Pyle (1980).

The possible occurrence of hyperacute BPF was reported in Tanzania. The diagnosis was based on the clinical signs and on the postmortem findings characterized by extensive hemorrhages throughout the tissues. However, the organisms were not demonstrated (Jaffery and Mwangota 1974). This diagnosis of BPF in Tanzania has been questioned by other workers.

There has been a case report of *E. ovina* in the mononuclear cells of sheep (Seneviratna and Jainudeen 1967) and of an *E. bovis*-like organism in cattle in Sri Lanka (Seneviratna and Dhanapala 1962).

Transmission

Ixodid ticks are the vectors of several Ehrlichiae species. Under natural conditions canine ehrlichiosis is transmitted transstadially by the common brown dog tick *R. sanguineus*. The ticks are infective during all stages and adults remain infective for at least 5 months. Ticks are a more important source epidemiologically than carrier dogs. Also, an important reservoir of *E. canis* is wild Canidae. Experimental transmission has been accomplished by a variety of parenteral routes with infected blood and its components. The vectors of the causative organism of equine ehrlichiosis and BPF are not known and presumed to be ticks. Wild ruminants of East Africa are reservoirs of *C. ondiri*. The rickettsia causing benign bovine and ovine ehrlichiosis is transmitted by a *Hyalomma* genus in cattle and in sheep by *R. bursa*. Experimentally the disease can be transmitted by blood and tissues.

Literature

The development of *E. canis* in *R. sanguineus* was studied in the adult tick by fluorescent microscopy and by infectivity. Intracytoplasmic inclusions containing 1 to 80 elementary bodies were observed in the cells of the midgut, salivary glands, and hemocytes. No evidence of multiplication was found in the ovary. Partial feeding of *R. sanguineus* was a prerequisite for infection of dogs with tissues from infected ticks (Smith *et al.* 1976, 1978). Adult *R. sanguineus* ticks were infective for dogs for 155 days after engorging as nymphs on dogs in the acute phase of ehrlichiosis. When ticks were fed during the chronic phase, infection was not transmitted (Lewis *et al.* 1977). Transmission occurred transstadially but not transovarially (Groves *et al.* 1975).

In Africa *E. canis* was transmitted to the wild dog (*Lycaon pictus*) and the black-backed jackal (*Canis mesomelas*). Van Heerden (1979) stated that several authors had mentioned outbreaks of disease in free-living wild dogs. The symptoms were anorexia, depression with anemia, leukopenia, and mild thrombocytopenia. Jackals (*C. mesomelas*) in

Kenya were also found to be infected using the peripheral leukocytes cell culture technique (Price and Karstad 1980). In North America, infections were transmitted transstadially by ticks *R. sanguineus* to the red fox (*Vulpex fulva*) and the gray fox (*Urocyon cinereoargenteus*) (Amyx and Huxsoll 1973).

It has been proposed that the carrier state in BPF occurs among wild ruminants. The bushbuck (*Tragelaphus scriptus*) could be experimentally infected and was a natural carrier (Snodgrass 1978). The African buffalo was also found to be susceptible to experimental infection, developing a parasitemia for 9 to 35 days, and was a species which could play a role in the epizootiology of the disease (Davies 1981). Multiplication of organisms also occurred after experimental infection in the impala, bushbuck, Thomson's gazelle, and wildebeest, but isolation could only be made from naturally infected bushbuck (Snodgrass *et al.* 1975). Trombiculid mites were not implicated in the epizootiology of BPF (Walker *et al.* 1974).

INFECTION

Ehrlichia canis infects monocytes, lymphocytes, and neutrophils. The morulae forms are observed predominantly in monocytes or granulocytes, depending upon the strain. Strains which have a predilection for granulocytes are less pathogenic. Reproduction is primarily by binary fission of either elementary or larger bodies. Animals recovered from clinical disease develop a carrier state which may persist for up to 3 years.

Ehrlichia equi parasitizes granulocytes. It is the only species of *Ehrlichia* which infects a wide range of mammalian hosts, including dogs, cats, cattle, sheep, goats, and primates. These species develop a mild or inapparent infection.

Cytoecetes ondiri is found in granulocytes. Following infection, the initial multiplication of *C. ondiri* occurs in the spleen. Peak titers are reached during the period of clinical illness. The greatest concentration of organisms are found in the lungs, spleen, bone marrow, blood, and liver. Latent infections are found in sheep and cattle for up to 4 weeks.

Ehrlichia bovis and *E. ovina* are found in monocytes.

Literature

In the USA a relatively avirulent strain of *E. canis* was found principally to infect circulating neutrophils and eosinophils, rather than lymphocytes and monocytes (Ewing *et al.* 1971; Carillo and Green 1978). Other strains from Nigeria and from the Netherlands Antilles also produced a similar mild clinical reaction with comparable hematological changes (Leeflang and Périe 1972).

Dogs, cats, rhesus macaques (*Macaca mulatta*), and baboons (*Papio anubis*) were susceptible to *E. equi*. Organisms were found in polymorphonuclear cells and the morula forms were persistent for 1 to 4 days. In dogs, infection resulted in slight evidence of disease with mild pyrexia, transient thrombocytopenia, and mild anemia (Lewis *et al.* 1975). Goats and sheep were also susceptible to experimental infection but did not develop any apparent clinical signs (Sells *et al.* 1976). Neither intact nor splenectomized vervet monkeys (*Cercopithecus pygerythrus*) could be infected (van Heerden and Goosen 1981).

In tissues of cattle and sheep infected with *Cytoecetes ondiri* the organisms were most consistently found in the spleen. Multiplication took place within 24 hours after inoculation, and during the highest titers organisms were demonstrable in circulating leukocytes (Snodgrass 1975a). Mugera and Kiptoon (1978), in addition to finding organisms in the circulating leukocytes, also observed them in the cells of the reticuloendothelial system, including the capillary endothelial cells, of various tissues and organs. A strain isolated from a relatively mild form of BPF was passaged in sheep and found to be comparable to the more classical strain causing acute disease (Dawe *et al.* 1970).

Mechanical transmission of *C. ondiri* by needle passage could be undertaken using a variety of tissues and various routes of infection. Passage resulted in loss of virulence and the organism could not be maintained by this method indefinitely (Danskin and Burdin 1963). It was found that in inducing experimental infections that about half the cattle were resistant. Experimental infections of sheep produced a disease similar to the mild form of disease seen in cattle, with development of fever and parasitemia but without hemorrhages. Sheep have been used in studies of the pathogenesis (Snodgrass 1978). Attempts to transmit the organism to rodents have not been successful even after splenectomy, irradiation, and cortisone treatment (Cooper 1973).

CLINICAL SIGNS

The four phases in canine ehrlichiosis are the incubation, febrile, subclinical, and chronic phases. The febrile phase is characterized by high temperature and associated with anorexia, vomiting, epistaxis, weight loss, enlarged lymph nodes, occasionally corneal opacity, conjunctivitis, respiratory malfunction, and edema of legs and scrotum. There is accompanying pancytopenia, particularly thrombocytopenia. Clinical signs last from 2 days to 3 weeks and are followed by the subclinical phase, during which there is clinical recovery but the hematological changes are still apparent. Death is associated with extensive tissue hemorrhages and secondary infections. Chronic forms of the disease have persistent hematological changes.

There appears to be a genetic predisposition of dogs, reflected in differences in breed susceptibility, to both mild and severe forms of ehrlichiosis. Uncomplicated ehrlichiosis, in some breeds, is considered to be a mild disease except in young puppies in which it may be fatal. Many of the earlier clinical studies on canine ehrlichiosis were complicated by *Babesia* infections which are the most common secondary complication infections. Tropical canine pancytopenia is a severe clinical form of the disease and has been initially reported from south Asia. Unilateral or bilateral epistaxis is a characteristic clinical sign and severe anemia, leukopenia, and thrombocytopenia develop.

Ehrlichia equi causes clinical signs which are characterized by fever, anorexia, depression, subcutaneous edema, and ataxia. The incubation period is 1 to 9 days, and is followed by a febrile clinical phase of 1 to 12 days which is characterized by edema of the legs, ventral abdomen, and prepuce. Presence of the organisms in the granulocytes is associated with hematological changes.

Cytoecetes ondiri also causes syndromes of varying severity. The incubation period is 5 to 14 days and is followed by a short febrile period of 4 to 5 days with onset of depression, muscular tremors, enlargement of superficial lymph nodes, edema of the eyelids, and petechiation of the buccal mucosa, conjunctiva, and mucous membranes of external genitalia. Blood may be present in the feces. The acute disease is associated with a decrease in circulating white blood cells (WBCs) and thrombocytes. Experimentally infected sheep and goats have only slight thermal reaction without any other clinical signs.

There is little information on the diseases caused by *E. bovis* and *E. ovina*. The clinical signs are difficult to detect and may consist only of irregular fever of several weeks' duration. The acute form is characterized by drooping and swelling of the ears with fever, loss of appetite, incoordination, and constipation. Infection is characterized by an extended latent period with animals becoming carriers for 10 months.

Literature

The severity and duration of canine ehrlichiosis were extremely variable and could persist for several weeks. Hematological changes preceded the appearance of clinical signs. Following the acute phase of 4 to 6 weeks the animal could become chronically affected with depression, anorexia, emaciation, pancytopenia, and hemorrhage. Severe chronic disease was thought to be due to an anaplastic anemia (Lewis and Huxsoll 1977). Severe clinical and hematological findings were described in epizootics of tropical canine pancytopenia in military dogs in Vietnam. The incubation period was approximately 11 days, followed by a febrile phase for 3 to 5 days with complete anorexia, severe weight loss, and weakness. After recovery from the major clinical signs, a subclinical phase ensued with persistent hematological changes which could terminate in death with either epistaxis or severe pancytopenia (Walker *et al.* 1970). Experimental tropical canine pancytopenia was comparable to the natural occurring disease (Huxsoll *et al.* 1970a, b, 1972). Clinical tropical canine pancytopenia was often not recognized until unilateral or bilateral epistaxis was observed. Prior to the onset of epistaxis the only evidence of disease was altered hemograms. The commonly observed clinical signs – which included mucosal, petechial, and ecchymotic hemorrhages of the genitalia, buccal cavity, and conjunctiva – accompanied epistaxis. The infection was detectable on day 20 and organisms were demonstrable for 29 months after infection (Ewing and Buckner 1965).

The clinical signs of equine ehrlichiosis were reported in four cases by Stannard *et al.* (1969) and in 46 cases by Madigan and Gribble (1982). Mortality was low and in younger animals the clinical signs were less severe. The characteristic signs were fever, depression, partial anorexia, edema of limbs, petechiation, icterus, ataxia, and reluctance to move.

Severity of BPF varies considerably between breeds and individual animals within a breed (Snodgrass 1975b). Of the approximately 1000 animals used in transmission experiments, only about half could be infected. The incubation period was 5 to 14 days and was followed by elevation of temperature with subsequent development of hemorrhages on the mucous membranes; occasionally blood was also found in the feces (Danskin and Burdin 1963). Depending on the severity of the disease, petechia were observed from 1 to 10 days of demonstrable infection and in a few cases the 'poached egg' eye developed, which was a swelling and protrusion of the conjunctiva of the eye as a result of edema and effusion of blood into the anterior chamber (Piercy 1953). In experimental infections, fever was followed in 2 days by dullness, harsh coat, and hemorrhages of external mucosa and mortality of 10% (Snodgrass 1978). After the disappearance of hemorrhages, some animals still died 2 to 3 weeks later with severe anemia (Danskin and Burdin 1963).

There is little recent information on clinical disease and pathological manifestation of the syndromes caused by *E. bovis* and *E. ovina*. The available earlier literature has been summarized by Smith and Ristic (1977).

PATHOLOGY

The hematological, gross, and microscopic changes depend on the species of *Ehrlichia*, the severity of the syndromes, and the duration of infection. In *E. canis* infection, decreases in the blood cellular components begin to occur during the incubation phase and progress into the febrile phase. Hematological changes consist of anemia, leukopenia, and thrombocytopenia, and there is elevated erythrocyte sedimentation with hypoalbuminemia and hypergammaglobulinemia. At this time the coagulation and prothrombin time are normal. The most characteristic feature is the reduction of platelet numbers which persist into the chronic stage in subclinically affected dogs. The accompanying macroscopic lesions consist of hemorrhages of the mucosal and serosal surfaces and subcutaneous tissue and lymphadenopathy. The dominant microscopic changes are perivascular inflammatory cell infiltrations in brain, lungs, and kidneys, and either hyperplastic or hypoplastic changes in lymphoid organs and bone marrow. During the early stages of infection there is bone-marrow hyperplasia, and during the later stages there is bone-marrow hypoplasia. Secondary bacterial infections often complicate the terminal phase.

In *E. equi* infection, the hematological changes consist of thrombocytopenia, leukopenia, mild anemia, and elevated plasma icterus index. At necropsy, edema, petechial and ecchymotic hemorrhages occur in the subcutaneous tissue and fascia of the legs. There may be jaundice and accumulation of fluid in the peritoneal and pericardial cavities. Microscopically, there is a vasculitis of small arteries and veins characterized by swelling of endothelial cells, thrombosis, and perivascular infiltration of monocytes and lymphocytes.

Bovine petechial fever is characterized by anemia, decrease in lymphocytes, neutrophils, and eosinophils. The gross lesions consist of extensive hemorrhages throughout the body and enlargement of lymph nodes and spleen. Microscopic lesions have not been fully described.

Literature

There has been relatively little information published on the pathogenesis of the various forms of ehrlichiosis in various species of animals. Most studies on hematological, gross, and microscopic changes have been undertaken on canine ehrlichiosis, but the basic mechanism of cell and tissue injury have not been demonstrated. Acute platelet destruction was observed within a few days after infection and contributed to the thrombocytopenia during the acute phase of the *E. canis* infection (Smith *et al.* 1974, 1975a). The pancytopenia in acute canine ehrlichiosis was not related to bone-marrow depletion. Reduced numbers of circulating platelets and leukocytes observed 6 to 10 weeks after infection were associated with marked depletion of megakaryocytes and early granulocyte precursors. Bone-marrow hypoplasia was important in the chronic phase (Buhles *et al.* 1975). Prolonged and incomplete recovery of the hematological parameter following termination of infection by tetracycline therapy indicated that aplastic anemia was involved in pathogenesis (Buhles *et al.* 1974).

Macroscopic and microscopic lesions observed in 100 dogs dying of ehrlichiosis were reported by Hildebrandt *et al.* (1971). The commonest gross changes were hemorrhages in the subcutaneous tissue and in various organs and tissue systems, generalized lymphadenopathy with mesenteric nodes being most commonly affected, and edema of the legs. Hemorrhages were most common in the heart, lungs, gastrointestinal system, and urogenital tract. Microscopically, there was encephalitis, pneumonitis, ischemic necrosis of the liver, and hypoplasia of bone marrow. Erythrophagocytosis and accompanying hemosiderosis was observed in the lymph nodes (Hildebrandt *et al.* 1973a, b). Chronic inflammation has been described in the brain, lungs, kidneys, lymph nodes, tonsils, spleen, and heart. In meningo-encephalitis, the lesion was characterized by the presence of large numbers of macrophages in the meninges, and in the lungs by a proliferative interstitial pneumonia, occasionally with acute catarrhal and fibrinous inflammation caused by secondary bacterial infection (van Dijk 1971). Perivascular inflammatory reactions including plasma cells have been described in parenchymatous organs (Hildebrandt *et al.* 1970). Mononuclear cells infected with *E. canis* were also found to adhere to the endothelial cells of the small blood vessels of the lungs (Simpson 1974). The severity of lesions in acute canine ehrlichiosis was reduced following immunosuppressive therapy. This was considered to indicate the possibility of immunogenically derived tissue injury playing a role in the pathogenesis (Reardon and Pierce 1981b). Complement consumption was found to occur in acute canine syndromes and coincided with the development of thrombocytopenia and altered platelet function (Lovering *et al.* 1980). Death has often been attributed to secondary bacterial infection (Carillo and Green 1978).

In *E. equi* infections, the subcutaneous edema and hemorrhages were associated with a vasculitis which was both proliferative and necrotizing, thrombosis, and perivascular accumulation of monocytes and neutrophils (Gribble 1969).

The main lesions in BPF were subcutaneous, submucosal, subserosal hemorrhages affecting the upper respiratory system, heart, and gastrointestinal tract (Danskin and Burdin 1963; Plowright 1962). The frequency of the mucosal hemorrhages in the buccal and nasal cavities were recorded in 25 cases and a high percentage of animals had petechia on the tongue. Death was due to massive internal and external bleeding. Lymph nodes and spleen were enlarged (Plowright 1962). The pathogenesis of the hemorrhage and edema was not determined, but it was considered that thrombocytopenia alone was unlikely to be responsible for these changes (Snodgrass 1978). Multiplying organisms were observed in the cells of the reticuloendothelial system of various organs, including the endothelial cells of small blood vessels, and caused vasculitis and thrombosis and extravasation of blood (Mugera and Kiptoon 1978).

IMMUNOLOGY

In canine ehrlichiosis, hypergammaglobulinemia occurs with increase of IgM, IgA, and IgG, and persists in the carrier state following recovery from clinical disease. The indirect fluorescent antibody (IFA) test is used in demonstrating the antibody response to infection. Although there is no evidence of antigenic variation, antigenic diversity is indicated by cross-protection tests. Immunity is dependent on state of premunition, with recovered animals being immune to reinfection.

There is little information on the immunology of other forms of ehrlichiosis.

Literature

Antibody production in experimental *E. canis* infection was examined using the IFA method. Seven days after infection, antibodies were in the IgM and IgA and at 21 days in the IgG classes. A decrease in the three classes occurred at time of death (Weisiger *et al.* 1975). Increased antibody titers reflected persistent infection (Buhles *et al.* 1974). The tropical canine pancytopenia syndrome was characterized by hypergammaglobulinemia, hypergammaglycoglobulinemia, and concomitant decrease in serum albumin value. The levels of gamma protein and glycoprotein fractions were correlated to the duration of the disease (Burghen *et al.* 1971). Cell-mediated responses were also observed in experimentally infected dogs (Nyindo *et al.* 1980).

The IFA test has been used to detect and titrate the antibodies to *E. canis* and was found to be specific (Ristic *et al.* 1972). The serological relationship between *R. sennetsu*, which causes rickettsiosis in man in Japan, and *E. canis* was demonstrated. This relationship was of interest because of the morphological uniqueness of the two agents and the lack of serological correlationship with other important rickettsial agents and *E. canis* (Nyindo *et al.* 1980).

Following infection by *E. canis*, incomplete protection to heterologous strains and complete protection to homologous challenge was observed (Leeflang and Périe 1972). Sterile immunity, following oxytetracycline treatment of dogs was found to occur (Leeflang 1971). However, other reports did not support the development of sterile immunity. Dogs were free of the infection following treatment and became infected with homologous strains and development of hyperglobulinemia (Amyx *et al.* 1971; Buhles *et al.* 1974).

There has been little information available on the immunology in other forms of ehrlichiosis. In BPF, effective immunity to homologous and heterologous strains was observed in cattle, and to homologous strains in sheep (Snodgrass 1975a). Recovered animals were immune to experimental challenge for at least 2 years (Danskin and Burdin 1963).

DIAGNOSIS

In enzootic regions, presumptive diagnosis can be made fairly accurately on some of the ehrlichiosis syndromes when characteristic clinical signs are present. Definitive diagnosis is based on finding the inclusions in the blood of infected animals, and at times it is difficult to demonstrate the typical morula forms which should be made from various tissues. In addition the distribution of organisms varies, as for example in the cytoplasma of the leukocytes. With some clinical syndromes of ehrlichiosis the organisms are difficult to find in the blood. Parasitemias are often high only during the febrile phase of the syndromes. The cytoplasmic granules, which commonly occur in unparasitized leukocytes, are not readily distinguishable from solitary elementary bodies on Giemsa stains. During the carrier stage, organisms are rarely observed and diagnosis is difficult, if not impossible. In these cases serological techniques have to be used. At postmortem, smears for the detection of *E. canis* in leukocytes are best made from the lungs.

Literature

Ehrlichia canis has been demonstrated by the direct immunofluorescent test in buffy-coat and in tissue smears, a method which was more efficient than examination of smears stained with Giemsa stain (Carter *et al.* 1971).

In the diagnosis of BPF, on the basis of clinical signs and the postmortem picture, the acute disease could be confused with other diseases which cause extensive hemorrhages. In addition to demonstrating organisms in smears of blood and tissues, other methods have been employed, including intravenous injection of sheep and goats with tissue suspensions, particularly of the spleen and lung tissues in which organisms were most numerous. Circulating WBCs from recipient animals were examined daily for 10 days for the presence of organisms (Snodgrass 1975a).

Direct and indirect fluorescent antibody tests have been used in canine ehrlichiosis (Carter *et al.* 1971; Ristic *et al.* 1972). These methods were more sensitive than those relying on the demonstration of organisms stained with Giemsa stain, especially in the more chronic cases.

CHEMOTHERAPY

Tetracyclines administered either orally or parenterally are the treatment of choice. Prolonged treatment is usually required to eliminate organisms in the carrier animals and in chronic syndromes. During severe clinical syndromes, supportive therapy is also required.

Literature

Dogs treated intramuscularly with 10 mg/kg for 4 consecutive days became free of the organisms (Leeflang 1971). Intravenously oxytetracycline at a dose of 10 mg/kg once daily had to be administered for at least 10 days (Immelman and Button 1973). A single oral dose of 100 mg/kg, once daily or divided into two doses, was found to yield blood levels of 1 μg/ml of oxytetracycline for 24 hours, and could be used in effectively treating the natural cases (Immelman 1975). Tetracycline hydrochloride, administered orally at 66 mg/kg for 14 days, also resulted in remission of clinical signs, but some of the dogs remained carriers (Amyx *et al.* 1971). In another study, oral treatment with tetracycline at 6.6 mg/kg daily for 14 days caused the remission of clinical signs and caused the disappearance of antibody in 60% of the dogs (Davidson *et al.* 1978). Doxycycline (alpha-6-deoxy-5-oxytetracycline hydrochloride), a synthetic derivative of methacycline, was used in the treatment of canine ehrlichiosis when relapses were observed with other therapeutic agents. At doses of 5 mg/kg once a day for 10 days it was effective in acute cases, while in chronic cases doses of 10 mg/kg daily for 10 days or 10 mg/kg intravenously once daily for 5 days were recommended (van Heerden and Immelman 1979).

Oxytetracycline in food prevented infection after challenge and was fed every 12 hours for 90 days at 1700 parts per million and calculated to exceed the therapeutic oral dose for dogs at 27.5 mg/kg body weight (Seamer and Snape 1972). Prophylactically, tetracycline could be used orally at doses of 5 to 6.6 mg/kg (Amyx *et al.* 1971; Davidson *et al.* 1978). The efficacy of imidocarb dipropionate and tetracycline hydroxide in the treatment of naturally occurring ehrlichiosis in dogs was compared: 5 to 7 mg/kg of imidocarb dipropionate intramuscularly in two doses 14 days apart was as effective in the control of clinical signs as 14 doses of oral tetracycline hydroxide at 66 mg/kg. Imidocarb had the advantage of also controlling secondary babesial infections. There were some transient toxic side effects with the imidocarb (Price and Dolan 1980). In another study, imidocarb dipropionate at 6 mg/kg in two subcutaneous injections 14 days apart, and also orally at 10 mg/kg for 10 days, did not result in clinical cure and failed to sterilize the infection (van Heerden and van Heerden 1981). In experimental infection, treatment with gloxazone (alpha-ethoxyethylglyoxaldithiosemicarbazone) at doses of 10 mg/kg body weight given by intravenous injections on the fourth, seventh, and tenth days after inoculation delayed infection (Seamer and Snape 1972).

There has been little information on the treatment and prophylaxis of other forms of ehrlichiosis with compounds effective against *E. canis*. In BPF successful treatment with oxytetracycline was possible only during the incubation period, but not during the clinical reaction. It was found to be more effective in treating experimental infections in sheep and cattle. Dithiosemicarbazone given intravenously at 5 mg/kg was more effective than two different tetracyclines given at 14 to 20 mg/kg by intramuscular injection (Snodgrass 1976).

BIBLIOGRAPHY

Amyx, H. L. and Huxsoll, D. L., 1973. Red and gray foxes – potential reservoir hosts for *Ehrlichia canis*, *J. Wildl. Dis.*, **9**: 47–50.

Amyx, H. L., Huxsoll, D. L., Zeiler, D. C. and Hildebrandt, P. K., 1971. Therapeutic and prophylactic value of tetracycline in dogs infected with the agent of tropical canine pancytopenia, *J. Am. vet. med. Ass.*, **159** (11): 1428–1774.

Boole, P. H., 1959. Studies on *Ehrlichia canis* (syn. *Rickettsia canis*), *Acta trop.*, **16**(2): 97–107.

Buhles, W. C. Jr, Huxsoll, D. L. and Hildebrandt, P. K., 1975. Tropical canine pancytopenia: role of aplastic anaemia in the pathogenesis of severe disease. *J. Comp. Path.*, **85**: 511–21.

Buhles, W. C. Jr, Huxsoll, D. L. and Ristic, M., 1974. Tropical canine pancytopenia: clinical, hematologic, and serologic response of dogs to *Ehrlichia canis* infection, tetracycline therapy, and challenge inoculation, *J. Infect. Dis.*, **130**(4): 357–67.

Burghen, G. A., Beisel, W. R., Walker, J. S., Nims, R. M., Huxsoll, D. L. and Hildebrandt, P. K., 1971. Development of hypergammaglobulinemia in tropical canine pancytopenia, *Am. J. vet. res.*, **32**(5): 749–56.

Carrillo, J. M. and Green, R. A., 1978. A case report of canine ehrlichiosis: neutrophilic strain, *J. Am. Anim. Hosp. Assoc.*, **14**: 100–4.

Carter, G. B., Seamer, J. and Snape, T., 1971. Diagnosis of tropical canine pancytopaenia (*Ehrlichia canis* infection) by immunofluorescence, *Res. vet. Sci.*, **12**: 318–22.

Cooper, J. E., 1973. Attempted transmission of the Ondiri disease (bovine petechial fever) agent to laboratory rodents, *Res. vet. Sci.*, **15**: 130–3.

Costa, J. O., Batista, J. A. Jr, Silva, M. and Guimaraes, M. P., 1973. *Ehrlichia canis* infection in dog in Belo Horizonte – Brazil, *Minas de Escola, Arquivos da Escola de Veterinaria, Universidade de Minas gerais*, **25**: 199–200.

Danskin, D. and Burdin, M. L., 1963. Bovine petechial fever, *Vet. Rec.*, **75**(14): 391–4.

Davidson, D. E. Jr, Dill, G. S. Jr, Tingpalapong, M., Premabutra, S., Nguen, P. L., Stephenson, E. H. and Ristic, M., 1975. Canine ehrlichiosis (tropical canine pancytopenia) in Thailand, *Southeast Asian J. Trop. Pub. Hlth*, **6**(4): 540–3.

Davidson, D. E. Jr, Dill, G. S. Jr, Tingpalapong, M., Premabutra, S., Nguen, P. L., Stephenson, E. H. and Ristic, M., 1978.

Prophylactic and therapeutic use of tetracycline during an epizootic of ehrlichiosis among military dogs, *J. Am. vet. med. Ass.*, **172**(6): 697–700.

Davies, F. G., 1981. Experimental infection of the African buffalo with *Cytoecetes ondiri, Trop. Anim. Hlth Prod.*, **13**: 165.

Dawe, P. S., Ohder, H., Wegener, J. and Bruce, W., 1970. Some observations on bovine petechial fever (Ondiri disease) passaged in sheep, *Bull. epiz. Dis. Afr.*, **18**: 361–8.

Ewing, S. A., 1969. Canine ehrlichiosis. In *Advances in Veterinary Science and Comparative Medicine*, C. A. Brandly, C. E. Cornelius. Academic Press (New York and London), vol. 13, pp. 331–53.

Ewing, S. A. and Buckner, R. G., 1965. Observations on the incubation period and persistence of *Ehrlichia* sp. in experimentally infected dogs, *Vet. Med./Small Anim. Clin.*, **60**: 152–5.

Ewing, S. A. and Philip, C. B., 1966. Ehrlichia-like rickettsiosis in dogs in Oklahoma and its relationship to *Neorickettsia helminthoeca, Am. J. vet. Res.*, **27**(116): 67–9.

Ewing, S. A., Roberson, W. R., Buckner, R. G. and Hayat, C. S., 1971. A new strain of *Ehrlichia canis, J. Am. vet. med. Ass.*, **159**(12): 1771–4.

Gribble, D. H., 1969. Equine ehrlichiosis, *J. Am. vet. med. Ass.*, **155**(2): 462–9.

Groves, M. G., Dennis, G. L., Amyx, H. L. and Huxsoll, D. L., 1975. Transmission of *Ehrlichia canis* to dogs by ticks (*Rhipicephalus sanguineus*), *Am. J. vet. Res.*, **36**(7): 937–40.

Haig, D. A. and Danskin, D., 1962. The aetiology of bovine petechial fever (Ondiri disease), *Res. vet. Sci.*, **3**: 129–38.

Harper, B. E., 1975. Four cases of naturally occurring canine ehrlichiosis, *Vet. Med./Small Anim. Clin.*, **70**: 1153–7.

Hemelt, I. E., Lewis, G. E. Jr, Huxsoll, D. L. and Stephenson, E. H., 1980. Serial propagation of *Ehrlichia canis* in primary canine peripheral blood monocyte cultures, *Cornell Vet.*, **70**: 37–42.

Henning, M. W., 1956. Rickettsiosis of dogs. In *Animal Diseases of South Africa*. Central News Agency (South Africa), pp. 1179–85.

Hildebrandt, P. K., Conroy, J. D., McKee, A. E., Nyindo, M. B. A. and Huxsoll, D. L., 1973a. Ultrastructure of *Ehrlichia canis, Infect. Immun.*, **7**(2): 265–71.

Hildebrandt, P. K., Huxsoll, D. L. and Nims, R. M., 1970. Experimental ehrlichiosis in young beagle dogs, *Fed. Proc.*, **29**: 754.

Hildebrandt, P. K., Huxsoll, D. L. and Nims, R. M., 1971. Tropical canine pancytopenia, *Proc. 19th World Vet. Congr., Mexico City*, **1**: 296–9.

Hildebrandt, P. K., Huxsoll, D. L., Walker, J. S., Nims, R. M., Taylor, R. and Andrews, M., 1973b. Pathology of canine ehrlichiosis (tropical canine pancytopenia), *Am. J. vet. Res.*, **34**(10): 1309–19.

Huxsoll, D. L., Amyx, H. L., Hemelt, I. E., Hildebrandt, P. K., Nims, R. M. and Gochenour, W. S. Jr., 1972. Laboratory studies of tropical canine pancytopenia, *Exp. Parasitol.*, **31**: 53–9.

Huxsoll, D. L., Hildebrandt, P. K., Nims, R. M., Amyx, H. L. and Ferguson, J. A., 1970a. Epizootiology of tropical canine pancytopenia, *J. Wildl. Dis.*, **6**: 220–5.

Huxsoll, D. L., Hildebrandt, P. K., Nims, R. M., Ferguson, J. A. and Walker, J. S., 1969. *Ehrlichia canis* – the causative agent of a haemorrhagic disease of dogs?, *Vet. Rec.*, **85**: 587.

Huxsoll, D. L., Hildebrandt, P. K., Nims, R. M. and Walker, J. S., 1970b. Tropical canine pancytopenia, *J. Am. vet. med. Ass.*, **157**: 1627–32.

Immelman, A., 1975. Die bestudering van faktore wat die absorpsie van oksitetrasiklin vanuit die maagdermkanaal van die hond mag beinvloed. M. Med. Vet. (Pharm et Tox.) thesis Univ. of Pretoria.

Immelman, A. and Button, C., 1973. *Ehrlichia canis* infection. (Tropical canine pancytopenia or canine rickettsiosis), *J. S. Afr. vet. med. Ass.*, **44**: 241–5.

Itard, J., 1957. A case of *Rickettsia canis* in Oubangui-Chari, French Equatorial Africa, *Rev. Elev. Méd. vét. Pays trop.*, **10**: 219–20.

Jaffery, M. S. and Mwangota, A. U., 1974. Hyperacute bovine petechial fever, *Vet. Rec.*, **95**: 212–13.

Klopfer, U. and Nobel, T. A., 1972. Canine ehrlichiasis (tropical canine pancytopenia) in Israel, *Refuah Vet.*, **29**: 24–9.

Krauss, H., Davies, F. G., Ødegaard, Ø. A. and Cooper, J. E., 1972. The morphology of the causal agent of bovine petechial fever, *J. Comp. Path.*, **82**: 241–6.

Leeflang, P., 1971. Relation between carrier-state oxytetracycline administration and immunity in *Ehrlichia canis* infections, *Vet. Rec.*, **90**: 703–4.

Leeflang, P. and Périe, N. M., 1972. A comparative study of the pathogenicities of Old and New World strains of *Ehrlichia canis*, *Trop. Anim. Hlth Prod.*, **4**: 107–8.

Lewis, G. E. Jr and Huxsoll, D. L., 1977. Canine ehrlichiosis. In *Current Veterinary Therapy Small Animal Practice*, ed. R. W. Kirk. W. B. Saunders Co. (Philadelphia, London, Toronto), vol. VI, pp. 1333–6.

Lewis, G. E. Jr, Huxsoll, D. L., Ristic, M. and Johnson, A. J., 1975. Experimentally induced infection of dogs, cats, and nonhuman primates with *Ehrlichia equi*, etiologic agent of equine ehrlichiosis, *Am. J. vet. Res.*, **36**(1): 85–8.

Lewis, G. E., Ristic, M., Smith, R. D., Lincoln, T. and Stephenson, E. H., 1977. The brown dog tick *Rhipicephalus sanguineus* and the dog as experimental hosts of *Ehrlichia canis, Am. J. vet. Res.*, **38**(12): 1953–5.

Lovering, S. L., Pierce, K. R. and Adams, L. G., 1980. Serum complement and blood platelet adhesiveness in acute canine ehrlichiosis, *Am. J. vet. Res.*, **41**(8): 1266–71.

Madigan, J. E. and Gribble, D. H., 1982. Equine ehrlichiosis: diagnosis and treatment. A report of 46 clinical cases, *Proc. Ann. Conv. A.H.E.D.*, pp. 305–12.

Mugera, G. M. and Kiptoon, J. C., 1978. Some observations of the morphology and infection of the agent of bovine petechial fever, *Bull. Anim. Hlth Prod.*, **26**: 101–5.

Nims, R. M., Ferguson, J. A., Walker, J. L., Hildebrandt, P. K., Huxsoll, D. L., Reardon, M. J., Varley, J. E., Kolaja, G. J., Watson, W. T., Shroyer, E. L., Elwell, P. A. and Vacura, G. W., 1971. Epizootiology of tropical canine pancytopenia in southeast Asia, *J. Am. vet. med. Ass.*, **158**(1): 53–63.

Nyindo, M., Huxsoll, D. L., Ristic, M., Kakoma, I., Brown, J. L., Carson, C. A. and Stephenson, E. H., 1980. Cell-mediated and humoral immune responses of German Shepherd dogs and beagles to experimental infection with *Ehrlichia canis, Am. J. vet. Res.*, **41**: 250–4.

Nyindo, M. B. A., Ristic, M., Huxsoll, D. L. and Smith, A. R., 1971. Tropical canine pancytopenia: *in vitro* cultivation of the causative agent – *Ehrlichia canis, Am. J. vet. Res.*, **32**(11): 1651–8.

Philip, C. B., 1959. Canine rickettsiosis in western United States and comparison with a similar disease in the Old World, *Arch. Inst. Pasteur de Tunis*, **36**: 595–603.

Philip, C. B., 1974. Ehrliceae. In *Bergey's Manual of Determinative Bacteriology*, eds R. E. Buchanan, N. E. Gibbons. Williams and Wilkins (Baltimore, Md.). pp. 893–5.

Pierce, K. R., 1971. *Ehrlichia canis*: a cause of pancytopenia in dogs in Texas, *SWest. Vet.*, **24**: 263–7.

Piercy, S. E., 1953. Bovine infectious petechial fever, *East Afr. Agric. J.*, **19**: 65–8.

Plowright, W., 1962. Some notes on bovine petechial fever (Ondiri disease) at Muguga, Kenya, *Bull. epiz. Dis. Afr.*, **10**: 499–505.

Price, J. E. and Dolan, T. T., 1980. A comparison of the efficacy of

imidocarb dipropionate and tetracycline hydrochloride in the treatment of canine ehrlichiosis, *Vet. Rec.*, **107**: 275–7.
Price, J. E. and Karstad, L. H., 1980. Free-living jackals (*Canis mesomelas*) – potential reservoir hosts for *Ehrlichia canis* in Kenya, *J. Wildl. Dis.*, **16**(4): 469–73.
Pyle, R. L., 1980. Canine ehrlichiosis, *J. Am. vet. med. Ass.*, **177**: 1197–9.

Raghavachari, K. and Reddy, A. M. K., 1958. *Rickettsia canis* in Hyderabad, *Indian vet. J.*, **35**: 63–8.
Reardon, M. J. and Pierce, K. R., 1981a. Acute experimental canine ehrlichiosis. I. Sequential reaction of the hemic and lymphoreticular systems, *Vet. Pathol.*, **18**: 48–61.
Reardon, M. J. and Pierce, K. R., 1981b. Acute experimental canine ehrlichiosis. II. Sequential reaction of the hemic and lymphoreticular systems of selectively immunosuppressed dogs, *Vet. Pathol.*, **18**: 384–95.
Ristic, M., Huxsoll, D. L., Tachibana, N. and Rapmund, G., 1981. Evidence of a serological relationship between *Ehrlichia canis* and *Rickettsia sennetsu*, *Am. J. trop. Med. Hyg.*, **30**(6): 1324–8.
Ristic, M., Huxsoll, D. L., Weisiger, R. M., Hildebrandt, P. K. and Nyindo, M. B. A., 1972. Serological diagnosis of tropical canine pancytopenia by indirect immunofluorescence, *Infect. Immun.*, **6**(3): 226–31.

Seamer, J. and Snape, T., 1970. Tropical canine pancytopenia and *Ehrlichia canis* infection, *Vet. Rec.*, **86**: 375.
Seamer, J. and Snape, T., 1972. *Ehrlichia canis* and tropical canine pancytopenia, *Res. vet. Sci.*, **13**: 307–14.
Sells, D. M., Hildebrandt, P. K., Lewis, G. E. Jr, Nyindo, M. B. A. and Ristic, M., 1976. Ultrastructural observations on *Ehrlichia equi* organisms in equine granulocytes, *Infect. Immun.*, **13**(1): 273–80.
Seneviratna, P. and Dhanapala, S. B., 1962. *Ehrlichia bovis*-like organisms in cattle in Ceylon, *Ceylon vet. J.*, **11**: 101.
Seneviratna, P. and Jainudeen, M. R., 1967. The presence of *Ehrlichia ovina*-like organisms in the mononuclear cells of sheep in Ceylon, *Ceylon vet. J.*, **15**(4): 141.
Simpson, C. F., 1972. Structure of *Ehrlichia canis* in blood monocytes of a dog, *Am. J. vet. Res.*, **33**(12): 2451–4.
Simpson, C. F., 1974. Relationship of *Ehrlichia canis*-infected mononuclear cells to blood vessels of lungs, *Infect. Immun.*, **10**(3): 590–6.
Smith, R. D., Hooks, J. E., Huxsoll, D. L. and Ristic, M., 1974. Canine ehrlichiosis (tropical canine pancytopenia): survival of phosphorus-32-labeled blood platelets in normal and infected dogs, *Am. J. vet. Res.*, **35**(2): 269–73.
Smith, R. D. and Ristic, M., 1977. Ehrlichiae. In *Parasitic Protozoa*, ed.

J. P. Kreier. Academic Press (New York), vol. IV, pp. 295–328.

Smith, R. D., Ristic, M., Huxsoll, D. L. and Baylor, R. A., 1975a. Platelet kinetics in canine ehrlichiosis: evidence of increased platelet destruction as the cause of thrombocytopenia, *Infect. Immun.*, **11**(6): 1216–21.

Smith, R. D., Sells, D. M., Lewis, G. E. and Ristic, M., 1978. Development and maintenance of *Ehrlichia canis* in its invertebrate and vertebrate hosts. In *Tick-borne Diseases and their Vectors*, ed. J. K. H. Wilde. Lewis Reprints (Tonbridge), pp. 517–18.

Smith, R. D., Sells, D. M., Stephenson, E. H., Ristic, M. and Huxsoll, D. L., 1976. Development of *Ehrlichia canis*, causative agent of canine ehrlichiosis, in the tick *Rhipicephalus sanguineus* and its differentiation from a symbiotic rickettsia, *Am. J. vet. Res.*, **37**(2): 119–26.

Smith, R. D., Small, E., Weisiger, R., Byerly, C. S. and Ristic, M., 1975b. Isolation in Illinois of a foreign strain of *Ehrlichia canis*, the causative agent of canine ehrlichiosis (tropical canine pancytopenia), *J. Am. vet. med. Ass.*, **166**(2): 172–4.

Snodgrass, D. R., 1975a. Pathogenesis of bovine petechial fever. Latent infections, immunity, and tissue distribution of *Cytoecetes ondiri*, *J. Comp. Path.*, **85**: 523–9.

Snodgrass, D. R., 1975b. Clinical response and apparent breed resistance in bovine petechial fever, *Trop. Anim. Hlth Prod.*, **7**: 213–18.

Snodgrass, D. R., 1976. Chemotherapy of experimental bovine petechial fever, *Res. vet. Sci.*, **20**: 108–9.

Snodgrass, D. R., 1978. Studies on bovine petechial fever. In *Tick-borne Diseases and their Vectors*, ed. J. K. H. Wilde. Lewis Reprints (Tonbridge), pp. 531–5.

Snodgrass, D. R., Karstad, L. H. and Cooper, J. E., 1975. The role of wild ruminants in the epidemiology of bovine petechial fever, *J. Hyg., Camb.* **74**: 245–50.

Stannard, A. A., Gribble, D. H. and Smith, R. S., 1969. Equine ehrlichiosis: a disease with similarities to tick-borne fever and bovine petechial fever, *Vet. Rec.*, **84**: 149–50.

Stephenson, E. H. and Osterman, J. V., 1980. Somatic cell hybrids of canine peritoneal macrophages and SV40-transformed human cells: derivation, characterization, and infection with *Ehrlichia canis*, *Am. J. vet. Res.*, **41**(2): 234–40.

Tuomi, J., 1975. Rickettsiae and immunisation against rickettsioses in animals. Rickettsial diseases of domestic animals, *Proc. 20th World Vet. Congr., Thessaloniki*, pp. 1320–6.

van Dijk, J. E., 1971. Studies on *Ehrlichia canis*, *Zbl. Vet. Med.*, **B18**: 787–803.

van Heerden, J., 1979. The transmission of canine ehrlichiosis to the

wild dog *Lycaon pictus* (Temminck) and black-backed jackal *Canis mesomelas* Schreber, *J. S. Afr. vet. med. Ass.*, **50**: 245–8.
van Heerden, J. and Goosen, D. J., 1981. Attempted transmission of canine ehrlichiosis to the vervet monkey (*Cercopithecus pygerythrus*), *Onderstepoort J. vet. Res.*, **48**: 127–8.
van Heerden, J. and Immelman, I., 1979. The use of doxycycline in the treatment of canine ehrlichiosis, *J. S Afr. vet med. Ass.*, **50**: 241–4.
van Heerden, J. and van Heerden, A., 1981. Attempted treatment of canine ehrlichiosis with imidocarb dipropionate, *J. S. Afr. vet. med. Ass.*, **52**: 173–5.

Walker, A. R., Cooper, J. E. and Snodgrass, D. R., 1974. Investigations into the epidemiology of bovine petechial fever in Kenya and the potential of trombiculid mites as vectors, *Trop. Anim. Hlth Prod.*, **6**: 193–8.
Walker, J. S., Rundquist, J. D., Taylor, R., Wilson, B. L., Andrews, M. R., Barck, J., Hogge, J. L. Jr, Huxsoll, D. L., Hildebrandt, P. K. and Nims, R. M., 1970. Clinical and clinicopathologic findings in tropical canine pancytopenia, *J. Am. vet. med. Ass.*, **157**(1): 43–55.
Weisiger, R. M., Ristic, M. and Huxsoll, D. L., 1975. Kinetics of antibody response to *Ehrlichia canis* assayed by indirect fluorescent antibody method, *Am. J. vet. Res.*, **36**(5): 689–94.
Wilkins, J. H., Bowden, R. S. T. and Wilkinson, G. T., 1967. A new canine disease syndrome, *Vet. Rec.*, **81**: 57–8.
Wilkinson, G. T., 1976. *Ehrlichia canis*, canine ehrlichiosis and tropical canine pancytopenia. Taxonomy. Canine rickettsiosis, *Proc. Course for Veterinarians* (*Univ. of Sydney*), **27**: 60–70.

Chapter

21

Heartwater

Contents

INTRODUCTION

Heartwater is a tick-borne, noncontagious disease of sheep, goats, cattle, and wild ungulates, caused by *Cowdria* (*Rickettsia*) *ruminantium* and characterized by septicemia, fever, and gastrointestinal and nervous symptoms. It is transmitted by the *Amblyomma* species of ticks and confined to Africa, Madagascar, Réunion, and some of the Caribbean islands.

Literature

Henning (1956) presented the history of the discovery of the disease in Africa and gave the most comprehensive review of the literature up to 1956. A brief summary on heartwater was presented by Choudary (1981). Uilenberg (1983) published the most comprehensive review on heartwater, and pointed out that it has continued to be a neglected disease in many African countries because it emerged as a significant disease in susceptible populations of ruminants introduced in enzootic regions. The severe disease has been most seen in imported exotic breeds of domestic ruminants.

ETIOLOGY

Cowdria ruminantium is the only species of rickettsiae of tropical veterinary importance which infects primarily the endothelial cells. It appears with light microscopy as relatively uniform spherical cocci, 0.2 to 0.5 μm in diameter, occurring in clumps and staining purple with Giemsa's stain. Comparable forms are found in the gut epithelial cells and in the gut lumen of ticks. Ultrastructural studies show pleomorphism of organisms in these colonies.

There is no information of the biochemical properties or metabolism of the causative agent. Only partial success has been reported in maintaining the organisms in kidney and tick cell cultures.

Literature

The ultrastructure of the organism was studied in the endothelial cells of the choroid plexus from experimentally infected sheep. The organisms were developed within the confines of a membrane-bound vacuole in the cytoplasm of cells, and pleomorphism was evident with four different forms of the organisms observed which differed in size and structure (Pienaar 1968, 1970). In mouse macrophages, and Kupffer cells, and bovine histiocytes, however, the organism was not separated from the cell cytoplasm by a limiting membrane (Du Plessis 1975).

Primary kidney cell cultures were established from goats infected with *C. ruminantium* and were infective to goats for periods of 5 to 31 days. The organism was observed in the culture, but whether it actually multiplied or was merely maintained in these cultures was not determined. The latter possibility appeared likely (Jongejan *et al.* 1980).

In monolayers of tick cells inoculated with infective sheep blood the organisms multiplied for 9 days and were infective for sheep (Andreasen 1974). In leukocyte cultures from infected goats, sheep, and cattle maintained for 5 days, organisms were demonstrated in the cytoplasm of cells (Sahu *et al.* 1983).

EPIZOOTIOLOGY

Heartwater is an important disease of imported breeds of cattle, sheep, and goats in Africa south of the Sahara. In indigenous domestic ruminants in enzootic areas it rarely induces clinical disease. Morbidity and mortality vary considerably from one region to another. The incidence depends on the prevalence of the vectors which are *Amblyomma* species of ticks, particularly *A. variegatum*. The organism is transmitted transstadially but not transovarially in ticks.

Literature

In the Sudan in approximately 46 000 sheep and goats morbidity was 10% and the mortality of sick animals was 50%. The disease was transmitted by *A. lepidum* (Karrar 1960, 1966). A peracute form of heartwater was observed to occur in Mozambique in the most susceptible cattle (Valadao 1969). Clinical disease was described in sheep, cattle, and goats in Madagascar (Uilenberg 1971).

Outside the African continent rickettsial diseases resembling heartwater have been described. There has been a preliminary note on rickettiosis in sheep and goats in India which resembled heartwater (Manjrekar 1951). A heartwater-like disease of goats in Yugoslavia was also described (Aleraj *et al.* 1956). There has been a report on the occurrence of heartwater in the French Antilles (Guadeloupe) and the Mascarene Islands (Réunion and Mauritius) (Perreau *et al.* 1980). Rickettsiosis in ruminants in Argentina was also reported (Ciprian *et al.* 1965).

Transmission of *C. ruminantium* by *A. variegatum* was transstadial and not transovarial (Ilemobade and Leeflang 1978). Transstadial experimental transmission was also possible by *A. maculatum*, and because of the widespread distribution of this species of tick a possibility exists of the spread of heartwater outside the African continent (Uilenberg 1982).

INFECTION

After a bite by an infected tick the organism first multiplies in the reticuloendothelial cells of lymph nodes and subsequently invades the endothelial cells of blood vessels in various organs. Blood infection develops most consistently during the early stages of infection, but may also be found during the carrier state. The organisms will infect mice without causing signs of disease. Intraperitoneal infection in this species is used as a method of maintaining the organism. Organisms from the majority of field isolates cannot be serially passaged through mice. There are exceptions and these isolates are utilized in laboratory procedures.

Literature

Multiplication of *C. ruminantium* first occurred in the reticulum cells of the lymph nodes several days prior to the appearance of the organisms in the endothelial cells. Thus, the developmental cycle in the mammalian host first began in the lymphoid organs (Du Plessis 1970). It was postulated that the organisms released from the lymphoid tissue infected endothelial cells where further multiplication took place by binary fission (Du Plessis 1975). Blood became infected and the infectivity was associated with red blood and not white blood cells, platelets, plasma, or serum (Fawi *et al.* 1977), an observation which has not been fully validated. Other investigations showed that in the blood the organism was present in the plasma and leukocytes, and not in the red blood cells component (Ilemobade and Blotkamp 1978a). Recent leukocyte culture technique verified the presence of intracytoplasmic organisms in circulating white blood cells (Sahu *et al.* 1983). In the peripheral circulation, the organism was present during the latter part of the incubation period for about 24 hours before the rise in temperature. After clinical recovery, the organism was found to persist for variable periods of time (Fawi *et al.* 1977). *Cowdria ruminantium* could be demonstrated from the blood for up to 40 days after clinical disease, both after spontaneous recovery and after therapy with oxytetracycline. Following challenge of immune animals, the organism could also be recovered for up to 50 days. It was concluded that recovery from a clinical syndrome was followed by a carrier state and that immune uninfected animals could also be reinfected and serve as carriers (Ilemobade 1978).

Cowdria ruminantium could be maintained for periods of up to 90 days in mice by intraperitoneal injection, but could not be passaged in this species. The organism did not multiply but merely survived for long periods of time (Haig 1952; Ramisse and Uilenberg 1971). Exceptions have been reported and some strains were serially passaged (Du Plessis and Kumm 1971). Of the other laboratory animals only the ferret has been shown to be susceptible to infection (Henning 1956).

Some attempts to preserve the infectivity of the organism at −70 °C have been inconclusive (Abdel Rahim and Shommein 1978a), but infectivity could be preserved with or without 10% of dimethyl sulfoxide at −85 and −196 °C (Ilemobade *et al.* 1975; Ramisse and Uilenberg 1970).

Differences in the virulence of strains have been observed and virulent strains could be used in immunization procedures (van Winkelhoff and Uilenberg 1981). Attempts at irradiation of *C. ruminantium* in the vector host *A. hebraeum* have not been successful in inducing attenuation, and doses of 20 to 30 krad were fatal to the organism (Spickett *et al.* 1981).

There have been only relatively few investigations of infectivity for wild species in Africa. Eland (*Taurotrachus oryx oryx*) were infected with blood from sheep and showed temperature elevation, but no other clinical signs were observed (Grosskopf 1958).

Experimental infection can be induced in domestic ruminants by inoculating blood from the febrile period of disease. The organisms were infective by intravenous injection of whole blood or mononuclear leukocytes and by subcutaneous injections of brain homogenates from infected animals (Ilemobade 1978).

CLINICAL SIGNS

Clinical syndromes are divided into peracute, acute, subacute, chronic, and mild forms. Imported breeds are more susceptible than indigenous stock and there is considerable difference between individual animals and between various breeds. Very young animals, particularly calves and to a lesser degree lambs and kids, possess high innate resistance to heartwater and infections cause mild clinical or subclinical syndromes. The incubation period also varies considerably. After intravenous injection of infected blood the incubation period is 7 to 14 days; after tick transmission it is 11 to 18 days. Under field conditions the incubation period is longer, 14 to 28 days. The peracute disease is characterized by high fever, sudden collapse, and the animal dies in convulsions. In the acute form the rise in temperature is followed by depression and loss of appetite, and as the disease advances nervous symptoms gradually appear. The nervous signs are characterized initially by high stepping and unsteady gait followed by progressive signs of encephalitis which include chewing movements, twitching of eyelids, walking in circles, aggressive attitude with blind charges, and final collapse with convulsions, galloping movements, and twitching of muscles. When the typical nervous symptoms of heartwater develop, the prognosis is unfavorable with mortality occurring in 50 to 90% of cases. In the subacute or chronic forms, the symptoms are less severe and may be characterized by diarrhea. In the mild form, only slight elevation of temperature is observed.

Literature

Neitz and Alexander (1941) showed that calves under 3 weeks of age could be infected intravenously but showed little clinical reaction and developed solid immunity. Severe clinical signs have rarely been seen in animals indigenous to a particular enzootic area. In imported animals the mortality could be 80% (Synge and Scott 1978). Only 60 to 70% of animals raised in heartwater-free areas reacted to experimental infection (Du Plessis and Bezuidenhout 1979). Differences in the susceptibility of the different local breeds and imported breeds of goats and cattle were observed in Nigeria (Ilemobade 1977). A case of peracute syndrome in a calf was reported from Nigeria and was characterized by sudden onset of nervous signs (Bida and Adams 1973). The disease in goats in Ghana was characterized by acute syndromes with central nervous system involvement (Hughes 1953).

PATHOLOGY

In all ruminants the lesions are fairly consistent but vary with the virulence of different strains. In the peracute form there are rarely any gross lesions. In less severe disease the most characteristic changes are ascites, hydrothorax, and hydropericardium. The amount of fluid in cavities varies from a few milliliters to several liters. The hydropericardium is a more characteristic lesion in small ruminants and in inconsistently and rarely seen in cattle. There may be reddening of the mucous membranes of the respiratory tract and edema of the lungs. Variable amounts of hemorrhage are evident on serosal surfaces. Mucous membranes of the abomasum in the small and large intestines are discolored and there may be hemorrhages. The lymph nodes and spleen are enlarged. The principal microscopic changes are leukostasis and perivascular infiltration in the liver and kidneys, and encephalitis. Varying degrees of anemia, leukopenia, and thrombocytopenia are occasionally reported.

Literature

There has been limited description of the lesions observed in various organ and tissue systems. Most information is available on microscopic changes found in the brain. In the majority of cases there was no gross abnormality in the brain. In a few instances petechial hemorrhages were observed on the surface. The microscopic lesions were characterized by degenerative and necrotic changes occurring in the blood vessels. In the neuropil, microcavitation, perivascular and meningeal mononuclear inflammatory cell infiltration, gliosis, perivascular accumulation of globules, and swelling of axis-cylinders occurred (Pienaar *et al.* 1966). Depletion of lymphocytes from lymph nodes and spleen was reported by Ilemobade and Blotkamp (1978b).

The hematological changes observed in goats infected with *C. ruminantium* consisted of a drop in hemoglobin, marked leukopenia due to lymphopenia and neutropenia, and a fall in total serum protein.

An increase in alpha globulins and a decrease in gamma globulins also occurred (Ilemobade 1978). Based on the observation made that the organism was associated with red blood cells, microcytic hyperchromic anemia was associated with the infection (Abdel Rahim and Shommein 1978b).

In acute fatal cases in sheep and cattle there were no changes in the blood chemistry. There was a drop in eosophils, hematocrit, and a decrease in terminal plasma volume (Clark 1962). Effects on respiratory and cardiac functions have been described by Owen *et al.* (1973).

IMMUNOLOGY

Antigenic differences are not considered to occur between different strains although research on this feature is limited. Following infection, immunity is not complete against all strains, suggesting possible differences in antigenic composition.

Literature

After recovery from the disease, sheep and goats are immune against homologous challenge and only partially against heterologous strains (Henning 1956). Postrecovery immunity consisted of a short period of premunition followed by a period of gradually decreasing sterile immunity. Challenge during the period of sterile immunity resulted in reinfection. Organisms were observed in the peripheral circulation of immune sheep whether or not clinical signs developed (Neitz *et al.* 1947).

A capillary flocculation test, using antigens prepared from infected bovine and caprine brain tissue, detected antibodies 1 to 2 weeks after clinical recovery, either spontaneous or after chemotherapy, and persisted for a period of 1 to 3 weeks (Ilemobade and Blotkamp 1976). The indirect fluorescent test, using the peritoneal cell of mice as antigen, detected antibodies in sheep and cattle. In sheep, antibodies were first observed 2 weeks after infection and peak levels were maintained for 8 to 10 days after febrile response. Low levels were still demonstrable at 18 months (Du Plessis 1981).

VACCINATION

To date no satisfactory vaccine for heartwater is available. Vaccination procedures involving infection and treatment methods are used in sheep, goats, and cattle only on a limited scale. Currently, tetracycline antibiotics are most commonly used and are administered either systemically or orally. Because of the inherent problems with the types of vaccination methods they are not widely applied.

Literature

Early immunization efforts in cattle, using infection and treatment methods have been reported from Swaziland (Fick and Schuss 1952; Barnard 1953). Clinical reactions caused by immunization by the infection and treatment method using terramycin were not different in various breeds of cattle (Sutton 1960). The treatment of cattle has to be started early in the reaction in highly susceptible imported breeds (Uilenberg 1971). In indigenous breeds, delay of treatment has been beneficial because the later the therapy is instituted during the febrile period the better the immunity. Selection of strain for its low virulence to diminish the high rate of postvaccinal mortality in sheep and goats has to be an important feature in any vaccination procedure (Erasmus 1976).

Observations were reported on approximately 2700 animals immunized using one or two doses of infected blood administered intravenously, and treatment simultaneously with intramuscular injection of 2 to 10 mg/kg of oxytetracycline and repeated within 24 hours whether or not elevation of temperature was observed. If the temperature persisted for longer than 48 hours, or if other clinical signs developed, a further dose of tetracycline was given intravenously. In cases when severe symptoms developed sulfadimidine sodium solution was also administered intravenously. It was found that 0.83% of the animals died as a result of these vaccination procedures, but the immunity was effective and animals withstood challenge (van der Merwe 1979). In another study, following immunization, animals were challenged at 3, 6, 12, and 24 months and there was a relationship between the levels of conglutinin and susceptibility to challenge (Du Plessis and Bezuidenhout 1979).

Investigations were undertaken earlier to develop the most cost-effective method of vaccination of sheep and goats. Treatment with chlortetracycline suspended in oil at 4.4 mg/kg body weight on the tenth and twelfth days after infection, and treatment with tetracycline in aqueous solution at 5.5 mg/kg on the tenth and eleventh days were both effective and economical (Poole 1962a). In another method, immunization of goats was undertaken using oxytetracycline at 6.6 mg/kg body weight (Thomas and Manvelt 1957). The use of oral antibiotics for 38 days under field conditions could be a practical method of immunization against the disease in sheep (Mare 1972). Synchronization of treatments in the immunization procedure in goats increased the efficiency of handling and decreased the cost of vaccination (Poole 1962b). In the highly susceptible Angora goats, treatment had to be undertaken on the first day rather than the second or third to prevent mortality, but resistance was poor (Du Plessis *et al.* 1983). Cross-immunity trials in goats demonstrated that strains of

C. ruminantium from Nigeria and South Africa cross-protected (van Winkelhoff and Uilenberg 1981).

CHEMOTHERAPY

Sulfonamide, chlortetracycline, and oxytetracycline administered orally and systemically to cattle, sheep, and goats are effective drugs, but to be effective must be given early in the course of febrile reaction before clinical signs appear.

Literature

Oxytetracycline in drinking water at 300 mg/11.3 kg body weight for goats, 200 mg/11.3 kg for sheep, and 200 to 250 mg/45.3 kg for cattle was effective, but treatment had to be started early in the thermal reaction (Karrar and El Hag Ali 1965). The prolonged oral administration to sheep of tetracyclines at doses varying from 100 to 200 mg per day per sheep modified the course of the disease, resulting in a symptomatic or mild form of disease (Mare 1972). Aureomycin at 5.5 mg/kg given intravenously during the period of incubation in sheep suppressed clinical signs, and and at 22 mg/kg clinical signs were completely eliminated (Weiss *et al.* 1952; Haig *et al.* 1954). Treatment of sheep with 8.8 mg/kg of oxytetracycline was also effective in controlling heartwater (Hurter 1967).

Comparison of the efficacy of different formulations of tetracyclines in the treatment of heartwater of sheep was undertaken. Administered at 4.4 mg/kg body weight, chlortetracycline hydrochloride suspension in oil was shown to be the most effective and required two or three treatments (Poole 1961a, b). Oxytetracycline was shown to be superior to chlortetracycline in treatment of cattle, but even this drug was not optimal because the therapeutic effect was slow and relapses were frequent (Uilenberg 1971). The bovine rickettsiosis reported from Senegal was treated with aureomycin given intravenously at 4 to 5 mg/kg for 4 to 5 days (Rioche 1966). Prophylactic treatment of cattle with oxytetracycline at 2.2 mg/kg intravenously for 2 days, and sulfamethazine at 55 mg/kg subcutaneously was used (Isoun *et al.* 1974).

DIAGNOSIS

Provisional diagnosis of heartwater can be made on history, clinical signs, and postmortem lesions. Definitive diagnosis requires demonstration of the rickettsiae in blood or endothelial cells. At postmortem examination the method of choice for making a definitive diagnosis is by examination of brain squash preparations stained with Giemsa stain. The organism can also stain with routine hematoxylin, but affinity to all dyes is quickly lost through autolysis.

Literature

Heartwater infection was confirmed by demonstrating the organism in smears and sections. Organisms stained with Giemsa stain and were pleomorphic, ranging in size from either 0.2 to 0.3 μm or 0.6 to 1.7 μm in diameter (Purchase 1945; Synge and Scott 1978). Other methods of choice included examination of smears and sections, the former were fixed with methyl alcohol and the latter with Carnoy's fluid, and staining with methyl green and pyronin Y (Burdin 1962). A method for sampling of the cerebral cortex through the foramen occipitale was described (Schreuder 1980). Until recently serological tests for the diagnosis of heartwater have not been available (Ilemobade and Blotkamp 1976). Recently the indirect fluorescent antibody test has shown promise in detecting serological responses to infection to up to 18 months (Du Plessis 1981).

CONTROL

The control measures are undertaken by immunization and partial tick control. Prophylactic methods are applicable only in selected circumstances. Vaccination is not extensively used because in addition to losses due to mortality the process is cumbersome, time consuming, expensive, and requires very close monitoring of animals after vaccination. This method may have to be used in those situations where exotic cattle are imported into an enzootic area because often all other precautions taken to limit infection are not effective. The control of the vector species of *Amblyomma* ticks is undertaken by regular dipping, but is rarely thorough enough to eradicate the vector completely. In most areas this process is also expensive, both in materials and time, is not warranted for heartwater alone, and has to be part of a general tick control program. In face of an outbreak, chemotherapy on a herd basis is undertaken.

BIBLIOGRAPHY

Abdel Rahim, A. I. and Shommein, A. M., 1978a. The infectivity of a strain of *Rickettsia ruminantium* maintained in −70 °C deep freezer and white mice, *Bull. Anim. Hlth Prod. Afr.*, **26**(2): 148–9.

Abdel Rahim, A. I. and Shommein, A. M., 1978b. Haematological studies in goats experimentally infected with *Rickettsia ruminantium*, *Bull. Anim. Hlth Prod. Afr.*, **26**(3): 232–5.

Aleraj, Z., Audi, S. and Topolnik, E., 1956. A disease of goats in Dalmatia resembling heartwater disease, *Vet. arhiv, Zagreb*, **26**(3–4): 111–19.

Andreasen, M. P., 1974. Multiplication of *Cowdria ruminantium* in monolayer of tick cells, *Acta path. microbiol. scand., Sect. B*, **82**: 455–6.

Barnard, W. G., 1953. Heartwater immunization under field conditions in Swaziland, *Bull. epiz. Dis. Afr.*, **1**: 300–13.

Bida, S. A. and Adams, E. W., 1973. Heartwater in a Bunaji calf: a case report, *Vet. Rec.*, **92**: 200–1.

Burdin, M. L., 1962. Selective staining of *Rickettsia ruminantium* in tissue sections, *Vet. Rec.*, **74**(48): 1371–2.

Choudary, Ch., 1981. Rickettsial disease in bovines (Review). 1. Heart water, *Livestock Adviser*, **6**(2): 37–9.

Ciprian, F., Epstein, B., Andreatta, J. N., Poetela, R. A., Menéndez, N. and Etcheverrigaray, M. E., 1965. Estudios experimentales de rickettsia patogenica de rumiantes comprobada recientemente en la Argentina, *Rev. Fac. C. Vet. La Plata*, **7**(17); 197–210.

Clark, R., 1962. The pathological physiology of heartwater (*Cowdria (Rickettsia) ruminantium* Cowdry, 1926), *Onderstepoort J. vet. Res.*, **29**(1): 25–33.

Daubney, R., 1930. Natural transmission of heart-water of sheep by *Amblyomma variegatum* (Fabricius 1794), *Parasitology*, **22**: 260–7.

Du Plessis, J. L., 1970. Pathogenesis of heartwater: I. *Cowdria ruminantium* in the lymph nodes of domestic ruminants, *Onderstepoort J. vet. Res.*, **37**(2): 89–96.

Du Plessis, J. L., 1975. Electron microscopy of *Cowdria ruminantium* infected reticulo-endothelial cells of the mammalian host, *Onderstepoort J. vet. Res.*, **42**(1): 1–14.

Du Plessis, J. L., 1981. The application of the indirect fluorescent antibody test to the serology of heartwater, *Proc. Int. Congr. on Tick Biology and Control*, Grahamstown, 1981, pp. 47–52.

Du Plessis, J. L. and Bezuidenhout, J. D., 1979. Investigations on the natural and acquired resistance of cattle to artificial infection with *Cowdria ruminantium*, *J. S. Afr. vet. med. Ass.*, **50**: 334–8.

Du Plessis, J. L., Jansen, B. C. and Prozesky, L., 1983. Heartwater in Angora goats. I. Immunity subsequent to artificial infection and treatment, *Onderstepoort J. vet. Res.*, **50**: 137–43.

Du Plessis, J. L. and Kumm, N. A. L., 1971. The passage of *Cowdria ruminantium* in mice, *J. S. Afr. vet. med. Ass.*, **42**(3): 217–21.

Erasmus, J. A., 1976. Heartwater: the immunisation of Angora goats, *J. S. Afr. vet. med. Ass.*, **47**(2):143.

Fawi, M. Y., Karrar, G., Obeid, H. M. and Campbell, R. S. F., 1977. Studies on the infectivity of heartwater using various blood components, *Bull. Anim. Hlth Prod.*, **25**(1): 45–7.

Fick, J. F. and Schuss, J., 1952. Heartwater immunisation under field conditions in Swaziland, *J. S. Afr. vet. med. Ass.* **23**(1):9–14.

Finelle, P., 1958. Rickettsiose à *Rickettsia bovis* en Oubangui-Chari, *Rev. Elev. Méd. vét. Pays trop.*, **11**: 291–2.

Grosskopf, J. F. W., 1958. Hartwaterimmunisasie van elande (*Taurotrachus oryx oryx*, Pallas), *J. S. Afr. vet. med. Ass.*, **29**(4): 329–30.

Haig, D. A., 1952. Note on the use of the white mouse for the transport of strains of heartwater, *J. S. Afr. vet. med. Ass.*, **23**(3): 167–70.

Haig, D. A., Alexander, R. A. and Weiss, K. E., 1954. Treatment of heartwater with terramycin, *J. S. Afr. vet. med. Ass.*, **25**(1): 45–8.

Henning, M. W., 1956. Heartwater, hartwater. In *Animal Diseases in South Africa. Being an Account of the Infectious Diseases of Domestic Animals*. Central News Agency (South Africa), pp. 1155–78.

Hughes, M. H., 1953. A rickettsial disease of goats in the Gold Coast, *Ann. trop. Med. Parasit.*, **47**: 299–303.

Hurter, L. R., 1967. Field research on the problem of heartwater: immunization of lambs and kids by the intraperitoneal route in the Potgietersrus area. 1964–1966, Final Report, *Agric. Res., Pretoria*, **1**: 52–3.

Ilemobade, A. A., 1977. Heartwater in Nigeria. I. The susceptibility of different local breeds and species of domestic ruminants to heartwater, *Trop. Anim. Hlth Prod.*, **9**: 177–80.

Ilemobade, A. A., 1978. The persistence of *Cowdria ruminantium* in the blood of recovered animals, *Trop. Anim. Hlth Prod.*, **10**: 170.

Ilemobade, A. A. and Blotkamp, C., 1978a. Heartwater in Nigeria. II. The isolation of *Cowdria ruminantium* from live and dead animals and the importance of routes of inoculation, *Trop. Anim. Hlth Prod.*, **10**: 39–44.

Ilemobade, A. A. and Blotkamp, C., 1978b. Clinico-pathological study of heartwater in goats, *Z. Tropenmed. Parasit.*, **29**: 71–6.

Ilemobade, A. A. and Blotkamp, J., 1976. Preliminary observations on the use of the capillary flocculation test for the diagnosis of heartwater (*Cowdria ruminantium* infection), *Res. vet. Sci.*, **21**: 370–2.

Ilemobade, A. A., Blotkamp, J. and Synge, B. A., 1975. Preservation of *Cowdria ruminantium* at low temperatures, *Res. vet. Sci.*, **19**: 337–8.

Ilemobade, A. A. and Leeflang, P., 1978. Experiments on the transmission of *Cowdria ruminantium* by the tick *Amblyomma variegatum*. In *Tick-borne Diseases and their Vectors*, ed. J. K. H. Wilde. Lewis Reprints (Tonbridge), pp. 527–30.

Isoun, T. T., Akpokodje, J. U., Ikede, B. O. and Fayemi, O., 1974. Heartwater in imported Brown Swiss breed of cattle in Nigeria, *Bull. Anim. Hlth Prod.*, **22**: 321–34.

Jongejan, F., van Winkelhoff, A. J. and Uilenberg, G., 1980. *Cowdria ruminantium* (Rickettsiales) in primary goat kidney cell cultures, *Res. vet. Sci.*, **29**: 392–3.

Karrar, G., 1960. Rickettsial infection (Heartwater) in sheep and goats in the Sudan, *Br. vet. J.*, **116**: 105–14.

Karrar, G., 1966. Further studies on the epizootiology of heartwater in the Sudan, *Sudan J. Vet. Sci. Anim. Husb.*, **6**: 83–5.

Karrar, G. and El Hag Ali, B., 1965. Oral treatment of heartwater with oxytetracycline (terramycin soluble powder), *Br. vet. J.*, **121**: 28–33.

Manjrekar, S. L., 1951. A preliminary note on rickettsiosis in sheep and goats in Bombay state, *Curr. Sci.*, **20**(3): 74–5.

Manjrekar, S. L., 1954. *Rickettsia* of domesticated animals (a short review), *Indian vet. Sci.*, **24**: 217–22.

Mare, C. J., 1972. The effect of prolonged oral administration of oxytetracycline on the course of heartwater (*Cowdria ruminantium*) infection in sheep, *Trop. Anim. Hlth Prod.*, **4**: 69–73.

Neitz, W. O. and Alexander, R. A., 1941. The immunisation of calves against heartwater, *J. S. Afr. vet. med. Ass.*, **12**: 103.

Neitz, W. O., Alexander, R. A. and Adelaar, T. F., 1947. Studies on immunity in heartwater, *Onderstepoort J. vet. Sci. Anim. Ind.*, **21**(2): 243–9.

Owen, N. C., Littlejohn, A., Kruger, J. M. and Erasmus, B. J., 1973. Physiopathological features of heartwater in sheep, *J. S. Afr. vet. med. Ass.*, **44**(4): 397–403.

Parrot, G., 1937. Les rickettsioses confèrent-elles l'immunité vraie ou la prémunition? *Archives de l'institut Pasteur d'Algeria*, **15**: 188–213.

Perreau, P., Morel, P. C., Barre, N. and Durand, P., 1980. Cowdriosis (heartwater) by *Cowdria ruminantium* in ruminants of French Indies (Guadeloupe) and Mascarene Islands (La Réunion and Mauritius), *Rev. Elev. Méd. vét. Pays trop).*, **33**(1): 21–2.

Pienaar, J. G. 1968. Electron microphotograph of a colony of *Cowdria ruminantium*: a new view of well-known parasite causing heartwater in ruminants, *J. S. Afr. vet. med. Ass.*, **39**: 12.

Pienaar, J. G., 1970. Electron microscopy of *Cowdria* (*rickettsia*) *ruminantium* (Cowdry, 1926) in the endothelial cells of the vertebrate host, *Onderstepoort J. vet. Res.*, **37**(1): 67–78.

Pienaar, J. G., Basson, P. A., van der Merwe, J. L. de B., 1966. Studies on the pathology of heartwater (*Cowdria* (*rickettsia*) *ruminantium*), Cowdry, 1926. I. Neuropathological changes, *Onderstepoort J. vet. Res.*, **33**(1): 115–38.

Poole, J. D. H., 1961a. Comparison of efficacy of different tetracycline antibiotics and different formulations of these antibiotics in the treatment of heartwater. I. Comparison of five tetracycline formulations in the treatment of heartwater in sheep, *J. S. Afr. vet. med. Ass.*, **32**(3): 361–5.

Poole, J. D. H., 1961b. Comparison of efficacy of different tetracycline antibiotics and different formulations of these antibiotics in the treatment of heartwater. II. Comparison of four liquid tetracycline formulations in the treatment of heartwater in sheep, *J. S. Afr. vet. med. Ass.*, **32**(4): 523–7.

Poole, J. D. H., 1962a. Flock immunisation of sheep and goats against heartwater: I. Investigations regarding routine flock immunisation of sheep, *J. S. Afr. vet. med. Ass.*, **32**(1): 35–41.

Poole, J. D. H., 1962b. Flock immunisation of sheep and goats against heartwater. II: preliminary experiments on flock immunisation of goats, *J. S. Afr. vet. med. Ass.*, **32**(3): 357–62.

Purchase, H. S., 1945. A simple and rapid method for demonstrating *Rickettsia ruminantium* (Cowdry, 1925) in heartwater brains, *Vet. Rec.*, **57**(36): 413–14.

Rake, G., Alexander, R. and Hamre, D. M., 1945. The relationship of the agent of heart-water fever – *Rickettsia rumimantium, Science*, **102**(2652): 424–5.

Ramisse, J. and Uilenberg, G., 1970. *Cowdria ruminantium* preservation by freezing, *Rev. Elev. Méd. vét. Pays trop.*, **23**(3): 313–16.

Ramisse, J. and Uilenberg, G., 1971. Studies on cowdriosis in Madagascar. Part III, *Rev. Elev. Méd. vét. Pays trop.*, **24**(4): 519–22.

Rioche, M., 1966. Bovine rickettsiosis in Senegal, *Rev. Elev. Méd. vét. Pays trop.*, **19**(4): 485–94.

Sahu, S. P., Dardiri, A. H. and Wool, S. H., 1983. Observation of *Rickettsia ruminantium* in leukocytic cell cultures from heartwater-infected goats, sheep and cattle, *Am. J. vet. Res.*, **44**(6): 1093–7.

Schreuder, B. E. C., 1980. A simple technique for the collection of brain samples for the diagnosis of heartwater, *Trop. Anim. Hlth Prod.*, **12**: 25–9.
Siegrist, J. J. and Hess, E., 1968. Rickettsiose chez les animaux domestiques, *Bull. Off. int. Epiz.*, **70**: 315–23.
Spickett, A. M., Bezuidenhout, J. D. and Jacobsz, C. J., 1981. Some effects of ^{60}CO irradiation on *Cowdria ruminantium* in its tick host *Amblyomma hebraeum* Koch (Acarina: Ixodidae), *Onderstepoort J. vet. Res.*, **48**: 13–14.
Sutton, G. D., 1960. Reactions to heartwater immunization shown by cattle, *J. S. Afr. vet. med. Ass.*, **32**(2): 285–8.
Synge, B. A. and Scott, G. R., 1978. The diagnosis of heartwater. In *Tick-borne Diseases and their Vectors*, ed. J. K. H. Wilde. Lewis Reprints (Tonbridge), pp. 519–22.

Thomas, A. D. and Manvelt, P. R., 1957. The immunization of goats against heartwater. *J. S. Afr. vet med. Ass.*, **28**(2): 163–8.

Uilenberg, G., 1971. Studies on cowdriosis in Madagascar. Part II, *Rev. Elev. Méd. vét. Pays trop.*, **24**(3): 355–64.
Uilenberg, G., 1982. Experimental transmission of *Cowdria ruminantium* by the Gulf Coast tick *Amblyomma maculatum*: danger of introducing heartwater and benign African theileriasis onto the American mainland, *Am. J. vet. Res.*, **43**: 1279–82.
Uilenberg, G., 1983. Heartwater (*Cowdria ruminantium* infection): current status, *Adv. Vet. Sci. Comp. Med.*, **27**: 427–80.

Valadao, F. G., 1969. A incidencia de formas fulminantes da hidropericardite infecciosa em Mocambique e o problema da premunicao contra esta doenca, *Anais dos Servicos de Vetrinaria de Mocambique*, **12/14**: 85–90.
van der Merwe, L., 1979. Field experience with heartwater (*Cowdria ruminantium*) in cattle, *J. S. Afr. vet. med. Ass.*, **50**: 323.
van Winkelhoff, A. J. and Uilenberg, G., 1981. Heartwater: cross-immunity studies with strains of *Cowdria ruminantium* isolated in West and South Africa, *Trop. Anim. Hlth Prod.*, **13**: 160–4.

Weiss, K. E., Haig, D. A. and Alexander, R. A., 1952. Aureomycin in the treatment of heartwater, *Onderstepoort J. vet. Res.*, **25**(4): 41–50.

Chapter

22

Q Fever

CONTENTS

INTRODUCTION

Q fever is a disease of man caused by *Coxiella burnetii* (*Rickettsia burnetii*); it is characterized by sudden onset, fever, severe headaches, and general malaise. Its importance in tropical veterinary medicine is that it is a widespread infection in wild and domestic mammals and birds, but without accompanying clinical signs.

Literature

Q fever has attracted relatively little interest in veterinary medicine. Babudieri (1959) presented an extensive review of the disease as a zoonosis, dealing in depth with its history, its geographical distribution on a country basis, etiology, epidemiology, and diagnosis. Infection in sheep and goats was briefly reviewed by Siegrist and Hess (1968). Behymer (1980) presented a comprehensive summary of information on the infection and the disease which was primarily of veterinary interest. More recently, Baca and Paretsky (1983) discussed the disease and its causative agent as a model for host–parasite interaction. They included a summary of the information on the history, epidemiology, biology, and pathology in man and animals.

ETIOLOGY

Coxiella burnetii is an obligate intracellular organism and has the general characteristics of *Rickettsia*, but also has important biological differences that justify its separation from this genus, and the creation of and its inclusion in a new genus, *Coxiella*. One important characteristic of the organism is its resistance to various environmental conditions such as drying, temperature and pH, and chemicals. It is able to survive at a temperature of 63 °C for 30 to 40 minutes and is resistant for hours to chemical agents such as formalin and phenol. With light microscopy it has a pleomorphic structure, varying from rod-like to cocco-bacillary forms, and stains readily either with Giemsa's, Gram's, or Macchiavello's stains. Depending on the modification of the Gram stain, it is either Gram-negative or Gram-positive. It multiplies, forming colonies which appear as large intracytoplasmic masses of tightly packed organisms about 20 to 30 μm in diameter. Electron microscopy reveals two forms – large and small cell types which have different internal structures and which suggest cellular differentiation of endospore formation.

Coxiella burnetii can be cultivated in a variety of primary and established cell cultures and is most easily grown in embryonated hen's eggs. It exists in two distinct growth phases, phases I and II, which appear following a variable number of passages in embryonated eggs and are distinguished antigenically. The existence of the two phases could be due to transformation or selection of these two different antigenic types in response to the host environment.

Literature

The resistance to *C. burnetii* to physical and chemical agents was found to be greater than that for other *Rickettsia* (Behymer 1980; Ransom and Huebner 1951).

The entry into the cell in tissue culture was a passive event taking place by phagocytosis and involved initial attachment of the organism to the cell wall. Unlike other rickettsiae, *C. burnetii* was found within phagolysosomes in the cytoplasm of the cell (Hackstadt and Williams 1981). The organism grew within these vacuoles and enlarged the cell (Baca and Paretsky 1983). The organism had a limiting membrane within which there was a granular region and a dense central body (Stoker *et al.* 1956). Recent studies have suggested that the development cycle in cells consisted of vegetative and sporogenic differentiation (McCaul and Williams 1981). Early electron-microscopic studies of phases I and II showed no fundamental differences (Nermut *et al.* 1968). Live and killed purified phase I and II organisms were phagocytosed by macrophages and neutrophils and had pronounced differences in nonspecific phagocytosis. Phase I was phagocytosed by only a low percentage of leukocytes. It was proposed that surface antigen, serologically characteristic of phase I, was a factor associated with virulence (Brezina and Kazár 1963, 1965; Kazár *et al.* 1975a, b). The immunologic and biologic characteristics of phases I and II have been recently studied and included maintaining the integrity of the morphology, and their isolation free of host cell components (Williams *et al.* 1981).

EPIZOOTIOLOGY

Geographic distribution

Coxiella burnetii is very widespread throughout temperate and tropical zones of the world. Infections have been demonstrated on many species of domestic animals including cattle, sheep, goats, camels, buffalo, horses, dogs, and swine as well as in some species of domestic birds such as pigeons, geese, and fowl. Under certain epizootiological conditions, infection can be transmitted from wild to domestic animals and often vice versa. In the tropics it is an important zoonosis, occasionally causing abortions but not known to cause significant economic losses in the livestock industry. Infection in wild animals and birds enables a wide geographic distribution. In man, particularly in the tropics, infection is probably much more prevalent than is shown in published information.

Literature

There is a considerable amount of information published on the epidemiology of Q fever, including serological surveys in domestic animals, game animals, and infections in a variety of ticks. Q fever, brucellosis, and leptospirosis have been regarded to be the three major zoonoses of human populations living in close association with cattle, sheep, and goats, and of those people who come in contact with some of the products of the livestock industry (Murphy and Magro 1980). Because Q fever has not been regarded as affecting the health and production of domestic animals, it has received relatively little attention in the veterinary literature (Burgdorfer 1975). The geographical distribution of Q fever in animals was reviewed by Kaplan and Bertagna (1955) and tables were presented on the occurrence in various continents, the serological tests used, and the species of animals affected. The distribution on a country basis in animals and arthropods was reviewed by Berge and Lennette (1953). A historical review of the literature on Q fever in various geographical regions was presented by Wentworth (1955). In the tropics, since much of the population lives in the rural areas, a large segment of the population comes in contact with a variety of domestic animals and Q fever should be regarded as a major problem. In the temperate zone, Q fever has been viewed as an important disease only of some occupational groups (Vanek and Thimm 1976). It is probably more prevalent but seldom recognized.

Serology in domestic animals and man indicated that infections were considerably more frequent in the tropics than in temperate climates (Vanek and Thimm 1976). Incidence of up to 17% was observed using the complement fixation (CF) test in man, cattle, sheep, goats, and game in Tanzania (Hummel 1976). An overall infection rate of 12% was found in camels (*Camelus dromedarius*) slaughtered in northern Nigeria (Addo 1980). In domestic ruminants an incidence of up to 12% was observed in Somalia, Egypt, and Jordan (Schmatz *et al*. 1978). In India, in a recent survey an overall incidence of 19% was found in goats, cattle, poultry, and in dairy cows it was 20% (Tanwani *et al*. 1979). In California, USA, 82% of cows were seropositive and 23% were shedding the organisms in milk (Biberstein *et al*. 1974). A high percentage of carrion-eating birds in California had agglutinating antibodies and it was proposed that these birds were involved in the epidemiology of the infections (Enright *et al*. 1971d). In wild mammals in the USA the distribution of infection, as based on the CF test, varied considerably with the species (Enright *et al*. 1971a).

Transmission

Coxiella burnetii is maintained in two cycles, one in wild mammals which probably involves ticks and the other in domestic animals where, although infection can be transmitted by ticks, it is probably most commonly spread by either inhalation or ingestion of material contaminated by secreta or excreta from infected animals including urine, feces, milk, and placental fluids. The major reservoirs of infection are dairy cows, sheep, and goats. Infections are prevalent in domestic animals of many countries where ticks are very rare. The importance of ticks in various tropical regions varies, but since *C. burnetii* can infect about 40 species of argasid and ixodid ticks in 12 genera this method of transmission could be important. The organism persists for remarkable periods of time in secretion and environment. Infection in the milk can persist for as long as 32 months, while soil and water may be contaminated for periods of up to 150 days. Large quantities of the organism are shed during parturition, and extensive contamination of the environment occurs by postparturient tissues of cows, sheep, and goats, being responsible for the transmission of the infection both to man and domestic animals. Most infections occur due to the inhalation of infectious aerosols. Another route is by ingestion of milk, but this is not infectious enough to cause clinical illness. Transmission from man to man by contact is extremely rare.

Literature

The organism was shed in various body secretions and particularly in birth fluids with parturition itself creating infective aerosols of considerable magnitude and duration (Welsh *et al.* 1958). A major source of infection for sheep in endemic areas was the organisms shed in the placenta of infected ewes (Enright *et al.* 1971b). Wool was also a source of infection (Abinanti *et al.* 1955) and organisms have been recovered from dust-laden air (DeLay *et al.* 1950). In cattle, infected milk was found to contain up to 10 000 infectious guinea pig doses per milliliter (Behymer 1980). Contamination of the udder by the organism did not induce infection through the teat canal (Stoenner and Lackmann 1952).

Henning (1956) presented a table of ticks found naturally infected with *C. burnetii*. Infections were usually contracted by the larval stage and persisted for successive stages. The fate of the organisms in the ticks varied greatly but generally multiplication took place, resulting in extraordinary numbers where, for example, 1 g of feces from *Rhipicephalus sanguineus* contained 10^8 to 10^{10} guinea pig infective doses (Babudieri 1959; Burgdorfer 1975). Inhalation of infected feces could be of importance in the transmission.

INFECTION

Following infection, rickettsiemia develops and the organism localizes in the placenta, mammary glands, and probably other organs of the cow, ewe, and goat. During parturition the organism proliferates, which results in its abundant emission with various secretions and excretions. Approximately half of chronically infected cows may shed the organisms in the milk during successive lactations throughout their productive life. Up to 90 to 95% of lactating cows may have a positive antibody titer and shed the organisms, and the higher the antibody titer the greater likelihood of recovering rickettsiae from the milk. The incidence varies with geographic location.

Literature

Following experimental infection in sheep, rickettsiemia was evident for a short period of time and the organism localized in the kidneys, udder, and placenta, and could be isolated from blood, milk, and urine only for a very short time (Babudieri and Ravaioli 1952; Jellison *et al.* 1950; Khera 1962). Following either the intratracheal or intravenous route of infection in sheep, the organism was not demonstrated in either milk, feces, urine, or oral and nasal secretions, but latent infections developed in various tissues. This period of quiescence ended abruptly at parturition with large numbers of organisms occurring in the placenta, and various secretions and excretions of the parturient animals (Abinanti *et al.* 1953b). In the placentas of naturally infected sheep infection occurred with equal frequency in serologically positive and serologically negative animals (Welsh *et al.* 1951). Levels of infection in the placenta of infected sheep have been recorded to be as high as 10^9 guinea pig infective doses per gram of tissue (Burgdorfer 1975). In the birth fluids, up to 10^5 hamster infective doses per milliliter have been observed (Abinanti *et al.* 1953a). The organism was found in various secretions for 2 weeks postpartum and rarely thereafter (Welsh *et al.* 1959). Organisms were present for at least 7 days in the feces of naturally infected sheep and at levels of 2×10^7 hamster infective doses per gram (Winn *et al.* 1953).

In dairy cows, *C. burnetii* has been commonly isolated from placentas of animals serologically positive (Luoto and Huebner 1950; Enright *et al.* 1971c). Organisms have been demonstrated in the milk, udder tissue, and in the supramammary lymph nodes, but not in blood and other tissues (Jellison *et al.* 1948). The organisms were present in colostrum as well as in milk and up to 10^4 infective guinea pig doses per milliliter were observed. The high temperature of commercial pasteurization processes killed the organisms (Behymer *et al.* 1975, 1977).

CLINICAL SIGNS

Little information is available on the symptomatology of natural infection in domestic animals. In the majority of cases, infections are considered to be clinically inapparent. Evidence of possible clinical involvement occurring in domestic animals is obtained from the study of experimental infection. Occasionally, infections are associated with abortion in sheep and goats and to a lesser degree in cattle. Losses from abortion in natural infections are usually not great enough to attract the attention of either the owners or the veterinarians. Guinea pigs are highly susceptible and are the experimental animals of choice, usually developing a mild clinical disease, but which may on occasion terminate in death in 1 to 3 weeks.

The clinical syndrome in man is characterized by severe headache, high fever, anorexia, malaise, general weakness, and interstitial pneumonia – a syndrome not readily distinguished from other nonspecific 'influenza'-like illnesses.

Literature

Behymer (1980) summarized the clinical manifestations in domestic animals. In cattle, the infection did not result in recognizable clinical signs or lesions. Although abortion could be induced by experimental infection, *C. burnetii* was not considered as a common cause of abortion. On occasion *C. burnetii* has been associated with abortions in goats, sheep, and cattle (Khera 1962). After intravenous infection, fever, rickettsiemia and seroconversion developed and infection persisted in tissue for up to 43 days. The occurrence of histological lesions was equivocal (Lennette *et al.* 1952). Although abortion in experimentally inoculated dairy cows was attributed to the organism, the direct relationship between the organism as the cause of the abortion was not established (Behymer *et al.* 1976). The occurrence of Q fever in Cyprus was reviewed recently by Polydorou (1981) and infections were associated with abortion and stillbirth in sheep and goats. The presence of large numbers of organisms, extensive lesions in fetal membranes, and the rising antibody titers supported this conclusion. Abortion in goats has been associated with *C. burnetii* in the USA (Waldhalm *et al.* 1978).

In most laboratory animals, *C. burnetii* did not cause specific clinical disease, lesions, or death. Guinea pigs have been the animals most commonly used in experimental work. In the cat, subcutaneous, oral, and by contact infections were associated with lack of appetite and lethargy (Gillespie and Baker 1952).

PATHOLOGY

Lesions are not associated with *C. burnetii* infections in domestic animals and have not been described in the rare cases of abortion which are reported. The pathology in man has not been studied as extensively as epidemiology and immunology. Information on pathogenesis is obtained from guinea pigs which often develop a mild syndrome. The occurrence of lesions depends on the virulence of a particular strain and involves tissue injury in the liver, lungs, spleen, and heart. In man, endocarditis is commonly observed and hepatomegaly and splenomegaly are found occasionally.

Literature

Necrotic foci have been observed in the liver, spleen, and heart of guinea pigs (Heggers *et al.* 1975). The necrotic and inflammatory lesions in the liver were often mild and did not appear to endanger the life of the animal or cause any detectable organ malfunction. Organisms did not appear actually to infect hepatocytes (Johnson and McLeod 1977).

Biochemical changes were associated with degenerative lesions in the liver characterized by hepatomegaly and fatty infiltration (Paretsky *et al.* 1964). *Coxiella burnetii* affected the synthesis of ribonucleic acid in guinea pig livers increasing protein synthesis (Paretsky *et al.* 1981; Thompson and Paretsky 1973). The authors summarized work which indicated that there was depletion of liver glycogen and fatty infiltration of the liver within 24 hours after infection (Paretsky *et al.* 1964; Paretsky and Stueckmann 1970; Stueckmann and Paretsky 1971; Tsung and Paretsky 1968; Bernier *et al.* 1974). The glycolytic activity was also assayed in infected yolk sacs (McDonald and Mallavia 1975). It was proposed that the organism produced an endotoxic substance which caused similar pathophysiological responses to those induced by the endotoxin of Gram-negative organisms (Baca and Paretsky 1983).

Recent work in human pathology has shown that the disease could be more widespread and more serious than previously recognized. Endocarditis has been identified as the characteristic lesion of Q fever in man (Haldane *et al.* 1983; Peacock *et al.* 1981; Marrie *et al.* 1982).

IMMUNOLOGY

Humoral and cellular immunity control *C. burnetii* infections in laboratory animals. The cellular component eliminates and the specific antibody accelerates elimination of organisms by phagocytosis by macrophages and polymorphonuclear cells.

Many serological tests are used in both experimental and field situations including: CF, agglutination, precipitation, and indirect fluorescent antibody tests. The value of each test depends on the purpose of the serological investigation and demonstrates different classes of antibodies. Intradermal allergic tests could be useful in surveys in both man and domestic animals, but as yet are not used widely because of the undesirable local and systemic reactions at large doses. The skin test is used routinely before vaccination in humans to avoid sterile abscesses.

Literature

Comparison of the CF test, standard, capillary and microscopic slide agglutination tests for detection and measurement of antibody to *C. burnetii* in naturally exposed sheep showed that the latter test was superior in sensitivity (Welsh *et al.* 1959). The agglutination tests have not been used by other workers. In cattle, colostrum containing complement-fixing antibodies fed to newborn calves transferred the antibodies (Winn and Elson 1952). A variety of more modern tests have been used in the diagnosis of infection in man and animals and include the microagglutination test (Fiset *et al.* 1969), the enzyme-linked immunosorbent assay (Field *et al.* 1983), and immunofluorescent procedures (Ascher *et al.* 1983c). The dermal cellular hypersensitivity induced by the organism has been investigated in man and guinea pigs (Ascher *et al.* 1983a, b, d).

Antibody responses in experimental animals varied depending on different models and alone did not appear to play a role in controlling infections. Passive transfer of immune serum did not influence the course of action in mice (Humphres and Hinrichs 1981). Using congenitally athymic mice, it was determined that the host defence mechanisms involved thymus-dependent cell-mediated immunity (Kishimoto *et al.* 1978). The role of these immunological responses in controlling infections in domestic animals has not been defined.

VACCINATION

Vaccination is used in the control of the infection in man and domestic animals. In cattle, phase I inactivated vaccines are effective in reducing the incidence of infections and the shedding of the organisms. In man, vaccines prepared from strains of killed *C. burnetii*, predominantly in phase I, have been shown to be effective in eliciting humoral antibodies. Local and systemic postvaccination reactions can occur.

Literature

Growth phases I and II influenced the immunity induced by the organisms. Vaccines prepared from phase I had protective potencies 100 to 300 times greater than those of phase II (Ormsbee *et al.* 1964). A phase I formalin-inactivated vaccine greatly reduced the shedding of *C. burnetii* in milk. Only 1% of cows vaccinated as calves shed the organisms as compared to 24% of nonvaccinated animals (Biberstein *et al.* 1977). Calves vaccinated at 6 months of age developed agglutinating antibodies which persisted for at least 20 months (Behymer *et al.* 1977). The phase I vaccine was used on naturally infected cattle and did not reduce the incidence of shedders (Schmittdiel *et al.* 1981). Vaccination of dairy calves with phase II vaccine was not ideal and was found to be only partially successful in preventing the shedding of the organisms in milk (Luoto *et al.* 1952).

In man, vaccination has been used in people in high-risk occupations. The protective efficacy of a killed, purified, phase I *C. burnetii* vaccine was tested in cynomolgus monkeys and provided only partial protection 12 months later against aerosol challenge. The clinical signs were milder and the rickettsiemia was of shorter duration (Kishimoto *et al.* 1981).

CHEMOTHERAPY

Various tetracycline combinations are occasionally used in attempts to reduce shedding in milk of *C. burnetii* in dairy cows.

In man, chloramphenicol and chlortetracycline alone or in combination are used against rickettsia.

Literature

Treatment of pregnant dairy cows chronically infected with *C. burnetii* with 8 mg/kg of chlortetracycline orally for 30 days during the dry period have been undertaken. Organisms were not recovered from mammary fluid after the second week of treatment. At parturition, organisms were not demonstrated in placenta, colostrum, or calf tissues. Intramammary infusion and IV (intravascular) treatment with aureomycin failed to eliminate *C. burnetii* from the milk of cattle (Behymer 1980).

DIAGNOSIS

The diagnostic tests used for Q fever in domestic animals and man depend on whether the objective is to detect the infection or to define the epidemiological situation, and involve either isolation of the organism or demonstration of the incidence of positive serological response. Shedding of dairy cows is determined by testing either individual or pooled milk samples.

In man the clinical syndrome cannot be readily differentiated from viral diseases, such as influenza, because of the nonspecific clinical signs.

Literature

Standard culture and serology have been undertaken in both domestic animals and man. A reliable method of demonstrating organisms in man was by inoculation of material in either mice, guinea pigs, or chick embryos (Burgdorfer 1975). The most common serological methods for diagnosis were the CF and agglutination tests. In most cases, the carrier and shedder animals had antibody titers while only a low percentage of serum negative animals excreted organisms (Babudieri 1959).

CONTROL

Control of infection in domestic animals depends on determining the incidence in a particular epizootiological situation. Prophylactic vaccination reduces rates of infection in animals. Use of large quantities of antibiotics in attempts to treat animals are not generally successful. Prevention of exposure of man to placental fluids and infected milk are important control measures.

BIBLIOGRAPHY

Abinanti, F. R., Lennette, E. H., Winn, J. F. and Welsh, H. H., 1953a. Q fever studies XVIII. Presence of *Coxiella burnetii* in the birth fluids of naturally infected sheep, *Am. J. Hyg.*, **58**: 385–8.

Abinanti, F. R., Welsh, H. H., Lennette, E. H. and Brunetti, O., 1953b. Q fever studies XVI. Some aspects of the experimental infection induced in sheep by the intratracheal route of inoculation, *Am. J. Hyg.*, **57**: 170–84.

Abinanti, F. R., Welsh, H. H., Winn, J. F. and Lennette, E. H., 1955. Q fever studies XIX. Presence and epidemiologic significance of *Coxiella burnetii* in sheep wool, *Am. J. Hyg.*, **61**: 326–70.

Addo, P. B., 1980. A serological survey for evidence of Q fever in camels in Nigeria, *Br. vet. J.*, **136**: 519–21.

Ascher, M. S., Berman, M. A., Parker, D. and Turk, J. L., 1983a. Experimental model for dermal granulomatous hypersensitivity in Q fever, *Infect. Immun.*, **39**(1): 388–93.

Ascher, M. S., Berman, M. A. and Ruppaner, 1983b. Initial clinical and immunologic evaluation of a new phase I Q fever vaccine and skin test in humans, *J. Infect. Dis.*, **148**(2): 214–300.

Ascher, M. S., Horwith, G. S., Thornton, M. F., Greenwood, J. R. and Berman, M. A., 1983c. A rapid immunofluorescent procedure for serodiagnosis of Q fever in mice, guinea pigs, sheep, and humans, *Diagnost. Immunol.*, **1**: 33–8.

Ascher, M. S., Williams, J. C. and Berman, M. A., 1983d. Dermal granulomatous hypersensitivity in Q fever: comparative studies of the granulomatous potential of whole cells of *Coxiella burnetii* phase I and subfractions, *Infect. Immun.*, **42**(3): 887–9.

Babudieri, B., 1959. Q fever: a zoonosis. In *Advances in Veterinary Science*, eds C. A. Brandly, E. L. Jungherr. Academic Press (New York and London), vol. V, pp. 81–182.

Babudieri, B. and Ravaioli, L., 1952. Infezione sperimentale della pecora con *Coxiella burnetii, Zooprofilassi Rivista Mensile di Scienza e Tecnica Veterinaria*, **7**(1): 1–21.

Baca, O. G., Akporiaye, E. T., Aragon, A. S., Martinez, I. L., Robles, M. V. and Warner, N. L., 1981. Fate of phase I and phase II *Coxiella burnetii* in several macrophage-like tumor cell lines, *Infect. Immun.*, **33**(1): 258–66.

Baca, O. G. and Paretsky, D., 1983. Q fever and *Coxiella burnetii*: a model for host–parasite interactions, *Microbiol. Rev.*, **47**(2): 127–49.

Behymer, D., 1980. Q fever. In *Bovine Medicine and Surgery*, ed. H. E. Amstutz. American Veterinary Publications (Santa Barbara, Calif.). vol. I, pp. 346–54.

Behymer, D. E., Biberstein, E. L., Riemann, H. P., Franti, C. E. and Sawyer, M., 1975. Q fever (*Coxiella burnetii*) investigations in dairy cattle: persistence of antibodies after vaccination, *Am. J. vet. Res.*, **36**(6): 781–4.

Behymer, D. E., Biberstein, E. L., Riemann, H. P., Franti, C. E., Sawyer, M., Ruppaner, R. and Crenshaw, G. L., 1976. Q fever (*Coxiella burnetii*) investigations in dairy cattle. Challenge of immunity after vaccination, *Am. J. vet. Res.*, **37**: 631–4.

Behymer, D., Rupanner, R., Riemann, H. P., Biberstein, E. L. and Franti, C. E., 1977. Observation on chemotherapy in cows chronically infected with *Coxiella burnetii* Q fever, *Folia Veterinaria Latina*, **7**(1): 64–70.

Berge, T. O. and Lennette, E. H., 1953. World distribution of Q fever: human, animal and arthropod infection, *Am. J. Hyg.*, **57**(2): 125–43.

Bernier, R. D., Haney, T. and Paretsky, D., 1974. Changes in lipids of liver and plasma during Q fever, *Acta virol.*, **18**: 75–80.

Biberstein, E. L., Behymer, D. E., Bushnell, R. B., Crenshaw, G. L., Riemann, H. P. and Franti, C. E., 1974. A survey of Q fever (*Coxiella burnetii*) in California in dairy cows, *Am. J. vet. Res.*, **35**: 1577.

Biberstein, E. L., Riemann, H. P., Franti, C. E., Behymer, D. E., Ruppanner, R., Bushnell, R. and Crenshaw, G. L., 1977. Vaccination of dairy cattle against Q fever (*Coxiella burnetii*): results of field trials, *Am. J. vet Res.*, **38**: 189–93.

Brezina, R. and Kazár, J., 1963. Phagocytosis of *Coxiella burnetii* and the phase variation phenomenon, *Acta virol.*, **7**: 476.

Brezina, R. and Kazár, J., 1965. Study of the antigenic structure of *Coxiella burnetii*. IV. Phagocytosis and opsonization in relation to the phases of *C. burnetii, Acta virol.*, **9**: 268–74.

Burgdorfer, W., 1975. Q fever. In *Diseases Transmitted from Animals to Man*, eds W. T. Hubbert, W. F. McCulloch, P. R. Schnurrenberger. Charles C. Thomas (Springfield, Ill.), pp. 387–92.

DeLay, P. D., Lennette, E. H. and DeOme, K. B., 1950. Q fever in California. II. Recovery of *Coxiella burnetii* from naturally infected air-borne dust, *J. Immunol.*, **65**: 211–20.

Enright, J. B., Franti, C. E., Behymer, D. E., Longhurst, W. M., Dutson, V. J. and Wright, M. E., 1971a. *Coxiella burnetii* in a wildlife–livestock environment. Distribution of Q fever in wild mammals, *Am. J. Epidemiol.*, **94**(1): 79–90.

Enright, J. B., Franti, C. E., Longhurst, W. M., Behymer, D. E., Wright, M. E. and Dutson, V. J., 1971b. *Coxiella burnetii* in a wildlife–livestock environment. Antibody response of ewes and lambs in an endemic Q fever area, *Am. J. Epidemiol.*, **94**(1): 62–71.

Enright, J. B., Longhurst, W. M., Franti, C. E., Behymer, D. E., Dutson, V. J. and Wright, M. E., 1971c. *Coxiella burnetii* in a wildlife–livestock environment. Isolations of rickettsiae from sheep and cattle, *Am. J. Epidemiol.*, **94**(1): 72–8.

Enright, J. B., Longhurst, W. M., Wright, M. E., Dutson, V. J., Franti, C. E. and Behymer, D. E., 1971d. Q-fever antibodies in birds, *J. Wildl. Dis.*, **7**: 14–21.

Field, P. R., Hunt, J. G. and Murphy, A. M., 1983. Detection and persistence of specific IgM antibody to *Coxiella burnetii* by enzyme-linked immunosorbent assay: a comparison with immunofluorescence and complement fixation tests, *J. Infect. Dis.*, **148**(3): 477–87.

Fiset, P., Ormsbee, R. A., Silberman, R., Peacock, M. and Spielman, S. H., 1969. A microagglutination technique for detection and measurement of rickettsial antibodies, *Acta virol.*, **13**: 60–6.

Gillespie, J. H. and Baker, J. A., 1952. Experimental Q fever in cats, *Am. J. vet. Res.*, **13**: 91–4.

Hackstadt, T. and Williams, J. C., 1981. Biochemical stratagem for obligate parasitism of eukoryotic cells by *C. burnetii*, *Proc. Natl. Acad. Sci.*, **78**: 3240–4.

Haldane, E. V., Marrie, T. J., Faulkner, R. S., Lee, S. H. S., Cooper, J. H., MacPherson, D. D. and Montague, T. J., 1983. Endocarditis due to Q fever in Nova Scotia: experience with five patients in 1981–1982, *J. Infect. Dis.*, **148**(6): 978–85.

Heggers, J. P., Billups, L. H., Hinrichs, D. J. and Mallavia, L. P., 1975. Pathologic features of Q fever-infected guinea pigs, *Am. J. vet. Res.*, **36**(7): 1047–52.

Henning, M. W., 1956. Q fever. In *Animal Diseases in South Africa*. Central News Agency (South Africa), pp. 1201–19.

Hummel, P. H., 1976. Incidence in Tanzania of CF antibody to *Coxiella burnetii* in sera from man, cattle, sheep, goats and game, *Vet. Rec.*, **98**: 501–5.

Humphres, R. C. and Hinrichs, D. J., 1981. Role for antibody in *Coxiella burnetii* infection, *Infect. Immun.*, **31**(2): 641–5.

Jellison, W. L., Ormsbee, R., Beck, M. D., Huebner, R. J., Parker R. R. and Bell, E. J., 1948. Q fever studies in southern California. V. Natural infection in a dairy cow, *Pub. Hlth Rep.*, **63**(5): 1611–18.

Jellison, W. L., Welsh, H. H., Elson, B. E. and Huebner, R. J., 1950. Q fever studies in southern California. XI. Recovery of *Coxiella burnetii* from milk of sheep, *Pub. Hlth Rep.*, **65**: 395–9.

Johnson, J. W. and McLeod, C. G. Jr, 1977. Lesions in guinea pigs infected with *Coxiella burnetii* strain M-44, *J. Infect. Dis.*, **135**(6): 995–8.

Kaplan, M. M. and Bertagna, P., 1955. The geographical distribution of Q fever, *Bull. Wld Hlth Org.*, **13**: 829–60.

Kazár, J., Brezina, R., Schramek, S., Palanova, A. and Tvrdá, B., 1981. Suitability of the microagglutination test for detection of post-infection and post-vaccination Q fever antibodies in human sera, *Acta virol.*, **25**: 235–40.

Kazár, J., Brezina, R., Skulktétyová, K., Kovácová, E. and Schramek, S., 1975a. Phase II and phase I conversion of *Coxiella burnetii* in immunosuppressed mice, *Acta virol.*, **19**: 359–63.

Kazár, J., Skulktétyová, E. and Brezina, R., 1975b. Phagocytosis of *Coxiella burnetii* by macrophages, *Acta virol.*, **19**: 426–31.

Khera, S. S., 1962. Rickettsial infection in animals: a review, *Indian J. vet. Sci.*, **32**: 283–301.

Kishimoto, R. A., Gonder, J. C., Johnson, J. W., Reynolds, J. A. and Larson, E. W., 1981. Evaluation of a killed phase I *Coxiella burnetii* vaccine in cynomolgus monkeys (*Macaca fascicularis*), *Lab. Anim. Sci.*, **31**: 48–51.

Kishimoto, R. A., Rozmiarek, H. and Larson, E. W., 1978. Experimental Q fever infection in congenitally athymic nude mice, *Infect. Immun.*, **22**(1): 69–71.

Lennette, E. H., Holmes, M. A. and Abinanti, F. R., 1952. Q fever studies XIV. Observations on the pathogenesis of the experimental infection induced in sheep by the intravenous route, *Am. J. Hyg.*, **55**: 254–67.

Luoto, L. and Huebner, R. J., 1950. Q fever studies in southern California IX. Isolation of Q fever organisms from parturient placentas of naturally infected dairy cows, *Pub. Hlth Rep.*, **65**: 541–4.

Luoto, L., Winn, J. F. and Huebner, R. J., 1952. Q fever studies in southern California XIII. Vaccination of dairy cattle against Q fever, *Am. J. Hyg.*, **55**: 190–202.

Manjrekar, S. L., 1954. *Rickettsia* of domestic animals (a short review), *Indian J. vet. Sci.*, **24**: 217–22.

Marrie, T. J., Haldane, E. V., Noble, M. A., Faulkner, R. S., Lee, S. H. S., Gough, D., Meyers, S. and Stewart, J., 1982. Q fever in Maritime Canada, *CMA Journal*, **126**: 1295–1300.

McCaul, T. F. and Williams, J. C., 1981. Development cycle of *Coxiella burnetii*: structure and morphogenesis of vegetative and sporogenic differentiations, *J. Bacteriol.*, **147**: 1063–76.

McDonald, T. L. and Mallavia, L. P., 1975. Host response to infection by *Coxiella burnetii*, *Can. J. Microbiol.*, **21**: 675–81.

Murphy, A. M. and Magro, L., 1980. IgM globulin response in Q fever (*Coxiella burnetii*) infections, *Pathology*, **12**: 391–6.

Nermut, M. V., Schramek, S. and Brezina, R., 1968. Electron microscopy of *Coxiella burnetii* phase I and II, *Acta virol.*, **12**: 446–52.

Ormsbee, R. A., Bell, E. J., Lackman, D. B. and Tallent, G., 1964. The influence of phase on the protective potency of Q fever vaccine, *J. Immunol.*, **92**: 404–12.

Paretsky, D., Downs, C. M. and Salmon, C. W., 1964. Some biochemical changes in the guinea pig during infection with *Coxiella burnetii*, *J. Bacteriol.*, **88**(1): 137–42.

Paretsky, D., Gonzalez, F. R. and Berquist, K., 1981. Temporal studies of factors associated with changes in transcription during Q fever, *J. Gen. Microbiol.*, **122**: 227–33.

Paretsky, D. and Stueckemann, J., 1970.Chemical and biochemical changes in subcellular fractions of guinea pig during infection with *Coxiella burnetii*, *J. Bacteriol.*, **102**: 334–40.

Peacock, M. G., Philip, R. N., Williams, J. C. and Faulkner, R. S., 1981. Serological evaluation of Q fever in humans: enhanced phase I titers of immunoglobulins G and A are diagnostic for Q fever endocarditis, *Infect. Immun.*, **41**(3): 1089–98.

Polydorou, K., 1981. Q fever in Cyprus: a short review, *Br. vet. J.*, **137**: 470–7.

Ransom, S. E. and Huebner, R. J., 1951. Studies on the resistance of *Coxiella burnetii* to physical and chemical agents, *Am. J. Hyg.*, **53**: 110–19.

Schmatz, H. D., Krauss, H., Viertel, P., Ismail, A. S. and Hussein, A. A., 1978. Seroepidemiological investigations in domestic ruminants from Egypt, Somalia and Jordan for the demonstration of complement fixing antibodies against *Rickettsia* and *Chlamydia*, *Acta trop.*, **35**: 101–11.

Schmittdiel, E., Bauer, K., Steinbrecher, H. and Justl, W., 1981. Vaccination of Q-fever infected cattle: the effect on excretion of *Coxiella burnetii, Tierarztl. Umschau*, **36**: 159–62.

Siegrist, J. J. and Hess, E., 1968. Rickettsiose chez les animaux domestiques, *Bull. Off. int. Epiz.*, **70**: 315–23.

Stoenner, H. G. and Lackmann, D. B., 1952. The role of the milking process in the intraherd transmission of Q fever among dairy cattle, *Am. J. vet. Res.*, **13**: 458–65.

Stoker, M. G. P., Smith, K. M. and Fiset, P., 1956. Internal structure of *Rickettsia burnetii* as shown by electron microscopy of thin section, *J. gen. Microbiol.*, **15**: 632–5.

Stueckemann, J. and Paretsky, D., 1971. Changes in hepatic glycogen, protein and ribonucleic acid synthesis, and some effects of cortisol, during Q fever, *J. Bacteriol.*, **106**: 920–4.

Tanwani, S. K., Sharma, S. N. and Yadav, R., 1979. A note on the seroprevalence of Q fever in domestic animals and poultry, *Haryana Vet.*, **18**: 50–2.

Thompson, H. A. and Paretsky, D., 1973. Ribonucleic acid and protein synthesis in guinea pig liver during Q fever, *Infect. Immun.*, **7**(5): 718–24.

Tsung, P-K. and Paretsky, D., 1968. Biochemical and ultrastructural changes in liver endoplasmic reticular fractions during Q fever, *Acta virol.*, **12**: 49–53.

Vanek, E. and Thimm, B., 1976. Q fever in Kenya. Serological investigations in man and domestic animals, *E. Afr. Med. J.*, **53**(12): 678–84.

Waldhalm, D. G., Stoenner, H. G., Simmons, R. E. and Thomas, L. A., 1978. Abortion associated with *Coxiella burnetii* infection in dairy goats, *J. Am. vet. med. Ass.*, **173**(12): 1580–1.

Welsh, H. H., Jensen, F. W. and Lennette, E. H., 1959. Q fever studies XX. Comparison of four serologic techniques for the detection and measurement of antibody to *Coxiella burnetii* in naturally exposed sheep, *Am. J. Hyg.*, **70**: 1–13.

Welsh, H. H., Lennette, E. H., Abinanti, F. R. and Winn, J. F., 1951. Q fever in California IV. Occurrences of *Coxiella burnetii* in the placenta of naturally infected sheep, *Publ. Hlth Rep.*, **66**: 1473–7.

Welsh, H. H., Lennette, E. H., Abinanti, F. R. and Winn, J. F., 1958.

Air-borne transmission of Q fever: the role of parturition in the generation of infective aerosols, *Ann. N.Y. Acad. Sci.*, **70**: 528–40.

Welsh, H. H., Lennette, E. H., Abinanti, F. R., Winn, J. F. and Kaplan, W., 1959. Q fever studies XXI. The recovery of *Coxiella burnetii* from the soil and surface water of premises harboring infected sheep, *Am. J. Hyg.*, **70**: 14–20.

Wentworth, B. B., 1955. Historical review of the literature on Q fever, *Bacteriol. Rev.*, **19**: 129–49.

Williams, J. C., Peacock, M. G. and McCaul, T. F., 1981. Immunological and biological characterization of *Coxiella burnetii*, phases I and II, separated from host components, *Infect. Immun.*, **32**: 840–51.

Winn, J. F. and Elson, B. E., 1952. Effects of feeding colostrum containing *Coxiella burnetii* antibodies to newborn calves of two categories, *Ann. J. trop. Med. Hyg.*, **1**: 821–5.

Winn, J. F., Lennette, E. H., Welsh, H. H. and Abinanti, F. R., 1953. Q fever studies XVII. Presence of *Coxiella burnetii* in the feces of naturally infected sheep, *Am. J. Hyg.*, **58**: 183–7.

PART

V

HELMINTHIC DISEASES

Chapter

23

Filariasis

CONTENTS

INTRODUCTION

Filariasis in mammals is caused by filarial nematodes in the families Filariidae, Dipetalonematidae and Stephanofilariidae. Each of these has numerous genera and species which infect a variety of species of domestic and wild animals. However, only relatively few cause sufficiently severe lesions to produce clinically recognizable syndromes. Filariasis is very complex, composed of a number of different diseases whose features depend on the species of filaria and species of host. A further complication is the lack of host specificity resulting in infections causing varying degrees of disease in heterogeneous hosts.

Those genera and species which are of veterinary importance – either on a clinical or economic basis – in domestic animals are described in this chapter. The primary objective is to present an introduction to these disease syndromes which occur in the tropics. Such aspects as morphology, transmission, cyclic development in the vector, and the geographic distribution are not discussed here because of the complexity of filariasis. In many forms of filariasis in domestic animals the available information is often incomplete and the economic importance is not determined.

Literature

A vast amount of medical literature has been available on various features of filariasis of man, and this overshadows what is known on the subject in veterinary medicine. There have been many comprehensive monographs and texts which have dealt with a single disease entity as, for example, the monographs published by the World Health Organization (WHO) on various aspects of onchocerciasis in man and the extent of the problem in various tropical countries. Although bovine onchocerciasis has been established to occur widely in many tropical and temperate regions, it has not been extensively investigated.

Levine (1968) presented a comprehensive and detailed description of filarial nematodes which included their incidence, economic importance, and the clinical diseases induced in domestic animals. In many types of filariasis the infections, lesions, and diseases have not been studied because of the relatively innocuous nature of the host–parasite relationship.

ETIOLOGY

The species which are of clinical importance in domestic animals are found in the genera *Parafilaria*, *Onchocerca*, *Stephanofilaria*, *Dipetalonema*, and *Brugia*.

In the genus *Parafilaria*, two species cause lesions: *P. bovicola* is found in cutaneous nodules in cattle and water buffalo, and *P. multipapillosa* occurs in the subcutaneous and intramuscular connective tissue of equines.

The *Onchocerca* genus has a number of species which infect cattle, buffalo, camels, and equines and there is considerable confusion in the literature regarding nomenclature. *Onchocerca gutturosa* occurs in cattle, water and African buffalo in various sites, including the ligamentum nuchae and around joints, and *O. lienalis* occurs in the gastrosplenic ligament; *Onchocerca gibsoni* is found on the brisket and hind legs; and *O. armillata* is located in the inner surface of the aorta. In the camel, *O. fasciata* is found in the nodules in the ligamentum nuchae. In equines, *O. reticulata* occurs in the tendons and ligaments of the front legs and *O. cervicalis* in the ligamentum nuchae and eyes.

Various species in the genus *Stephanofilaria* cause dermatitis in different regions. In cattle and buffalo, *S. stilesi* is found on the ventral surface of cattle, *S. assamensis* on the hump, *S. kaeli* on the lower legs of cattle, and *S. zaheeri* on the ears of buffalo.

In the genus *Eleaophora*, *E. poeli* occurs in the aorta of cattle and buffalo, while *E. schneideri* is found in various arteries in sheep. Another species, *Deraiophoronema evansi*, occurs in various arteries in the camel.

In the genus *Dirofilaria*, the species *D. immitis* is found in the heart and blood vessels while *D. repens* occurs in the subcutaneous tissue of dogs, cats, and other wild carnivores. The *Dipetalonema* genus is important in differential diagnosis from dirofilariae and one species, *D. reconditum*, is found in the subcutaneous connective and perirenal tissues.

In the genus *Brugia*, which has species infecting primarily man, *B. pahangi*, *B. patei*, and *B. ceylonensis* also infect cats, dogs, and wild animals, and are found in lymph nodes.

Literature

Levine (1968) reviewed in detail the morphology of the species infecting domestic animals. Additional information has been published on some species; for example, on *P. bovicola* (Nelsen *et al.* 1962) and on *Onchocerca* species with 17 types having been described, the most economically important species being considered to be *O. gibsoni* and *O. armillata* in cattle and *O. reticulata* and *O. cervicalis* in horses (Supperer 1966). The morphology of the embryonated eggs and microfilaria *O. gibsoni* and their distribution in the worm nodule was also described in cattle (Isshiki 1964a, b, c). The three established species in cattle, *O. gibsoni*, *O. gutturosa*, and *O. lienalis* could be distinguished on morphology of the females, host–parasite relationship, and distribution in the host (Ottley and Moorhouse 1979). In studies on *O. gutturosa*, *O. lienalis*, and *O. stilesi* in cattle, considerable controversy and confusion was evident on the taxonomic status of these species. Before classification was possible a complete morphological study of all forms was necessary (Eberhard 1979). The microfilariae in the skin of the species, *O. volvulus*, *O. gutturosa*, and *O. reticulata*, could be distinguished on the basis of form, size, and arrangement of caudal nuclei (Gibson 1952). However, overlap in structural components in the skin microfilariae of *O. cervicalis*, *O. gutturosa*, and *O. volvulus* was evident, which made their identification and taxonomic classification difficult (Mellor 1974). The problems of identifying various species in the *Onchocerca* species have been discussed by Mueller (1979).

EPIZOOTIOLOGY

Incidence and geographical distribution

Filariasis in domestic animals is enzootic and common in most tropical countries but, because of the relatively innocuous nature of many of the syndromes, relatively little attention is given in veterinary medicine to the clinical manifestations and economic importance. What information is available on the incidence of infections is usually incomplete and depends largely on methods of survey, particularly on the techniques used to demonstrate microfilariae and to search for adult worms. Dissection techniques used to find adult worms are tedious, difficult, often unrewarding, and as a result are rarely undertaken. Prevalence rates reported often depend on the extent of the meat inspection procedures undertaken in various tropical regions. The lesions which are recorded as of significance in one region may be disregarded in another. Therefore, great variability occurs in the prevalence reported from various tropical regions and countries.

Literature

Levine (1968) presented in considerable detail the geographic distribution of the various genera of *Filaria* and the incidences of infection in various species of domestic animals, and included those species which were associated with lesions and those which were asymptomatic. In many regions and countries comprehensive surveys have not been undertaken to define the incidences of filariasis in various species of livestock. In a study from East Africa, filarial infections in man, wild and domestic animals, and mosquitoes on the Kenyan coast were described (Nelson *et al*. 1962). More recently there have been a few reports from other countries on incidence of specific species of worms in some species of domestic animals. A direct relationship between the occurrence of filariasis in cattle and buffalo and hot weather has been observed, and was related to transmission of the infections by the vectors (Khamis *et al*. 1973).

The history of the worldwide spread of *P. bovicola* was reviewed by Nevill (1975). An extensive survey for bovine parafilariasis on 32 000 cattle was undertaken in southern Africa and the prevalence, distribution, and economic importance were discussed. Considerable variation occurred between the different regions. Economic losses were due to downgrading, trimming, and condemnation and the disease was responsible for 33% of all carcass condemnations (Carmichael and Koster 1978). Lesions were caused by mature worms migrating through subcutaneous and intramuscular connective tissue and resulted in condemnation of approximately 6 kg of meat in affected animals. The incidence was seasonal, affecting primarily animals on pasture and mainly those in the 1- to 2-year age group. There has been relatively little recent information on parafilariasis from other regions of Africa. Occasionally in temperate zones, for example in Canada, *P. bovicola* has been detected in imported cattle (Niilo 1968; Webster and Wilkins 1970).

More information has been available on onchocerciasis in African cattle. Bwangamoi (1970) reported the occurrence of *O. gutturosa* in cattle in Uganda. The presence of this species was demonstrated in Sudanese cattle by detecting microfilariae in the skin (Elbihari and Hussein 1978) and there has been a preliminary report on bovine onchocerciasis from Nigeria (Amakiri 1972). In Kenya about 8% of cattle were infected with *O. gutturosa* and 2% with *O. armillata*, but *O. lienalis* and *O. gibsoni* were not observed (Clarkson 1964). A 90% incidence of *O. armillata* was reported in Sudanese cattle (Malek 1958). Patnaik (1962) summarizes the available information on the occurrence of *O. armillata* in cattle, and an incidence of 90% was common in various regions of the world, particularly in countries of Africa.

In Australia, incidence in cattle of worms in nodules caused by *O. gibsoni* were reported; the prevalence of *O. lienalis* in the gastrosplenic ligament was 33% overall (Beveridge *et al.* 1979, 1980). In a large survey of 5712 cattle an infection rate of 86% with *O. gibsoni* and development of nodules in the brisket was reported; information on the prevalence of lesions with regard to age, sex, breed, and seasons was also included (Ladds *et al.* 1979).

There have been several reports from India on the occurrence of filarial infections in cattle and buffalo. Lesions due to *O. armillata* and *O. gutturosa* were found to be widely prevalent in buffalo and associated with prominent lesions (Chauhan and Pande 1972; Shastri 1973). The occurrence of *O. armillata* was also reported in buffalo calves (Srivastava and Pande 1965) and in cattle (Patnaik 1962).

There have been fewer reports on the incidence in cattle and buffalo of other filarial worm infections. In Thailand *O. sweetae* occurred in buffalo (Bain *et al.* 1980). In Pakistan, *S. assamensis* was associated with hump sore and had an infection rate of 25% (Rahman 1957).

High incidences of equine onchocerciasis due to *O. cervicalis* in North America have been reported (Collins 1973; Marcoux *et al.* 1977; Rabalais *et al.* 1974). The incidence of infections increased with age, ranging from 10% in horses less than a year of age to 90% in horses 16 years of age. In old horses, infections were associated with granulomas and mineralization around adult worms (Schmidt *et al.* 1982a). In Iran filarial infections of equines were reported with *O. cervicalis*, *P. multipapillosa*, and *E. bohmi* (Mirzayans and Maghsoodloo 1977).

The most numerous reports from various countries on filariasis have been of the incidence of *Dirofilaria* and *Dipetalonema* infections in dogs. *Dirofilaria immitis* is widely distributed throughout the world both in the tropics and subtropics, and is an important pathogen. At least 11 species of filarial worms have been reported to occur naturally in dogs worldwide. Otto (1969) summarized the geographical distribution of vectors and the life cycle of *Dirofilaria*. In the USA information has been available on incidence in various regions (Healy and Kagan 1960; Kazacos 1978; Walters *et al.* 1981). An overall incidence of *D. immitis* and *Dipetalonema reconditum* in Hawaii was about 45% and the distribution and periodicity were determined (Gubler 1966). The occurrence in the USA of dog filariasis caused by species other than *D. immitis* was first described by Newton and Wright in 1956. At this time *Dipetalonema reconditum* was identified and it was conclusively shown that more than one filaria species infected dogs in the USA. Morphological differences of the microfilariae and of the adult worms identify the two species (Korkejian and Edeson 1978). In Chile an incidence of *Dipetalonema* was reported (Alcaino *et al.* 1977). *Dipetalonema reconditum* and *D. grassii* were reported in Brazil (Costa and Freitas 1962). In Malaysia incidences of *D. immitis* were 25.8 and 32% of microfilariae and adult worms (Kan *et al.* 1977; Retnasabapathy and San 1976). In the Philippines an incidence of 90% was reported (Cabrera *et al.* 1970). The occurrence of other species has not been well documented. Adults of *Brugia pahangi*, a species resembling *B. malayi* in man, were found in dogs and cats in Malaya (Buckley and Edeson 1956). Microfilariae resembling *B. malayi* were also detected in dogs and cats in East Africa (Nelson and Heisch 1957) while *B. patei* was observed in cats and dogs on Pate Island, Kenya (Buckley *et al.* 1958).

Transmission

Transmission of filarial infections in cattle depends upon the ecology and habits of the vectors. Information is available on the vectors and the life cycle in these invertebrate hosts for various filarial species of medical importance, but less of veterinary interest is known on the species. In most cases it is anticipated that numerous intermediate hosts are present for any one species of filarial worms and that the life cycle in the vector is complex. Filarial worms are transmitted by biting arthropods, either ectoparasites or free-flying. Ecological and environmental factors rather than phylogenetic properties govern the rate of development and transmission. Microfilariae in the appropriate intermediate arthropod host reach an infective stage after a period of 7 to 14 days. The presence of numerous filarial species in vectors is of epidemiological importance in human filariasis because it requires differentiation between the species infecting man and those infecting animals. This is a problem because of morphological similarities between these species and it is a serious complication in determining the intensity of challenge to man.

Literature

Nelson (1964) reviewed the factors which influence the development and behaviour of filarial worms in vectors.

In South Africa flies of the species *Musca* (subgenus *Eumusca*) were vectors of *P. bovicola*. Ingested microfilariae developed after 14 days into infective third-stage larvae which after injection into the host took up to 10 months to develop into adult worms (Bech-Nielsen *et al*. 1982a, b).

Black flies are vectors of *Onchocerca* species and the epizootiology is affected by the behavioral characteristics of the various species. In general, simulium flies have been difficult to feed and thus maintain under laboratory conditions. A method has been described for feeding flies with blood infected with *O. gutturosa* (McMahon 1968).

Relatively more information has been available on the transmission of *D. immitis*. About 30 different species of mosquito have been infected in the laboratory and shown to support development of the worms (Tolbert and Johnson 1982). Ingested microfilariae made their way to the Malpighian tubules where development took place through first-, second-, and third-stage larvae. The last stage migrated to the mouth parts of the mosquito (Otto and Bauman 1959; Otto 1969). Transplacental transmission of *D. immitis* was also possible but was infrequently observed (Todd and Howland 1983).

INFECTION

Most filarial worms have fairly strict specificity for their definitive mammalian hosts. There are some exceptions, especially *B. malayi*, which is found in a wide range of hosts which includes primates, carnivores, rodents, edentates, and insectivores. In man, eight species are host-specific and very rarely cause natural infection of animals.

Most of the filarial worms are well adapted to their hosts, causing little tissue damage. Even those species which infect the blood vessels, such as *D. immitis* in dogs and *Deraiophoronema evansi* in camels, are in most cases well tolerated. The worm burden is of primary importance in the pathogenesis, and the life span of both microfilariae and adult worms which is relatively long also plays a significant role in development of tissue injury. Occasionally, aberrant heterogeneous infections cause considerable damage to vital tissue, such as the brain, and result in severe clinical signs.

Tissue distribution of adults and microfilariae varies with the species of worm. Adults are found in various body tissues and organs including blood vessels, heart, lymphatics, skeletal muscles, connective tissues, and serous cavities. The worms are viviparous and the microfilariae are found either in the blood, skin, or lymph. Marked periodicity is evident with some species in the numbers of circulating microfilariae, and increases coincide with periods most favorable for maximum contact with suitable vectors.

The distribution of adult worms varies with the species. *Parafilaria bovicola* in cattle and buffalo is found in cutaneous nodules, while *P. multipapillosa* occurs in subcutaneous and intramuscular connective tissues of equines. The females pierce the skin, and eggs, microfilariae, and blood exude from the lesions on to the skin.

Various species of *Onchocerca* are ubiquitous in cattle, buffalo, and horses and are rarely recognized as causing disease. In the mammalian host, the third-stage larvae transmitted by the arthropod migrate to a preferential tissue site where molting and development into adult worms takes place. Females become fertilized, and microfilariae are released into the bloodstream and migrate to the skin. In cattle, *O. gutturosa* is found in the nuchal ligament and *O. lienalis* is found in the gastrosplenic ligament; microfilariae are abundant in the skin where occasionally they cause dermatitis characterized by pruritis. *Onchocerca gibsoni* produces nodular swellings of the skin and of the brisket. Obvious lesions in the aorta are caused by *O. armillata* with the adults present in and around the walls. The microfilariae are found in the skin and occasionally in the blood. Microfilaria of various *Onchocerca* species localizing in the skin have different distributions over the body depending on the site of the adult worm and the migrating properties of immature worms. Microfilariae of *O. gibsoni* are found around the brisket and umbilical region, those of *O. lienalis* also localize around the umbilicus, and *O. gutturosa* microfilaria are distributed mainly, but not exclusively, on the dorsal surface of the host. In horses, *O. reticulata* localizes in the suspensory ligaments of the fetlock while *O. cervicalis* is found in the ligamentum nuchae. Microfilaria of *O. reticulata* are found in the skin and those of *O. cervicalis* in skin and eyes. The distribution of microfilariae in the skin is an evolving adaptation to coincide with the biting behavior of the vectors.

The microfilaria of various species of *Stephanofilaria* localize in different regions in the skin of cattle. *Elaeophora poeli* localizes in the aorta of cattle and *E. schneideri* in the arteries of sheep, with the microfilariae localizing in the skin on the poll region and face.

Adults of *Dirofilaria immitis* are found in the heart and pulmonary blood vessels and microfilariae are present in the blood.

Adults of *B. pahangi* occur in lymph vessels and lymph nodes of cats and dogs, and microfilariae are found in the blood.

Literature

Levine (1968) discussed the various features of filarial infections caused by different species in cattle, sheep, goats, buffalo, camels, pigs, horses, dogs, and cats. For each species of host the available information on the life cycle and pathogenesis were discussed. Scholtens (1975) tabulated the information on filarial infections in domestic and wild mammals and included 41 species which infected domestic animals. The host species infected, geographical distribution, vectors, and the tissue location of adults and of microfilariae were presented. A brief summary of filariasis in domestic animals was presented by Mortelmans (1961).

The distribution of adults of the three species of *Onchocerca* infecting cattle in Australia has been described. *Onchocerca gutturosa* was found in the ligamentum nuchae, on the scapular cartilage, and on the hips, stifle, and shoulder region; *O. gibsoni* was found on the brisket, stifle, and hip regions; while *O. lienalis* occurred along the gastrosplenic ligament and above the xiphisternum (Ottley and Moorhouse 1978a). The distribution of microfilariae in the skin of cattle was related to a pattern corresponding to biting habits of the vectors (Venkataratnam and Kershaw 1961). In the UK the distribution of the microfilariae of *O. gutturosa* (now known to be *O. lienalis*) in the skin of cattle was primarily in the lower part of the body (Eichler and Nelson 1968), while in Sudanese cattle the highest incidence was found to be in the region of the hump (Elbihari and Hussein 1978).

In horses, *O. cervicalis* localized in the ligamentum nuchae, and *O. reticulata* on the suspensory ligament of the forelegs (Rabalais *et al.* 1974). Equine onchocerciasis in Australia was caused by *O. cervicalis* and, to a lesser degree, by *O. gutturosa* and *O. reticulata* infections. It was concluded that *O. cervicalis* was the predisposing factor in the etiology of equine nucheal disease seen clinically as fistulous withers. *Onchocerca gutturosa,* although a cattle parasite, also infected and was well tolerated by horses (Ottley *et al.* 1983; Ottley and Moorhouse 1978a, b). The normal habitat of the adult *D. immitis* was the right ventricle and pulmonary artery (Jackson *et al.* 1962), and the life cycle has been more extensively studied than in other forms of filariasis (Kotani and Powers 1982; Kume and Itagaki 1955). After injection through the bite of an infected vector, larvae underwent further development in subcutaneous muscle, adipose tissues, and subserosal veins. In 2 to 3 months larvae began to arrive in the right side of the heart or adjacent vessels. After maturing, microfilariae were released into the blood after a period of 6 months. Adult worms persisted for years in the host. The first established population of worms was small but grew considerably in length, and in the case of the females became 35 times longer than the initial young adults (Otto and Bauman 1959; Otto 1969). Marked periodicity occurred in the numbers of microfilariae in the peripheral circulation. High parasitemia was observed in the early evening and at night. Host's body temperature did not appear to play a role in the periodicity (Hawking *et al.* 1967). Mechanisms which affected the level of circulating microfilariae were studied but could not be defined (Wong 1964) and could not be described by mathematical analysis (Church *et al.* 1976).

In a general review of human filariasis in Malaysia caused by *B. malayi,* Wilson (1961) mentioned that natural infections caused by this species were found in a variety of domestic and wild carnivores. Edeson (1962) presented a list of wild and domestic animals surveyed for *Brugia* infections; *B. malayi* was considered to occur primarily in man while *B. pahangi* was found in dogs and cats. Experimental infections in cats could be produced with *B. malayi, B. pahangi,* and *B. patei,* and these three species occurred naturally in cats with adult worms localizing in lymphatics, closely mimicking the *B. malayi* and *Wuchereria bancrofti* in man (Denham 1979).

Most filarial infections in animals have not been considered as important zoonoses. Those filariae which have on occasion infected man were discussed and were regarded as rare and atypical forms of filariasis. The dirofilariae infection of dogs is the most common important form of zoonosis of all domestic animal filariasis (Dissanaike 1979; Nelson 1965b).

CLINICAL SIGNS

In the tropics localized skin lesions in cattle, buffalo, horses, and camels are a common finding and it is often difficult to determine the etiology. Adults and microfilaria can cause a variety of clinical syndromes characterized by dermatitis, nodules, and ulcers. Location of the lesions and their severity varies both with the species of filarial worms and the species of host. A direct correlation between development of lesions, clinical signs, and presence of infections is often not clearly established. In the majority of instances there are no accompanying systemic signs. The skin lesions are usually chronic, develop slowly, are most frequently in order animals, and often regress spontaneously. Following infection, the prepatent period varies considerably and development of lesions depends on prior sensitization of the host by previous filarial infections and the immune status of the host. On occasion a species which is nonpathogenic in one species causes severe clinical signs in abnormal hosts by its localization in certain tissues such as the central nervous system.

Parafilaria bovicola, *P. multipapillosa*, and *P. sahaii* cause seasonal hemorrhagic dermatitis in cattle, horses, and buffalo, characterized by development of nodules on the head, neck, withers, shoulders, and sides which periodically ooze a bloody exudate. These lesions are occasionally complicated by secondary infection causing abscesses.

Relatively little attention is given to the clinical and pathological manifestations of bovine and equine onchocerciasis. Lesions are most commonly caused either by microfilariae or by adult worms localizing in the skin. The larvae may cause dermatitis characterized by pruritis. At times it is difficult to determine the cause of a particular skin lesion because many infections are asymptomatic and multiple infections may occur. Whether the dermatitis is due to the microfilariae or due to a hypersensitivity to the actual bite of the vector is still not clearly established. In cattle and buffalo the adults of *O. gutturosa* may cause small fibrous nodules around joints, resulting in a proliferative inflammatory reaction around tendons and ligaments. *Onchocerca gibsoni* and *O. sweetae* cause nodules in the skin on the brisket, shoulders, flanks, and hind legs. In camels, *O. gibsoni* causes lesions the same as those in cattle. *Onchocerca armillata* causes atheromata in the aorta and *E. poeli* induces nodules in the aorta. It is not clear what circulatory malfunction can be associated with these lesions. In sheep, infection by *E. schneideri* causes a clinical syndrome characterized by facial dermatitis.

In horses, at least four distinct pathological conditions are at times associated with *O. cervicalis* infection. Poll evil and fistulous withers are chronic inflammatory conditions of the ligamentum nuchae and thought to be caused by adult worms. Recurring seasonal dermatitis with pruritis, scaly alopecia, and periodic ophthalmia are caused by microfilariae in the skin. Microfilariae of *O. cervicalis* are frequently found in the eyes of horses and are associated with severe ophthalmia. Although onchocerciasis in man is a common cause of blindness, relatively little attention has been given to the development of ocular onchocerciasis in domestic animals. Adults of *O. reticulata* cause swellings of the suspensory ligament of the fetlock and microfilariae also cause dermatitis.

In cattle and buffalo, various *Stephanofilaria* species cause chronic dermatitis in different parts of the body. *Stephanofilaria stilesi* usually causes lesions on the ventral surface along the midline of the abdomen, but may be found in other parts of the body; *S. dedoesi* is found on the sides of the neck, withers, dewlap, and shoulders; *S. assamensis* occurs on the hump, while *S. kaeli* causes small sores on the legs. *Stephanofilaria zaheeri* occurs only in the buffalo and causes dermatitis on the ears.

Central nervous system involvement is observed in abnormal *Setaria digitata* infections in sheep, goats, and horses. This parasite of cattle causes focal encephalomyelomalacia resulting in severe clinical signs of central nervous system involvement by migrating larvae through the brain and spinal cord.

Dirofilaria immitis causes a well-defined clinical syndrome in dogs with systemic signs usually developing 8 or 9 months after infection which initially consist of the observation that dogs tire, even collapse, after exercise. In advanced cases associated with circulatory system malfunction, ascites and anasarca are present. Clinical signs result from the presence of large numbers of worms in the right ventricle and pulmonary vessels, causing cardiac decompensation and passive congestion. Inflammatory lesions are also found in skin and eyes associated with localization of microfilariae.

In man, three species are responsible for major disease problems affecting large populations in various parts of the world. *Wuchereria bancrofti* and *B. malayi* cause disease of lymphatics while *O. volvulus* causes skin and eye lesions.

Literature

In cattle and buffalo the clinical development of dermatitis and skin ulcers associated with filarial infections has not been described in any detail. This probably could be due to the usual mild form of the lesion which does not come to veterinary attention. Occasionally new syndromes have been reported as with *Stephanofilaria zaheeri* which was associated with skin lesions on ears in the buffalo in India (Agrawal and Dutt 1976; Agrawal *et al.* 1978). Minor differences in the distribution of lesions have been noted between species of hosts, with nodules caused by *O. sweetae* in water buffalo being found intradermally as opposed to those of *O. gibsoni* in cattle which were subcutaneous and in the musculature of the brisket (Spratt and Moorhouse 1971).

In sheep, an unusual filarial disease was reported from North America caused by *E. schneideri*, an infection which was characterized by dermatitis, stomatitis, rhinitis, and keratitis. Microfilariae were found in these inflammatory lesions, and the adult worms were localized in the arteries which include those that supply the affected tissues of the head as well as the aorta and the anterior mesenteric artery (Jensen and Seghetti 1955). In camels, infection with *Deraiophoronema evansi* in the spermatic vessels has been associated with orchitis.

Pathogenesis of *Onchocerca* infections in horses has not been well established. Several clinical syndromes, for example periodic ophthalmia and fistulous withers, have been associated with the presence of adult worms and microfilaria. But often it has been difficult to relate infection to tissue damage (Collins 1973). McMullan (1972) compared the onchocerciasis of man to the syndromes seen in horses. Examination of a large number of horses with periodic ophthalmia revealed that microfilariae of *O. cervicalis* were present in a high percentage and were considered to be the causative agents (Bohm and Supperer 1954). However, a number of predisposing factors were necessary for infections to cause lesions (Roberts 1963). In one survey of equine ocular onchocerciasis, 40 out of 368 normal eyes examined contained microfilariae in the conjunctiva without any clinical abnormalities (Schmidt *et al.* 1982b). In another study, a high incidence of microfilariae was found in 266 of 431 horses, localized in the cornea without development of lesions. It was proposed that the relationship between the clinical onchocerciasis of skin and eyes must take into account the prevalence of infections without clinical signs (Marolt *et al.* 1966). Adult *O. cervicalis* in the ligamentum nuchae of 120 horses were of minor importance and, although either small calcified or caseous nodules were sometimes found, poll evil and fistulous withers were not detected (Mellor 1973). The allergic dermatitis of horses, known as Queensland itch and thought to be due to skin infection caused by *O. reticulata* microfilariae, was in fact the result of hypersensitivity to bites of midges (Riek 1954).

Various clinical signs have been closely monitored in *Dirofalaria immitis* infections. Pulmonary vascular malfunction resulting in pulmonary hypertension developed due to the presence of adult parasites and microfilariae, and the severity varied widely from case to case (Rawlings 1978, 1980). Scintigraphic evaluations of pulmonary perfusion in dogs were poorly correlated to vascular abnormalities as detected by thoracic radiographs and circulatory deficits (Thrall *et al.* 1979a). Pulmonary hypertension has also been evaluated during treatment (Rawlings 1980). In addition to the classical disease described, other manifestations were occasionally observed and one was characterized by a rapidly fatal course of 12 to 24 hours' duration, resulting in the presence of adult worms in the vena cava and associated with hemoglobinuria and bilirubinuria (Jackson *et al.* 1962). Another syndrome was characterized by the absence of circulating microfilariae. This could be induced by repeated injections of microfilariae, with adult worms occurring in the heart and the microfilariae being trapped in the granulomatous lesions in the lung (Wong 1974a). Nodular skin lesions have also been associated with microfilariae in the skin blood vessels (Scott 1979). Ocular dirofilariasis has also been reported (Guterbock *et al.* 1981; Lavers *et al.* 1969). Cerebral vascular lesions have resulted in neurological disturbances (Segedy and Hayden 1978).

PATHOLOGY

Pathogenesis is dependent mainly on site of tissue and organ localization in the host by the adults and microfilariae. Longevity of worms and the immune status of the host play significant roles. The damage caused is usually associated with a chronic inflammatory reaction around dead adults and microfilariae. Live parasites appear to induce little tissue damage. Circulating live microfilariae do not cause damage and may survive for long periods of time – in fact for years as in the case of infections in man. No relationship exists between injury, severity of host response, and the size of the worm. In animals, the relatively mild forms of filariasis may be due to the short survival of these species in the host. In man the severe response may be related to persistence of adult infections for years.

Adults of the majority of filarial species found in the subcutaneous tissue usually cause little reaction. Adults of *Onchocerca* species are an exception, becoming encapsulated to form fibrous nodules which contain either live or dead worms. In the internal tissue habitats, granulomatous lesions also occur at the site of localization of the adult worms. Members of *Parafilaria* and *Stephanofilaria* species produce open skin lesions through which the microfilariae escape to the surface in exudates. The microfilariae of *Onchocerca* species are found in intact skin and may cause severe dermatitis. A characteristic anatomical pattern of distribution of microfilariae occurs in the skin. The development and severity of lesions is dependent on the level of infection. In cattle and horses onchocerciasis in the majority of the infections is characterized by lack of lesions. *Onchocerca armillata* causes granulomous nodules in the aorta. *Brugia* species infect the lymph nodes and lymphatics in dogs and cats.

Extensive lesions occur in dogs infected with *D. immitis*. Infection of the right ventricle, right auricle, and pulmonary arteries results in a severe villous obliterative endarteritis and right heart failure, with chronic pulmonary congestion, hepatomegaly, ascites, and death. In addition to changes in the blood vessels, granulomatous nodules containing microfilariae are found in lung parenchyma. Another intravascular species of filarial worms, *Deraiophoronema evansi*, is found in the heart and spermatic vessels of camels and, in heavy infestation, causes arteriosclerotic lesions which lead to development of orchitis with aneurysms.

Literature

A comprehensive review of the pathology of filarial diseases was presented by Nelson (1965a). Control to the pathogenesis was the diversity of tissue environments infected by the different species of filarial worms resulting in lesions which were tabulated. Microfilariae localized either in the blood or the skin. Adult worms were found in the skin, subcutaneous tissue, eye, lymph nodes and lymphatics, cardiovascular system, peritoneal cavity, central nervous system, spleen, and the urinary organs.

In cattle, adult *P. bovicola* caused streaks of bloody exudate on the skin and slimy bruise-like lesions in the subcutaneous tissue. These lesions could be confused with contusions occurring during transport to slaughter (Bech-Nielsen *et al.* 1982a). Female worms perforated the skin causing nodules and a trickle of blood (Nevill 1975). Comparable lesions occurred in mules (Deorani and Dutt 1967). Skin lesions due to parafilariasis have been reported in elephants (Ramanujachari and Alwar 1954).

Lesions caused by *O. armillata* and *O. gutturosa* infections in cattle have not been described in detail. Quantitative histopathology of the nodules caused by *O. gibsoni* in the brisket of cattle was investigated (Nitisuwirjo and Ladds 1980). The histopathology of skin in *O. gutturosa* infections and their association with ulcerative dermatitis was reported in cattle (Herin and Fain 1955). The pathology of the skin lesions on the legs of cattle caused by *S. kaeli* has also been reported (Loke and Ramachandran 1967).

Lesions in the aorta caused by *O. armillata* consisted of focal nodular thickening of the intima and adventitia, resulting in tortuous tunnels, calcified plaques, and occasionally small intimal ulcerations, and were associated with partial thrombosis. These lesions contained male and female worms and the tissue reaction varied from slight inflammation to extensive fibrous response and calcification (Cheema and Ivoghli 1978; Zak 1975; Chodnik 1958). The pig has also been found as a possible host for an *Onchocerca* species which caused lesions resembling those of *O. armillata* in bovines (Ramanujachari and Alwar 1953). Another vascular lesion has been caused by *E. poeli* in aortas of cattle and buffalo and consisted of corrugated migratory tracts and nodular lesions (Prasad and Bhalla 1977).

In horses periodic ophthalmia has been associated with the

microfilariae lodged in the cornea and sclera. In addition to inflammation in the cornea and sclera, exudative iritis, cylitis, and chorioiditis have been observed (Bohm and Supperer 1954).

Systemic effects due to filariasis do not occur in domestic ruminants. Microfilariae primarily of *Setaria cervi* and *O. armillata* species were associated with increased levels of erythrocyte sedimentation and low hemoglobin levels, and various other hematological parameters were also affected (Singh *et al.* 1972, 1973). However, the significance of these hematological changes was quesioned and the general statement that microfilariae in the circulation were asymptomatic still held (Singh *et al.* 1972).

Live adult *Dirofilaria immitis* caused pulmonary endarteritis characterized by villous endarterial fibrosis and obstructive fibrosis. Embolic adult dirofilarial worms occasionally led to thrombosis and extensive granulomatous response (Adcock 1961; Hennigar and Ferguson 1957). Peripheral pulmonary arterial lesions have also been associated with mature larvae and were similar to the endarteritis caused by adult worms (Atwell 1980). Ultrastructural studies have been undertaken and connected with pulmonary vascular malfunction (Schaub and Rawlings 1980; Schaub *et al.* 1980). Hemoglobinuria was reported to result from chronic intravascular hemolysis and increase erythrocyte fragility (Ishihara *et al.* 1978, 1981). The glomerulosclerosis observed was not associated with immune complexes (Shirota *et al.* 1979), but in another study kidney lesions were thought to be induced by the deposit of immune complexes on the glomerular basement membrane (Abramowsky *et al.* 1981; Aikawa *et al.* 1981). Hepatic lesions resulted from cardiac failure with development of characteristic central lobular necrosis (von Lichtenberg *et al.* 1962). Comparable lesions have also been observed in the fox (*Vulpes bengalensis*) (Rao and Acharjyo 1971). In dogs with massive infections of *D. repens*, lesions were occasionally observed in association with the adult worms as well as with microfilariae (Mandelli and Mantovani 1966).

In experimental infection of cats and dogs, lymphadenitis and lymphengitis was caused by the mature and larval stages of *B. pahangi* (Schacher and Sahyoun 1967). In multiple infections of cats by this species, the main histological lesions were in the lymph nodes and consisted of hyperplasia of both thymic and nonthymic dependent areas which was followed by depletion of the lymphocytes and fibrous tissue proliferation (Rogers *et al.* 1975).

Pathological aspects of human onchocerciasis, primarily the dermal and ocular lesions, were reviewed by Gibson *et al.* (1980) and by Rodger (1962). One of the main effects of the dead parasite was in the blood vessels, causing vascular atrophy resulting in local tissue anoxia. The role of allergic responses in the development of the skin lesions has not been clearly defined.

IMMUNOLOGY

In most forms of filariasis in domestic animals there is relatively little information on immunological responses, their involvement in development of resistance, and the role of cellular and humoral components in the pathogenesis. A considerable amount of literature has been published on the immunology of human filariasis and the experimental models.

To some extent, features of the immunology of the disease caused by *Dirofilaria immitis* in dogs are available. One factor which probably plays a major role in immunity is the continuous exposure of man and domestic animals in the tropics to a variety of heterogenous filarial infections which may induce heterogenous immunity and be of importance in modifying the susceptibility and pathogenesis. There is circumstantial evidence that resistance develops in man following initial infection to subsequent challenge.

Literature

Various aspects of the immunology of human filariasis including immunodiagnosis, role of immunity in resistance, immunopathology, and prophylaxis were briefly summarized in a report from a WHO scientific working group on filariasis (1981). The immunological diagnostic methods for human filariasis were presented by Kagan (1963).

Dogs chronically infected with *D. immitis* had an increase in IgG and IgE antibodies, but there were no changes in the cellular responses. These immunological responses were not correlated with the worm burden (Weil *et al.* 1981), but in another study depression of responses of peripheral lymphocytes to phytohemagglutinin was observed (Grieve *et al.* 1979). Following treatment with diethylcarbamazine, the IgG and IgE levels were decreased in those dogs which showed severe to moderate adverse reactions, but did not decline in nonreacting dogs (Desowitz *et al.* 1978). Quantitative fluorescent tests have been used to measure antibody responses in experimentally infected dogs and were compared with enzyme-linked immunosorbent assays (Gittelman *et al.* 1981).

DIAGNOSIS

Skin ulcers, nodules, inflammatory exudates, and chronic dermatitis in domestic animals are common in the tropics and are a diagnostic problem. Filariasis has to be differentiated from localized lesions caused by other agents, particularly by mycotic, bacterial, and viral infections. One major difficulty is the frequent occurrence in the blood and tissues of microfilariae of nonpathogenic filarial worms. Single and multiple infections of pathogenic and nonpathogenic species further complicate the diagnosis, requiring careful examination of the worm morphology. For example, diagnosis of dirofilariasis in the dog is a problem in some regions because of the frequency of *Dipetalonema* and *Brugia* microfilaria in the blood.

Accuracy of the diagnosis of filarial infections depends on techniques used to find the adults and microfilariae in blood and tissues. Detection of lesions caused by adult worms depends on the care taken to find the location of the worms and their migration. Microfilariae are also often difficult to demonstrate. The Knott technique is most often used to search for microfilariae in the blood. It consists of mixing 1 ml of blood with 9 ml of 2% formalin solution, centrifugation, and examination of the sediment stained with aqueous methylene blue solution. This technique is a relatively old but proven method, but it has been generally replaced by filtration techniques using either millipore or nucleopore filters. With those species which localize in solid tissues other methods are employed. *Parafilaria bovicola* infections are diagnosed by detecting the microfilariae in the hemorrhagic exudate, while microfilariae of other species are looked for in deep scrapings or biopsies of skin.

Literature

Gradient centrifugation of peripheral blood was described for the concentration of microfilariae (Jones *et al.* 1975). The early filter techniques were found not to be useful for isolation and detection of microfilariae in dogs with *Dirofilaria immitis* infection (Palumbo and Perri 1972). Now standard procedure has been to use either 3 or 5 μm nucleopore membrane filters (G. S. Nelson, personal communication). In addition to morphological methods, various histochemical staining techniques were used to help identify microfilariae of man and domestic animals, and the acid-phospatase activity is a useful method (van Veen and Blotkamp 1978).

Diagnosis of dirofilariasis in dogs in the early literature was confused in that all microfilariae found were considered to be *D. immitis*. In 1956 microfilariae of *D. conditum* were identified and differentiated from *D. immitis* based on stained specimens. Microfilariae of *D. immitis* were longer and wider, with the most conspicuous feature being a pointed straight tail as compared to that of the *Dipetalonema* which ended in a sharp bend (Otto and Bauman 1959). Histochemical stains have also been used and differentiation of these two species described (Acevedo *et al.* 1981). Methods of preservation and storage of blood samples influenced the morphology of the microfilariae, particularly the size of the worms (Sawyer *et al.* 1963). Dirofilariasis without circulating microfilariae has been a diagnostic problem, and in these cases a persistent eosinophilia and the presence of serum antibodies to the microfilariae have been useful. Histological examination has revealed dead microfilariae in the lungs of these aparasitemic cases (Wong *et al.*

1973). Immunological tests have also been used in the diagnosis of canine dirofilariasis. Four kinds of filarial antigens were prepared from intrauterine microfilariae and had high sensitivity and specificity (Hayasaki 1981). The indirect fluorescent antibody test has been used to detect occult forms of dirofilariasis (Wong and Suter 1979). The sensitivity of *in vitro* lymphocyte proliferative responsiveness using antigen purified by affinity chromatography was found to be greater than that of serological tests (Welch and Dobson 1981). In filariasis of other domestic animals immunological tests have not been used extensively. A slide agglutination test has also been adapted for the diagnosis of *Deraiophoronema evansi* in camels with the antigen being prepared from microfilariae (Michael and Saleh 1977).

CHEMOTHERAPY

Antimonials are used to control some forms of filariasis in domestic ruminants in some countries, particularly in Asia. In many cases, because of the relatively mild nature of clinical signs, chemotherapy is usually not undertaken in the tropics. Canine dirofilariasis is controlled by arsenical thiacetarsamide, and the currently recommended treatment consists of two components, administration of the drug to kill the adult worms, and 6 weeks later a microfilaricide is given to eliminate the circulating microfilariae.

Literature

Levine (1968) reviewed the control and therapy of various forms of animals filariasis.

A recent summary of information on the control of human filariasis was published by Nelson (1981), and various advances in chemotherapy and needs for research were outlined. The use of diethylcarbamazine and a few of the new compounds for the treatment of filariasis in man was reviewed by Hawking (1979). He concluded that although many compounds are active against filarial worms, the only compound of practical general use in man continued to be diethylcarbamazine with Suramin being used specifically for onchocerciasis. Methods for testing compounds against filaricidal activity were presented by Denham (1979). The characteristics of ideal models of infections to be used for screening of drugs were discussed and included *Dirofilaria immitis* in the dog, *Brugia* species in the cat, and *Onchocerca* species in cattle. *Onchocerca gutturosa* infection in cattle was proposed as a possible tertiary screen for testing drugs against *O. volvulus* in man because, although it was not ideal, it was much more available than the more expensive *O. volvulus* lower primate models (Denham and Mellor 1976). The efficacy of new antifilarial drugs was evaluated on the basis of its effect on the migration of the larval stages of *D. immitis* (Kotani and Powers 1982).

A number of compounds have been tested for their filaricidal effects against *P. bovicola*. Levamisole hydrochloride, Nitroxynil, and Fenbendazole, at various doses and routes of administration, gave promising results with a 90% reduction of lesions (Viljoen 1976; Viljoen and Boomker 1977). Nitroxynil at doses of 20 mg/kg given twice 72 hours apart was found to be effective (Wellington 1978). Sodium antimony tartrate given twice a week intravenously for 3 weeks at doses of 20 ml of 2% solution was also effective (Sahai *et al.* 1965).

Two formulations of levamisole were used in Japan for treatment of chronic inflammatory lesions on the muzzle and teats of cattle caused by *S. okinawaensis*. Oral administration of either levamisole hydrochloride at doses of 7.5 g/100 kg body weight or with levamisole phosphate solution injected subcutaneously at doses of 364 mg/45 kg body weight were effective (Ueno and Chibana 1980). Hump sores caused by *S. assamensis* were treated with repeat application of Neguvon ointment (Srivastava and Malviya 1968).

McMullan (1972) reviewed the treatments which have been used in onchocerciasis in horses. Diethylcarbamazine in *O. cervicalis* infections at doses of 2 mg/0.45 kg of body weight for 21 days or longer relieved the pruritis and inflammation. Ivermectin at 2 mg|kg eliminated microfilariae from the skin 4 to 33 days after treatment, with clinical improvement occurring within 2 to 3 weeks. In 10 to 15% of the horses an edematous reaction occurred following injection at the site and on the lower portion of the abdomen (Herd and Donham 1983). Ivermectin was also effective against adult *S. equina* as well as microfilariae of *O. cervicalis* (Klei *et al.* 1980).

The treatment of canine dirofilariasis with thiacetarsamide sodium has been widely undertaken. Recommended doses of thiacetarsamide were 2.2 mg/kg given over 2 days (Keith *et al.* 1983a) and 0.75 mg/kg given intravenously for 3 days (Otto and Bauman 1959), but a variety of doses have been tested (Aubrey 1964). Diethylcarbamazine citrate has also been used successfully in prophylaxis at 200 mg/4.5 kg body weight for 3 days administered every 3 months (Aubrey 1964). Avermectins, an antiparasitic macrocyclic lactone, was evaluated and shown to suppress circulating microfilariae but had no effect against adults (Campbell and Blair 1978; Kotani and Powers 1982). Destruction of the adult worms resulted in resolution of the lesions if the dog survived the first month of treatment (Rawlings *et al.* 1983). The most severe sequelae to the therapy was pulmonary thromboembolism caused by dead adult worms being carried to the distal branches of pulmonary arteries (Keith *et al.* 1983b). The severity of these post-therapy adverse reactions were also related to the level of microfilaremia (Palumbo *et al.* 1981). Administration of aspirin and prednisolone affected the development of lesions, a significant decrease in the severity being observed with aspirin (Keith *et al.* 1983b). Surgical treatment of heartworm disease has been undertaken, but it is not a practical solution and is used only in special cases (Jackson 1969).

BIBLIOGRAPHY

Abramowsky, C. R., Powers, K. G., Aikawa, M. and Swinehart, G., 1981. *Dirofilaria immitis*. 5. Immunopathology of filarial nephropathy in dogs, *Am. J. Pathol.*, **104**: 1–12.

Acevedo, R. A., Theis, J. H., Kraus, J. F. and Longhurst, W. M., 1981. Combination of filtration and histochemical stain for detection and differentiation of *Dirofilaria immitis* and *Dipetalonema reconditum* in the dog, *Am. J. vet. Res.*, **42**(3): 537–40.

Adcock, J. L., 1961. Pulmonary arterial lesions in canine dirofilariasis, *Am. J. vet. Res.* **22**: 655–62.

Agrawal, M. C. and Dutt, S. C., 1976. Sex ratio in *Stephanofilaria zaheeri* Singh 1958, infection in buffaloes, *Indian vet. J.*, **53**: 475–6.

Agrawal, M. C., Vegad, J. L. and Dutt, S. C., 1978. Pathology of naturally occurring *Stephanofilaria zaheeri* Singh, 1958 infection in buffaloes, *Indian J. Anim. Sci.*, **48**(4): 261–5.

Aikawa, M., Abramowsky, C., Powers, K. G. and Furrow, R., 1981. Dirofilariasis. IV. Glomerulonephropathy induced by *Dirofilaria immitis* infection, *Am. J. trop. Med. Hyg.*, **30**(1): 84–91.

Alcaino, H., Gorman, T., Torres, C. and Montes, G., 1977. Canine filariasis in the metropolitan area, Chile, *Arch. Med. Vet.*, **9**(1): 23–8.

Amakiri, S. F., 1972. Bovine filariasis in Nigeria – a preliminary report, *Bull. epiz. Dis. Afr.*, **21**(2): 123–8.

Atwell, R. B., 1980. Early stages of disease of the peripheral pulmonary arteries in canine dirofilariasis. *Aust. vet. J.*, **56**: 157–9.

Aubrey, J. N., 1964. Treatment of canine dirofilariasis in northern Australia, *Aust. vet. J.*, **40**: 161–2.

Bain, O., Chabaud, A.-G., Wanantasamruad, P. and Nabhitabhata, J., 1980. *Onchocerca sweetae* occurring in the buffalo in Thailand, *Ann. Parasitol. (Paris)*, **55**(2): 253–9.

Bech-Nielsen, S., Bornstein, S., Christensen, D., Wallgren, T.-B., Zakrisson, G. and Chirico, J., 1982a. *Parafilaria bovicola* (Tubangui 1934) in cattle: epizootiology – vector studies and experimental transmission of *Parafilaria bovicola* to cattle, *Am. J. vet. Res.*, **43**(6): 948–54.

Bech-Nielsen, S., Sjogren, U. and Lundquist, H., 1982b. *Parafilaria bovicola* (Tubangui 1934) in cattle: epizootiology – disease occurrence, *Am. J. vet. Res.*, **43**(6): 945–7.

Beveridge, I., Kummerow, E. and Wilkinson, P., 1979. The prevalence of *Onchocerca lienalis* in the gastrosplenic ligament of cattle in northern Queensland, *Aust. vet. J.*, **55**: 204–5.

Beveridge, I., Kummerow, E. L. and Wilkinson, P., 1980. Observations on *Onchocerca gibsoni* and nodule development in naturally infected cattle in Australia, *Z. Tropenmed. Parasit.*, **31**: 75–81.

Bohm, L. K. and Supperer, R., 1954. Weitere untersuchungen uber mikrofilarien als erreger der periodischen augenentzundung der Pferde, *Tierarztl. Monatsschr.*, **41**(3): 129–39.

Buckley, J. J. C. and Edeson, J. F. B., 1956. On the adult morphology of *Wuchereria* sp. (*malayi*?) from a monkey (*Macaca irus*) and from cats in Malaya, and on *Wuchereria pahagi* n.sp. from a dog and cat, *J. Helminthol.*, **30**(1): 1–20.

Buckley, J. J. C., Nelson, G. S. and Heisch, R. B., 1958. On *Wuchereria patei* n.sp. from the lymphatics of cats, dogs and genet cats on Pate Island, Kenya, *J. Helminthol.*, **32**(1–2): 73–80.

Bwangamoi, O., 1970. *Onchocerca guttorosa* in cattle in Uganda, *Vet. Rec.*, **86**: 286–7.

Cabrera, B. D., Arambulo, P. V. III. and Tongson, M. S., 1970. A preliminary note on the examination of native dogs for microfilaria of the subcutaneous filariid (*Dipetalonema*), *J. Phil. Vet Med. Ass.*, **2**(4): 116–18.

Campbell, W. C. and Blair, L. S., 1978. Efficacy of avermectins against *Dirofilaria immitis* in dogs, *J. Helminthol.*, **52**: 308–10.

Carmichael, I. H. and Koster, S., 1978. Bovine parafilariosis in southern Africa: a preliminary report, *Onderstepoort J. vet. Res.*, **45**: 213–14.

Chauhan, P. P. S. and Pande, B. P., 1972. Onchocercal lesions in aorta and ligamentum nuchae of buffaloes and bullocks: a histological study, *Indian J. Anim. Sci.*, **42**(10): 809–13.

Cheema, A. H. and Ivoghli, B., 1978. Bovine onchocerciasis caused by *Onchocerca armillata* and *O. guttorosa*, *Vet. Pathol.*, **15**: 495–505.

Chodnik, K. S., 1958. Histopathology of the aortic lesions in cattle infected with *Onchocerca armillata* (filariidae), *Ann. trop. Med. Parasit.*, **52**: 145–8.

Church, E. M., Georgi, J. R. and Robson, D. S., 1976. Analysis of the microfilarial periodicity of *Dirofilaria immitis*, *Cornell Vet.*, **66**: 333–46.

Clarkson, M. J., 1964. The species of *Onchocerca* in cattle in Kenya and Somalia, *Ann. Trop. Med. Hyg.*, **58**: 153–8.

Collins, R. C., 1973. Onchocerciasis of horses in southeastern Louisiana, *J. Parasitol.*, **59**(6): 1016–20.

Costa, H. M. A. and Freitas, M. G., 1962. *Dipetalonema reconditum* (Grassi, 1890) e *Dipetalonema grassii* (Noé, 1907) em caes de minas gerais (Nematoda: Filarioidea), *Arq. Esc. Vet.*, **14**: 91–101.

Denham, D. A., 1979. A review of methods for testing compounds for filaricidal activity, *J. Helminthol.*, **53**: 175–87.

Denham, D. A. and Mellor, P., 1976. The anthelmintic effects of a new compound 'E' (Friedheim) on *Onchocerca guttorosa* in the cow – a possible tertiary screening system for drug action against *O. volvulus* in man, *J. Helminthol.*, **50**: 49–52.

Deorani, V. P. S. and Dutt, S. C., 1967. Histopathology of parafilariasis in mules, *Curr. Sci.*, **36**: 240–1.

Desowitz, R. S., Barnwell, J. W., Palumbo, N. E., Una, S. R. and Perri, S. F., 1978. Rapid decrease of precipitating and reaginic antibodies in *Dirofilaria immitis*-infected dogs which develop severe adverse reactions following treatment with diethylcarbamazine, *Am. J. Trop. Med. Hyg.*, **27**(6): 1148–51.

Dissanaike, A. S., 1979. Zoonotic aspects of filarial infections in man, *Bull. Wld Hlth Org.*, **57**(3): 349–57.

Eberhard, M. L., 1979. Studies on the *Onchocerca* (Nematoda: Filarioidea) found in cattle in the United States. I. Systematics of *O. guttorosa* and *O. lienalis* with a description of *O. stilesi* sp.n., *J. Parasitol.*, **65**(3): 379–88.

Edeson, J. F. B., 1962. The epidemiology and treatment of infection due to *Brugia malayi*, *Bull. Wld Hlth Org.*, **27**: 529–41.

Eichler, D. A. and Nelson, G. S., 1968. The distribution of microfilariae of *Onchocerca guttorosa* in the skin of cattle and laboratory rat, *Trans. R. Soc. trop. Med. Hyg.*, **62**(1): 9–10.

Elbihari, S. and Hussein, H. S., 1978. *Onchocerca guttorosa* (Neumann, 1910) in Sudanese cattle. I. The microfilariae, *Rev. Elev. Méd. vét. Pays trop.*, **31**(2): 179–82.

Gibson, C. L., 1952. Comparative morphology of the skin-inhabiting microfilariae of man, cattle, and equines in Guatemala, *Am. J. Trop. Med. Hyg.*, **1**: 250–61.

Gibson, D. W., Heggie, C. and Connor, D. H., 1980. Clinical and pathological aspects of onchocerciasis, *Pathol. Ann.*, **15**(2): 195–240.

Gittelman, H. J., Grieve, R. B., Hitchings, M. M., Jacobson, R. H. and Cypess, R. H., 1981. Quantitative fluorescent immunoassay for measurement of antibody to *Dirofilaria immitis* in dogs, *J. Clin. Microbiol.*, **13**(2): 309–12.

Grieve, R. B., Gebhardt, B. M. and Bradley, R. E. Sr, 1979. *Dirofilaria immitis*: cell-mediated and humoral immune responses in experimentally infected dogs, *Int. J. Parasitol.*, **9**: 275–9.

Gubler, D. J., 1966. A comparative study on the distribution incidence and periodicity of the canine filarial worms *Dirofilaria immitis* Leidy and *Dipetalonema reconditum* Grassi in Hawaii, *J. Med. Ent.*, **3**(2): 159–67.

Guterbock, W. M., Vestre, W. A. and Todd, K. S. Jr, 1981. Ocular dirofilariasis in the dog, *Mod. Vet. Pract.*, **62**: 45–7.

Hawking, F., 1979. Diethylcarbamazine and new compounds for the treatment of filariasis, *Adv. Pharmacol. Chemother.*, **16**: 129–94.

Hawking, F., Moore, P., Gammage, K. and Worms, M. J., 1967.

Periodicity of microfilariae XII. The effect of variations in host body temperature on the cycle of *Loa loa, Monnigofilaria setariosa, Dirofilaria immitis* and other filariae, *Trans. R. Soc. trop. Med. Hyg.*, **61**(5): 674–83.

Hayasaki, M., 1981. Indirect hemagglutination test for diagnosis of canine filariasis, *Jap. J. vet. Sci.*, **43**: 21–6.

Healy, G. R. and Kagan, I. G., 1960. The prevalence of filariasis in dogs from Atlanta, Georgia, *J. Parasitol.*, **47**: 90.

Hennigar, G. R. and Ferguson, R. W., 1957. Pulmonary vascular sclerosis as a result of *Dirofilaria immitis* infection in dogs, *J. Am. vet. med. Ass.*, **131**: 136–340.

Herd, R. P. and Donham, J. C., 1983. Efficacy of ivermectin against *Onchocerca cervicalis* microfilarial dermatitis in horses, *Am. J. vet. Res.*, **44**(6): 1102–5.

Herin, V. and Fain, A., 1955. Filarioses des bovidés au Ruanda-Urundi. II. Etude histopathologique, *Ann. Soc. Belge. Med. Trop.*, **35**: 523–33.

Ishihara, K., Kitagawa, H., Ojima, M., Yagata, Y. and Suganuma, Y., 1978. Clinicopathological studies on canine dirofilarial hemoglobinuria, *Jap. J. vet. Sci.*, **40**: 525–37.

Ishihara, K., Kitagawa, H., Yokoyama, S. and Ohashi, H., 1981. Studies on hemolysis in canine dirofilarial hemoglobinuria lipid alterations in blood serum and red cell membrane, *Jap. J. vet. Sci.*, **43**: 1–11.

Isshiki, O., 1964a. Studies on bovine onchocerciasis in Korea. II. Morphological characters of the female of *Onchocerca gibsoni* Cleland and Johnston, 1910, with special reference to its body wall structure, *Jap. J. vet. Sci.*, **26**: 151–8.

Isshiki, O., 1964b. Studies on bovine onchocerciasis in Korea. III. Comparison of embryonated eggs *in utero* between *Onchocerca gibsoni*, Cleland and Johnston, 1910 and *O. guttorosa*, Neumann, 1910, *Jap. J. vet. Sci.*, **26**: 259–66.

Isshiki, O., 1964c. Studies on bovine onchocerciasis in Korea. IV. Morphology of microfilariae of *Onchocerca gibsoni* Cleland and Johnston, 1910 and their distribution in the nodule, *Jap. J. vet. Sci.*, **26**: 285–94.

Jackson, R. F., von Lichtenberg, F. and Otto, G. F., 1962. Occurrence of adult heartworms in the venae cavae of dogs, *J. Am. vet. med. Ass.*, **41**: 117–21.

Jackson, W. F., 1969. Surgical treatment of heartworm disease, *J. Am. vet. med. Ass.*, **154**: 383–4.

Jensen, R. and Seghetti, L., 1955. Elaeophoriasis in sheep, *J. Am. vet. med. Ass.*, **127**: 499–505.

Jones, T. C., Mott, K. and Pedrosa, L. C., 1975. A technique for isolating and concentrating microfilariae from peripheral blood by gradient centrifugation, *Trans, R. Soc. trop. Med. Hyg.*, **69**(2): 243–6.

Kagan, I. G., 1963. A review of immunologic methods for the diagnosis of filariasis, *J. Parasitol.*, **49**(5): 773–98.

Kan, S. P., Rajah, K. V. and Dissanaike, A. S., 1977. Survey of dirofilariasis among dogs in Seremban, Malaysia, *Vet. Parasitol.*, **3**: 177–81.

Kazacos, K. R., 1978. The prevalence of heartworm (*Dirofilaria immitis*) in dogs from Indiana, *J. Parasitol.*, **64**(5): 959–60.

Keith, J. C., Rawlings, C. A. and Schaub, R. G., 1983a. Treatment of canine dirofilariasis: pulmonary thromboembolism caused by thiacetarsamide – microscopic changes, *Am. J. vet. Res.*, **44**(7): 1272–7.

Keith, J. C., Rawlings, C. A. and Schaub, R. G., 1983b. Pulmonary thromboembolism during therapy of dirofilariasis with thiacetarsamide: modification with aspirin or prednisolone, *Am. J. vet. Res.*, **44**(7): 1278–83.

Khamis, Y., Helmy, N. and Fahmy, L., 1973. Filariasis in buffaloes and cattle, *Vet. Med. Rev.*, No. 4: 305–18.

Klei, T. R., Torbert, B. J. and Ochoa, R., 1980. Efficacy of ivermectin (22, 23-dihydroavermectin B_1) against adult *Setaria equina* and microfilariae of *Onchocerca cervicalis* in ponies, *J. Parasitol.*, **66**(5): 859–61.

Korkejian, A. and Edeson, J. F. B., 1978. Studies on naturally occurring filarial infections in dogs in Lebanon, I. *Dipetalonema reconditum, Ann. Trop. Med. Parasitol.*, **72**(1): 65–78.

Kotani, T. and Powers, K. G., 1982. Developmental stages of *Dirofilaria immitis* in the dog, *Am. J. vet. Res.*, **43**(12): 2199–206.

Kume, S. and Itagaki, S., 1955. On the life-cycle of *Dirofilaria immitis* in the dog as the final host, *Br. vet. J.*, **3**: 16–24.

Ladds, P. W., Nitisuwirjo, S. and Goddard, M. E., 1979. Epidemiological and gross pathological studies of *Onchocerca gibsoni* infection in cattle, *Aust. vet. J.*, **55**: 455–62.

Lavers, D. W., Spratt, D. M. and Thomas, C., 1969. *Dirofilaria immitis* from the eye of a dog, *Aust. vet. J.*, **45**: 284–6.

Levine, N. D., 1968. Filarial nematodes. In *Nematode Parasites of Domestic Animals and Man*. Burgess Publishing Co. (Minneapolis, USA), pp. 436–518.

Loke, Y. W. and Ramachandran, C. P., 1967. The pathology of lesions in cattle caused by *Stephanofilaria kaeli* Buckley, 1937, *J. Helminthol.*, **41**(2–3): 161–6.

Malek, E. A., 1958. Occurrence of *Onchocerca armillata* Railliet and Henry, 1909, in Sudanese cattle, *Bos indicus, J. Parasitol.*, **44**(2): 30–1.

Mandelli, G. and Mantovani, A., 1966. Study of a case of massive infestation of *Dirofilaria repens* in a dog, *Parasitologia*, **8**(1): 21–8.

Marcoux, M., Fréchette, J. L. and Morin, M., 1977. Infection by *Onchocerca cervicalis* in Québec: clinical signs and diagnostic method, *Can. Vet. J.*, **18**(4): 108–10.

Marolt, J., Zuković, M. and Molan, M., 1966. Equine onchocerciasis. A. Contribution to the etiology of lameness and diseases of the skin and eyes, *Tierarztl. Wchschr.*, **73**(6): 130–4.

McMahon, J. P., 1968. Artificial feeding of *Simulium* vectors of human and bovine onchocerciasis, *Bull. Wld Hlth Org.*, **38**: 957–66.

McMullan, W. C., 1972. Onchocercal filariasis, *Swest. Vet.*, **25**(3): 179–91.

Mellor, P. S., 1973. Studies on *Onchocerca cervicalis* Railliet and Henry 1910: II. Pathology in the horse, *J. Helminthol.*, **47**(2): 111–18.

Mellor, P. S., 1974. Studies on *Onchocerca cervicalis* Railliet and Henry 1910: III. Morphological and taxonomic studies on *Onchocerca cervicalis* from British horses, *J. Helminthol.*, **48**(2): 145–53.

Michael, S. A. and Saleh, S. M., 1977. The slide agglutination test for the diagnosis of filariasis in camels, *Trop. Anim. Hlth Prod.*, **9**: 241–4.

Mirzayans, A. and Maghsoodloo, H., 1977. Filarial infection of equidae in the Tehran area of Iran, *Trop. Anim. Hlth Prod.*, **9**: 19–20.

Mortelmans, J., 1961. Aperçu des filarioses animales, *Ann. Soc. Belge. Méd. Trop.*, **4**: 307–322

Mueller, R., 1979. Identification of *Onchocerca*. In *Problems in the Identification of Parasites and their Vectors*, Seventeenth Symp. Br. Soc. of Parasitology, eds. E. R. Taylor, R. Mueller. Oxford and Blackwell Scientific Publications, vol. 17, pp. 175–206.

Nelson, G. S., 1964. Factors influencing the development and behavior of filarial nematodes in their arthropodan hosts. In *Host Parasite Relationships in Invertebrate Hosts*. Second Symp. Br. Soc. of Parasitology, ed. E. R. Taylor. Oxford and Blackwell Scientific Publications, pp. 75–119.

Nelson, G. S., 1965a. The pathology of filarial infections, *Helminthol. Abstr.*, **35**(4): 311–36.

Nelson, G. S., 1965b. Filarial infections as zoonoses, *J. Helminthol.*, **39**(2–3): 220–50.

Nelson, G. S., 1970. Onchocerciasis, *Adv. Parasitol.*, **8**: 173–224.

Nelson, G. S., 1981. Issues in filariasis – a century of enquiry and a century of failure, *Acta trop.*, **38**: 197–204.

Nelson, G. S. and Heisch, R. B., 1957. Microfilariae like those of *Wuchereria malayi* in dogs and cats in East Africa, *Trans. R. Soc. trop. Med. Hyg.*, **51**: 90.

Nelson, G. S., Heisch, R. B. and Furlong, M., 1962. Studies in filariasis in East Africa. II. Filarial infections in man, animals, and mosquitoes on the Kenya coast, *Trans. R. Soc. trop. Med. Hyg.*, **56**(3): 202–17.

Nevill, E. M., 1975. Preliminary report on the transmission of *Parafilaria bovicola* in South Africa, *Onderstepoort J. vet. Res.*, **42**(1): 41–8.

Newton, W. L. and Wright, W. H., 1956. The occurrence of a dog filariid other than *Dirofilaria immitis* in the United States, *J. Parasitol.*, **42**: 246–58.

Niilo, L., 1968. Bovine hemorrhagic filariasis in cattle imported into Canada, *Can. Vet. J.*, **9**(6): 132–7.

Nitisuwirjo, S. and Ladds, P. W., 1980. A quantitative histopathological study of *Onchocerca gibsoni* nodules in cattle, *Z. Tropenmed. Parasit.*, **31**: 467–74.

Ottley, M. L., Dallemagne, C. and Moorhouse, D. E., 1983. Equine onchocerciasis in Queensland and the Northern Territory of Australia, *Aust. vet. J.*, **60**(7): 200–3.

Ottley, M. L. and Moorhouse, D. E., 1978a. Bovine onchocerciasis: aspects of carcase infection, *Aust. vet. J.*, **54**: 528–30.

Ottley, M. L. and Moorhouse, D. E., 1978b. Equine onchocerciasis, *Aust. vet. J.*, **54**: 545.

Ottley, M. L. and Moorhouse, D. E., 1979. *Onchocerca* (Nematoda: Filarioidea) from Queensland cattle: a redescription of *Onchocerca gibsoni* (Cleland and Johnston) and *O. lienalis* (Stiles), *Zool. Anz.*, **203**(5–6): 369–77.

Otto, G. F., 1969. Geographical distribution, vectors, and life cycle of *Dirofilaria immitis, J. Am. vet. med. Ass.*, **154**: 370–3.

Otto, G. E. and Bauman, P. M., 1959. Canine filariasis, *Vet. Med.*, **54**: 87–96.

Palumbo, N. E., Desowitz, R. S. and Perri, S. F., 1981. Observations on the adverse reaction to diethylcarbamazine in *Dirofilaria immitis*-infected dogs, *Tropenmed. Parasit.*, **32**: 115–18.

Palumbo, N. E. and Perri, S. F., 1972. Some observations on diagnosis of canine filariasis, *J. Am vet. med. Ass.*, **160**(5): 715–19.

Patnaik, B., 1962. Onchocerciasis due to *O. armillata* in cattle in Orissa, *J. Helminthol.*, **36**(3): 313–26.

Prasad, M. C. and Bhalla, N. P., 1977. Pathology of aortic elaeophoriasis in Indian water buffaloes (*Bubalus bubalis*), *Indian vet. J.*, **54**: 97–101.

Rabalais, F. C., Eberhard, M. L., Ashley, D. C. and Platt, T. R., 1974. Survey for equine onchocerciasis in the mid-western United States, *Am. J. vet. Res.*, **35**(1): 125–6.

Rahman, M. H., 1957. Observations on the mode of infection of the hump of cattle by *Stephanofilaria assamensis* in East Pakistan, *J. Parasitol.*, **43**: 434–5.

Ramanujachari, G. and Alwar, V. S., 1953. Indian pig (*Sus scrofa domestica*) as a host for *Onchocerca* sp. and *Enterobius vermicularis*, *Indian vet. J.*, **29**(4): 329.

Ramanujachari, G. and Alwar, V. S., 1954. Further observations on parafilariasis (?) of elephants, *Indian vet. J.*, **31**(3): 206–9.

Rao, A. T. and Acharjyo, L. N., 1971. Histopathological changes in some of the organs in heartworm infection in an Indian fox (*Vulpes bengalensis*), *Indian vet. J.*, **48**(4): 342–4.

Rawlings, C. A., 1978. Pulmonary vascular response of dogs with heartworm disease, *Can. J. comp. Med.*, **42**(4): 452–9.

Rawlings, C. A., 1980. Cardiopulmonary function in the dog with *Dirofilaria immitis* infection: during infection and after treatment, *Am. J. vet. Res.*, **41**(3): 319–25.

Rawlings, C. A., Losonsky, J. M., Schaub, R. G., Greene, C. E., Keith, J. C. and McCall, J. W., 1983. Post-adulticide changes in *Dirofilaria immitis*-infected beagles, *Am. J. vet. Res.*, **44**(1): 8–15.

Retnasabapathy, A. and San, K. T., 1976. Incidence of canine heartworm (*Dirofilaria immitis*) in Malaysia, *Vet. Rec.*, **98**(4): 68–9.

Riek, R. F., 1954. Studies on allergic dermatitis (Queensland itch) of the horse: the aetiology of the disease, *Aust. J. Agric. Res.*, **5**(1): 109–28.

Roberts, S. R., 1963. Etiology of equine periodic ophthalmia, *Am. J. Ophthal.*, **55**: 1049–55.

Rodger, F. C., 1962. A review of recent advances in scientific knowledge of the symptomatology, pathology and pathogenesis of onchocercal infections, *Bull. Wld Hlth Org.*, **27**: 429–48.

Rogers, R., Denham, D. A., Nelson, G. S., Guy, F. and Ponnudurai, T., 1975. Studies with *Brugia pahangi*. III. Histological changes in the affected lymph nodes of infected cats, *Ann. trop. Med. Parasit.*, **69**(1): 77–84.

Sahai, B. N., Singh, S. P. and Srivastava, V. K., 1965. Chemotherapy of parafilariasis in bovines, *Indian vet. J.*, **42**: 881–3.

Sawyer, T. K., Weinstein, P. P. and Bloch, J., 1963. Canine filariasis – the influence of the method of treatment on measurements of microfilariae in blood samples, *Am. J. vet. Res.*, **24**(100): 395–401.

Schacher, J. F. and Sahyoun, P. F., 1967. A chronological study of the histopathology of filarial disease in cats and dogs caused by *Brugia pahangi* (Buckley and Edeson, 1956), *Trans. R. Soc. trop. Med. Hyg.*, **61**(2): 234–43.

Schaub, R. G. and Rawlings, C. A., 1980. Pulmonary vascular response during phases of canine heartworm disease; scanning electron microscopic study, *Am. J. vet. Res.*, **41**(7): 1082–9.

Schaub, R. G., Rawlings, C. A. and Stewart, G. J., 1980. Scanning electron microscopy of canine pulmonary arteries and veins, *Am. J. vet. Res.*, **41**(9): 1441–6.

Schmidt, G. M., Krehbiel, J. D., Coley, S. C. and Leid, R. W., 1982b. Equine ocular onchocerciasis: histopathologic study, *Am. J. vet.* midwestern U.S. horses, *Vet. Pathol.*, **19**: 16–22.

Schmidt, G. M., Krehbiel, J. D., Coley, S. C. and Leid, R. W., 1982b. Equine ocular onchocerciasis: histopathologic study, *Am. J. vet. Res.*, **43**(8): 1371–5.

Scholtens, R. G., 1975. Filarial infections – with a note on dracunculiasis. In *Diseases Transmitted from Animals to Man*, eds W. T. Hubbert, W. F. McCulloch, P. R. Schnurrenberger. Charles C. Thomas (Springfield, Ill.), pp. 572–83.

Scott, D. W., 1979. Nodular skin disease associated with *Dirofilaria immitis* infection in the dog, *Cornell Vet.*, **69**: 233–40.

Segedy, A. K. and Hayden, D. W., 1978. Cerebral vascular accident caused by *Dirofilaria immitis* in a dog, *J. Am. Anim. Hosp. Ass.*, **14**(6): 752–6.

Shastri, U. V., 1973. A preliminary note on filarial infections in cattle (*Bos indicus*) and buffaloes (*Bubalus bubalis*) in Maharashtra, *Indian J. Anim. Hlth.*, **49**: 193–5.

Shirota, K., Takahashi, R., Fujiwara, K. and Hasegawa, A., 1979. Canine interstitial nephritis with special reference to glomerular lesions and filariasis, *Jap. J. vet. Sci.*, **41**: 119–29.

Singh, D. V., Joshi, H. C. and Shivnani, G. A., 1972. Blood chemical changes in and chemotherapy of microfilariasis of buffaloes, *Phil. J. Vet. Med.*, **11**(2): 101–9.

Singh, D. V., Joshi, H. C. and Shivnani, G. A., 1973. Biochemical and haematological studies in microfilariasis of buffaloes, *Indian J. Exp. Biol.*, **11**: 336–7.

Spratt, D. M. and Moorhouse, D. E., 1971. *Onchocerca sweetae* sp.nov. (Nematoda: Filarioidea), a parasite of the water buffalo (*Bubalus bubalis*) from northern Australia, *Zool. Anz.*, **186**(1–2): 147–53.

Srivastava, H. D. and Malviya, H. C., 1968. Treatment of 'humpsore' in cattle caused by *Stephanofilaria assamensis*, *Indian vet. J.*, **45**: 484–8.

Srivastava, S. C. and Pande, B. P., 1965. Occurrence of aortic onchocerciasis and spirocercosis in buffalo-calves with a note on the reports in other domestic animals, *Indian J. vet. Sci.*, **34**(4): 222–31.

Supperer, R., 1966. Onchocerosis in animals, *Berl. Münch. Tierarztl. Wochenschr.*, **79**(1): 10–14.

Thrall, D. E., Badertscher, R. R., Lewis, R. E. and McCall, J. W., 1979a. Scintigraphic evaluation of pulmonary perfusion in dogs experimentally infected with *Dirofilaria immitis*, *Am. J. vet. Res.*, **40**(10): 1426–32.

Thrall, D. E., Badertscher, R. R. II., McCall, J. W. and Lewis, R. E., 1979b. The pulmonary arterial circulation in dogs experimentally infected with *Dirofilaria immitis*: its angiographic evaluation, *J. Am. Vet. Radiol. Soc.*, **20**: 74–8.

Todd, K. S. Jr and Howland, T. P., 1983. Transplacental transmission of *Dirofilaria immitis* microfilariae in the dog, *J. Parasitol.*, **69**(2): 371.

Tolbert, R. H. and Johnson, W. E., Jr., 1982. Potential vectors of *Dirofilaria immitis* in Macon County, Alabama, *Am. J. vet. Res.*, **43**(11): 2054–6.

Ueno, H. and Chibana, T., 1980. Clinical and parasitological evaluations of levamisole as a treatment for bovine stephanofilariasis, *Vet. Parasitol.*, **7**: 59–68.

van Veen, T. W. S. and Blotkamp, J., 1978. Histochemical differentiation of microfilariae of *Dipetalonema, Dirofilaria, Onchocerca* and *Setaria* spp. of man and domestic animals in the Zaria area (Nigeria), *Z. Tropenmed. Parasit.*, **29**(1): 1–136.

Venkataratnam, A. and Kershaw, W. E., 1961. Distribution of the microfilariae of onchocerca in the skin of cattle, *Ann. Soc. Belge Méd. Trop.*, **41**(4): 323–8.

Viljoen, J. H., 1976. Studies on *Parafilaria bovicola* (Tubangui 1934). 1. Clinical observations and chemotherapy, *J. S. Afr. vet. med. Ass.*, **47**(3): 161–9.

Viljoen, J. H. and Boomker, J. D. F., 1977. Studies on *Parafilaria bovicola* Tubangui, 1934. 2. Chemotherapy and pathology, *Onderstepoort J. vet. Res.*, **44**(2): 107–12.

von Lichtenberg, F., Jackson, R. F. and Otto, G. F., 1962. Hepatic lesions in dogs with dirofilariasis, *J. Am vet. med. Ass.*, **141**(1): 121–8.

Walters, L. L., Lavoipierre, M. M. J., Timm, K. I. and Jahn, S. E., 1981. Endemicity of *Dirofilaria immitis* and *Dipetalonema reconditum* in dogs of Pleasants Valley, northern California, *Am. J. vet. Res.*, **42**(1): 151–4.

Webster, W. A. and Wilkins, D. B., 1970. The recovery of *Parafilaria bovicola* Tubangui, 1934 from an imported Charolais bull, *Can. Vet. J.*, **11**(1): 13–14.

Weil, G. J., Ottesen, E. A. and Powers, K. G., 1981. *Dirofilaria immitis*: parasite-specific humoral and cellular immune responses in experimentally infected dogs, *Exp. Parasitol.*, **51**: 80–6.

Welch, J. S. and Dobson, C., 1981. Imunodiagnosis of parasitic zoonoses: sensitivity and specificity of *in vitro* lymphocyte proliferative responsiveness using nematode antigens purified by affinity chromatography, *Trans. R. Soc. trop. Med. Hyg.*, **75**(1): 5–14.

Wellington, A. C., 1978. The effect of nitroxynil on *Parafilaria bovicola* infestations in cattle, *J. S. Afr. vet. med. Ass.*, **49**(2): 131–2.

Wilson, T., 1961. Filariasis in Malaya – a general review, *Trans. R. Soc. trop. Med. Hyg.*, **55**(1): 107–29.

Wong, M. M., 1964. Studies on microfilaremia in dogs, *Am. J. Trop. Med. Hyg.*, **13**: 57–77.

Wong, M. M., 1974a. Experimental dirofilariases in macaques. Susceptibility and host responses to *Dirofilaria immitis*, the dog heartworm, *Trans. R. Soc. trop. Med. Hyg.*, **68**(6): 479–90.

Wong, M. M., 1974b. Experimental occult dirofilariasis in dogs with reference to immunological responses and its relationship to tropical eosinophilia in man, *Southeast Asian J. Trop. Med. Pub. Hlth*, **5**(4): 480–6.

Wong, M. M. and Suter, P. F., 1979. Indirect fluorescent antibody test in occult dirofilariasis, *Am. J. vet. Res.*, **40**(3): 414–20.

Wong, M. M., Suter, P. F., Rhode, E. A. and Guest, M. F., 1973. Dirofilariasis without circulating microfilariae; a problem in diagnosis, *J. Am. vet. med. Ass.*, **163**(2): 133–9.

World Health Organization Scientific Working Group on Filariasis, 1981. The immunology of filariasis, *Bull. Wld Hlth Org.*, **59**(1): 1–8.

Zak, F., 1975. Parasite aortopathy due to *Onchocerca armillata* in cattle, *Path Microbiol.*, **43**: 150.

Chapter

24

Fascioliasis (*Fasciola gigantica*)

CONTENTS

INTRODUCTION

Fascioliasis is a disease caused by flukes and is widely distributed throughout the world. A large volume of literature has been published on various *Fasciola* species and those disease syndromes which occur in nontropical regions. This chapter is limited to presentation and discussion of information on a tropical form of fascioliasis, the liver disease caused by *F. gigantica*, a species of particular importance in Africa and Asia. The focus is on the features of *F. gigantica* and the disease it causes which are specific to this species. In the tropics *F. hepatica* is commonly observed in the cooler regions found at higher elevations while *F. gigantica* is primarily found in the lowlands. The distribution of the two species overlap in many tropical areas.

Literature

There is a considerable amount of literature published on *F. hepatica*, while information of *F. gigantica* is incomplete. Fascioliasis in ruminants, including the syndrome caused by *F. gigantica* was reviewed by Malek (1980). Other published reviews include a report on experimental fascioliasis caused by *F. hepatica* in Australia (Boray 1969), and the invasive stages of this species in a mammalian host (Dawes and Hughes 1964). Schillhorn van Veen (1980) published a comprehensive short review specifically on the syndrome in West Africa caused by *F. gigantica*. El-Azazy and Schillhorn van Veen (1983) reviewed the most recent information on animal fasciolisasis and schistosomiasis in Egypt and the Sudan.

ETIOLOGY

Fasciola gigantica is longer and slightly narrower than *F. hepatica*. The life cycle in the snail and vertebrate host is similar in both species.

Relatively few metabolic studies on *F. gigantica* are available, but it is likely that most features of the basic physiology of this species are comparable to that of *F. hepatica* on which information is available.

Literature

The morphology of *F. gigantica* as observed in India was investigated to determine the validity of reclassifying the parasite found in this region as *F. indica*. It was concluded that on a morphological basis there were no grounds for classifying it as another species (Malviya 1967). The morphology of *Fasciola* worms found in buffalo, cattle and sheep in Egypt was also studied (Haiba and Selim 1960a).

The carbohydrate reserves of *F. gigantica* were in glycogen and most of the energy was derived in an aerobic environment (Goil 1961a; Al-Barwari and Abdel-Fattah 1975–76), and was affected by temperature and pH (Al-Barwari 1975–76). The rate of oxygen consumption and hemoglobin contents was also studied (Goil 1961b, c). Enzymes of *F. gigantica* have been investigated histochemically (Michael and Awadalla 1976). Specific and nonspecific cholinesterose activity of homogenate whole flukes were studied by Durrani *et al.* (1982).

EPIZOOTIOLOGY

Geographic distribution and incidence

The two species, *F. hepatica* and *F. gigantica*, have worldwide distribution, with *F. hepatica* having a wider range than *F. gigantica*. Fascioliasis caused by the latter species is widespread through Africa, Asia, and Hawaii and in many countries both species occur.

Fascioliasis accounts for serious economic losses in Africa due to reduced productivity and condemnation of large numbers of infected livers. The incidence varies depending on the climatic conditions, availability of permanent water, and particularly on grazing practices. Considerable differences in prevalence of infections and severity of disease syndromes are evident in various geographical regions. Incidences of severe infections are usually available from records which, however, are not always reliable in slaughter facilities. Frequency of infections depends on source of water, and in irrigation schemes with large snail populations 90 and 100% of cattle, sheep, and buffalo have the parasites. Cases of severe acute disease are observed 6 to 8 months after the end of the wet season.

In addition to domestic ruminants, rodents, pigs, equines, carnivores, and primates including man can be infected. The host range is probably as wide as that for *F. hepatica* and wild herbivores may serve as reservoirs. *Fasciola gigantica* is better adapted as a parasite of cattle than *F. hepatica* and also differs in its ability to infest laboratory animals.

Literature

The incidence of *F. gigantica* in various African countries was summarized by Malek (1980). The disease in West Africa, with particular reference to the major epizootic aspects related to the distribution of the intermediate host, *Lymnaea natalensis*, was reviewed by Schillhorn van Veen (1980). As an example of the high rate of infection between 1973 and 1977 the incidence was 65.4% in cattle, 40.8% in sheep, and 17.6% in goats, with the incidence being highest during and just after the rainy season (Schillhorn van Veen *et al.* 1980). In southern Nigeria the incidence on parasitological examination in cattle was 2.5%, with a mortality rate of 1% and a liver condemnation rate of 7% (Ogunrinade and Ogunrinade 1980). Additional information on prevalence was presented from Nigeria based on abattoir records from 1971 to 1976 (Ogunrinade *et al.* 1981). The incidence in trade cattle in eastern Nigeria was also reported by Ikeme and Obioha (1973). Variations in prevalence could have been due to differences in the quality of meat inspection, and whether indeed slaughter records or other data were used.

In eastern Africa, reports on prevalence are available from several countries. In an abattoir survey undertaken in Kenya from 1972 to 1975, 13 to 21% of livers were condemned (Preston and Castelino 1977). Breed differences were observed, with Boran cattle (*Bos indicus*) having lower infection rates and fluke burdens than *B. taurus* cattle. Aberdeen Angus had a lower infestation rate than Friesian–Boran crosses and Herefords (Castelino and Preston 1979). The small Zebu type cattle also had a level of infection lower than the exotic and large Zebu breeds. An association was made between the incidence and the level of rainfall in different regions of Kenya (Bitakaramire 1973a). In Zambia, the incidence in cattle over a number of years was also high, from 80 to 90% as determined by numbers of condemned livers (Silangwa 1973). In Malawi, the incidence varied from 10 to 60% from one district to another. The incidence of immature flukes was highest in the rainy season, September to December, and of mature flukes from December to March (Mzembe and Chaudhry 1981). Fascioliasis was considered to be one of the most important parasitic diseases in Zimbabwe with high rates of liver condemnations (Condy 1962). Economic losses as determined by abattoir surveys have been estimated in Kenya (Preston and Castelino 1977), Uganda (Coyle 1956), South Africa (Purchase 1957), Mozambique (Alves 1970), the Sudan (Eisa and Dalil 1963; Magzoub and Adam 1977), and Ethiopia (Gemechu and Mamo 1979).

In wild ruminants, *F. gigantica* has been found either in bile ducts or in gall bladders in approximately 50% of the following animals: African buffalo (*Syncerus caffer*), Uganda kob (*Adenota* (*Kobus*) *kob*) and hartebeest (*Alcelaphus buselaphus jacksoni*) (Bindernagel 1972). This species of fluke has also been found in the liver of the Indian rhinoceros (*Rhinoceros unicornis*) (Bhattacharjee and Halder 1971) and in the warthog (*Phacochoerus aethiopicus*) (Troncy *et al.* 1973).

Outside Africa, surveys of *F. gigantica* infestation among animals slaughtered have been reported from Iraq (Al-Barwari 1977), Jordan (Ismail *et al.* 1978), Turkmenia (Kibakin 1968), Israel (Nobel *et al.* 1972), Egypt (Zaki 1960) and Saudi Arabia, where the prevalence in cattle and camels was higher in those areas which had increased rainfall and/or irrigation schemes (Magzoub and Kasim 1978). Reports were also available from Indonesia on rates of infection in water buffalo and cattle (Edney and Muchlis 1963; Rivai 1979; Soesetya 1975).

Transmission

In many tropical regions the search for feed and water results in migratory livestock-raising methods. This often exposes animals to high levels of infestation by metacercaria in areas of limited and crowded watering sources.

In the water, development of eggs takes place under optimal temperatures for 10 to 15 days. A fully developed miracidium leaves the egg and swims actively to invade species of snails in the family Lymnaeidae. Sporocysts develop from each miracidium and progress through the rediae stages to cercariae. The rate of development in snail hosts is also affected by environmental factors, particularly temperature. Cercariae develop into metacercariae and are ingested by the mammalian host through drinking or eating infested water and grasses. Transmission can also occur when grasses are harvested from watersides and are fed as hay or straw. Development in the snails to the metacercarial stage takes 2 to 3 months, and in cattle 1 to 2 months are required for acute clinical signs to develop.

The intermediate hosts and *F. gigantica* have features in their life cycle which make them adaptable to tropical environments. *Lymnaea natalensis* is the common species which serves as the intermediate host in Africa. A very high degree of intermediate host specificity occurs with different species of *Fasciola*. Within a species of flukes, biologically distinct races can be distinguished to some degree by their ability to select different species and subspecies of lymnaeid snails.

Literature

Kendall (1965) presented a comprehensive review of the relationships between various species of *Fasciola* and their snail hosts. Cross-infection by *F. gigantica* and *F. hepatica* in some species of *Lymnaea* have also been reported (El Harith 1980b). The geographical distributions of fascioliasis, including other trematode infections of veterinary importance, were presented by Over (1982).

Distributions of *L. natalensis* as a potential host of *F. gigantica* was reported in Ghana (McCullough 1965) and Togo (Séguin 1976). The levels of infestation of watering sources for livestock depended on prevalence of snails, their levels of infection, and the seasonal temperatures. In Malawi, snail infections were high in April and May with the release of most metacercariae occurring in August and October (Mzembe and Chaudhry 1979). Seasonally low temperatures in Kenya delayed the larval development (Dinnik and Dinnik 1963).

Outside Africa other species of lymnaeid snails have been identified to transmit *F. gigantica,* and their geographical distribution was reviewed by Over (1982). The distribution in a region of India and the ecology of *L. auricularia* var. *rufescens* as intermediate host of *F. gigantica* was described (Patnaik and Ray 1968). Both *L. peregra* and *L. auricularia* (*gedrosiana*) were the intermediate hosts for *F. gigantica* in Iran

(Massoud and Sadjadi 1980). In the Philippines, *L. rubiginosa* was the principal snail vector of fascioliasis (Dumag *et al.* 1976).

A laboratory method has been described for the maintenance of *L. natalensis* and the mass production of *F. gigantica* metacercariae (Kendall and Parfitt 1965; El Harith 1980b; Madsen and Monrad 1981).

In the Philippines, it was found that metacercariae of *F. gigantica* were able to exist on almost any kind of grass, particularly rice plants, and that feeding of rice straw during the dry season spread the infection (Dumag *et al.* 1976). At 20 °C and 12% relative humidity metacercariae could be destroyed after 6 minutes on the infested straw (Kimura *et al.* 1980). In laboratory studies the effect on infectivity of metacercariae was tested at different freezing temperatures (Boray and Enigk 1964).

INFECTION

The life cycle of *F. gigantica* in cattle is similar to that of *F. hepatica*, with a difference that the metacercariae of the *F. gigantica* have relatively slower maturation and hepatic invasion and migration into bile ducts than *F. hepatica*. The migration of the flukes starts with penetration of the duodenum, then takes place through the peritoneal cavity, across the liver capsule, and into the liver parenchyma. The maturing flukes pass through the liver parenchyma into the bile ducts causing considerable tissue damage. In nonfatal acute cases the liver regenerates quickly and its function returns almost to normal. Acute fascioliasis is associated with migration of large numbers of flukes through the liver, and the chronic form is caused by localization in bile ducts of mature worms. After the flukes have entered the bile ducts the infection becomes patent, as determined by passage of eggs in feces. Up to this stage the duration of the cycle is from 90 to 100 days. The numbers of eggs passed in feces increase for up to 7 to 10 weeks and reflects the level of infection, but thereafter counts cannot be associated with degree of infestation and egg production may be low even in heavy infestations. The infection is self-limiting with the numbers of adult flukes in the bile ducts decreasing soon after patency, eventually reaching very low numbers.

Mice, rats, rabbits, and guinea pigs have varying degrees of susceptibility to infection and have been used as useful models in the study of fascioliasis. The variation is susceptibility is probably due to innate immunity.

Literature

Review articles have been published primarily on *F. hepatica* infestations in domestic ruminants and these have been cited in the introduction to this chapter. Sewell and Hammond (1974) discussed the pathogenesis of fascioliasis and pointed out differences between infections caused by *F. gigantica* and *F. hepatica*. *Fasciola gigantica* had a greater infectivity, less preference for the ventral lobe of the liver, a longer prepatent period of 12 to 13 weeks as compared with 8 to 9 weeks for *F. hepatica*, and less rapid reduction and elimination of mature flukes. In cattle, this was attributed to a lower resistance to infection by this species.

Various features of fascioliasis caused by *F. gigantica* have been studied experimentally to a limited degree in sheep and laboratory animals. Experimental chronic infections in sheep have been investigated (Kendall and Parfitt 1953; Hammond 1973). The flukes entered bile ducts from 60 to 70 days after infestation and infections were prepatent from day 90 to day 120. Up to 60% of metacercariae used in causing the infections matured to adult worms. There have been relatively few studies on *F. gigantica* infection of small laboratory animals. Most common laboratory species (except the rat) were susceptible; lesions developed in livers, and mortality occurred. However, the flukes did not become fertile (Gerber *et al.* 1974). Infections have also been established in mice (Hanna and Jura 1976) and rabbits (Graber 1971). The susceptibility varied with the species, decreasing in the following order: hamsters, guinea pigs, mice, and then rabbits (Mango *et al.* 1972). In guinea pigs the migration of immature flukes took place through the duodenal wall and via the peritoneal cavity into the liver, a route comparable to that observed in ruminants (Srivastava and Singh 1972).

CLINICAL SIGNS

Three partially overlapping clinical syndromes are observed in cattle and small ruminants and include: the acute disease caused by immature worm migration through the liver; the subacute form characterized by anemia caused by the young adult flukes emerging from the liver into the bile ducts; and a chronic stage which is a wasting disease with the presence of flukes in the bile ducts. Regular use of anthelmintics results in prevalence of the chronic form of disease as well as many cases of asymptomatic infections. When seasonal conditions enable massive infestation of water sources by metacercariae, and these are ingested over a short period of time, outbreaks of acute and subacute fascioliasis can result in considerable mortality. The severity of syndromes is related to the number of flukes which are migrating, the size of the population established in the bile ducts, and to the immunological and nutritional status of the host.

There are no pathognomonic clinical signs, but symptoms in an acute syndrome differ from those observed in chronic forms. In the acute disease, death is often the first evidence of a problem in a herd. Other animals are depressed and lethargic and occasionally jaundiced. In the chronic form debility and anemia occur, with subcutaneous edema developing on the face and lower regions of the abdomen and thorax.

Literature

Although *F. gigantica* infestation of cattle is of considerable economic loss in Asia and Africa, relatively little detailed information has been published on the clinical disease and on the pathogenesis (Bitakaramire and Bwangamoi 1969). Large numbers of metacercariae were required to produce an acute syndrome experimentally. Ingestion of 20 000 metacercariae gave rise to 7000 young flukes in the liver which in turn caused mortality in 11 weeks (Sewell 1966). From doses ranging from 500 to 10 000 metacercariae, 12 to 40% matured to adults. The severity and mortality of the syndromes was directly related to the numbers of flukes ingested. Development of acute clinical disease has been observed in chronic fascioliasis in undernourished animals, especially in native herds at the end of the dry season (Graber 1971).

PATHOLOGY

The pathogenesis of the diseases caused by *F. gigantica* and *F. hepatica* is similar. Lesions induced by *Fasciola* in all species of animals are also similar but vary in severity. Major damage to the liver occurs between 12 and 15 weeks after infection. The course of the disease depends on the number of metacercariae ingested and on their infectivity. When metacercariae penetrate the intestine some tissue damage results, but the most extensive injury occurs from the trauma and inflammation produced during migration through the liver parenchyma and when the flukes finally localize in the bile ducts and gall bladder. Acute hepatic insufficiency is associated with extensive traumatic lesions caused by young flukes eating their way through the liver. Migrating worms initially cause small 1 to 2 mm hemorrhagic spots in the liver capsules, then, as the young flukes grow, tortuous traumatic tracts increase in size, finally resulting in larger areas of necrosis. These traumatic lesions are accompanied by hyperplasia of small bile ducts, and jaundice is evident in the latter stages of acute syndromes with an increase in both total and direct serum bilirubin concentrations. This liver malfunction results in loss of weight and rapid development of progressive anemia.

Characteristic chronic lesions consist of dilatation and thickening of bile ducts with periportal fibrosis and infiltration of eosinophils, lymphocytes, and macrophages. The most important lesion in pathogenesis is the extent of liver fibrosis following the establishment of flukes in the biliary system. Fibrosis, hyperplasia, and calcification of bile ducts is particularly severe in *F. gigantica* infestations as compared to *F. hepatica* infections. In enzootic regions it is not uncommon to find evidence of both chronic and acute lesions in the same animal.

The bile duct lesions are associated with hypoalbuminemia and chronic anemia which is normocytic and normochromic and appears to be caused by blood loss. Other biochemical and cellular changes in the blood depend on the stage and severity of the syndrome. The mechanisms responsible for anemia are multifactorial and depend on the stage of infection. Ingestion of blood by the migrating flukes, hepatic malfunction, hemorrhage into the bile ducts, and possibly interference in the erythropoiesis all play a role. Proline, which is an amino acid released by flukes, is involved in the production of anemia and induction of fibrosis around bile ducts.

Literature

Pathological, hematological, and biochemical aspects of naturally occurring bovine fascioliasis caused by *F. gigantica* were investigated in 228 cases by Haroun and Hussein (1975). The authors compared their observations with those of others made on both *F. gigantica* and *F. hepatica* infections. Earlier, Sewell (1966) reviewed the pathogenesis of acute and subacute fascioliasis caused by *F. gigantica* in Zebu cattle and discussed similarities and differences between syndromes caused by *F. hepatica*.

Lesions related to the invasive stages of *F. hepatica* in the intestinal wall, abdominal cavity, liver, and the final change in the biliary system were reviewed in experimental and natural infections (Dawes and Hughes 1964; El-Harith 1980a). Comparable changes occurred in *F. gigantica* infections with young worms burrowing their way through the liver by feeding on hepatic cells. The damage to the liver and severity of the disease depended on the size and number of migrating immature flukes (Bitakaramire 1967a; Magzoub and Adam 1977).

The majority of information on the pathology has been on chronic forms of the disease. Haroun and Hussein (1975) presented a comprehensive description of the gross and microscopic lesions in the chronic form caused by *F. gigantica*. Carcasses were emaciated and there was subcutaneous edema and serous effusion into body cavities. Livers were enlarged, fibrosed, pale gray or grayish-yellow color, with prominent lobulations and occasionally fibrous capsular adhesions. Areas of hemorrhage and telangiectasis were scattered throughout the parenchyma. Bile ducts and gall bladder were dilated, thickened, fibrosed, calcified, and contained a thick greenish-gray exudate containing flukes and their remnants, and occasionally biliary calculi. Microscopically the bile ducts were hyperplastic with an occasional adenomatous type of proliferation, and these changes were associated with extensive inflammatory cell infiltration. The most extensive biliary lesions resulted in pseudo-lobulation of parenchyma with lobules being surrounded by fibrous tissue. Black pigment and hemosiderin were observed both in Kupffer's cells and extracellularly. Fluke eggs were surrounded by foreign body type of granulomas. Hepatic arteries and portal veins were hypertrophied with endothelial cell hyperplasia and extensive perivascular inflammatory reactions. Hepatic lymph nodes were enlarged, nodular, and edematous with dark yellowish-brown or greenish discoloration. Histologically there was follicular enlargement, hyperplasia, hemosiderosis, and hypertrophy of the medullary arteries. The sequential development of lesions in experimental infection of cattle with *F. gigantica* consisted of an initial parenchymal necrosis followed by bile duct proliferation and then by calcification (Bitakaramire and Bwangamoi 1970). Occasionally, in addition to the typical liver changes, lesions were observed in the lungs and pancreas. In certain regions of the world pulmonary fascioliasis has been reported to be common, as for example in some outbreaks in water buffalo (*Bubalus bubalis*) (Dwivedi and Singh 1965). Lesions in livers of cattle infested with *F. gigantica* observed in slaughterhouses have been often described. Microabscesses contained larvae or eggs, interlobular fibrosis, proliferation of bile ducts, and peribiliary fibrosis have been reported (Jha *et al.* 1977; Uzoukwu and Ikeme 1978).

In species of domestic ruminants other than cattle, lesions were comparable to those observed in cattle. In buffalo, the numerous hemorrhagic tracts in the early stages were followed by hyperplasia and hypertrophy of bile ducts (Sengupta and Iyer 1968). In goats and sheep the lesions were also comparable to those seen in cattle (Arora and Iyer 1973). In West African dwarf sheep, pregnancy appeared to enhance the pathogenicity of *F. gigantica* (Ogunrinade 1979a; Schillhorn van Veen 1979).

Hematology and blood chemistry have been studied extensively in *F. hepatica* and different observations reported by various workers could probably be related to the severity and the stages of infection which were investigated. Anemia and hypoproteinemia have been regarded to be common features of fascioliasis. The pathogenesis of anemia has not been determined. Ingestion of blood flukes, loss through hemorrhage in bile ducts, toxic components, and hemapoietic tissue malfunction have all been proposed as the mechanism involved (Maclean *et al.* 1976; Ogunrinade *et al.* 1980; Ogunrinade and Anosa 1981). The severity of anemia in *F. gigantica* infection has been associated with the level of infection and was related to blood meals taken by the flukes (Ogunrinade 1981; Ogunrinade and Bamgboye 1980). In sheep, anemia occurred 10 to 12 weeks after infection at the time when adult flukes were present in the bile ducts and decreased erythrocyte survival occurred (Ogunrinade and Anosa 1981). In another study in experimental infection of sheep a decrease in erythrocyte counts and hematocrit values was observed at both 6 and 10 weeks after infection respectively, while eosinophilia developed between 2 and 4 weeks after infection (Kadhim 1976a). *Fasciola gigantica* took longer to reach maturity in the liver than *F. hepatica*, this being associated with delays in hematological changes (El Harith 1980a). Changes in serum proteins mainly consisted of hypoalbuminemia and hyperglobulinemia, without noticeable changes in the total protein values (Weinbren and Coyle 1960). In buffalo, hematological and biochemical changes were comparable to those of cattle (Dessouky and Moustafa 1976). Additional information on other biochemical changes in blood associated with *F. gigantica* infections has not been available.

A consistent effect on enzymes which could be used to demonstrate liver malfunction has not been observed. There has not been a consistent relationship between infection and bilirubinemia. It has been proposed that glutamate oxalate transaminase levels were the only reliable indicator of chronic fascioliasis even at low levels of infection in cattle (Ogunrinade *et al.* 1980). Biochemical composition of the bile and serum of buffalo, cattle, and sheep with fascioliasis was reported (Haiba and Selim 1960b). A significant decrease in the serum and bile calcium levels, but not in phosphorus and magnesium, were observed in buffalo (Haiba *et al.* 1964). In large numbers of buffalo reduction of hemaglobin and total serum proteins was associated with increase in various serum enzymes (Kumar *et al.* 1982a). Comparable studies in cattle showed similar changes in enzymes (Kumar *et al.* 1982b).

Proline is an amino acid released in large quantities by adult *F. hepatica* and has been shown to cause increased red blood cell lysis which results in anemia (Isseroff *et al.* 1979). The role of proline in the bile duct hyperplasia was considered to be more important than that induced by the mechanical stimulation by the presence of worms in the lumen (Isseroff *et al.* 1977).

IMMUNOLOGY

Resistance of cattle to infections by *Fasciola* species following an initial exposure is due to the development of resistance in the liver to reinfection. This is probably due to an immunological process. This resistance reduces the numbers of mature and immature flukes which develop. The mechanism by which *Fasciola* species evade the host defense mechanisms is not known. Resistance can be induced experimentally in cattle, and to some extent in sheep, by *F. hepatica* and this has given rise to the possibility of artificially producing resistance to infections. Comparable studies are not available on *F. gigantica*.

Differences in acquired immunity among the various species of host are evident. Sheep show little resistance to reinfection while cattle become significantly refractory. A decreased susceptibility is also apparent in several laboratory animal models. Resistance to infection is measured by monitoring the liver enzyme glutamate dehydrogenase.

Various components of juvenile and adult worms are used as antigens to investigate acquired resistance. High serum levels of immunoglobulins occur and react with various secretory and excretory antigens of the flukes. A high level of antibody response to antigens of the tegument is often observed. Serological tests are increasingly used in diagnosis of fascioliasis.

Literature

Serum protein in sheep infested with *F. gigantica* was increased mainly due to the globulin fraction with a decrease occurring in albumin. The overall protein concentration was also influenced by blood loss and degree of liver malfunction (Kadhim 1976b). Evidence of acquired resistance occurring in experimental *F. hepatica* infection in laboratory animals was summarized by Malek (1980). The suppressed development of young flukes in reinfection and self-cure could be indicative of immunological-mediated resistance (Sewell 1966; Hammond and Sewell 1975). Heterologous resistance induced by schistosome infections (to *F. hepatica*) have also been reported (Sirag *et al.* 1981; Monrad *et al.* 1981).

VACCINATION

Attempts have been made to induce immunity to *F. hepatica* by active immunization and by passively administering antiserum. In the active immunization, various tissue antigens as well as secretions and excretions of mature and immature forms were used. Vaccination with irradiated metacercariae has also been tried. Further laboratory and field investigations are necessary to explore the possibility of using immunization procedures to enhance resistance to infections and to development of clinical syndromes.

Literature

Attempts at vaccination have been reported (Blancou *et al.* 1975; Ogunrinade 1979b; Bitakaramire 1973b). The results are variable and required more in-depth studies to define the effect of using irradiated infections as a form of vaccination.

CHEMOTHERAPY

Fasciolicides should be used in heavy infestation, but time of treatment is critical in producing a benefical effect. Treatment against immature flukes is particularly important in order to prevent development of severe lesions and mortality and avoid contamination of pastures. However, no anthelmintic is fully effective and safe against acute fascioliasis. Several drugs are able to kill the migrating parenchymal forms, but at high dosage these drugs are usually toxic.

Literature

Berger (1971) summarized the therapies used against *F. gigantica.* A variety of commercially available compounds and new developmental compounds have been tested. The efficiency of five fasciolicides –

carbon tetrachloride, hexachlorophene, Oxyclozanide, Nitroxynil, and Niclopholan – was compared using various dose levels administered at different stages of infection. Treatments with either 0.2 ml/kg carbon tetrachloride or 20 mg/kg of Nitroxynil were useful when given 6 to 8 weeks after challenge. Treatment with the other compounds involved prohibitive costs and increased chances of dangerous toxicity. At 8 weeks the choice of drugs widened to include hexachlorophene at 20 mg/kg and Niclopholan at 6 mg/kg. At 11 weeks, carbbon tetrachloride gave total clearance and other compounds such as hexachlorophene, Nitroxynil, and Niclopholan were all efficient at standard doses. In general, fasciolicides were progressively more efficient as doses were increased and as a time of administration after infection was extended (Qadir 1981).

Common anthelmintics used against *Fasciola* infestations in West Africa were carbon tetrachloride, hexachlorophene and hexachlorothane. During the last 15 years other drugs have been tried, the most common being bithionol sulfoxide, Bromphenophos, Niclopholan, Nitroxynil, and Rafoxanide. All animals should be treated twice at the beginning of the dry season and again at the beginning of the wet season (Schillhorn van Veen 1980).

Nitroxynil at doses of 10 mg/kg in cattle, buffalo, and sheep was 100% effective against liver flukes 6 weeks or more after infection (Roy and Reddy 1969). In Zimbabwe, treatment with nitroxynil or rafoxanide at regular intervals of 8 to 12 weeks had obvious beneficial economic affects only on occasion. Economically beneficient treatment was most obvious against the immature forms but not the adult worms (Needham 1977). Rafoxanide was effective at 10 mg/kg in sheep and 10 to 15 mg/kg in cattle (Graber 1979; Horak *et al.* 1972; Snijders *et al.* 1971). The compound was also tested against a variety of mature and immature forms of trematode and nematode infections of cattle (Schroder *et al.* 1977). Dirian, a thiobenzamide, at doses of 15 to 20 mg/kg was active against immature and mature stages (Karrasch *et al.* 1975). Niclosulide was also effective in treatment of cattle (Federis and Tongson 1977). Experimentally infected sheep treated with Hilomid, a bistrichlormethylbenzol, at 30 mg/kg between 10 and 16 weeks after infection had progressively reduced the worm burden (Hildebrandt 1968). After 75 days of infection an effect was observed on both immature and mature worms when the drug was administered at doses of between 150 and 155 mg/kg (Hildebrandt 1967). The activity of a fasciolicide, Acedist, has been investigated in *F. gigantica* infection in goats (Qadir 1981).

DIAGNOSIS

Chronic fascioliasis is diagnosed by demonstrating the characteristic eggs in the feces using either smear or concentration techniques to examine feces. Quantitative methods are used to estimate levels of infection but the reliability of interpretation is questionable.

Serodiagnosis techniques are necessary during prepatent periods and when the egg output is low. Numerous serological tests are available; however, the source of the antigen and the specificity of a serological test must be clearly defined before the value of a test can be determined. The tests tried in *F. hepatica* infections include indirect hemagglutination, counterimmune electrophoresis, double immunodiffusion, enzyme-linked immunosorbent assay, and precipitation tests. Their application in *F. gigantica* infections is not determined.

Literature

Serological and parasitological diagnostic procedures used in *F. hepatica* infection could be applied to *F. gigantica*, but there has been relatively little information confirming their usefulness. Standard methods separating eggs from feces and making counts were used to determine levels of *F. gigantica* infection in cattle (Bitakaramire 1967b). Radioimmunoassays have been used to detect *F. gigantica* infections in cattle (Bitakaramire *et al.* 1971). Fluorescent antibody techniques using single and multiple whole-fluke antigens were not useful in detecting chronic infections (Schillhorn van Veen and Buys 1979). Intradermal tests with crude antigen have been used in developing diagnostic procedures but their reliability has been questionable (Abdou *et al.* 1966).

CONTROL

Control of fascioliasis is dependent on the epizootiology of both infections and diseases and the level of infestation of water sources. Various factors such as grazing patterns, water sources, population levels of intermediate hosts and their seasonal variations can influence the severity of the problem and vary from one region to another, and have to be assessed in order to apply rational, economic, and feasible control programs. One or more measures are undertaken and involve control of snails, eradication of adult worms, and reduction of the chances of infection by adequate livestock management of grazing and watering by such techniques as drainage and fencing to ensure provision of uncontaminated feed and water. These procedures are expensive, often uneconomic, and are difficult to institute. Limited application of chemotherapy is often the only possible practical control measure which can be undertaken.

Literature

The ecological basis for the control of trematodes, particularly liver flukes, was reviewed by Over (1982).

BIBLIOGRAPHY

Abdou, A. H., El-Sherrif, A. and El-Sawi, A. F., 1966. Intradermal diagnosis of *Fasciola* infection, *J. Arab Vet. Med. Ass.*, **26**: 255–60.

Al-Barwari, S. E., 1975–76. The role of carbohydrates in the biology of the liver fluke, *Fasciola gigantica*: effects of temperature and pH upon glucose uptake, *Bull. Endem. Dis.*, **16**(1–2): 87–94.

Al-Barwari, S. E., 1977. A survey on liver infections with *Fasciola gigantica* among slaughtered animals in Iraq, *Bull. Endem. Dis.*, **18**(1–4): 75–92.

Al-Barwari, S. E. and Abdel-Fattah, R. F., 1975–76. The role of carbohydrates in the biology of the liver fluke, *Fasciola gigantica*: glycogen content, its utilization and resynthesis by starved flukes. *Bull. Endem. Dis.*, **16**(1–2): 57–70.

Alves, R. M. R., 1970. Subsidios para o conhecimento da epizootologia da fasciolose bovina em Moçambique (1), *Rev. Cienc. Vet.*, **3**(2): 147–71.

Arora, R. G. and Iyer, P. K. R., 1973. Studies on the pathology of fascioliasis in sheep and goats, *Indian J. Anim. Sci.*, **43**(8): 720–3.

Berger, J., 1971. A comparison of the activity of some fasciolicides against immature *Fasciola gigantica* in experimentally infected calves, *Bull. epiz. Dis. Afr.*, **19**: 37–44.

Bhattacharjee, M. L. and Halder, B. R., 1971. The occurrence of *Fasciola gigantica* in the liver of an Indian rhinoceros (*R. unicornis*), *Br. vet. J.*, **127**(5): vii–viii.

Bindernagel, J. A., 1972. Liver fluke *Fasciola gigantica* in African buffalo and antelopes in Uganda, East Africa, *J. Wildl. Dis.*, **8**: 315–17.

Bitakaramire, P. K., 1967a. Bovine fascioliasis in Kenya, *Vet. Med. Rev.*, pp. 77–84.

Bitakaramire, P. K., 1967b. A new technique for the recovery of *Fasciola gigantica* eggs from cattle faeces, *Bull. epiz. Dis. Afr.*, **15**: 389–91.

Bitakaramire, P. K., 1973a. The incidence of fascioliasis in different breeds of cattle in Kenya. *Bull. epiz. Dis. Afr.*, **21**(2): 145–52.

Bitakaramire, P. K., 1973b. Preliminary studies on the immunization of cattle against fascioliasis using gamma-irradiated metacercariae of *Fasciola gigantica*, *Proc. Res. Coordination Meet. FAO/ILEA Int. Atomic Energy Agency Vienna*, pp. 23–32.

Bitakaramire, P. K. and Bwangamoi, O., 1969. Experimental infection

of calves with *Fasciola gigantica, Exp. Parasitol.*, **25**: 353–7.
Bitakaramire, P. K. and Bwangamoi, O., 1970. The pathology of experimental infection of cattle with *Fasciola gigantica, Bull. epiz. Dis. Afr.*, **18**: 149–57.
Bitakaramire, P. K., Movsesijan, M. and Castelino, J. B., 1971. Radioimmunoassay of *Fasciola gigantica* infection in cattle, *Bull. epiz. Dis. Afr.*, **19**: 353–6.
Blancou, J.-M., Bouchet, A. and Daynes, P., 1975. Trials to induce an acquired immunity against the infestation by *Fasciola gigantica, Rev. Elev. Méd. vét. Pays trop.*, **28**(2): 133–6.
Boray, J. C., 1969. Experimental fascioliasis in Australia, *Adv. Parasitol.*, **7**: 95–210.
Boray, J. C. and Enigk, K., 1964. Laboratory studies on the survival and infectivity of *Fasciola hepatica*- and *Fasciola gigantica*-metacercariae, *Z. Tropenmed. Parasit.*, **15**(3): 324–31.

Castelino, J. B. and Preston, J. M., 1979. The influence of breed and age on the prevalence of bovine fascioliasis in Kenya, *Br. vet. J.*, **135**: 198–203.
Condy, J. B., 1962. Fascioliasis – a disease of major economic importance, *Rhod. Agric. J.*, **59**: 259–262, 269.
Coyle, T. J., 1956. Liver fluke in Uganda, *Bull. epiz. Dis. Afr.*, **4**: 47–55.

Dawes, B. and Hughes, D. L., 1964. Fascioliasis: the invasive stages of *Fasciola hepatica* in mammalian hosts, *Adv. Parasitol.*, **2**: 97–168.
Dessouky, M. I. and Moustafa, I. H., 1976. Some haematological and biochemical studies on *Fasciola* infected buffaloes, *Vet. Med. J.*, **3**(5): 179–87.
Dinnik, J. A. and Dinnik, N. N., 1963. Effect on the seasonal variations of temperature on the development of *Fasciola gigantica* in the snail host in the Kenya Highlands, *Bull. epiz. Dis. Afr.*, **11**: 197–207.
Dumag, P. U., Batalos, J. A., Escandor, N. B., Castillo, A. M. and Gajudo, C. E., 1976. The encystment of *Fasciola gigantica* metacercariae on different pasture grasses, *Philipp. J. Anim. Ind.*, **31**(1–4): 72–86.
Durrani, M. S., Nawaz, M. and Chaudhary, N. I., 1982. Studies on specific inhibitors and substrates of cholinesterases of *Fasciola gigantica* from cattle and buffaloes, *Zbl. Vet. Med.* **B29**: 636–41.
Dwivedi, J. N. and Singh, C. M., 1965. The occurrence of *Fasciola gigantica* in the lungs of Indian buffaloes (*Bos bubalis*), *Indian vet. J.*, **42**: 662–3.

Edney, J. M. and Muchlis, A., 1963. Fascioliasis in Indonesian livestock, *Comm. Vet. Bogor*, **6**(2): 49–62.

Eisa, A. M. and Dalil, E. A. M., 1963. Incidence of parasites in bovine livers, *Sudan J. Vet Sci. Anim. Husb.*, **4**(2): 72–6.

El-Azazy, O. M. E. and Schillhorn van Veen, T. W., 1983. Animal fascioliasis and schistosomiasis in Egypt and Sudan, *Helminth. Abstr.-A*, **52**(8): 421–8.

El-Harith, A., 1980a. Studies on animal fascioliasis: comparative development and pathogenesis of *Fasciola gigantica* and *Fasciola hepatica* in sheep, *Sudan J. Vet. Sci. Anim. Husb.*, **21**(2): 86–99.

El-Harith, A., 1980b. The influence of the alternative intermediate host '*Lymnaea truncatula*' on the development and pathogenesis of *Fasciola gigantica* infection in sheep, *Sudan J. Vet. Sci. Anim. Husb.*, **21**(1): 16–25.

Federis, M. T. and Tongson, M. S., 1977. Anthelmintic efficacy of niclosulide in natural *Fasciola gigantica* infection of cattle and carabao, *Philipp. J. Anim. Ind.*, **32**(1–4): 94–114.

Gemechu, B. and Mamo, E., 1979. A preliminary survey of bovine fascioliasis in Ethiopia, *Eth. J. Agr. Sci.*, **1**: 1–12.

Gerber, H.-Ch., Horchner, F. and Oguz, T., 1974. (*Fasciola gigantica*-infection in small laboratory animals), *Berl. Münch. Tierarztl. Wschr.*, **87**(11): 207–10.

Goil, M. M., 1961a. Physiological studies on trematodes – *Fasciola gigantica* carbohydrate metabolism, *Parasitology*, **51**: 335–7.

Goil, M. M., 1961b. Physiological studies on trematodes – *Fasciola gigantica* rate of oxygen consumption, *Z. Parasitenkd.*, **20**: 568–71.

Goil, M. M., 1961c. Haemoglobin in trematodes. 1. *Fasciola gigantica*. 2. *Cotylophoron indicum*, *Z. Parasitenkd.*, **20**: 572–5.

Graber, M., 1971. Role du facteur alimentaire dans la distomatose bovine et ovine a *Fasciola gigantica*, *Bull. epiz. Dis. Afr.*, **19**: 45–60.

Graber, M., 1979. (Treatment, in tropical Africa, of sheep and cattle fascioliasis with refoxanide), *Rev. Elev. Méd. vét. Pays trop.*, **32**(1): 11–17.

Haiba, M. H., El-Rawii, K. A. and Osman, H. G., 1964. A comparative study on the levels of Ca, inorganic P and Mg in the blood serum and bile of the normal healthy buffalo (*Bos bubalus*) and those of buffaloes infested with liver fluke (*Fasciola gigantica*), *Z. Parasitenkd.*, **23**: 527–31.

Haiba, M. H. and Selim, M. K., 1960a. Detailed study on the morphological status of *Fasciola* worms infesting buffaloes, cows and sheep in Egypt, *Z. Parasitenkd.*, **19**: 525–34.

Haiba, M. H. and Selim, M. K., 1960b. A comparative preliminary biochemical study on the effect of *Fasciola* infestation in bile and serum of Egyptian buffaloes, cows and sheep, *Z. Parasitenkd.*, **19**: 535–40.

Hammond, J. A., 1973. Experimental chronic *Fasciola gigantica* infection in sheep, *Trop. Anim. Hlth Prod.*, **5**: 12–21.

Hammond, J. A. and Sewell, M. M. H., 1975. Experimental infections of cattle with *Fasciola gigantica*: numbers of parasites recovered after varying periods of infection, *Trop. Anim. Hlth Prod.*, **7**: 105–13.

Hanna, R. E. B. and Jura, W., 1976. *In vitro* maintenance of juvenile *Fasciola gigantica* and their use to establish infections in mice, *Res. vet. Sci.*, **21**: 244–6.

Haroun, E. M. and Hussein, M. F., 1975. Clinico-pathological studies on naturally ocurring bovine fascioliasis in the Sudan, *J. Helminthol.*, **49**: 143–52.

Hildebrandt, J., 1967. The effect of Hetol on immature and mature stages of *Fasciola gigantica* in artificially infected sheep, *Berl. Münch. Tierarztl. Wschr.*, **80**: 369–71.

Hildebrandt, J., 1968. Dibromosalicylanilide tribromosalycylanide. Effect against immature and mature stages of *Fasciola gigantica* in artificially infested sheep, *Vet. Rec.*, **82**: 699–700.

Horak, I. G., Snijders, A. J. and Louw, J. P., 1972. Trials with rafoxanide 5. Efficacy studies against *Fasciloa hepatica, Fasciola gigantica, Paramphistomum microbothrium* and various nematodes in sheep, *J. S. Afr. vet. med. Ass.*, **43**(4): 397–403.

Ikeme, M. M. and Obioha, F., 1973. *Fasciola gigantica* infestations in trade cattle in eastern Nigeria, *Bull. epiz. Dis. Afr.*, **21**(3): 259–64.

Ismail, N. S., Saliba, E. K. and Lutfy, R. G., 1978. Fascioliasis in Azraq Oasis, Jordan. I. Incidence and degree of infection in cows and buffaloes, *Acta Parasitological Polonica*, **25**(39): 333–40.

Isseroff, H., Sawma, J. T. and Reino, D., 1977. Fascioliasis: role of proline in bile duct hyperplasia, *Science*, **198**: 1157–9.

Isseroff, H., Spengler, R. N. and Charnock, D. R., 1979. Fascioliasis: similarities of the anemia in rats to that produced by infused proline, *J. Parasitol.*, **65**: 709–14.

Jha, S. N., Singh, C. D. N., Jha, G. J. and Sinha, B. K., 1977. Studies on the pathology of liver diseases in bovines. (1) Parasitic diseases, *Kerala J. Vet. Sci.*, **8**(1): 119–25.

Kadhim, J. K., 1976a. Haematological changes during the course of experimental infection with *Fasciola gigantica* in sheep. In *Pathophysiology of Parasitic Infections*, ed. E. J. L. Soulsby. Academic Press (New York), pp. 105–14.

Kadhim, J. K., 1976b. Changes in serum protein values of sheep infected with *Fasciola gigantica*, *Am. J. vet. Res.*, **37**(2): 229–31.

Karrasch, A. W., Horchner, F. and Bohnel, H., 1975. (Efficacy of Dirian against *Fasciola gigantica* and paramphistomes in naturally infected cattle from Madagascar), *Berl. Münch. Tierarztl. Wschr.*, **88**: 348–51.

Kendall, S. B., 1965. Relationship between the species of *Fasciola* and their molluscan hosts, *Adv. Parasitol.*, **3**: 59–98.

Kendall, S. B. and Parfitt, J. W., 1953. Life-history of *Fasciola gigantica* Cobbold 1856, *Nature*, **171**: 1164–5.

Kendall, S. B. and Parfitt, J. W., 1965. The life-history of some vectors of *Fasciola gigantica* under laboratory conditions, *Ann. trop. Med. Parasit.*, **59**: 10–16.

Kibakin, V. V., 1968. The epizootiology of sheep fascioliasis in Turkmenia. In *Natural Nidality of Diseases*, eds N. Levine, F. K. Plous. Illinois Press (Chicago), pp. 273–5.

Kimura, S., Shimizu, A. and Kawano, J., 1980. Extermination of *Fasciola gigantica* metacercariae, *J. Parasitol.*, **66**(4): 699–700.

Kumar, M., Maru, A. and Pachauri, S. P., 1982a. Changes in blood cellular components, serum protein concentrations and serum enzyme activities in buffaloes infested with *Fasciola gigantica*, *Res. vet. Sci.*, **33**: 260–1.

Kumar, M., Pathak, K. M. L. and Pachauri, S. P., 1982b. Clinico-pathological studies on naturally occurring bovine fascioliasis in India, *Br. vet. J.*, **138**: 241–6.

Maclean, J., Holmes, P. H., Dargie, J. D. and Mulligan, W., 1976. Pathophysiology of *Fasciola hepatica* infections. In *Pathophysiology of Parasite Infections*, ed. E. J. L. Soulsby. Academic Press (New York), pp. 117–23.

Madsen, H. and Monrad, J., 1981. A method for laboratory maintenance of *Lymnaea natalensis* and for mass production of *Fasciola gigantica* metacercariae, *J. Parasitol.*, **67**(5): 735–7.

Magzoub, M. and Adam, S. E. I., 1977. Laboratory investigations on natural infection in Zebu cattle with *Fasciola gigantica* and *Schistosoma bovis*, *Zbl. Vet. Med.*, **B24**: 53–62.

Magzoub, M. and Kasim, A. A., 1978. The prevalence of fascioliasis in Saudi Arabia, *Trop. Anim. Hlth Prod.*, **10**(4) 205–6.

Malek, E. A., 1980. Fascioliasis. In *CRC Handbook Series in Zoonoses*, ed. J. H. Steele. CRC Press (Boca Raton, Fla.), vol. 2, pp. 131–70.

Malviya, H. C., 1967. Morphological observations on *Fasciola gigantica* Cobbold, 1855, with remarks on the validity of *Fasciola indica* Varma, 1953, *Indian J. vet. Sci.*, **37**(2): 67–77.

Mango, A. M., Mango, C. K. A. and Esamal, D., 1972. A preliminary note on the susceptibility, prepatency and recovery of *Fasciola gigantica* in small laboratory animals, *J. Helminthol.*, **46**(4): 381–6.

Massoud, J. and Sadjadi, S., 1980. Susceptibility of different species of *Lymnaea* snails to miracidia of *Fasciola gigantica* and *F. hepatica* in Iran, *J. Helminthol.*, **54**: 201–2.

McCullough, F. S., 1965. *Lymnaea natalensis* and fascioliasis in Ghana, *Ann. trop. Med. Parasit.*, **59**: 320–6.

Michael, A. I. and Awadalla, H. N., 1976. A histochemical study of some enzymes of *Fasciola gigantica*, *J. Egypt. Vet. Med. Ass.*, **35**(4): 9–16.

Monrad, J., Christensen, N. Ø., Nansen, P. and Frandsen, F., 1981. Resistance to *Fasciola hepatica* in sheep harbouring primary *Schistosoma bovis* infections, *J. Helminthol.*, **55**: 261–71.

Mzembe, S. A. T. and Chaudhry, M. A., 1979. The epidemiology of fascioliasis in Malawi: 1. The epidemiology in the intermediate host, *Trop. Anim. Hlth Prod.*, **11**: 246–50.

Mzembe, S. A. T. and Chaudhry, M. A., 1981. The epidemiology of fascioliasis in Malawi. II. Epidemiology in the definitive host, *Trop. Anim. Hlth Prod.*, **13**: 27–33.

Needham, A. J. E., 1977. Observations on the economics of treatment of *Fasciola gigantica* infestation in cattle in Rhodesia, *Rhod. vet. J.*, **8**: 14–20.

Nobel, T. A., Klopfer, U. and Neuman, M., 1972. An outbreak of fascioliasis (*Fasciola gigantica*) in a nature reserve in Israel, *Refuah Vet.*, **29**(1): 33–4.

Ogunrinade, A., 1979a. A preliminary observation on the pathogenicity of *Fasciola gigantica* in pregnant West African dwarf ewes, *Rev. Elev. Méd vét. Pays trop.*, **32**(3): 247–9.

Ogunrinade, A., 1979b. Assessment of the attenuation produced by irradiation of *Fasciola gigantica* metacercariae in hamsters, *Res. vet. Sci.*, **27**: 238–9.

Ogunrinade, A., 1981. Bovine fascioliasis in Nigeria. III. Haemoglobin polymorphism in infected zebu cattle, *Veterinarski Arhiv.*, **51**(3): 129–34.

Ogunrinade, A. F., Adenaike, F. A., Fajnimi, J. L. and Bamgboye, E. A., 1980. Bovine fascioliasis in Nigeria. II. Blood chemistry and its correlation with worm burdens in chronic fascioliasis, *Zbl. Vet. Med.*, **B27**: 622–30.

Ogunrinade, A. F. and Anosa, V. O., 1981. Red blood cell survival and faecal clearance in sheep infected with *Fasciola gigantica*, *J. Comp. Path.*, **91**: 381–5.

Ogunrinade, A. F. and Bamgboye, E. A., 1980. Bovine fascioliasis in Nigeria. I. Haematological indices and their correlation with worm burden in chronic fascioliasis, *Br. vet. J.*, **136**: 457–62.

Ogunrinade, A. F., and Ogunrinade, B. I., 1980. Economic importance of bovine fascioliasis in Nigeria, *Trop. Anim. Hlth Prod.*, **12**(3): 155–60.

Ogunrinade, A. F., Okon, E. D. and Fasanmi, E. F., 1981. The prevalence of bovine fascioliasis in Nigeria. A 5-year analysis of abattoir records, *Bull. Anim. Hlth Prod. Afr.*, **29**: 381–7.

Over, H. J., 1982. Ecological basis of parasite control: trematodes with special reference to fascioliasis, *Vet. Parasitol.*, **11**: 85–97.

Patnaik, M. M. and Ray, S. K., 1968. Studies on geographical distribution and ecology of *Lymnaea auricularia* var. *rufescens*, the intermediate host of *Fasciola gigantica* in Orissa, *Indian J. Vet. Sci. Anim. Husb.*, **38**(3): 484–508.

Preston, J. M. and Castelino, J. B., 1977. A study of the epidemiology of bovine fascioliasis in Kenya and its control using *N*-tritylmorpholine, *Br. vet. J.*, **133**(6): 600–8.

Purchase, H. S., 1957. How important is 'liver fluke disease' in South Africa? *S. Afr. vet. med. Ass.*, **28**(4): 337–40.

Qadir, A. N. M. A., 1981. Anthelmintic efficiency of Acedist, a new fasciolicide against immature *Fasciola gigantica* in goats, *Indian vet. J.*, **58**: 197–8.

Rivai, M., 1979. Losses caused by *Fasciola hepatica* in infected cattle and buffaloes slaughtered at Padang Panjang abattoir, *Vet. Parasitol.*, **5**(1): 81.

Roy, R. M. and Reddy, N. R., 1969. Study on the activity of nitroxynil (M.B. 10.755) on buffaloes, cattle and sheep naturally infected with *Fasciola gigantica*, *Vet. Rec.*, **85**(4): 85–7.

Schillhorn van Veen, T. W., 1979. Ovine fascioliasis (*Fasciola gigantica*) on the Ahmadu Bello University farm, *Trop. Anim. Hlth Prod.*, **11**: 151–6.

Schillhorn van Veen, T. W., 1980. Fascioliasis (*Fasciola gigantica*) in West Africa: a review, *Vet. Bull.*, **50**(7): 529–33.

Schillhorn van Veen, T. W. and Buys, J., 1979. The serodiagnosis of chronic fascioliasis (*Fasciola gigantica*) using a fluorescent antibody technique with single and multiple whole-fluke antigens, *Z. Tropenmed. Parasit.*, **30**: 194–7.

Schillhorn van Veen, T. W., Folaranmi, D. O. B., Usman, S. and Ishaya, T., 1980. Incidence of liver fluke infections (*Fasciola gigantica* and *Dicrocoelium hospes*) in ruminants in northern Nigeria, *Trop. Anim. Hlth Prod.*, **12**: 97–104.

Schroder, J. Honer, M. R. and Louw, J. P., 1977. Trials with rafoxanide. 8. Efficacy of an injectable solution against trematodes and nematodes in cattle, *J. S. Afr. vet. med. Ass.*, **48**(2): 95–7.

Séguin, D., 1976. Considerations sur les distomatoses hepato-biliares des ruminants domestiques au Togo *Ann. Univ. Bénin, Togo*, **2**(1): 43–54.

Sengupta, U. and Iyer, P. K. R., 1968. Studies on the pathology of buffalo livers infested with *Fasciola gigantica*, *Indian J. Anim. Hlth*, **7**: 111–19.

Sewell, M. M. H., 1966. The pathogenesis of fascioliasis, *Vet. Rec.*, **78**(3): 98–105.

Sewell, M. M. H. and Hammond, J. A., 1974. A comparison of infections of cattle with *Fasciola gigantica* and *F. hepatica*, *Proc. 3rd Int. Congr. Parasitol.*, **1**: 500–1.

Silangwa, S. M., 1973. Incidence of liver flukes (*Fasciola gigantica*) in Barotse cattle, Zambia, *Bull. epiz. Dis. Afr.*, **21**(1): 11–17.

Sirag, S. B., Christensen, N. Ø., Nansen, P., Monrad, J. and Frandsen, F., 1981. Resistance to *Fasciola hepatica* in calves harbouring primary patent *Schistosoma bovis* infections, *J. Helminthol.*, **55**: 63–70.

Snijders, A. J., Louw, J. P. and Serrano, F. M. H., 1971. Trials with rafoxanide. 1. *Fasciola gigantica* in cattle in Angola, *J. S. Afr. vet. med. Ass.*, **42**(3): 249–51.

Soesetya, R. H. B., 1975. The prevalence of *Fasciola gigantica* infection in cattle in East Java, Indonesia, *Mal. Vet. J.*, **6**: 5–8.

Srivastava, P. S. and Singh, K. S., 1972. Early migration of *Fasciola gigantica* Cobbold, 1855, in guinea-pig, *Indian J. Anim. Sci.*, **42**(1): 63–71.

Troncy, P. M., Graber, M. and Thal, J., 1973. *Phacochoerus aethiopicus* (Pallas), a new host of *Fasciola gigantica* Cobbold, 1855, *Bull. Soc. Path. Exp.*, **66**(1): 129–33.

Uzoukwu, M. and Ikeme, M. M., 1978. Hepatic changes in natural *Fasciola gigantica* infestations of the Fulani zebu, *Bull. Anim. Hlth Prod. Afr.*, **25**: 162–7.

Weinbren, B. M. and Coyle, T. J., 1960. Uganda zebu cattle naturally infected with *Fasciola gigantica* with special reference to changes in the serum proteins, *J. Comp. Path.*, **70**: 176–81.

Zaki, H., 1960. Ovine endoparasites of Egyptian sheep and pastures with special reference to fascioliasis, *J. Egypt. Vet. Med. Ass.*, **20**: 157–72.

Chapter

25

Schistosomiasis

CONTENTS

INTRODUCTION

Schistosomiasis is a snail-borne trematode infection of man and domestic and wild animals. The sexually dimorphic adult worms localize in blood vessels of the liver, lungs, gastrointestinal and urogenital tracts, and the nasal cavity of the final host following infection by cercariae which penetrate the skin.

In man a number of species cause severe clinical syndromes which are of major public health importance in most tropical regions. On the other hand, schistosomiasis of domestic animals, although prevalent in Asia, Africa, and other tropical and subtropical regions, is only occasionally responsible for clinical disease. This may have limited the interest in schistosomiasis of animals. Schistosomal infections of livestock may involve a single species although mixed infections, including those primarily occurring in man and wild animals are frequently found.

Literature

The literature on schistosomiasis in man is extensive and that published between 1963 and 1974 has been abstracted in a comprehensive bibliography (Warren 1973a; Warren and Hoffman 1977). Comprehensive general descriptions of human schistosomiasis were presented by Malek (1980) and Nelson (1975).

There are considerably fewer publications on schistosomiasis in domestic animals. Hussein and Amin (1973) and Hussein (1973) reviewed the life cycle, clinical aspects, and pathogenesis of animal schistosomiasis in Africa caused by *Schistosoma bovis* and *S. mattheei,* while Lawrence (1978a) reviewed bovine schistosomiasis in southern Africa. Christensen *et al.* (1983) reviewed the biology and transmission of species infecting cattle in Africa and these included *S. bovis, S. mattheei, S. margrebowiei,* and *S. leiperi,* the latter two species being primarily parasites of wild ruminants. Schistosomiasis in Africa as an important zoonosis was reviewed by Nelson (1960).

ETIOLOGY

Identification of schistosomes which infect domestic animals is based primarily on the morphology of the adults and the eggs, and to a lesser degree the species of snail infected. Because this information is incomplete, identification of species in domestic and wild animals may be difficult.

A number of species are recognized as causing infestations in domestic animals. In Africa *S. bovis* and *S. mattheei* are reported in cattle, sheep, goats, and horses. In addition, pigs and camels are infected with *S. bovis*. However, the similar morphology of *S. bovis* and

S. mattheei have raised problems in classification, and the shape of eggs is the most useful criterion for differentiation of the two species. *Schistosoma spindale* is found in India and southeast Asia in buffalo, cattle, goats, and sheep. In this region *S. incognitum* infects horses, pigs, and dogs, and *S. indicum* is found in horses and occasionally in cattle. *Schistosoma nasalis* is located in the veins of the nasal mucosa of cattle, buffalo, and occasionally in small domestic ruminants. In the Far East *S. japonicum* is an important parasite of cattle, dogs, and pigs. *Ornithobilharzia turkestanicum* is distributed in the Middle East and central Asia, and although not pathogenic for cattle, horses, and camels, may cause severe lesions in sheep and goats. *Heterobilharzia americana* is one of two species that parasitize mammals in North America. It is found in dogs, nutria, and raccoons and occasionally causes clinical disease in dogs.

Some species of schistosomes are not strictly host specific and cross-infections occur between domestic and wild animals and man, resulting in a very complex etiology involving single and multiple infections. This is important in zoonosis because various species infecting man are also found in a variety of wild and domestic animals which serve as reservoirs. This applies particularly to *S. japonicum*.

Literature

A checklist tabulating the extensive literature on the definitive hosts of the species in the genus *Schistosoma* which occur naturally in Africa and the Middle East in wild and domestic species was published by Pitchford (1977).

Some workers have considered *S. bovis* and *S. mattheei* as members of the same species. Others have separated the two on the basis of morphology, specificity of intermediate host, the range of definitive hosts, and pathology. Eggs have been regarded as either uniform with each proposed species and therefore distinguishable, or as pleomorphic and indistinguishable between the two species. *Schistosoma bovis* has generally been considered to be a parasite primarily of cattle, but it also infects sheep and goats, and occasionally camels, horses, and donkeys. *Schistosoma mattheei* has a wider range, infecting various domestic and wild ruminants and also man. It has been suggested that *S. bovis* was introduced into Africa with the migration of people and cattle while *S. mattheei* was an indigenous parasite of African wild ruminants (Dinnik and Dinnik 1965). Within *S. bovis* distinct strains were thought to exist based on biological characteristics of growth rates, maturation rates, egg production, and infectivity in both intermediate and definitive hosts. One has been identified in North Africa, some Mediterranean islands, and the Middle East, and another was found in western Kenya (Southgate and Knowles 1975a; Ross *et al.* 1978). These biological types of *S. bovis* were all different from *S. matthei*. Isoelectric focusing of enzymes from the adult worms has assisted in the identification of species, but could not be used to identify strain (Southgate *et al.* 1980; Ross *et al.* 1978).

On the west coast of Africa the life cycle of the parasite *S. curassoni* was described and shown to be the causative agent of urinary schistosomiasis both in man and cattle (Grétillat 1962a, b). Although morphological differences between *S. bovis* and *S. curassoni* have been reported (Grétillat 1964), the validity of this latter species has not been established.

Schistosomiasis of domestic animals in India is caused by *S. spindale*, *S. nasalis*, *S. indicum*, and *S. incognitum* (Kalapesi and Purohit 1954). *Schistosoma incognitum* has been regarded as a common parasite of pigs and dogs in India and its life cycle was defined in the intermediate and definitive host (Krishnamurthi 1956; Sinha and Srivastava 1960).

Nasal schistosomiasis was common in cattle and buffalo in India but was uncommon in goats and sheep (Sen and Ray 1969; Muraleedharan *et al.* 1973).

Heterobilharzia americana was first reported in a dog in the USA in 1961; previously it was known to occur only in wild animals (Pierce 1963).

Schistosoma japonicum has been recorded to infect cattle, dogs, pigs, rats, and man and has been widely distributed in various species of wild animals (Schneider *et al.* 1975).

EPIZOOTIOLOGY

Incidence and geographic distribution

In the epizootiology of schistosomiasis in domestic animals, the prevalence of infection and incidence of clinical disease must be differentiated. The prevalence of infections reported are related to circumstances under which studies are undertaken and depend on the various techniques used to detect infections, such as fecal counts and examination of abattoir material. Prevalence in most tropical regions is probably much greater than that currently reported.

Outbreaks of disease in sheep, goats, cattle, and buffalo are reported from various parts of the world, but as with other helminthiases losses due to overt clinical disease are probably only a fraction of those which result from the much more prevalent subclinical infections. Recently, more attention has been given to the importance of schistosomiasis in livestock and its impact on the industry. The rates of infection and occurrence of clinical signs depend on the distribution of intermediate hosts and local environmental conditions which affect the level of infestations making up the challenge.

In Africa *S. bovis* and *S. mattheei* are widely distributed and both are thought to cause significant economic losses. Prevalence in Africa may be as high as 90% and appears to be increasing in cattle, but varies considerably from one region to another. *Schistosoma mattheei* is found in the southern half of Africa while *S. bovis* is found in East and North

Africa. This species is also reported in the Middle East, southern Europe, the Mediterranean islands, and western Asia. With the development of various tropical regions involving establishment of large irrigation projects and increased numbers of livestock, the pattern of schistosomiasis in livestock is changing and appears to be increasing in importance.

There is relatively less information available on the incidence of infections and diseases caused by other schistosome species in animals in various parts of the world. The incidences of schistosomiasis in both cattle and buffalo and small ruminants are variable.

Schistosomiasis is one of the most widespread parasitic diseases with 500 million people being exposed to four main species in Africa, the Middle East, South America, and the Orient.

Literature

A map of the distribution of various species of *Schistosoma* in domestic animals in East and South Africa was presented by Dinnik and Dinnik in 1965. Recently the distribution of species causing bovine schistosomiasis has been published by Christensen *et al.* (1983).

A number of outbreaks in Africa of clinical disease in cattle, sheep, and goats have been reported primarily from South Africa and Zimbabwe. Mortality in sheep and goats was recorded in South Africa (Strydom 1963; Hurter and Potgieter 1967). Surveys in Zimbabwe showed 50 to 70% infection rates in cattle and sheep, but these were not related to obvious economic losses (Condy 1960; Lawrence and Condy 1970; Lawrence 1977a; McKenzie 1970; McKenzie and Grainge 1970). In the Sudan, bovine schistosomiasis caused by *S. bovis* is of increasing economic importance with the occurrence of severe epizootics (Malek 1960, 1969). Prevalence as determined by fecal egg counts was higher during the hot summer months, with 90% of 1- to 2-year-old cattle affected, but a lower frequency was observed in older animals (Majid *et al.* 1980a; Eisa 1966; Magzoub and Adam 1977). The losses from *S. bovis* were due to mortality, delayed growth, and decreased calf production and occurred primarily in the 6- to 13-month age group (McCauley *et al.* 1983). The incidence of *S. bovis* in regions of Nigeria was relatively low during drought conditions and was dependent on the establishing of water reservoirs (Pugh *et al.* 1980). Reports have been made on the occurrence of *S. bovis* from other countries including the Congo (Schwetz 1955), Ethiopia (Lo and Lemma 1975), Egypt (Soliman 1956), Israel (Klopfer *et al.* 1977), Iran (Arfaa *et al.* 1965), Spain (Martin 1972), and Sardinia (Coluzzi *et al.* 1966). The epidemiology of schistosomiasis in cattle, goats, and sheep has also been reported in Senegal and Mauritania (Marill 1961; Grétillat 1963).

The prevalence of *S. japonicum* in domestic animals was monitored for several years in Japan (Okoshi 1958) where in dairy cattle it varied from 5 to 40% (Yokogawa *et al.* 1971).

Ornithobilharzia turkestanicum has been reported from Russia, China, India, and various countries around the Mediterranean. In Iran, the prevalence varied from 2 to 30% in sheep, goats, and buffalo, and infections were associated with less severe clinical syndromes than those observed with *S. bovis* (Massoud 1973a, b).

Epizootiology of nasal schistosomiasis has been reported from various regions of India in both cattle and buffalo (Biswas and Subramanian 1978; Biswal 1956; Varma 1954). The overall rates of infection in cattle and buffalo ranged from approximately 2 to 30% of animals examined (Muraleedharan *et al.* 1976a). Prevalence was greater in cattle than in buffalo, and in older animals as compared with young. Nasal schistosomiasis in goats and sheep has also been described (Achuthan and Alwar 1973).

Malek (1980) presented tables on the geographic distribution and hosts of the zoonotic schistosomes in domestic animals. Iarotski and Davis (1981) presented the magnitude of the world problem of schistosomiasis in man based on surveys undertaken by the World Health Organization and the control programs conducted in 103 countries. Human and animal schistosomiasis do not necessarily occur in the same region; for example, infections in man have been very common in the islands of Mauritius, Madagascar, and Egypt, but animal schistosomiasis has not been described. Conversely, on the islands of Corsica and Sardinia *S. bovis* has been shown to be common but human schistosomiasis is not present (Pitchford 1963).

Transmission

Transmission of schistosomes is complex, involving contact between animals and water containing infective cercarial stages. Eggs excreted by the mammalian host and in contact with fresh water will remain viable for at least 5 days. Ciliated miracidia emerge from the egg under the influence of environmental factors which include osmotic effects, temperature, and agitation, and are viable for 15 to 30 hours. These free-living larval stages are attracted chemotactically by mucous secretions to an aquatic snail, and after penetration of the foot of a suitable intermediate host develop through two generations of sporocyst. Cercariae develop within a daughter sporocyst and are released from the snail to infect the mammalian host transdermally. The optimal cycle in the snail is about 4 to 5 weeks but is variable depending on the temperature. During winter the incubation period is lengthened to 3 to 4 months and even longer in colder areas. On leaving the snail cercariae remain viable for up to 40 hours.

Literature

There has been relatively little detailed information available in schistosomiasis of domestic animals on transmission, species of snails, and cyclic development in the intermediate hosts. *Schistosoma bovis* has been transmitted by *Bulinus* spp. in the africanus, forskali, and truncatus groups, and *S. mattheei* by species in the africanus and forskali groups (Southgate and Knowles 1975a, b). A study on distribution of snails of medical and veterinary importance has been undertaken in Nigeria (Smith 1982).

INFECTION

Sexual reproduction occurs in the final host which is infected by the cercariae which penetrate the skin or mucous membranes aided by vigorous movement and secretion of enzymes. The organisms are changed anatomically, physiologically, and biochemically into schistosomula which leave the skin within 24 to 48 hours. Migration takes place through blood and lymphatic vessels, first to the lungs then to the liver where they mature into adult worms, mate, and then pass to their final habitat in the blood vessels of various tissues depending on the species of schistosome. In the blood vessels, fertilized females produce large numbers of eggs, with a potential of 3000 eggs per day depending on the immune response of the host. A miracidium develops within the egg which, aided by its spine and the excretion of proleolytic enzyme, passes out of the venules through the tissue into either the lumen of the intestine and urinary bladder or the nasal cavity. Up to 50% of the eggs laid remain within the body of the definitive host.

The basic host–parasite relationship during infection is similar for *S. mattheei* and *S. bovis*. Cattle are more adapted for the survival of *S. bovis*. In sheep, *S. mattheei* is more pathogenic than in cattle. The predilection site of mature worms varies with the species of schistosome, and in some cases with the duration of infection. Mature *S. mattheei* and *S. bovis* inhabit the portal, common mesenteric, submucosal, and subserosal intestinal veins, pancreatic and sometimes splenic and gastropiploic veins, and pulmonary vessels. The distribution is, in part, dependent on the level of infestation, being more widely disseminated in heavy infestations. *Schistosoma mattheei* and rarely *S. bovis* occasionally affect the urinary bladder and uterus. There is relatively little definitive information on the life cycle and tissue distribution of other schistosomes of veterinary importance.

The effect of infections and the severity of the pathogenic responses are related to levels of adult infestations and the presence of eggs in the tissue. The level of infection to which an animal is exposed depends on the system of husbandry, season, and water supply. Numbers of cercariae in the water and the time an animal spends in contact with infected water govern the level of infection.

The majority of schistosome species infect a relatively wide range of mammalian hosts, the susceptibility of a host to infection and the pathogenicity of a species varying with the degree of innate and acquired resistance of the host. Infection with more than one species may give rise to hybrids.

A variety of laboratory animals are used as models of schistosomiasis of man and domestic animals. One important feature which was observed with passage of *S. mattheei* in a laboratory animal was reduction of pathogenicity for the natural host.

Literature

The relationship between life cycle, tissue tropism, level of infestation with schistosomes, and pathogenesis has been discussed and summarized by Warren (1973a, 1978, 1982). The amount of information available on the different aspects of infection varies with the species, but generally there has been less research into those schistosomes which are of veterinary importance as compared with those infecting man.

Most available information on the various stages of infection relates to *S. mattheei*. The pathogenesis and pathology of infection in cattle and sheep have been studied quite extensively, particularly by Lawrence and co-workers. In cattle, the schistosomula migrate from the lung to the mesentery and although not proven it is proposed to be by active migration against the bloodstream along the pulmonary arteries, heart, and caudal vena cava and hepatic vein into the liver (Lawrence 1978a; Kruger *et al.* 1969). In the hepatic portal vein the worms mated and migrated to the final site, the mesenteric veins. The predilection site for paired adult worms was the small intestine and proximal large intestine, with egg-laying tending to be most intense in the terminal ileum, cecum, and proximal colon. Following the acute clinical phase of infestation occurring shortly after patency at 8 to 9 weeks, there was a temporary shift of the parasite to the distal colon and rectum and further migration at 18 weeks of the worms from the intestine to the veins of the urinary bladder and stomach (Lawrence 1974a, 1977b, 1978a). Bladder lesions occur in about 10.5% of naturally infected cattle. There is a shift of infestation from the intestine to the bladder during the latter stages of infestation (Lawrence 1974a). Alves (1953) presented evidence that *S. bovis* also produced infection in the urinary bladder in cattle. As the parasite invoked an immunological response in the host the adult worms became reduced in length and were eliminated between 18 and 40 weeks after infestation. However, in spite of this hostile host response parasites survived for up to 2 years (Lawrence 1978a). In contrast, the population of parasites in sheep remained at constant levels during the first year (Lawrence 1974b).

Females penetrated into the smaller veins, usually of the intestine, to lay their eggs. Anywhere from 600 to 3000 eggs were deposited and up to 80% passed into the feces. The eggs penetrated the blood vessels and moved through the intestine into the lumen. The prepatent period was usually 6 to 9 weeks and egg-laying was very active from about 8 weeks onward, but was sharply reduced to low levels by 10 to 14 weeks when acute clinical signs subsided. Immunological response governed the egg-laying ability of the worm and limited the pathogenic effect of the parasite (Lawrence 1973a, 1977a, 1978a). As the immunological reaction to adult worms increased, the worms withdrew from the deeper layers of the intestine and eggs were localized in the adventitia and muscle layers of the blood vessels. Eggs deposited in the submucosa of the intestinal tract persisted for 4 to 5 weeks and then were broken down and phagocytosed. During this latter stage of infection a large proportion of eggs laid in the mesenteric vein was carried to the liver. However, passage of eggs in the feces still continued for up to 18 months. Because of variations in daily fecal counts of eggs, no correlation with the levels of infections could be established (Lawrence 1974b, 1978a). Lawrence (1977b) summarized the information on the wide distribution of eggs in various organs in bovine schistosomiasis caused by *S. mattheei*. In sheep, *S. mattheei* were also found in the mesenteric vessels as well as in the vasculature of the rumen and urinary bladder (Hurter and Potgieter 1967; McCully and Kruger 1969).

Relatively little information is available on other schistosomes of veterinary interest. *Schistosoma incognitum*, after entry of the final host through the mouth, skin, and mucous membranes, developed into the adult in hepatic portal mesenteric veins in 36 days (Sinha and Srivastava 1960). Pulmonary involvement by this species has also been found in pigs (Singh and Rajya 1978).

In an experimental *S. nasalis* infestation of buffalo calves, the worms migrated to the lungs before reaching nasal veins. Eggs appeared in nasal discharge after 24 days with nodules developing in the mucosa after 6 months (Muraleedharan *et al.* 1976c).

Relatively light infection with *S. mattheei* and *S. bovis* produced little effect, while heavy infestation caused clinical disease and death (Dinnik and Dinnik 1965; Lawrence 1973b). Pathogenicity was related to number of worms present and usually was limited to levels of infection which could be well tolerated by the host. Clinical signs developed in isolated instances involving large numbers of worms (Lawrence 1978a). At low levels of infection the parasites survived in a steady state with pathogenicity regulated by the host's defense mechanisms (Lawrence 1973b).

Age has been found to affect the susceptibility of sheep to *S. mattheei* infection with young animals having a higher incidence and level of infection. This was maintained on the basis of the numbers of parasites observed at different stages of infections in different age groups and breeds of sheep (van Wyk *et al.* 1976). *Schistosoma bovis* infection in cattle was also shown to have a relationship to age (Bushara *et al.* 1980). Ninety percent of 2-year-old cattle were infected and this rate fell to a level of 30% in 10-year-old animals (Hussein 1980).

The incidences of *S. nasalis* infection in cattle have been reported to be higher than in buffalo, and in the latter species infections were more apt to be asymptomatic. In experimental infections, cattle excreted two to three times more eggs than did buffalo (Rao and Devi 1971). However, cross-infection between cattle and buffalo did occur (Koshy *et al.* 1975).

In the laboratory, natural hosts and various laboratory animals have been used to study infections and pathogenesis. Various methods of inducing experimental infection in sheep with *S. mattheei* have been compared (van Wyk *et al.* 1975; van Wyk and Groeneveld 1973). An apparatus used to apply *S. mattheei* cercariae to the skin of cattle and sheep has been described (Lawrence and Joannou 1975).

Frandsen (1981) gave an up-to-date account of the maintenance and mass production of *S. mansoni* in the laboratory to be used for chemotherapy trials in mice. Mice and hamsters have also been used for the study of *S. bovis* infections. In the hamsters, mortality occurred between 58 and 64 days after infection with cercaria (Lengy 1962). Following several passages of *S. mattheei* in hamsters the pathogenicity of the strain was reduced for sheep (Taylor *et al.* 1977). The postcercarial development of *S. incognitum* has been investigated in mice (Ahluwalia 1971). Experimentally, hamsters and mice could be infected with *H. americana* while rabbits, guinea pigs, and cats exhibited some degree of host resistance. Albino rats and rhesus monkeys were totally resistant (Lee 1962).

Infectivity and pathogenicity of six species of African schistosomes and their hybrids were compared in mice and hamsters, and significant differences were observed between hybrids and the parental species (Taylor and Andrews 1978). Development of hybrids between *S. mattheei* and *S. hematobium* and other species could be important because hybrids were capable of not only infecting laboratory animals but cattle, sheep, and man (Pitchford 1963).

CLINICAL SIGNS

In domestic animals, schistosomiasis is characterized clinically by anorexia, diarrhea, dysentery, emaciation, dehydration, edema, anemia, muscular weakness, and abdominal pain. Clinical signs and associated lesions are dependent on the distribution of the mature worms and on the eggs deposited in tissues. Severity of clinical signs and the extent of the lesions are related to the level of infection and the intensity of host responses, and can be modified by a number of factors including nutrition and other complicating diseases.

Acute disease is most frequently observed in animals experiencing first exposure to schistosomes which usually occurs at an early age. In cases of heavy infestation, there is a rapid onset of clinical signs often followed by spontaneous remission. In the more common light infections the disease is usually chronic with few detectable signs, although infected animals are probably more susceptible to other diseases.

Clinical syndromes associated with *S. mattheei* and *S. bovis* infection are comparable and usually appear as chronic diseases with no distinctive or characteristic clinical signs. With *S. mattheei* infections, two forms are recognized in cattle: an intestinal syndrome caused by extensive deposition of eggs in the walls of the intestine, and a chronic hepatic syndrome caused by immunological response to the adult worms. The disease is less important in cattle than in sheep and tends to be less severe than that caused by *S. bovis*. Acute and severe forms have been studied but information on the subtle mild chronic forms is not well documented. Severe clinical signs are most often associated with the periods of heaviest egg-laying.

In domestic animals, little is known of the severity of cutaneous response caused by the penetrating cercariae but it is generally considered to be of little importance.

Species of schistosomes which occur in domestic animals outside Africa cause a variety of syndromes in a number of domestic species. Clinical signs are not well described and appear to vary with both the species of worms and species of host. Nasal schistosomiasis in cattle and buffalo is characterized by frequent sneezing and discharge of thick mucus from nostrils. As the disease progresses, the discharge becomes fetid, mucipurulent, and contains blood, with the sneezing becoming more pronounced and progressing to snoring. The breathing may become difficult and interfere with feeding. In buffalo, the signs and associated lesions are usually much less apparent than in cattle. Buffalo are thought to be naturally resistant to nasal schistosomiasis and rarely exhibit clinical signs in any form.

Literature

Descriptions of clinical syndromes caused by *S. mattheei* in cattle and sheep have been published from southern Africa. Lawrence and McKenzie (1972) presented a brief review of the outbreaks of schistosomiasis in sheep and cattle between 1967 and 1971 in Zimbabwe. Field outbreaks of *S. mattheei* in some regions of southern Africa have been acute, resulting from very high levels of infection (van Wyk *et al.* 1974). The most common syndrome was the intestinal form caused by *S. mattheei* (Lawrence 1976a, b, 1977c, 1978a). It was characterized by acute diarrhea or dysentery developing 7 to 8 weeks after infection associated with the onset of heavy egg-laying in the intestinal mucosa. This was accompanied by anorexia, loss of condition, and reduction of growth rates. The severity and duration of clinical signs was related to the level of infection. Clinical signs usually abated and recovery was spontaneous. Occasionally the acute syndrome was followed by unthriftiness without diarrhea (Lawrence 1977c, 1978a; Hurter and Potgieter 1967). The chronic hepatic syndrome was characterized by progressive hepatic fibrosis resulting in liver insufficiency and loss of condition. Acute terminal hepatic failure provoked nervous signs such as ataxia and mania (Lawrence 1976b, 1978a).

In experimental studies in cattle, a single large infection of *S. mattheei* usually resulted in an acute intestinal syndrome with death occurring within 2 weeks. Hemorrhage was observed from the large intestine (Lawrence 1976b). Following repeated experimental infections, death occurred after 74 weeks of progressive hepatic failure accompanied by severe eosinophilia and hypergammaglobulinemia (Lawrence 1977d). Sheep were more susceptible than cattle to *S. mattheei* and developed more severe clinical manifestations of the disease. In sheep the experimental clinical syndrome was progressive for the first 25 weeks, with mortality occurring in some animals; then the disease became chronic with no evidence of recovery up to 67 weeks (Lawrence 1980).

The disease in cattle caused by *S. bovis* has been reported to be more severe than that caused by *S. mattheei*. A morbidity rate of 100% and a mortality rate of 50% have been reported in one district of the Sudan. The severity of the disease varied with age, being most pronounced in calves (Hussein and Nelson 1968). Experimental exposure of calves to heavy challenge with *S. bovis* resulted in severe hemorrhagic diarrhea about 7 weeks after infection. The animals became weak and listless with a staring coat, anorexia, and loss of weight (Taylor *et al.* 1980). During primary infection, fecal egg counts were the best indicator of clinical disease which could be related to the level of infection. Under field conditions, however, with occurrence of multiple infections and infections of long duration, fecal counts were not indicative of the severity of the disease (Dargie 1980).

There have been only occasional reports of clinical disease caused by primarily human species. Desert sheep in the Sudan were found to be susceptible to *S. mansoni* infestation resulting in anorexia, soft feces, progressive weakness, and loss of wool. Because of this susceptibility and development of patent infection the species was regarded as a carrier of *S. mansoni* (Adam and Magzoub 1976). Experimental infestations by *S. mansoni* in the goat have also resulted in inappetance, diarrhea, anemia, dyspnea, and wasting. These clinical signs were associated with characteristic lesions observed in the intestine and liver (Adam and Magzoub 1977).

There is only limited information on clinical signs of natural and experimental infection with schistosomal species occurring outside Africa. Unusual outbreaks of *S. spindale* infection characterized by high mortality in cattle have been reported. Buffalo were found to be more refractory than cattle. In these outbreaks, in addition to the usual sites of localization of adult worms in portal and mesenteric veins, large numbers of worms were present in the heart, aorta, vena cava, lungs, liver, and spleen. Eggs were also widely disseminated in various tissues including the liver, brain, kidneys, heart, and lungs (Kulkarni *et al.* 1954).

Vashista *et al.* (1981) reported clinical observations associated with a natural outbreak of *S. indicum* infestation in sheep in India with a mortality of 10 to 33%. Pulmonary lesions in sheep and goats have been associated with *S. indicum* (Sharma and Dwivedi 1976). In another outbreak pulmonary lesions were observed in sheep, the morbidity being 21% and mortality 8% among animals from 1.5 to 4 years of age (Lodha *et al.* 1981). Cirrhosis caused by this species in the liver of horses was common in India (Raghavan 1958).

Schistosoma incognitum has been reported to cause a severe disease in dogs characterized by emaciation, severe anemia, respiratory distress, and hemorrhagic diarrhea (Tewari and Singh 1977). Experimental infestation resulted in death in 10 to 12 weeks in some animals, with lesions occurring in the lungs, liver, and intestine (Tewari *et al.* 1966). Clinical signs in pigs consisted of dysentery, periodic fever, anorexia, and general malaise with blood and mucus present in the feces (Ahluwalia and Dutt 1972).

With nasal schistosomiasis, variable susceptibility to infestation and clinical signs was observed in cattle and buffalo (Rao and Naik 1957). Incidences and severities of infestations in both cattle and buffalo depended on the particular geographic region, and occasionally infections were more prevalent in buffalo than in cattle (Rajamohanan and Peter 1972). The granulomatous growths in the nasal cavity resulted in discharges and snoring (Rao and Devi 1971). A correlation between level of infection and the severity of gross lesions and clinical signs was not necessarily observed. A low percentage of cattle was found to have eggs in the discharge but were clinically negative. A larger percentage of positive buffalo did not exhibit either gross lesions or clinical symptoms (Muraleedharan *et al.* 1976b; Rao and Mohiyuddeen 1955). In another study in buffalo there were no clinical signs and lesions were mild, while in cattle the lesions were more extensive, granulomatous, and associated with obvious clinical signs (Rajamohanan and Peter 1972). Relationship between egg count, types of gross lesions, and nature of nasal discharge were investigated. A majority of cases showed low egg count although the severity of lesions varied. Serous discharge was predominant in cases of nodular lesion, mucoid or mucopurulent with cauliflower-like growths and bloody discharge with advanced stages of the disease (Muraleedharan *et al.* 1976b, c).

Heterobilharzia americana infections in dogs caused a syndrome similar to bovine schistosomiasis with anorexia, emaciation, and diarrhea containing mucus and blood (Thrasher 1964; Goff and Ronald 1980). In addition, severe dermatitis has been reported in dogs (Pierce 1963). The first report of canine schistosomiasis in the Western Hemisphere was reported by Malek *et al.* (1961). Adult worms were found in both small and large intestine and intrahepatic portal veins. Granulomas were found in the liver and in the wall of the intestines as well as in the lungs, kidneys, and spleen.

PATHOLOGY

Characteristic lesions are granulomatous reactions due to the presence of schistosomes and ova in blood vessels and tissues. Veins which contain adult schistosomes have periphlebitis with proliferative inflammatory reactions extending into surrounding tissue. Dead adults cause thrombosis, extensive granulomatous reaction, and localized lymphoid tissue proliferation. Ova cause granulomatous reactions which on occasion are referred to as pseudotubercles. The pathogenesis is attributed primarily to the widely disseminated eggs and the accompanying granulomatous reactions within tissue and vessels, particularly in the alimentary tract, liver, and lungs, and partially to the presence of dead worms. Accompanying these lesions in the tissues are hyperplastic, hypertrophic, and granulomatous reactions in the local drainage lymph nodes.

The pathogenesis of *S. mattheei* infections varies between the acute and chronic syndromes. In the former the changes are due to tissue damage and characterized by intestinal lesions, anemia, hypoalbuminemia, and high fecal egg counts. Deposition of the eggs in the intestinal mucosa is the most important feature and is responsible for the gastrointestinal malfunction, which usually results in diarrhea containing blood and mucus. In the chronic syndrome the lesions are regenerative and proliferative in the intestines, liver, and lung, and associated with eosinophilia, hyperglobulinemia, and lower egg counts.

The intestinal syndrome caused by *S. mattheei* lesions varies from acute enteritis, with hemorrhage and acute inflammatory exudate. The mucosa is coated with thick mucous exudate and occasionally is pigmented grayish-black. Histologically, in the mucosa there is an infiltration of eosinophils and mononuclear cells with an increase in the goblet cells in the granular mucosa. A major factor in the severity of the syndrome in sheep is the intestinal bleeding caused by passage of eggs through the bowel wall. In the chronic form, granulomas are present on the mucosal and serosal surfaces and appear as raised foci. Granulomatous inflammatory reaction is found in the mucosa, lamina propria, and submucosa. The significance of hepatic and pulmonary lesions in the clinical syndrome is often not clear. Hepatosplenomegaly is not a feature of *S. bovis* or *S. mattheei* in cattle or sheep, but chronic infection may cause periportal fibrosis and a decrease in size of the liver with surface irregularities. Gray pigmentation is usually an indication of heavy infection. Microscopically, there is fibrosis of portal veins, granulomatous reaction around eggs, and lymphoid nodule formation. Thrombosis of blood vessels also occurs with adult worms being present in the thrombi. Lesions occur in the lungs in heavily infected animals, and consist of disseminated granulomas and discoloration by grayish-black pigment. Infarcts may also be found in the lungs and are associated with dead worms. The pancreas is another site of lesions and, in addition to the characteristic granulomatous and vascular changes, there are areas of adipose tissue necrosis, acinar atrophy, and fibrosis. Characteristic lesions develop in the bladder in the latter stages of heavy infestation with *S. mattheei*.

Early and late clinical signs in cattle are associated with hematological changes. Normochromic and normocytic anemia, hypoalbuminemia, and lymphopenia occur. Neutrophilia is present only during acute illness and is followed by neutropenia. Hemoglobin and serum albumin levels decrease as the result of intestinal hemorrhage and loss of plasma into the intestine. During the latter stages of the acute infestation there is an increase in eosinophils and immunoglobulins. The eosinophils reflect the degree of inflammatory response, and an increase occurs 6 to 10 weeks after infection and is associated with the deposition of eggs. Serological changes include a decrease in levels of albumin and beta globulin, and a marked increase in alpha and gamma globulins.

The pathogenicity of *S. nasalis* depends on the severity, duration of infection, and the response of the host. Lesions are less extensive in buffalo than in cattle and are in the mucous membranes in the anterior part of the nasal cavity, varying from a few pimple-like eruptions to cauliflower-like masses of well-vascularized granulation tissue. The initial nasal discharge and sneezing are associated with redness of the mucosa and the development of edema with subsequent nodule formation. Histologically the acute inflammatory reaction is around eggs, progressing to granulation tissue reaction and ulceration.

Literature

The pathology of African schistosomiasis in domestic animals was summarized by Hussein and Amin (1973). Comprehensive summaries of the pathology and pathobiology of schistosomiasis were presented by Warren (1973a, 1978, 1982) and included observations made in domestic animals. Pathogenesis was related to the distribution of the adult worms within blood vessels and the numbers of eggs retained in the veins and tissues. The host granulomatous response to these antigenic foreign bodies was critical in causing tissue malfunction and was related to the cell-mediated type of response. These large granulomatous formations and fibrosis caused destruction in liver parenchyma, resulting in obstruction to portal blood flow. Recently, the specific antigens responsible for the delayed type of hypersensitivity have been identified. In acute and chronic syndromes it has been postulated that the hypersensitivity of immediate and delayed types and deposition of immune complexes played a role in tissue injury.

The basic lesion in blood vessels was a phlebitis due to the dead adult parasites lodging in blood vessels in the liver, lungs and intestine. The characteristic microscopic picture was hypertrophy, hyperplasia, and the development of extensive lymphoid nodules and follicles in the affected tissues (Hussein 1971). The histology of lesions caused by *S. mattheei* observed in cattle and sheep was described in detail by McCully and Kruger (1969). Globule leukocytes containing large acidophilic granules have been detected in the inflammatory lesions caused by *S. mattheei* infestation in cattle and have been associated with an immune response (Lawrence 1977e).

In experimental schistosomiasis of cattle infected with *S. bovis* and *S. mattheei*, various features of pathogenesis and pathology were similar. The pathology of *S. mattheei* in cattle has been attributed to the eggs causing lesions. Well-developed granulomas were found around eggs in the liver, intestinal tract, pancreas, lungs, forestomachs, and local drainage lymph nodes. Inflammation was caused primarily by immunological responses to the antigens released by eggs and the dead worms (Lawrence 1977c, 1978c). In the large intestine the early mucosal lesions were hemorrhagic due to the hypersensitivity to the migrating eggs. As the infection progresses, concentrations of eggs in the intestinal wall decrease and the distribution of eggs between mucosa and submucosa muscle layers alter. In the latter stages of the infection the inflammatory response was primarily granulomatous (Lawrence 1978b).

Early lesions in mucosa of the urinary bladder consisted of petechial hemorrhages associated with an immediate type of allergic reaction, with chronic lesions appearing as greenish-gray nodules coalescing to form large raised areas (Condy 1960). These lesions have also been described as either granular or polypoidal patches, or polyps (Bartsch and van Wyk 1977).

The degree of clinical pathology in cattle was related to levels of *S. mattheei* infection. Anemia, lymphopenia, and hypoalbuminemia developed during the acute phase. With clinical recovery, eosinophilia and hypergammaglobulinemia appeared (Lawrence 1977f; Taylor *et al.* 1980). Similar changes were also observed in *S. mattheei* infections in sheep (Dargie *et al.* 1973; Malherbe 1970; Preston *et al.* 1973a; van Zyl 1973, 1974). Anemia was associated with hemodilution, gastrointestinal hemorrhage, and dyshemopoiesis (Preston *et al.* 1973b; Preston and Dargie 1974; Dargie and Preston 1974). Each of these factors had a varying effect on different stages throughout the progression of clinical disease (Preston and Dargie 1975). A good correlation was observed between the severity of the anemia, reduction of red blood cell survival, and magnitude of intestinal hemorrhage.

Severity of the acute clinical syndromes caused by *S. bovis* in cattle depended on the level of infection, the reproductive activities of worms, and the age of the host. Main lesions were in the small and large intestines resulting in hemorrhage and loss of fluid into the lumen. Malfunction in digestion and absorption resulted in reduction in intake and feed utilization efficiency, which was accompanied by diarrhea, anemia, hyperglobulinemia, and hypoalbuminemia (Dargie 1980). In naturally ocurring bovine schistosomiasis, lesions were found in the intestinal tract, liver, and other organs. These were characterized by formation of granulomas, periportal inflammatory infiltration, fibrosis, pigmentation of Kupffer cells, medial hypertrophy of portal veins, and lymphoid nodule formation (Hussein *et al.* 1975). The presence of *S. bovis* eggs in the lungs of cattle and sheep resulted in pseudotubercles, gray pigmentation, and increased mucus production (Deiana 1953). Differences have been observed between calves, sheep, and goats infected experimentally with *S. bovis*. The lesions in calves had a pronounced medial hypertrophy of portal veins. Sheep had proliferative endophlebitis and abundant eosinophil infiltration, and the goats had large numbers of eggs surrounded by stellate-shaped accumulations of eosinophilic antigen–antibody material (Massoud 1973b).

Infected calves became clinically ill around the seventh week after exposure, with clinical signs persisting for 2 to 3 months. The animals became progressively anemic, hypoalbuminemic, hyperglobulinemic, and developed eosinophilia which was most prominent during the 2 months when egg levels were highest (Arru and Parriciatu 1960; Hussein and Tartour 1973; Saad *et al.* 1980). Comparable observations on hematological changes were made in sheep infected with *S. bovis* (Holmes *et al.* 1975; Monrad *et al.* 1982) and *S. indicum* (Pandey *et al.* 1979).

In massive *S. curassoni* infestation in cattle, sheep, and goats the lesions were comparable to those found with *S. mattheei* and *S. bovis* and consisted of extensive hepatic fibrosis and pigmentation of the lungs (Grétillat and Picart 1964).

Schistosoma indicum has been observed to cause hepatic and intestinal lesions in horses, donkeys, sheep, goats, and cattle. Pulmonary lesions due to schistosomiasis were relatively rare (Arora and Iyer 1968; Dhodapkar *et al.* 1964; Krishnamurthi 1956; Sharma and Dwivedi 1976; Sreekumaran and Chaubal 1975; Srivastava *et al.* 1964).

Ornithobilharzia turkestanicum produced less severe lesions in cattle, sheep, and goats than *S. bovis*, the liver being less affected and lesions being observed in the duodenum in association with eggs (Massoud 1971).

Natural infection in pigs with *S. incognitum* resulted in lesions in the liver, intestine, and lungs (Ahluwalia 1959; Shrivastav and Dubey 1969; Singh and Rajya 1978). In experimental infections, pseudotubercles developed in lungs and liver by 2 months and extensive fibrosis was evidenced by 12 months (Ahluwalia 1972a).

The comparative pathology of nasal schistosomiasis in buffalo and cattle has been studied. In both species lesions developed around eggs. In cattle, the gross lesions were pathopneumonic with the nodular growths being extensive in advanced cases. In buffalo the lesions were generally scanty and inconspicuous (Biswal and Das 1956; Krishnamurthi 1956; Muraleedharan *et al.* 1976b; Sankar and Anantaraman 1974). In experimental infestation of laboratory animals, kids, and lambs, lesions were observed in the portal triads with degenerative changes in the hepatic cells and inflammatory cell infiltrations. Parasites were present in the lumen of hepatic vessels (Sahay and Sahai 1976; Sahay *et al.* 1977).

Reports of the lesions caused by schistosomes in game animals of Africa are few. McCully *et al.* (1967) reported on observations made on hippopotami (*Hippopotamus amphibius linnaeus*) and found lesions primarily in the lungs and liver and to a lesser extent in other tissues and organs, including the heart. Adult *S. hippopotami* were widely disseminated in the blood vessels.

IMMUNOLOGY

Innate and acquired immunity to schistosomes occur in animals. Innate immunity depends on genetic constitution and is primarily responsible for defining the range of hosts susceptible to infections. Acquired immunity is induced and governed by prior exposure to either homologous or heterologous infections. Immunity is induced by adult worms and larvae resulting in partial protection against invading schistosomular stages. Exposure to one species of schistosome may confer some degree of immunity against challenge by another species but, as with most helminth infestations, the degree of protection is incomplete. Immunity is manifested by a decrease in the number of adult parasites which develop, size of the adult worms, number of eggs laid, and ability to withstand superinfection. Heterologous immunity is considered to play a role in limiting the severity of schistosomiasis in man, although it is probably of very limited importance in domestic animals. Infections in man and domestic animals are common in the young. As animals get older, there is a decrease in production of eggs and infections become asymptomatic, suggesting a gradual development of resistance by the young. Immunity may take years to become pronounced and during the initial stages is only partially effective.

There is relatively little information on humoral and cellular immunological responses in schistosomiasis in domestic animals. Antigens are isolated from both adults and cercariae for serological tests. Complement fixation (CF), immunodiffusion, indirect hemagglutination, indirect fluorescent, and intradermal tests are used commonly in schistosomiasis of man and occasionally in animals.

Literature

Compared to the literature available on schistosomiasis in man, there has been little information on the immunological responses in various domestic animals. Advances in the immunology of schistosomiasis in man and experimental animals have been summarized in a number of reviews (Capron *et al.* 1982; Smithers 1972; Smithers and Terry 1969).

Various extraction methods have been used to prepare the antigen from schistosomes, both adults and cercaria of *S. mattheei* and *S. bovis* (Du Plessis and van Wyk 1972; Duffus *et al.* 1975; Preston and Duffus 1975).

The indirect fluorescent antibody (IFA) test and indirect hemagglutination test were observed to have high specificity in detecting *S. mattheei* infection in cattle. Other immunological methods including intradermal sensitivity and immunodiffusion were not so satisfactory. Complement fixation showed a high degree of cross-reaction with other helminths (Lawrence 1974c). Antibodies detected by CF and indirect fluorescent tests rose to a peak at about 25 weeks, then fell. The indirect hemagglutination antibodies rose more slowly and remained high for a longer period of time. Peaks of indirect hemagglutination and IFAs were proportional to the level of infection (Lawrence 1977g).

Other tests have been used to a limited degree in animal schistosomiasis. Circum-oval precipitin and intradermal tests were found to be positive in pigs infected with *S. incognitum* (Ahluwalia 1972b, c). The Cercarien–Hullen reaction – characterized by development of an envelope around living cercariae when placed in homologous immune serum – was also used to detect development of antibody 18 days postinfection (Ahluwalia 1972a; Bhatia and Rai 1974). The rise and fall of antibody titers was detected by the passive hemagglutination test and found to be related to the course of infection, decreasing as the infection progressed, the egg count becoming low (Subramanian *et al.* 1973).

Cattle and, to a lesser extent, sheep developed heterologous immunity to *S. bovis* following infection with other schistosome species, with a reduction of 30 to 40% in number of adult worms and lower egg burdens in tissues. In sheep, the immunity was less remarkable (Massoud and Nelson 1972). In cattle, naturally acquired immunity developed to *S. bovis* and was clearly demonstrated by the differences in body weight, hematological measurement, histopathological and pathophysiological responses, as well as worm and egg counts (Bushara *et al.* 1980). In cattle infected with *S. mattheei* the immunological response could eliminate infection and suppress egg-laying by reducing the reproductive activity. These mechanisms limited the pathogenic effects. It was postulated that acquired immunity was responsible for the low levels of infestation observed in various parts of Africa (Lawrence 1978a). Substantial resistance to heterologous challenge with *Fasciola hepatica* was also demonstrated in sheep harboring *S. bovis* infection with a reduction in fluke burden of 70 to 93%. This resistance was also evidenced by the presence of less severe lesions and lower fecal egg counts (Monrad *et al.* 1981).

VACCINATION

Animals living in enzootic areas may develop solid resistance to schistosomiasis as a result of repeated infections. Based on epidemiological evidence and experimental studies in animals, immunization to schistosomiasis is considered a possibility. The key issue in the use of vaccines is their cost effectiveness as based on the potential economic losses in the region. The successful development of vaccines and their application will also depend on their stability, ease of attenuation, degree of protection, ability to increase the weak natural immunity, and safety. There is an increasing interest in developing a practical field vaccine against schistosomiasis of ruminants in Africa. Effective protection with minimal side effects has been produced using a vaccine developed by attenuating cercariae or schistosomula by high levels of radiation.

Literature

Nelson (1974) suggested that reversed zooprophylaxis could be of importance in the livestock industry in animals, enabling development of resistance to schistosomiasis. Zooprophylaxis was defined as the prevention or control of the severity of the disease in man as a result of previous exposure to heterologous infection of animal origin. In both filariasis and schistosomiasis, zooprophylaxis was considered to play an important role because of the frequency of cross-infection between species of infections in man and domestic animals in a tropical environment.

It has been shown that sheep and cattle can be protected against serious effects of *S. mattheei* and *S. bovis* by previous exposure to human schistosomes (Nelson 1974). Calves and sheep exposed to cercariae of *S. mansoni* and then challenged with *S. mattheei* developed resistance, as demonstrated by reduction in egg production and adult worm burden (Hussein *et al.* 1970; Preston *et al.* 1972). Following single infection and challenge of sheep and cattle with *S. mattheei*, the only evidence of acquired resistance was in the reduction of the length of the adult worms (Preston and Webbe 1974), but after repeated infection a very active immunological response has been observed (Lawrence 1976c). Attempts to induce immunity by transfer of hyperimmune serum, inoculation of dead schistosome material, or inoculation of eggs have generally been unsuccessful in domestic animals (Hussein and Bushara 1976).

A relatively nonpathogenic laboratory strain of *S. mattheei* was developed by passage through hamsters. This strain protected sheep against acute schistosomiasis on challenge with a homologous virulent strain. Following challenge of vaccinated sheep, elevation of gamma globulins was observed earlier, clinical signs were milder, and there was a reduction in worm population as well as in the fecundity of the worms (Dargie *et al.* 1977).

Recently in Africa, particularly in the Sudan, work has been undertaken on the use of an irradiated vaccine and the subject has been reviewed by Hussein (1980). A symposium on the development and testing of a vaccine in cattle was held in the Sudan (Nelson 1980). Hoffman *et al.* (1981) reported on another workshop on the development of vaccines against schistosomiasis. Irradiated larval vaccine against *S. bovis* in cattle was investigated and was highly immunogenic. Single exposure to *S. mansoni* cercariae induced partial resistance against *S. bovis* which after vaccination was higher at 24 than at 8 weeks. Sheep vaccinated with irradiated *S. bovis* cercariae were resistant to challenge with *S. bovis* (Hussein and Bushara 1976). Calves immunized with irradiated *S. bovis* cercaria had significantly higher growth rate, lower fecal egg output, lower tissue egg and adult worm counts, and milder lesions (Bushara *et al.* 1978). Use of the irradiated *S. bovis* vaccine under field conditions resulted in lower mortality rate, lower rate of reinfection, and lower egg counts. Vaccinated animals had a 60 to 70% reduction in adult worms (Majid *et al.* 1980b). Similar results were found in sheep vaccinated against *S. mattheei* and *S. bovis* using irradiated schistosomula. As in cattle, vaccinated sheep had fewer worms developing after challenge and lower density of eggs in tissue (Bickle *et al.* 1979; Taylor *et al.* 1979). Irradiated *S. incognitum* cercaria injected into dogs also caused significant reduction in the number of challenge flukes which developed to maturity (Tewari and Singh 1977). McCauley *et al.* (1983) concluded that in development and application of vaccines, cost of effective production techniques and favorable returns from improved livestock production have to be taken into account to evaluate the benefit of this control measure.

CHEMOTHERAPY

In Africa, where ruminant schistosomiasis is becoming an increasingly important verterinary problem, drugs are now being considered for mass treatment. However, the migratory husbandry practices in tropical livestock industry often make effective control impossible. Application of molluscicides is difficult and expensive. Preventing or limiting exposure of animals to contaminated water sources and providing a good plane of nutrition and good management are beneficial in controlling disease. Chemotherapy is often not beneficial and may be toxic. Multiple administration of tartar emetic and antimonial compounds has been used in cattle but found to be only partially effective. Tartrates are toxic and too irritant for use other than by intravenous injection, making their use difficult. Stibophen and Lucanthone are effective, but occasionally cause deaths. Organophosphates are tolerated when administered intramuscularly but are toxic orally.

Literature

The most frequently used drugs in man have been Niridazole, Stibophen, and Lucanthone. These drugs have been used to a limited degree in sheep and cattle with some success but the costs are prohibitive for wide use. Treatment trials on *S. mattheei* infection in sheep with Stibophen, Lucanthone, and Niridazole were reported by Lawrence and co-workers. Treatment of sheep experimentally infected with *S. mattheei* with Lucanthone at 50, 40, and 30 mg/kg body weight on 3 consecutive days was moderately effective and useful in field outbreaks. Treatment with the other two drugs was ineffective (Lawrence 1968, 1976a). Hycanthone administered intramuscularly in a single dose at 3 mg/kg was also moderately effective and at 6 mg/kg was highly effective (Lawrence and McKenzie 1970). In *S. bovis* infection eight treatments at intervals of 3 to 4 days with Trichlorfon (metrifonate) at

100 to 120 mg/kg body weight was found to be effective, resulting in clinical improvement and elimination of the worms (Medda 1970). In cattle infected with *S. mattheei*, treatments with Stibophen at 7.5 mg/kg daily for 6 days and Lucanthone at 30 mg/kg on each of 3 alternate days were effective in removing the parasites and in the alleviation of clinical signs (Lawrence and Schwartz 1969). Repeated doses of Trichlorfon, an organophosphate, at 75 mg/kg given orally, with intervals of a few days between each treatment, were successful but the number of treatments required varied between animals (Dinnik 1967). Trichlorfon has also been used in sheep, goats, and white mice infected with *Orientobilharzia dattai* at various doses given either orally or subcutaneously (Singh and Ahluwalia 1977).

Antimony salts, potassium tartrate, and sodium tartrate have been used in the treatment of *S. incognitum* in pigs and caused toxicity (Ahluwalia 1972d). The comparative efficacy of Trichlorfon, Niradazole, and sodium antimony tartrate against nasal schistosomiasis in cattle was investigated. Administration of trichlorfon at doses of 30, 40, and 50 mg/kg body weight for 4 to 8 days effected a cure or resulted in a decrease in the symptoms and lesions of some animals, but was also complicated by toxic effect and death. Niradazole was not effective. Intravenous administration of sodium antimony tartrate was effective at doses of 1.5 mg/kg body weight given twice daily for 2 consecutive days or once daily for 4 days (Alwar 1959, 1962; Biswal and Das 1956; Muraleedharan *et al.* 1977). Doses of 2, 2.5, and 3 mg/kg per day for 4 consecutive days given intravenously gave 100% cure, but at higher doses the drug was toxic (Anandan and Lalitha 1979a). Treatment with lithium antimony thiomalate was effective when administered over a prolonged period of time in a variety of schedules (Rao and Gopalakrishnamurthy 1964). The distribution of *S. nasalis* in internal organs in treated cattle was reported, and worms were in the liver, nasal mucosa, and lungs (Anandan and Lalitha 1979b).

Praziquantel, probably the current drug of choice for treatment of schistosomiasis in man, has been evaluated in ruminants. Oral treatment of cattle at a dose rate of 20 mg/kg body weight 9 and 14 weeks after experimental infection with *S. bovis*, reduced fecal egg counts to near zero and caused a 98.9% reduction in adult worm burdens (Bushara *et al.* 1982). This suggests that Praziquantel will also be useful for the treatment of clinical schistosomiasis in livestock.

DIAGNOSIS

Although clinical signs, in association with grazing history and local epizootiology of schistosomiasis, may be useful in diagnosis of severe clinical disease, diagnosis is usually based on the demonstration of characteristic eggs in feces. Smears, sedimentation, and incubation methods are used. Demonstration of eggs in feces is not such a reliable method in ruminants, particularly in chronic infections when fecal egg counts are reduced. Rectal biopsy is another method which is used and a piece of mucous membrane is compressed between two slides for microscopic examination. Because of the absence of lesions in many cases of schistosomiasis in ruminants, postmortem diagnosis based on demonstration of adult worms, which may be seen by holding the bowel and mesentery up to the light, is often missed. The worms in vessels are up to 2 cm in length and are readily recognized by the black streak of digested blood in their gut. Retrograde perfusion methods are used for recovery of worms from the blood vessels.

Relatively little information is available on the use of serological tests in diagnosis of schistosomiasis in domestic animals. A variety of methods have been tried in man. The CF and hemagglutination tests are regarded to be good serological techniques for diagnosis of human schistosomiasis. Other tests which are used are agglutination, precipitation, the Cercarien–Hullen reaction, and fluorescent antibody techniques. The indirect hemagglutination test is the one serological method which may be useful in ruminant schistosomiasis.

Literature

The diagnosis of schistosomiasis in ruminants was reviewed by Martin (1973). Methods involved examination of fecal samples and rectal scrapings, and isolation of miracidia. Following washing of eggs from infected feces with saline and resuspension in fresh water the miracidia hatched within minutes, but were difficult to detect in the debris. A method was described which involved concentration of eggs by sedimentation, hatching of schistosome miracidia, and examination of the sediment (Dinnik and Dinnik 1963).

The IFA technique was found to be applicable in the diagnosis of bovine schistosomiasis. There was cross-serological reaction between *S. bovis*, *S. mattheei*, *S. spindale*, and *S. mansoni*. It was concluded that more research was necessary to evaluate the usefulness of this technique (Hussein 1972). *Schistosoma bovis* in cattle was also diagnosed by the indirect hemagglutination test and there was no apparent cross-reaction with cattle infected with other helminths. The test was validated by an extensive epizootiological survey in Kenya and correlated well with postmortem examination. The indirect hemagglutination test was proposed as a simple, sensitive, and reproducible method (Preston and Duffus 1975). In *S. incognitum* infections in pigs, the miracidial immobilization test was described, but was found to be of limited application in the early stages of infestations (Hajela *et al.* 1976).

In cases of nasal schistosomiasis, scrapings and nasal washings have been used in diagnosis. Tissue samples have to be ground up to release the eggs (Biswal and Das 1956).

CONTROL

Control of schistosomiasis in domestic animals by chemotherapy and molluscicides, in general, is impractical. However, the disease can be prevented and controlled by limiting or preventing exposure of animals to infested waters. Seasonal grazing, fencing of infested water bodies, effective drainage, and provision of a freshwater supply may be useful under some husbandry conditions. Such provisions, which will also aid in the control of fascioliasis and paramphistomiasis, are more viable as farming in the tropics becomes more intensive.

BIBLIOGRAPHY

Achuthan, H. N. and Alwar, V. S., 1973. A note on the occurrence of nasal schistosomiasis in sheep and goats in Tamil Nadu, *Indian vet. J.*, **50**(10): 1058–9.

Adam, S. E. I. and Magzoub, M., 1976. Susceptibility of desert sheep to infection with *Schistosoma mansoni* of northern Sudan, *Vet. Pathol.*, **13**: 211–15.

Adam, S. E. I. and Magzoub, M., 1977. Clinico-pathological changes associated with experimental *Schistosoma mansoni* infection in the goat, *Br. vet. J.*, **133**: 201–10.

Ahluwalia, S. S., 1959. Studies on blood flukes of domestic animals. II. Observations on natural infection in pig with *Schistosoma incognitum* Chandler 1926, *Indian J. vet. Sci.*, **29**(2–3): 40–8.

Ahluwalia, S. S., 1971. Post-cercarial development of *Schistosoma incognitum* in a mammalian host, *Indian J. Anim. Sci.*, **41**(12): 1130–4.

Ahluwalia, S. S., 1972a. Cercarien–Hullen reaction (CHR) in pigs infected with *Schistosoma incognitum, Indian J. Anim. Sci.*, **42**(12): 1029–31.

Ahluwalia, S. S., 1972b. Intradermal test in pigs infected with *Schistosoma incognitum, Indian J. Anim. Sci.*, **42**(9): 729–31.

Ahluwalia, S. S., 1972c. Circum-oval precipitin test in pigs infected with *Schistosoma incognitum, Indian J. Anim. Sci.*, **42**(11): 955–6.

Ahluwalia, S. S., 1972d. Chemotherapy of *Schistosomiasis incognitum* in pig. I. Antimony potassium tartrate and antimony sodium tartrate: a note, *Indian J. Anim. Sci.*, **42**(12): 1054–6.

Ahluwalia, S. S., 1972e. Experimental schistosomiasis incognitum in pigs, *Indian J. Anim. Sci.*, **42**(9): 723–9.

Ahluwalia, S. S. and Dutt, A., 1972. Clinical study on *Schistosoma incognitum* infection of the domestic pig. *Indian vet. J.*, **49**: 863–7.

Alves, W., 1953. Urinary bilharziasis in an ox in southern Rhodesia, *Trans. R. Soc. trop. Med. Hyg.*, **47**: 272.

Alwar, V. S., 1959. Intensive treatment of nasal schistosomiasis in cattle. A preliminary report, *Indian vet. J.*, **36**: 56–65.

Alwar, V. S., 1962. Further studies on intensive treatment of nasal schistosomiasis in cattle, *Indian vet. J.*, 33–9.

Anandan, R. and Lalitha, C. M., 1979a. Chemotherapeutic trials against nasal schistosomiasis. I. Efficacy of different schistosomicides, *Chieron*, **8**(3): 187–92.

Anandan, R. and Lalitha, C. M., 1979b. Chemotherapeutic trials against nasal schistosomiasis. II. Distribution of *Schistosoma nasale* worms in the internal organs of treated animals, *Cheiron*, **8**(4): 212–14.

Arfaa, F., Sabbaghian, H. and Bijan, H., 1965. Studies on *Schistosoma bovis* in Iran, *Trans. R. Soc. trop. Med. Hyg.*, **59**(6): 681–3.

Arora, R. G. and Iyer, P. K. R., 1968. Observations on the pathology of ovine and caprine livers infested with *Schistosoma indicum* Montgomery (1906), *Indian J. Anim. Hlth*, **7**: 67–74.

Arru, E. and Parriciatu, A., 1960. Siero di bovini con schistosomiasi all'esame elettroforetico, *Parasitologia*, **2**(1–2): 7–11.

Bartsch, R. C. and van Wyk, J. A., 1977. Studies on schistosomiasis. 9. Pathology of the bovine urinary tract, *Onderstepoort J. vet. Res.*, **44**(2): 73–94.

Bhatia, B. B. and Rai, D. N., 1974. Cercarien–Hullen reaction in early phase of experimental infection with *Schistosoma incognitum* in pigs, *Indian J. Exp. Biol.*, **12**(6): 576–7.

Bickle, Q. D., Taylor, M. G., James, E. R., Nelson, G. S., Hussein, M. F., Andrews, B. J., Dobinson, A. R. and Marshall, T. F. de C., 1979. Further observations on immunization of sheep against *Schistosoma mansoni* and *S. bovis* using irradiated–attenuated schistosomula of homologous and heterologous species, *Parasitology*, **78**(2): 185–93.

Biswal, G., 1956. Incidence of nasal schistosomiasis in buffaloes in Orissa, preliminary report, *Indian vet. J.*, **32**: 360–1.

Biswal, G. and Das, L. N., 1956. Observations on the treatment of nasal schistosomiasis in cattle and buffaloes in Orissa, *Indian vet. J.*, **33**: 204–16.

Biswal, G. and Subramanian, G., 1978. A note on the incidence of nasal schistosomiasis in Bareilly District, Uttar Pradesh, *Indian J. Anim. Sci.*, **48**(7): 544–5.

Bushara, H. O., Hussein, M. F., Saad, A. M., Taylor, M. G., Dargie, J. D., Marshall, T. F. de C. and Nelson, G. S., 1978. Immunization of calves against *Schistosoma bovis* using irradiated cercariae or schistosomula of *S. bovis*, *Parasitology*, **77**: 303–11.

Bushara, H. O., Hussein, M. F., Majid, A. A. and Taylor, M. G., 1982. Effects of praziquantel and metrifonate on *Schistosoma bovis* in Sudanese cattle, *Res. vet. Sci.*, **33**: 125–6.

Bushara, H. O., Majid, A. A., Saad, A. M., Hussein, M. F., Taylor, M. G., Dargie, J. D., Marshall, T. F. de C. and Nelson, G. S., 1980. Observations on cattle schistosomiasis in the Sudan, a study in comparative medicine. II. Experimental demonstration of naturally acquired resistance to *Schistosoma bovis*, *Am. J. trop. Med. Hyg.*, **29**(3): 442–51.

Capron, A., Dessaint. J–P., Capron, M., Joseph, M. and Torpier, G., 1982. Effector mechanisms of immunity to schistosomes and their regulation, *Immunological Rev.*, **61**: 41–66.

Christensen, N. Ø., Metani, N. A. and Frandsen, F., 1983. Review of the biology and transmission ecology of African bovine species of the genus *Schistosoma*, *Z. Parasitenkd.*, **69**: 551–70.

Coluzzi, A., Orecchia, P., Paggi, L. and Nuvòle, A., 1966. Study on the incidence of *S. bovis* and on the geographical distribution of *B. truncatus* in Sardinia, *Proc. 1st Int. Congr. Parasit.*, Rome, 1964, p. 738.

Condy, J. B., 1960. Bovine schistosomiasis in southern Rhodesia, *Cent. Afr. J. Med.*, **69**(9): 381–4.

Dargie, J. D., 1980. The pathogenesis of *Schistosoma bovis* infection in Sudanese cattle, *Trans. R. Soc. trop. Med. Hyg.*, **74**(5): 560–2.

Dargie, J. D., Berry, C. I., Holmes, P. H., Reid, J. F. S., Breeze, R., Taylor, M. G., James, E. R. and Nelson, G. S., 1977. Immunization of sheep against a virulent strain of *Schistosoma mattheei* using a strain of *S. mattheei* attenuated by hamster passage, *J. Helminthol.*, **51**: 347–57.

Dargie, J. D., MacLean, J. M. and Preston, J. M., 1973 Pathophysiology of ovine schistosomiasis. III. Study of plasma protein metabolism in experimental *Schistosoma mattheei* infections, *J. Comp. Path.*, **83**: 543–57.

Dargie, J. D. and Preston, J. M., 1974. Patho-physiology of ovine schistosomiasis. VI. Onset and development of anaemia in sheep experimentally infected with *Schistosoma mattheei* – ferrokinetic studies, *J. Comp. Path.*, **84**: 83–91.

Deiana, S., 1953. Bronco-polmonite da *Schistosoma bovis* (Sonsino, 1876) nei ruminanti (Rilievi anatomosed istopatologici), *Riv. Parassit.*, **14**(3): 181–90.

Dhodapkar, B. S., Pandit, C. N. and Awadhiya, R. P., 1964. A note on the lesions produced by ova of *Schistosoma indicum* in caprine liver, *J. Vet. Anim. Husb. Rev.*, **8**: 117–18.

Dinnik, J. A. and Dinnik, N. N., 1963. A method for the simultaneous diagnosis of schistosomiasis, fascioliasis and paramphistoliasis in cattle, *Bull. epiz. Dis. Afr.*, **11**: 29–36.

Dinnik, J. A. and Dinnik, N. N., 1965. The schistosomes of domestic ruminants in eastern Africa, *Bull. epiz. Dis. Afr.*, **13**: 341–59.

Dinnik, N. N., 1967. The effect of Neguvon on *Schistosoma bovis* in naturally infected cattle, *Vet. Med. Rev., Leverkusen*, **1**: 76–8.

Duffus, W. P. H., Preston, J. M. and Staak, C. H., 1975. Initial fractionation of adult *Schistosoma bovis* antigen for diagnosis of infection in cattle, *J. Helminthol.*, **49**: 1–7.

Du Plessis, J. L. and van Wyk, J. A., 1972. Studies on schistosomiasis. 3. Detection of antibodies against *Schistosoma mattheei* by the indirect immuno-fluorescent method, *Onderstepoort J. vet. Res.*, **39**(3): 179–80.

Eisa, A. M., 1966. Parasitism – a challenge to animal health in the Sudan, *Sudan J. Vet. Sci. Anim. Husb.*, **7**(2): 85–98.

Frandsen, F., 1981. Cultivation of schistosomes for chemotherapeutic studies, *Acta pharmacol. toxicol.*, **49**(5): 118–22.

Goff, W. L. and Ronald, N. C., 1980. Miracidia hatching technique for diagnosis of canine schistosomiasis, *J. Am. vet. med. Ass.*, **177**(8): 699–700.

Grétillat, S., 1962a. Parasitologie Recherches sur le cycle évolutif du schistosome des ruminants domestiques de l'Ouest-Africain (*Schistosoma curassoni* Brumpt, 1931), *CR Acad. Sci., Paris*, **225**: 1657–9.

Grétillat, S., 1962b. Parasitologie. Une nouvelle zoonose, la 'Bilharziose Ouest-Africain' *Schistosoma curassoni* Brumpt, 1931, commune à l'homme et aux ruminants domestiques, *CR Acad. Sci., Paris*, **255**: 1805–7.

Grétillat, S., 1963. Epidémiologie de certaines affections à trématodes des animaux domestiques en Corse (Bilharziose bovine et Distomatose bovine et ovine), *Ann. Parasit. Hum. Comp.*, **38**: 471–81.

Grétillat, S., 1964. Morphological difference between *Schistosoma bovis* (Khartoum strain) and *Schistosoma curassoni* (Mauritania strain), *Rev. Elev. Méd. vét. Pays trop.*, **17**(3): 429–32.

Grétillat, S. and Picart, P., 1964. Preliminary observations on the lesions caused in ruminants heavily infected by *Schistosoma curassoni, Rev. Elev. Méd. vét. Pays trop.*, **17**(3): 433–40.

Hajela, S. K., Bhatia, B. B. and Rai, D. N., 1976. A note on miracidial immobilization test in *Schistosoma incognitum* infection in pigs, *Indian J. Anim. Sci.*, **46**(3): 157–8.

Hoffman, D. B., Phillips, S. M. and Cook, J. A., 1981. Vaccine development for schistosomiasis: report of a workshop, *Am. J. trop. Med. Hyg.*, **30**(6): 1247–51.

Holmes, P. H., Mamo, E. and Lemma, A., 1975. Preliminary studies on albumin metabolism in Ethiopian sheep infected with *Schistosoma bovis*. In *Nuclear Techniques in Helminthological Research*. International Atomic Energy Agency (Vienna), pp. 115–20.

Hurter, L. R. and Potgieter, L. N. D., 1967. Schistosomiasis in small stock in the Potgietersrus veterinary area, *J. S. Afr. vet. med. Ass.*, **38**(4): 444–6.

Hussein, M. F., 1971. The pathology of experimental schistosomiasis in calves, *Res. vet. Sci.*, **12**: 246–52.

Hussein, M. F., 1972. Preliminary observations on the use of the indirect fluorescent antibody technique in the diagnosis of bovine schistosomiasis, *Sudan J. Vet. Sci. Anim. Husb.*, **13**(1): 21–6.

Hussein, M. F., 1973. Animal schistosomiasis in Africa; a review of *Schistosoma bovis* and *Schistosoma mattheei*, *Vet. Bull.*, **43**: 341–7.

Hussein, M. F., 1980. Prospects for the control of *Schistosoma bovis* infection in Sudanese cattle, *Trans. R. Soc. trop. Med. Hyg.*, **74**(5): 559–62.

Hussein, M. F. and Amin, M. B. A., 1973. Pathology and immunology of animal schistosomiasis in Africa. In *Isotopes and Radiation in Parasitology*. International Atomic Energy Agency (Vienna), vol III, pp. 91–100.

Hussein, M. F. and Bushara, H. O. 1976. Investigations on the development of an irradiated vaccine for animal schistosomiasis. In *Nuclear Techniques in Animal Production and Health*. International Atomic Energy Agency (Vienna), pp. 421–31.

Hussein, M. F. and Nelson, G. S., 1968. Observations on the pathology of natural and experimental bovine schistosomiasis, *Trans. R. Soc. trop. Med. Hyg.*, **62**: 9.

Hussein, M. F., Saeed, A. A. and Nelson, G. S., 1970. Studies on heterologous immunity in schistosomiasis, *Bull. Wld Hlth Org.*, **42**: 745–9.

Hussein, M. F. and Tartour, G., 1973. Serum protein changes and eosinophilia in experimental schistosomiasis in calves, *Br. vet. J.*, **129**: 94–6.

Hussein, M. F., Tartour, G., Imbabi, S. E. and Ali, K. E., 1975. The pathology of naturally occurring bovine schistosomiasis in the Sudan, *Ann. Trop. Med. Parasitol.*, **69**(2): 217–25.

Iarotski, L. S. and Davis, A., 1981. The schistosomiasis problem in the world: results of a WHO questionnaire survey, *Bull. Wld Hlth Org.*, **59**(1): 115–27.

Kalapesi, R. M. and Purohit, B. L., 1954. Observations on histopathology of morbid tissues from a case of natural infection with *Schistosoma spindalis* in a bovine, *Indian vet. J.*, **30**: 336–40.

Klopfer, U., Neumann, M., Perl, S., Gros, U. and Nobel, T. A., 1977. An outbreak of paramphistomiasis and schistosomiasis in cattle, *Refuah Vet.*, **34**(4): 141–3.

Koshy, T. J., Achuthan, H. N. and Alwar, V. S., 1975. Cross transmissibility of *Schistosoma nasale* (Rao, 1933) infection between cattle and buffaloes, *Indian vet. J.*, **52**: 216–18.

Krishnamurthi, C. R., 1956. The pathology of schistosomiasis in

animals, *Madras Vet. Coll. Annual*, **14**: 19–23.
Kruger, S. P., Heitman, L. P., van Wyk, J. A. and McCully, R. M., 1969. The route of migration of *Schistosoma mattheei* from the lungs to the liver in sheep, *J. S. Afr. vet. med. Ass.*, **40**(1): 39–43.
Kulkarni, H. V., Rao, S. R. and Chaudhari, P. G., 1954. Unusual outbreaks of schistosomiasis in bovines due to *Schistosoma spindalis* associated with heavy mortality in Bombay State, *Bombay Vet. Coll. Magazine*, **4**: 3–15.

Lawrence, J. A., 1968. Treatment of *Schistosoma mattheei* infestation in sheep, *J. S. Afr. vet. med. Ass.*, **39**(4): 47–51.
Lawrence, J. A., 1973a. *Schistosoma matttheei* in cattle: variations in parasite egg production, *Res. vet. Sci.*, **14**: 402–4.
Lawrence, J. A., 1973b. *Schistosoma mattheei* in cattle: the host–parasite relationship, *Res. vet. Sci.*, **14**: 400–2.
Lawrence, J. A., 1974a. *Schistosoma mattheei* in cattle: variations in parasite distribution, *Proc. Third Int. Congr. Parasitol.*, Munich, **2**: 832.
Lawrence, J. A., 1974b. *Schistosoma mattheei* in sheep: the host–parasite relationship, *Res. vet. Sci.*, **17**: 263–4.
Lawrence, J. A., 1974c. *Schistosoma mattheei* in cattle: immunological diagnosis techniques, *Proc. Third Int. Congr. Parasitol.*, Munich, **3**: 1216–17.
Lawrence, J. A., 1976a. The toxicity of trichlorphon in the treatment of sheep infested with *Schistosoma mattheei*, *Rhod. vet. J.*, **7**(2): 35–7.
Lawrence, J. A., 1976b. *Schistosoma mattheei* in the ox: clinical aspects, *Rhod. vet. J.*, **7**(3): 48–51.
Lawrence, J. A., 1976c. *Schistosoma mattheei* in the ox. Ph.D. thesis, University of Rhodesia.
Lawrence, J. A., 1977a. *Schistosoma mattheei* in the ox: observations on the parasite, *Vet. Parasitol.*, **3**: 291–303.
Lawrence, J. A., 1977b. *Schistosoma mattheei* in the ox: distribution of the parasite in the host, *Vet. Parasitol.*, **3**: 305–15.
Lawrence, J. A., 1977c. *Schistosoma mattheei* infestation in the ox: the intestinal syndrome, *J. S. Afr. vet. med. Ass.*, **48**(1): 55–8.
Lawrence, J. A., 1977d. *Schistosoma mattheei* in the ox: the chronic hepatic syndrome, *J. S. Afr. vet. med. Ass.*, **48**(2): 77–83.
Lawrence, J. A., 1977e. The globule leukocyte in bovine schistosomiasis, *Res. vet. Sci.*, **23**: 239–40.
Lawrence, J. A., 1977f. *Schistosoma mattheei* in the ox: clinical pathological observations, *Res. vet. Sci.*, **23**: 280–7.
Lawrence, J. A., 1977g. *Schistosoma mattheei* in the ox: the serological response, *Res. vet. Sci.*, **23**: 288–92.
Lawrence, J. A., 1978a. Bovine schistosomiasis in South Africa, *Helminthol. Abstr.*, **A49**(7): 261–70.
Lawrence, J. A., 1978b. The pathology of *Schistosoma mattheei* infection in the ox. 1. Lesions attributable to the eggs, *J. Comp. Path.*, **88**: 1–14.

Lawrence, J. A., 1978c. The pathology of *Schistosoma mattheei* infection in the ox. 2. Lesions attributable to the adult parasite, *J. Comp. Path.*, **88**: 15–29.
Lawrence, J. A., 1980. The pathogenesis of *Schistosoma mattheei* in sheep, *Res. vet. Sci.*, **29**: 1–7.
Lawrence, J. A. and Condy, J. B., 1970. The developing problem of schistosomiasis in domestic stock in Rhodesia, *Cent. Afr. J. Med.*, **16**(7): 19–22.
Lawrence, J. A. and Joannou, J., 1975. An apparatus for the infestation of large animals with schistosomes, *Rhod. vet. J.*, **5**(4): 64–5.
Lawrence, J. A. and McKenzie, R. L., 1970. Treatment of *Schistosoma mattheei* infestation in sheep: further observations, *J. S. Afr. vet. med. Ass.*, **41**(4): 298–306.
Lawrence, J. A. and McKenzie, R. L., 1972. Schistosomiasis in farm livestock, *Rhod. agric. J.*, **69**(4): 79–83.
Lawrence, J. A. and Schwartz, W. O. H., 1969. Treatment of *Schistosoma mattheei* infestation in cattle, *J. S. Afr. vet. med. Ass.*, **40**(2): 129–36.
Lee, H.-F., 1962. Susceptibility of mammalian hosts to experimental infection with *Heterobilharzia americana*, *J. Parasitol.*, **48**(5): 740–5.
Lengy, J., 1962. Studies on *Schistosoma bovis* (Sonsino, 1876) in Israel. II. The intra-mammalian phase of the life cycle, *Bull. Res. Counc. Israel*, **10E**: 73–96.
Lo, C. T., and Lemma, A., 1975. Studies on *Schistosoma bovis* in Ethiopia, *Ann. trop. Med. Parasit.*, **69**(3): 375–82.
Lodha, K. R., Raisinghani, P. M., Sharma, G. D., Pant, U. V., Arya, P. L. and Vyas, U. K., 1981. Note on an outbreak of ovine pulmonary schistosomiasis in the arids of Rajasthan, *Indian J. Anim. Sci.*, **51**(3): 382–5.

Magzoub, M. and Adam, S. E. I., 1977. Laboratory investigations on natural infection in Zebu cattle with *Fasciola gigantica* and *Schistosoma bovis*, *Zbl. Vet. Med.*, **B24**: 53–62.
Majid, A. A., Marshall, T. F. de C., Hussein, M. F., Bushara, H. O., Taylor, M. G., Nelson, G. S. and Dargie, J. D., 1980a. Observations on cattle schistosomiasis in the Sudan, a study in comparative medicine. I. Epizootiological observations on *Schistosoma bovis* in the White Nile Province, *Am. J. Trop. Med. Hyg.*, **29**(3): 435–41.
Majid, A. A., Bushara, H. O., Saad, A. M., Hussein, M. F., Taylor, M. G., Dargie, J. D., Marshall, T. F. de C. and Nelson, G. S., 1980b. Observations on cattle schistosomiasis in the Sudan, a study in comparative medicine. III. Field testing of an irradiated *Schistosoma bovis* vaccine, *Am. J. Trop. Med. Hyg.*, **29**(3): 452–5.
Malek, E. A., 1960. Human and animal schistosomiasis in Khartoum Province, Sudan, *J. Parasitol.*, **46**: 111.
Malek, E. A., 1969. Studies on bovine schistosomiasis in the Sudan,

Ann. trop. Med. Parasit., **63**(4): 501–13.
Malek, E. A., 1980. Schistosomiasis. In *Snail-transmitted Parasitic Diseases*. CRC Press (Boca Raton, Fla).
Malek, E. A., Ash, L. R., Lee, H. F. and Little, M. D., 1961. *Heterobilharzia* infection in the dog and other mammals in Louisiana, *J.Parasitol.*, **47**: 619–23.
Malherbe, W. D., 1970. A clinico-pathological study of bilharziasis in sheep, *Onderstepoort J. vet. Sci.*, **37**(1): 37–44.
Marill, F.-G., 1961. Diffusion de la bilharziose chez les bovins, ovins, et caprins en Mauritanie et dans la vallée du Sénégal, *Bull. Acad. Nat. Méd.*, **145**: 147–50.
Martin, V. R., 1972. Contribucion al estudio epizootiologico de la esquistosomiasis bovina (*Schistosoma bovis*) en la provincia de Salamanca, *Rev. Iber. Parasitol.*, **32**(3–4): 207–46.
Martin, V. R., 1973. Treatment and diagnostic test in the schistosomiasis of ruminants, *General de Colegioas Veterinarios Espana Boletin Consejo informativo y Supplemento Cientifico*, **195**: 7–20.
Massoud, J., 1971. The pathology of *Ornithobilharzia turkestanicum* and *Schistosoma bovis* in cattle, sheep and goats in Iran, *Trans. R. Soc. trop. Med. Hyg.*, **65**(4):431.
Massoud, J., 1973a. Studies on the schistosomes of domestic animals in Iran: I. Observations on *Ornithobilharzia turkestanicum* (Skrjabin, 1913) in Khuzestan, *J. Helminthol.*, **47**(2): 165–80.
Massoud, J., 1973b. Parasitological and pathological observations on *Schistosoma bovis* Sonsino, 1876, in calves, sheep and goats in Iran, *J. Helminthol.*, **47**(2): 155–64.
Massoud, J. and Nelson, G. S., 1972. Studies on heterologous immunity to schistosomiasis. 6. Observations on cross-immunity to *Ornithobilharzia turkestanicum*, *Schistosoma bovis*, *S. mansoni*, and *S. haematobium* in mice, sheep, and cattle in Iran, *Bull. Wld Hlth Org.*, **47**: 591–600.
McCauley, E. H., Majid, A. A. and Tayeb, A., 1983. Economic evaluation of the production impact of bovine schistosomiasis and vaccination in the Sudan, *Am J. trop. Med. Hyg.*, **32**: 275–81.
McCully, R. M. and Kruger, S. P., 1969. Observations on bilharziasis of domestic ruminants in South Africa, *Onderstepoort J. vet. Res.*, **36**(1): 129–62.
McCully, R. M., van Niekerk, J. W. and Kruger, S. P., 1967. Observations on the pathology of bilharziasis and other parasitic infestations of *Hippopotamus amphibius* Linnaeus, 1758, from the Kruger National Park, *Onderstepoort J. vet. Res.*, **34**(2): 563–618.
McKenzie, R. L., 1970. Investigations into schistosomiasis in sheep in Mashonaland, *Cent. Afr. J. Med.*, **16**, Suppl. to No. 7: 27–8.
McKenzie, R. L. and Grainge, E. B., 1970. *Schistosoma mattheei* infestation in sheep in Mashonaland, *Rhod. agric. J.*, **67**(3): 66.
Medda, A., 1970. Neguvon for therapy in schistosomiasis of sheep, *Vet. Med. Rev. Lever*, **4**: 307.
Monrad, J., Christensen, N. Ø., Nansen, P. and Frandsen, F., 1981.

Resistance to *Fasciola hepatica* in sheep harbouring primary *Schistosoma bovis* infections, *J. Helminthol.*, **33**: 261–71.

Monrad, J., Christensen, N. Ø., Nansen, P. and Frandsen, F., 1982. Clinical pathology of *Schistosoma bovis* infection in sheep, *Res. vet. Sci.*, **33**: 382–3.

Muraleedharan, K., Kumar, S. P., Hegde, K. S. and Alwar, V. S., 1976a. Studies on the epizootiology of nasal schistosomiasis bovines. I. Prevalence and incidence of infection, *Mysore J. agric. Sci.*, **10**: 105–17.

Muraleedharan, K., Kumar, S. P., and Hegde, K. S., 1976b. An efficient egg counting technique for nasal schistosomiasis, *Indian vet. J.*, **53**: 143–6.

Muraleedharan, K., Kumar, S. and Hegde, K. S., 1976c. Studies on the epizootiology of nasal schistosomiasis of bovines. 2. Intensity and severity of infection, *Mysore J. agric. Sci.*, **10**: 463–70.

Muraleedharan, K., Kumar, S. P., Hegde, K. S., and Alwar, V. S., 1973. Incidence of *Schistosoma nasale*, Rao, 1933, infection in sheep, *Indian vet. J.*, **50**(10): 1056–7.

Muraleedharan, K., Kumar, S. P., Hegde, K. S. and Alwar, V. S., 1977. Comparative efficacy of Neguvon, Ambilhar and sodium antimony tartrate against nasal schistosomiasis in cattle, *Indian vet. J.*, **54**: 703–8.

Nelson, G. S., 1960. Schistosome infections as zoonoses in Africa, *Trans. R. Soc. trop. Med. Hyg.*, **54**: 301–16.

Nelson, G. S., 1974. Zooprophylaxis with special reference to schistosomiasis and filariasis. In *Parasitic Zoonoses. Clinical and Experimental Studies*, ed. E. J. L. Soulsby. Academic Press. (New York, San Francisco, London), pp. 273–85.

Nelson, G. S., 1975. Schistosomiasis. In *Diseases Transmitted from Animals to Man*, eds W. T. Hubbert, W. F. McCulloch, P. R. Schnurrenberger. Charles C. Thomas (Springfield, Ill.), pp. 620–40.

Nelson, G. S. 1980. Schistosomiasis in the Sudan: the development and testing of a vaccine in cattle, *Trans. R. Soc. trop. Med. Hyg.*, **74**(5): 557–8.

Okoshi, S., 1958. The schistosomiasis japonica in domestic animals, *Bull. Off. int. Epiz.*, **49**: 593–9.

Pandey, G. S., Sharma, R. N. and Iyer, P. K. R., 1979. Serum protein changes in ovine and caprine hepatic schistosomiasis due to *Schistosoma indicum*, *Indian J. vet. Path.*, **1**(1): 64–8.

Pierce, K. R., 1963. *Heterobilharzia americana* infection in a dog, *J. Am. vet. med. Ass.*, **143**(5): 496–9.

Pitchford, R. J., 1963. Some brief notes on schistosomes occurring in animals, *J. S. Afr. vet. med. Ass.*, **34**(4): 613–18.

Pitchford, R. J., 1977. A check list of definitive hosts exhibiting evidence of the genus *Schistosoma* Weinland, 1858 acquired naturally in Africa and the Middle East, *J. Helminthol.*, **51**: 229–52.

Preston, J. M. and Dargie, J. D., 1974. Patho-physiology of ovine schistosomiasis. V. Onset and development of anaemia in sheep experimentally infected with *Schistosoma mattheei* – studies with Cr-labelled erythrocytes, *J. Comp. Path.*, **84**: 73–81.

Preston, J. M. and Dargie, J. D., 1975. Mechanisms involved in ovine schistosomal anaemia. In *Nuclear Techniques in Helminthological Research*. International Atomic Energy Agency (Vienna), pp. 121–6.

Preston, J. M. Dargie, J. D. and MacLean, J. M., 1973a. Patho-physiology of ovine schistosomiasis. I. A clinico-pathological study of experimental *Schistosoma mattheei* infections, *J. Comp. Path.*, **83**: 401–15.

Preston, J. M., Dargie, J. D., and MacLean, J. M., 1973b. Patho-physiology of ovine schistosomiasis. II. Some observations on the sequential changes in blood volume and water and electrolyte metabolism following a simple experimental infection of *Schistosoma mattheei*, *J. Comp. Path.*, **83**: 417–28.

Preston, J. M. and Duffus, W. P. H., 1975. Diagnosis of *Schistosoma bovis* infection in cattle by indirect hemagglutination test, *J. Helminthol.*, **49**: 9–17.

Preston, J. M., Nelson, G. S. and Saeed, A. A., 1972. Studies on heterologous immunity in schistosomiasis. 5. Heterologous schistosome immunity in sheep, *Bull. Wld Hlth Org.*, **47**: 587–90.

Preston, J. M. and Webbe, G., 1974. Studies on immunity to reinfection with *Schistosoma mattheei* in sheep and cattle, *Bull. Wld Hlth Org.*, **50**: 566–8.

Pugh, R. N. H., Schillhorn van Veen, T. W. and Tayo, M. A., 1980. Malumfashi endemic diseases research project. *Schistosoma bovis* and *Fasciola gigantica* in livestock, *Ann. trop. Med. Parasit.*, **74**(4): 447–53.

Raghavan, R. S., 1958. Nodular cirrhosis of liver in equines, *Indian vet. J.*, **35**: 387–90.

Rajamohanan, K. and Peter, C. T., 1972. Studies on nasal schistosomiasis in cattle and buffaloes, *Indian vet. J.*, **49**: 1063–5.

Rao, N. S. K. and Mohiyuddeen, S., 1955. Nasal schistosomiasis in buffaloes, *Indian vet. J.*, **31**: 356–9.

Rao, N. S. K. and Naik, R. H., 1957. Nasal schistosomiasis in buffaloes, *Indian vet. J.*, **34**: 341–3.

Rao, P. L. N. and Gopalakrishnamurthy, K., 1964. Treatment of nasal schistosomiasis in cattle, *Indian vet. J.*, **41**: 289–93.

Rao, P. V. R. and Devi, T. I., 1971. Nasal schistosomiasis in buffaloes. In *Pathology of Parasitic Diseases*, eds S. M. Gaafar, G. M. Urquhart,

J. Euzeby, E. J. L. Soulsby, G. Lammer. Purdue University Studies (Lafayette, Ind.), pp. 303–7.
Ross, G. C., Southgate, V. R. and Knowles, R. J., 1978. Observations on some isoenzymes of strains of *Schistosoma bovis, S. mattheei, S. margebowiei*, and *S. leiperi*, *Z. Parasitenkd.*, **57**: 49–56.

Saad, A. M., Hussein, M. F., Dargie, J. D., Taylor, M. G. and Nelson, G. S., 1980. *Schistosoma bovis* in calves: the development and clinical pathology of primary infections, *Res. vet. Sci.*, **28**: 105–11.
Sahay, M. N. and Sahai, B. N., 1976. Histopathology of experimental nasal schistosomiasis in laboratory animals, kids and lambs, *Indian J. Anim. Hlth*, **15**: 93–5.
Sahay, M. N., Sahai, B. N. and Prasad, G., 1977. Histochemical observations on liver, lung and heart of laboratory animals, kids and lambs in experimental nasal schistosomiasis, *Indian J. Anim. Sci.*, **47**(12): 814–18.
Sankar, D. G. and Anantaraman, M., 1974. On comparative pathology of nasal schistosomiasis in buffaloes and cattle in India, *Proc. Third Int. Congr. Parasitol.*, Munich, **2**: 846.
Schneider, C. R., Kitikoon, V., Sornmani, S. and Thirachantra, S., 1975. Mekong schistosomiasis. III. A parasitological survey of domestic water buffalo (*Bubalus bubalis*) on Khong island, Laos, *Ann. trop. Med. Parasit.*, **69**(2): 227–32.
Schwetz, J., 1955. Recherches sur la bilharziose des bovidés (*Schistosoma bovis*) dans le Haut-Ituri (Région de Bunia-Irumu), *Bull. Agric. Congo Belge*, **46**(6): 1444–54.
Sen, T. L. and Ray, N. B., 1969. Nasal schistosomiasis in Black-Bengal goats, *Indian vet. J.*, **46**: 455.
Sharma, D. N. and Dwivedi, J. N., 1976. Pulmonary schistosomiasis in sheep and goats due to *Schistosoma indicum* in India, *J. Comp. Path.*, **86**: 449–54.
Shrivastav, H. O. P. and Dubey, J. P., 1969. Schistosomal cirrhosis in pigs in Jabalpur, M. P., *Curr. Sci.*, **38**(6): 147–8.
Singh, B. P. and Ahluwalia, S. S., 1977. Efficacy of Neguvon (Bayer) against *Orientobilharzia dattai* in sheep, goat and white mice, *Indian vet. J.*, **54**: 859–61.
Singh, K. P. and Rajya, B. S., 1978. A note on pulmonary schistosomiasis in pigs, *Indian J. Anim. Sci.*, **48**(10): 764–8.
Sinha, P. K. and Srivastava, H. D., 1960. Studies on *Schistosoma incognitum* Chandler, 1926 II. On the life history of the blood fluke, *J. Parasitol.*, **46**: 629–41.
Smith, V. G. F., 1982. Distribution of snails of medical and veterinary importance in an organically polluted water course in Nigeria, *Ann. trop. Med. Parasit.*, **76**(5): 539–46.
Smithers, S. R., 1972. Recent advances in the immunology of schistosomiasis, *Br. med. Bull.*, **28**(1): 49–54.
Smithers, S. R. and Terry, R. J., 1969. The immunology of schistosomiasis, *Adv. Parasitol.*, **7**: 41–93.

Soliman, K. N., 1956. The occurrence of *Schistosoma bovis* (Sonsino, 1876) in the camel, *Camelus dromedarius*, in Egypt, *J. Egyptian Med. Ass.*, **39**(3): 171–81.

Southgate, V. R. and Knowles, R. J., 1975a. Observations on *Schistosoma bovis* Sonsino, 1876, *J. nat. Hist.*, **9**: 273–314.

Southgate, V. R. and Knowles, R. S., 1975b. The intermediate hosts of *Schistosoma bovis* in western Kenya, *Trans. R. Soc. trop. Med. Hyg.*, **69**(3): 356–7.

Southgate, V. R., Rollinson, D., Ross, G. C. and Knowles, R. J., 1980. Observations on an isolate of *Schistosoma bovis* from Tanzania, *Z. Parasitenkd.*, **63**: 241–9.

Sreekumaran, P. M. and Chaubal, S. S., 1975. Schistosomiasis in equines, *J. of the Remount and Veterinary Corps*, **14**(1): 15–21.

Srivastava, H. D., Muralidharam, S. R. G. and Dutt, S. C., 1964. Pathogenicity of experimental infection of *Schistosoma indicum* Montgomery (1906) to young sheep, *Indian vet. J.*, **34**(1): 35–40.

Strydom, H F., 1963. Bilharziasis in sheep and cattle in the Piet Retief district, *J. S. Afr. vet. med. Ass.*, **34**(1): 69–72.

Subramanian, G., Verma, J. C., Verma, T. K. and Singh, K. S., 1973. Time course of antibody response in experimental *Schistosoma incognitum* infection in pigs, *Indian J. Anim. Sci.*, **43**(3): 223–5.

Taylor, M. G. and Andrews, B. J., 1978. Comparison of the infectivity and pathogenicity of six species of African schistosomes and their hybrids 1. Mice and hamsters, *J. Helminthol.*, **47**(4): 439–53.

Taylor, M. G., James, E. R., Bickle, W., Hussein, M. F., Andrews, B. J., Dobinson, A. R. and Nelson, G. S., 1979. Immunization of sheep against *Schistosoma bovis* using an irradiated schistosomular vaccine, *J. Helminthol.*, **53**: 1–5.

Taylor, M. G., James, E. R., Nelson, G. S., Bickle, Q., Dunne, D. W., Dobinson, A. R., Dargie, J. D., Berry, C. I. and Hussein, M. F., 1977. Modification of the pathogenicity of *Schistosoma mattheei* for sheep by passage of the parasite in hamsters, *J. Helminthol.*, **51**: 337–45.

Taylor, M. G., Nelson, G. S., Marshall, T. F. de C., Hussein, M. F., Bushara, H. O., Majid, A. A., Saad, A. M. and Dargie, J. D., 1980. Cattle schistosomiasis in the Sudan, a study in comparative medicine, *Trans. R. Soc. trop. Med. Hyg.*, **74**(1): 117–18.

Tewari, H. C., Dutt, S. C. and Iyer, P. K. R., 1966. Observations on the pathogenicity of experimental infection of *Schistosoma incognitum* Chandler (1926) in dogs, *Indian J. vet. Sci.*, **36**: 227–31.

Tewari, H. C., and Singh, K. S., 1977. Acquired immunity in dogs against *Schistosoma incognitum*, *J. Parasitol.*, **63**(5): 945–6.

Thrasher, J. P., 1964. Canine schistosomiasis, *J. Am. vet. med. Ass.*, **144**(10): 1119–26.

van Wyk, J. A., Bartsch, R. C., van Rensburg, L. J., Heitmann, L. P.

and Goosen, P. J., 1974. Studies on schistosomiasis. 6. A field outbreak of bilharzia in cattle, *Onderstepoort J. vet. Res.*, **41**(2): 39–50.

van Wyk, J. A. and Groeneveld, H. T., 1973. Studies on schistosomiasis. 5. Sampling methods for estimating the numbers of cercariae in suspension with special reference to the infestation of experimental animals, *Onderstepoort J. vet. Res.*, **40**(4): 157–74.

van Wyk, J. A., Heitmann, L. P. and van Rensburg, L. J., 1975. Studies on schistosomiasis. 7. A comparison of various methods for the infestation of sheep with *Schistosoma mattheei*, *Onderstepoort J. vet. Res.*, **42**(2): 71–4.

van Wyk, J. A., van Rensburg, L. J. and Heitmann, L. P., 1976. Studies on schistosomiasis. 8. The influence of age on the susceptibility of sheep to infestation with *Schistosoma mattheei*, *Onderstepoort J. vet. Res.*, **43**(2): 43–54.

van Zyl, L. C., 1973. Serum protein fractions obtained by cellular acetate electrophoresis in *Schistosoma mattheei* infested sheep, *Agri. Res.*, Dept. of Agricultural Technical Service, Rep. of S. Africa, Pretoria.

van Zyl, L. C., 1974. Serum protein fractions as determined by cellulose acetate electrophoresis in *Schistosoma mattheei* infested sheep, *Onderstepoort J. vet. Res.*, **41**: 7–14.

Varma, A. K., 1954. Studies on the nature, incidence, distribution and control of nasal schistosomiasis and fascioliasis in Bihar, *Indian J. vet. Sci.*, **24**: 11–31.

Vashista, M. S., Pant, U. V., Kulshrestha, T. S., Singh, N. and Singh, J., 1981. Gist of some clinical experiences in a natural outbreak of *Schistosoma indicum* infection in sheep in Rajasthan and that of clinical trial of tartar emetic, *Livestock Adviser*, **6**: 39–41.

Warren, K. S., 1973a. The pathology of schistosome infections, *Helminthol. Abstr.*, **42**(8): 591–633.

Warren, K. S., 1973b. *Schistosomiasis. The Evaluation of a Medical Literature. Selected Abstracts and Citations, 1952–1972*. MIT Press (Cambridge, Mass.).

Warren, K. S., 1978. The pathology, pathobiology and pathogenesis of schistosomiasis, *Nature*, **273**(5664): 609–12.

Warren, K. S., 1982. The secret of the immunopathogenesis of schistosomiasis: *in vivo* models, *Immunol. Rev.*, **61**: 189–213.

Warren, K. S. and Hoffman, D. B., 1977. *Schistosomiasis III: Abstracts of the Complete Literature 1963–1974*, 2 vols. Halstead Press.

Yokogawa, M., Sano, M., Kojima, S., Araki, K., Ogawa, K., Yamada, T., Shimotokube, A., Iijima, T., Higuchi, K. and Hayasaka, S., 1971. An outbreak of *Schistosoma* infection among dairy cows in the Tone River basin in Chiba Prefecture, *Jap. J. Parasitol.*, **20**(6): 507–11.